Handbook
of
Sensory Physiology

Volume VII/1

Photochemistry of Vision

E. W. Abrahamson · Ch. Baumann · C. D. B. Bridges
F. Crescitelli · H. J. A. Dartnall · R. M. Eakin
G. Falk · P. Fatt · T. H. Goldsmith · R. Hara
T. Hara · S. M. Japar · P. A. Liebman · J. N. Lythgoe
R. A. Morton · W. R. A. Muntz · W. A. H. Rushton
T. I. Shaw · J. R. Wiesenfeld · T. Yoshizawa

Edited by

Herbert J. A. Dartnall

With 296 Figures

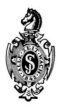

Springer-Verlag Berlin · Heidelberg · New York 1972

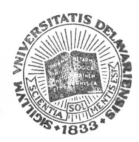

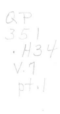

ISBN 3-540-05145-7 Springer-Verlag, Berlin · Heidelberg · New York
ISBN 0-387-05145-7 Springer-Verlag, New York · Heidelberg · Berlin

Typesetting, printing and binding: Brühlsche Universitätsdruckerei Gießen

Preface

Radiation can only affect matter if absorbed by it. Within the broad range of 300–1000 nm, which we call "the visible", light quanta are energetic enough to produce excited electronic states in the atoms and molecules that absorb them. In these states the molecules may have quite different properties from those in their dormant condition, and reactions that would not otherwise occur become possible.

About 80 % of the radiant energy emitted by our sun lies in this fertile band, and so long as the sun's surface temperature is maintained at about 6000° C this state of affairs will continue. This and the transparency of our atmosphere and waters have allowed the generation and evolution of life. Before life began the atmosphere probably also transmitted much of the solar short-wave radiation, but with the rise of vegetation a new product – oxygen – appeared and this, by a photochemical reaction in the upper atmosphere, led to the ozone layer that now protects us from the energetic "short-wave" quanta that once, perhaps, took part in the generation of life-molecules.

Light is an ideal sensory stimulus. It travels in straight lines at great speed and, consequently, can be made to form an image from which an animal can make "true", continuous and immediate assessments of present and impending events. It is no surprise then that the visual sense is found in nearly every division of the animal kingdom – from the hawk to the jumping spider, from man to blow-fly maggot, from the octopus to the rotifer.

In the visual apparatus an image of the environment is focused by the eye on a sensitive surface made up of photoreceptive cells – the rods and cones of vertebrates, and the retinulae of invertebrates. These cells contain photosensitive pigments whose prime function is to absorb light. The spectral regions visible to an animal are, indeed, determined by the light-absorbing properties of its visual pigments. Some insects, for example, are equipped with an ultraviolet-absorbing visual pigment by which they see honey-guide markings in certain flowers that to us seem of a uniform hue. Fishes of freshwaters having light climates biased towards the red, possess pigments absorbing in that spectral region. Deep-sea fishes, on the other hand, have blue-sensitive visual pigments, thus making good use of the dim, slim band of solar radiation that filters down to them. Some animals change their visual pigments on changing their habitat, as the amphibia do when they metamorphose to live on land, and as the migratory fishes do when they switch from the river to the sea, or vice versa, on their spawning runs. Changes in visual pigments can even occur in some sedentary species of freshwater fishes, presumably in response to seasonal variation in their light environment.

In spite of these differing situations, severally calling for visual sensitivity to any part of the spectrum from the near ultraviolet to the near infrared, all known visual pigments are built to a common molecular pattern. Whether derived from vertebrates or invertebrates, they are photosensitive chromoproteins consisting of a chromophoric group, based on vitamin A, that is intimately joined to one of a family of proteins called opsins. Moreover, so far as is known, the chromophoric group is always in the 11-*cis* conformation, and the photochemical change that occurs on absorption of a photon is the mere isomerisation of this group from the *cis* to the *trans* form. But the consequences of this simple change are momentous. Released in this way from the embrace of its chromophoric group, the protein moiety relaxes to expose the hitherto concealed active groups. These initiate in the visual cells the electrical changes that are transmitted to the higher visual centres.

The theme of this volume — The Photochemistry of Vision — has been interpreted in a catholic sense, and the Contributors come from many different disciplines. A substantial part of the account is, indeed, directly concerned with the chemistry and photochemistry of the visual pigments. — What is the nature of the linkage between chromophoric group and opsin ? : — How can such a variety of light-absorptive properties be reconciled with such apparently homogeneous chemical and photochemical properties ? : — What is the nature of the photochemical change and what is its quantum efficiency ? : — How many stages are there in the cascade of thermal reactions that follows the photochemical event — and which of them is the visual trigger ? : — How do these reactions differ in vertebrates and invertebrates — and why ? : — How is the visual pigment molecule reconstituted after bleaching ? The answers to these and many other questions are attempted.

But in addition to this photochemical approach the subject is also treated on the broader basis of photobiology. A description of the visual pigments and of the cells containing them is given for the whole animal kingdom from invertebrates to vertebrates, and treated from both taxonomic and ecological standpoints. Here the reader will find attempts to answer such questions as — What is the ancestral photoreceptor ? : — How long does it take for a species to evolve a new visual pigment ? : — Can a visual pigment help to decide an animal's taxonomic position ? Supporting data for the ecological approach is provided by descriptions of the light climate in such diverse situations as the open land at sea-level, underneath a canopy of vegetation, below the surface in rivers, lakes, estuaries and coastal waters, and at various depths of the open seas. Peripheral data relevant to the quality of light reaching the visual pigments, namely, the optical properties of oil droplets and other pre-retinal media, and of tapeta, are given and, likewise, the spectral qualities of bioluminescence — frequently more intense than the attenuated light of the sun at quite moderate depths in murky coastal waters, and the only source of light in the abyssal depths of the oceans.

The study of visual pigments prepared by extractive procedures has provided much information about the scotopic pigments but has not been very successful with cone pigments. Here the methods of retinal densitometry and, more recently, of microspectrophotometry have helped to provide some of the missing information.

Apart from the satisfaction of bringing together such a diverse assortment of material, this volume has been produced with two main objects: to seduce the honours graduate into a study of vision, and to provide a source book for the research worker. With the latter in mind, the contributors have not hesitated to quote their unpublished material, to speculate, and to draw attention to neglected areas that could be fruitful. These parts of the text are duly logged in the subject index under "Problems, unsolved".

Falmer, November, 1971   H. J. A. DARTNALL

Contents

Acknowledgments

Many of the illustrations in this volume have been reproduced from the Literature. Where practicable the permissions of the Authors have been obtained, and also of the Editors and/or Proprietors of the relevant Journals and Books. Acknowledgment to the authors is given in each figure or table caption, and the reference lists at the end of each Chapter give the full titles and particulars of the sources. In addition, the following formal acknowledgments are made.

Journals

Vision Research (Pergamon Press Ltd.):

Figs. 7, 8 and Table 1, Chapter 4; Fig. 3, Chapter 6; Figs. 2, 3, Chapter 9; Figs. 5—8, 14, 22—33, 36 and Tables 1, 6—8, Chapter 11; Figs. 5, 11, Chapter 12; Figs. 2, 4, Chapter 13; Figs. 14, 16, 18, Chapter 14.

Nature, London (Macmillan Journals Ltd.):

Fig. 3, Chapter 2; Fig. 3, Chapter 3; Figs. 5, 7, 9, 18, 19 and Table 1, Chapter 5; Fig. 4, Chapter 6; Fig. 6, Chapter 9; Fig. 4, Chapter 10; Figs. 19, 35, Chapter 11; Figs. 54, 55, Chapter 16; Figs. 1, 5, 7, 9—14, Chapter 18

Zeitschrift für Zellforschung und mikroskopische Anatomie (Springer Verlag):

Figs. 4, 23, 27, 28, 30, 36, 38—40, 46—49, 51, 53, Chapter 16

Publications of the American Chemical Society:

1. Biochemistry

    Figs. 4—8, 15—17, Chapter 3; Fig. 2, Chapter 11

2. Journal of the American Chemical Society

    Fig. 10, Chapter 1; Figs. 5—7, Chapter 2; Fig. 6, Chapter 6

3. Analytical Chemistry

    Fig. 9, Chapter 1

Journal of Ultrastructure Research (Academic Press Inc.):

Fig. 2, Chapter 8; Figs. 8, 29, 31, 41, 45, 52, 57, 58, Chapter 16

Journal of the Optical Society of America (American Institute of Physics):

Fig. 3, Chapter 12; Figs. 1, 2, 6, 11 and Table 2, Chapter 14

Journal of General Physiology (The Rockefeller Institute Press):

Fig. 23, Chapter 8; Figs. 1—3, Chapter 10; Fig. 1, Chapter 17

Proceedings of the National Academy of Sciences of the U.S.A. (National Academy of Sciences, Washington):

Figs. 1, 2, 5, Chapter 6; Fig. 5, Chapter 16

Journal of Physiology (The Physiological Society, published by Cambridge University Press):

Fig. 2, Chapter 7; Figs. 4, 5, 10, Chapter 9

Photochemistry and Photobiology (Pergamon Press Ltd.):

Fig. 13, Chapter 3; Figs. 9, 11, 12, Chapter 9

Journal of Cell Biology (The Rockefeller University Press):

Figs. 10, 18, 33, Chapter 16

Quarterly Journal of Microscopical Science (The Company of Biologists Ltd.):
   Figs. 9, 20, 50, Chapter 16

Journal of Cellular and Comparative Physiology (The Wistar Institute of Anatomy and Biology):
   Figs. 24—26, Chapter 16

Canadian Journal of Zoology (National Research Council of Canada, Ottawa):
   Figs. 16—18, Chapter 11

Biochemical Journal (Cambridge University Press):
   Figs 1, 2, 4, Chapter 2

Helvetica Chimica Acta:
   Fig. 8 and Tables 3, 4, Chapter 2

Zeitschrift für Vergleichende Physiologie (Springer-Verlag):
   Figs. 3, 5, 6, Chapter 17

Bulletin of the Johns Hopkins Hospital:
   Figs. 9, 10, Chapter 3 and Fig. 19, Chapter 16 (from H. V. Zonana's article "Fine structure of the Squid Retina" in Vol. 109, Number 5 (1961) pages 185—205. © The Johns Hopkins Press)

Annals of the New York Academy of Sciences:
   Figs. 7, 8, Chapter 9

Acta Zoologica:
   Figs. 7, 8, Chapter 8

Protistologica (Centre Nationale de la Récherche Scientifique, Paris):
   Figs. 43, 56, Chapter 16

Journal of Cell Science (Cambridge University Press):
   Figs. 2, 3, Chapter 16

Japanese Journal of Ophthalmology (University of Tokyo):
   Fig. 6, Chapter 18

Biochimica et Biophysica Acta (Elsevier):
   Table 2, Chapter 3

Progress in Biophysics and Molecular Biology (Pergamon Press Ltd.):
   Table 7, Chapter 3

Archiv für Mikrobiologie (Springer-Verlag):
   Fig. 11, Chapter 16

Experimental Cell Research (International Society for Cell Biology: Academic Press Inc.):
   Fig. 6, Chapter 13

Journal of Experimental Biology (Cambridge University Press):
   Fig. 9, Chapter 17

British Medical Bulletin (Medical Department, The British Council):
   Fig. 1, Chapter 11

Advances in Electronics and Electron Physics (Academic Press Inc.):
   Fig. 3, Chapter 14

Ecology:
   Fig. 5, Chapter 14

Journal of the Marine Biological Association (U.K.) (Cambridge University Press):
    Fig. 9, Chapter 14

Izvestiya Akadamii nauk SSSR (Geofiz.), Leningrad:
    Fig. 12, Chapter 14

Compte Rendu de l'Académie des Sciences (Institut de France, Académie des Sciences):
    Fig. 7, Chapter 16

Science (American Association for the Advancement of Science):
    Fig. 12, Chapter 2

Optica Acta:
    Fig. 5, Chapter 10

Books

Comprehensive Biochemistry (Eds. FLORKIN, M. and STOTZ, E. H.). Vol. 27, Photobiology, Ionizing Radiations. Amsterdam-London-New York: Elsevier 1965.
    (Fig. 9, Chapter 2; Fig. 3, Chapter 11 from article by BRIDGES, C. D. B. entitled "Biochemistry of Visual Processes")

The Visual Pigments by DARTNALL, H. J. A. London: Methuen and Co. Ltd, New York: John Wiley & Sons Inc. 1957.
    (Fig. 1, Chapter 4)

The Functional Organization of the Compound Eye (Ed. BERNHARD, C. G.). Symposium Publications Division, Oxford-London-Edinburgh-New York-Toronto-Sydney-Paris-Braunschweig: Pergamon Press 1966.
    (Fig. 22, Chapter 16, from article by EGUCHI, E. and WATERMAN, T. H. entitled "Fine Structure Patterns in Crustacean Rhabdoms"; Figs. 2, 7, Chapter 17, from article by GOLDSMITH, T. H. and FERNÁNDEZ, H. R. entitled "Some Photochemical and Physiological Aspects of Visual Excitation in Compound Eyes")

Fundamentals of Limnology by RUTTNER, R. (Trans. FREY, D. G. and F. E. J.). Toronto: University of Toronto Press, 1953.
    (Fig. 10, Chapter 11)

Evolutionary Biology, Vol. II (Eds. DOBZHANSKY, T., HECHT, M. K., STEERE, W. C.). New York: Appleton-Century-Crofts 1968.
    (Fig. 37, Chapter 16, from article by EAKIN, R. M. entitled "Evolution of Photoreceptors").

Molecular Bases of Biological Functions (Biophysics, Vol. 6). Kyoto: Yoshioka 1965.
    (Fig. 4, Chapter 18, from article by HARA, T. entitled "Vision and Rhodopsin")

Visual Problems of Colour, Vol. 1. National Physical Laboratory Symposium No. 8. London: Her Majesty's Stationery Office, 1958.
    (Figs. 4 and 5, Chapter 4)

The Vertebrate Eye and its Adaptive Radiation by WALLS, G. L. New York-London: Hafner Publishing Co. 1963.
    (Fig. 5, Chapter 13)

Color Science: Concepts and Methods, Quantitative Data and Formulas by WYSZECKI, G. and STILES, W. S. New York-London-Sydney: John Wiley & Sons, Inc. 1967.
    (Table 1, Chapter 4; Fig. 14, Chapter 13)

Optical Oceanography by JERLOV, N. G. Amsterdam-London-New York: Elsevier 1968.
    (Figs. 7, 8, 10 and Table 4, Chapter 14)

The Retina. Morphology, Function and Clinical Characteristics (Eds. STRAATSMA, B. R., HALL, M. O., ALLEN, R. A., CRESCITELLI, F.), U.C.L.A. Forum in Medical Sciences No. 8. Berkeley and Los Angeles: University of California Press 1969.

(Figs. 1, 2, Chapter 3, from article by COHEN, A. I. entitled "Rods, Cones and Visual Excitation". Permission to reprint granted by The Regents of the University of California)

Cold Spring Harbor Symposia on Quantitative Biology, Vol. 30. Published by The Long Island Biological Association, New York, 1965.

(Fig. 10, Chapter 2, from article by WALD, G. and BROWN, P. K. entitled "Human Vision and Colour Blindness": Figs. 12, 20 and Table 5 from article by BRIDGES, C. D. B. entitled "Absorption Properties, Interconversions and Environmental Adaptation of Pigments from Fish Photoreceptors")

Advances in Comparative Physiology, Vol. 1. (Ed. LOWENSTEIN, O.). Academic Press Inc., 1962.

(Fig. 4, Chapter 14, from article by NICOL, J. A. C. entitled "Animal Luminescence", pp. 217—273)

Persons

The following persons have kindly donated original material or supplied unpublished information used as indicated.

R. DUNN
From Ph. D. Thesis, University of California, Los Angeles (1965) entitled "Electron Microscopy Studies on the Photoreceptor Cells of the Gecko, *Coleonyx variegatus.*"

(Fig. 18, Chapter 8)

J. M. CULLEN   (Fig. 10 and Table 3, Chapter 13)

P. E. KING-SMITH   (Fig. 12, Chapter 13)

R. NISHIOKA   (Fig. 35, Chapter 16)

C. GREUET   (Fig. 42, Chapter 16)

Editor's Acknowledgments

I record my appreciation of the support given and forbearance shown to me by the Contributors — of the cheerful industry of my secretary, Mrs Patricia Chatfield — and of the courtesy and uncomplaining efficiency of the Staff of Springer-Verlag.

H. J. A. DARTNALL

List of Contributors

ABRAHAMSON, Edwin W., Department of Chemistry, Case Western Reserve University, Cleveland, Ohio 44106, USA

BAUMANN, Christian, William G. Kerckhoff-Institut der Max-Planck-Gesellschaft, D-6350 Bad Nauheim, Germany

BRIDGES, C. D. B., Department of Ophthalmology, New York University Medical Center, New York, New York 10016, USA

CRESCITELLI, Frederick, Department of Zoology, University of California, Los Angeles, California 90024, USA

DARTNALL, Herbert James Ambrose, Medical Research Council's Vision Unit, School of Biological Studies, The University of Sussex, Falmer, Brighton, BN1 9QY, Great Britain

EAKIN, Richard M., Department of Zoology, University of California, Berkeley, California 94720, USA

FALK, Gertrude, Department of Biophysics, University College London, London, WC1E 6BT, Great Britain

FATT, P., Department of Biophysics, University College London, London, WC1E 6BT, Great Britain

GOLDSMITH, Timothy H., Department of Biology, Yale University, New Haven, Connecticut 06520, USA

HARA, Reiko, Department of Biology, Nara Medical University, Kashihara, Nara, Japan

HARA, Tomiyuki, Department of Biology, Nara Medical University, Kashihara, Nara, Japan

JAPAR, Steven M., Division of Pure Physics, National Research Council, Ottawa, Canada

LIEBMAN, Paul A., Department of Anatomy, School of Medicine, University of Pennsylvania, Philadelphia, Pennsylvania 19104, USA

LYTHGOE, John Nicholas, Medical Research Council's Vision Unit, School of Biological Studies, The University of Sussex, Falmer, Brighton, BN1 9QY, Great Britain

MORTON, Richard Alan, Department of Zoology, The University of Liverpool, Liverpool, L69 3BX, Great Britain

MUNTZ, W. R. A., Laboratory of Experimental Psychology, The University of Sussex, Falmer, Brighton, BN1 9QY, Great Britain

RUSHTON, William A. H., Trinity College, Cambridge, Great Britain

SHAW, Trevor Ian, Department of Zoology and Comparative Physiology, Queen Mary College, University of London, London E. 1, Great Britain

WIESENFELD, John R., Department of Physical Chemistry, The University of Cambridge, Cambridge, Great Britain

YOSHIZAWA, Tôru, Department of Biology, Faculty of Science, Osaka University, Toyonaka, Osaka, 560 Japan

Chapter 1

Principles of the Interaction of Light and Matter

By

Edwin W. Abrahamson and S. M. Japar, Cleveland, Ohio (USA)

With 15 Figures

Contents

I. Introduction

This chapter deals with those principles of spectroscopy and photochemistry that form the logical basis for a molecular approach to photophysiological processes. It is a familiar fact that most plants operate through a photosynthetic apparatus that stores light energy, absorbed by chlorophyll, as chemical energy in the form of carbohydrates produced from carbon dioxide and water. There are also other light-mediated processes in the plant kingdom, such as phototropism (bending of organisms) and phototaxis (locomotion of organisms), which arise from a spatial imbalance of a growth hormone (auxin), and, in many species of plants, the processes of flowering, seed germination, and other photoperiodic effects appear to be controlled by a photosensitive hormone, phytochrome. In the animal kingdom photoperiodism is also observed, but the principal photophysiological process here is vision, and it is largely this process that has guided the development of this chapter.

Most photophysiological processes use visible light to produce excited electronic states of chromophoric molecules. In general the excited electronic states of molecules bear little or no resemblance to ground states existing at physiological temperatures in the dark. An electronically excited molecule can have not only an electronic distribution but also a geometry and a whole host of properties, such as absorbance spectra, acidity, and general reactivity that differ from those of the ground state. We must view the electronically excited molecule as a separate molecule, therefore, with an entire chemistry of its own. We must also recognize that excited molecules have a singular property not found in the ground state, very short lives which under physiological conditions may vary over the broad range from ten picoseconds to one-tenth of a millisecond. Electronic excitation by light, then, results not merely in the accretion of energy by a system but, more importantly, in the generation of new and reactive molecular species from dormant ground-state molecules.

II. Light and Matter — The Development of Concepts

If we follow the evolution of scientific concepts we find that all of them have their origin in our immediate conscious experiences. If we carry over these concepts, derived from the macroscopic world, to the submicroscopic molecular domain beyond our direct sensory experiences, we quite often find that they are no longer adequate to describe the full range of submicroscopic behavior. As we generally do not possess the imagination to penetrate this perceptual barrier, we resort quite naturally to a description of molecular events in terms of hybrid concepts. Nowhere is this process more clearly exemplified than in the development of our modern concepts of light and matter.

A. The Wave and Photon Theories of Light

The latter part of the 17th century was marked by a polemic between Sir Isaac Newton and Christian Huygens as to the nature of light. The former deduced, from its rectilinear propagation, that light was a stream of particles, while the latter, on the basis of the non-interference of crossed beams, concluded that light was a wave. But it was not until the early 19th century that Thomas Young and Augustin Fresnel showed that light manifested the clearly undulatory and non-particulate property of diffraction, thus firmly establishing the wave theory.

Fresnel furnished us with a mathematical description of the light wave and adequately accounted for most of its known properties such as reflection, refraction, polarization, and dispersion into colors. His plane polarized light wave was a transverse wave travelling in space and time (Fig. 1) characterized by a wavelength, λ, and a frequency, ν, related by the equation

$$\nu\lambda = c \tag{1}$$

in which c is the velocity of light in vacuo, equal to 0.299 gigameters/sec.

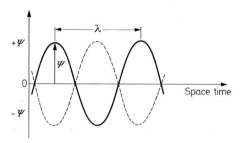

Fig. 1. FRESNEL's picture of a transverse light wave polarized in the plane of the page and travelling in space and time. The continuous curve represents the wave in space at an instant in time. The dashed curve represents this same wave as it moves in time when viewed at the fixed point O in space

The amplitude Ψ of the light wave was described by the equation

$$\Psi = A \sin 2\pi \, (z/\lambda - \nu t) \tag{2}$$

in which A is an arbitrary constant. From this is derived by double differentiation of Ψ with respect to space (z) and time (t) the fundamental equation of a transverse wave motion,

$$\frac{d^2\Psi}{dz^2} = \frac{1}{c^2} \frac{d^2\Psi}{dt^2} \,. \tag{3}$$

The FRESNEL description, however, had nothing to say about the physical nature of the amplitude function Ψ. It represented an unknown force producing a displacement in matter. To accommodate this unknown force in empty space the so-called luminiferous ether was postulated to react to the force field.

The nature of the amplitude Ψ was not apparent until 1864 when JAMES CLARK MAXWELL published his famous equations of the electromagnetic field relating the electric and magnetic phenomena studied earlier by FARADAY and OERSTED. By a simple mathematical operation these equations gave rise to two new equations of the form of (3)

$$\frac{\partial^2 E}{\partial z^2} = \frac{1}{c^2} \frac{\partial^2 E}{\partial t^2} \,, \tag{4}$$

$$\frac{\partial^2 H}{\partial z^2} = \frac{1}{c^2} \frac{\partial^2 H}{\partial t^2} \tag{5}$$

describing plane polarized electric (E) and magnetic (H) waves propagated in empty space (along the z axis) and in time. These were further related by equations of the form (6).

$$\frac{\partial E_y}{\partial z} = \frac{\partial H_x}{\partial t} \text{ and } \frac{\partial E_x}{\partial z} = \frac{\partial H_y}{\partial t} \,. \tag{6}$$

The electromagnetic wave that MAXWELL ascribed to light is shown in Fig. 2.

1*

Although Maxwell had correctly predicted and described electromagnetic radiation, it was not until 20 years later that Heinrich Hertz succeeded in producing the first detectable, though not visible, electromagnetic wave ($\lambda \sim 0.3$ m). He did this by discharging electrical energy stored in a condenser through an inductance-capacitance circuit. Using a simple planar wire loop with a small spark gap placed some twenty feet away from the generator, he was able to detect an electromagnetic wave during the discharge by means of a visible spark. From this

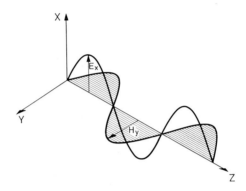

Fig. 2. A plane polarized electromagnetic wave propagated in space (along the Z-axis)

demonstration arose the concept of an accelerated charge as the source of electromagnetic radiation. Maxwell's electromagnetic wave was a structureless entity, i.e., the energy was assumed to be continuously distributed in the wave. This implied that the radiation field could lose or gain energy in any arbitrary quantity. The first hint that there might be some structure to the radiation field came in 1902 from Max Planck's analysis of the frequency distribution of radiation from socalled black bodies, which could absorb and emit the full radiation spectrum. He was able to account for this frequency spectrum by assuming that the radiation was emitted by electric oscillators in matter, not continuously, but rather in discrete quantities of energy. These quantities were integral multiples of a basic quantum of energy, hν; where ν is the oscillator frequency in hertz and h is Planck's constant, equal to 6.626×10^{-27} erg seconds.

This suggestion that energy was introduced into the radiation field in discrete quanta posed the question whether the field itself was structured energetically. The answer was provided by Einstein in 1905 in his analysis of Lenard's data on the photoelectric effect. Lenard had noted two rather puzzling observations made with reference to this effect: (i) when the photocathode was irradiated with very low light intensities, a photocurrent was produced immediately and (ii) a current could be detected only when the frequency of light exceeded a certain value ν_0. Assuming radiation to be continuously distributed in the field, one would predict that at low light intensities there would be an appreciable time lag in the photocurrent before the electron could gain sufficient energy to free itself from the cathode surface. From this Einstein concluded that the energy in the radiation field must be structured into small particles called photons. The frequency-dependence of electron emission led him to the conclusion that the energy of a photon was identical to PLANCK's quantum, $h\nu$. This particulate property of the photon was later (1923) dramatically demonstrated by the Compton effect, i.e., the scattering of X-rays by electrons. EINSTEIN then proposed to relate the mass property (momentum p) and the wave property (wavelength λ) of the electron by the simple equation

$$\lambda = h/p . \tag{7}$$

In this manner the hybrid, wave-particle concept of light developed. The wave aspect was manifest in scattering phenomena such as reflection, refraction, dispersion and interference while the particle or photon was manifest in the absorption and emission of radiation. In its modern formulation, electromagnetic radiation is viewed as a collection of particulate photons of momentum $h\nu/c$ guided by a wave. No longer is the ether necessary to account for its propagation in free space now that (scientific) man is reconciled to the wave-particle concept.

B. The Dual Nature of Matter

The atomistic theory of matter harks back to ancient Greece and the philosopher DEMOCRITUS. But it was not until the early nineteenth century that FARADAY, whose experimental work was the foundation of MAXWELL's electromagnetic theory of light, provided the key to the structure of the atom with his demonstration that electrically charged ions could be produced in the electrolysis of metals. This prompted the later experiment of the ionization of gases in the Crookes ray tube, leading to the discovery of the electron and the proton.

The quantitative measurement of the charge-to-mass ratio of the electron was made by J. J. THOMSON at the close of the nineteenth century. This measurement, together with a subsequent study of the scattering of X-rays by electrons, allowed him to determine the size of the atom as approximately 10 pm in diameter. It was not until 1912, however, that RUTHERFORD and SODDY in their study of the scattering of nuclear α particles by metal foils gave us what is essentially our modern picture of the atom. They were able to show that the mass of the atom was concentrated in a minuscule positively charged nucleus approximately 1 fm in diameter, about which swarmed the negatively charged electrons.

It was apparent from RUTHERFORD's experiments that the electrons in the atom had a dynamical character that was not in accord with the prediction of classical electromagnetic theory. If the electrons were indeed in some sort of angular motion about the nucleus, as was apparent from the diameter of the atom, they should, by their accelerated motion, lose energy as radiation and eventually collapse into the nucleus. In the following year (1913) NIELS BOHR realized that this classical picture of the atom would have to be drastically modified. He proposed, therefore, that in the normal ground state atoms the electrons were confined to motion in discrete orbits without energy loss. These orbits were characterized by a constant angular momentum, and energy gain or loss could occur only when an electron underwent a transition from one discrete orbit to another. Thus, even at a temperature of absolute zero, electrons would, by this model, possess kinetic and potential energy of orbital motion, referred to as the zero point energy.

The Bohr theory developed in the next dozen years to a point where it could rationalize practically all aspects of atomic spectra. Its classical trappings, however, finally led to quantitative failures, even for the hydrogen atom. But its principal shortcoming was clearly its inadaptability to molecules.

In 1923 Louis de Broglie laid down the philosophical foundations of the new theory of matter. On the basis of Einstein's explanation of the photoelectric effect as a consequence of the particle nature of the light wave, he suggested that particulate matter might have, reciprocally, a wave character, the two aspects being related by the same Eq. (7) that Einstein had used to describe a photon. Thus, the electron would have a wavelength, λ, related to its momentum by $\lambda = h/p$.

Experimental verification of de Broglie's hypothesis was obtained in 1926 when Davison and Germer and Thomson demonstrated that electrons having a fixed velocity and, therefore, constant de Broglie wavelength, were diffracted by crystalline matter in the same manner as X-rays. Furthermore, the diffraction pattern was identical to that obtained for X-rays having the same wavelength as that of the de Broglie wave as calculated from Eq. (7). The possibility that the diffracted electron beam might, in fact, have been X-rays produced by electron bombardment of the matter was discounted by Thomson who showed that the diffracted beam could be effectively blocked by material that readily absorbed electrons but was transparent to X-rays. Eventually much heavier particles such as atoms and even small molecules were shown to be diffracted in a wave pattern. Thus, the wave character of matter was quite firmly established.

C. The Uncertainty Principle

Another fundamental aspect of matter emerged when Compton demonstrated that electrons undergo a change in their speed and direction (more precisely their momentum) on collision with high energy X-ray photons. This led to the famous uncertainty principle of Heisenberg, which formally set forth the inherent impossibility of simultaneously measuring the position and momentum of a particle with absolute precision.

A measurement of position or momentum of a particle requires that it be illuminated and this means that the particle will be disturbed by photon bombardment. Any attempt to measure either of these quantities with absolute precision would render the measurement of the other imprecise. Thus, in order to minimize the uncertainty of the momentum of the particle due to its collision with a photon, very low energy photons, or light of long wavelength must be used. However, a law of optics states that the position of a particle can be measured with no greater precision than the wavelength of the light used. Therefore, by making the momentum measurement more precise, the measurement of the position of the particle becomes less precise. Conversely, the use of short wavelength, high energy photons for the precise measurement of position renders the momentum more uncertain by the Compton effect. By a very simple argument Heisenberg was able to show that the product of the measured uncertainties in the position (Δq) and momentum (Δp) was the order of magnitude of Planck's constant, h, or more precisely,

$$\Delta p \cdot \Delta q = h/2\pi . \tag{8}$$

Wave mechanics carries this notion even further by saying that irrespective of whether or not a measurement is performed, it is impossible for a particle to have, simultaneously, a precisely defined position and momentum.

An important consequence of the uncertainty principle is the existence of an electronic zero point energy, a point first apparent in the Bohr theory of the hydrogen atom. If the electron were to behave as a classical charge, it would gradually lose energy in the form of radiation as it spiralled into the nucleus and came to rest there. The electron's position would then be precisely defined at the nucleus, and its momentum would be precisely zero, in contradiction to the Uncertainty Principle. Since the average kinetic energy $\bar{T}$ is a function of the momentum p,

$$\bar{T} = p^2/2m \tag{9}$$

where m is the mass of the electron, and the average potential energy $\bar{V}$ is a function of r, the distance between the two charge centers

$$\bar{V} = Ze^2/r \tag{10}$$

where Ze is the charge of the nucleus and e that of the electron, it is obvious that $\varDelta p$ and $\varDelta q$ cannot both be zero and hence the total energy $E = \bar{T} + \bar{V}$ cannot be just the potential energy of the static system of a proton and an electron in contact with each other. The system must be dynamic, i.e., the electron must be in motion with respect to the proton, thus possessing both kinetic and potential energy, called the zero point energy, which is compatible with Eq. (8).

It is perhaps worth elaborating how the Uncertainty Principle and the molecular zero point energy relate to the chemical bond. Consider, for example, the simplest molecule, the hydrogen molecule ion, H_2^+, which has a one-electron chemical bond. The molecule can be viewed as consisting of classical charges — two positively charged protons and a negatively charged electron situated between them, all in some dynamical relationship to one another. The electron could be pictured as moving in some periodic fashion in a region between the two massive protons whose vibration along the internuclear axis would have a frequency several orders of magnitude smaller than that of electronic motion. But, as was shown earlier, classical charges in accelerated motion lose energy through radiation, and on this basis the charge system should collapse eventually to a linear triad, the electron in contact with the two protons, held together by a considerable coulombic binding energy of about 16 nanoergs. The uncertainty principle, however, prevents this extreme localization, for the position and momentum of the charged particles would then be precisely defined in the collapsed state. Instead the dynamical character of the system is maintained, the internuclear distance being on the average 100 pm with the consequence that the binding energy is very much smaller, i.e. about 4.3 picoergs. The difference in energy between this and the energy of the collapsed state is the zero point energy. When taken on a molar basis this is about 230,000 kcal as compared to the actual molar binding energy of 64.5 kcal, i.e., the energy necessary to separate H_2^+ into a proton and a hydrogen atom.

From the example of the hydrogen molecule ion it should be apparent that it is not the stability or binding energy that presents any difficulty in understanding the nature of the chemical bond, for this is for the most part coulombic. Rather it is the factors that control the bond distance and the electronic zero point energy. In the one-electron case described this is the uncertainty principle but in polyelectronic systems another principle, to be discussed later, comes into play, called the Pauli principle. It is this principle that governs the correlated motion of the electrons, and hence their coulombic repulsion energy.

III. The Wave Mechanical Descriptions of Atoms and Molecules

A. The One-Electron System — the Hydrogen Atom

The DE BROGLIE picture of the matter wave is adequate for particles traveling in straight lines but is inadequate when applied to an electron moving about a positively charged nucleus since such a wave would be forced to bend continuously about a path no longer than its own wavelength. Plane light waves do not behave in this way but are, instead, diffracted as spherical waves. In 1926, a more viable 3-dimensional wave-mechanical description of electron movement was provided by SCHRÖDINGER. SCHRÖDINGER's system of dynamics differs in both aims and methods from the classical approaches of NEWTON and his followers. Instead of searching for equations that would allow a prediction of the exact positions and velocities of the particles of a system in a certain state of motion, he devised a method of calculating a function of the coordinates of the system and the time, with which probable coordinate values and dynamical quantities could be predicted for the system. Thus, the SCHRÖDINGER wave equation and its auxiliary postulates allow one to determine a wave amplitude function Ψ, which is a function of the coordinates of a system and time. A system that is isolated, i.e. not exchanging energy with the surroundings, is characterized by a number of discrete stationary states of constant energy E and a time-independent wave function, ψ, which is a function of spatial coordinates only.

An intuitive way of making the transition from classical to wave mechanics is to start with our simple wave Eq. (2) for a transverse wave and remove the time dependency.

$$\psi = A \sin 2\pi z/\lambda \tag{11}$$

Differentiating twice with respect to space (z) yields

$$\frac{\partial^2 \psi}{\partial z^2} = - \frac{4\pi^2}{\lambda^2} \psi. \tag{12}$$

Using the DE BROGLIE relation, (7), to introduce the particle aspect (momentum) into the equation one obtains

$$\frac{\partial^2 \psi}{\partial z^2} = \frac{-4\pi^2 p^2}{h^2} \psi \tag{13}$$

from which it follows that

$$p^2\psi = - \frac{h^2}{4\pi^2} \frac{\partial^2}{\partial z^2} (\psi). \tag{14}$$

Clearly, the momentum p is no longer a simple number but takes on a new aspect, that of a mathematical operator given by

$$p_{\text{op}} = - \frac{h}{2\pi \sqrt{-1}} (\partial/\partial_z) \tag{15}$$

which in three dimensions becomes

$$p_{\mathrm{op}} = \frac{h}{2\pi\sqrt{-1}}\,\nabla\,. \tag{16}$$

One can derive from (16) other wave mechanical operators merely by substituting in the classical expression. Thus for the total stationary state energy we have the Hamiltonian operator, H_{op}, given as

$$H_{\mathrm{op}} = \frac{p_{\mathrm{op}}^2}{2m} + V(x, y, z) = \frac{-h^2}{8\pi^2}\sum_i \frac{1}{m_i}\nabla^2 + V(x, y, z) \tag{17}$$

where the summation is over all particles i of mass m_i and $V(x, y, z)$ is the classical potential energy. The SCHRÖDINGER equation simply expresses the result of operating with the total stationary state energy (Hamiltonian) operator on the wave function of a system,

$$H_{\mathrm{op}}\psi_n = E_n\psi_n\,. \tag{18}$$

The problem in wave mechanics is, therefore, to find the correct mathematical form of ψ_n, the eigenfunction of a given state n of a system, which yields the correct value of the energy or eigenvalue of this state, E_n.

For the case of the hydrogen atom, neglecting any kinetic energy of translation and any relativistic corrections, the SCHRÖDINGER equation in cartesian coordinates takes the form

$$\left(-\frac{h^2}{8\pi^2 m}\nabla_{x,y,z}^2 - \frac{Ze^2}{\sqrt{x^2 + y^2 + z^2}} - E\right)\psi = 0\,. \tag{19}$$

But one can more readily solve (19) if one expresses it in spherical polar coordinates (Fig. 3) in which case it becomes

$$\frac{1}{r^2}\frac{\partial}{\partial r}\left(r^2\frac{\partial}{\partial r}\right) + \frac{1}{r^2\sin\theta}\frac{\partial}{\partial\theta}\left(\sin\theta\frac{\partial}{\partial\theta}\right)$$
$$+ \frac{1}{r^2\sin^2\theta}\frac{\partial^2}{\partial\varphi^2} + \frac{8\pi^2 m}{h^2}\left(E + \frac{Ze^2}{r}\right) = 0\,. \tag{20}$$

The mathematical solution (21) to (20) is an exact one expressed as the product of three separate functions each involving only one of the simple variables defined in Fig. 3.

$$\psi(r, \theta, \varphi) = R_{n,\,l}(r) \cdot \Theta_{l,\,m}(\theta) \cdot \Phi_m(\varphi)\,. \tag{21}$$

Implicit in the solution are the integer quantum numbers n, l, and m which define the *state* of the hydrogen atom, i.e. each state has a different set of quantum numbers. The radial function $R(r)$ contains both the principal quantum number n and the azimuthal quantum number l which determine its form. $R(r)$ is defined only for values of $n = 1,2,3,\ldots$, and for values of $l = 0,1,2,\ldots n-1$. The angular functions Θ and Φ, on the other hand, are spherically symmetric and therefore unity

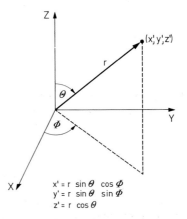

x' = r sin θ cos Φ
y' = r sin θ sin Φ
z' = r cos θ

Fig. 3. Conversion of the Cartesian co-ordinates (x', y', z') to spherical polar co-ordinates (r, Θ, Φ)

when l and m are zero, and develop angular dependency only when they are non-zero. In Table 1 are given the mathematical forms of the state functions for the lower energy states of the hydrogen atom. The corresponding graphical descriptions of these functions are shown in Fig. 4.

Table 1. *Hydrogenic wave functions*

Z — *nuclear charge;* $a_0 = 0.529 \times 10^{-8}$ *cm;*
r — *distance of electron from nucleus*

K Shell

$n = 1, l = 0, m = 0$ $\qquad 1s = \dfrac{1}{\sqrt{\pi}} \left(\dfrac{Z}{a_0}\right)^{3/2} \exp{-\dfrac{Z}{a_0} r}$

L Shell

$n = 2, l = 0, m = 0$ $\qquad 2s = \dfrac{1}{4\sqrt{2\pi}} \left(\dfrac{Z}{a_0}\right)^{3/2} \left(2 - \dfrac{Z}{a_0} r\right) \exp\left(-\dfrac{Z}{2a_0} r\right)$

$n = 2, l = 1, m = 0$ $\qquad 2p_z = \dfrac{1}{4\sqrt{2\pi}} \left(\dfrac{Z}{a_0}\right)^{3/2} \dfrac{Z}{a_0} r \exp\left(-\dfrac{Z}{2a_0} r\right) \cos\theta$

$n = 2, l = 1, m = \pm 1^a$ $\quad 2p_x = \dfrac{1}{4\sqrt{2\pi}} \left(\dfrac{Z}{a_0}\right)^{3/2} \dfrac{Z}{a_0} r \exp\left(-\dfrac{Z}{2a_0} r\right) \sin\theta \cos\varphi$

$\qquad\qquad\qquad\qquad\quad 2p_y = \dfrac{1}{4\sqrt{2\pi}} \left(\dfrac{Z}{a_0}\right)^{3/2} \dfrac{Z}{a_0} r \exp\left(-\dfrac{Z}{2a_0} r\right) \sin\theta \sin\varphi$

[a] The function $\Phi(\varphi) = \dfrac{1}{\sqrt{\pi}} e^{\sqrt{-1}m\varphi}$ is imaginary. But a *real* representation can be given by taking a sum and difference combination of Φ's with some absolute value of m. This yields two *real* functions. $\Phi_{|m|}(\varphi)_x = \dfrac{1}{\sqrt{\pi}} \cos_{|m|}$ and $\Phi_{|m|}(\varphi)_y = \dfrac{1}{\sqrt{\pi}} \sin_{|m|} \varphi$.

An instructive analogy to hydrogenic Schrödinger waves can be reached by considering the sort of standing sound waves that can be established in a thin-walled sphere filled with a gas. Such a sphere with a suitable perturbation could be made to resonate at certain frequencies corresponding to the fixed normal mode vibrations of the gas confined in the sphere. These normal mode vibrations would produce regions of high and low gas density relative to that of the resting state, corresponding to the crests (positive) and troughs (negative) of transverse waves. Now the normal mode vibrations for the sound waves would have qualitatively the same amplitude pattern obtained for the hydrogenic state wave functions of Fig. 4, the primary difference being that the amplitude, ψ, of the sound wave would not be defined beyond the wall of the sphere while for all Schrödinger waves ψ approaches zero as the distance r approaches infinity. But as ψ decreases sharply with increasing r its value beyond a few tenths of a nanometer is minuscule.

Though the physical significance of the amplitude of a sound wave is readily apparent in terms of gas density, the amplitude of the Schrödinger equation has no physical significance *per se*. But, as Max Born showed, the product of the square of the amplitude of a hydrogenic state wave function and a unit volume of configuration space, $\psi^2 dv$, where $dv = dxdydz$, could be interpreted as the probability that the electron would be found in that particular unit volume. In quantum mechanics it is convenient to normalize the total position probability to unity via Eq. (22)[1]

$$A^2 \int_{-\infty}^{+\infty} \psi^2 \, dv = 1 \qquad (22)$$

which requires that the amplitude function, ψ, be multiplied by a constant normalizing factor A. The wave hydrogenic functions given in Table 1 are normalized.

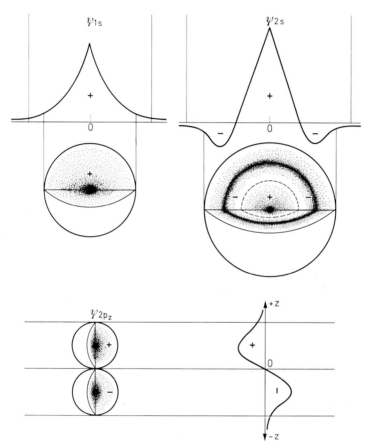

Fig. 4. Graphical representations of some of the hydrogenic wave functions shown in Table 1. Nodal points are represented by dotted lines. The magnitude of ψ is indicated by the density of shading

B. Absorption and Emission of Radiation

When the absorption and emission spectra of the hydrogen atom are examined, it is noted that the observed lines correspond to relatively few of the total possible

---

[1] $\psi^2 \, dv$ should properly be given as $\psi^*\psi \, dv$ where ψ^* is the complex conjugate of ψ in which $\sqrt{-1}$ is replaced by $-\sqrt{-1}$. Thus $\psi^*\psi$ will always be real.

electronic transitions. This would imply that there are selection rules governing electronic transitions. Referring to our model of a gas confined to a sphere, which we assume is vibrating in the $1s$ normal mode (Fig. 4), let us consider what would happen if one beat the sphere with a drumstick in the direction of the x-axis. If the beating force were delivered with a frequency ν_l that was the difference in normal mode frequencies, $\nu_{2p} - \nu_{1s}$, one would find, after an amount of energy had been absorbed by the sphere equivalent to the energy difference, $E_{2p} - E_{1s}$, that the sphere would be vibrating in the $2p_x$ mode. Had we, instead, applied a spherically symmetric 'squeeze' force to the sphere at the same frequency ν_l, the ν_{2s} mode, which is degenerate (having the same energy and frequency) with ν_{2p}, would have been gradually excited.

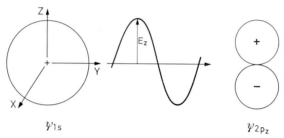

$$\psi_{1s} \qquad\qquad\qquad \psi_{2p_z}$$

Fig. 5. Electronic excitation of the hydrogen atom with plane polarized light (electric vector directed along the Z-axis)

Consider now the oscillating electric field vector E_z of a plane polarized light wave acting on the hydrogen atom in the $1s$ state (Fig. 5). The linear electric force field acts much like the drumstick when applied to our electron distribution. It sets the electronic charge cloud in motion, generating a transition dipole moment $\mu_z = ez$ along the z axis. Unlike the drumstick beating on the gas-filled sphere, however, energy is not delivered continuously to the system even though the charge cloud is set in motion. Only after approximately one million oscillations of the electric field vector of the wave at a frequency of about 10^{15} hertz does the hydrogen atom suddenly absorb energy from the field in a single oscillation as a photon, $h\nu$, where $\nu = (E_{2p} - E_{1s})/h$. Having once been excited the hydrogen atom will remain so for approximately a nanosecond, or approximately one million oscillations of the light wave, before a photon of the same frequency is emitted, unless the excitation energy is removed during this period by collision with other atoms or molecules.

Electronic transitions in wave mechanical terms are best understood in terms of the symmetry properties of the stationary state wave functions. Wave functions that are functions of the coordinates x, y, and z have the property that their amplitude remains unchanged in magnitude (but not necessarily in sign) when the coordinates are transformed in certain ways. For example, the symmetry operation of reflection in the xy plane is equivalent to exchange of z and $-z$. When this, or any, operation is performed on ψ_{1s}, neither magnitude nor sign changes. Therefore, ψ_{1s} is symmetric (S) to all such operations. On the other hand, ψ_{2p_z} changes sign, but not magnitude, when z is replaced by $-z$, and is antisymmetric (A) to reflection in the xy plane. However, it is symmetric to reflection in the xz and yz planes.

A fundamental law of wave mechanics states that all observable events, such as spectroscopic transitions, must be totally symmetric events, i.e., symmetric to all symmetry operations that leave the magnitude unchanged. The probability or allowedness of the spectroscopic transition $\psi_{1s} \to \psi_{2p_z}$ $(\Delta l = 1)$ will be governed by the magnitude of the square of the integral

$$\int_{-\infty}^{+\infty} (\psi_{1s}^* \mu_z \psi_{2p_z}) \; dx\,dy\,dz.$$

This integral will be non-zero only if the product of the symmetries of the wave functions and the transition dipole moment are symmetric to the exchange of all coordinates. All quantities within the parenthesis are symmetric to the exchange of y and $-y$ or of x and $-x$, but ψ_{1s} is symmetric and ψ_{2p_z} antisymmetric to the exchange of z and $-z$. Furthermore, the transition dipole μ_z, which is a vector pointing along the z-axis, has the same symmetry as the z-axis and is, therefore, antisymmetric to the last exchange. Since symmetries multiply together like algebraic signs, $(\psi_{1s}^* \mu_z \psi_{2p_z})$ has the symmetry product $(S \cdot A \cdot A) = S$ for the exchange of z and $-z$ and can have a non-zero value. The transition $\psi_{1s} \to \psi_{2p_z}$ is, therefore, an observable or allowed transition. Similar descriptions of transitions where $\Delta l = 0 (\psi_{1s} \to \psi_{2s})$ or $\Delta l = 2 (\psi_{1s} \to \psi_{3d})$ will show that the analogous symmetry products are antisymmetric for exchange of at least one of the coordinates, and the transitions are not allowed.

Further development of the theory of spectroscopy for large molecules will show that the definition of allowedness remains unchanged, although the actual selection rules may change depending on the type of molecule involved.

C. Polyelectronic Systems

1. Atoms with More than one Electron — the Pauli Principle

The total wave function Ψ for polyelectronic systems, which can be used to calculate the energy and other properties of the system, must describe all the electrons of the system. Considering the physical interpretation of $\psi^2 dv$ as the probability that a single electron occupies a given region in space of volume dv, $\Psi^2 dv$ can be considered as the probability that i electrons have a distribution in space such that electron 1 is confined to a region dv_1, electron 2 to another region dv_2, etc. Since the probability of a number of events occurring simultaneously is the product of the probabilities of the single events, the probability that i electrons have a given distribution is simply the product of the single electron probabilities.

$$\Psi^2 dv = \prod_i \psi_i^2 dv_i = \psi_1^2 \cdot \psi_2^2 \ldots \psi_i^2 (dv_1 dv_2 \ldots dv_i) . \tag{23}$$

In any polyelectronic system there is a contribution to the potential energy from the mutual electrostatic repulsion of the electrons. Therefore, the electrons are not completely independent of each other, and an exact mathematical expression for the total wave function cannot be obtained. However, "approximate" wave functions can be constructed for the system by taking the product of one-electron functions, as in Equation (23). These one-electron wave functions will not be identical to hydrogen atom wave functions, but they will retain the latter's qualitative features.

Electron spin becomes an important factor in polyelectronic atoms and must be accounted for in the wave function. The Pauli Exclusion Principle states that no two electrons in the same atom can have all four quantum numbers, n, l, m, and the spin quantum number, s, the same.

The first three quantum numbers mentioned above are embodied in the one-electron orbital wave function but, to account for the spin quantum number s, a separate spin wave function must be introduced. As there is no proper classical description of electron spin and no knowledge of the coordinates of its wave function, it can only be denoted symbolically using α as the wave function for an electron with spin $+ 1/2$ and β for spin $- 1/2$. The total one-electron functions may now be written as spin-orbital wave functions. For example, the ground state of helium has two electrons with the same one-electron orbital function but different spin functions. An approximate wave function for this system can be given in terms of spin-orbital functions as

$$\Psi = \psi_{1s'\alpha}(1) \cdot \psi_{1s'\beta}(2) \tag{24}$$

where $\psi_{1s'\alpha}(1)$ is a one-electron spin-orbital function in which electron 1 has an orbital wave function similar to the hydrogenic $1s$ orbital function and an α spin wave function.

In one-electron systems such as the hydrogen atom, the spin of the electron has only a negligible effect on the energy of the system, but in polyelectronic systems the total electron spin substantially affects the energy. Electrons having the same spin tend to "avoid" one another to a much greater degree than do electrons having the opposite spin. This tendency is most marked when a pair of electrons have almost identical quantum numbers. In the case of a pair of electrons with the same n, l, and m, which therefore occupy the same configuration space, it is not possible for them, as in the case of the ground state of helium, to have the same spin quantum number. This is what is implied by the statement of the Pauli Exclusion Principle given above. Should the pair of electrons on the atom have the same, n, and l but differ in m, their spin quantum numbers can be either the same, yielding a triplet state $[2S + 1 = 2 (+ 1/2 + 1/2) + 1 = 3]$, or opposed, yielding a singlet state $[2S + 1 = 2(+ 1/2 - 1/2) + 1 = 1]$. The greater tendency of the triplet pair of electrons to avoid one another leads to a smaller positive electron repulsion energy and hence a lower (more negative) total energy for triplet states as opposed to singlet states having the same orbital configuration.

The solution of the Schrödinger equation for polyelectronic atoms and molecules is a much more complex process than for one-electron atoms. The inclusion of electron repulsion terms $\sum_{i<j} e^2/r_{ij}$ in the Hamiltonian operator does not permit an exact solution for the wave function. One must therefore use laborious approximation methods to obtain quantitatively meaningful one-electron wave functions such as in Equation (24). There is also an important criterion for the total wave function Ψ for any polyelectronic system imposed by the Pauli Principle and that is that the total wave function must be antisymmetric with respect to exchange of coordinates. This can be accomplished by expressing Ψ as an appropriate linear combination of product terms such as in (24) in which the electrons are exchanged among the spin-orbital function. Thus the antisymmetrized form of (24) would be

$$\Psi = \sqrt{\frac{1}{2}}\, [\psi_{1s'\alpha}(1) \cdot \psi_{1s'\beta}(2) - \psi_{1s'\alpha}(2) \cdot \psi_{1s'\beta}(1)] . \tag{25}$$

To insure that the proper linear combination is made, Ψ may be expressed in the form of a Slater determinant (26), which expands to (25)

$$\Psi = \sqrt{\frac{1}{2}} \begin{vmatrix} \psi_{1s'\alpha}(1) & \psi_{1s'\alpha}(2) \\ \psi_{1s'\beta}(1) & \psi_{1s'\beta}(2) \end{vmatrix}. \tag{26}$$

2. Molecular Wave Functions

a) The Total Wave Function and the Born-Oppenheimer Approximation. In addition to electronic motion, molecules have quantized nuclear motions of vibration and rotation. A frequency can be assigned to electronic motion in a stationary state that is of the order of 10^{16} hertz. Vibrations of atomic nuclei in molecules have frequencies of the order of 10^{13} hertz while rotational frequencies of molecules are of the order of 10^{10} hertz. The threefold order of magnitude difference in their respective frequencies makes these three motions essentially independent of each other. Thus many cycles of electronic vibrations are completed in a time in which intermolecular distances have changed negligibly in the course of a nuclear vibration. This allows us, as shown by BORN and OPPENHEIMER, to write a total wave function for a molecule in the gas phase in terms of the product of respective wave functions for electronic, vibrational and rotational motion of a molecule,

$$\Psi_{e,v,r} = \Psi_e \cdot \psi_v \cdot \psi_r. \tag{27}$$

In solutions or solid phases common to biological media, however, quantized rotational motion is impeded by neighboring molecules and can, therefore, be eliminated from consideration.

b) The Electronic Wave Function. The Schrödinger equation for the electronic motion in a molecule is written simply as

$$H_{op} \Psi = E\Psi. \tag{28}$$

The Hamiltonian operator H_{op} is given as

$$H_{op} = -\frac{h^2}{8\pi^2} \sum_i \frac{1}{m_i} \nabla_i^2 - \sum_{i,n} \frac{Z_n e^2}{r_{in}} + \sum_{i<j} \frac{e^2}{r_{ij}} \tag{29}$$

where the first term on the right is the sum of kinetic energy operators for all i electrons in the molecule, the second term the summation of all the electron-nuclear attractive potential energies, Z_n being the nuclear charge and r_{in}, the electron-nuclear distance, and the last term is the interelectron repulsion energies.

The total electronic wave function Ψ, as in the case of polyelectronic atoms, is conveniently represented as the product of one-electron spin-orbital wave functions antisymmetrized via a Slater determinant (30) for n electrons occupying n one-electron spin-orbital functions.

$$\Psi = \frac{1}{\sqrt{n}} \begin{bmatrix} \phi_1(1)\,\phi_2(1) \cdots \phi_n(1) \\ \vdots \qquad\qquad \vdots \\ \phi_1(n) \text{------} \phi_n(n) \end{bmatrix} \tag{30}$$

The chief problem in molecular wave mechanics is the construction of one-electron orbital functions. Most widely used is the molecular orbital method developed by Hund and Mulliken, which makes use of the fact that the one-electron orbital function should have much the same character as the constituent atomic orbital function in the neighborhood of the atomic nuclei. Thus one can, to a good approximation, construct one-electron molecular orbital functions. This is referred to as the LCAO-MO method. The criterion for judging the quality of a set of one-electron wave functions is how close the energy of the molecule, as calculated by the resulting Schrödinger equation, comes to the experimental energy. The energy of the molecule is most conveniently calculated by Eq. (31).

$$E_{\text{exp.}} \leqq E_{\text{calc.}} = \frac{\int\limits_{-\infty}^{+\infty} \Psi^* H_{\text{op}} \Psi \, dv}{\int\limits_{-\infty}^{+\infty} \Psi^* \Psi \, dv} . \tag{31}$$

This is an alternative formulation of the Schrödinger equation embodying the variation principle, which implies that any wave function arbitrarily chosen for the lowest energy state of a molecule will always yield calculated energies that will be equal to, or greater than, the true or experimental energy.

The one-electron molecular orbital functions ϕ_i of the total wave function (30) are written as a linear combination of j atomic orbital functions ψ_j located on the constituent atoms of the molecule (32).

$$\phi_i = \sum_j c_j \psi_j . \tag{32}$$

Generally, there is more than one atomic orbital function on each atom. A simple, one-term hydrogenic representation of these atomic orbital functions (Table 1) will yield a qualitatively correct picture of the molecular wave function, but for a quantitative calculation of the energy a better representation is needed. This can be accomplished by adding to the basic one-term hydrogenic (or equivalent) functions a small admixture of higher order (higher n, l, m) hydrogenic functions so that, in general, the atomic orbital functions ψ_j can be expressed as a linear combination of terms from the zeroth order set of atomic hydrogenic wave functions or their equivalent (33).

$$\psi_j = \sum C_{j l} \psi_l^o . \tag{33}$$

The constant coefficient terms c_j in (32) must be chosen to give a minimum value of the calculated energy. This is done by differentiating Eq. (31) with respect to each coefficient c_j separately, i.e. $dE/dc_j = 0$ at the energy minimum. A set of j simultaneous equations is obtained by this process and are collectively called the secular equation. This equation is solved to yield a set of j molecular orbitals with known energies (eigenvalues) and coefficients c_j (eigenvectors).

IV. Molecular Orbital Calculations

The calculation of the molecular wave function can be approached in several different ways, but most techniques in current use, ranging from simple qualitative estimates to refined *ab initio* methods, are based on the Hund-Mulliken one-electron molecular orbital concept.

A. Hückel Molecular Orbitals

The Hückel molecular orbital method is the simplest of all molecular orbital techniques and is widely used by organic chemists. It is usually applied only to the π electron system of linear and cyclic conjugated polyenes. Starting with the one-electron molecular orbital as a linear combination of the j atomic $2p$ orbitals, (32), on the carbon atoms of the π electron skeleton, it generates a set of π molecular orbitals, j in number, of the form given in (32). By introducing (32) directly into (31) and minimizing the energy with respect to each coefficient c_j, viz $dE/dc_j = 0$, a set of j simultaneous equations (the secular equation) is obtained. In the case of butadiene (Fig. 6) the secular equation takes the form of (34)

$$(\alpha_{11}-ES_{11})c_1 + (\beta_{12}-ES_{12})c_2 + (\beta_{13}-ES_{13})c_3 + (\beta_{14}-ES_{14})c_4 = 0,$$
$$(\beta_{21}-ES_{21})c_1 + (\alpha_{22}-ES_{22})c_2 + (\beta_{23}-ES_{23})c_3 + (\beta_{24}-ES_{24})c_4 = 0,$$
$$(\beta_{31}-ES_{31})c_1 + (\beta_{32}-ES_{32})c_2 + (\alpha_{33}-ES_{33})c_3 + (\beta_{34}-ES_{34})c_4 = 0, \qquad (34)$$
$$(\beta_{41}-ES_{41})c_1 + (\beta_{42}-ES_{42})c_2 + (\beta_{43}-ES_{43})c_3 + (\alpha_{44}-ES_{44})c_4 = 0,$$

where

$$\alpha_{jj} = \int_{-\infty}^{+\infty} \psi_j^* \, H_{op} \, \psi_j \, dv \,, \quad \beta_{ij} = \beta_{ji} = \int_{-\infty}^{+\infty} \psi_i^* \, H_{op} \, \psi_j \, dv \,, \quad \text{and} \quad S_{ij} = \int_{-\infty}^{+\infty} \psi_i^* \, \psi_j \, dv \,.$$

For the carbon atoms all the coulomb integrals, α_{jj}, are equal. The resonance integrals, β_{ij}, are zero except for adjacent carbon atoms and the overlap integral S_{ij} is unity for $i = j$ but taken as zero for $i \neq j$. For the secular equation (34) to be generally true the determinantal equation of the coefficients of c_1, c_2, c_3, and c_4 must be equal to zero. With the simplifications just given this becomes

$$\begin{vmatrix} \alpha-E & \beta & 0 & 0 \\ \beta & \alpha-E & \beta & 0 \\ 0 & \beta & \alpha-E & \beta \\ 0 & 0 & \beta & \alpha-E \end{vmatrix} = 0 . \qquad (35)$$

The solution of the determinantal equation is considerably simplified if it can be reduced to block form in which only the terms along or adjacent to the leading diagonal, i.e. 1,1 to 4,4, are non-zero. This can oftentimes be accomplished by making use of the symmetry properties of the molecular orbitals. From Fig. (6) it is apparent that carbon atoms 1 and 4, and 2 and 3 are equivalent, which means that for the set of four molecular orbitals $c_1 = \pm c_4$ and $c_2 = \pm c_3$. This set of four will consist of two symmetric (S) molecular orbitals in which $c_1 = c_4$ and $c_2 = c_3$, and two antisymmetric (A) molecular orbitals in which $c_1 = -c_4$ and $c_2 = -c_3$. Combining terms in (34) the determinantal equation (35) reduces to two 2×2 determinants (36)

$$\begin{vmatrix} \alpha-E & \beta & 0 & 0 \\ \beta & \alpha-E+\beta & 0 & 0 \\ 0 & 0 & \alpha-E-\beta & \beta \\ 0 & 0 & \beta & \alpha-E \end{vmatrix} = 0 \qquad (36)$$

which expand to two quadratic equations each with two roots yielding a total of four eigenvalues (energies). These energies are not given explicitly but rather in the relative terms of the constants α and β, both of which are negative quantities. The molecular orbitals corresponding to these energies are obtained by substituting each energy value E into (34) and solving for the eigenvector coefficients c_1, c_2, c_3 and c_4.

The Hückel method makes no attempt to construct an antisymmetrized product function like (30) for the total molecular wave function. Instead, each one-electron molecular orbital is considered to hold two electrons with opposite spins. In the ground state, therefore, only the lower energy $j/2$ molecular orbitals are fully occupied. Absorption of a photon will promote an electron from a filled to a higher-energy empty orbital. But this gives only a qualitative picture, as the excited orbital configuration does not distinguish energetically between the singlet and triplet states belonging to the same orbital configuration.

From this qualitative picture one can obtain a reasonable pattern of the electronic charge distribution in the ground and excited states merely by summing the respective c_j^2 over the fully and partially occupied molecular orbitals. This charge density correlates very well with the reactivity of such molecules toward electrophilic reagents. The spectral absorbance intensity pattern can also be predicted reasonably well by this method from the value of the transition moment

$$\int\limits_{-\infty}^{+\infty} \phi_{\pi*}^{*} \, \mu_{x,\,y,\,z} \, \phi_{\pi} \, dv \tag{37}$$

integral (37). Thus, in butadiene the electronic transition from ϕ_2 to ϕ_3 yields a finite value for (37) while for ϕ_2 to ϕ_4 (37) is zero. In the former transition (involving no change in electron spin) (37) is symmetric and therefore electric-dipole-allowed, while for the latter (37) is antisymmetric and therefore forbidden.

B. *Ab initio* Methods

In contrast to the simple Hückel method, *ab initio* methods make a complete calculation on all electrons in the molecule using the full Hamiltonian including the electron repulsion interaction. Such a calculation is a formidable task requiring the evaluation of well in excess of 100,000 integrals for a molecule with as few as 8 electrons, and is feasible only with the larger computing machines.

The method most used is one formulated by ROOTHAAN based on a method originally developed for polyelectronic atoms by HARTREE and FOCK. A total molecular wave function is constructed as the antisymmetrized product of one-electron spin-orbitals. To make the calculation tractable the Hamiltonian is approximated in one-electron terms by treating the electron repulsion as a static condition assuming each electron to be acted on by an average static field of all other electrons. This average field of each electron is obtained from the square of the molecular orbital wave function, ϕ_i^2. Thus the Hamiltonian contains the one-electron molecular orbital functions implicitly as part of the potential energy operator. Under these conditions the solution of Eq. (31) can be arrived at by a method of successive approximations. One first uses a trial set of molecular orbital functions in the Hamiltonian (29) to approximate the electron repulsion terms, which in turn yields a new set of molecular orbitals on solution of (31) differing in eigenvectors from the initial trial set. Substituting this new set in (29) the iteration procedure is continued until the eigenvectors are self-consistent, i.e. remain constant on iteration.

The accuracy of *ab initio* methods depends on the type and size of the basis set of orbitals chosen for the calculation, i.e., the number of terms in (33). If the Slater type atomic orbitals (STO), which resemble the hydrogenic ones, are used, usually two to three terms are included in each atomic orbital function, making the basis set about two and one half times the number of atoms in the molecule.

C. Semi-Empirical Methods

There are a number of semi-empirical molecular orbital methods that have been developed to handle specific problems in molecular quantum mechanics. Most of these use the basic ROOTHAAN formalism of the *ab initio* method but the size of the calculation is markedly reduced by making a number of simplifying approximations as to the value of the integrals arising from Eq. (31).

One such method which has been widely used to calculate the spectra of many aromatic and heterocyclic compounds is the Pariser, Parr, Pople method. It treats only the π electrons of molecules, considering them to be in a fixed potential field of all sigma electrons, i.e. those associated with single bonds, and atomic nuclei. The total π electronic wave function for the ground state is antisymmetrized and a set of self-consistent field (SCF) molecular orbitals are obtained from the calculation.

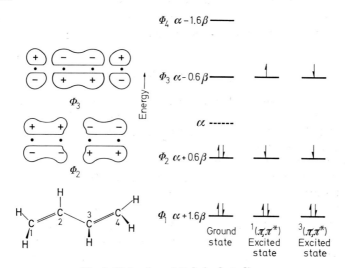

Fig. 6. Molecular orbitals for butadiene

The unfilled (virtual) SCF molecular orbitals of the ground state are used to construct electronically excited configurations, such as in Fig. 6 for butadiene. Those excited configurations that have the same symmetry are then subjected to a configuration interaction that mixes their individual wave functions, the interaction energy being the electron repulsion. For example, let us say that there

2*

are two excited states of the same symmetry, and for simplicity let us assume that they are degenerate. Then, if Ψ_1 and Ψ_2 are the total wave functions of the two states, one can make a linear combination of the two wave functions and obtain two new non-degenerate states whose wave functions are given in Fig. 7a. Should the two states be non-degenerate as in Fig. 7b, configuration interaction can still occur but the relative energy lowering and raising will depend largely on the difference in energy of the initial and final states, Ψ_1 and Ψ_2.

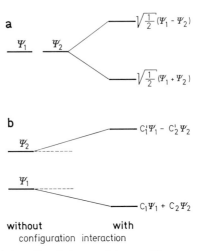

Fig. 7. Configuration interaction between states. a, The case of degenerate states. b, The case of non-degenerate states

It was pointed out previously that triplet states generally have lower energies than singlet states of the same orbital configuration in consequence of the Pauli "avoidance" by electrons of the same spin. In *ab initio* calculations based on the Hartree-Fock, one-electron Hamiltonian, the two states differ in energy by twice a quantity called the exchange integral, K_{ij}, which for a (π, π^*) excited configuration such as in Fig. 6 takes the form,

$$K_{ij} = \int\limits_{-\infty}^{+\infty} \phi_{\pi^*}^*(1)\,\phi_\pi(1)\,\frac{e^2}{r_{12}}\,\phi_\pi^*(2)\,\phi_{\pi^*}(2)\,dv_1,\,dv_2\,. \tag{38}$$

V. The Spectra of Polyenes

A. Radiative Transitions and the Franck-Condon Principle

Most molecules of photobiological interest are derived from linear or cyclic polyenes and their heteroatomic conjugates. Generally, they have a characteristic absorption in the ultraviolet and visible regions of the spectrum and many of them, when excited under the proper conditions, will emit radiation as fluorescence or phosphorescence. The former is a radiative transition between states of the same spin multiplicity while the latter refers to a radiative transition between states of different spin multiplicity.

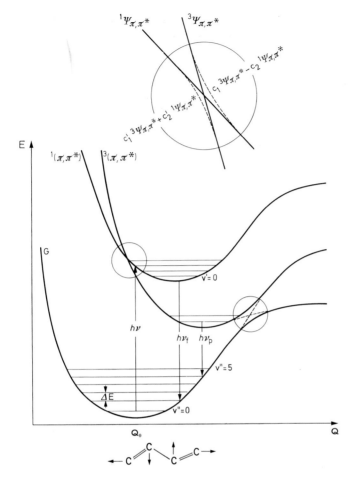

Fig. 8. Variation of electronic state energies along the normal co-ordinate Q. Intersection of two state curves along a normal vibrational co-ordinate. (Two regions, where interactions of potential energy surfaces permit radiationless transitions, are encircled)

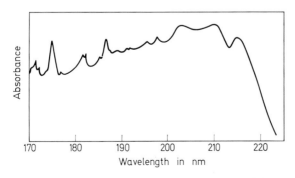

Fig. 9. Absorbance spectrum of 1,3-Butadiene. (Jones and Taylor, 1955)

It is convenient to describe electronic states of molecules and the transitions between them in terms of diagrams that show how the energy of a molecule varies with the distance between the constituent atomic nuclei. This is expressed as a displacement along a normal vibration coordinate. For example, *trans*-butadiene has a normal stretching coordinate Q for the carbon skeleton, which is represented in Fig. 8, and a frequency that is associated with this vibration in the excited $^1(\pi, \pi^*)$ state appears as structure in the absorption band (Fig. 9). The horizontal lines in each parabolic energy curve represent quantum states of vibration in the normal mode Q for each particular electronic state, the energy difference ΔE between the levels being a measure of the frequency of the vibration, ν_i, in a given electronic state, i.e., $\Delta E = h\nu_i$. Transitions from the $v=0$ to $v=1$ vibrational level of the ground state can usually be observed in the infra-red region of the spectrum.

In the ground state at room temperature, essentially all molecules are vibrating in the $v=0$ vibrational level. When a molecule like butadiene absorbs a photon of light of the proper frequency, it is promoted from the ground state to the excited singlet state $^1(\pi, \pi^*)$. But because vibration along coordinate Q is comparatively slow, having a period of about 100 femto seconds, there will be essentially no change in the relative positions of the atomic nuclei (displacement along Q) during the transition, an effect known as the Franck-Condon principle. Excited electronic state energy curves are generally displaced toward larger values of Q relative to the ground state in consequence of their weaker binding between constituent atoms. Because the vibrating molecule in the ground state has its greatest position probability in the $v=0$ level at the minimum of the energy curve, Q_0, the absorption spectrum will show a maximum extinction corresponding to promotion from the $v=0$ level of Q_0 to higher vibrational levels ($v' > 0$) of the excited state.

Ideally, the absorbance spectrum should consist of a series of sharp lines indicative of rotational and vibrational transitions and indeed, certain molecular gases at low pressures show this structure. But collisions between molecules in gases at higher pressures 'broaden' these lines, destroying the rotational structure and smoothing out the vibrational structure to some degree. In solution, solvation effects further enhance this smoothing so that the vibrational structure in absorption bands is often not evident.

B. Radiationless Transitions

As molecules can remain electronically excited for a nanosecond or longer, they usually lose their excess vibrational energy through collisions and are rapidly degraded to the lowest vibrational level ($v' = 0$) of the excited state before they emit radiation. Emission is predominantly to the higher vibrational levels of the ground state because of the Franck-Condon principle, giving rise to a mirror image relationship between the absorption and emission spectra from a given excited state. There is a region of overlap between the two spectra, called the 0—0 band, corresponding to the transition between the respective zero vibration levels of the ground and excited state, i.e., $v=0 \leftrightarrow v'=0$.

Comparatively few polyatomic molecules fluoresce or phosphoresce since the predominant path for loss of excitation energy is via radiationless transitions. A radiationless transition can occur when two curves intersect or closely approach each other along a normal vibrational coordinate Q as shown in the encircled regions in Fig. 8. Thus radiationless transitions can occur from the $^1(\pi, \pi^*)$ to the $^3(\pi\ \pi^*)$ state in the region where the two intersect, or between the $^3(\pi, \pi^*)$ and the ground state at somewhat larger values of Q where the latter states are in close proximity.

A radiationless transition is brought about by a small perturbation, usually within the molecule, which mixes the two electronic states in the region of intersection so that the dotted rather than the unperturbed solid line paths are followed. Such transitions between states of the same spin multiplicity are called internal conversions, and are usually brought about by vibronic perturbations that arise from the interaction of electrons with the electric dipole moments generated by the vibrating molecule. Weaker, spin-orbit perturbations, arising from the magnetic force on electrons by virtue of their motion in the electric field of positively charged atomic nuclei, are responsible for radiationless transitions between states of different spin multiplicity, which are called intersystem crossings.

There is always a finite probability that a radiationless transition can occur whenever the molecule, during the course of vibration along Q, passes through the region of interaction of two states. This probability will depend principally on the magnitude of the mixing perturbation and the relative positions of the energy curves of the two states. Internal conversions can occur in the course of a single vibration (one tenth of a picosecond) while intersystem crossings may require as long as one hundred nanoseconds. Polyatomic molecules containing N atoms have $3N - 6$ normal modes of vibration, and along each one of these normal vibrational coordinates there is usually a region of appreciable interaction of electronic state energy curves. This would appear to be the reason for the ubiquity of radiationless transitions in such molecules.

C. The Spectra of the Retinals

All visual pigments known in the animal kingdom appear to be based on two chromophoric molecules, 11-*cis*-retinal and its 3-dehydro derivative (Chapter 3). In Fig. 10 are shown the absorbance spectra of the *trans* and 11-*cis* isomers of retinal together with the fluorescence spectrum of the *trans* isomer. The mirror image relationship between absorption and fluorescence is clearly evident, as is the $0-0$ overlap region. No vibrational structure is apparent in the spectrum at room temperature in hydrocarbon solvents, though at low temperatures in rigid solvents there is some indication of a stretching vibration.

The *trans*-isomer shows a single absorption peak with an extinction coefficient, ε, equal to 40,000 litre/cm/mole. Polyene aldehydes like retinal have another singlet state lying usually at somewhat lower energies than the $^1(\pi, \pi^*)$. This is the so-called $^1(n, \pi^*)$ state which arises from the promotion of an electron, one of a lone pair, located in an atomic $2p$ orbital on the oxygen atom (Fig. 11). This is a formally forbidden transition and usually has a very low extinction coefficient ($\varepsilon \sim 50$). The transition from the ground state to the $^1(n, \pi^*)$, i.e. $^1(n, \pi^*) \leftarrow G$, is not apparent in the absorbance spectrum of any of the isomers of retinal, presumably because it is masked by the very intense $^1(\pi, \pi^*) \leftarrow G$ absorption. However, it may be clearly seen in the spectrum of polyene aldehydes with fewer carbon atoms.

The spectrum of the 11-*cis* isomer shows three distinct absorbance maxima, the two higher energy transitions presumably arising from its non-linear geometry which renders them electric-dipole-allowed in contrast to the *trans* isomer where they are forbidden by the essentially linear character of the π electron system. Fig. 11 illustrates how these spectroscopic transitions are interpreted within the framework of molecular orbital theory. Self-consistent field molecular orbital eigenvectors as calculated by WIESENFELD and ABRAHAMSON (1968) for *cis*-retinal are shown for the two lowest energy unoccupied orbitals along with the atomic $2p$ orbital of the oxygen atom of the carbonyl group. Promotion of an electron from π_1 to π_1^* accounts

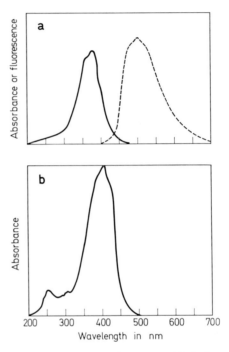

Fig. 10. a, Absorbance (continuous curve) and fluorescence (dashed curve) spectra of all-trans-retinal at $77°$ K. b, Absorbance spectrum of 11-*cis*-retinal at $77°$ K. (BALKE and BECKER, 1967)

for the allowed transition to the $^1(\pi, \pi^*)$ singlet state in both isomers. Transitions of an electron from π_1 to π_2^* or from π_2 to π_1^* appear to be degenerate, i.e. of equal energy. But configuration interaction between these two singlet states $^1(\pi_1 \pi_2^*)$ and $^1(\pi_2 \pi_1^*)$ removes their degeneracy in the manner shown in Fig. 6, giving rise to the two higher energy absorption bands. The energies of these states have been calculated by the Pariser, Parr, Pople method and are described in Chapter 3.

Singlet-triplet transitions are not normally seen in the absorbance spectra of polyenes as they are electric-dipole-forbidden. But under high pressures of oxygen a singlet-triplet absorption band with its 0—0 band at 905 nm has been detected for the π-electron skeleton of retinal in its close relative, dodeca-2,4,6,8,10-pentenal (EVANS, 1960). This corresponds to the absorptive transition $^3(\pi, \pi^*) \leftarrow G$. As yet, phosphorescence emission from the lowest $^3(\pi, \pi^*)$ states has not been observed.

Native visual pigments contain the 11-*cis* retinylidene group bound to the amino group of a lipoprotein moiety, and the spectra of such Schiff base complexes are very much like those of the corresponding retinals (see Chapter 3). The Schiff base, however, is protonated, which produces a considerable red (bathochromic) shift in the $^1(\pi, \pi^*) \leftarrow G$ transition. But this bathochromic shift is not sufficient to account for the spectral range of visual pigments observed in native pigments, which have the retinylidene group as chromophore. Various mechanisms have been proposed to account for this controlled bathochromic shift and are discussed at length in Chapter 3.

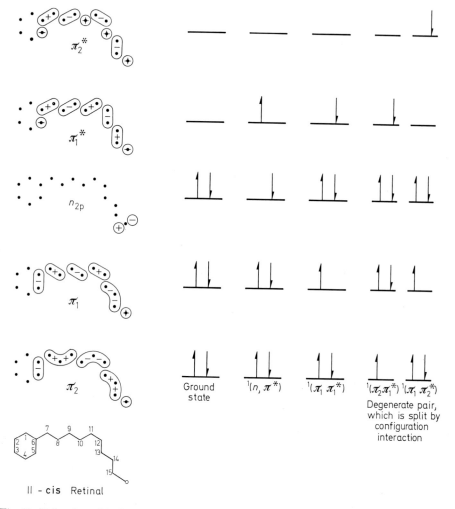

11 - cis Retinal

Fig. 11. Molecular orbitals for the polyene aldehyde 11-*cis*-retinal. The π orbitals are formed from atomic 2p orbitals directed normal to the plane of the page. Only those π amplitude lobes that lie above the plane of the page are shown. The sign of the π lobe lying below the plane of the page is opposite to that shown

VI. Photochemistry

Chemical and physical processes involving electronically excited molecules are generally so closely related that both fall within the purview of photochemistry. Electromagnetic radiation producing such excited molecules covers the broad spectral region extending from the far vacuum ultraviolet ($\sim$ 50 nm) to the near infra red ($\sim$ 1000 nm). Photophysiology on this planet is confined to the low energy end ($\lambda > 300$ nm) which is the region of transparency of our atmosphere to solar radiation. The principal photophysiological chromophores are the linear and cyclic tetrapyrroles (phytochromes and chlorophylls) and the linear polyenes (the carotenoids and the visual pigments). So far, our discussion has dealt with the spectra and the quantum mechanical description of complex molecules, in particular the parent chromophore of the visual pigments, retinal. In this section, principles and certain techniques of photochemistry are discussed within the framework of retinal photochemistry largely to provide a background for the discussion of the behavior of visual pigments given in Chapter 3.

A. Principles

Fundamental to photochemistry is the law of GROTTHUS and DRAPER which states that only light absorbed by a substance is capable of producing a physical or chemical change within it. Fifty years later a basis for measurement was provided by BEER and LAMBERT who demonstrated the proportionality of the amount of light absorbed per unit thickness of material (BEER) and the amount of light absorbed per unit concentration of absorbing material (LAMBERT) to the initial light intensity. Taken together these relations constitute the Beer-Lambert law which in integrated form defines the absorbance as

$$\log I_i/I_t = \varepsilon c l \qquad (39)$$

where I_i and I_t are the incident and emergent light intensities respectively after passage through a light path of l centimeters in a medium where the concentration of absorbing molecules is c moles/liter. The constant ε is the molar absorbance (or extinction) coefficient.

A further quantitative dimension was added to photochemistry by EINSTEIN with his introduction of the photon concept. This took the form of the Law of Photochemical Equivalence which states that a photochemical reaction is the consequence of the absorption of a single photon of energy, $h\nu$, by a molecule. The *einstein*, $\mathscr{E}$, the energy of a mole of monochromatic photons, became the measure of absorbed light intensity

$$\mathscr{E} = N_0 h\nu = N_0 hc/\lambda \text{ ergs/mole} \qquad (40)$$

where N_0 is AVOGADRO's number (6.02×10^{23} molecules/mole). With this concept it was possible to relate absorbed light energy to the molar thermodynamic quantities, ΔF, the change in free energy, and ΔH, the change in enthalpy. For example, for the process of breaking a carbon-carbon single bond in a typical hydrocarbon ΔH, which is a measure of the bond energy, is about 80 kcal. According to Eq. (40) this is equivalent to light of wavelength 365 nm. This represents the long wavelength limit of light that could possibly effect such a process, given an appropriate electronic transition in the molecule whose energy could be so utilized. Usually, however, higher photon energies are required since a substantial fraction of the absorbed light energy is dissipated by other paths. The law of photochemical equivalence has had to be modified in consequence of the recent development of intense monochromatic laser beams, which have revealed multiphotonic processes.

In the usual photochemical process only a fraction of the total monochromatic photons absorbed lead to reaction. This fraction, expressed as the number of moles of reactant that undergo reaction per einstein of absorbed radiation, is known as the quantum yield, γ, of the process. Some photochemical processes have an overall quantum yield that is greater than unity. This arises from the thermal (dark) reactions of species produced in the primary photochemical process with the parent light absorbing molecule. The primary photochemical process, which embodies excitation and the reaction of the electronically excited molecule, has a quantum yield that does not exceed unity.

B. The Isomerization of the Retinals

HUBBARD, BOWNDS and YOSHIZAWA (1966) have studied the thermal isomerization of 11-*cis* to all-*trans*-retinal in a variety of solvents. The kinetic data can best be interpreted in terms of Absolute Reaction Rate Theory which pictures chemical and certain physical processes as proceeding from reactants to products via a transition state. That part of the process leading from reactants to the transition state is described in terms of pseudo-thermodynamic parameters, $\Delta H^{\pm}$, $\Delta S^{\pm}$ and $\Delta F.^{\pm}$ $\Delta H^{\pm}$, the enthalpy of activation can be considered as the energy gained or lost by the making or breaking of chemical bonds, or changes in solvent-solute interaction in achieving the transition state. $\Delta S^{\pm}$, the entropy of activation, is a measure of the change in the degree of order or probability accompanying the formation of the transition state, a negative $\Delta S^{\pm}$ indicating the transition state to be more ordered, or a more improbable, state than that of the reactants. These two parameters are related to the free energy of activation, $\Delta F^{\pm}$ by Eq. (41), where T is the absolute temperature.

$$\Delta F^{\pm} = \Delta H^{\pm} - T \Delta S^{\pm} . \tag{41}$$

The activation parameters can be calculated from the kinetic data if the rate constant k is determined at several different temperatures. Thus the rate constant k is related to $\Delta F^{\pm}$ by Eq. (42).

$$k = \frac{RT}{N_0 h} \exp(-\Delta F^{\pm}/RT) . \tag{42}$$

Putting (42) into logarithmic form, (43),

$$\log_{10} k \bigg/ \frac{RT}{N_0 h} = \Delta S^{\pm}/2.3R - \Delta H^{\pm}/2.3R \left(\frac{1}{T}\right) \tag{43}$$

and plotting the logarithm term containing k against $1/T$, one obtains the (assumed) temperature-independent $\Delta H^{\pm}$ as the slope of the linear curve. $\Delta S^{\pm}$ can be obtained from (41).

In a *cis-trans* isomerization, where no formal chemical bonds are broken, $\Delta H^{\pm}$ can be interpreted as the energy barrier to rotation about the formal double bond. HUBBARD, BOWNDS, and YOSHIZAWA (1966) found that the $\Delta H^{\pm}$ for the thermal isomerization was 21.7 kcal in 1-propanol and 25.5 kcal in n-heptane. In aqueous 1% digitonin the $\Delta H^{\pm}$ for isomerization was 23.8 kcal suggesting that the digitonin micelle provided an essentially hydrocarbon environment for the retinal.

The $\Delta S^{\pm}$ for the isomerization was -21.4 cal/deg in 1-propanol which increased to -10.0 cal/deg in heptane and to -12.5 cal/deg in aqueous digitonin. These pronounced negative entropies of activation indicate that passage through the transition state is a very improbable process, the improbability being associated with the intersystem-crossing transition from the ground singlet to the lowest triplet state of retinal. The reader is here referred to Chapter 3 for a discussion of behavior of these two states on torsion about the 11—12 bond of retinal.

In the presence of iodine the rate of thermal isomerization in n-heptane is considerably enhanced. This is reflected in a decrease in $\Delta H^{\pm}$ by 2.1 kcal and a rather marked increase in $\Delta S^{\pm}$ from -10 to $+0.7$ e.u. A logical interpretation of these results is that a complex is formed between retinal and iodine. The formation of this complex results in an admixture of the two heavy iodine atoms into the molecular wave function. This not only markedly increases the spin-orbit mixing of the ground singlet and the lowest triplet state (and hence the intersystem-crossing probability between the two) but also lowers by approximately 2 kcal the energy of the lowest triplet state and hence the energy barrier to isomerization.

In an initial study of the photoisomerization of retinal isomers HUBBARD (1956) found the 11-*cis* isomer to be the most photolabile. Quantitative measurements on the photoisomerization of retinal isomers is very difficult because of the spectral similarity of the isomers. Recently, KROPF and HUBBARD (1970) have made a quantitative measurement of the photoisomerization of the 11-*cis* to the all-*trans* isomer, making use of the singular *cis* absorption peak of the former. For this process they found a quantum yield of approximately 0.1. The significance of this value relative to the pathway of the photoisomerization will be discussed in the next section.

C. The Flash Photolysis of Retinal

Conventional photochemistry employs steady sources of light whose output in usable bandwidths seldom exceeds 10 micro-einsteins/sec. Short-lived intermediates such as electronically excited molecules whose lifetime is less than a millisecond are clearly not detectable under these conditions. The flash photolysis technique, however, allows one to introduce as much as 10 micro-einsteins of actinic light into a system in a single flash lasting less than 10 μsec. Under these conditions measurable concentrations of short lived intermediates can be produced, and their decay kinetics can be followed by rapid spectrophotometric methods.

The flash photolysis apparatus in current use in our laboratory has been employed for the study of retinal and visual pigments and is shown in Fig. 12. It consists of a pair of xenon-filled quartz flash tubes with tungsten electrodes mounted symmetrically within a polished aluminium reflector about a cylindrical photolysis cell. Electrical energy stored in high voltage capacitors (10 kV) is discharged through the flash tubes by means of a triggered thyratron connected in series with them. The light flash so produced is absorbed by the solution contained in the thermostatted photolysis cell. In the optical path there is, in sequence, a steady source of continuous radiation, a shutter (to shield the photolysis cell) that opens when the flash is triggered, the photolysis cell, a baffle system to minimize scattered light from the flash entering the optical path, and a beam splitter that divides the scanning beam and passes it through two separate monochromators set to pass different wavelengths of radiation. At the exit slits of both monochromators are multiplier phototubes whose responses are recorded on a dual beam cathode ray oscilloscope. With this system rapid changes in light transmission, and hence absorbance, can be studied simultaneously in two different regions of the spectrum.

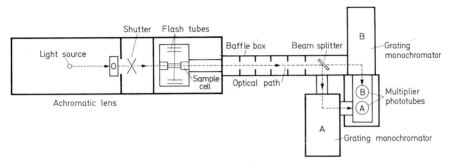

Fig. 12. Dual-beam flash photolysis unit

The first flash photolysis studies on retinal were made by ABRAHAMSON, ADAMS, and WULFF (1959) who flash-illuminated oxygen-free solutions of *trans*-retinal in methylcyclohexane. Immediately on flashing they observed the ground state retinal absorbance peak at 380 nm to disappear and to be replaced by a new intermediate absorbing maximally at 456 nm. This new absorbance peak was observed to decay at room temperature as a first order process with a rate constant of $k = 8.85 \times 10^4 \sec^{-1}$, which is equivalent to a lifetime $\tau = 1/k$ of $11.3 \mu sec$. The growth and decay of this new intermediate shown in Fig. 13 is a typical oscillogram showing the change in light transmission in wavelengths associated with the ground state and the new intermediate. Fig. 14 shows the relative absorbances of both species.

Small amounts of oxygen in the solution were found to markedly enhance the decay rate of the intermediate, and as excited triplet states are readily quenched by molecular oxygen, which itself is a triplet molecule in the ground state, the new intermediate absorbing at 456 nm was assigned to the lowest $^3(\pi, \pi^*)$ of retinal. This assignment was further supported by the intense molar absorbance at 456 nm (80,000), characteristic of triplet-triplet transitions.

No triplet state population was observed on flash illuminating vitamin A (retinol) or the protonated Schiff base of retinal and p-aminobenzoic acid. Neither of these two compounds has an (n, π^*) singlet-triplet pair of states lying lower in energy than the lowest $^1(\pi, \pi^*)$ state, which requires that the $^3(\pi, \pi^*)$ must be populated by a direct radiationless intersystem crossing from the $^1(\pi, \pi^*)$. The spin-orbit operator only rarely has the proper symmetry to mix a $^1(\pi, \pi^*)$ with its $^3(\pi, \pi^*)$ (EL-SAYED, 1963), and as this perturbation governs intersystem crossing, the failure to populate the $^3(\pi, \pi^*)$ in these two cases is understandable. When an $^1(n, \pi^*)$ state lies intermediate in energy between the $^1(\pi, \pi^*)$ and $^3(\pi, \pi^*)$ a vibronic perturbation can usually effect a radiationless internal conversion from the $^1(\pi, \pi^*)$ to the $^1(n, \pi^*)$ in times of the order of one tenth of a nanosecond (El-Sayed, 1963), but further internal conversion to the ground state is very improbable because of the forbidden character of such a transition. This provides ample opportunity for

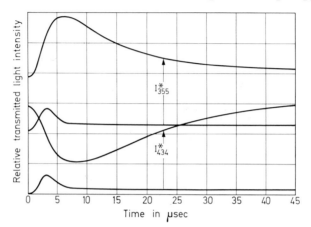

Fig. 13. Simultaneous dual-beam oscilloscope traces for 434 nm and 355 nm responses from trans-retinal in methylcyclohexane. The base lines for the two traces show the profile of the scattered light from the flash

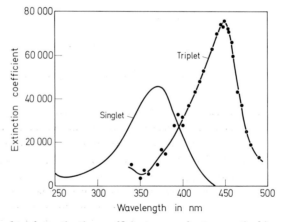

Fig. 14. Singlet and triplet extinction coefficient curves for trans-retinal in methylcyclohexane

intersystem crossing from the $^1(n, \pi^*)$ to the $^3(\pi, \pi^*)$ by a spin-orbit perturbation (El-Sayed, 1963). Thus it is the intermediate $^1(n, \pi^*)$ state in retinal that provides a favorable radiationless pathway into the lowest triplet state. This is illustrated in Fig. 15.

Grellman, Memming, and Livingston (1962) observed that in oxygen-free alcoholic solvents, both the population and the decay rate of the retinal triplet were substantially reduced. Dawson and Abrahamson (1962) showed that this could be attributed to the formation of a complex between the alcohol and retinal in which the lone pair of electrons on the carbonyl oxygen atom of retinal was hydrogen-bonded to the hydroxylic hydrogen atom of alcohol. They reasoned that such a complex would raise the energy of the $^1(n, \pi^*)$ state well above the $^1(\pi, \pi^*)$ removing it from the radiationless pathway to the $^3(\pi, \pi^*)$. They were able to establish that such a hydrogen-bonded complex did, in fact, exist, by infra-red spectral studies of retinal and methanol in carbon tetrachloride.

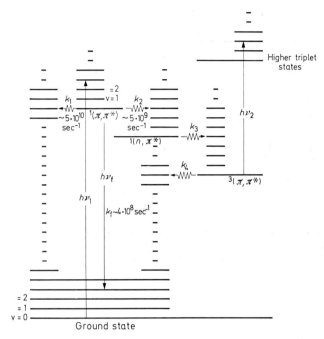

Fig. 15. Radiative ($\longrightarrow$) and radiationless ($\cdots\!\cdots\!\rightarrow$) paths in retinal

To account for the decrease in the observed rate constant for the decay of the retinal triplet in alcohol, they made studies of the triplet decay in mixed methyl-cyclohexane-methanol solvents of varying composition. They concluded that the triplet state of retinal also could hydrogen-bond to the alcohol, producing a complex whose decay rate constant was approximately one-half that of the retinal triplet. The equilibrium constant for the formation of the triplet retinal-methanol complex was determined from their data to be the same as the ground state retinal-methanol complex measured in carbon tetrachloride. This confirmed the identification of the lowest triplet as $^3(\pi, \pi^*)$ rather than $^3(n, \pi^*)$, for the latter, having only a single electron in the orbital available for hydrogen bonding, would hardly be expected to show the same hydrogen-bonding capacity as would a pair of electrons.

A few remarks are in order relative to the rate constants of the various processes shown in Fig. 15. An absolute quantum yield measurement for retinal fluorescence has not been reported but a preliminary measurement in the authors' laboratory indicates that it is approximately 0.01 at room temperature in hydrocarbon solvents. The intrinsic or radiative lifetime $\tau\ (= 1/k)$ for a given excited electronic state, i.e. the lifetime in the absence of quenching or radiationless decay processes, can be approximated as $10^{-5}/\varepsilon_{max}$, where ε_{max} is the maximum extinction coefficient associated with the optical absorptive transition to that state. For the $^1(\pi, \pi^*)$ state of *trans*-retinal τ is approximately 2.5 nanoseconds making the fluorescence rate constant $k_f = 4 \times 10^8$ sec^{-1}. Assuming a fluorescence yield of 0.01 the actual lifetime τ' is given as

$$\tau' = 0.01\,\tau = \frac{1}{k_f + k_1 + k_2}. \tag{44}$$

Since $k_2 \sim 0.11\,k_1$, values for the radiationless rate constants are $k_1 \sim 5 \times 10^{10}$ sec^{-1} and $k_2 \sim 5 \times 10^9$ sec^{-1}.

The above discussion and Figure 15 also provide some insight into the mechanism of photoisomerization. The fact that the quantum yield for this process is essentially the same as for triplet population clearly indicates that photoisomerization occurs via the triplet state. This would suggest that under conditions where (n, π^*) states do not mediate the population of the lowest $^3(\pi, \pi^*)$, the photoisomerization must occur by a much less favorable pathway energetically, and hence with a much smaller quantum yield.

Acknowledgment

We record our thanks to the National Institute of Neurological Diseases and Blindness and to the Eye Institute of the National Institute of Health for supporting the work of our laboratory reported herein.

References
General

CALVERT, J. G., PITTS, J. N., JR.: Photochemistry. New York-London-Sydney: John Wiley & Sons 1966.

KAUZMANN, W.: Quantum chemistry: an introduction. New York: Academic Press 1957.

KING, G. W.: Spectroscopy and molecular structure. New York-Chicago-San Francisco-Toronto-London: Holt, Rinehart and Winston 1965.

PARR, R. G.: Quantum theory of molecular electronic structure. New York: Benjamin 1963.

PAULING, L., WILSON, E. B., JR.: Introduction to quantum mechanics with application to chemistry. New York: McGraw-Hill 1935.

SUZUKI, H.: Electronic absorption spectra and geometry of organic molecules. An application of molecular orbital theory. New York-London: Academic Press 1967.

Text References

ABRAHAMSON, E. W., ADAMS, R., WULFF, V. I.: Reversible spectral changes in retinene solutions following flash illumination. J. Phys. Chem. **63**, 441—443 (1959).

BALKE, D. E., BECKER, R. S.: Spectroscopy and photochemistry of all-trans-retinal and 11-cis-retinal. J. Amer. chem. Soc. **89**, 5061—5062 (1967).

DAWSON, W. R., ABRAHAMSON, E. W.: Population and decay of the lowest triplet state of polyenes with conjugated heteroatoms: retinene. J. Phys. Chem. **66**, 2542—2547 (1962).

EL-SAYED, M. A.: Spin-orbit coupling and the radiationless processes in nitrogen heterocycles. J. Chem. Phys. **38**, 2834—2838 (1963).

EVANS, D. F.: Magnetic perturbation of singlet-triplet transitions. Part IV. Unsaturated compounds. J. chem. Soc. 1735—1745 (1960).

GRELLMANN, K. H., MEMMING, R., LIVINGSTON, R.: Some flash-photolytic and photochemical studies of retinene and related compounds. J. Amer. chem. Soc. **84**, 546—548 (1962).

HUBBARD, R.: Geometrical isomerization of vitamin A, retinene and retinene oxide. J. Amer. chem. Soc. **78**, 4662—4667 (1956).

— BOWNDS, D., YOSHIZAWA, T.: The chemistry of visual photoreception. Cold Spr. Harb. Symp. quant. Biol.: 1965; **30**, 301—315 (1966).

JONES, L. C., JR., TAYLOR, L. W.: Far ultraviolet absorption spectra of unsaturated and aromatic hydrocarbons. Anal. Chem. **27**, 228—237 (1955).

KROPF, A., HUBBARD, R.: The photoisomerization of retinal. Photochem. Photobiol. **12**, 249—260 (1970).

PLATT, J. R.: Electronic structure and excitation of polyenes and porphyrins. In: Radiation biology. Vol. III: Visible and near-visible light, 71—123. New York: McGraw-Hill 1956.

WIESENFELD, J. R., ABRAHAMSON, E. W.: Visual pigments: their spectra and isomerizations. Photochem. Photobiol. **8**, 487—493 (1968).

Chapter 2

The Chemistry of the Visual Pigments

By

R. A. Morton, Liverpool (Great Britain)

With 12 Figures

Contents

I. Introduction

My postgraduate studies under E. C. C. Baly began in October 1921 and among those attracted to Liverpool by the professor's reputation as a spectroscopist was Selig Hecht, holding a National Research Fellowship. It was from Hecht that Baly's group first heard of visual purple and dark adaptation, and of the special place of the Journal of General Physiology under Loeb. I was one of Hecht's subjects in a classical study of 'The visibility of monochromatic radiation and the absorption spectrum of visual purple' (Hecht and Williams, 1922). Hecht was a very adaptable and resourceful conversationalist and he kept his 'victims' entertained during the preparatory half hour in darkness. In carrying out his researches he oscillated between the Chemistry Department where he studied visual purple and the Physics Laboratory where he measured visual responses. My interests were in absorption spectrophotometry and I little thought then that I should myself work on visual pigments.

In an early paper Hecht (1921), writing from Creighton University, Omaha, summarised his ideas on 'the photochemistry of the sensitivity of animals to light' based on papers that had already appeared in the Journal of General Physiology (1919—1920).

Hecht and Williams (1922) had a clear and direct approach:

"When the visible spectrum is reduced to a very low intensity, and is viewed by a dark-adapted eye, it appears colourless. The different portions of the spectrum, however, possess different degrees of brightness, the centre being much brighter than the ends. Apparently a given quantity of light energy will produce a quantitatively different effect depending on its frequency."

Reviewing earlier work they added:

"It might therefore seem superfluous for us to have undertaken this work, and to add another to the already overwhelming number of papers on vision."

Was there a vein of irony in that sentence?

The basic measurement was the relative energy, in different (monochromatic) portions of the spectrum, needed to produce a colourless sensation. The reciprocal of this relative energy at any wavelength was regarded as proportional to the absorbance coefficient of a sensitive substance in the eye. The curve representing the visibility of the spectrum at very low intensities had the same shape as that for the visibility at high intensities involving colour vision, but the curve at high intensities was 48 nm further toward the red (see Hyde, Forsythe, and Cady, 1918).

The absorbance spectrum of visual purple (from one human retina) was first measured by Koenig (1894) using a modified Vierordt spectrophotometer, then very new. The solution was cloudy but the maximum was found to be near 500 nm. Hecht noted that:

"The extended and fantastic theories which Koenig developed as a result of his measurements with this single retina are open for him to read who will. It is not for us to dwell too harshly on these lapses."

The careful work of Köttgen and Abelsdorff (1896) on monkey, cat, rabbit and frog, showed that the absorbance (difference) spectrum of visual purple extracted into bile salt solution was reproducible with a maximum near 503 nm. The maximum of the scotopic sensitivity spectrum was some 8 nm nearer the red. Hecht attributed this shift to the greater density and refractive index of the rods in the eye as compared with water. He toyed with the idea that the displacement of the curve for colour vision was due to the same pigment affected to an even greater degree by the cone 'environment'.

Even as a young man Hecht's historical sense was acute, and his appreciation of the work of the pioneers was generous. Writing from Columbia University, Hecht (1942) noted Boll's (1876) observation that the pink colour of a fresh frog retina slowly faded in the light. He commented on Kühne's (1878, 1879) extraction of the pigment by bile salts and went on:

"Kühne did a prodigious amount of experimentation with visual purple; indeed much of the subsequent work by others merely carried out with precision those experiments which he made by rough methods, and the meaning of which he appreciated fully. In spite of this, interest in visual purple declined rapidly. One reason was that Kühne's industry and acumen had pushed the investigation to the margin of contemporary knowledge and therefore it had to await the general growth of chemistry. Another reason was that visual purple was found only in the rods and not in the cones. Since the region of sharpest vision contains only cones and no rods, visual purple could not be considered essential for good vision. Moreover, frogs whose visual purple had been completely bleached by sunlight were still capable of most accurate vision."

Some twenty years were to elapse before photochemical ideas seriously began to impinge on the subject (Lasareff, 1913; Pütter, 1918; Hecht, 1919). Three steps were postulated: (1), a primary photochemical process; (2), a dark reaction that replaced the decomposed photosensitive material, either from its products or from other precursors; and (3), a second 'dark' process by which the primary photo-products, alone or with other substances, initiated a nerve impulse. This picture dominated Hecht's effort for many years. His work was neatly summarised in a Harvey Lecture (Hecht, 1938). The duplicity theory of vision (Schultze, 1866) in which the cones are regarded as the receptors for colour perception and high-intensity vision, and the rods the mediators of achromatic, low-intensity vision, had been neglected until Parinaud (1881) rediscovered it. Hecht and his collaborators did much to validate the theory, embracing in their experiments a wide range of phenomena such as flicker and intensity discrimination. The reality of discontinuous rod-cone transitions was fully verified (see Hecht, 1942).

The state of knowledge just before the Second World War was full of interest. It was agreed that visual purple was a conjugated protein with a detachable prosthetic group. Kühne (1879) had found that after 'bleaching' by light the pigment could be regenerated. Many attempts to discover an extractable photo-sensitive cone pigment, however, had failed. The first success was reported by Wald (1937b). Digitonin extracts from chick retinas contained two light sensitive substances with maxima at 510 nm and 575 nm respectively (see also, Bliss, 1946). The chick retina contained far more cones than rods but surprisingly there seemed to be much more of visual purple ($\lambda_{max} = 510$ nm) in the extract than of the new cone pigment iodopsin ($\lambda_{max} = 575$ nm).

II. The Vitamins A

A. In Vivo Tests for Vitamin A

In the middle thirties Wald (1935a, b; 1936) made the new observation that on bleaching or fading, visual purple produced a 'carotenoid', retinene, that could give rise to vitamin A. This was the beginning of a link between the *chemistry* of vision and nutritional night blindness resulting from vitamin A deficiency.

Vitamin A_1 (retinol) and vitamin A_2 (3-dehydroretinol) are related to the carotenoids, an important example of which is β-carotene, $C_{40}H_{56}$. The carotenoids, very numerous and widely distributed in Nature, are generally yellow to red in colour. All are polyisoprenoid compounds linked 'head to tail' except in the middle of the molecule. This can be clearly seen in the open-chain, tomato pigment lyco-

3*

pene, $C_{40}H_{56}$, the structural formula of which,

lycopene

shows its relationship to the isomeric β-carotene,

β -carotene

a molecule that is likewise symmetrical about the 15 : 15′ double bond (Karrer and Jucker, 1948).

Many centuries before the vitamin concept had been formulated, defective dim-light vision had been recognised as a manifestation of dietary deficiency; moreover the ingestion of liver had been found to have a very beneficial effect. Fridericia and Holm (1925), building on the work of McCollum, Hopkins, and others (see McCollum, 1956) had induced experimental night blindness in rats deprived of vitamin A. The experiments of Holm (1925) revealed differences in behaviour in dim light between normal rats and deprived rats, consistent with poor scotopic vision for the latter, and subsequent provision of vitamin A caused a marked improvement in the behaviour of the deprived animals. Fridericia and Holm associated dim-light vision with retinal rods and the presence of pigment. They observed that the vitamin A-deficient rats had little visual purple and, after exposure to bright light, almost colourless retinas. A more recent study (Dowling and Wald, 1965) carried out on weanling rats illustrates the present day approach to the relationship between vitamin A deficiency and night blindness.

Steenbock and Gross (1919) found that certain yellow-red foods (e.g. carrots) contained something that relieved the symptoms of vitamin A deficiency. Steenbock and Boutwell (1920a, b) expressed the conviction that although carotene was not vitamin A it was in some way related to it. They separated carotenes (hydrocarbons) from 'xanthophylls' (hydroxylated hydrocarbons) and found the vitamin A-replacing effect to belong to the former but not the latter. They compared various butter samples and found that vitamin A responses did not run parallel with carotenoid pigment concentration.

Palmer and Kempster (1919) had already carried out careful experiments on white leghorn chicks reared on a diet virtually carotenoid-free. After six weeks the chicks pined but were restored by adding pig liver to the diet. (Pig liver contains practically no carotenoid but is a source of the almost colourless vitamin A). The hens laid many eggs and, though the yolks contained no yellow carotenoids, viable chicks were hatched from them. Stephenson (1920) removed pigment from yellow butter fat (dissolved in light petroleum) by shaking with charcoal. Although all pigment was absent, the colourless butter fat still gave a vitamin A response. Palmer and Kennedy (1922) showed that the vitamin A of cod liver oil was distinct from carotene.

B. In Vitro Tests for Vitamin A

Cod liver oil was known to be a useful source of vitamin A, and biological assays had verified that, on saponification, the active principle passed quantitatively into the non-saponifiable fraction, from which cholesterol had been removed by crystallisation at —60°. It had been observed (ROSENHEIM and DRUMMOND, 1925) that liver oils and extracts gave a strong blue colour with arsenic trichloride, the intensity apparently varying with vitamin A content. CARR and PRICE (1926) found that a saturated solution of anhydrous antimony trichloride in chloroform was a more convenient reagent, and gave a similar blue colour. WOKES (1928) studied the colour tests by spectroscopic methods.

PEACOCK (1926) had suggested that vitamin A was decomposed by light. MORTON and HEILBRON (1928a, b) made quantitative determinations of the spectral absorbance in the ultraviolet of a variety of products, mainly from fish livers. A close correlation was observed between the absorbances at 328 nm and the corresponding colour test intensities with the Carr-Price reagent. Comparison of biological activities with the ultraviolet absorbances and the colour test intensities provided convincing evidence that the 328 nm absorption band was indeed due to vitamin A (COWARD, DYER, MORTON, and GADDUM, 1931, 1932). This led to the examination of the liver oils from a wide range of fish species, and it soon became clear that many fish liver oils were very much richer in vitamin A than was cod liver oil. This discovery made available much richer concentrates and eventually led to the isolation of the vitamin in a state of purity (see TAKAHASHI and KAWAKAMI, 1923; KARRER, MORF and SCHÖPP, 1931; VON EULER and KARRER, 1931; HEILBRON, HESLOP, MORTON, WEBSTER, REA, and DRUMMOND, 1932; HAMANO, 1935, 1937; HOLMES and CORBETT, 1937a, b; BAXTER and ROBESON, 1940).

The determination of structure resulted from work done in the schools of KARRER, HEILBRON, MILAS, and others but it is only necessary here to note the outcome. Vitamin A (retinol) is a primary alcohol $C_{20}H_{29}OH$ with the structure:

Vitamin A (retinol)

C. Precursors of Vitamin A

Once it was established that vitamin A was quite distinct from carotene, and could be recognised by its ultraviolet absorption the way forward was clear. Crucial experiments were carried out by MOORE (1929, 1930) when he administered nearly pure carotene to vitamin A-deficient young rats and demonstrated that their livers acquired a store of true vitamin A. VON EULER, VON EULER, and HELLSTRÖM (1928) had confirmed STEENBOCK's view that carotene gave rise to the vitamin. Just as ergosterol had been shown to be a *photochemical* precursor of vitamin D, carotene had been recognised as a *metabolic* provitamin A. In fact all those carotenoids that contained one half of the symmetrical β-carotene molecule proved to be provitamins A. CAPPER, MCKIBBIN, and PRENTICE (1931) using MOORE's methods, extended his findings on rats to chickens.

Many workers tried without any definite success to show that liver tissue *in vitro* would convert carotene to vitamin A. Belief persisted that in the whole animal the site of conversion was liver, despite failure to prove it.

In studies on the distribution of vitamin A in fishes (EDISBURY, MORTON, SIMPKINS, and LOVERN, 1938; LOVERN, MORTON, and IRELAND, 1939; LOVERN and MORTON, 1939) it was found that in many species relatively large amounts of vitamin occurred in the alimentary tract, particularly in the pyloric caecae. These appendages occur, for example, in cod, herring, halibut, salmon, trout and sturgeon and, together with the absorptive part of the gut, they yield oil very much richer in vitamin A than the corresponding liver oil. In fact more than half the total vitamin A of the halibut may be found in the lipids of intestinal mucosae. The intestines of mammals, however, contain little or no vitamin and the main store is in the liver.

Soon after the War vitamin A aldehyde was fed to rats and was found to be converted to vitamin A in the intestinal wall. The conversion of carotene to vitamin A also occurred in intestinal mucosae (BALL, GLOVER, GOODWIN, and MORTON, 1947; GLOVER, GOODWIN, and MORTON, 1947, 1948; MATTSON, MEHL, and DEUEL, 1947). GOODWIN and GREGORY (1948) showed that, in the goat, conversion of carotene to vitamin A occurred in the gut of the intact animal. Similar results were obtained by KON's group at about the same time (THOMPSON, GANGULY, and KON, 1947, 1949; THOMSON, BRAUDE, COATES, COWIE, GANGULY, and KON, 1950) and extended to pigs. Although conversion of carotene to vitamin A may possibly occur at other body sites the intestinal epithelium is by far the major locus.

D. Discovery of Vitamin A₂ (3-dehydroretinol)

The blue colour produced by the interaction of vitamin A and antimony trichloride is characterised by a sharp absorption band near 617 nm, and vitamin A determinations may be made by measuring the absorbance at that wave length. Much of the early work was done by means of a direct vision spectrophotometer of the Hilger-Nutting type. In tests on fish liver oils, or concentrates derived therefrom, additional peaks at 690—700 nm and 635—655 nm were often seen (HEILBRON, GILLAM, and MORTON, 1931) and as further experience was gained a colour test maximum at 693 nm was linked with a vitamin A congener. This was clearly not a carotenoid. In liver oils from salt-water fishes the 617 nm band due to vitamin A greatly predominated (ca. 10 : 1) over the 693 nm band. Subsequently it was found that in some freshwater-fish livers the 693 nm chromogen was dominant. No mammalian liver oil or concentrate showed any evidence of the 693 nm chromogen, but EDISBURY, MORTON, and SIMPKINS (1937) found it to be predominant in the eyes of goldfish and in the livers of trout. They suggested that the 693 nm chromogen should be designated vitamin A₂ because its distribution suggested that it might replace vitamin A₁ in some fresh-water fishes. LEDERER and ROSANOVA (1937) independently observed the 693 nm chromogen in fishes caught in Russian rivers (see also GILLAM, HEILBRON, LEDERER and ROSANOVA, 1937; EDISBURY, MORTON, SIMPKINS, and LOVERN, 1938; GILLAM, HEILBRON, JONES and LEDERER, 1938). The non-saponifiable extract from goldfish eyes showed ultraviolet maxima at 350 nm and 288 nm which are characteristic of vitamin A_2 (Fig. 1). The proportions of vitamins A_1 and A_2 occurring in fish livers are highly variable; moreover both vitamins may in some species co-exist in retinas, giving rise to two types of visual pigment.

This is not the place to detail the proof of structure; it must suffice to say that vitamin A_2 is 3-dehydroretinol, and that both vitamins A_1 and A_2 are now available as synthetic products.

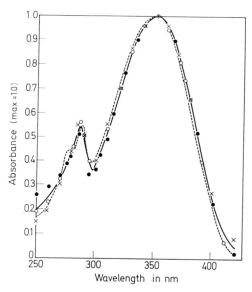

Fig. 1. The spectral absorbance in ethanol of vitamin A_2 (3-dehydroretinol) from several sources, the mean being given by the continuous curve. Filled circles, from preparations obtained by reduction of retinene$_2$ (3-dehydroretinal) *in vivo*; plain circles, from preparations reduced by the Pondorff method *in vitro*; dotted curve from preparations reduced by lithium aluminium hydride; crosses, vitamin A_2 from fish liver oil, according to CAMA, DALVI, MORTON, and SALAH (1952). (CAMA, DALVI, MORTON, SALAH, STEINBERG, and STUBBS, 1952)

III. Structure of Visual Pigments

A. The Retinenes and their Relation to the Vitamins A

As already mentioned, WALD (1933, 1934, 1935a, b, 1936) carried out revealing experiments with frog eyes. He observed that when dark-adapted retinas were treated in the dark with light petroleum the visual pigment remained unchanged and was not extracted. Subsequent treatment with chloroform denatured the rhodopsin and a new substance was then extracted. Designated *retinene*, it was readily soluble in organic solvents and gave a blue colour with the antimony trichloride reagent. The spectrum of the blue solution showed a very sharp band with its centre near 665 nm. The chloroform extract displayed a broad and intense band with maximum near 390 nm. In petroleum ether the peak was displaced towards shorter wave-lengths.

Somewhat later WALD (1937) noticed that the retinas of freshwater fishes often contained a visual pigment (extractable by 1 % aqueous digitonin) displaying an absorbance peak on the long wave side of the rhodopsin maximum. The new pigment was called *porphyropsin* (λ_{max} originally given as 522 ± 2 nm but now known to range, in different species, from 512 to 543 nm at least). When denatured by chloroform (or bleached under conditions that produced retinene from rhodopsin) the pigment gave rise to a new product that showed a colour test maximum near 700 nm and a broad absorption band with $\lambda_{max} = 407$ nm in the chloroform solution. This compound was given the name retinene$_2$, and its analogue, formerly known as retinene, became retinene$_1$ (WALD, 1939).

Further progress was no doubt held up by the War. In any case the amounts of material obtainable from retinas were then quite insufficient for chemical characterisation of the retinenes. It was later shown (MORTON, 1944; MORTON and GOODWIN, 1944; BALL, GOODWIN, and MORTON, 1948) that retinene$_1$ was the aldehyde corresponding with vitamin A$_1$ (retinol), and retinene$_2$ the aldehyde corresponding with vitamin A$_2$ (3-dehydroretinol). By that time vitamin A was available in a state approaching purity and its structure was known. The hypothesis that retinene$_1$ was an aldehyde had great spectroscopic appeal, but the smooth conversion of an alcohol containing five conjugated double bonds to the unsaturated aldehyde seemed difficult. Trials in which potassium permanganate was used as the oxidising agent produced small amounts of a substance giving an absorption band in the colour test with a 664 nm peak. In some experiments manganese dioxide was formed in the course of the oxidation and this led to a test with the oxide itself. Vitamin A (retinol) dissolved in light petroleum was converted to the aldehyde in high yield at room temperature merely by contact with manganese dioxide. This surprisingly effective process has since been used very widely on a whole range of alcohols (EVANS, 1951).

Fish liver oil concentrates containing mixtures of vitamin A$_1$ and vitamin A$_2$ were available but the separation of the two vitamins could not at that time be effected. However, the two vitamins yielded mixtures of the corresponding aldehydes on standing in light petroleum over manganese dioxide, and it proved possible to separate the aldehydes by chromatography (CAMA, DALVI, MORTON, and SALAH, 1952; CAMA, DALVI, MORTON, SALAH, STEINBERG, and STUBBS, 1952). During the War, vitamin A fish liver oils sent to England under the Lend-Lease arrangement with the U.S. Government were tested at Liverpool, and we were particularly interested in ling cod liver oil. This was extremely rich in vitamins A and, although the A$_1$/A$_2$ ratio was about 7/1, the oil was still a very good source of vitamin A$_2$. Some of the ling cod liver oil was used after the War to prepare very rich unsaponifiable fractions. These were oxidised over manganese dioxide, and the two aldehydes were separated by chromatography on alumina and finally crystallised.

Pure retinene$_2$ was reduced by the Ponndorf method and also by the use of lithium aluminium hydride, and vitamin A$_2$ was obtained in practically the pure state (CAMA, DALVI, MORTON, SALAH, STEINBERG, and STUBBS, 1952). The structure of vitamin A$_2$ is,

(Morton, Salah, and Stubbs, 1947a, b; Farrer, Hamlet, Henbest, and Jones, 1952).

Today, when synthetic vitamin A acetate is commercially available as a pure substance, vitamin A alcohol, prepared by careful alkaline hydrolysis, is transferred to pure light petroleum and almost quantitatively converted to retinene$_1$ over manganese dioxide. Retinene$_1$ is dehydrogenated to retinene$_2$ in good yield by means of N-bromosuccinimide. Retinene$_2$ can be reduced to vitamin A$_2$ by means of lithium aluminium hydride (Henbest, Jones, and Owen, 1955).

Adequate supplies of retinene$_1$ and retinene$_2$ permitted new experimental ventures. It was soon shown that the aldehydes could be enzymically reduced to the alcohols (vitamins A$_1$ and A$_2$) and that the classical NAD-dependent alcohol dehydrogenase catalysed the reaction, the equilibrium in the reversible process being well on the alcohol side (Wald, 1949, 1950). Reference has already been made to the reduction of retinene to retinol in the gut wall (p. 38).

B. Indicator Yellow and Schiff's Bases

The aldehyde retinene readily combines with some substances that contain amino groups, and in order to appreciate the significance of this it is necessary to refer to the work of Lythgoe and his colleagues at University College London done some thirty years ago. Lythgoe (1937) and Lythgoe and Quilliam (1938) prepared good quality rhodopsin solutions displaying λ_{max} near 500 nm. Exposure of such solutions to bright light resulted in a displacement of λ_{max} to 470—480 nm. This was attributed to the formation of a derived pigment, *transient orange*. This decomposed at room temperature to give *indicator yellow*, which was pale yellow in

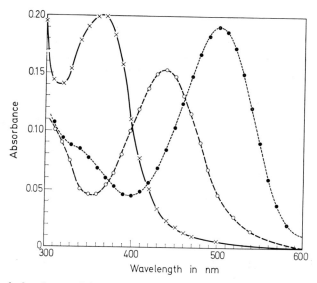

Fig. 2. Spectral absorbance of frog rhodopsin (curve through filled circles) and of the acid indicator yellow (curve through plain circles) and alkaline indicator yellow (curve through crosses) derived therefrom. All curves have been corrected for irrelevant "absorption" due to scattering. (Collins and Morton, 1950b)

alkaline solutions and deep yellow in acid (Fig. 2). BRODA and GOODEVE (1941) found that when rhodopsin in a glycerol-water medium was strongly cooled, the transient orange produced by exposure was stable, but on warming the preparation to room temperature, indicator yellow and retinene were formed.

It was shown by the Liverpool group (BALL, COLLINS, MORTON, and STUBBS, 1948; BALL, COLLINS, DALVI, and MORTON, 1949; COLLINS, 1953, 1954; COLLINS and MORTON, 1950a, b), that retinene entered into combination with many compounds containing amino groups to give Schiff's bases:

$$*C_{19}H_{27}CHO + RNH_2 \rightarrow H_2O + C_{19}H_{27}CH = NR \underset{OH^-}{\overset{H^+}{\rightleftarrows}} C_{19}H_{27}CH = \overset{+}{N}HR .$$

alkaline form   acid form
Schiff's bases

* or $C_{19}H_{25}CHO$ in the case of 3-dehydroretinal (retinene$_2$)

These had spectroscopic properties resembling those of indicator yellow (λ_{max}440 nm in acid, 365 nm in alkaline solutions). The experiments suggested the possibility that retinene, if liberated as the free aldehyde, might unite with the free amino groups of proteins, so that 'indicator yellow' could be an artifact having no necessary or direct relationship to rhodopsin. However COLLINS (1953) showed that if rhodopsin solutions were 'bleached' by light in the presence of 10 M formaldehyde, 'alkaline' indicator yellow still resulted. He argued that as the formaldehyde blocked amino groups the indicator yellow could not be a secondary 'artifact', and hence that the C—N link in the true indicator yellow must have been present in rhodopsin itself. Moreover when rhodopsin was photochemically decomposed in the presence of acid, the deep yellow form of indicator yellow resulted. No free retinene was detected and in any case the Schiff's base would not have been formed under acid conditions.

C. Nature of Prosthetic Group-Protein Linkage

At this point it is convenient to follow WALD's nomenclature. Visual pigments are made up of specific proteins — *opsins* (scotopsins for rod pigments, photopsins for cone pigments) — united with a prosthetic group based on one or other of the vitamin A aldehydes, namely retinal or 3-dehydroretinal. The multiplicity and variability of visual pigments is due both to the alternative aldehydes and to a plurality of opsins. The opsins can be obtained by extracting visual pigments with a detergent solution (1 % digitonin), detaching the aldehyde by a mild reagent, and removing it by extraction with an organic solvent, to leave the undenatured protein in the aqueous phase. The opsins are insoluble in pure water and are readily denatured. The prototype, rhodopsin, is a lipoprotein containing a considerable proportion of phospholipid.

MORTON and PITT (1955) found that on addition of acid to rhodopsin to bring the pH quickly to about 1.0, N-retinylidene opsin was formed with the retinylidene group still attached to nitrogen. This had the same spectrophotometric characteristics as retinylidene-methylamine which had been prepared and studied carefully.

$$C_{19}H_{27}CHO + H_2N \cdot CH_3 \rightarrow C_{19}H_{27}CH{=}N \cdot CH_3 + H_2O .$$

From what has already been said rhodopsin can thus be regarded as related to an N-retinylidene opsin. It has recently been shown (BOWNDS and WALD, 1965; BOWNDS, 1967; AKHTAR, BLOSSE, and DEWHURST, 1965, 1967) that sodium borohydride will not affect rhodopsin but will reduce the N-retinylidene opsin produced as an intermediate on irradiating rhodopsin. The product is a retinyl opsin in which the prosthetic group is still attached to the protein.

$$C_{19}H_{27}CH = N\text{-opsin} \rightarrow C_{19}H_{27}CH_2NH\text{-opsin}.$$

N-retinylidene opsin   *N-retinyl opsin*

BOWNDS (1967) and AKHTAR, BLOSSE, and DEWHURST (1967) independently proved that the retinyl group is attached to the protein at an ε-amino group of a lysyl residue.

Thus BOWNDS (1967) obtained rhodopsin solutions in 2 % digitonin, and exposed them to light at pH 8 in the presence of sodium borohydride. The sequence of thermal reactions (p. 56) following the exposure proceeded under these conditions to metarhodopsin II ($\lambda_{max} = 380$ nm), which the borohydride then reduced to N-retinylopsin, ($\lambda_{max} = 333$ nm). At this point the solution was dialysed against water at 4° to remove excess borate. Alkaline hydrolysis (100° for 6 hours) then yielded a mixture, which on chromatographic analysis (silica gel) gave two fluorescent fractions. These were examined by thin layer chromatography using fifteen synthetic N-retinylaminoacids as markers.

The compound from N-retinyl opsin could not be distinguished from N-retinyl-lysine or N-retinyl-ornithine. The latter might have come from N-retinyl-arginine, and N-retinyl-lysine was shown to undergo rearrangement between the α- and

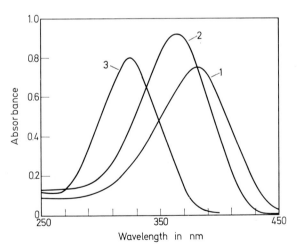

Fig. 3. Synthesis of an N-retinyl amino acid. Curve 1 is the spectral absorbance of all-trans retinal in 60 per cent aqueous methanol (1.75×10^{-5} M; $\lambda_{max} = 383$ nm). A 200-fold molar excess of alanine was then added, and the pH adjusted to 9.5 by adding 1N sodium hydroxide solution. After 20 mins the retinal had been converted to the Schiff base N-retinylidenealanine, $C_{19}H_{27}CH = N - C(CH_3)HCOO^-$ (curve 2, $\lambda_{max} = 367$ nm). Addition of 10 mg of powdered sodium borohydride reduced this to the corresponding secondary amine, $C_{19}H_{27}CH_2NHC(CH_3)HCOO^-$ (curve 3, $\lambda_{max} = 328$ nm). (BOWNDS, 1967)

ε-amino groups of lysine. Accordingly N-retinylopsin (in digitonin solution) was exposed to pronase (a mixture of proteases from *Streptomyces griseus*) with the result that small N-retinylpeptides were formed. Chromatographic isolation of N-retinylpeptides was followed by acid hydrolysis (6 N. HCl, 24 hours) or alkaline hydrolysis. All the fluorescent peptides yielded N-retinyl lysine on hydrolysis. The smallest peptide contained lysine, phenylalanine (2) and alanine; and the largest corresponded with a decapeptide (phe₃ ala, ileu, pro, thr and ε-N-retinyl-lys). The following residues must, therefore, occur quite near to the lysyl residue, which binds the retinyl group: lysine, phenylalanine, threonine, isoleucine and proline.

AKHTAR, BLOSSE, and DEWHURST (1967) reduced 11-*cis*-retinal with tritiated borohydride to give tritiated retinol, which was oxidised (MnO₂) to tritiated retinal. This was incubated with bovine scotopsin to give labelled rhodopsin, and excess retinal was removed as oxime. The labelled rhodopsin was irradiated in the presence of sodium borohydride, and the product ($\lambda_{\mathrm{max}} = 335$ nm) was freeze-dried. The solid was mixed with carrier ε-N-retinyl lysine (i.e. retinylidene-lysine reduced by borohydride) and the mixture was hydrolysed (5 N NaOH). The hydrolysate was neutralised and freeze-dried, and retinylamino-acid was extracted from it with a chloroform-methanol mixture (70 : 30 v/v). Chromatography of the extract showed that activity was in ε-N-retinyl-lysine, and after reduction (palladium-charcoal) to ε-N-perhydroretinyl-lysine the activity persisted. Experiments with dinitrofluorobenzene discriminated clearly in favour of ε-N-perhydroretinyl-lysine as against α-N-perhydroretinyl-lysine. AKHTAR, BLOSSE, and DEWHURST, following the ideas of MULLIKEN, explained the 500 nm band of rhodopsin as due to a charge transfer complex. Bonding is regarded as due to resonance i.e.,

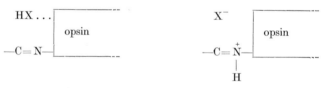

... = bond due to van der Waal's forces   Electrostatic polarization

The resistance of rhodopsin to attack by borohydride suggests that in the intact visual pigment the nature of the attachment between prosthetic group and opsin prevents the —C=N-group from being reduced. There is quite independent evidence that the retinal grouping is not exposed, inasmuch as lipoxidase fails to attack rhodopsin, although it will act on free retinal. BOWNDS argues that at the lysine point of attachment the relevant region of the protein is probably hydrophobic as a result of predominantly non-polar aminoacid side-chains.

D. Analysis of Rhodopsin

It is difficult to obtain rhodopsin solutions entirely free from irrelevant absorption, some of it due to other proteins, but the best preparations are now made by a standard procedure. Dark-adapted retinas are carefully removed under dim red illumination into saline. Moderate shaking removes the rod outer segments, which contain all the pigment. The suspension is stirred into concentrated sucrose solution (40—45 %) and centrifuged, whereupon the rod outer segments remain suspended while the retinal debris sediments. The supernatant sucrose solution is withdrawn from debris and then diluted with water and centrifuged to throw down the rod outer segments. The sediment is washed free from sucrose and finally extracted with 1 % digitonin (see MORTON and PITT, 1957). The full analysis of rhodopsin is quantitatively a little uncertain because a true 'dry weight' is difficult to reach.

COLLINS, LOVE, and MORTON (1954) reported 31.9 % phospholipid, 38.5 % protein and 7 % of minor constituents with water probably accounting for most of the remainder. FLEISCHER and McCONNELL (1966) studied the lipids of bovine retinal outer segment discs and found the lipid content to be unusually high for an organelle from animal tissue. Ultrasonic disintegration has been effectively used to obtain small particles from rod outer segments (BARER and SIDMAN, 1953; MORTON, PETERSON, and PITT, 1957). The best preparations of rhodopsin have three regions of selective absorption (see Fig. 4), and the peak at 275 nm belongs

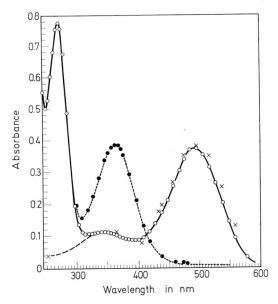

Fig. 4. The spectral absorbance of a nearly-pure extract of cattle rhodopsin at pH 9.2 (curve through plain circles); and of the bleached extract (curve through filled circles). Crosses give the photosensitivities of frog rhodopsin (according to GOODEVE, LYTHGOE, and SCHNEIDER) adjusted to correspond to the absorbance curve at 500 nm. The dashed interpolation gives the probable contribution to absorbance below 320 nm by the rhodopsin chromophore.
(COLLINS, LOVE, and MORTON, 1952)

to the protein moiety of opsin. If the ratio of the absorbance at 275 nm to that at 500 nm is much over 2.0 the preparation is significantly contaminated by extraneous protein. The relative absorbances at 400 nm and 500 nm lie around 0.21—0.24 to 1, and haemoglobin as impurity raises this ratio. The molecular weight of rhodopsin from cattle is not more than 40,000 Hubbard (1954) and may be nearer to 32,000 (Krinsky, 1958a, b) made up as to polypeptide, 18,000 and phospholipid, 14,000. Shields (1967) concluded that the molecular weight of the protein moiety was 21,000, and Abrahamson and Ostroy (1967) obtained similar results.

IV. Cis-Trans Isomerism

Some of the early samples of retinene₁ (retinal) were made by the manganese dioxide method from vitamin A concentrates prepared from fish liver oil. These retinal preparations were effective in producing rhodopsin when incubated with opsin. When retinal was prepared by the same method from synthetic vitamin A, however, synthesis of visual pigment did not take place. Nevertheless, if the synthetic retinene were first exposed to light, formation of rhodopsin then occurred readily. A distinction was thus drawn between 'active' and inactive forms of retinal (Hubbard and Wald, 1952a, b, c).

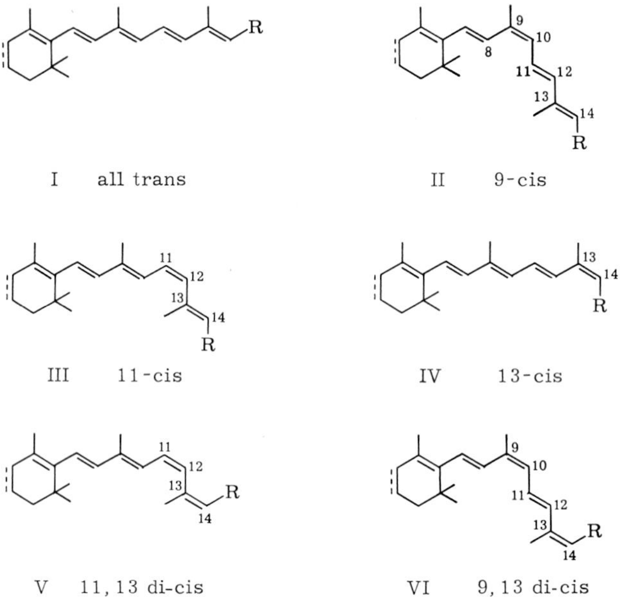

Fig. 5. Structural formulae for the isomeric forms of retinols and 3-dehydroretinols ('R' is CH₂OH) and the retinals and 3-dehydroretinals ('R' is CHO). The 3-dehydro derivatives have an additional double bond in the ring structure (position indicated by dotted line)

It is well known that carotenoids, and polyenes generally, undergo *cis-trans* changes on irradiation particularly with iodine as catalyst (Zechmeister, 1944, 1954). Moreover there was evidence already that the vitamin A of fish liver oils was a mixture of very closely related substances, and the hypothesis of *cis-trans* isomerism provided a plausible explanation for the neovitamins A. Dieterle and Robeson (1954) succeeded in separating and crystallising an isomeride of vitamin A aldehyde which they designated neoretinene b, and Brown and Wald (1956) obtained the neo-b isomers of both retinol and retinal. The 'active' aldehyde was readily reduced to the corresponding alcohol by lithium aluminium hydride or sodium borohydride. The ultraviolet spectra of both the neo-b retinol and neo-b retinal were consistent with *cis* forms. The antimony trichloride colour test ($\lambda_{max} = 664$ nm) for the retinal had the normal intensity. Irradiation of the *cis* compounds gave mixtures similar to those produced by the action of light on the synthetic (all-*trans*) materials (HUBBARD, GREGERMAN, and WALD, 1953).

It was not at all clear, however, precisely how the 'active' retinal differed from all-*trans* retinal. PAULING (1939, 1949) had considered the possible *cis* forms of vitamin A in the light of current concepts of steric hindrance. According to his argument some *cis* isomerides of isoprenoid compounds would be improbable as a result of twists in the chain produced by the methyl groups. The double bonds at positions 7 and 11 of retinol and retinal would not readily assume *cis* configurations and the 7-*cis* or 11-*cis* isomers should be 'hindered' and quite unstable. The more likely, i.e. more stable, isomerides should thus be all-*trans*, 9-*cis*, 13-*cis* and 9-13 di-*cis*.

Table 1. *Spectral properties of cis-trans isomers of retinol (vitamin A_1) in ethanol. (Source references in* MORTON *and* PITT, *1957)*

Isomer	Formula (Fig. 5)	λ_{max} (nm)	ε_{max} (litre cm⁻¹ mole⁻¹)
All-*trans*	I	325	52,800
9-*cis*	II	323	42,300
11-*cis*	III	319	34,900
13-*cis*	IV	328	48,300
11,13 di-*cis*	V	311	26,200
9,13 di-*cis*	VI	324	39,500

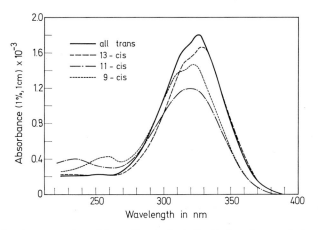

Fig. 6. The absorbance spectra of four vitamin A_1 (retinol) stereoisomers in hexane. Note that the main bands of the unhindered isomers (all-trans, 13-cis, 9-cis) show fine structure while the main band of the hindered 11-cis isomer is symmetrical, and has a flat peak. Note also that the 9-cis isomer has a "cis peak" at 259 nm, and that the 11-cis isomer has a raised absorbance in the "cis peak" region and a subsidiary band at 233 nm. (HUBBARD, 1956)

Now the preponderating natural form of vitamin A appeared to be the all-*trans* isomeride and the main congener, known to biochemists and analysts as neo-vitamin A, was eventually to be identified as 13-*cis* (MEUNIER and JOUANNETEAU, 1948; ROBESON and BAXTER, 1947). The corresponding aldehyde was known (DALVI and MORTON, 1951). Another form, probably 9-*cis* retinal, had also been described (GRAHAM, VAN DORP, and ARENS, 1949). The most surprising development, however, was the discovery in the laboratories of Distillation Products Industries of *five* isomeric forms of retinal (ROBESON, BLUM, DIETERLE, CAWLEY, and BAXTER, 1955). There was then nothing for it but to undertake unambiguous stereo-specific syntheses.

This is not the place to describe in detail the elegant synthetic work that finally fixed the structures; it will suffice to give references. The central problem in the present context was the structure of neo-retinene b, the form active in the synthesis of rhodopsin. It was at first thought to be 11 : 13 di-*cis*, then either 7-*cis* or 11-*cis*. The latter was a courageous idea due primarily to OROSHNIK (OROSHNIK and MEBANE, 1954; OROSHNIK, 1956; OROSHNIK, BROWN, HUBBARD, and WALD, 1956) and eventually the structure was unambigously shown to be

Table 2. *Spectral properties of cis-trans isomers of retinal (retinene₁) in ethanol. (Source references in* MORTON *and* PITT, *1957)*

Isomer	Formula (Fig. 5)	λ_{max} (in nm)	ε_{max} (litre cm⁻¹ mole⁻¹)
All-*trans*	I	381	43,400
9-*cis*	II	373	36,100
11-*cis*	III	376.5	24,900
13-*cis*	IV	375	35,800
11,13 di-*cis*	V	373	19,900
9,13 di-*cis*	VI	368	32,400

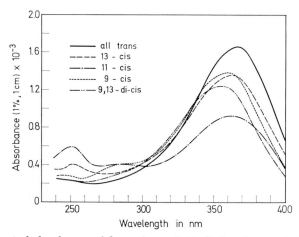

Fig. 7. The spectral absorbances of five retinene₁ (retinal) stereoisomers in hexane. Note that the 9-cis isomer has a "cis peak" (282.5 nm); the 11-cis isomer both a "cis peak" and a strong subsidiary band (251 nm); and the 13-cis isomer a raised absorbance in the "cis peak" region and a weak subsidiary band (252 nm). (HUBBARD, 1956)

11-*cis*. The unusual feature of this story is that PAULING'S studies, though widely verified in other instances, were wrong in this one. But it must be admitted that the existence, as a relatively stable substance, of the 11-*cis* isomer in the retinol, retinal, 3-dehydroretinol, 3-dehydroretinal series has few if any parallels.

WALD (1953) considered that some of his retinene$_2$ (3-dehydroretinal) preparations contained two *cis* isomers. The "*cis*$_1$" fraction, when incubated in darkness with opsin from the eyes of a freshwater fish, gave a porphyropsin of $\lambda_{max} = 523$ nm, while the "*cis*$_2$" isomer gave a pigment with $\lambda_{max} = 507$ nm (isoporphyropsin). There is good evidence that "*cis*$_1$" is the 11-*cis* form. Similarly 11-*cis* retinal incubated with chick opsin produces a pigment with $\lambda_{max} = 562$ nm, consistent with its being an iodopsin or cone pigment (WALD, 1953). There is also evidence that the 11-*cis* dehydroretinal will unite with chick opsin to form a 620 nm pigment 'cyanopsin' but the status of this compound has remained uncertain until recently, when a convincing paper by LIEBMAN and ENTINE (1967) appeared. In the frog *Rana pipiens* the rods and cones use retinene$_2$ at the tadpole stage, but on meta-

Table 3. *Spectral properties of cis-trans isomers of 3-dehydroretinol (vitamin A$_2$) in ethanol (from* V. PLANTA, SCHWIETER, CHOPARD-DIT-JEAN, RÜEGG, KOFLER *and* ISLER, *1962)*

Isomer	Formula (Fig. 5)	λ_{max} (in nm)			ε_{max} (litre cm^{-1} mole^{-1})		
		a	b	c	a	b	c
All-*trans*	I	350	286	276	41,300	20,300	15,800
9-*cis*	II	348	287	277	32,500	26,100	21,800
11-*cis*	III	344	286	278	28,100	16,100	14,000
13-*cis*	IV	352	288	277	39,000	18,400	14,000
11,13 di-*cis*	V	337	290	277	25,700	13,100	13,300
9,13 di-*cis*	VI	350	288	280	29,300	21,600	18,000

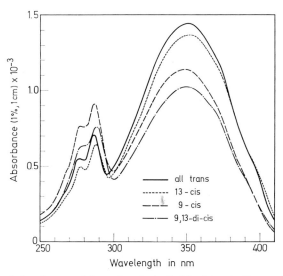

Fig. 8. The spectral absorbances of four vitamin A$_2$ (3-dehydroretinol) stereoisomers in ethanol. (V. PLANTA, SCHWIETER, CHOPARD-DIT-JEAN, RÜEGG, KOFLER, and ISLER, 1962)

morphosis only retinene₁ occurs in the adult eye. Porphyropsin is replaced by rhodopsin, and microspectrophotometry on cones shows that cyanopsin (620 nm) is replaced by an iodopsin (570 nm). A freshwater tortoise (*Pseudemys scripta*) also has the 620 nm pigment in its cones.

The commercial procedure for the synthesis of retinol from citral has been described (Wagner and Folkers, 1964; Isler, Kofler, Huber, and Ronco, 1946, 1947; Isler, 1951). The hindered 11-*cis* retinol and 11,13 di-*cis* retinol are made by the condensation of *cis*-or *trans*-3-methyl-2-penten-4-yn-1-ol, (*a*), with 4-(1,6,6-trimethyl-1-cyclohexen-1-yl)-2-methyl-2-buten-1-al, (*b*).

$$HC \equiv C - \underset{\underset{CH_3}{|}}{C} = CH - CH_2OH$$

(*a*)   (*b*)

The *cis* form of (*a*) resulted in 11,13 di-*cis* retinol, and the *trans* form in 11-*cis* retinol.

Table 4. *Spectral properties of cis-trans isomers of 3-dehydroretinal (retinene₂) in ethanol (from* v. Planta, Schwieter, Chopard-dit-Jean, Rüegg, Kofler *and* Isler, *1962)*

Isomer	Formula (Fig. 5)	λ_{max} (in nm)			ε_{max} (litre cm⁻¹ mole⁻¹)		
		a	b	c	a	b	c
All-*trans*	I	401	314		41,500	11,100	
9-*cis*	II	391	315		34,100	19,000	
11-*cis*	III	393	321	252	24,900	14,400	12,700
13-*cis*	IV	395	314		33,300	11,600	
11,13 di-*cis*	V	386	269	261	27,200	11,000	11,000

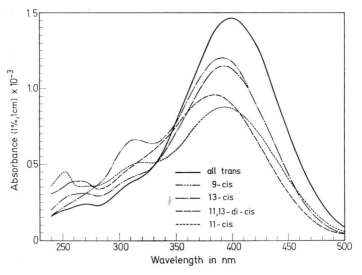

Fig. 9. The spectral absorbances of five retinene₂ (3-dehydroretinal) stereoisomers in ethanol. (After Bridges, 1967, from data supplied by F. Hoffmann-LaRoche, Basel)

HUBBARD and WALD (1952) found that the 9-*cis* isomer of retinal (as well as the 11-*cis*) would combine with opsins to form light-sensitive pigments. In every case these *iso* pigments have their peak absorbances at somewhat shorter wavelengths than the normal pigments derived from 11-*cis* retinal. The *iso* pigments have not been encountered in the retina under physiological conditions.

V. Recapitulation

At this stage the emerging picture can be summarized. In the herbivorous animal, for example, ingested β-carotene is metabolised to a significant extent in the gut wall to yield retinol, probably via retinal. Esterified retinol is stored in the liver but free retinol exists in the blood at the level of about 1 international unit per ml. The circulating retinol is mainly the all-*trans* form. Conversion of retinol to retinal is catalysed by alcohol dehydrogenase, which occurs in the retina (BLISS, 1949) and at other sites. The cofactor may be either NAD or NADP (FUTTERMAN, 1963). The pigment epithelium of the eye contains a store of esterified retinol, mainly palmitate (KRINSKY 1958a, b,; DOWLING, 1960; ANDREWS and FUTTERMAN, 1964). When rhodopsin is decomposed by light retinal is liberated in the all-*trans* form and is open to attack by alcohol dehydrogenase.

Regeneration of visual pigment involves oxidation of retinol to all-*trans* retinal and isomerisation of the latter to 11-*cis* retinal. As BLISS (1951) observed, the equilibrium of the retinol-retinal system greatly favours retinol, and if retinal is to be formed in significant amounts it must be removed rapidly. The trapping of retinal by opsin to form rhodopsin is conditional, however, on conversion of the all-*trans* to the 11-*cis* form. Just how this occurs has not been fully explained. It is clear that the retina possesses an isomerase (HUBBARD, 1955) that, in the absence of light, allows about 5 % of the retinal to become 11-*cis*. In dim light possibly one-third becomes 11-*cis*. There is evidence (FISHER, KON, and THOMPSON, 1952) that some crustaceans store their vitamin A in the eye mainly as the 11-*cis* isomer. Vertebrates too have a store of 11-*cis* retinol in eye tissues (KRINSKY, 1958a, b). It is a little difficult to think that light is itself responsible for the formation of 11-*cis* retinal, but assuming this isomeride is also necessary for photopic vision the enzymic isomerisation must otherwise be an extremely rapid process. A further complication arises over vitamin A acid (retinoic acid),

Retinoic acid

ARENS and VAN DORP (1946) showed that the acid could replace vitamin A in promoting growth in rats on a vitamin A-deficient diet. The sequence of events in the deprived animal is a gradual depletion of liver reserves of vitamin esters followed, as the level approaches zero, by a fall in blood retinol concentration. When this falls to below half the normal level defective scotopic vision results. By this time young rats have ceased to gain weight and, after a period on a weight plateau, xerophthalmia appears; there is then a rather rapid weight loss and the

4*

animal dies. Retinoic acid at dosages comparable with effective prophylaxis by retinol permits normal growth, and the animals remain in vigorous health, but scotopic vision fails and eventually blindness ensues.

For young rats retinoic acid displays biological activity equal to that of retinol but there is no storage. Discontinuance of dosing quickly results in symptoms of deficiency. The failure to replace retinol in visual processes is explained by the fact that the reaction

$$\text{X—CHO} \longrightarrow \text{X—COOH}$$

retinal	retinoic acid
or 3-dehydroretinal	or 3-dehydroretinoic acid

$$(\text{X} = C_{19}H_{27} \text{ or } C_{19}H_{25})$$

is not reversible.

DOWLING and WALD (1958, 1966) observed that "the failure to form visual pigments also has specific anatomical consequences; the outer segments of the visual cells deteriorate followed by the loss of almost all the cells themselves in an otherwise normal retina." They concluded that "the only function vitamin A may perform directly is to supply the prosthetic group of its visual pigments. All other functions, growth, general tissue maintenance are served equally well by vitamin A acid".

The situation is, however, more complicated than this. It was observed at Liverpool (HOWELL, THOMPSON, and PITT, 1963, 1964a, b) that rats on a vitamin A-deficient diet with a retinoic acid supplement grew well and appeared to have normal health but became blind and barren. Female rats on the retinoic acid diet displayed normal sexuality until the third week of pregnancy when the foetuses were resorbed, necrosis at the edge of the placental disc being seen. Retinol added to the diet prevented the lesion, and normal litters were born. Male rats on the retinoic acid diet showed a failure of spermatogenesis, and this too was reversed by retinol. The reproductive failure was not prevented by administering the follicle stimulating hormone (FSH) nor by testosterone, oestrone and progesterone, separately or in combination.

Guinea pigs fed on a vitamin A-free diet with a methyl retinoate supplement exhibited reproductive failure and became night-blind, but the degeneration of the retinas seen in rats did not occur. Vision was speedily restored by a retinol supplement (HOWELL, THOMPSON, and PITT, 1967).

Experiments on domestic fowls showed that chicks reared on a retinoic acid diet slowly went blind. In males spermatogenesis appeared normal, and semen used to inseminate normal hens resulted in normal fertility. Egg production by hens fed on a diet supplemented by retinoic acid was nearly normal, but the eggs fertilised by semen from normal cocks developed normally for only 48 hours on incubation. Thereupon the embryos became disorganised and died (THOMPSON, HOWELL, PITT, and HOUGHTON, 1965).

The overall position is thus somewhat open and contradictory. One hypothesis is that when in certain circumstances retinoic acid fails and retinol succeeds this is merely a matter of a breakdown in transport; retinol may enter the relevant tissue and even, perhaps, act only after conversion to retinoic acid by a two-stage enzymic process:

$$R \cdot CH_2OH \rightarrow R \cdot CHO \rightarrow R \cdot COOH \, .$$

Another hypothesis is that retinol *per se* has functions not possessed by retinoic acid. A third hypothesis is that retinol is a precursor of an active metabolite that cannot be made *in vivo* from retinoic acid.

From the standpoint of the chemistry of vision the most disturbing aspect of the evidence is that in some species retinoic acid sustains the morphological and chemical integrity of the rod outer segments, including opsin biosynthesis, whereas in other species this does not happen.

JUNGALVALA and CAMA (1965) have found that retinol 5,6 epoxide (a) gives rise to 5,6 epoxyretinal, which can be converted to a 5,8 epoxy (furanoid) compound (b)

CH$_2$OH

(a)

CH$_2$OH

(b)

These compounds also combine with opsin to give "visual pigments" under appropriate experimental conditions *in vitro*. The observations are of great interest but their direct bearing on vision is dubious.

We now return to retinal, which remains central. We still do not know how a high concentration of the 11-*cis* isomer is maintained against an unfavourable thermodynamic background. Moreover the high specificity of the 11-*cis* configuration has to be accounted for, and we must distinguish between what is actually proved and what is highly plausible.

DARTNALL (1957) discussed the arguments for and against the ideas that in rhodopsin the prosthetic group retinal is bound to opsin through nitrogen (Liverpool view) or sulphur (Harvard view). DARTNALL considered the evidence to favour the nitrogen link. He also suggested that the 11-*cis* form of retinal fitted snugly into the opsin moiety and that photoisomerisation to all-*trans* retinal resulted in a partial disengagement of the prosthetic group from the protein, with resulting exposure of sulphydryl and other active groups. HUBBARD (1958) and HUBBARD and KROPF (1959) accepted the N-retinylidene concept of MORTON and PITT (1955) and, in pictorial representations of opsin, they, too, envisaged the 11-*cis* form as fitting into the protein very closely, 9-*cis* fitting less closely, and all-*trans* retinal so loosely as to be readily detachable.

As a net effect (whatever the intermediate stages) illuminated rhodopsin yields opsin plus all-*trans* retinal. In addition under certain circumstances the protein itself undergoes re-arrangement, and sulphydryl groups are "exposed" and might even be concerned in visual excitation. It is, perhaps, necessary to look at this more closely. WALD and BROWN (1952) investigated the regeneration of rhodopsin at different pH values and concluded that the pH optimum favoured the condensation of retinal with sulphydryl groups rather than amino groups. Moreover they found that sulphydryl blocking reagents inhibited regeneration. They saw sulphydryl groups as directly concerned in the binding of the aldehyde group or with a possible alternative that the sulphydryl groups could appear as a result of reductive fission of a disulphide group, -S—S-. Later work on the attachment to a lysyl residue via the ε-amino group (p. 44) suggests, however, that the photochemical change merely exposes masked but pre-existing sulphydryl groups.

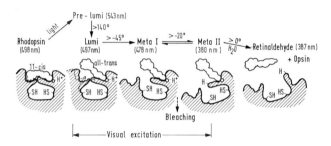

Fig. 10. A diagrammatic interpretation of stages in the photolysis and thermal decomposition of rhodopsin. The prosthetic group (11-cis) of rhodopsin fits closely a section of the opsin structure. The action of light is to isomerize the prosthetic group to the all-trans configuration (prelumirhodopsin). Then the structure of opsin opens up progressively (lumi- and the metarhodopsins) and finally retinaldehyde is hydrolysed from opsin. Bleaching (i.e. loss of colour) occurs in the transition from metarhodopsin I to II, and visual excitation must have occurred by this stage. The opening-up of opsin exposes new chemical groups, including one hydrogen-ion-binding and two sulphydryl groups. The absorbance maxima shown are for prelumirhodpsin at —190° C; for lumirhodopsin at —65° C; and for the other pigments at room temperature. (Wald and Brown, 1965)

The overall situation is seen as follows:

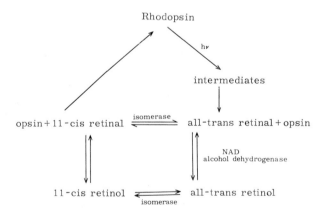

The molar extinction-coefficients of all-*trans* retinal and 11-*cis* retinal are known, and the firmest evidence in support of Wald's scheme is that the retinal resulting from the photochemical 'bleaching' of rhodopsin has a peak absorbance 1.5 times that of the retinal entering the system to form the pigment. The values of ε_{max} for all-*trans* retinal and 11-*cis* retinal are in the ratio 1.7 to 1 (Brown and Wald, 1956).

VI. Photochemical Considerations

A. Vertebrate Rhodopsin

WALD has repeatedly committed himself to the statement that so far as we know *the only thing that light does in vision is to isomerise the retinal chromophore.* This has been a legitimate view since it emphasised the initial act as leading to a whole series of thermal effects, and it had the additional merit of simplicity. That isomerisation of the chromophore occurs cannot be doubted, but the effect of light may not be quite so simple (WULFF, ADAMS, LINSCHITZ and KENNEDY, 1958). Photoregeneration can occur, and light may isomerise the retinals. It was observed by BRIDGES (1961, 1967) that irradiation of frog rhodopsin resulted in a thermally stable fraction with $\lambda_{max} = 494$ nm made up of about half isorhodopsin and half rhodopsin. Incidentally, the experiments of COLLINS and MORTON (1950a, b, c) on cattle rhodopsin point in a similar direction. These effects do not invalidate WALD'S generalisation, but perhaps there should be greater emphasis on "so far as we know".

The photochemical decomposition of rhodopsin is still not fully understood. In the present context it is of considerable interest that ultraviolet light (276 nm) absorbed by the aromatic amino-acid residues in opsin bleaches the pigment, the process apparently displaying a quantum efficiency of 0.24 (KROPF, 1967) as compared with 0.5—0.6 at 500 nm (ABRAHAMSON and OSTROY, 1967). DARTNALL (1968) has discussed in detail the photosensitivities of visual pigments in the presence of hydroxylamine. The original elegant work of DARTNALL, GOODEVE, and LYTHGOE (1936, 1938) and of SCHNEIDER, GOODEVE, and LYTHGOE (1939) indicated, on photochemical bases, a quantum efficiency between 0.6 and 1.0. DARTNALL (1968) has now established for seven retinal-based pigments (rhodopsins) and for five dehydroretinal-based pigments (porphyropsins) that the quantum efficiencies are very close to 0.65 when modern data for molar extinction coefficients are used. DARTNALL (loc. cit.) has also pointed out that KROPF (1967) had implicitly assumed that the quanta of ultraviolet were absorbed exclusively by the aromatic amino-acids of the protein in his suggestion that the energy was transferred intra-molecularly to the retinal moiety. This ignores the possibility that the prosthetic group may itself absorb at 276 nm, and KROPF'S quantum efficiency (0.24) is, therefore, questionable. So far as human vision is concerned the 'protein' absorbance of rhodopsin is physiologically irrelevant because no radiation shorter than about 295 nm normally reaches the earth and still less the retina. Nevertheless, in the laboratory, the ultraviolet irradiation appears to 'bleach' rhodopsin by isomerising the retinal chromophoric group from 11-*cis* to all-*trans*. The spectral absorbance of rhodopsin (see TAKAGI, 1963) allows the 350 nm inflexion to be attributed to the *cis* absorption, but some energy transfer may nevertheless occur after a large quantum (275 nm) has been absorbed by phenylalanine, tyrosine and tryptophan residues. The statement that the sole action of light on rhodopsin is to isomerise the chromophore may here need to be qualified.

The course of the photochemical change has been much studied at low temperatures and brief comment is necessary here, although the whole matter is discussed

fully by YOSHIZAWA in Chapter 5. It is highly probable that the major photochemical change is the initial formation of prelumirhodopsin, the subsequent
changes being thermal (YOSHIZAWA, KITO, and ISHAGAMI, 1960; GRELLMAN,
LIVINGSTON, and PRATT, 1962; YOSHIZAWA and WALD, 1963; PRATT, LIVINGSTON,
and GRELLMAN, 1964), but at very low temperatures there appears to be a steady
state involving prelumirhodopsin and (11-*cis*) rhodopsin.

GUZZO and POOL (1968) studied the fluorescence of freeze-dried outer segments
and also of rhodopsin in digitonin solution. The 'solid' preparation illuminated by
490—500 nm radiation at —196° gave a definite fluorescence with λ_{max} = 600 nm.
The quantum efficiency was only 0.005. The 'dissolved' rhodopsin at 3° and pH 6.7,
when illuminated by 490 nm light, fluoresced with a well marked peak at 575 nm.
The emission was abolished by bleaching at —196°. When the reaction, rhodopsin
to prelumirhodopsin, was effected by light of wave-length 440 nm, an equilibrium
was set up and the fluorescence reduced by half. Irradiation with light of wavelength
600 nm regenerated rhodopsin, and the fluorescence reappeared. The absorbance
peak of prelumirhodopsin is at 543 nm and no satisfactory explanation of the shift
from 500 nm to 543 nm has been offered. For that matter no entirely convincing
explanation of the *position* of the 500 nm peak for rhodopsin or the 560 nm peak
for iodopsin has been advanced. Moreover the relevance of findings at —140° to the
processes occurring in the living animal is perhaps uncertain (ABRAHAMSON and
OSTROY, 1967). Equally fair, however, would be to ask how closely rhodopsin-
digitonin micelles in 'solution' correspond with physiological conditions. A scheme
due to OSTROY, ERHARDT, and ABRAHAMSON (1966) included much that was due
to MATTHEWS, HUBBARD, BROWN, and WALD (1963), which in turn replaced to
some extent the pioneer work of LYTHGOE and QUILLIAM (1938):

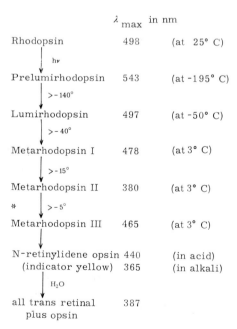

	λ_{max} in nm	
Rhodopsin	498	(at 25° C)
↓ hν		
Prelumirhodopsin	543	(at -195° C)
↓ >-140°		
Lumirhodopsin	497	(at -50° C)
↓ >-40°		
Metarhodopsin I	478	(at 3° C)
↓ >-15°		
Metarhodopsin II	380	(at 3° C)
* ↓ >-5°		
Metarhodopsin III	465	(at 3° C)
↓		
N-retinylidene opsin	440	(in acid)
(indicator yellow)	365	(in alkali)
↓ H_2O		
all trans retinal	387	
plus opsin		

---

* OSTROY, RUDNEY and ABRAHAMSON (1966) have shown that it is at this stage that
—SH groups are released (or exposed).

Many suggestions have been put forward to account for the positions of absorbance maxima in the whole decomposition sequence (DARTNALL, 1957; KROPF and HUBBARD, 1958; HUBBARD and KROPF, 1958, 1965; AKHTAR, BLOSSE, and DEWHURST, 1965; ISHIGAMA, MAEDA, and MISHIMA, 1966; MIZUNO, OSAWA, and KUNO, 1966), but no view commands assent. The multiplicity of pigments involving retinal or 3-dehydroretinal means that the protein opsins must be variable in the detailed structure at the active site. Moreover the opsins themselves undergo change during photodecomposition. The selective absorption near 235 nm (TAKAGI, 1963), the optical rotatory dispersion and circular dichroism (CRESCITELLI, MOMMAERTS, and SHAW, 1966; HUBBARD, BOWNDS, and YOSHIZAWA, 1965; KITO and TAKEZAKI, 1966) all display changes as a result of irradiation, and the iso-electric point is also altered (RADDING and WALD, 1956a, b). Free opsin, which is partly 'unfolded', may refold under the action of 11-*cis* retinal, and light may re-form the active isomer of retinal from all-*trans* retinal (SEKOGUTI, TAKAGI, and KITO, 1964). TAKAGI has offered evidence that the major alteration in protein configuration occurs after the formation of metarhodopsin I. There are very significant differences between different Schools in the interpretation of evidence concerning changes in opsin itself and much remains to be done.

ROSENBERG (1966) takes the view that after 80 years of study not one solid piece of evidence relates the bleaching theory directly to visual excitation. "Indeed the more we understand the photochemical process the less likely it is that it will provide the definitive answer". He considers that light initiates the release from the excited chromophore of a mobile electron. The movement of the charge through the 'solid' phase of the rod, shielded from water, sets up a current that changes the voltage across a membrane some distance away, and initiates a nerve impulse. It is true that β-carotene (ROSENBERG, 1961a, b) and protonated retinyl-idene Schiff's bases are photoconductive (ROSENBERG and KRIGAS, 1967) and that light 'generates a mobile electronic charge'. The 11-*cis* isomer of retinal is much more photoconductive than all-*trans* retinal. ROSENBERG'S ideas are of consider-able interest but they leave large tracts of experimentation unexplained, and are therefore vulnerable.

B. Invertebrate Rhodopsin

Squid 'rhodopsin' is a visual pigment that is photosensitive but does not undergo 'bleaching'. Apparent analogues of the normal prelumirhodopsin and lumirhodopsin are formed (HUBBARD and ST. GEORGE, 1958; YOSHIZAWA and WALD, 1967) but squid metarhodopsin exhibits $\lambda_{\max}$ at 500 nm in neutral or slightly acid solutions, and at 380 nm in alkaline solution. In this it differs from mammalian metarhodopsin. Squid rhodopsin has some importance in the history of the subject because its peculiarity of not being bleached permitted HUBBARD and ST. GEORGE to establish the primacy of the 11-*cis* to all-*trans* isomerisation. SEKOGUTI, TAKAGI, and KITO (1964) showed that the protein component of squid rhodopsin changed in configuration on irradiation. It seems clear that the funda-mental difference between vertebrate rhodopsin and cephalopod rhodopsin is in the protein moiety (Fig. 11). It may be doubted whether the term metarhodopsin is appropriate for the squid rhodopsin decomposition product (cf p. 113).

This raises another issue. It seems likely that 11-*cis* retinal is needed in photopic pigments just as much as in rhodopsin and porphyropsin. This means that the picture of 11-*cis* retinal nestling snugly in a pre-determined space in the protein molecule (Fig. 10) and being eased out as photolysis proceeds becomes a shade inadequate, if on forming prelumirhodopsin ($\lambda_{max} = 543$ nm) or prelumi-iodopsin ($\lambda_{max} = 640$ nm) the fit becomes better (as indicated by the longer λ_{max}). Moreover the plurality of photopic pigments must mean either coexisting opsins or alternative sites of attachment.

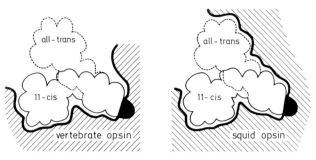

Fig. 11. Hypothetical diagrams of the prosthetic-group sites on vertebrate and squid opsins. Both opsins complement the shape of the 11-cis chromophore all the way from the Schiff-base linkage, shown on the right of each diagram by the black patch, to the β-ionone ring on the left. But while squid opsin also complements the shape of the all-trans chromophore, vertebrate opsin does not

Further complications arise from the work of HARA and his associates (HARA and HARA, 1965, 1967; HARA, HARA, and TAKEUCHI, 1967) on vision in octopus and squid (see Chapter 18). The squid (*Ommastrephes sloani pacificus* Steenstrup) contains in its retina two photopigments A and B. A is a rhodopsin ($\lambda_{max} = 480$ nm) with 11-*cis* retinal as its chromophore. At acid pH and up to 20° there is no photochemical bleaching but a mixture ($\lambda_{max} = 488$ nm) of acid metarhodopsin and rhodopsin is formed. Pigment B ($\lambda_{max} = 495$ nm) bleaches at any pH and behaves rather like vertebrate rhodopsin. Pigment A is extracted from the rhabdomes while pigment B is obtained from rhabdome-free retinas, and is designated retinochrome. Rhabdomes were separated from black pigment fragments, and methods for obtaining rhabdome-free retinas were worked out. Retinochrome in alkaline digitonin solution showed λ_{max} at 490 nm and 370 nm (at pH 10). At pH 7.0 the 490 nm band became stronger and the 370 nm peak disappeared. On bleaching, the long wave band disappeared, with a compensating rise in absorption near 370 nm. The wavelengths (λ_{max}) for which the cephalopod rhodopsins and retinochromes have maximum absorbance are given in Chapter 18.

Rhodopsin is the first photoreceptive substance for vision, but retinochrome is sufficiently *more* photosensitive to respond to the feeble light that passes through the rhabdomes and the dense layer of black pigment. HARA and HARA (1967) concluded that the prosthetic group in unbleached retinochrome was all-*trans* while that of the photoproduct was in the *cis*-configuration. The retinal liberated by photolysis of retinochrome was 11-*cis*, so the light effected an isomerisation all-*trans* to 11-*cis*!

The coexistence of two different kinds of photopigment is *not* here a sign of colour vision. Rather is it associated with a quite different physiological function.

"Rhodopsin is in the forward part of the visual cell where the incident light iso-merises its chromophore from 11-*cis* to all-*trans*, so converting rhodopsin to the all-*trans* chromoprotein [via prelumirhodopsin and metarhodopsin ?]". On the other hand retinochrome, occurring just behind the rhabdomes surrounded by black pigment granules may be decomposed even by faint light and liberate the 11-*cis* retinal required for rhodopsin regeneration. The illuminated retinochrome can remove all-*trans* retinal from metarhodopsin and regenerate retinochrome. Retino-chrome seems to be the prosthetic group of a retinene isomerase.

C. Iodopsin

YOSHIZAWA and WALD (1967) prepared a mixture of rod and cone outer seg-ments from light-adapted chicken retinas and, by extraction (2 % digitonin pH 6.5), obtained mixed rod and cone opsins in solution. On incubating the mixture in the dark with excess 11-*cis* retinal a mixture of rhodopsin and iodopsin was obtained, but if a little less retinal was added than that needed to 'saturate' the cone opsin, only iodopsin was formed. Similarly if the mixed opsins were incubated with 9-*cis* retinal, iso-iodopsin was formed exclusively if the amount of isomeric retinal was insufficient for the synthesis of both iso-iodopsin and isorhodopsin. The 'yields' in terms of absorbance (optical density 0.3) were only moderate and, by centrifuging overnight, the pigment-digitonin micelles could be spun down to a watery gel. This was mixed with an equal volume of glycerol and stored at —15°C.

Spectral absorbance curves were recorded at —195°C or —78°C. The following scheme summarises the findings. (See also, Chapter 5 by YOSHIZAWA, p. 146).

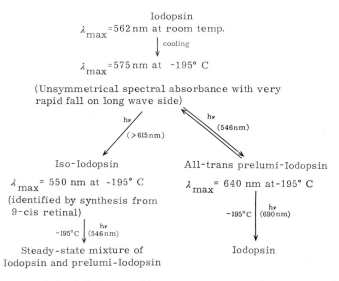

"That iodopsin and iso-iodpsin on this treatment go to the same steady state is plain evidence that all three pigments differ only in the configuration of the chromo-phore". Only prelumi-iodopsin absorbs deep red light and on irradiation by wave-lengths near 690 nm iodopsin is reformed at —195°C, i.e. the all-*trans* chromophore re-isomerises to 11-*cis* in preference to 9-*cis*.

All transformations from iodopsin to iso-iodopsin are seen as two-quantum isomerisations with prelumi-iodopsin an obligatory intermediate. It is possible to begin with iso-iodopsin and go through a similar sequence. Prelumi-iodopsin behaves differently from prelumirhodopsin on warming up in darkness. Ox prelumirhodopsin at temperatures above $-140°$ goes to lumirhodopsin and then to other all-*trans* 'bleach' products. Prelumi-iodopsin on warming in the dark reverts to iodopsin, i.e. the chromophore returns from the all-*trans* to the 11-*cis* configuration (complete at $-140°C$). In other words, prelumi-iodopsin can revert to iodopsin equally well by a photochemical or a thermal process at low temperature. Irradiation of *iso*-iodopsin at $-78°$ with light of wavelength 546 nm surprisingly converts it to iodopsin via prelumi-iodopsin, which goes thermally to iodopsin. At $-78°$, 546 nm-irradiation of iodopsin effects no overall change; the photochemically formed prelumi-iodopsin being very rapidly reconverted to iodopsin by a thermal process.

Lumi-iodopsin ($\lambda_{max} = 515$ nm) is formed slowly at $-78°$ by irradiation with long wavelength light (> 595 nm). On irradiation with green light (546 nm) iodopsin is re-formed. The spectral absorbance of prelumi-iodopsin ($\lambda_{max} = 640$ nm) was obtained by an indirect method and it should, of course, be a blue pigment. This substance is unusually unstable, its molar absorbance is high, and it has a strong tendency to revert to iodopsin in the dark. YOSHIZAWA and WALD state: "the essential point is that prelumi-iodopsin is virtually an excited molecule stabilised only by the low temperature and the rigidity of the solvent . . . apparently needing little further energy for electronic excitation its absorption spectrum lies far over on the red".

Iodopsin is formed because of a close fit between 11-*cis* retinal and a particular configuration of opsin, and iso-iodopsin depends on a somewhat similar relationship between 9-*cis* retinal and the same opsin configuration, the 'fit' being less close and λ_{max} going from 575 nm to 550 nm. "In prelumi-iodopsin there is a highly strained condition, the 'fit' may be even better as the exalta- tion of spectrum (both in position and intensity) sug- gests that it is under ten- sion." It should be noted that the strained chromophore is all-*trans* and the configuration of the opsin is unchanged.

The differences between prelu- mirhodopsin and prelumi-iodopsin are explained by supposing that in the former the protein changes its conformation more readily than the chromophore, whereas in prelumi- iodopsin the reverse is the case. This latest work continues to build on earlier studies involving meta- iodopsins.

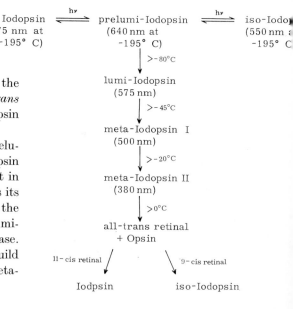

Iodopsin (575 nm at $-195°$ C) $\overset{h\nu}{\rightleftharpoons}$ prelumi-Iodopsin (640 nm at $-195°$ C) $\overset{h\nu}{\rightleftharpoons}$ iso-Iodop (550 nm at $-195°$ C)

prelumi-Iodopsin $\downarrow$ > $-80°$C

lumi-Iodopsin (575 nm) $\downarrow$ > $-45°$C

meta-Iodopsin I (500 nm) $\downarrow$ > $-20°$C

meta-Iodopsin II (380 nm) $\downarrow$ > $0°$C

all-trans retinal + Opsin

11-cis retinal $\swarrow$ $\searrow$ 9-cis retinal

Iodpsin   iso-Iodopsin

These complicated investigations and arguments have implications. RUSHTON (1957, 1958) devised methods for the direct measurement of difference spectra of photopic pigments with light reflected from the fundus of living human eyes. The fovea contains only cones, and the properties of foveal pigments of normal and colour blind persons are of direct relevance. Thus protanopes have a single pigment with $\lambda_{max} = 540$ nm. Persons with normal colour vision possess this pigment together with a 590 nm pigment revealed by partial bleaching with deep red light. The first pigment is called chlorolabe and the other erythrolabe. Deuteranopes also possess both, perhaps in single cones (see Chapter 9 by RUSHTON).

Direct microspectrophotometry (BROWN and WALD, 1963) confirmed the existence of two pigments, red-sensitive ($\lambda_{max} = 565$—570 nm) and green-sensitive ($\lambda_{max} = 535$—540 nm) respectively. Measurements on single parafoveal cones established three types of cones with $\lambda_{max} = 565$—570, 520—530 and 440—450 nm respectively. WEALE (1959) using a different approach found evidence for two cone pigments (C.P.); C.P. 540 and C.P. 600.

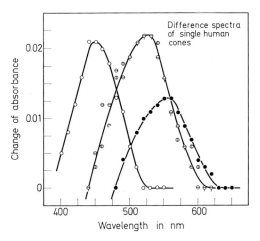

Fig. 12. Difference spectra of the visual pigments in single cones of the human parafovea. Spectra of unbleached cones were recorded from 650 nm to 380 nm, then again after bleaching with a flash of yellow light. The differences between these spectra are shown. They represent a blue-sensitive cone ($\lambda_{max} = $ c. 450 nm), a green-sensitive cone ($\lambda_{max} = $ c. 525 nm; two sets of measurements) and a red-sensitive cone ($\lambda_{max} = $ c. 555 nm). (BROWN and WALD, 1964)

MARKS, DOBELLE, and MACNICHOLL (1964) were pioneers in microspectrophotometric work on single cones. They found λ_{max} clustering around the wavelengths 445, 535 and 570 nm in primates. BROWN and WALD (1963, 1964) in their survey of human colour vision concluded that the summation of the spectra of all the photosensitive cone pigments accounts precisely for the foveal sensitivity curve. It is perhaps an accident that this also resembles the chick iodopsin curve. The analogous photopic pigments that are based on vitamin A_2 have λ_{max} near 450, 525 and 630 nm (MARKS, 1965).

D. Conclusion

If at this stage we take stock, it is evident that the chemistry of visual pigments has reached the point that very great advances have been made but numerous and serious difficulties remain. On the credit side the participation of retinol and 3-dehydroretinol is established. The corresponding aldehydes are formed under the action of alcohol dehydrogenase and are removed from the sphere of action by union with opsin at an ε-amino group of a lysyl residue. Formation of most visual pigments in Nature seems to depend on enzymic isomerisation of all-*trans* retinal to 11-*cis* retinal. Photodecomposition of rhodopsin involves conversion of an 11-*cis* retinal moiety to an all-*trans* moiety without hydrolysis. Under certain circumstances combined 11-*cis* retinal is formed from other isomers by absorption of light.

There seems to be no doubt that the opsins themselves undergo changes in conformation. Clearly if 11-*cis* retinal is common to rhodopsin and to mammalian cone pigments, and 11-*cis* dehydroretinal is common to porphyropsin and the related cone pigments it may be concluded (a) that the extra double bond in 3-dehydroretinal exerts displacements of pigment maxima that present little difficulty in respect of spectroscopic theory; (b) that in species that have rods and cones, and that display both scotopic vision and colour vision, at least four localised opsins ("scotopsin" and three "photopsins") must be postulated (c) that if initial effects, e.g. formation of prelumirhodopsin, prelumi-iodopsin, etc. involve formation of new unstable pigments with their peaks displaced substantially in the direction of longer wave-lengths, despite isomerisation to the all-*trans* configuration, the concept of perfect fit in the opsin-aldehyde pigment needs to be propped up. The fact must be reiterated that the positions of $\lambda_{\max}$ in the rhodopsin series as well as the porphyropsin series have not really been explained in terms of chemical structure. No doubt changes in the aminoacids in the vicinity of the lysyl residue offer a possible partial explanation, and changes in folding may add to it, but it is difficult to resist the conclusion that some quite important idea is missing.

Acknowledgment

I thank the Leverhulme Trust for the award of an Emeritus Fellowship.

References

Abrahamson, E. W., Ostroy, S. E.: The photochemical and macromolecular aspects of vision. Progr. Biophys. molec. Biol. **17**, 179—215 (1967).

Akhtar, M., Blosse, P. T., Dewhurst, P. B.: The reduction of a rhodopsin derivative. Life Sci. **4**, 1221—1226 (1965).

— — — The active site of the visual protein, rhodopsin. Chem. Commun. **13**, 631—632 (1967).

Andrews, J. S., Futterman, S.: Metabolism of the retina V. The role of microsomes in vitamin A esterification in the visual cycle. J. biol. Chem. **239**, 4073 (1964).

Arens, J. F., van Dorp, D. A.: Synthesis of some compounds possessing vitamin A activity. Nature (Lond.) **157**, 190—191 (1946).

Ball, S., Collins, F. D., Dalvi, P. D. Morton, R. A.: Studies in vitamin A. 11. Reactions of retinene$_1$ with amino compounds. Biochem. J. **45**, 304—307 (1949).

— — Morton, R. A., Stubbs, A. L.: Chemistry of visual processes. Nature (Lond.) **161**, 424—426 (1948).

— Glover, J., Goodwin, T. W., Morton, R. A.: Conversion of retinene$_1$ to vitamin A *in vivo*. Biochem. J. **41**, 14 (1947).

BALL, S., GOODWIN, T. W., MORTON, R. A.: Studies on vitamin A. 5. The preparation of retinene₁-vitamin A aldehyde. Biochem. J. **42**, 516—523 (1948).

BARER, R., SIDMAN, R. L.: Absorption spectrum of rhodopsin in solution and in intact rods. J. Physiol. (Lond.) **129**, 60 P (1953).

BAXTER, J. G., ROBESON, C. D.: Crystalline vitamin A palmitate and vitamin A alcohol. Science **92**, 203—204 (1940).

BLISS, A. F.: The chemistry of daylight vision. J. gen. Physiol. **29**, 277—297 (1946).

— Reversible enzymic reduction of retinene to vitamin A. Biol. Bull. **97**, 221—222 (1949).

— The equilibrium between vitamin A alcohol and aldehyde in the presence of alcohol dehydrogenase. Arch. Biochem. **31**, 197—204 (1951).

BOLL, F.: Zur Anatomie und Physiologie der Retina. Mber. Berlin. Akad. **41**, 783—787 (1876).

BOWNDS, D.: Site of attachment of retinal in rhodopsin. Nature (Lond.) **216**, 1178—1181 (1967).

— WALD, G.: Reaction of the rhodopsin chromophore with sodium borohydride. Nature (Lond.) **205**, 254—257 (1965).

BRIDGES, C. D. B.: Studies on the flash photolysis of visual pigments. I. Pigments present in frog rhodopsin solution after flash irradiation. Biochem. J. **79**, 128—134 (1961 a).

— Studies on the flash photolysis of visual pigments. II. Production of thermally stable photosensitive pigments in flash irradiated solutions of frog rhodopsin. Biochem. J. **79**, 135—143 (1961 b).

— Biochemistry of visual processes. In: Comprehensive biochemistry. Vol. 27, (FLORKIN, M., STOTZ, E. H., Eds.). Amsterdam: Elsevier 1967.

BRODA, E. E., GOODEVE, C. F.: The behaviour of visual purple at low temperature. Proc. roy. Soc. A. **179**, 151—159 (1941).

BROWN, P. H., WALD, G.: The neo-b isomer of vitamin A and retinene. J. biol. Chem. **222**, 865—877 (1956).

— — Visual pigments in human and monkey retina. Nature (Lond.) **200**, 37—43 (1963).

— — Visual pigments in single rods and cones of the human retina. Science **144**, 45—52 (1964).

CAMA, H. R., DALVI, P. D., MORTON, R. A., SALAH, M. K.: Studies in vitamin A. 20 and 21. Properties of retinene₂ and vitamin A₂. Biochem. J. **52**, 540—542, 542—547 (1952).

— — — — STEINBERG, G. R., STUBBS, A. L.: Studies on vitamin A. 19. Preparation and properties of retinene₂. Biochem. J. **52**, 535—540 (1952).

CAPPER, N. S., I. M. W. McKIBBIN, PRENTICE, J. H.: Conversion of carotene to vitamin A in chickens. Biochem. J. **25**, 205—274 (1931).

CARR, F. H., PRICE, E. A.: Colour reactions attributed to vitamin A. Biochem. J. **20**, 497—501 (1926).

COLLINS, F. D.: Rhodopsin and indicator yellow. Nature (Lond.) **171**, 469—471 (1953).

— The chemistry of vision. Biol. Rev. **29**, 453 (1954).

— LOVE, R. M., MORTON, R. A.: Studies in rhodopsin. 4: Preparation of rhodopsin. Biochem. J. **51**, 292—298 (1952).

— — — The preparation of rhodopsin and the chemical composition of rod outer sements. Biochem. J. **56**, 493—498 (1954).

— MORTON, R. A.: Studies on rhodopsin. 1: Methods of extraction and the absorption spectrum. Biochem. J. **47**, 3—10 (1950a).

— — Studies on rhodopsin. 2: Indicator yellow. Biochem. J. **47**, 10—17 (1950b).

— — Studies in rhodopsin. 3: Rhodopsin and transient orange. Biochem. J. **47**, 18—24 (1950c).

COWARD, K. H., DYER, F. J., MORTON, A. R., GADDUM, J. H.: The determination of vitamin A in cod liver oils (a) biologically (b) chemically (c) physically, with a statistical examination of the results. Biochem. J. **25**, 1102—1120 (1931).

— — — Further evidence that the intensity of absorption at 328 nm gives the best agreement with the biological measure of vitamin A in liver oils. Biochem. J. **26**, 1593—1600 (1932).

CRESCITELLI, F., MOMMAERTS, W. H. F. M., SHAW, T. I.: Circular dichroism of visual pigments in the visible and ultraviolet spectral regions. Proc. nat. Acad. Sci. (Wash.) **56**, 1729—1734 (1966).

DALVI, P. I., MORTON, R. A.: Preparation of neovitamin A esters and neoretinene₁. Biochem. J. **50**, 43—48 (1951).

DARTNALL, H. J. A.: The visual pigments. London: Methuen 1957.
— The photosensitivities of visual pigments in the presence of hydroxylamine. Vision Res. 8, 339—358 (1968).
— GOODEVE, C. F., LYTHGOE, R. J.: The quantitative analysis of the photochemical bleaching of visual purple solutions in monochromatic light. Proc. roy. Soc. A. 156, 158—170 (1936).
— — — The effect of temperature on the photochemical bleaching of visual purple solutions. Proc. roy. Soc. A. 164, 216—230 (1938).
DIETERLE, J. M., ROBESON, C. D.: Crystalline neoretinene-b. Science 120, 219—226 (1954).
DOWLING, J. E.: Chemistry of visual adaptation in the rat. Nature (Lond.) 188, 114—118 (1960).
— WALD, G.: Nutritional night blindness. Ann. N. Y. Acad. Sci. 74, 256—265 (1958).
— — On the mechanism of vitamin A deficiency and night blindness. Fourth International Congress of Biochemistry. Vol. XI. 185—197 (1965).
— — The biological functions of vitamin A acid. Proc. nat. Acad. Sci. (Wash.) 46, 587—608 (1966).
DRUMMOND, J. C., MORTON, R. A.: Observations on the assay of Vitamin A. Biochem. J. 23, 785—802 (1929).
EDISBURY, J. R., MORTON, R. A., SIMPKINS, G. W.: A possible vitamin A₂. Nature (Lond.) 140, 234 (1937).
— — — LOVERN, J. A.: The distribution of vitamin A and factor A₂. I. Biochem. J. 32, 118—140 (1938).
EVANS, R. H.: Oxidation by manganese dioxide in neutral media. Chem. Soc. Quarterly Rev. XIII, 61—70 (1951).
FARRER, K. R., J. C. HAMLET, H. B. HENBEST, H. B., JONES, E. R. H.: Studies in the polyene series. Part XLIII. The structure and synthesis of vitamin A₂ and related compounds. J. chem. Soc. 1952, 2657.
FISHER, L. R., KON, S. K., THOMPSON, S. Y.: Vitamin A and carotenoids in certain invertebrates: Marine crustaceae. J. marine biol. Ass. U.K. 31, 229—258 (1952).
FLEISCHER, S., McCONNELL, D. G.: Lipids of bovine retinal outer segment discs. Nature (Lond.) 212, 1366 (1966).
FRIDERICIA, L. S., HOLM, E.: Experimental contribution to the study of the relation between night blindness and malnutrition. Influence of deficiency of fat soluble A-vitamin in the diet on the visual purple in the eyes of rats. Amer. J. Physiol. 73, 63—78 (1925).
FUTTERMAN, S.: Metabolism of the retina. VI. The role of reduced triphosphopyridine nucleotide in the visual cycle. J. biol. Chem. 238, 1145—1150 (1963).
GILLAM, A. E., HEILBRON, I. M., JONES, E. R. H., LEDERER, E.: On the occurrence and constitution of the 693 nm chromogen (vitamin A₂?) of fish liver oils. Biochem. J. 32, 405—416 (1938).
— — LEDERER, E., ROSANOVA, V. A.: Differences in the chromogenic properties of freshwater and marine fish liver oils. Nature (Lond.) 140, 233 (1937).
GLOVER, J., GOODWIN, T. W., MORTON, R. A.: Conversion of β-carotene to vitamin A in the intestine of the rat. Biochem. J. 41, (1947). Biochem. J. 43, 512—518 (1948).
GOODWIN, T. W., GREGORY, R. A.: Studies on vitamins. 7. Carotene metabolism in herbivores. Biochem. J. 43, 505—518 (1948).
GRAHAM, W. D., VAN DORP, D. A., ARENS, J. F.: Synthesis of a cis-isomer of vitamin A aldehyde. Rec. Trav. chim. Pays-Bas 68, 609—612 (1949).
GRELLMAN, K. H., LIVINGSTON, R., PRATT, D.: A flash photolytic investigation of rhodopsin at low temperatures. Nature (Lond.) 193, 1258—1262 (1962).
GUZZO, A. V., POOL, G. L.: Visual pigment fluorescence. Science 159, 312—314 (1968).
HAMANO, S.: A crystalline derivative of vitamin A. Sci. Papers Inst. phys. chem. Res. Tokyo 26, 82—86 (1935).
— Crystalline esters of vitamin A. J. agric. chem. Soc. Japan 13, 502—506 (1937).
HARA, T., HARA, R.: New photosensitive pigment found in the retina of the squid Ommastrephes. Nature (Lond.) 206, 1331—1334 (1965).
— — — Rhodopsin and retinochrome in the squid retina. Nature (Lond.) 214, 573—575 (1967).
— — TAKEUCHI, M.: Vision in octopus and squid. Nature (Lond.) 214, 572—573 (1967).
HECHT, S.: The dark adaptation of the human eye. J. gen. Physiol. 2, 499—517 (1919).
— The photochemistry of the sensitivity of animals to light. J. opt. Soc. Amer. 5, 227—231 (1921).
— The nature of the visual process. Bull. N. Y. Acad. Med. 14, 21—43 (1938).

HECHT, S.: The chemistry of visual substances. Ann. Rev. Biochem. 11, 465—496 (1942).
— WILLIAMS, R. E.: The visibility of monochromatic radiation and the absorption spectrum of visual purple. J. gen. Physiol. 5, 1—33 (1922).
HEILBRON, I. M., GILLAM, A. E., MORTON, R. A.: Specificity in tests for vitamin A. A new conception of the chromogen constituents of fresh and aged liver oils. Biochem. J. 25, 1352—1366 (1931).
— HESLOP, R. N., MORTON, R. A., WEBSTER, E. T., REA, J. L., DRUMMOND, J. C.: Characteristics of highly active vitamin A preparations. Biochem. J. 26, 1179—1193 (1932).
HENBEST, H. B., JONES, E. R. H., OWEN, T. C.: Conversion of vitamin A_1 into vitamin A_2. J. chem. Soc. 1955, 2765.
HOLM, E.: Demonstration of hemeralopia in rats nourished on food devoid of fat soluble vitamins. Amer. J. Physiol. 13, 79—84 (1925).
HOLMES, H. N., CORBET, R. E.: A crystalline vitamin A concentrate. Science 85, 103 (1937a).
— — The isolation of crystalline vitamin A. J. amer. chem. Soc. 59, 2042—2047 (1937b).
HOWELL, J. McC., THOMPSON, J. N., PITT, G. A. J.: Histology of the lesions produced in the reproductive tract of animals fed a diet deficient in vitamin A alcohol but containing vitamin A acid. 1. The male rat. J. Reprod. Fertil. 5, 159—167 (1963).
— — — Histology of the lesions produced in the reproductive tract of animals fed a diet deficient in vitamin A alcohol but containing vitamin A acid. II. The female rat. J. Reprod. Fertil. 7, 251—258 (1964a).
— — — Vitamin A and reproduction in rats. Proc. roy. Soc. B. 159, 510—535 (1964b).
— — — Changes in the tissues of guinea-pigs fed on a diet free from vitamin A but containing methyl retinoate. Brit. J. Nutr. 21, 37—44 (1967).
HUBBARD, R.: The molecular weight of rhodopsin and the nature of the rhodopsin-digitonin complex. J. gen. Physiol. 37, 381—390 (1954).
— Retinene isomerase. J. gen. Physiol. 39, 935—962 (1955).
— Geometrical isomerization of vitamin A, retinene and retinene oxime. J. amer. chem. Soc. 78, 4662—4667 (1956).
— On the chromophores of the visual pigments. In: Visual problems of colour, National Physical Lab. Symposium No. 8. pp. 153—169. London: H. M. Stationery Office 1958.
— BOWNDS, D., YOSHIZAWA, T.: The chemistry of visual photoreception. Cold Spr. Harb. Symp. quant. Biol. 30, 301—315 (1965).
— HUBBARD, R., GEORGE, R. C. C. St.: The rhodopsin system of the squid. J. gen. Physiol. 41, 501—528 (1958).
— GREGERMAN, R. J., WALD, G.: Geometrical isomers of retinene. J. gen. Physiol. 36, 415—429 (1953).
— KROPF, A.: The action of light on rhodopsin. Proc. nat. Acad. Sci. (Wash.) 44, 130—139 (1958).
— — Molecular aspects of visual excitation. Ann. N. Y. Acad. Sci. 81, 388—398 (1959).
— — On the colours of visual pigment chromophores. J. gen. Physiol. 49, 381—385 (1965).
— WALD, G.: Cis-trans isomers of vitamin A and retinene in the rhodopsin system. Fed. Proc. 11, 233 (1952a). Science 115, 60—63 (1952b). J. gen. Physiol. 36, 269—315 (1952c).
HYDE, E. P., FORSYTHE, W. E., CADY, F. E.: The visibility of radiation. Astrophys. J. 18, 65—88 (1918).
ISHIGAMI, M., MAEDA, Y., MISHIMA, K.: A retinene-tryptophan complex. Biochim. biophys. Acta (Amst.) 112, 372—375 (1966).
ISLER, O.: Synthesis of Vitamin A. Chem. Eng. News 29, 3962 (1951).
— KOFLER, M., HUBER, W., RONCO, A.: Synthesis of vitamin A. Experentia (Basel) 2, 31 (1946).
— — — — Synthese des vitamin A. Helv. chim. Acta. 30, 1911—1927 (1947).
JUNGALVALA, F. B., CAMA, H. R.: Preparation and properties of 5,6-monoepoxy vitamin A acetate, 5,6-monoepoxy vitamin A alcohol, 5,6-monoepoxy vitamin A aldehyde and their corresponding 5,8-monoepoxy (furanoid) compounds. Biochem. J. 95, 17—26 (1965).
KARRER, P., JUCKER, E.: Carotenoide, Basel, Birkhäuser 1948.
— MORF, R., SCHÖPP, K.: Zur Kenntnis des Vitamins A aus Fischtranen. Helv. chim. Acta. 14, 1036—1044 (1931).
KITO, Y., TAKEZAKI, M.: Optical rotation of irradiated rhodopsin solution. Nature (Lond.) 211, 197—198 (1966).

Koenig, A.: Über den menschlichen Sehpurpur und seine Bedeutung für das Sehen. S.-B. Akad. Wiss. Kl. med. Wiss. **1894**, 577—598.

Köttgen, E., Abelsdorff, G.: Absorption und Zersetzung des Sehpurpurs bei den Wirbeltieren. Z. Psychol. Physiol. Sinnesorg. **12**, 161—184 (1896).

Krinsky, N. I.: The lipoprotein nature of rhodopsin. Arch. Opthal. **60**, 688—694 (1958a).

— The enzymatic esterification of vitamin A. J. biol. Chem. **232**, 881—894 (1958b).

Kropf, A.: Intramolecular energy transfer in rhodopsin. Vision Res. **7**, 811—818 (1967).

— Hubbard, R.: The mechanism of bleaching rhodopsin. Ann. N.Y. Acad. Sci. **74**, 266—280 (1958).

Kühne, W.: On the photochemistry of the retina and on visual purple. (Ed. Michael Foster) London: Macmillan 1878.

— Chemische Vorgänge. In: Die Netzhaut, Handbuch der Physiologie. (Ed. L. Hermann) **3**, pt. 1, 225—342. Leipzig: Vogel 1879.

Lasareff, P.: Theorie der Lichtreizung der Netzhaut beim Dunkelsehen. Pflügers Arch. ges. Physiol. **154**, 459 (1913).

Lederer, E., Rosanova, V. A.: Studies on vitamin A fish liver oils. An abnormal reaction of Carr and Price. Biokhimiya **2**, 293—303 (1937).

Liebman, P., Entine, G.: Cyanopsin, a visual pigment of retinal origin. Nature (Lond.) **216**, 501—503 (1967).

Lovern, J. A., Morton, R. A.: The distribution of vitamins A and A$_2$ III. Biochem. J. **33**, 330—337 (1939).

— — Ireland, J.: The distribution of vitamins A and A$_2$. II. Biochem. J. **33**, 325—329 (1939).

Lythgoe, R. J.: The absorption spectra of visual purple and of indicator yellow. J. Physiol. (Lond.) **89**, 331—358 (1937).

— Quilliam, J. P.: The relation of transient orange to visual purple and indicator yellow. Physiol. (Lond.) **94**, 390—410 (1938).

Marks, W. B.: Visual pigments of single goldfish cones. J. Physiol. (Lond.) **178**, 14—32 (1965).

— Dobelle, W. H., MacNichol, E. F.: Visual pigments of single primate cones. Science **143**, 1181—1183 (1964).

Matthews, R. G., Hubbard, R., Brown, P. K., Wald, G.: Tautomeric forms of rhodopsin. J. gen. Physiol. **47**, 215—239 (1963).

Mattson, F. H., Mehl, J. W., Deuel, H. J.: Studies on carotenoid metabolism. VII. The site of conversion of carotene to vitamin A. Arch. Biochem. **15**, 65—73 (1947).

McCollum, E. V.: Chap. XV in A history of nutrition. Boston: Stoughton Mifflin 1956.

McConnell, D. G.: The isolation of retinal outer segments. J. cell. Biol. **27**, 459—473 (1965).

Meunier, P., Jouanneteau, J.: Recherches sur l'isomerie *cis-trans* dans la série de la vitamin A (axerophthol). Bull. Soc. Chim. biol. (Paris) **30**, 260—264 (1948).

Mizuno, K., Osawa, K., Kuno, Y.: Synthesis of some coloured products related to rhodopsin and its degradation products. Exp. Eye Res. **5**, 276—285 (1966).

Moore, T.: Vitamin A and carotene. I. The association of vitamin A activity with carotene in the carrot root. Biochem. J. **23**, 803—811 (1929).

— Vitamin A and carotene. V. The absence of the liver oil vitamin A from carotene. VI. The conversion of carotene to vitamin A *in vivo*. Biochem. J. **24**, 692—702 (1930).

Morton, R. A.: Chemical aspects of the visual process. Nature (Lond.) **153**, 69—71 (1944).

— Goodwin, T. W.: Preparation of retinene *in vitro*. Nature (Lond.) **153**, 405—406 (1944).

— Heilbron, I. M.: The absorption spectrum of vitamin A. (a) Nature (Lond.) **122**, 10 (1928); (b) Biochem. J. **22**, 987—996 (1928).

— Peterson, H., Pitt, G. A. J.: Quoted in Morton and Pitt (1957).

— Pitt, G. A. J.: pH and the hydrolysis of indicator yellow. Biochem. J. **59**, 128—134 (1955).

— — Visual pigments. In: Fortschr. Chem. organ. Naturstoffe XIV. 244—316. Vienna: Springer 1957.

— Salah, M. K., Stubbs, A. L.: Retinene$_2$ and vitamin A$_2$. Nature (Lond.) **159**, 744 (1947a).

— — — Conversion of retinene$_2$ to vitamin A$_2$ *in vivo*. Biochem. J. **41**, 24., p. (1947b).

Oroshnik, W.: The synthesis and configuration of neo-b-vitamin A and neoretinene-b. J. Amer. chem. Soc. **78**, 2651—2652 (1956).

— Brown, P. K., Hubbard, R., Wald, G.: Hindered *cis* isomers of vitamin A and retinene: the structure of the neo-b isomer. Proc. nat. Acad. Sci. (Wash.) **42**, 578—580 (1956).

OROSHNIK, W., MEBANE, A. D.: Isoprenoid polyenes containing sterically hindered *cis* configurations. J. Amer. chem. Soc. **76**, 5719—5736 (1954).

OSTROY, S. E., ERHARDT, F., ABRAHAMSON, E. W.: Protein configuration changes in the photolysis of rhodopsin. II. The sequence of intermediates in the thermal decay of cattle rhodopsin *in vitro*. Biochim. biophys. Acta. (Amst.) **112**, 265—277 (1966).

— RUDNEY, H., E. W. ABRAHAMSON: Sulfhydryl groups of rhodopsin. Biochim. biophys. Acta. (Amst.) **126**, 409—412 (1966).

PALMER, L. S., KEMPSTER, H. L.: Relation of plant carotenoids to growth, fecundity and reproduction in fowls. J. biol. Chem. **39**, 299—312 (1919).

— and KENNEDY: Growth and reproduction of rats on whole milk as the sole diet. Proc. Soc. exp. Biol. (N. Y.) **20**, 506—508 (1922).

PARINAUD, H.: L'héméralopie et les fonctions du poupre visuel. C. R. Acad. Sci. (Paris) **93**, 286—287 (1881).

PAULING, L.: Recent work on the configuration and electron structure of molecules, with some applications to natural products. Fortschr. Chem. org. Naturst. **3**, 203—235 (1939); also: Helv. chim. Acta. **32**, 2241—2246 (1949).

PEACOCK, P. R.: Action of light on cod liver oil. Lancet **1926 II**, 328—330.

PITT, G. A. J., COLLINS, E. D., MORTON, R. A., STOK, P.: Studies on rhodopsin. 8. Retinylidene methylamine an indicator yellow analogue. Biochem. J. **59**, 122—128 (1955).

PRATT, D. C., LIVINGSTON, R., GRELLMAN, K. H.: Flash photolysis of rod particle suspensions. Photochem. Photobiol. **3**, 121—127 (1964).

PÜTTER, A.: Studien zur Theorie der Reizvorgänge. Pflügers Arch. ges. Physiol. **171**, 201—261 (1918).

RADDING, C. M., WALD, G.: Acid-base properties of rhodopsin and opsin. J. gen. Physiol. **39**, 909—922 (1956a).

— — The stability of rhodopsin and opsin. J. gen. Physiol. **39**, 923—933 (1956b).

ROBESON, C. D., BAXTER, J. G.: Neovitamin A. J. Amer. chem. Soc. **69**, 136—141 (1947).

— BLUM, W. P., DIETERLE, J. M., CAWLEY, J. D., BAXTER, J. G.: Geometrical isomers of vitamin A aldehyde and an isomer of its α-ionone analog. J. Amer. chem. Soc. **77**, 4120—4125 (1955).

ROSENBERG, B.: The effect of oxygen adsorption on photo- and semiconduction of β-carotene. J. chem. Phys. **34**, 812—819 (1961a).

— Photoconduction in a hindered *cis-trans* isomer of β-carotene in its relation to a theory of the visual receptor process. J. opt. Soc. Amer. **51**, 238—240 (1961b).

— In: Advances in Radiation Biology. Vol. II. (Ed. L. G. AUGENSTEIN, R. MASON, M. S. ZEILE) 193—241. New York: Academic Press 1966.

— KRIGAS, T. M.: Spectral shifts in retinal Schiff base complexes. Photochem. Photobiol. **6**, 769—773 (1967).

ROSENHEIM, O., DRUMMOND, J. C.: A delicate colour reaction for the presence of vitamin A. Biochem. J. **19**, 753—756 (1925).

RUSHTON, W. A. H.: Physical measurement of cone pigment in the living human eye. Nature (Lond.) **179**, 571—573 (1957).

— Visual pigments in the colour blind. Nature (Lond.) **182**, 690—692 (1958).

SCHNEIDER, E. E., GOODEVE, C. F., LYTHGOE, R. J.: The spectral variation of the photosensitivity of visual purple. Proc. roy. Soc. A. **170**, 102—112 (1939).

SCHULTZE, M.: Zur Anatomie und Physiologie der Retina. Arch. mikr. Anat. **2**, 175—286 (1866). See also: A Manual of histology (Ed. S. STRICKER). New York. Wm. Wood 1872.

SEKOGUTI, Y., TAKAGI, M., KITO, Y.: The reversible transconformation of rhodopsin. A. R. Sci. Works. Fac. Sci. Osaka Univ. **12**, 67—81 (1964).

SHIELDS, J. E.: Cited by ABRAHAMSON and OSTROY, 1967.

STEENBOCK, H., BOUTWELL, P. W.: Fat soluble vitamine. V. Thermostability of the fat soluble vitamine in plant materials. J. biol. Chem. **41**, 163—171 (1920a).

— — Fat soluble vitamine. VI. The extractability of the fat soluble vitamine from carrots, alfalfa and yellow corn by fat solvents. J. biol. Chem. **42**, 131—152 (1920b).

— GROSS, E. G.: Fat soluble vitamine. II. The fat soluble vitamine content of roots together with some observations on their water-soluble vitamin contents. J. biol. Chem. **40**, 501—531 (1919).

Stephenson, M.: A note on the differentiation of the yellow plant pigments from the fat-soluble vitamin. Biochem. J. 14, 715—720 (1920).

Takagi, M.: Studies on the ultraviolet spectral displacements of cattle rhodopsin. Biochem. biophys. Acta (Amst.) 66, 328—340 (1963).

Takahashi, K., Kawakami, Z.: Chemistry of vitamin A. Separation of the active constituent of cod liver oil and its properties. J. chem. Soc. Japan 44, 580—605 (1923).

Thompson, J. N., Howell, J. McC., Pitt, G. A., Houghton, C. I.: Biological activity of retinoic acid ester in the domestic fowl: production of vitamin A deficiency in the early chick embryo. Nature (Lond.) 205, 1006—1007 (1965).

Thompson, S. Y., Braude, R., Coates, M. E., Cowie, A. T., Ganguly, J., Kon, S. K.: Further studies on the conversion of β-carotene to vitamin A in the intestine. Brit. J. Nutr. 4, 398—421 (1950).

— Ganguly, J., Kon, S. K.: The intestine as a possible seat of conversion of carotene to vitamin A in the rat and the pig. Brit. J. Nutr. 1, 5—6 (1947).

— — — The conversion of β-carotene to vitamin A in the intestine. Brit. J. Nutr. 3, 50—78 (1949).

Von Euler, B., von Euler, H., Hellström, H.: A-Vitaminwirkungen der Lipochrome. Biochem. Z. 203, 370—384 (1928).

von Euler, H., Karrer, P.: Zur Kenntnis des Vitamins A aus Fischtranen. Helv. chim. Acta 14, 1036—1044 (1931).

v. Planta, C., Schwieter, U., Chopard-dit-jean, L., Rüegg, R., Kofler, M., Isler, O.: Synthesen in der Vitamin-A₂-Reihe. 4. Physikalische Eigenschaften von isomeren Vitamin-A- und Vitamin-A₂-Verbindungen. Helv. chim. Acta 45, 548—561 (1962).

Wagner, A. F., Folkers, K.: Chap. XV. In: Vitamins and coenzymes. New York-London. Interscience, Pub. 1964.

Wald, G.: Vitamin A in the retina. Nature (Lond.) 132, 316—317 (1933).

— Carotenoids and the vitamin A cycle in vision. Nature (Lond.) 134, 65 (1934).

— Vitamin A in eye tissues. J. gen. Physiol. 18, 905—915 (1935a).

— Carotenoids and the visual cycle. J. gen. Physiol. 19, 351—371 (1935b).

— Pigments in the retina. I. The frog. J. gen. Physiol. 19, 781—795 (1936).

— Visual purple system in fresh-water fishes. Nature (Lond.) 139, 1017—1018 (1937a).

— Photolabile pigments of the chick retina. Nature (Lond.) 140, 545—546 (1937b).

— The porphyropsin visual system. J. gen. Physiol. 22, 775—794 (1939).

— The chemical evolution of vision. Harvey Lect. 41, 117—160 (1947).

— The enzymatic reduction of the retinenes to vitamin A. Science 109, 482—483 (1949).

— The interconversion of the retinenes and vitamin A in vitro. Biochim. biophys. Acta 4, 215—228 (1950).

— Vision. Fed. Proc. 12, 606—611 (1953).

— The receptors of human colour vision. Science 145, 1007—1017 (1964).

— Brown, P. K.: The role of sulfhydryl groups in the bleaching and synthesis of rhodopsin. J. gen. Physiol. 35, 797—821 (1952).

— — Human color vision and color blindness. Cold Spr. Harb. Symp. quant. Biol. 30, 345—361 (1965).

Weale, R. A.: Photosensitive reactions in foveae of normal and cone monochromatic observers. Opt. Acta 6, 158—174 (1959).

Wokes, F.: Studies on colour tests for sterols and vitamin A. A spectroscopic study of the colour tests attributed to vitamin A. Biochem. J. 22, 997—1006 (1928).

Wulff, V. J., Adams, R. G., Linschitz, H., Kennedy, D.: The behaviour of flash illuminated rhodopsin in solution. Arch. Ophthal. 60, 695—701 (1958).

Yoshizawa, T., Kito, Y., Ishagami, M.: Studies in the metastable states in the rhodopsin cycle. Biochem. biophys. Acta (Amst.) 43, 329—334 (1960).

— Wald, G.: Prelumirhodopsin and the bleaching of visual pigments. Nature (Lond.) 197, 1279—1286 (1963).

— — Photochemistry of iodopsin. Nature (Lond.) 214, 566—571 (1967).

Zechmeister, L.: Cis-trans isomerization and stereochemistry of carotenoids and dipenyl-polyenes. Chem. Rev. 34, 267—344 (1944).

— Some stereochemical aspects of polyenes. Experientia (Basel) 10, 1 (1954).

Chapter 3

The Structure, Spectra, and Reactivity of Visual Pigments

By

Edwin W. Abrahamson and John R. Wiesenfeld, Cleveland, Ohio (USA)

With 18 Figures

Contents

I. Introduction

Recent chemical and physical studies have clearly shown that visual pigments are an integral part of a lipoprotein membrane whose apparent role is to initiate cation exchange flow across its boundaries, when illuminated, giving rise, thereby, to a neural receptor potential. As membrane structures visual pigments are unique in that they contain, as the principal prosthetic group, a chromophore whose rather singular absorption spectrum serves as a sensitive probe of its molecular environment and whose spectral changes provide an essentially non-perturbative method of monitoring molecular events occurring within the membrane.

In this chapter we discuss visual pigments largely with reference to their membrane milieu. Accordingly, in the first section we consider the gross anatomical structure of the receptor cell, then the structure and composition of the pigment membrane and finally the molecular structure of the visual pigment itself. In the second section we discuss the spectroscopy of visual pigments from a theoretical point of view with particular emphasis on the type of environmental conditions within the membrane that can give rise to, and control, the massive spectral adaptation required to fit the visual pigment to its physiological function of color discrimination. In the third section we deal with the character of the intermediates and intermediate processess in the photolytic cycle.

II. Structure of Visual Pigments

A. The Photoreceptor Cell in Vertebrates

The vertebrate retina is often referred to as "inverted" because it develops embryologically by way of an ectodermal evagination of the forebrain. As a consequence the rod and cone photoreceptor cells are found in the posterior region of the retina where light must pass through several layers of neurons, as well as the inner cell bodies of the receptor cells, before reaching their outer distal segments containing the visual pigment. Rod cells, being about 20 times more numerous than cone cells and more easily obtained, have been studied more thoroughly. But what is known comparatively of the two types of cells leads us to assume that on a molecular level they are much the same in their structure and behavior. Anatomically, however, they do differ as their names suggest. Rod outer segments are cylindrical in shape, on the average about 50 μm in length and 5 μm in diameter, while the cones are somewhat shorter and more conical in shape (Figs. 1 and 2). Both outer segments are connected to the main body of the cell via a cilium, a group of filaments, about nine in number in primates, that appear to terminate near the median point (Cohen, 1969).

Both rod and cone outer segments appear to be evaginations of the plasma membrane of the main cell body, derived, perhaps, directly from the cilium (Dowling, 1967). In the mature outer segment the highly infolded membranes pinch off into a stack of contiguous but separate circular to rosette-like discs or sacs, each with its own membrane. In the rod cell and the cone cells of higher vertebrates there is an outer, relatively-permeable sheath or plasma membrane enclosing the outer segment that joins the sac membrane near the cilium.

The rod sacs can be readily separated from the stack by sonication. These contain the visual pigment rhodopsin in a lipoprotein matrix. A dry weight analysis of frog rod outer segments shows the protein content to be about 57.4 % and the

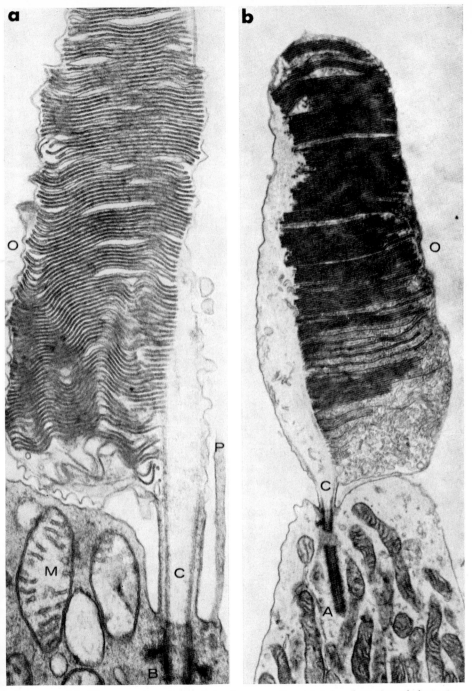

Fig. 1a and b. Electron micrographs of the human retina. a) A basal portion of the outer segment (*O*) of a rod joined to the inner segment by the cilium (*C*), a calycal process of the inner segment (*P*), the generative centriole or basal body (*B*), and a mitochondrion (*M*); × 44,400. b) An outer segment (*O*) of a peripheral cone joined by a cilium (*C*) to the inner segment; below the basal body are traces of rootlet fibrils and a large accessory centriole (*A*); × 15,800. (COHEN, 1969)

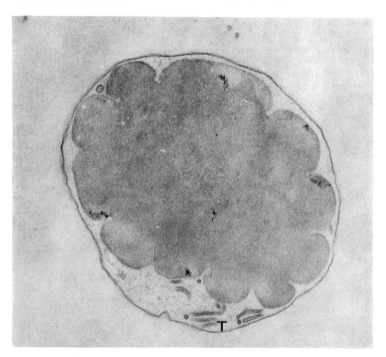

Fig. 2. Cross section of the outer segment of a human rod, with one to two saccules superimposed in the section; note scalloped saccule perimeter and the microtubular elements (T)
derived from the cilium; $\times$ 57,000 (Cohen, 1969)

lipid about 40.6 % (Eichberg and Hess, 1967). Electron microscopy and X-ray
diffraction of frog rods (Sjöstrand, 1961; Blasie, Worthington, and Dewey,
1969) place the rhodopsin molecules on the surface of the sac membrane where they
form a square array with a center-to-center distance ranging from 4 to 5 nm.
Blasie and Worthington (1969), on the basis of the temperature-broadening and
amplitude-decrease of the low angle X-ray diffraction maxima, view the rhodopsin
molecules as lying in an ordered planar liquid arrangement with, perhaps, some
mobility in the plane of the membrane surface.

Although the pigment molecule may have some degree of freedom within the
surface of the rod sac, the plane of the chromophore remains parallel to the surface,
which is appropriate since only light whose electric vector is parallel to this plane
is absorbed (Schmidt, 1938; Denton, 1954; Liebman, 1962; Wald, Brown, and
Gibbons, 1963). If one takes Liebman's value for the pigment concentration in
the rod outer segment of 2—2.5 mM (Liebman, 1962), then it would appear that
the pigment molecules are confined to one surface of the membrane.

The cross sectional structure of the discal sac membrane has been studied by
Blaurock and Wilkins (1969) and by Gras and Worthington (1969) using
X-ray diffraction. The picture that emerges from these studies is that of a typical
bilayer (protein-lipid-protein) membrane enclosing an intrasaccular aqueous cavity.
Fig. 3 shows the density pattern across the membrane surface.

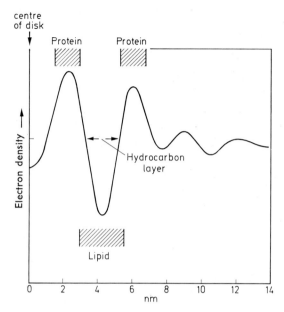

Fig. 3. Fourier synthesis map showing the possible distribution of electron density projected on to a line perpendicular to the disk. The disk is symmetrical about a mirror plane at the origin. The diagram shows, at one side of the centre of the disk, a bilayer membrane profile. There is another (not shown) on the left of the centre. The equivalent (unhydrated) thicknesses. derived from the optical measurements, of the membrane protein and lipid, are shown. Also, for comparison with the low density trough on the profile, the estimated width of the hydrocarbon layer is indicated by arrows. (BLAUROCK and WILKINS, 1969)

B. Vertebrate Visual Pigments as Lipoproteins

Almost a century ago KÜHNE (1879) had shown that the visual pigment of the frog retina was "bleached" by light from pink to yellow. That this same color change could be brought about by solutions now known to contain proteolytic enzymes (AYRES, 1882) was the first indication that visual pigments were proteins. Many years later MIRSKY (1936) suggested that the photobleaching reaction was a reversible protein denaturation similar to that observed for the chromoprotein, "old yellow enzyme."

When the rod pigment rhodopsin is extracted as an aqueous micellar suspension from the retina, with either bile salts or detergents such as digitonin, the protein character is clearly evident. Electrophoretic mobility of frog rhodopsin-digitonin micelles was first demonstrated by BRODA and VICTOR (1940) and later by RADDING and WALD (1958). Spectral studies of frog rhodopsin-digitonin micelles in aqueous solution (COLLINS, LOVE, and MORTON, 1952a) showed an absorbance maximum at 278 nm, typical of aromatic amino acids; and WALD and BROWN (1952) demonstrated that the photolysis of the micelles exposed several sulfhydryl groups, a phenomenon that often accompanies protein denaturation.

Similar preparations of frog rhodopsin at neutral pH had been shown by LYTHGOE and QUILLIAM (1938) to undergo a thermal bleaching at temperatures above 50° C. They observed a half life of 100 minutes, and from their data an enthalpy of activation, $\Delta H^{\pm}$, of 44 kcal/mole, and an entropy of activation, $\Delta S^{\pm}$, of 56 cal/mole/degree can be calculated; values that, again, are typical of protein denaturation.

Hubbard (1959) reported a $\Delta H^{\pm}$ of 100 kcal/mole and a $\Delta S^{\pm}$ of 225.3 cal/ degree mole for aqueous digitonin micelles of bovine rhodopsin at this same pH. In a recent study by Williams and Milby (1968), however, different values for the energy of activation for different rhodopsins were found at pH = 7, i.e. $E^* = 61.5$ kcal/mole for frog, and $E^* = 79.0$ kcal/mole for bovine rhodopsin. They concluded that the activation parameters are sensitive to the temperature range as well as to the pH range over which the thermal decomposition is studied. The same laboratory reports that the thermal stability of micellar rhodopsin depends on the detergent used, digitonin micelles being the most thermally-stable (Johnson and Williams, 1969).

Shields, Dinovo, Henriksen, Kimbel, and Millar (1967) were first to characterize that part of the total protein of bovine rhodopsin that could be solubilized in aqueous detergent micelles. From the amino acid analysis (Table 1) they determined this protein to be a single unit with a molecular weight of 28,600. Similar results were later found by Azuma and Kitô (1967), Heller (1968a) and Shichi, Lewis, Irreverre, and Stone (1969), and are compared in Table 1. Only 9 % of the total dry weight protein of bovine rod outer segments can be accounted

Table 1. *Amino acid analyses of native bovine rhodopsin*

	Number of residues per mole according to			
	a	b	c	d
Aspartic acid	18	16	15	19
Threonine	20	18	17	25
Serine	17	4	12	15
Glutamic acid	21	29	21	25
Proline	19	15	13	16
Glycine	19	19	16	21
Alanine	22	21	20	25
Cysteine	6	4	5	6
Valine	20	17	20	15
Isoleucine	14	13	13	10
Leucine	22	20	20	20
Tyrosine	11	11	11	10
Phenylananine	21	21	19	22
Lysine	13	6	10	8
Histidine	6	3	4	4
Arginine	10	6	6	6
Methionine	8	8	8	8
Tryptophan	—	7	5	—
Mol. wt.	28,600	—	26,400	27,700

[a] Shields, Dinovo, Henriksen, Kimbel, and Millar (1967).

[b] Azuma and Kitô (1967). (Their data were reported as moles/100 g protein $\times$ 10^2 but are presented here on the basis of 8 moles methionine/mole of protein.)

[c] Heller (1968a).

[d] Shichi, Lewis, Irreverre, and Stone (1969).

for in the detergent micelle (POINCELOT and ABRAHAMSON, 1970a, b). The remainder consists of two, or possibly three, fractions distinguishable by gel electrophoresis (FAGER, 1970) but not otherwise characterized as yet.

Other vertebrate rhodopsins that have been characterized in terms of the amino acid content and molecular weight of their detergent-soluble proteins are the frog and rat (AZUMA and KITÔ, 1967; HELLER, 1969). HELLER (1969) found the amino acid contents and molecular weights of the frog, rat and bovine proteins in CTAB micelles to be almost identical. BOWNDS (1970), on the other hand, has found that the micelle-bound protein constitutes as much as 50 % of the total dry-weight protein of frog and rat rhodopsin in contrast to the bovine case.

Free amino groups on the micelle-bound protein may feasibly serve as binding sites for the prosthetic group. Since no terminal N amino groups were found by ALBRECHT (1957), nor by SHIELDS, DINOVO, HENRIKSEN, KIMBEL, and MILLAR (1967), it would appear that the dibasic acids, lysine, and arginine are the only logical candidates for chromophoric-group binding sites on the protein. They found 13 lysine and 10 arginine residues, somewhat more than found in the later studies (Table 1). It would appear that the available numbers of binding sites for the chromophoric group on the protein range from 12 to 23.

Turning now to the other major constituent of the rod outer segments, the lipids, BRODA (1941) was the first to report lipid phosphorus in frog rhodopsin. COLLINS, LOVE, and MORTON (1952b) estimated that bovine ROS had approximately 30 % phospholipid on a dry weight basis while KRINSKY (1958) estimated 45 % phospholipid. Recently, ADAMS (1967) found 38.93 % lipid for bovine ROS agreeing closely with the value of 38.2 % found later by POINCELOT and ZULL (1969). Assuming an average phosphorus content in phospholipid of 4 %, the later data indicated that 26.3 % of the dry weight of ROS was phospholipid. From this and the phospholipid composition, bovine ROS were calculated to have 10.1 % phosphatidyl ethanolamine (PE), 1.9 % phosphatidyl serine (PS), 13.6 % phosphatidyl choline (PC) and 0.4 % sphingomyelin (SM). On this basis there is a total of 95 moles of phospholipid per mole of rhodopsin, of which 37 moles are PE and 49 moles are PC.

Hexane extracted approximately 26 % of the phospholipids in native bovine ROS (POINCELOT and ABRAHAMSON, 1970b) leaving 70 moles of phospholipid per mole of rhodopsin bound to the ROS; of these, 24 moles were PE and 42 were PC. The main bulk of PC, therefore, appears to be more firmly bound to the rod structure than does PE. Similar behavior was observed when the lipids of erythrocytes were extracted (ROELOFSON, DEGIER, and VAN DEENEN, 1964).

Phosphorus-free lipids account for almost 12 % of the dry weight of bovine ROS, but only 3 % is cholesterol (BORGGREVEN, DAEMEN, and BONTING, 1970). The remaining 9 % would appear to be glycolipid (FLEISCHER and McCONNELL, 1966), as found by EICHBERG and HESS (1967) for frog ROS.

When the ROS are extracted with detergents the backbone protein is removed together with a fraction of the total lipid that appears to depend on the type of detergent used. KRINSKY (1958) reports 20 moles of phospholipid per mole of prosthetic group in digitonin micelles of bovine rhodopsin. POINCELOT and ABRAHAMSON (1970a) find emulphogene micelles of rhodopsin to contain 31 moles of phospholipid, of which 15 are PE, 13 are PS and 3 are PC.

SHIELDS, DINOVO, HENRIKSEN, KIMBEL, and MILLAR (1967), in their amino acid analysis of digitonin micelles of bovine rhodopsin, found a non-amino acid fraction that was later identified as ethanolamine. This was equivalent to about 11 moles of phosphatidyl ethanolamine per mole of rhodopsin. One notes also that AZUMA and KITÔ's (1967) value for phosphatidyl serine is much lower than the other values reported in Table 1. This may be accounted for if one assumes the low value as due only to serine in the protein, the higher values of the other investigations reflecting phosphatidyl serine in addition to protein serine.

To obtain some notion of the amount of phospholipid intimately associated with, and essential to, the maintenance of the spectral integrity of native rhodopsin, POINCELOT and ABRAHAMSON (1970a) used the ammonium sulphate treatment of SHICHI, LEWIS, IRREVERRE, and STONE (1969) to remove the detergent from emulphogene micelles of bovine rhodopsin. Of the 31 molecules of phospholipid that the detergent-free preparation contained, 8 molecules were retained after washing with hexane. These can be considered as tightly bound to the protein. Of these 8, 5 were PE, 2 were PS 1 was PC. DAEMEN (1969), by treating ROS with phospholipase C was able to reduce the tightly bound phospholipid to 1 mole of PE and 2 of PS without destroying the spectral integrity of the native rhodopsin.

In contrast to the results quoted above, HELLER (1968a) reports less than 2 % phospholipids in an alcohol-ether extract of aqueous CTAB micelles of rhodopsin, and concludes that the CTAB micelle of bovine rhodopsin after purification on sephadex G-200 is essentially lipid free. But it is quite likely that in HELLER's procedure, significant amounts of phospholipid were retained by the micelle residue in the aqueous layer. Their extraction method (HESS and THEILHEIMER, 1965) was meant for tissue slices and not cationic detergent micelles which, especially in the presence of a large excess of detergent, should tightly bind the bulk of the phospholipid to the micelles. A single portion of ethanol-ether (3:1) would hardly be expected to remove more than a small fraction of the phospholipid present under these conditions.

Recently, HALL and BACHARACH (1970) injected frogs with ^{32}P phosphate and reported less than one mole of phosphorus per mole of protein in their rhodopsin fraction as purified by HELLER's method. But they made the assumption that all phospholipid in the membrane had the same ^{32}P turnover rate and made no distinction between tightly and loosely bound phospholipids (POINCELOT and ABRAHAMSON, 1970a), which would not be expected to have the same turnover rate.

In contrast to DAEMEN's earlier finding the Nijmegen Laboratory recently reported the preparation of phospholipase C-treated bovine rhodopsin that had between 3.5 and 4.4 moles of lipid phosphorus per mole of rhodopsin, of which only 0.24 was PE (BONTING, 1970). But here again the extraction procedure for removal of phospholipids may leave significant amounts of phospholipids or their breakdown products still bound to the proteinaceous residue. Clearly a definitive study in which a decisive phosphorus and ethanolamine analysis of the de-lipidated protein will be necessary to settle the question of whether a truly lipid-free vertebrate rhodopsin maintaining its spectral integrity can be prepared.

POINCELOT and ABRAHAMSON (1970b), as well as BORGGREVEN, DAEMEN, and BONTING (1970), have carried out analyses of the fatty acid groups of the phospholipids of bovine ROS. These results are shown in Table 2. The predominant saturated groups (attached to the β carbon of the glyceryl backbone) are C 16 and C 18 while the α group is predominantly a highly unsaturated fatty acid having

Table 2. *Fatty acid content of bovine rod outer segments, individual phospholipids and rhodopsin* (POINCELOT *and* ABRAHAMSON, *1970b*)

Fatty acid[a]	Content (wt. %)		PE[c]	PS[c]	PC[c]	Rhodopsin
	Rod outer segments					
	1	2				
12:0	Trace		Trace	0.4	Trace	Trace
14:0	0.2	< 16:0 0.6	0.3	1.4	1.2	0.2
15:0	Trace		0.5	1.7	0.5	0.5
16:0	18.6	19.4	15.3	11.8	26.2	20.1
16:1	0.1	0.8	0.2	3.7	2.3	0.3
17:0	Trace	0.6	0.3	2.1	0.2	0.3
18:0	23.5	23.1	19.4	14.3	22.7	19.9
18:1	7.6	6.4	6.4	8.5	8.9	9.9
18:2	0.8	1.4	1.0	1.2	0.9	1.6
18:3	0.2	—	1.4	1.4	1.6	0.4
20:0	0.2	—	1.7	2.5	0.3	0.4
20:1	0.2	—	Trace	0.8	Trace	Trace
20:2	3.2	—	Trace	0.4	Trace	0.2
20:3	1.0	—	1.1	0.4	0.3	0.5
20:4	7.0	6.0	9.4	4.7	8.2	8.3
22:0	0.6	—	0.7	0.8	Trace	0.4
22:1	0.3	—	Trace	0.4	1.0	0.6
22:2[b]	0.4	—	Trace	12.8	0.9	0.8
22:4	—	1.5[b]	—	—	—	—
22:5	—	1.2[b]	—	—	—	—
22:6	22.6	34.3	29.3	16.8	16.6	25.7
24:0	1.5	—	Trace	1.2	Trace	0.3
24:1[b]	5.0	—	3.9	2.3	2.3	3.4
24:2	6.7	—	8.0	3.6	5.7	5.1
Unidentified	0.2	4.7	0.9	6.8	0.0	1.0

Abbreviations: PE, phosphatidyl ethanolamine; PS, phosphatidyl serine; PC, phosphatidyl choline.
[a] Number of carbons: number of double bonds.
[b] Tentatively identified.
[c] Derived from outer segments.
1. POINCELOT and ABRAHAMSON (1970b).
2. BORGGREVEN, DAEMEN, and BONTING (1970).

22 carbons and 6 largely non-conjugated double bonds. This distribution holds both for the loosely bound phospholipids in the ROS as well as for the 8 tightly-bound phospholipids associated with the emulphogene-stripped rhodopsin after hexane extraction.

Pertinent data on the protein and lipid composition of bovine and frog rhodopsin are summarized in Table 3.

Table 3. *Comparative compositions of bovine and frog rod outer segments as determined by various investigators*

	Bovine						Frog
	1[a, b]	2[c]	3[d]	4[e]	5[f]	6[g]	7[h]
Dry weight percentage of rod outer segments							
Total lipid	37.3	39.0	38.9	38.8	—	—	40.6
Phospholipid[i]	25.8	31.5	—	31.5	—	28	26.6
Retinal	0.10	0.14	—	—	0.098	—	—
Cholesterol	—	3.1	—	0.9	—	—	1.7
Glycolipid	—	—	—	—	—	—	9.5
Total protein	62.7[j]	61.0[j]	61.1[j]	61.2[j]	—	70[k]	59.4[k]
Rhodopsin as lipoprotein[l]	14.0	19.6	—	—	14.0	—	—
Protein portion only[m]	9.0	12.6	—	—	9.0	—	50.0[p]
Percentage of total lipid phosphorus							
Phosphatidyl ethanolamine[n]	37.5	39.2		51.0			25.2
Phosphatidyl serine	7.3	11.2		11.7			9.5
Phosphatidyl choline[n]	51.3	36.4		31.0			49.4
Sphingomyelin	1.5	1.0		6.3			1.8
Other phospholipids	2.5	8.6[o]		—			9.2

[a] Poincelot and Zull (1969).
[b] Poincelot and Abrahamson (1970a).
[c] Borggreven, Daemen, and Bonting (1970).
[d] Adams (1967).
[e] Sjöstrand (1959).
[f] Hubbard (1954).
[g] Collins, Love, and Morton (1952b).
[h] Eichberg and Hess (1967).
[i] In calculating phospholipid content, average P percentage in phospholipids was assumed to be 4%.
[j] By difference.
[k] By protein analysis.
[l] Calculated on chromophore basis, using molecular weight (40,000) of rhodopsin as lipoprotein isolated by digitonin extraction.[f]
[m] Based in molecular weight of lipid-free denatured rhodopsin (Shields, Dinovo, Henriksen, Kimbel, and Millar, 1967; Heller, 1968; Shichi, Lewis, Irreverre, and Stone, 1969).
[n] Contains lyso and plasmalogen froms.
[o] Contaminated with unknown amount of lyso-phosphatidyl ethanolamine.
[p] Recent measurement of Bownds (1970).

C. The Chromophoric Group

Wald (1933) isolated from photobleached rhodopsin a yellow-colored pigment ($\lambda_{max} = 385$ nm) that amounted to about 0.3% of the dry weight of the ROS (Poincelot and Abrahamson, 1970b). He named this substance *retinene* on the assumption that it was related in some way to the polyene vitamin A present in the retina. Morton and Goodwin (1944) subsequently showed by direct synthesis that retinene was the aldehyde of vitamin A alcohol. The IUPAC system of nomenclature now refers to the various geometric isomers of retinene as *retinals*, and to the corresponding vitamin A derivatives as *retinols*. There are six known geometric isomers of retinal (Robeson, Blum, Dieterle, Cawley, and Baxter, 1955;

OROSHNIK, 1956). The ones of physiological importance, however, are the 11-*cis* and the *trans* isomers. The former, which can be extracted directly from heat-denatured rhodopsin (HUBBARD, 1959), is the physiologically-active isomer in native visual pigments. On illumination the *trans* configuration is produced.

D. The Binding Site of the Chromophoric Group in Vertebrates

From studies of the behavior of model Schiff bases of retinal with simple amines in MORTON's Liverpool laboratory (PITT, COLLINS, MORTON, and STOK, 1955; MORTON and PITT, 1955), it was concluded that in the visual pigment molecule, 11-*cis* retinal was bound to an amino group in the lipoprotein via a protonated Schiff base linkage. Such model protonated Schiff bases have spectral maxima at 440 nm, i.e. near the short-wave limit of the λ_{max} range of visual pigments built from 11-*cis* retinal.

The preponderance of protein properties exhibited by rhodopsin quite naturally led most investigators in the field to assume that the chromophoric group was bound to the protein, opsin. It was not unexpected, therefore, when BOWNDS and WALD (1965) reported that aqueous digitonin micelles of bovine rhodopsin could be reduced by $NaBH_4$ when illuminated and that subsequent hydrolysis showed the retinylidene chromophore to be attached to lysine residue (BOWNDS, 1967; AKHTAR, BLOSSE, and DEWHURST, 1967).

This finding appeared to settle the question of the binding site of the chromophoric group to the satisfaction of the investigators. There are two points, however, that make such a conclusion premature. First, both workers had carried out the $NaBH_4$ reduction at near neutrality, BOWNDS at pH = 8 and AKHTAR, BLOSSE, and DEWHURST at pH = 6.4. These are conditions under which MORTON and his colleagues (PITT, COLLINS, MORTON, and STOK, 1955; MORTON and PITT, 1955) as well as ourselves (POINCELOT, MILLAR, KIMBEL, and ABRAHAMSON, 1969, 1970) have found that simple-amine Schiff bases of retinal readily hydrolyze and undergo imine exchange. This being the case, there was the distinct possibility that the retinylidene chromophoric group could have migrated during the course of the reduction. But a more serious objection to the notion that the native binding site of the chromophoric group was a lysyl unit arose from the fact that the reduction could be effected only after the rhodopsin suspension had been *illuminated*. Clearly, as mentioned by BOWNDS (1967), this pointed to the occurrence of the reduction at some intermediate stage in the photolytic cycle, and not in native rhodopsin. If, as suggested by BONTING and BANGHAM (1967), the chromophoric group could migrate during the photolytic cycle, then the lysyl unit to which the chromophore was bound after illumination may not have been the native binding site.

In our laboratory ERHARDT (1963) had also demonstrated that digitonin micelles of rhodopsin could be reduced by $NaBH_4$ on illumination and that the chromophoric group was reductively affixed to the protein backbone under these conditions. However, the fact that native rhodopsin could not be directly reduced under these conditions left the question of the native binding site open, particularly in view of KRINSKY's (1958) reference to an earlier statement by WALD (1938) that "retinene extracted from rhodopsin solutions and brought into an organic solvent still, like bleached rhodopsin, is a pH indicator." Such indicator properties are characteristic of Schiff bases of retinal and not of retinal itself.

Our subsequent studies of the native binding site dealt with rod outer segments and CTAB micelles of bovine rhodopsin in the *unilluminated* native state (POINCE-LOT, MILLAR, KIMBEL, and ABRAHAMSON, 1969, 1970; POINCELOT and ABRAHAM-SON, 1970a). The decision to study rhodopsin at these two levels of organization was prompted by two questions often raised: (1) Is the spectral integrity maintain-ed at these two levels sufficient evidence that the local structural integrity of rhodopsin, i.e. the chromophoric group's binding site, is maintained? and (2) Is there an essential discontinuity in the two conditions that would vitiate general conclusions based on the study of only one?

Our initial approach was the extraction of lyophilized bovine ROS (Fig. 4) and CTAB micelles of bovine rhodopsin in the dark with absolute (dry) methanol.

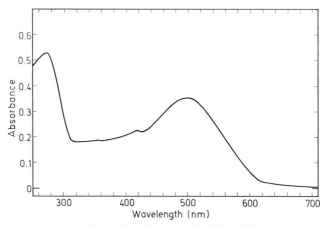

Fig. 4. Powder spectrum of native ROS taken after dark-lyophilization. (POINCELOT, MILLAR, KIMBEL and ABRAHAMSON, 1970)

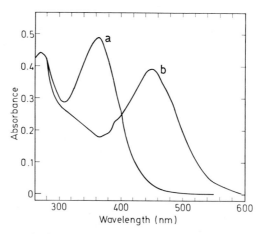

Fig. 5. Solution spectra of alkaline (*a*) and acidic (*b*) forms of the N-retinylidene Schiff base extracted in methanol. (POINCELOT, MILLAR, KIMBEL and ABRAHAMSON, 1970)

After an initial extraction with hexane to remove retinol and traces of retinal, both aggregates were homogenized in absolute (dry) methanol, which removed the chromophoric group almost quantitatively as the free base of a Schiff base complex (Fig. 5) with indicator properties.

The question of the identity of the substance to which the retinylidene chromophoric group was bound was answered in the following way (POINCELOT, MILLAR, KIMBEL, and ABRAHAMSON, 1969, 1970; POINCELOT and ABRAHAMSON, 1970). The methanolic solution was reduced with excess NaBH$_4$ to affix the chromophoric group to its binding site, and then purified on a Sephadex G-100 column. From the temporal elution pattern it was apparent that it had a molecular weight consistent with a retinyl complex of a phospholipid, either phosphatidyl ethanolamine or phosphatidyl serine. Hydrolysis of a portion of the methanol extract of the non-reduced chromophoric material with 6 N-HCl, and amino acid analysis showed ethanolamine to be present in the same molar percentage as the retinyl chromophore.

As a cross check both N-retinyl phosphatidyl ethanolamine (N-RH$_2$PE) and N-retinyl phosphatidyl serine (N-RH$_2$PS) were synthesized and chromatographed. The temporal elution pattern of the synthetic N-RH$_2$PE on Sephadex LH-20 was identical to that of the reduced chromophoric material. Co-chromotography of the synthetic N-RH$_2$PE with the reduced chromophoric material on thin layer plates (TLC) in three different solvent systems was further proof that the two were identical. Finally, when the NaBH$_4$-reduced chromophoric material was further reduced with hydrogen over Pd/charcoal, and hydrolyzed to remove the phospho-glyceride residue, the resulting material was shown by gas chromatography and elemental analysis to be identical with synthetic N-perhydroretinyl ethanolamine.

Although the original dry methanol extracts of ROS and CTAB micelles of rhodopsin most certainly contained the bulk of the chromophoric material as N-retinylidene phosphatidyl ethanolamine this, by itself, did not constitute evidence for the native binding site, for it was found that under these conditions it was possible for the retinylidene group to migrate. This was shown by the addition of aniline to a solution of N-retinylidene butylamine in dry methanol ($\lambda_{max} = 360$ nm). Immediately upon addition of aniline a new absorbance peak ($\lambda_{max} = 385$ nm) appeared, characteristic of the retinylidene Schiff base of aniline. The addition of HCl gas to the methanol solution before addition of aniline, however, stabilized the butylamine complex in the form of a protonated Schiff base. A concentration 10$^{-3.5}$ M in HCl was found to be sufficient to stabilize the retinylidene linkage against imine exchange, and to permit reduction with NaBH$_4$. It was assumed that such conditions would also preclude imine exchange in ROS and CTAB micelles of rhodopsin.

When the ROS and CTAB micelles of rhodopsin were treated in the dark with acid methanol the chromophoric moiety was extracted almost quantitatively as the 11-*cis* isomer of the protonated N-retinylidene phosphatidyl ethanolamine (N$-$R$_c$H$^+$PE). This was proved by subsequent analysis in the way described above. In contrast to the neutral Schiff base of the 11-*cis* isomer (N$-$R$_c$PE, which has its long wave maximum at 360 nm) the protonated Schiff base, N$-$R$_c$H$^+$PE, has maxima at 435 nm and at 397 nm (Fig. 6). The exact nature of the 397 nm-absorbing material is unknown at the present time.

When ROS and CTAB micelles of rhodopsin were simultaneously extracted with acid methanol and reduced with $NaBH_4$, the chromophoric moiety appeared largely as the 11-*cis* isomer of N-retinyl phosphatidyl ethanolamine (N—R_cH_2PE), with maximum at 330 nm. Small amounts of retinol were also observed.

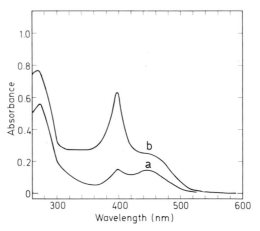

Fig. 6. Solution spectrum of the N-retinylidene Schiff base extracted in methanol containing $10^{-3.5}$ M HCl gas (*a*) and 0.1 M HCl gas (*b*). (Poincelot, Millar, Kimbel and Abrahamson, 1970)

Although the experiments done in acid methanol appeared to provide ample proof that in the native rhodopsin the chromophore is bound to phosphatidyl ethanolamine (Fig. 7), we decided as an additional check to reductively affix the chromophoric group to its binding site under aqueous conditions comparable to

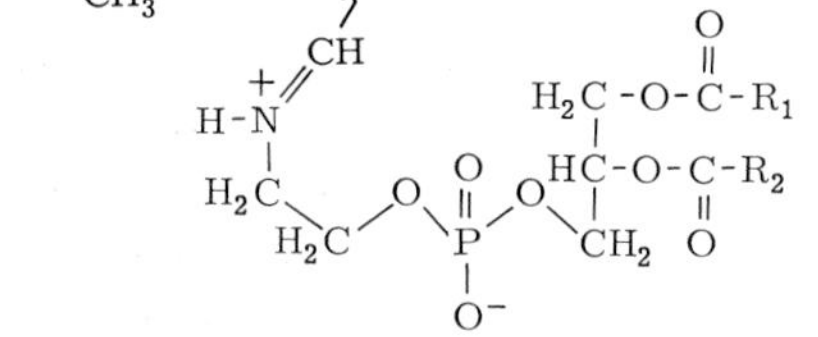

Fig. 7. Structure of protonated N-retinylidene phosphatidyl ethanolamine. R_1 and R_2 represent C 16 to C 22 chains containing zero to six double bonds. (Poincelot, Millar, Kimbel and Abrahamson, 1970)

those used by Bownds and by Akhtar. Accordingly, ROS and CTAB micelles were suspended in an aqueous solution, buffered at pH 4.5 to ensure that the chromophoric group would not migrate. The solutions were then heated at 66° for several hours in the presence of $NaBH_4$ during which time reduction of the binding site occurred. After lyophilization and solution of the solid material in methanol an absorbance maximum of 330 nm was observed (Fig. 8). Subsequent analysis proved the chromophoric group to be present quantitatively as $N-RH_2PE$.

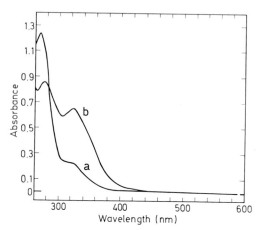

Fig. 8. Solution spectra of the organic soluble N-retinyl compound isolated from heat denatured, acid-buffered ROS (*a*) and CTAB-rhodopsin (*b*). (Poincelot, Millar, Kimbel and Abrahamson, 1970)

Subsequent experiments performed recently in Bonting's laboratory (Daemen, 1969) confirm our identification of the chromophoric-group binding site in vertebrate rhodopsin as phosphatidyl ethanolamine. It was found that under markedly alkaline conditions (pH = 10) CTAB micelles of rhodopsin release the chromophoric group as $N-R_cPE$. Reduction with $NaBH_4$, however, was carried out at pH = 8 which, as in Bownd's case, leaves open the question of chromophoric-group migration. It should, perhaps, be pointed out that in Schiff base complexes the imine linkage is more labile to attack by nucleophilic reagents when it is protonated. One would expect, therefore, that the acid condition would favor reaction of Schiff bases; and so it does in mildly acid conditions. But in moderately or strongly acid solutions the nucleophilic reagents present are effectively tied up by protons, rendering them inactive. Therefore, either moderately acid or alkaline solutions are sufficient to ensure the integrity of the binding site. The acid condition, however, is required for the $NaBH_4$-reduction of the imine linkage.

Further support for the phosphatidyl ethanolamine binding site in bovine rhodopsin is inherent in the work of Kitô, Suzuki, Azuma, and Sekoguti (1968), who showed that treatment of an aqueous digitonin solution of bovine rhodopsin at room temperature with 0.1 M trichloroacetic acid caused a shift in the spectral absorbance curve from a 500 to 440 nm-maximum. The original position could be almost quantitatively restored, however, by freezing the solution to $90-100°$ K. Akhtar and Hertenstein (1969) reported that when this trichloroacetic acid solution of rhodopsin was reduced with tritiated $NaBH_4$ and then lyophilized, about 60 % of the radioactivity was extractable in methanol, and approximately 70 % of the activity of the methanol-soluble material appeared as N-retinylphosphatidyl ethanolamine.

So far only two pieces of published evidence, both originating from the same laboratory, appear to contradict the notion of a phospholipid binding site for vertebrate rhodopsin; (1) Heller's (1968a, b) claim to have prepared an essentially lipid-free bovine rhodopsin as CTAB micelles and (2) Hall and Bacharach's report (1970) that ^{32}P labelled frog rhodopsin contains insufficient ^{32}P label to account for such a site. As has been already pointed out, the first claim is based on a questionable phosphorus analysis and the second on questionable assumptions relative to the incorporation of ^{32}P in frog ROS. A third piece of evidence in the form of an unpublished report from Bonting's laboratory (Bonting, 1970) suggests that there is insufficient PE in phospholipase C-treated rhodopsin to bind the chromophore. But evaluation of this claim must await publication of the details of the analysis.

The evidence from our own laboratory (Poincelot, Millar, Kimbel, and Abrahamson, 1969, 1970) quite clearly supports a PE binding site for the chromophoric group in native rhodopsin, as do the experiments of Akhtar and Hertenstein (1969). Of particular significance is the fact that in native bovine rhodopsin conditions (neutral pH in aqueous media) favorable to the affixation of the chromophore to binding sites other than PE (such as the lysyl group of the protein), have been tried but in no instance has there been even the slightest indication of a binding site other than PE. On the other hand when illuminated rhodopsin has undergone thermal reaction to the intermediate metarhodopsin$_{380}$II, the chromophore is clearly found to be attached to a lysyl group of a protein under the same conditions that yielded N—RPE in native, unilluminated rhodopsin (Section IV C, p. 102). If PE were not the chromophoric-group binding site in native bovine rhodopsin then it would be difficult to reconcile the vastly different behaviors of native rhodopsin and metarhodopsin$_{380}$II, with respect to acid methanol extraction and NaBH$_4$ reduction.

E. Visual Pigments of Cephalopods

The so-called "normal" retina of the invertebrate cephalopod, in contrast to the vertebrate retina, develops as an ectodermal invagination of the head region, so that light is directly incident on the outer segments of the photoreceptor retinula cells (Fig. 9) which form the larger anatomical units called rhabdomes. The squid (Loligo pealii) has been perhaps the most intensively studied of the invertebrates in terms of its fine structure and visual pigment chemistry, although by no means comparable in this respect to vertebrates such as the frog.

Electron micrographs (Wolken, 1958; Zonana, 1961) of the outer segments of the retinula cells, which are much larger than in vertebrates (being about 300 μm in length) reveal a composite fine structure which is shown in Fig. 10. The same basic lamella-pattern exhibited by all photoreceptors is present here but it differs from the vertebrate case in that the plasma membrane develops as hexagonal arrays of tubular extensions called microvilli. These microvilli, which contain the visual pigment rhodopsin, measure approximately 1 μm in length by 0.1 μm across, and are constricted at their base to about one-half their diameter.

There appear to be two types of retinula outer segments (Fig. 10). Type 1 are circular while Type 2 are elliptical. Each Type 1 segment is surrounded by four of

Type 2 and they occur in the ratio of 7 of Type 2 to 3 of Type 1. The microvilli of a single outer segment form two parallel rows oriented perpendicular to the intra-cellular space. A count of the outer segments reveals that there are $5-6 \times 10^4/\text{cm}^2$. The number of microvilli per cell are about 2×10^5 for Type 1 and 7×10^5 for Type 2.

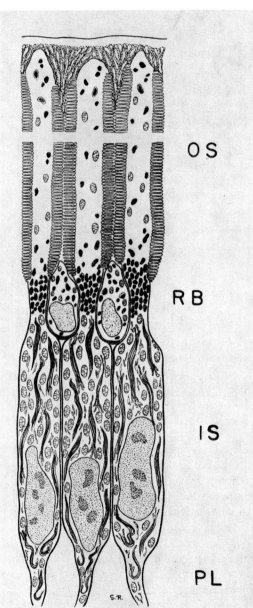

Fig. 9. Composite schematic representation of a longitudinal section through the squid retina. The major subdivisions are labelled: *OS* outer segment; *RB* rod base; *IS* inner segment; *PL* plexiform layer. (ZONANA, 1961)

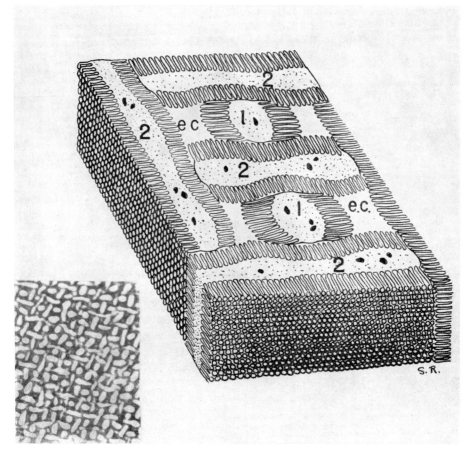

Fig. 10. Schematic three dimensional reconstruction of the rod outer segments. The extra-cellular space (*ec*) has been exaggerated for clarity. The rod types are labelled *1* and *2*. The microvilli are also seen to form a hexagonal array in cross section. (Zonana, 1961)

The visual pigment, rhodopsin, appears to be located in the cylindrical con-joined membrane surfaces, which measure approximately 10 nm in thickness. Nothing is known definitely about the orientation of the pigment in the membrane surface, but one may speculate that the perpendicular arrangement of the micro-villi of the separate cells along their surface of contact may possibly facilitate the detection of polarized light (Moody and Parris, 1960).

According to Hara and Hara (1965, 1967, 1968) there are two pigment systems, both based on the retinal, in the squid, octopus and cuttle fish. The pig-ment located in the outer segments of the retinula cells is called rhodopsin. The other pigment, retinochrome, appears to be localized in the myeloid bodies of the inner segment (Fig. 9) (Zonana, 1961; Yamamota, Tasaki, Sugawara, and Tonosaki, 1965). Squid rhodopsin, like the visual pigments of the vertebrates, has the 11-*cis* retinylidene chromophoric group (Hubbard and St. George, 1958). Retinochrome, on the other hand, has a *trans* retinylidene chromophoric group. In the five kinds of cephalopod rhodopsin studied by HARA and HARA (1967) the rhodopsins have λ_{max} in aqueous digitonin micelles that range from 490—522 nm while the corresponding retinochromes have λ_{max} displaced 15—20 nm towards longer wavelengths.

Much of the basic work on the photolytic behavior of squid *(Loligo pealii)* rhodopsin has been done in the Harvard Laboratory of WALD (HUBBARD and ST. GEORGE, 1958; BROWN and BROWN, 1958; KROPF, BROWN and HUBBARD, 1959; YOSHIZAWA and WALD, 1964). It was shown in these studies that squid rhodopsin, had the 11-*cis* retinylidene chromophoric group in protonated form (as in vertebrate rhodopsin) and that light converted it to the *trans* isomer. But, unlike vertebrate rhodopsin, the end product of the photolysis appeared to be a stable metarhodopsin in which the chromophoric group remained attached to a binding site on the opsin. Retinochrome, however, readily generates free 11-*cis* retinal on photolysis and there has been some speculation (HARA and HARA, 1968) that this pigment may play the role of a photosensitive isomerase (see Chapter 18). This would presumably involve a transimination exchange of the 11-*cis* and *trans* retinylidene groups between the two pigments during *in vivo* photolysis.

Nothing is known at the present time about the composition of retinochrome, but recent work in the writers' laboratory has shown that squid *(Loligo pealii)* rhodopsin, as vertebrate rhodopsin, is a lipoprotein. Aqueous digitonin will extract a lipoprotein micelle from the rhabdomes in which the chromophoric group has $\lambda_{max} = 490$ nm and an ε_{max} of 48,000 liter/cm mole (KROPF, BROWN, and HUBBARD, 1959). As in vertebrate preparations this micelle has a substantial lipid content and a single protein, but this protein has a molecular weight of 70,200 which is almost three times that of vertebrate rhodopsin (KIMBEL, FAGER, and ABRAHAMSON, 1970). An amino acid analysis of this protein (Table 4) shows that it has a composition quite different from vertebrate rhodopsin; all but four of the amino acids differ by more than 20 % from the bovine analysis.

Perhaps the most striking difference between squid and bovine rhodopsin is in the binding site of the chromophoric group. In bovine, and probably in all vertebrate rhodopsins the weight of evidence suggests that the chromophoric group is bound to the lipid phosphatidyl ethanolamine, but in the squid our experiments (KIMBEL, FAGER, and ABRAHAMSON, 1970) show the native rhodopsin to be a lysyl unit of the pigment-associated protein.

The binding site was determined by making use of the unique solubility in methanol of the squid chromolipoprotein and the acid stabilization of the chromophoric Schiff base linkage. When either lyophilized rhabdomes or lyophilized detergent micelles of native or light-exposed squid rhodopsin were extracted with absolute methanol 10^{-2} M in HCl gas, an orange solution was obtained that had an absorbance maximum at 445 nm, characteristic of protonated retinylidene Schiff bases. On reduction by $NaBH_4$, or on standing, the chromoprotein was precipitated essentially free of lipids, less than five percent of the chromophoric moiety being left in solution. After alkaline hydrolysis of the reduced retinyl protein, the retinyl group was shown, by thin layer chromatography in three different solvent systems, to be attached to a lysine residue. The implication of this finding relative to the comparative behavior of vertebrate and invertebrate visual pigments is discussed in Section IV.

Table 4. *Amino acid analysis of native squid rhodopsin* (Kimbel, Fager, and Abrahamson, 1970)

Amino acid	Probable number of residues	Mole fraction	Mole fraction (avg.) bovine rhodopsin
Lysine	34	0.05	0.04
Histidine	7	0.01	0.02
Arginine	16	0.03	0.03
Aspartic acid	50	0.08	0.07
Threonine	22	0.03	0.08
Serine	44	0.07	0.06
Glutamic acid	71	0.11	0.09
Proline	60	0.09	0.06
Glycine	49	0.08	0.08
Alanine	67	0.11	0.09
Valine	27	0.04	0.08
Isoleucine	44	0.07	0.05
Leucine	38	0.06	0.08
Tyrosine	28	0.04	0.04
Phenylalanine	32	0.05	0.08
Cysteine	9	0.01	0.02
Methionine	30	0.05	0.03
Tryptophan	10		
Mol. wt.	70,200		

III. Photochemistry of the Visual Pigments

A. Common Features of the Absorbance Spectra

The spectra of visual pigments, even though they are derived from widely differing species, have certain common features (Dartnall and Lythgoe, 1965). The most obvious is that each of the visual pigments displays several absorbance maxima. The absorption band lowest in energy lies in the visible region of the spectrum, its location ranging (in the retinal series) from 433 nm in the green rods of the frog (Dartnall, 1967) to 575 nm in its cones (Liebman and Entine, 1968). This band, having its maximum from 3,000 to 8,000 cm^{-1} to the red of the 11-*cis* retinal band and a molar extinction coefficient near to 41,000, is of the greatest importance to vision. The band next higher in energy though much lower in extinction — the so-called β-peak — absorbs in the near-ultraviolet region with location ranging between 350 nm (Collins, Love, and Morton, 1952a) and 370 nm (Wald, Brown, and Smith, 1955). Since 11-*cis* retinal displays similar absorbance maxima in somewhat higher energy regions (285 and 255 nm), it might be assumed that the β-band in visual pigments arises from the 11-*cis* configuration of the chromophoric group.

Another very intense band occurs at 278 nm. This has as its principal source the aromatic amino acids, tryptophan and tyrosine (Collins, Love, and Morton, 1952a, b). Finally, a complex system of bands appears in the vicinity of 250 nm. This contributes substantially to the 278 nm maximum but can be ascribed to lipids, and perhaps to nucleotides, present in the extracts studied (Poincelot and Abrahamson, 1970a, b). These are present both as integral parts of the rhodopsin molecule, i.e. tightly bound phospholipids, and as impurities extracted from the outer segments by the detergent solutions used.

The maximum absorbances of visual pigments in the long wavelength band are generally 40 % higher at room temperature than that of 11-*cis* retinal from which they are derived. The cause of this intensification is not known, but it is well to bear in mind that visual pigments are protonated Schiff base polyenes in a quasi solid-state environment, rather than polyene aldehydes in organic solvents. For this reason their spectral behavior may be markedly different in many respects. Nevertheless this enhancement could be explained on the same basis as the observed increase in the long wavelength absorbance of 11-*cis* retinal upon cooling. JURKO-WITZ (1959) attributes the increase to the molecule's assuming a more planar configuration at the lower temperature. This reasoning is apparently based on the notion that the out-of-plane twist occasioned by the steric interference of the C 13 methyl group with the C 10 hydrogen atom is confined only to formal single bonds. NASH (1969), who has tried to evaluate torsional potentials about the single bonds adjacent to the C 11—C 12 formal double bond within the framework of a simple Hückel molecular orbital calculation coupled with empirical non-bonded torsional potential functions, comes to the same conclusion. But it is apparent from the spectra of BALKE and BECKER (1967) (see Fig. 10 in Chapter 1, p. 24) that this increase in absorbance is accompanied by a decrease in absorbance in the two higher energy bands of 11-*cis* retinal. According to the molecular orbital calculations (Pariser-Parr-Pople method) of WIESENFELD and ABRAHAMSON (1968, 1970) twisting about the C 11—C 12 formal single bond will decrease the absorbance not only of the long-waveband but also that of the so-called "cis" peak at 255 nm. On the other hand, they find that twisting about the C 11—C 12 *double* bond will result in an increase in absorbance and a small red shift of all bands, as is actually observed when 11-*cis* retinal is cooled (BALKE and BECKER, 1967).

PATEL (1969), who has recently studied the 220 MHz NMR spectrum of 11-*cis* retinal, concludes that the twist is distributed over the entire C 11—C 14 region. He bases this conclusion in part on the fact that C 11 has a much greater π-electron density in the 11-*cis* isomer than in the *all-trans* one. Twisting about the C 12—C 13 single bond would give this result but so also would twisting about the adjacent C 11—C 12 double bond (WIESENFELD and ABRAHAMSON, 1968). Furthermore, the calculations of WIESENFELD and ABRAHAMSON (1969) predict that although the overall torsional barrier about the single bond C 12—C 13 is lower than that about the C 11—C 12 double bond, the π-energy difference within the first 30° is almost an order of magnitude greater for the former. This, coupled with the fact that models predict that the steric hindrance between the hydrogen atom on C 10 and the methyl group on C 13 would be relieved by a much smaller torsional displacement about the C 11—C 12 double bond than about the C 12—C 13 single bond, suggests that the twist in the C 11—C 14 region is heavily weighted in the C 11—C 12 double bond.

Another line of evidence suggests that steric hindrance is not the principal factor controlling the character of the spectral absorbance curve of 11-*cis* retinal. NELSON, DE RIEL, and KROPF (1970) have synthesized a series of retinal homologs and find that the absorbance maxima of the 11-*cis* isomers of retinal and 13-desmethyl retinal (the C 13 methyl group is here replaced by a hydrogen atom so that there is no intrinsic steric hindrance) are comparable. This may mean that the low temperature phenomenon of Jurkowitz could be attributed to a dramatic enhancement of the Franck-Condon factors (vibrational overlap integral between the ground and excited electronic state) of 11-*cis* retinal in the rigid environment of the organic glass at low temperatures, as has been suggested by Thompson (1969) for the same phenomenon in retinol isomers.

Sperling and Rafferty (1969) in their polarized-light studies of 11-*cis* retinal in stretched films suggest that the 255 nm band is not the "cis" peak as is generally assumed. They find a slight increase in the absorbance of light (presumably polarized perpendicular to the long axis of the molecule in the second transition) with a maximum at 285 nm which they take as evidence that it is the "cis" peak. As pointed out in Chapter 1 for the case of butadiene, the molecular orbital picture predicts that the second excited configuration, being doubly degenerate, should split by configuration interaction into two bands, the lower energy one having a transition dipole moment perpendicular to the long axis of the molecule. Applied symmetrical polyenes this would support the Sperling and Rafferty assignment. Wiesenfeld and Abrahamson (1969), however, have found in their calculations on 11-*cis* retinal that the 285 nm and 255 nm bands both have a mixed polarization which arises from the unsymmetrical character of the polyene chain and the presence of the terminal carbonyl group. On this basis both high-energy bands may be characterized as "cis" peaks.

The visual pigments that incorporate 3-dehydroretinal as the chromophoric group are known as porphyropsins (Wald, 1937, 1939). They absorb maximally at longer waves than the analogous rhodopsins formed when the same lipoproteins (opsins) react with 11-*cis* retinal (see Bridges, 1965). For example, cattle rhodopsin absorbs maximally at 500 nm while the porphyropsin made by incubating 11-*cis*-3-dehydroretinal with cattle opsin absorbs at 523 nm (see Bridges, 1967). Other characteristics of porphyropsin spectra are reduced absorbance and a pronounced high-energy tail (Bridges, 1965).

The bathochromic shift of the porphyropsin spectra relative to those of the rhodopsins is due largely to the nature of the respective chromophoric groups. The additional double bond present in 3-dehydroretinal increases the length of the conjugated polyene chain, with a concomitant shift to lower energies in the electronic transitions. This does not account, however, for the rather small difference in λ_{max} between rhodopsins and the corresponding porphyropsins that absorb in the blue, as opposed to the much larger differences observed for those that absorb in the red region of the spectrum (Dartnall and Lythgoe, 1965; Liebman and Entine, 1968). Several explanations of this phenomenon have been advanced, most of them dealing with the increased steric hindrance between the C 1 methyl group and the C 8 hydrogen atom in the *s-trans* configuration (Bridges, 1965; Liebman and Entine, 1968). But these arguments may be invalid for 3-dehydroretinal since it may well exist in the s-*cis* configuration, as does retinol (Stam and MacGillavry, 1963). The high-energy tail displayed by porphyropsins could be due to impurities unique to the extraction of these pigments, although it is more probably caused by some added distortion in the 3-dehydro polyene such as a torsional twist about the C 6—C 7 single bond. This could also explain the reduced absorbance of porphyropsins.

B. The Quantum Yield of Photolysis

Both rhodopsins and porphyropsins are very light-sensitive. Several studies to determine the quantum yield of the primary process have been made (e.g. DART-NALL, GOODEVE, and LYTHGOE, 1936, 1938; KROPF, 1967). Because intermediates in the thermal cycle can absorb light and regenerate rhodopsin, such studies are fraught with experimental difficulties (see DARTNALL, Chapter 4, p. 135). These obstacles can in principle be overcome by the use of low light intensities and temperatures in excess of $20°$ C, for under these conditions metarhodopsin $_{478}$I,the first intermediate seen above $0°$ C, will rapidly decay to metarhodopsin$_{380}$ II which does not absorb an appreciable amount of the visible light used.

The earliest investigations in this area were carried out on detergent micelles of frog rhodopsin. The rate of bleaching at 506 nm was measured and the "photo-sensitivity" was reported as 23,000 (litre/cm mole) (DARTNALL, GOODEVE, and LYTHGOE, 1936, 1938). From later measurements showing the ε_{max} of frog rhodopsin to be about 40,600 l/cm mole, the quantum yield of photobleaching was calculated to be about 0.5 (WALD and BROWN, 1953). The original studies were soon extended over a wide spectral range (SCHNEIDER, GOODEVE, and LYTHGOE, 1939; GOODEVE, LYTHGOE, and SCHNEIDER, 1942) and similarly indicated an average quantum yield of 0.58, with no significant variation in the visible. DARTNALL (1968) has recently found a somewhat higher value, near 0.66, for a variety of rhodopsins (and por-phyropsins) in the presence of hydroxylamine. WILLIAMS (1965), on the other hand, interprets his flashing light experiments on aqueous digitonin extracts of rhodopsin as favoring a quantum yield of unity.

In the excised rabbit eye HAGINS (1957) finds a quantum yield near 0.5 but RIPPS and WEALE (1969) report a value of unity for the living human eye. It would appear that the actual quantum yield is somewhere between 0.66 and 1.0 (see Chapter 4 for discussion).

Recently, studies have been undertaken to determine the quantum efficiency of irradiation in the lipoprotein absorption region at 278 nm (KROPF, 1967). These reveal that the quantum yield is about 1/2 to 3/4 that in the visible region. This reduced quantum efficiency may be accounted for by assuming that the high-energy β band of the chromophore makes a partial contribution to the absorbance in this region, funneling the energy by radiationless processes into the lowest singlet state (see Chapter 1). It might also be assumed, as KROPF does, that some process occurs whereby the energy absorbed by the lipoprotein is transferred radiationlessly to the chromophoric group, which then isomerizes to initiate the sequence of thermal decay. Again, the absorbed energy might initiate the proper sort of configurational change in the lipoprotein without any involvement of the chromophoric group.

C. Explanations of the Spectra

As previously mentioned, the visual pigments containing the 11-*cis* retinylidene chromophoric group range in λ_{max} from 430 to 575 nm (DARTNALL and LYTHGOE, 1965; LIEBMAN and ENTINE, 1968). We have already shown in vertebrates (POINCE-LOT, MILLAR, KIMBEL, and ABRAHAMSON, 1969) that the essential native visual pigment is N-11-*cis* retinylidene phosphatidyl ethanolamine stabilized in the

Zwitterionic form at near neutral pH (DAEMEN and BONTING, 1969). This has a long-wave absorbance maximum at 435—440 nm. Thus the lipoprotein environment must in some way produce the additional bathochromic shift necessary to fit the pigment to its physiological role.

There are numerous ways in which a controlled perturbation of the retinylidene system might be achieved. One is by an environmentally-imposed twist about some essential double bond in the retinylidene structure. Another way, first suggested by KROPF and HUBBARD (1958), would involve negatively charged groups, such as phosphate or carboxylate, positioned in the environment so as to lie close to the polyene chain. These are models very difficult to test out experimentally, but we have been able to develop theoretical quantum mechanical methods with which to test their feasibility (WIESENFELD and ABRAHAMSON, 1968, 1969; WIESENFELD, LEWIS, and ABRAHAMSON, 1970).

The Pariser-Parr-Pople (PPP) method (PARISER and PARR, 1953; POPLE, 1955) (see Chapter 1) treats only the π-electron system, by considering it to be in a fixed potential field of the nuclei and all other σ electrons. In order to test the applicability of this method to linear polyene systems we carried out a number of calculations on retinal and 3-dehydroretinal isomers whose spectra are well known. Of particular interest were the 11-*cis* and *trans* isomers. Calculations (WIESENFELD and ABRAHAMSON, 1969) show (Table 5) that the *trans* and 11-*cis* isomers are more stable when the C 6—C 7 bond adopts the s-*cis* position shown in Fig. 11. This is

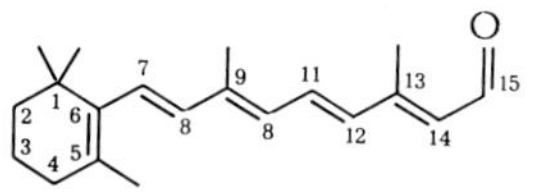

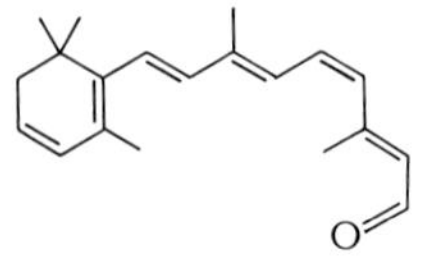

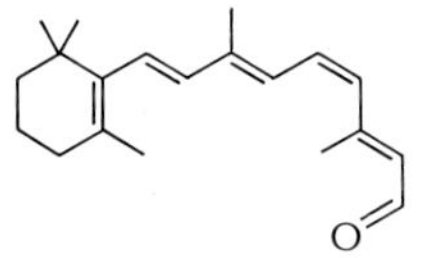

Fig. 11. Structures of (a) *trans* (6,14-s-*dicis*) retinal, (b) 11-*cis* (6,14-s-*dicis*) 3-dehydroretinal, and (c) 11-*cis* (6,14-s-*dicis*) retinal

also borne out by X-ray crystallography (STAM and MACGILLAVRY, 1963). The C 14—C 15 bond is also shown in the s-*cis* position. The principal reason for this assignment is based on high-resolution NMR data (PATEL, 1969) of various retinal isomers, which show a significant increase in the chemical shift for the C 13 methyl group in C 13 *cis* isomers. Such a shift can be associated with the enhanced deshielding caused by the proximity of the aldehydic oxygen atom. Only in the case of isomers with a 13-*cis* double bond would the C 13 methyl group be removed from the neighborhood of the oxygen atom, when a smaller chemical shift would be expected. Another reason for the s-*cis* assignment to the C 14−C 15 bond arises from the photochemical behavior at low temperatures (JURKOWITZ, 1959; BALKE and BECKER, 1967) when a photoproduct, believed to be a photo-enol of 11-*cis* retinal, is formed. Such a product could form intramolecularly if the carbonyl oxygen and the C 13 methyl group were close enough, as they are in the s-*cis* isomer, for hydrogen abstraction to occur.

Table 5. *Comparison of calculated and experimental parameters of absorption*

		$\lambda_{max(nm)}$	f	μ_x	μ_y
trans (6,14-s-*dicis*) retinal experimental (hexane)	$^1(\pi, \pi^*)$	372 375	1.99	2.27	1.27
	$^1(n, \pi^*)$	396			
11-*cis* (6,14-s-*dicis*) retinal experimental (hexane)	$^1(\pi, \pi^*)$	375 364 (375[a])	1.72	2.35	0.68
experimental (hexane)	$^1(\pi, \pi^*)'$	279 285	0.10	0.39	0.36
experimental (hexane)	$^1(\pi, \pi^*)''$	258 255	0.57	0.61	1.00
	$^1(n, \pi^*)$	384			
11-*cis* (6,14-s-*dicis*) 3-dehydroretinal experimental	$^1(\pi, \pi^*)$	399 393	1.67	2.31	0.92
trans (6,14-s-*dicis*) retinylidene imine experimental	$^1(\pi, \pi^*)$	371 366	2.05	2.29	1.33
trans (6,14-s-*dicis*) retinylidene iminium ion experimental (methanol)	$^1(\pi, \pi^*)$	428 435	1.79	2.31	1.32
11-*cis* (6,14-s-*dicis*) retinylidene iminium ion experimental (methanol)	$^1(\pi, \pi^*)$	441 435	1.34	2.30	0.43

[a] Absorbance maximum at 77° K.

Table 5 lists the calculated λ_{max}, oscillator strengths, f, and the in-plane, transition dipole-moment components, μ_x and μ_y, for various isomers of retinal and compares them with experimental data where known. Also included are the retinylidene Schiff base, its protonated form, and the retinylidene iminium ion, which is the basic model of visual pigments. The agreement with the experimental λ_{max} is, in general, quite satisfactory — sufficient in any respect to use the PPP method as a basis for perturbation studies. INUZUIKA and BECKER (1968), SUZUKI, TAKIZAWA, and KATO (1970) and LANGLET, PULLMAN, and BERTHOD (1970) have also carried out PPP calculations on retinal isomers with results similar to ours.

Although the PPP method is designed for π-electrons with a fixed nuclear framework and constant σ-electron potential, it has been used satisfactorily to investigate the effect of twisting about essential double bonds, even though a constant "core" potential is not maintained in the process (BORRELL and GREENWOOD, 1967). We therefore decided to investigate the effect on the spectra of twisting about the C 11−C 12 essential double bond in the protonated Schiff base, i.e. the retinylidene iminium ion. The torsional potential curves are shown in Fig. 12. A twist angle of 45° from the planar 11-*cis* configuration results in a 3500 cm^{-1} red shift in the long-wave λ_{max}. This is about the torsional limit one could expect and it only accounts for somewhat less than 50 % of the total energy range spanned by the visual pigments using the 11-*cis* retinylidene chromophoric group.

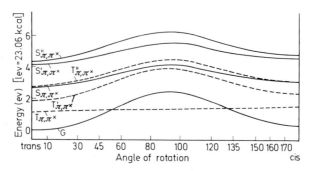

Fig. 12. Torsional potential curves for the rotation about the C 11—C 12 double bond of the 11-*cis*-N-retinylidene iminium ion G, ground state; $S\,\pi$, π^*, lowest singlet $(\pi,\,\pi^*)$ state; $T\,\pi$, π^*, lowest triplet $(\pi,\,\pi^*)$ state

The use of simple potential functions to represent the variation of the resonance integral with the angle of torsion, i.e. $\beta_\theta = \beta_0 \cos \theta$ as well as the perturbation of the σ-core potential hardly justifies using the torsional potential curves (Fig. 12) in other than a qualitative fashion. Nevertheless, it would appear that torsion about the C 11—C 12 bond alone cannot account for the full range of λ_{max}.

Next we investigated the effect of anionic groups using negative point charges placed at various positions with respect to the 11-*cis* retinylidene-iminium ion and its 3-dehydro derivative. The coulomb integral (see Chapter 1), which in the PPP method is taken as the sum of the ionization potential and the electron affinity of the (trivalent) carbon atom, was then corrected for each carbon atom in the π-electron system for the presence of the negative point charge. The calculated λ_{max} are given in Table 6 for negative point charges placed above each carbon atom in the conjugated system in a plane 0.45 nm above the plane of the molecule. The calculated bathochromic shift of 4100 cm^{-1} is more than 80 % of the total range (5100 cm^{-1}) of λ_{max} spanned by visual pigments based on the 11-*cis* retinylidene-iminium chromophoric group. For the 3-dehydro retinylidene-iminium case the calculated bathochromic shift is about 70 % of the total range observed. Had the charges been placed somewhat closer to the plane of the molecule or had several charges been used, it is quite likely that the full spectral range could have been covered in both systems. It is also interesting to note that point charges placed near the nitrogen shift the spectrum hypsochromically. This could account for the ultraviolet-absorbing pigments observed in insects (see MORTON and PITT, 1969).

DARTNALL and LYTHGOE (1965) have pointed out that the λ_{max} of visual pigments derived from retinal tend to cluster about positions in the spectrum separated by intervals of about 7 nm. This suggests that perhaps two types of perturbation are involved in the control of λ_{max} *in vivo*, which may be viewed as coarse and fine tuning. In terms of the model studied by us (WIESENFELD, LEWIS, and ABRAHAMSON, 1968, 1970) one can consider charge perturbation as the coarse tuning and an environmentally controlled torsion about the C 11—C 12 double bond as the fine tuning perturbation.

Another property of the retinal/3-dehydroretinal visual pigment system noted by DARTNALL and LYTHGOE (1965) is that the energy difference between the λ_{max} in the two systems is large in the red region of the spectrum but tends to approach zero in the blue. LIEBMAN and ENTINE (1968) and BLATZ, PIPPERT, and BALA-SUBRAMANIYAN (1968) assign this phenomenon to a controlled torsion about the C 6—C 7 single bond, which would tend to interrupt resonance between the cyclohexa(di)ene ring and the polyene side chain. As the long wave region of the spectra would be controlled largely by the polyene side chain, which is the same in both pigment systems, they reason that there is substantial torsion about the C 6—C 7 bond in both pigment systems that absorb in the blue region of the spectrum.

Examination of Table 6 shows that for the same charge position the energy difference between the two systems does not show the trend noted by DARTNALL

Table 6. *Calculated effects of a negative point-charge on the λ_{max} of retinylidene- and 3-dehydro-retinylidene iminium ions. (Charge placed 0.45 nm above the plane of the molecule at various positions as indicated)* (WIESENFELD, LEWIS and ABRAHAMSON, hitherto unpublished)

Charge position		Calculated λ_{max} (nm)			
		11-*cis* (6,14-s-*dicis*) retinylidene iminium ion		11-*cis* (6-14-s-*dicis*) 3-dehydroretinylidene iminium ion	
Carbon atom	3	—		558	
	4	—		547	
	5	530	518[a]	533	544[a]
	6	518		520	
	7	501		505	
	8	480		487	
	9	471		476	
	10	460		461	
	11	437		444	
	12	421		433	
	13	410		414	
	14	395		401	
	15	377		387	
Nitrogen atom	16	356	360[a]	368	362[a]

[a] Torsion angle of 30° about C 6—C 7 bond.

and Lythgoe. But if the molecule is twisted about the C 6—C 7 bond by approximately 30° with the charge at position 5 the calculated λ_{max} of 11-*cis* retinal shifts from 530 to 518 nm while that for the 3-dehydro derivative shifts from 533 to 544 nm. On the other hand if the charge is at position 16, 11-*cis* retinal shifts from 356 to 360 nm and the 3-dehydro derivative from 368 to 362 nm. Thus torsion about the C 6—C 7 single bond does apparently favor the observed trend.

Another model of rhodopsin holds that the chromophoric group is attached to the lipoprotein by an unprotonated Schiff base linkage (Dartnall, 1957; Bridges, 1962). "Secondary bonding" then occurs because of the presence of an anion-cation pair of charged groups on the lipoprotein situated near the polyene chain. It was originally supposed (Dartnall, 1957) that this interaction was sufficiently strong to localize an extra π-electron at one carbon atom producing a "π-hole" at another. As the energy required to perform such a task is indeed considerable, it was suggested that rather than actually causing the localization of electrons in the π-system, the formal charges of the lipoprotein induce a permanent dipole (Dartnall and Lythgoe, 1965) in the highly polarizable electron cloud associated with polyenes of such length (Platt, 1959). The fact that the protonated Schiff base of N-11-*cis* retinylidene phosphatidyl ethanolamine is stable at near neutral pH would tend to discount this picture (vide infra). Hubbard (1969) also provides evidence supporting the protonated Schiff base linkage.

There is another mode of controlled spectral perturbation, possibly operative in visual pigments, which involves a dispersive interaction between the molecule and its environment. For highly polarizable molecules with large transition dipole moments, such as Brooker dyes, this interaction may be quite appreciable in a highly polarizable solvent environment (Bayliss and McRae, 1954; Platt, 1959). Platt (1959) pointed this out with reference to visual pigments and recently Erickson and Blatz (1968) and Irving, Byers, and Leermakers (1969) have provided some experimental foundation for this notion. Thus quaternary salts of the retinylidene iminium ion vary in λ_{max} from 452 nm in polar solvents of low polarizability, such as methyl cyanide, to 497 nm in highly polarizable solvents such as 1,2,dichloroethane.

In the case of visual pigments Irving, Byers, and Leermakers invoke a dispersive interaction between the transition dipole of the chromophoric group and the "microenvironment", which they envision as optimally positioned groups of high polarizability on the associated protein, i.e., phenylalanine, tyrosine and tryptophan. Their data and those of Erickson and Blatz (1968) show the expected increase in bathochromic shift of λ_{max} with increasing size of the anion, a point implicit in the calculations of Wiesenfeld and Abrahamson (1968, 1970).

Although plausible in a qualitative sense, solvent spectra do not provide a proper experimental test for this theory. One should test the theory with a microenvironment of known composition and structure — ideally the microenvironment of the native visual pigment. This knowledge, however, is likely to be some time in arriving. Meanwhile it might be worthwhile to test the dispersive interaction theory in a theoretical way, such as was done for the charge perturbation model. Admittedly, however, this will be a much more difficult and sizeable task.

Two recent communications (Adams, 1967 and Adams, Jennings, and Sharpless, 1970) point to the possibility that an interaction of unsaturated linkages on the side-chain fatty acids of the phospholipids could be responsible for the bathochromic shift in visual pigment. They isolate a PE-retinal complex absorbing at 500 nm. The $\pi - \pi^*$ interaction they invoke as responsible for the shift may also be viewed as a dispersive interaction.

Although a number of other theories have been presented to account for the spectra of visual pigments, such as charge-transfer interaction (GALINDO, 1967) and retinal-protein complexes involving a thio-substituted aldimine linkage (MIZUNO, KUNO, and OZAWA, 1966; HELLER, 1968b), these can be ruled out as being inconsistent with the spectral or chemical properties of visual pigments (ABRAHAMSON and OSTROY, 1967). At the present time the charge-perturbation and dispersive-interaction theories seem the only plausible ones. It is quite possible that both these effects contribute to the spectral control of visual pigments in a way in which we can only understand when the microenvironment is known.

IV. Reactivity of the Visual Pigments

A. The Primary Photochemical Process

It has been established for a number of visual pigments that the retinylidene polyenic group, on the absorption of light, undergoes a photoisomerization from the 11-*cis* to the *trans* isomeric configuration (HUBBARD and KROPF, 1958). There has been a question, however, as to whether the primary photochemical process involves only photoisomerization or whether photoisomerization is accompanied by a more chemical change. MIRSKY (1936) long ago drew the analogy between the photobleaching of rhodopsin and protein denaturation, and more recent work (ABRAHAMSON, MARQUISEE, GAVUZZI, and ROUBIE, 1960) has pointed to the occurrence of rather substantial protein configuration changes in at least one of the thermal reactions of the bleaching sequence.

DARTNALL (1957) has suggested that the primary process must involve the disengagement of some "linch pin" that maintains the structural integrity of the visual pigment, thereby initiating the thermal changes that follow. Photochemical thinking would suggest that a substantial fraction of the 57 kcal of electronic excitation energy would be channelled into severing the linch pin. In principle this could be accomplished in several ways. One might envision proton or electron transfer from the excited chromophore to a suitable group in the immediate environment, but both these processes are energetically unfavorable; the first because the excited protonated retinylidene group is a weaker acid than when in its ground state, and the second because transfer of an electron would leave a bipositive charge on the polyene (ABRAHAMSON and OSTROY, 1967). There is also the possibility that an electron could be transferred to the excited dye from a suitable source such as an RS^- anion, a process reported by FUJIMORI (1964) for the photolysis of the cationic dye 3',6'-dichlorofuran. FUJIMORI observed a distinct electron-spin resonance (ESR) absorption accompanying this process, which he assigned to the pair of free radicals generated. Both KROPF (unpub.) and the authors (LUCKHURST and ABRAHAMSON, 1965; GOETZ, WIESENFELD, and ABRAHAMSON, 1967) have looked carefully for ESR signals on the illumination of ROS and digitonin micelles

of bovine rhodopsion at 77° K and higher temperatures, but have been unable
observe any signal that could be assigned to radical products derived from t
photolysis of rhodopsin.

In an earlier review (ABRAHAMSON and OSTROY, 1967) it was suggested th
the linch pin might consist of the coulombic interaction of a pair of charges, t
cationic nitrogen of the retinylidene group and an anionic group in the environme
positioned near the cyclohexa(di)ene ring, with the induced dipole so generated
the polyene system between them. Photoisomerization, of course, would remo
this coulombic bridge thereby breaking the linch pin. The advantage of this model
that a dual role is played by the anionic group, that of controlling the λ_{max} as w
as maintaining the linch pin.

As photoisomerization appears to be the primary process it is instructive to s
what insight into this process is forthcoming from comparable studies on mod
chromophoric systems. The closest systems to the retinylidene-iminium ion prot
type that have been studied are the retinal isomers (KROPF and HUBBARD, 197(
The range of values (0.06—0.2) reported for the quantum quield of the phot
isomerization of *trans*-retinal to mono *cis* isomers (KROPF and HUBBARD, 197
encompasses the quantum yield of 11 % found by DAWSON and ABRAHAMS(
(1962) for the population of the triplet state of retinal. This suggests that t
photoisomerization may take place via the $^3(\pi, \pi^*)$ state of retinal.

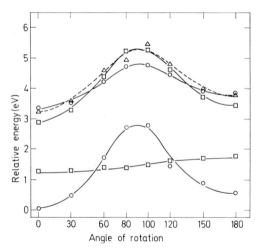

Fig. 13. Potential energy curves for ground and lower excited states of retinal. Singlet (π, π
circles; singlet (n, π^*), triangles; triplet (π, π^*), squares. (WIESENFELD and ABRAHAMSON, 196

Some insight into the pathway for photoisomerization in retinal is provided
the torsional potential curves about its C 11—C 12 formal double bond as calculat
by WIESENFELD and ABRAHAMSON (1968) (Fig. 13). It is apparent from Fig.
that the $^1(n, \pi^*)$ state of retinal is almost isoenergetic with the $^1(\pi, \pi^*)$ state, whi
is the one principally populated on light absorption. This being the case the pathw
to the $^3(\pi, \pi^*)$ state would logically involve a radiationless transition first to t
$^1(n, \pi^*)$ and from this state to the $^3(\pi, \pi^*)$ (ABRAHAMSON, ADAMS, and WULF

1959; DAWSON and ABRAHAMSON, 1962). The alternate path of isomerization by torsion about the C 11—C 12 bond while remaining in the $^1(\pi, \pi^*)$ state, appears to offer a higher energy barrier than the pathway through the $^1(n, \pi^*)$ and $^3(\pi, \pi^*)$ states.

In the case of the retinylidene-iminium ion prototype of the rhodopsin molecule no such $^1(n, \pi^*)$ state lies close in energy to the $^1(\pi, \pi^*)$ as a convenient pathway into the triplet, and the molecule would appear to have no other choice than to surmount the torsional barrier in the $^1(\pi, \pi^*)$ state (Fig. 13) in order to undergo isomerization. The torsional barriers shown in Fig. 13 have only a qualitative significance in view of the nature of the calculation (WIESENFELD and ABRA-HAMSON, 1968) and are probably lower than indicated. Furthermore one must bear in mind that electronic excitation will predominately populate the stretching vibrational modes of the polyene system, and that the normal mode torsional vibrational modes will, in some degree, involve torsion about all bonds in the carbon skeleton. For these reasons it is difficult to predict just what the size of the energy barrier to isomerization would be even if an accurate energy barrier for the C 11—C 12 torsion were known for the retinylidene group.

The situation is even more obscure for the polyene system of visual pigments in the lipoprotein matrix of their native microenvironment, for in this case the micro-environment will probably be the principal factor governing the form of the torsional potential curves (ABRAHAMSON and OSTROY, 1967). This is borne out by the much higher quantum yield for visual pigment photolysis (vide supra) as compared to *cis* retinal, as well as its independence of wavelength throughout the principal absorption band.

B. Intermediates in the Bleaching of Vertebrate Rhodopsin

In the bleaching of vertebrate rhodopsin, as typified by bovine micellar rhodop-sin, there are six intermediates. These have been characterized by their properties (MATTHEWS, HUBBARD, BROWN and WALD, 1963; OSTROY, ERHARDT and ABRAHAM-SON, 1966). They are shown in the scheme of Fig. 14. The first product, originally identified by YOSHIZAWA and KITÔ (1958) has been named prelumirhodopsin[1] by YOSHIZAWA and WALD (1963). Its λ_{max} lies at 543 nm, a considerable bathochromic shift relative to rhodopsin, and it is stable in aqueous glycerol below $-140°$ C. At higher temperatures it rapidly reverts to another intermediate, lumirhodopsin, first seen by BRODA and GOODEVE (1941). Lumirhodopsin is stable at $-50°$ C in aqueous glycerol and has λ_{max} at 497 nm, a 5 nm hypsochromic shift relative to rhodopsin at that temperature ($\lambda_{max} = 502$ nm). The extinction coefficient of lumirhodopsin is almost 10 % greater than rhodopsin, which is taken to indicate that the retinylidene chromophoric group is in the *trans* configuration (HUBBARD and KROPF, 1958).

ABRAHAMSON and OSTROY (1967) in agreement with YOSHIZAWA and WALD (1963) suggest that prelumirhodopsin is trapped in a form torsionally distorted about the C 11—C 12 bond, and held in this position by the low temperature

---

[1] Now called bathorhodopsin to distinguish it from hypsorhodopsin; see YOSHIZAWA, Chapter 5, p. 148.

microenvironment of the lipoprotein matrix. The thermal conversion of prelumi t
lumirhodopsin, in this view, merely completes the isomerization process.

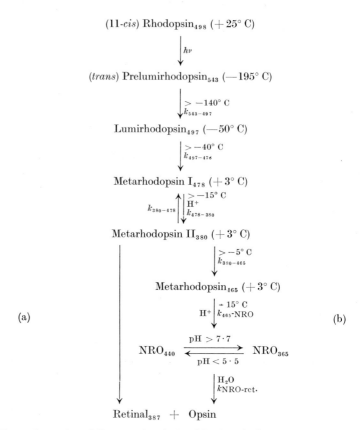

Fig. 14. Thermal reactions following photolysis of bovine rhodopsin. (a) Route according †
Matthews, Hubbard, Brown, and Wald (1963) (Metarhodopsin$_{465}$ is also known as Par
rhodopsin. NRO denotes N-retinylidene opsin). (b) Route according to Ostroy, Erhardt, an
Abrahamson (1966). (Figures in brackets are the temperatures at which the λ_{max} we
measured)

At temperatures above $-40°$ C lumirhodopsin is thermally converted to a
intermediate with λ_{max} at 478 nm, first seen by Broda and Goodeve (1941) an
more recently named metarhodopsin I by Matthews, Hubbard, Brown, an
Wald (1963). Ostroy, Erhardt, and Abrahamson (1966) prefer to add a subscri
to designate the λ_{max}, calling it metarhodopsin$_{478}$ or metarhodopsin$_{478}$I. Th
process was originally postulated to involve the exposure of two sulfhydryl grou
and the consumption of a hydrogen ion (Wald, Brown, and Gibbons, 1963) b
these events were subsequently shown by Erhardt, Ostroy, and Abrahamso
(1966) to occur at a later stage in the photolysis cycle, which is in keeping with th
fact that the sequence of thermal processes terminating in metarhodopsin$_{478}$I occ
in dried ROS or rhodopsin micelles (Kimbel, Poincelot, and Abrahamson, 1970

At temperatures above approximately $-5°$ C, metarhodopsin$_{478}$I is thermally converted to metarhodopsin$_{380}$II by a process requiring H_2O and H_3O^+, and at these temperatures a pseudo equilibrium can be observed between the two (MATTHEWS, HUBBARD, BROWN, and WALD, 1963; OSTROY, ERHARDT, and ABRAHAMSON, 1966). The equilibrium constant is best characterized by the following equation:

$$K_{I \to II} = \frac{[\text{Metarhodopsin}_{380}\text{II}]}{[\text{Metarhodopsin}_{478}\text{ I}]\,[H_3O^+]^{1/2}} .$$

Both groups of workers are in general agreement as to the thermodynamic parameters; $\Delta H = 10$ kcal/mole and $\Delta S = 34$ cal/degree mole.

Beyond the metarhodopsin$_{380}$II stage, however, there is a disagreement between the groups as to the intermediates in the main sequence. MATTHEWS, HUBBARD, BROWN, and WALD postulate a direct thermal conversion of metarhodopsin$_{380}$II to retinal and the protein opsin, while OSTROY, ERHARDT, and ABRAHAMSON expand the sequence as shown in Fig. 14 to include metarhodopsin$_{465}$ and N-retinylidene opsin (NRO$_{365}$), which is an acid-base indicator. This latter intermediate, originally identified by LYTHGOE and QUILLIAM (1938) and characterized by COLLINS (1953) as the *trans*-retinylidene group bound to an amino group on the protein opsin, was also included in the sequence scheme of MORTON and PITT (1957). In the view of MATTHEWS, HUBBARD, BROWN, and WALD (1963), however, metarhodopsin$_{465}$ — as implied by WALD's name for it, *pararhodopsin* (WALD, 1968) — lies outside the main stream of events. Similarly they regard NRO$_{365}$ as a product formed from liberated retinal and random amino sites on the protein opsin.

Evidence provided by HAGINS (1957) on the flash photolysis of excised albino rabbit eyes as well as by EBREY (1967) on rat retinae, suggest that in the physiological process parallel paths succeed metarhodopsin II, i.e., approximate both schemes shown in Fig. 14. In the frog retina DONNER and REUTER (1969) postulate two forms of metarhodopsin$_{380}$II; one leading to retinal + opsin, and another that is in equilibrium with metarhodopsin$_{478}$I. They regard metarhodopsin$_{465}$, which absorbs maximally at 470—480 nm in the frog retina, as regenerated metarhodopsin$_{478}$I.

WILLIAMS (1970) interprets his flash photolysis studies on bovine micellar rhodopsin as indicating more than one form of metarhodopsin$_{478}$I. The evidence that he cites, however, is based on spectra taken after a rather long (2 msec) flash which, in his terminology, produces photoequilibrium between rhodopsin and metarhodopsin$_{478}$I. At high temperatures this photoequilibrium appears to favor metarhodopsin$_{478}$I, which he rationalizes in terms of two forms of metarhodopsin$_{478}$I, one that readily regenerates rhodopsin and one that does not.

The sequences shown in Fig. 14 are apparently dependent on the pretreatment of micellar rhodopsin. Thus when aqueous digitonin micelles of bovine rhodopsin are treated with the sulfhydryl reagent Aq(tris)$_2^+$, as many as four sulfhydryl groups are complexed in the dark with no accompanying change in the 500-nm absorbance peak. On illumination, however, metarhodopsin$_{380}$II is the first detectable intermediate. The subsequent decay to metarhodopsin$_{465}$ appears to proceed normally and an additional 1—2 sulfhydryl groups are titratable at this stage (OSTROY, RUDNEY, and ABRAHAMSON, 1966). Incubation with weaker sulfhydryl reagents such as Ellman's (5,5'dithiobis-(2-nitrobenzoic acid)) complexes only one sulfhydryl group[2] immediately, in agreement with Heller's (1968a) later finding and 1—2 additional groups are further exposed on illumination. Prolonged in cubation in the dark, however, exposes 4—5[2] sulfhydryl groups (Ostroy, Rudney and Abrahamson, 1966).

Incubation of micellar rhodopsin in 8-molar urea, or with the sulfhydryl reagent parachloromecuribenzoate (PCMB) in a 1:20 mole ratio, near room temperature for two hours followed by illumination, produced metarhodopsin$_{465}$ as the first observable product (Ostroy, Erhardt, and Abrahamson, 1966). These observations indicate that blocking of sulfhydryl groups before illumination markedly affects the intermediate sequence, particularly the metarhodopsin$_{478}$ → metarhodopsin$_{380}$II process, which appears to be a key one in the initiation of neural impulse.

C. Apparent Changes in the Binding Site of the Chromophoric Group during Bleaching

The observations made by Bownds (1967) and Akhtar, Blosse, and Dewhurst (1967) that the NaBH$_4$-reduction of illuminated rhodopsin caused a substantial fraction of the retinylidene chromophoric group to be reductively affixed to a lysine residue of the protein, suggested that the retinylidene group had undergone transimination early in the bleaching sequence. In order to test this hypothesis we carried out the following experiments (Poincelot, Millar, Kimbel, and Abrahamson, 1969; Kimbel, Poincelot, and Abrahamson, 1970).

Bovine ROS and cetyltrimethylammonium bromide (CTAB) micelles of bovine rhodopsin were separately lyophilized and then illuminated to produce meta rhodopsin$_{478}$I (Fig. 15), which is the terminal product of bleaching in the dry state. Each of these preparations was then divided into two portions. One portion of each was extracted with absolute methanol, or absolute methanol 10$^{-3.5}$ M in HCl gas, as was done for the dried native pigments (Poincelot, Millar, Kimbel, and Abrahamson, 1969; Poincelot and Abrahamson, 1970a). The spectrum of the extract was identical to that of the protonated form of N-retinylidene phosphatidyl ethanolanine (NRPE) obtained previously, and in each case more than 90 % of the chromophoric group originally present in the sample was extracted as N—RPE. Reduction of each extract with NaBH$_4$ produced a material with spectrum identical to N-retinyl-phosphatidyl ethanolamine (N-RH$_2$PE) (Fig. 8). Analysis of each of the extracted and reduced materials by means of thin layer and gas chromato graphy as employed for the native material (Poincelot and Abrahamson, 1970a) confirmed the identification of the extracted material as N-RPE and of the reduced material as N-RH$_2$PE.

The second portions of the dried metarhodopsin$_{478}$I from ROS and CTAB micelles of bovine rhodopsin were converted to metarhodopsin$_{380}$II by wetting each material with a small amount of buffered (pH 4.5) water at 4° C. Each slurry was promptly re-dried after the yellow color of metarhodopsin$_{380}$II developed. The

---

[2] In Ostroy, Rudney and Abrahamson (1966) this result was reported as twice the value given here following Ellman (1959). However, Wasserman and Major (1969) show Ellman's value to be too large by a factor of 2.

difference spectrum relative to metarhodopsin$_{478}$I confirmed the identification of metarhodopsin$_{380}$II (Fig. 16) in each case.

When lyophilized metarhodopsin$_{380}$II derived both from ROS and from CTAB micelles was extracted with methanol only a small amount of N-RPE, less than 10 % of the total chromophoric group present in the powder, was obtained. On the

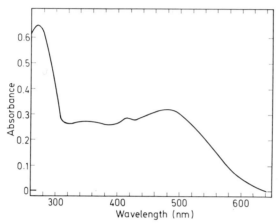

Fig. 15. Powder spectrum of lyophilized metarhodopsin$_{478}$I from ROS. (KIMBEL, POINCELOT and ABRAHAMSON, 1970)

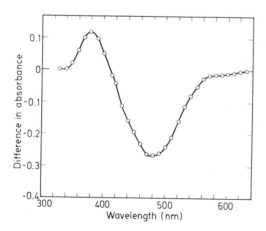

Fig. 16. Difference spectrum between metarhodopsin$_{478}$I and metarhodopsin$_{380}$II from ROS. (KIMBEL, POINCELOT and ABRAHAMSON, 1970)

other hand reduction of the metarhodopsin$_{380}$II powder with NaBH$_4$ in aqueous slurry buffered at pH 4.5 followed by extraction with aqueous CTAB yielded a material containing 82 % of the chromophoric group and spectrally identical to N-retinylopsin (Fig. 17). After alkaline hydrolysis the material was chromatograph-ed and the chromophoric group material identified as N-retinyl lysine by thin layer chromatography in two solvent systems.

The above results clearly suggest that the retinylidene group is transferred from the lipid PE to a lysyl group on the protein during the change from metarhodopsin$_{478}$I to metarhodopsin$_{380}$II. The small amount of N-RPE found in the metarhodopsin$_{380}$II powder can easily be accounted for as from rhodopsin, isorhodopsin and small quantities of metarhodopsin$_{478}$I in equilibrium with metarhodopsin$_{380}$II.

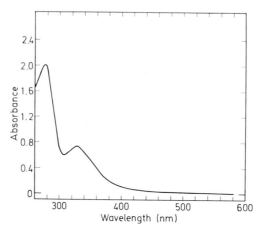

Fig. 17. N-retinylopsin as produced by NaBH$_4$ reduction (pH 4.5) of metarhodopsin$_{380}$II. (KIMBEL, POINCELOT and ABRAHAMSON, 1970)

One might assume, however, that the retinylidene group in metarhodopsin$_{478}$I is attached to the same protein (lysine) binding site as found in metarhodopsin$_{380}$II. But this raises the perplexing question of why it artifactually transiminates to PE in substantial measure at one intermediate stage but not the other when the same amount of PE is present.

The binding site of the chromophoric group at later stages in the bleaching sequence have not as yet been studied. Of particular interest in this respect is metarhodopsin$_{465}$. There is some suggestion that in this intermediate the group may again be bound to a lipid. This is based largely on DONNER and REUTER's (1969) identification of this material with regenerated metarhodopsin$_{478}$I, and the fact that incubation of rhodopsin with FCMB or urea, prior to illumination, yields metarhodopsin$_{465}$ as the first identifiable intermediate. The aforementioned dependence of this intermediate on the regeneration of rhodopsin suggests that it may in some way be involved in isomerase activity.

D. Kinetics of the Intermediate Processes

The kinetics of the intermediate processes have received rather limited attention because either rapid-reaction or low-temperature techniques are required for the study of the more important ones. Most studies of this kind have relied on measurements in the visible region of the spectrum. Although this is a very sensitive technique, in view of the rather large extinction coefficients of visual pigment intermediates in this region, it has disadvantages. In the first place, the spectral changes reflect changes only in the immediate environment of the chromophoric group, and equally significant changes occuring in the macromolecular milieu of the pigment may not be detected at all, or only indirectly. Moreover, a number of chemical species may contribute to the absorption at the wavelength at which the kinetic measurements are made, thus making analysis somewhat ambiguous. On the other hand changes in the conductivity of aqueous suspensions of visual pigments, changes that presumably reflect hydrogen-ion uptake or release by the pigment at some point other than the chromophoric binding site, do correlate with the kinetics of the spectral changes (FALK and FATT, 1966).

The intermediates already discussed have been characterized by their visible spectra, and the kinetics discussed in this section are based on spectral changes in this region. The first of such measurements made on micellar rhodopsin dealt with the metarhodopsin$_{478}$I $\rightarrow$ metarhodopsin$_{380}$II reaction (LINSCHITZ, WULFF, ADAMS, and ABRAHAMSON, 1957; WULFF, ADAMS, LINSCHITZ, and ABRAHAMSON, 1958). Rather complex kinetics, typical of many biological processes, were found initially for this process, and the simplest scheme of analysis of the kinetics seemed to be in terms of simultaneous first order processes. Since the other intermediate processes appeared to be similar in character, this same treatment was also applied to them by ourselves and others (ABRAHAMSON, MARQUISEE, GAVUZZI, and ROUBIE, 1960; GRELLMAN, LIVINGSTON, and PRATT, 1962; PRATT, LIVINGSTON, and GRELLMAN, 1964; ERHARDT, OSTROY, and ABRAHAMSON, 1966; OSTROY, ERHARDT, and ABRAHAMSON, 1966). In the more recent kinetic studies in our laboratory other treatments have been used and these, in some cases, yield more plausible molecular mechanisms than the earlier schemes (RAPP, WIESENFELD, and ABRAHAMSON, 1969, 1970).

The kinetics of the various thermal processes are discussed below in order of their appearance in the sequence of Fig. 14. It has been our practice to characterize these processes in terms of the parameters of Absolute Reaction Rate Theory, i.e., the free energy of activation, $\Delta F^{\pm}$; the enthalpy of activation, $\Delta H^{\pm}$; and the entropy of activation, $\Delta S^{\pm}$ (ABRAHAMSON, MARQUISEE, GAVUZZI, and ROUBIE, 1960; ERHARDT, OSTROY, and ABRAHAMSON, 1966; OSTROY, ERHARDT, and ABRAHAMSON, 1966). Although the theoretical significance of these parameters in such complex macromolecular processes as occur in the decompositon of visual pigments may be obscure, the fact that in many similar processes, such as the denaturation of enzymes, the parameters $\Delta H^{\pm}$ and $\Delta S^{\pm}$ are sensible fractions of their thermodynamic counterparts (BRAY and WHITE, 1957) justifies their use as an empirical measure of the configurational changes occurring.

1. Conversion of Prelumirhodopsin$_{543}$ to Lumirhodopsin$_{497}$

This thermal process has been studied both in aqueous glycerol extracts of bovine rhodopsin and in bovine ROS by LIVINGSTON and coworkers using a flash photolysis technique adapted to low temperatures (GRELLMAN, LIVINGSTON, and PRATT, 1962; PRATT, LIVINGSTON, and GRELLMAN, 1964). They chose to treat their kinetic data in the same manner as WULFF, ADAMS, LINSCHITZ, and ABRAHAMSON (1958) for the metarhodopsin$_{478}$I $\rightarrow$ metarhodopsin$_{380}$II process, i.e., by resolving it into three simultaneous first-order processes (Table 7). On this model, all three processes had much the same enthalpy of activation both for micellar rhodopsin and for the ROS, although the latter had somewhat higher entropies of activation which are reflected in their greater rate constants.

As pointed out previously this process probably represents an environmental relaxation about the chromophoric polyene, thus removing the torsional strain in the C11—C12 bond. One might invoke in the extracts three different forms of prelumirhodopsin to relate to the three simultaneous first-order processes, but it is difficult to do so in rod segments. One could, perhaps, suppose that there is some local inhibitory effect in the ROS but this again is difficult to visualize in molecular terms. Second-order processes might also be considered but these seem unlikely at the low temperatures used in the study. Whatever the molecular mechanism of this thermal process it is rather unlikely that its $\Delta H^{\pm}$ or $\Delta S^{\pm}$ will differ substantially from the values reported in Table 7.

Table 7. *Thermal decay of prelumirhodopsin$_{543}$* (Abrahamson *and* Ostroy, *1967*)

(i) Grellman, Livingston, and Pratt (1962)

Rhodopsin solutions	Rate constants (sec^{-1}) (—50° C)	(—67° C)	$t_{1/2}$ (38° C)[a] (sec)	$\Delta H^{\pm}$ kcal/mole	log A	$\Delta S^{\pm b}$ (e.u.)
k_1	3960	1270	1.5×10^{-7}	10 ± 2	13.7	5
k_2	715	219	8.6×10^{-7}	10 ± 2	12.9	0.9
k_3	251	53	3.8×10^{-5}	10 ± 2	12.2	—2

(ii) Pratt, Livingston, and Grellman (1964)

Rod particles	—50° C	—65° C				
k_1		2580	1.3×10^{-8}	12.5 ± 3	16.5	18
k_2	5180	417	7.8×10^{-8}	12.5 ± 3	15.7	14
k_3	1026	118	2.8×10^{-7}	12.5 ± 3	15.2	12

[a] Calculated from Arrhenius equation.
[b] Log A was reported. $\Delta S^{\pm}$ calculated for $T = $ —60° C.

2. Conversion of Lumirhodopsin$_{497}$ to Metarhodopsin$_{478}$I

Kinetic studies of this process in digitonin micelles have been rather difficult to carry out as the spectra of the two intermediates are very much alike. The early measurements made in our laboratory (Erhardt, 1963; Erhardt, Ostroy, and Abrahamson, 1966) are rather imprecise, for they relied on the "0 to 1.0" absorbance scale of the Cary recording spectrophotometer. But even the more recent measurements with a higher precision slide wire ("0 to 0.1") and temperature control, still did not yield very reproducible data. Furthermore, the treatment of the kinetic data in terms of two or more simultaneous first order processes (see Erhardt, Ostroy, and Abrahamson, 1966, for the method) was not very successful particularly in the early stages of the reaction.

The most recent data of Rapp (1970) are compared in Table 8 with the earlier data from the same laboratory (Erhardt, Ostroy, and Abrahamson, 1966) and with data obtained in the Harvard laboratory of GEORGE WALD (HUBBARD, BOWNDS, and YOSHIZAWA, 1965). The rate constants obtained on the two occasions in our laboratory do not differ radically from one another, considering the usual poor reproducibility of such measurements, though the derived kinetic parameters show substantial differences in the two slower processes. On the other hand, the rate constants from the Harvard laboratory based on a single first order process are smaller by almost two orders of magnitude and the derived kinetic parameters are radically different from those obtained in our laboratory. These results reflect the complexity of this process in detergent micelles and suggest that the multiform first order analysis, which places principle emphasis on the terminal stages of the reaction, may not be a proper treatment of the kinetic data for this process.

Table 8. *The thermal decay of lumirhodopsin$_{497}$ treated as simultaneous first order processes*

	Process	Temp. °C	k sec^{-1}	$\Delta F^{\ddagger}$ kcal/mole	$\Delta H^{\ddagger}$ kcal/mole	$\Delta S^{\ddagger}$ cal/ degree mole
RAPP (1970) 66% glycerol in aqueous digitonin (pH = 7)	k_2	—13.8	0.0635	16.5	17.6	4.0
	k_3		0.0046	17.9	18.4	1.9
	k_2	—20.0	0.0224	16.6		
	k_3		0.0020	17.9		
	k_2	—30.7	0.0061	16.6		
	k_3		0.0038	17.9		
ERHARDT, OSTROY, and ABRAHAMSON (1966). 50% glycerol in aqueous digitonin (pH = 7)	k_1	—21.4	0.03	16.9	16.3	—2.3
	k_2		0.0097	17.0	3.60	—53.0
	k_3		0.0015	17.9	5.29	—52.0
MATTHEWS and WALD as quoted by HUBBARD, BOWNDS, and YOSHIZAWA (1965). Treated as simple first-order process	k	—20.0	0.00045	19.0	60	+160

A picture more in keeping with our recent binding-site studies is obtained if the data are analyzed as a bimolecular reaction of the form of Eq. (1) (RAPP, WIESENFELD, and ABRAHAMSON, 1970)

$$L + E \rightarrow \text{metarhodopsin}_{478} I , \qquad (1)$$

where L represents the chromolipid lumirhodopsin, and E represents some other substrate. For such a process a plot of log L/E against time should be linear, the rate constant k_{LE} being obtained from the slope, which is given by Eq. (2). L_0 and E_0 are the molar concentrations of L and E respectively.

$$\text{slope} = \frac{(L_0 - E_0) k_{LE}}{2.303} . \qquad (2)$$

L_0 and L can be obtained from the light transmittance data (knowing the amount of rhodopsin photolyzed) and E_0 is so chosen as to yield a linear plot of log L/E vs time for the entire course of the reaction. The rate constants for this process, both in detergent micelles and in sonicated suspensions of ROS, are given in Table 9 along with the derived activation parameters. In both cases linear plots were obtained for $L_0/E_0 = 1.05$. The rate constants in the ROS were about two orders of magnitude greater on a comparable basis than those for the digitonin micelles, a point reflected in the larger positive $\Delta S^{\ddagger}$ for the ROS. When the same process was studied at temperatures above $0°$ C using the rapid measuring flash photolytic unit described in Chapter 1 entirely different kinetic parameters were obtained (Table 9). In contrast to the high $\Delta H^{\ddagger}$ and $\Delta S^{\ddagger}$ of the low-temperature process, indicative of the substantial configuration changes in the bimolecular formation of metarhodopsin$_{478}$I, the process at physiological temperatures appears to involve little if any such changes. Furthermore a tenfold smaller value of L_0/E_0 was necessary to obtain linearity of log L/E vs time.

Table 9. *The thermal decay of lumirhodopsin treated as a second order process according to Eq. (1) (p. 107)*

	Temp. ° C	$k \times 10^{-3}$ liters/mole sec	$\Delta F^{\ddagger}$ kcal/mole	$\Delta H^{\ddagger}$ kcal/mole	$\Delta S^{\ddagger}$ cal/ degree mole
66% glycerol-aqueous digi-	—13.8	13.5	10.2	25.1	57.3
tonin, pH = 7,	—20.0	3.74	10.6		
$L_0/E_0 = 1.05$	—31.0	0.486	11.1		
ROS in 66% glycerol-aqu-	—42.0	10.9	9.55	25.3	70.3
eous buffer, pH = 7,	—46.2	3.49	9.56		
$L_0/E_0 = 1.05$	—50.0	2.23	9.53		
ROS in 66% glycerol-aqu-	3.0	51.5	5.12	3.51	—5.8
eous buffer, pH = 7,	9.9	63.0	5.15		
$L_0/E_0 = 0.10$	27.1	94.5	5.25		
	35.9	115.0	5.31		

The simple second order process of Eq. (1) when applied to the decay of lumi-rhodopsin$_{497}$ in ROS sac membranes suggests that photoisomerization renders the chromolipid lumirhodopsin mobile in the membrane surface. Thus it could undergo collisions with protein molecules in the surface, each protein molecule apparently having 10 equally available and independent lysyl amino-group sites for reaction at physiological temperatures. At lower temperatures, near $-40°$ C, the configuration of the protein could be such that only one amino group site is available for reaction. Applied to the micellar process, the second-order picture is somewhat more awkward to interpret in that the chromolipid in the monodispersed pigment micelles must either migrate from micelle to micelle in the course of reaction or suffer collision with another micelle in order that the proper conformation of chromolipid with its protein in the micelle characteristic of metarhodopsin$_{478}$I is achieved. A crude estimate (Rapp, Wiesenfeld, and Abrahamson, 1970) suggests that between 500 and 1000 micelle collisions can occur for each molecule that reacts in the aqueous-glycerol medium, even at low temperatures.

The reaction mechanism derived from the second order treatment of Eq. (1) is probably oversimplified, but it nevertheless provides a working hypothesis for the decay of lumirhodopsin$_{497}$ that is more in harmony with our recent binding-site studies than is the earlier postulated mechanism of several simultaneous first-order processes.

3. Conversion of Metarhodopsin$_{478}$I to Metarhodopsin$_{380}$II

The decay of metarhodopsin$_{478}$I was the first intermediate process whose kinetics were studied in aqueous digitonin. Treatment of the rate data as simultaneous first order processes led naturally to the postulate of several different forms of metarhodopsin$_{478}$I (WULFF, ADAMS, LINSCHITZ, and ABRAHAMSON, 1958). On the basis of the large enthalpies and entropies of activation associated with the decay of these multiforms of metarhodopsin$_{478}$I, these processes were further postulated to involve very substantial configuration changes in the lipoprotein similar to those observed in reversible protein denaturation (ABRAHAMSON, MARQUISEE, GAVUZZI, and ROUBIE, 1960). Kinetic data for several studies of this process are given in Table 10.

In distinction to the kinetic data for the decay of lumirhodopsin there is reasonable agreement in the rate constants and kinetic parameters for the data obtained

Table 10. *Kinetic data for the conversion of micellar bovine metarhodopsin$_{478}$I to metarhodopsin$_{380}$II treated as simultaneous first order processes*

(i) WULFF, ADAMS, LINSCHITZ, and ABRAHAMSON (1958)		Rate constants (sec^{-1})			$\Delta F^{\ddagger}$ kcal/ mole	$\Delta H^{\ddagger}$ kcal/ mole	$\Delta S^{\ddagger}$ cal/degree mole
		28° C		36.7° C			
Aqueous digitonin	k_1	3300		22,000	12.5	36.2	78
pH = 7	k_2	120		2,700	14.5	50.2	119
	k_3	21.0		200	15.8	43.0	90
(ii) ABRAHAMSON, MARQUISEE, GAVUZZI, and ROUBIE (1960)		6.7° C	10.2° C	15.8° C			
Aqueous digitonin	k_1	577					
pH = 7	k_2	45.5	87.5	303.0	15.0	37.1	76.5
	k_3	0.88	1.59	9.9	15.6	43.1	95.2
(iii) OSTROY, ERHARDT, and ABRAHAMSON (1966)		—13.7° C		—9.2° C			
33% glycerol-aqueous digitonin. pH = 5.85	k_2	0.0051		0.0353		59.9	162
pH = 4.5	k_2	0.0121		0.0836		58.7	159
(iv) PRATT, LIVINGSTON, and GRELLMAN (1964)		5° C	15° C	25° C	37° C		
33% glycerol-aqueous	k_1		126	550			
digitonin pH = 7	k_2	0.45	10	126	12,000	43	97
	k_3	0.09	0.18	17	250	41	83
(v) Data of MATTHEWS and WALD as reported by HUBBARD, BOWNDS, and YOSHIZAWA (1965) for single first-order process		Rate constants not reported			19	60	160

at temperatures above 0° C using the flash photolysis technique (Chapter 1). At the lower temperatures, however, there is some disagreement. Whereas Ostroy Erhardt, and Abrahamson (1966) could resolve two first order processes, Wald and Matthews (Hubbard, Bownds, and Yoshizawa, 1965) obtained only a single first order process. The kinetic parameters, $\Delta H^{\pm}$ and $\Delta S^{\pm}$, however, are not too different and present essentially the same molecular picture as do the flash photolysis studies.

The quasi equilibrium between metarhodopsin$_{478}$I and metarhodopsin$_{380}$II discovered by Matthews, Hubbard, Brown, and Wald (1963) has the associated thermodynamic parameters, $\Delta H = 10$ kcal/mole and $\Delta S = 34$ cal/degree mole. These are much smaller than would be expected on the basis of the kinetic activation parameters, $\Delta H^{\pm}$ and $\Delta S^{\pm}$ (Bray and White, 1957). This may be due, however, to the fact that the measured equilibrium constant, representing a summation of the concentrations of the several forms of metarhodopsin$_{478}$I and metarhodopsin$_{380}$II, has no meaning relative to the equilibrium constants for the individual processes (Ostroy, Erhardt, and Abrahamson, 1966). The apparent dependence of the observed equilibrium on the square root of the hydrogen ion concentration would further support this notion.

The apparent incongruity between the kinetic parameters and their thermodynamic counterparts as well as the non-integral dependence of the equilibrium constant on the hydrogen ion concentration can be rationalized in terms of multiform first-order processes, or they may suggest as do the studies of Williams (1970) an even more complex kinetic scheme for the decay of micellar metarhodopsin$_{478}$I.

In contrast to the micellar process, the conversion of metarhodopsin$_{478}$I to metarhodopsin$_{380}$II in rod segment suspensions or in intact eyes appears to be much simpler. The data of Table 11 show only a single first order decay process in

Table 11. *Kinetic data for the decay of metarhodopsin I in rod particles and intact eyes treated as first order process*

	Rate constants (sec^{-1})	$\Delta F^{\pm}$ kcal/mole	$\Delta H^{\pm}$ kcal/mole	$\Delta S^{\pm}$ cal/ degree mole
(i) Pratt, Livingston, and Grellman (1964)	$k_1 = 6.0$ at 10° C 50 at 20° C	35	28	70
Bovine rod particles. Treated as two simultaneous first order processes	$k_2 = 1.3$ at 10° C 12 at 20° C	37	29	74
(ii) Rapp (1970) Sonicated bovine rod segments	19.1 at 13° C 41.4 at 18° C 310.0 at 28.1° C 1480 at 39.4° C	14—15	30.7	54.8
(iii) Hagins (1957) Excised rabbit eye	30.0 at 12° C 600 at 26° C	13.0	37.6	80.0
(iv) Ebrey (1967) Rat rhodopsin *in situ*. Measured as the decay of ERP	~ 3.5 at 6.0° C ~ 28 at 13.0° C	14.7	41 ± 8	91 ± 20

these conditions (apart from the observation by PRATT, LIVINGSTON, and GRELL-
MAN (1964) of two simultaneous first-order processes in the rods). The data of RAPP
(1970) for optically-clear sonicated rod segment suspensions, however, appear to
be the more precise and accurate. Considering the imprecision in such kinetic
measurements on intact eyes, the agreement between RAPP's single first-order rate
constants and those of HAGINS (1957) and of EBREY (1967) is quite remarkable. The
activation parameters are also in reasonable agreement, which is even more remarkable considering the different species of rhodopsin. Their magnitude quite clearly
attests to significant configurational changes occuring to lipoprotein in the process.
It will be interesting to see whether an equilibrium between metarhodopsin$_{478}$I and
metarhodopsin$_{380}$II is detectable in rod segments and if so whether the thermodynamic parameters derived from the equilibrium constant are more in harmony
with the kinetic activation parameters than in the case of micellar rhodopsin.

At the present time the several forms of metarhodopsin$_{478}$I manifest in micellar
rhodopsin have no convincing explanation. The suggestion put forward some years
ago (ABRAHAMSON, MARQUISEE, GAVUZZI, and ROUBIE, 1960) that these forms
involved different isomers of the retinylidene chromophore hardly seems tenable
vis-à-vis the results on sonicated ROS. There remains the possibility that the different micellar forms represent different degrees of partial denaturation of the
lipoprotein. On this basis it would appear that the membrane of the rod disc
provides a more stabilizing environment for the rhodopsin molecule than does the
detergent micelle.

The molecular mechanism suggested for the conversion of metarhodopsin$_{478}$I to
metarhodopsin$_{380}$II by spectral changes, kinetic studies in rod segments and intact
eyes, and also by binding site studies, is a transimination of the chromophore
from a protonated lipid Schiff base to an unprotonated protein (lysine) Schiff base,
a process that requires hydrogen ion, and results in significant protein configuration
changes besides the release of phospholipid (POINCELOT and ABRAHAMSON, 1970a).
Consideration that this process is the first in the intermediate sequence to involve
water, and occurs at physiological temperatures in times of less than a millisecond,
and, in addition, correlates temporally with the early receptor potential (EBREY,
1967) suggests that it is the key process in the generation of a neural receptor
potential in vertebrate rod cells.

4. The Thermal Decay of Metarhodopsin$_{380}$II

There are two different views regarding the normal physiological pathway for
this process. OSTROY, ERHARDT, and ABRAHAMSON (1966) maintain that meta-
rhodopsin$_{380}$II decays quantitatively to metarhodopsin$_{465}$ which in turn decays to
N-retinylidene opsin (NRO). Hydrolysis of this latter intermediate then yields retinal
and free opsin. MATTHEWS, HUBBARD, BROWN, and WALD (1963), however, claim
that metarhodopsin$_{380}$II decays directly to retinal and opsin in the main sequence,
metarhodopsin$_{465}$ (pararhodopsin in WALD's nomenclature) being a side product.
The earlier study of this process in the excised eye of an albino rabbit by HAGINS
(1957) and later studies by EBREY (1967) and by DONNER and REUTER (1969) suggest that both pathways may be followed in situ.

OSTROY, ERHARDT, and ABRAHAMSON (1966) had to work in acid media in order
to study the kinetics of the decay of metarhodopsin$_{380}$II in digitonin micelles, and

even under these conditions only the initial rate, which was assumed to be firs order, was resolvable. The activation parameters derived from the rate dat (Table 12) suggest that this conversion is in some measure a reversal of the meta rhodopsin$_{478}$I to metarhodopsin$_{380}$II process, in keeping with the notions of DON NER and REUTER (1969). It would be of interest in this regard to determine th binding site in metarhodopsin$_{465}$.

HUBBARD, BOWNDS, and YOSHIZAWA (1965) interpreted the findings of MATTH EWS, HUBBARD, BROWN, and WALD (1963) and calculated activation parameter for the decay of metarhodopsin$_{380}$II to retinal and opsin. From the reported ΔF it is apparent that the rate is much the same as given by OSTROY, ERHARDT, an ABRAHAMSON (1966) (Table 12) but $\Delta H^{\pm}$ and $\Delta S^{\pm}$ are quite different. EBRE (1967) reporting on what he considers to be the same process in the excised rat ey as monitored by the amplitude of the early receptor potential (ERP), finds para meters similar to those of HUBBARD.

Table 12. *The thermal decay of metarhodopsin$_{380}$II*

	Temp. ° C	k sec^{-1}	$\Delta F^{\pm}$ kcal/mole	$\Delta H^{\pm}$ kcal/mole	$\Delta S^{\pm}$ cal/ degree mo
(i)OSTROY, ERHARDT, and ABRA-HAMSON (1966). Conversion to meta-rhodopsin$_{465}$ in 2% aqueous digitonin, pH = 5.1	3.8 9.0 19.6	7.7×10^{-5} 1.0×10^{-4} 1.7×10^{-4}	21.4 21.7 22.2	7.47	—50.4
(ii) HUBBARD, BOWNDS, and YOSHI-ZAWA (1965) with reference to MATT-HEWS, HUBBARD, BROWN, and WALD (1963). Conversion to retinal + opsin in aqueous digitonin	No rate data given		21	19	— 7
(iii) EBREY (1967). Decay of meta-rhodopsin$_{380}$II based on ERP measurements on the excised eye of an albino rat	37.0	4.29×10^{-3}	18.8 ± 0.2	16 ± 5	$-10 \pm 1C$

5. Conversion of Metarhodopsin$_{465}$ to N-Retinylidene Opsin (NRO)

OSTROY, ERHARDT, and ABRAHAMSON (1966) have shown this process to be single first-order process in digitonin micelles. Although the rate is much slowe

Table 13. *The conversion of metarhodopsin$_{465}$ to N-retinylideneopsin*

	Temp. ° C	k sec^{-1}	$\Delta F^{\pm}$ kcal/mole	$\Delta H^{\pm}$ kcal/mole	$\Delta S^{\pm}$ cal/ degree mo
(i) OSTROY, ERHARDT, and ABRA-HAMSON (1966). In 2% aqueous digitonin solution, pH = 7	3.0 12.7	6.28×10^{-7} 6.44×10^{-6}	24.0 23.5	37.3	48.4
(ii) EBREY (1967). Based on ERP measurements on the excised eye of an albino rat	37.0	5.45×10^{-4}	27.7	$32 \begin{Bmatrix} -4 \\ +12 \end{Bmatrix}$	$30 \begin{Bmatrix} -10 \\ +40 \end{Bmatrix}$

the process resembles the conversion of metarhodopsin$_{478}$I to metarhodopsin$_{380}$II in terms of its activation parameters (Table 13). This may be indicative of a second transfer of the chromophoric group from a lipid to a protein binding site. EBREY (1967) has studied this process in the excised eye of the rat and finds rates and activation parameters comparable to those found by OSTROY, ERHARDT, and ABRAHAMSON (1966).

E. Intermediates in the Photolysis of Cephalopod Rhodopsin

In contrast to the findings of our laboratory concerning the binding sites in vertebrate bovine rhodopsin and its photolytic intermediates (POINCELOT, MILLAR, KIMBEL, and ABRAHAMSON, 1969, 1970; KIMBEL, POINCELOT, and ABRAHAMSON, 1970) our more recent studies on cephalopod (squid) rhodopsin (KIMBEL, FAGER, and ABRAHAMSON, 1970) indicate that a lysine unit on the digitonin-extractable protein is the binding site both in the native rhodopsin and also in the terminal intermediates, acid and alkaline metarhodopsin. In the regeneration phase there may be a transmigration of the *trans* and 11-*cis* retinylidene groups between metarhodopsin and retinochrome as suggested by HARA and HARA (1965, 1967) but this has yet to be established.

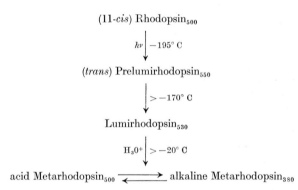

Fig. 18. Intermediate processes in the photolysis of squid rhodopsin

The course of the photolysis of squid *(Loligo pealii)* rhodopsin in 2 : 1 glycerol-aqueous extract as found by the Harvard Group (HUBBARD and ST. GEORGE, 1958; KROPF, BROWN, and HUBBARD, 1959; YOSHIZAWA and WALD, 1964) is shown in Fig. 18. Since the molar absorbances of the intermediates are about 1.5 times that of rhodopsin it seems likely that they all contain the chromophoric group in the *trans* configuration. The primary photochemical process, therefore, as in the vertebrate case appears to be the photoisomerization of the retinylidene group from the 11-*cis* to the *trans* form, although there may be some torsional displacement about the C11—C12 double bond at the prelumi stage.

Save for prelumirhodopsin the intermediates formed in the photolysis of squid rhodopsin have different λ_{max} from their nominal counterparts in the bovine system. Further differences are apparent when one compares the change from lumirhodopsin to metarhodopsin in the two cases. Whereas the reaction does not require water in the bovine system and appears to involve only minimal configuration changes, the process in squid requires water and is acid catalyzed. Furthermore, low temperature photolysis, shows this process to be of the first order, with activation parameters $\Delta H^{\neq} = 40$ kcal/mole and $\Delta S^{\neq} = 90$ e.v./mole, suggesting that it is the analog of the bovine metarhodopsin$_{478}$I to metarhodopsin$_{380}$II reaction. But this change in the squid apparently involves no lipid-to-protein transimination as does, by our evidence, the metarhodopsin$_{478}$I to metarhodopsin$_{380}$II change in the bovine case.

Another point of difference lies in the behavior of squid metarhodopsin. The conversion from acid to alkaline metarhodopsin bears no relationship to the metarhodopsin$_{478}$I → metarhodopsin$_{380}$II process in the vertebrate system but rather is analogous to the interconversion of acid and alkaline N-retinylidene opsin (NRO) in that system. But here again there is a significant difference, for NRO readily hydrolyzes to yield free retinal and opsin, while squid metarhodopsin is stable to hydrolysis under normal conditions.

V. The Emerging Picture

The most significant fact emerging from recent work on visual pigments is that they are not merely chromoproteins of unknown organization existing in the outer segments of the rod and cone cells but rather that they form an integral part of a lipoprotein membrane structure. In the vertebrate rod these membranes have the form of a flattened disc-like sac enclosing an internal aqueous space. In structure and composition these sac membranes resemble other cell membranes but their unique feature appears to be the regular mosaic-like pattern of visual pigment molecules in their external surface. In the invertebrate case the pigment-containing membrane appears to have a different structure, forming the boundaries of tubular microvilli, but no structural studies on these units comparable to the vertebrate rod outer segment have as yet been reported.

Regarding the structure and microenvironment of visual pigments, recent evidence suggesting a phospholipid binding site for the chromophoric group in vertebrate visual pigments points the need for a major revision in the general concept of their structure. Formerly, the view of a protein-binding site for the chromophoric group defined the structure problem as involving a determination of the amino acid sequence and an X-ray study of the tertiary structure of the "crystallized" pigment. Now the problem must be viewed in a larger context even if the chromophoric group in vertebrates is eventually shown to be on the protein. The fact that it appears on phosphatidylethanolamine on extraction or reductive affixation of the native visual pigment or the early intermediate metarhodopsin$_{478}$I, but on a lysine unit of the protein at the metarhodopsin$_{380}$II stage, clearly points to the phospholipid as playing a major structural role. Thus the protein structure problem remains but it must now be modified to answer the further questions of which lipids are germane to the maintenance of the native structure, and what their conformation is relative to the protein. Indeed, "opsin", which earlier was regarded as a protein, now takes on a broader meaning.

In the squid, and perhaps in all invertebrate pigments the binding site of the chromophoric group appears to be on a protein, and one very different from that of vertebrate rhodopsin. This suggests a more profound difference between vertebrate and invertebrate pigments than originally assumed. However, although the problem here would appear to be one of the secondary and tertiary structure of a protein, the presence of a substantial lipid fraction in detergent micelles of squid rhodopsin suggests that lipids here again play a key role in the maintenance of the structure of native invertebrate visual pigments.

The enigmatic problem of how nature can generate a large number of visual pigments covering a very broad range of the spectrum ($\lambda_{max} = 430-620$ nm) from only two chromophoric sources, 11-*cis* retinal and its 3-dehydro derivative, has now been given two plausible solutions. Quantum mechanical calculations suggest that spectral control over this wide range can be achieved by properly positioned charged groups in the microenvironment of the conjugated polyene chromophore, possibly coupled with controlled torsion about key bonds in the system. An alternative model involving a dispersive interaction of the chromophore with highly polarizable groups in the lipoprotein microenvironment has been given some experimental foundation. Either or both of these effects could be operative physiologically but the actual situation can only be determined after the structures and microenvironments of the pigments are known. The fact that invertebrate and vertebrate pigments exhibit the same spectral behavior suggest a common type of microenvironment for the chromophoric group. This is a point favoring a common (protein) binding site, although different binding sites could be quite readily reconciled within the framework of both the environmental charge perturbation and polarizability interaction theories.

All intermediates in the vertebrate photolytic sequence have apparently been identified, and some have been provisionally characterized as regards the binding site of the chromophoric group. There is still some question as to the proper physiological sequence in the longer-lived intermediates, and there is some indication that metarhodopsin$_{465}$ plays a role in the regeneration of rhodopsin. The weight of chemical evidence to date suggests that the chromophore is transferred from a lipid- to a protein-binding site in the early and rapid conversion of metarhodopsin$_{478}$I to metarhodopsin$_{380}$II, a process involving extensive protein configuration changes. Kinetic studies of the intermediate processes in vertebrate pigments, particularly in sonicated bovine rod outer segment suspensions, indicate that the early intermediate sequence beginning with lumirhodopsin and terminating in metarhodopsin$_{380}$II is quite consistent with a transimination of the chromophoric group.

Intermediates in the invertebrate (squid) sequence are fewer in number and bear only a superficial spectral similarity to those of vertebrates. A second photosensitive pigment (retinochrome), present in the inner segments of the retinula cells, may play the role of a photoisomerase but this has yet to be demonstrated both *in vivo* and *in vitro* (see Chapter 18).

There appear to be only two features common to vertebrate and invertebrate visual pigments: the primary photochemical process, involving photoisomerization of the 11-*cis* retinylidene chromophoric group, and an acid-catalyzed first-order process involving significant protein configuration changes. This latter thermal process is sufficiently rapid in both cases to be temporally involved in the generation of a membrane receptor potential. In the vertebrate case there is evidence supporting a direct correlation between this process and the early receptor potential of the electroretinogram, which is a precursor to the membrane receptor potential.

In summary the chief problems of current concern from a molecular viewpoint are (1) The elucidation of the structure of visual pigment molecules and their membrane milieu and (2) The establishing of the chain of events relating key processes, such as lipoprotein configuration change, to the receptor membrane potential.

Acknowledgment

We record our thanks to the National Institute of Neurological Diseases and Blindness and the Eye Institute of the National Institute of Health for supporting the work of our laboratory reported herein.

References

Abrahamson, E. W., Adams, R. G., Wulff, V. J.: Reversible spectral changes in retinene solutions following flash illumination. J. phys. Chem. **63**, 441—443 (1959).
— Marquisee, J., Gavuzzi, P., Roubie, J.: Flash photolysis of visual pigments. Z. Elektrochem. **64**, 177—180 (1960).
— Ostroy, S. E.: The photochemical and macromolecular aspects of vision. Progr. Biophys. molec. Biol. **17**, 179—215 (1967).
Adams, R. G.: Effect of light on the extraction of lipid from retinal rods. J. Lipid Res. **8**, 245—248 (1967).
— Jennings, W. H., Sharpless, N. E.: Phospholipid-retinal complex. Nature (Lond.) **226**, 270—272 (1970).
Akhtar, M., Blosse, P. T., Dewhurst, P. B.: The active site of the visual protein, rhodopsin. Chem. Commun. **13**, 631—632 (1967).
— Hertenstein, M.: The chemistry of the active site on rhodopsin. Biochem. J. **115**, 607—608 (1969).
Albrecht, G.: Acetylrhodopsin. Science **125**, 70—72 (1957).
Ayres, W. C.: Zum chemischen Verhalten des Sehpurpurs. Untersuch. Physiol. Inst. Univ. Heidelberg **2**, 444—447 (1882).
Azuma, M., Kitô, Y.: Studies on optical rotation, circular dichroism and amino acid composition of rhodopsin. Ann. Rep. Biol. Works Fac. Sci. Osaka Univ. **15**, 59—69 (1967).
Balke, D. E., Becker, R. S.: Spectroscopy and photochemistry of *all-trans* retinal and 11-*cis* retinal J. amer. chem. Soc. **89**, 5061—5062 (1967).
Bayliss, N. S., McRae, E. G.: Solvent effects in organic spectra: Dipole forces and the Franck-Condon principle. J. phys. Chem. **58**, 1002—1006 (1954).
Blasie, J. K., Worthington, C. R.: Planar liquid-like arrangement of photopigment molecules in frog retinal receptor disc membranes. J. molec. Biol. **39**, 417—439 (1969).
— — Dewey, M. M.: Molecular localisation of frog retinal receptor photopigment by electron microscopy and low angle X-ray diffraction. J. molec. Biol. **39**, 407—416 (1969).
Blatz, P. E., Pippert, D. K., Balasubramaniyan, V.: Absorption maxima of cations related to retinal and their implication to mechanisms for bathochromic shift in visual pigments. Photochem. Photobiol. **8**, 309—315 (1968).
Blaurock, A. E., Wilkins, M. H. F.: Structure of frog photoreceptor membranes. Nature (Lond.) **223**, 906—907 (1969).
Bonting, S. L.: Abstract Iscerg Symposium, September 7th—12th, Pisa, Italy (1970).
— Bangham, A. D.: On the biochemical mechanism of the visual process. Exp. Eye Res. **6**, 400—413 (1967).
Borggreven, J. M. P. M., Daeman, F. J. M., Bonting, S. L.: Biochemical aspects of the visual process VI. The lipid composition of native and hexane-extracted cattle rod outer segments. Biochim. biophys. Acta (Amst.) **202**, 374—381 (1970).

BORRELL, P., GREENWOOD, H. H.: The photochemistry of stilbene. Some S.C.F. molecular orbital calculations. Proc. roy. Soc. A **298**, 453—466 (1967).

BOWNDS, D.: Site of attachment of retinal in rhodopsin. Nature (Lond.) **216**, 1178—1181 (1967).
— Private communication (1970).
— WALD, G.: Reaction of the rhodopsin chromophore with sodium borohydride. Nature (Lond.) **205**, 254—257 (1965).

BRAY, H. G., WHITE, K.: Kinetics and thermodynamics in biochemistry. New York: Academic Press 1957.

BRIDGES, C. D. B.: Studies on the flash photolysis of visual pigments. III. Interpretation of the slow thermal reactions following flash irradiation of frog rhodopsin solutions. Vision Res. **2**, 201—214 (1962).
— Absorption properties, interconversions, and environmental adaptation of pigments from fish photoreceptors. Cold Spr. Harb. Symp., quant. Biol. **30**, 317—334 (1965).
— Biochemistry of the visual process. In: Comprehensive biochemistry. **27** (FLORKIN, M., STOTZ, E. H., eds.) Amsterdam: Elsevier 1967.

BRODA, E. E.: The role of the phospholipid in visual purple solutions. Biochem. J. **35**, 960—964 (1941).
— GOODEVE, C. F.: The behaviour of visual purple at low temperature. Proc. roy. Soc. A **179**, 151—159 (1941).
— VICTOR, E.: The cataphoretic mobility of visual purple. Biochem. J. **34**, 1501—1506 (1940).

BROWN, P. K., BROWN, P. S.: Visual pigments of octopus and cuttlefish. Nature (Lond.) **182**, 1288—1290 (1958).

COHEN, A. I.: Rods, cones and visual excitation. In: The retina. (Eds., STRAATSMA, B. R., HALL, M. O., ALLEN, R. A., CRESCITELLI, F.) Los Angeles: Univ. California Press Berkeley 1969.

COLLINS, F. D.: Rhodopsin and indicator yellow. Nature (Lond.) **171**, 469—471 (1953).
— LOVE, R. M., MORTON, R. A.: Studies in rhodopsin 4. Preparation of rhodopsin. Biochem. J. **51**, 292—298 (1952a).
— — — Studies in rhodopsin 5. Chemical analysis of retinal material. Biochem. J. **51**, 669—673 (1952b).

DAEMEN, F. J. M.: Private communication (1969).
— BONTING, S. L.: Internal protonation in retinylidene phosphatidylethanolamine and the red shift in rhodopsin. Nature (Lond.) **222**, 879—881 (1969).

DARTNALL, H. J. A.: The visual pigments. Methuen, London. New York: John Wiley 1957.
— The visual pigment of the green rods. Vision Res. **7**, 1—16 (1967).
— The photosensitivities of visual pigments in the presence of hydroxylamine. Vision Res. **8**, 339—358 (1968).
— GOODEVE, C. F., LYTHGOE, R. J.: The quantitative analysis of the photochemical bleaching of visual purple solutions in monochromatic light. Proc. roy. Soc. A **156**, 158—170 (1936).
— — — The effect of temperature on the photochemical bleaching of visual purple solutions in monochromatic light. Proc. roy. Soc. A **164**, 216—230 (1938).
— LYTHGOE, J. N.: The spectral clustering of visual pigments. Vision Res. **5**, 81—100 (1965).

DAWSON, W. R., ABRAHAMSON, E. W.: Population and decay of the lowest triplet state in polyenes with conjugated heteroatoms: Retinene. J. phys. Chem. **66**, 2542—2547 (1962).

DENTON, E. J.: On the orientation of molecules in the visual rods of *Salamandra maculosa*. J. Physiol. (Lond.) **124**, 17—24 (1954).

DONNER, K. P., REUTER, T.: The photoproducts of rhodopsin in the isolated retina of the frog. Vision Res. **9**, 815—847 (1969).

DOWLING, J. E.: The organization of vertebrate visual receptors. In: Molecular organization and biological function, (ALLEN, J. M., ed.), pp. 186—210. New York: Harper and Row 1967.

EBREY, T.: The thermal decay of the intermediates of rhodopsin *in situ*. Thesis, University of Michigan (1967).

EICHBERG, J., HESS, H. H.: The lipid composition of frog retinal rod outer segments. Experientia (Basel) **23**, 993—994 (1967).

ELLMAN, G. L.: Tissue sulfhydryl groups. Arch. Biochem. **82**, 70—77 (1959).

ERHARDT, F.: Unpublished observations (1963).

Erhardt, F., Ostroy, S. E., Abrahamson, E. W.: Protein configuration changes in the photolysis of rhodopsin. 1. The thermal decay of cattle lumirhodopsin *in vitro*. Biochim. biophys. Acta (Amst.) **112**, 256—264 (1966).

Erickson, J. O., Blatz, P. E.: N-retinylidene-1-amino-2-propanol: A Schiff base analog for rhodopsin. Vision Res. **8**, 1367—1375 (1968).

Fager, R.: Private communication (1970).

Falk, G., Fatt, P.: Rapid hydrogen uptake of rod outer segments and rhodopsin solutions on illumination. J. Physiol. (Lond.) **183**, 211—224 (1966).

Fleischer, S., McConnell, D.: Preliminary observations on the lipids of bovine retinal outer segment discs. Nature (Lond.) **212**, 1366—1367 (1966).

Fujimori, E.: Photoinduced electron transfer in dye-sulphydryl protein complex. Nature (Lond.) **201**, 1183—1185 (1964).

Fukami, I.: On the electrophoresis of cattle rhodopsin. J. Physiol. (Japan) **10**, 666—672 (1960).

Galindo, I. G.: A charge transfer process in visual pigments. Bull. math. Biophys. **29**, 677—690 (1967).

Goetz, D., Wiesenfeld, J., Abrahamson, E. W.: Unpublished observations (1967).

Goodeve, C. F., Lythgoe, R. J., Schneider, E. E.: The photosensitivity of visual purple solutions and the scotopic sensitivity of the eye in the ultra-violet. Proc. roy. Soc. B **130**, 380—395 (1942).

Gras, W. J., Worthington, C. R.: X-ray analysis of retinal photoreceptors. Proc. nat. Acad. Sci. (Wash.) **63**, 233—238 (1969).

Grellman, K. H., Livingston, R., Pratt, D. C.: A flash-photolytic investigation of rhodopsin at low temperatures. Nature (Lond.) **193**, 1258—1260 (1962).

Hagins, W. A.: Rhodopsin in the mammalian retina. Thesis, Univ. of Cambridge (1957).

Hall, M. O., Bacharach, A. D. E.: Linkage of retinal to opsin and absence of phospholipids in purified frog visual pigment$_{500}$. Nature (Lond.) **225**, 637—638 (1970).

Hara, T., Hara, R.: New photosensitive pigment found in the retina of the squid, *Ommastrephes*. Nature (Lond.) **206**, 1331—1334 (1965).

— — Rhodopsin and retinochrome in the squid retina. Nature (Lond.) **214**, 573—575 (1967).

— — Regeneration of squid retinochrome. Nature (Lond.) **219**, 450—454 (1968).

Heller, J.: Structure of visual pigments. I. Purification, molecular weight and composition of bovine visual pigment$_{500}$. Biochemistry **7**, 2906—2913 (1968a).

— Structure of visual pigments. II. Binding of retinal and conformational changes on light exposure in bovine visual pigment$_{500}$. Biochemistry **7**, 2914—2920 (1968b).

— Comparative study of a membrane protein. Characterization of bovine, rat and frog visual pigments$_{500}$. Biochemistry **8**, 675—678 (1969).

Hess, H. H., Theilheimer, C.: Extraction and partition of lipids and assay of nucleic acids. Neurochemistry **12**, 193—198 (1965).

Hubbard, R.: The molecular weight of rhodopsin and the nature of the rhodopsin-digitonin complex. J. gen. Physiol. **37**, 381—399 (1954).

— The thermal stability of rhodopsin and opsin. J. gen. Physiol. **42**, 259—280 (1959).

— Absorption spectrum of rhodopsin: 500 nm absorption band. Nature (Lond.) **221**, 432—435 (1969).

— Bownds, D., Yoshizawa, T.: The chemistry of visual photoreception. Cold Spr. Harb. Symp. quant. Biol. **30**, 301—315 (1965).

— Kropf, A.: The action of light on rhodopsin. Proc. nat. Acad. Sci. (Wash.) **44**, 130—139 (1958).

— St. George, R. C. C.: The rhodopsin system of the squid. J. gen. Physiol. **41**, 501—528 (1958).

Inuzuika, R., Becker, R.: Mechanisms of photoisomerization in the retinals and implications in rhodopsin. Nature (Lond.) **219**, 383—385 (1968).

Irving, C. S., Byers, G. W., Leermakers, R. A.: Effect of solvent polarizability on the absorption spectrum of all-trans-retinylpyrrolidiniminium perchlorate. J. amer. chem. Soc. **91**, 2141—2143 (1969).

— Leermakers, P. A.: Spectroscopic behavior of all-trans retinal and its Schiff bases in various media. The role of conformational perturbation. Photochem. Photobiol. **7**, 665—670 (1968).

Johnson, R., Williams, T. P.: Private communication (1969).

JURKOWITZ, L.: Photochemical and stereochemical properties of carotenoids at low temperatures. 1. The photochemical behaviour of retinene. Nature (Lond.) **184**, 614—617 (1959).

KIMBEL, R. L., FAGER, R., ABRAHAMSON, E. W.: Unpublished observations (1970).

— POINCELOT, R. P., ABRAHAMSON, E. W.: Chromophore transfer from lipid to protein in bovine rhodopsin. Biochemistry **9**, 1817—1820 (1970).

KITÔ, Y., SUZUKI, T., AZUMA, M., SEKOGUTI, Y.: Absorption spectrum of rhodopsin denatured with acid. Nature (Lond.) **218**, 955—956 (1968).

KRINSKY, N. I.: The lipoprotein nature of rhodopsin. Ann. med. Ass. Ophthal. (Chic.) **60**, 688—694 (1958).

KROPF, A.: Intramolecular energy transfer in rhodopsin. Vision Res. **7**, 811—818 (1967).

— HUBBARD, R.: The photoisomerization of retinal. Photochem. and Photobiol. **12**, 249—260 (1970).

— BROWN, P. K., HUBBARD, R.: Lumi- and meta-rhodopsins of squid and octopus. Nature (Lond.) **183**, 446—447 (1959).

— HUBBARD, R.: The mechanism of the bleaching of rhodopsin. Ann. N. Y. Acad. Sci. **74**, 266—280 (1958).

— — The quantum yield of retinal isomerization. Photochem. and Photobiol. In press (1970).

KÜHNE, W.: Chemische Vorgänge in der Netzhaut. In: Handbuch der Physiologie der Sinnesorgane (Ed. HERMAN, L.) Vol. 3, pt. 1, S. 235—342. Leipzig: Vogel 1879.

LANGLET, J., PULLMAN, B., BERTHOD, H.: Étude quantique de l'isomérisation *s-cis-s-trans* de l'anneau cyclohexène rapport à la chaine polyénique dans le rétinal et l'acide β-ionylidène crotonique. J. molec. Structure **6**, 139—144 (1970).

LIEBMAN, P. A.: *In situ* microspectrophotometric studies on the pigments of single retinal rods. Biophys. J. **2**, 161—178 (1962).

— ENTINE, G.: Visual pigments of frog and tadpole. Vision Res. **8**, 761—775 (1968).

LINSCHITZ, H., WULFF, V. J., ADAMS, R. G., ABRAHAMSON, E. W.: Light initiated changes of rhodopsin in solution. Arch. Biochem. **68**, 233—236 (1957).

LUCKHURST, G., ABRAHAMSON, E. W.: Unpublished observations (1965).

LYTHGOE, R. J., QUILLIAM, J. P.: The thermal decomposition of visual purple. J. Physiol. (Lond.) **93**, 24—38 (1938).

MATTHEWS, R. G., HUBBARD, R., BROWN, P. K., WALD, G.: Tautomeric forms of metarhodopsin. J. gen. Physiol. **47**, 215—240 (1963).

MIRSKY, A. E.: The visual cycle and protein denaturation. Proc. nat. Acad. Sci. (Wash.) **22**, 147—149 (1936).

MIZUNO, K., KUNO, Y., OZAWA, K.: Studies on models of rhodopsin and its degradation intermediates. Jap. J. Oph. **10** 85—93 (1966)

MOODY, M., PARRIS, J.: Discrimination of polarized light by octopus. Nature (Lond.) **186**, 839—840 (1960).

MORTON, R. A., GOODWIN, T. W.: Preparation of retinene *in vitro*. Nature (Lond.) **153**, 405—406 (1944).

— PITT, G. A. J.: Studies on rhodopsin. 9: pH and the hydrolysis of indicator yellow. Biochem. J. **59**, 128—134 (1955).

— — Visual pigments. Fortschr. Chem. org. Naturst. **14**, 244—316 (1957).

— — Aspects of visual pigment research. Advan. Enzymology **32**, 97—171 (1969).

NASH, H. A.: The stereoisomers of retinal. J. theor. Biol. **22**, 314—324 (1969).

NELSON, R., DE RIEL, J. K., KROPF, A.: 13-Desmethyl rhodopsin and 13-desmethyl isorhodopsin: Visual pigment analogues. Proc. nat. Acad. Sci. (Wash.) **66**, 531—538 (1970).

OROSHNIK, W. P.: The synthesis and configuration of neo-b vitamin A and neoretinene b. J. amer. chem. Soc. **78**, 2651—2652 (1956).

OSTROY, S. E., ERHARDT, F., ABRAHAMSON, E. W.: Protein configuration changes in the photolysis of rhodopsin. II. The sequence of intermediates in the thermal decay of cattle rhodopsin *in vitro*. Biochim. biophys. Acta (Amst.) **112**, 265—277 (1966).

— RUDNEY, H., ABRAHAMSON, E. W.: The sulphydryl groups of rhodopsin. Biochim. biophys. Acta (Amst.) **126**, 409—412 (1966).

PARISER, R., PARR, R. G.: A semi-empirical theory of the electronic spectra and electronic structure of complex unsaturated molecules. I. J. chem. Phys. **21**, 466—471 (1953).

Patel, D.: 220 MHz proton nuclear magnetic resonance spectra of retinals. Nature (Lond.) **221**, 825—828 (1969).

Pitt, G. A. J., Collins, F. D., Morton, R. A., Stok, P.: Studies on rhodopsin. 8. Retinyl-idene-methylamine, an indicator yellow analogue. Biochem. J. **59**, 122—128 (1955).

Platt, J. R.: Carotene-donor-acceptor complexes in photosynthesis. Science **129**, 372—374 (1959).

Poincelot, R. P., Abrahamson, E. W.: Phospholipid composition and extractability of bovine rod outer segments and rhodopsin micelles. Biochemistry **9**, 1820—1825 (1970a).

— — Fatty acid composition of bovine rod outer segments and rhodopsin. Biochim. biophys. Acta (Amst.) **202**, 382—385 (1970b).

— Millar, P. G., Kimbel, R. L., Abrahamson, E. W.: Lipid to protein chromophore transfer in the photolysis of visual pigments. Nature (Lond.) **221**, 256—257 (1969).

— — — — Determination of the chromophoric binding site in native bovine rhodopsin. Biochemistry **9**, 1809—1816 (1970).

— Zull, J. E.: Phospholipid composition and extractability of light and dark adapted bovine retinal rod outer segments. Vision Res. **9**, 647—651 (1969).

Pople, J. A.: The electronic spectra of aromatic molecules II. A theoretical treatment of excited states of alternant hydrocarbon molecules based on self-consistent molecular orbitals. Proc. phys. Soc. A **68**, 81—89 (1955).

Pratt, D. C., Livingston, R., Grellman, K. H.: Flash photolysis of rod particle suspensions. Photochem. Photobiol. **3**, 121—127 (1964).

Radding, C. M., Wald, G.: The action of enzymes on rhodopsin. J. gen. Physiol. **42**, 371—383 (1958).

Rapp, J.: Thesis, Case Western Reserve University (1970).

— Wiesenfeld, J. R., Abrahamson, E. W.: The rapid lipid to protein chromophore transfer in the photolysis of the visual pigment membrane. Biophys. J. A **9**, 89 (1969).

— — — The kinetics of intermediate processes in the photolysis of rhodopsin. 1. A re-examination of the decay of bovine lumirhodopsin. Biochim. biophys. Acta (Amst.) **201**, 119—130 (1970).

Ripps, H., Weale, R. A.: Flash bleaching of rhodopsin in the human retina. J. Physiol. (Lond.) **200**, 151—159 (1969).

Robeson, C. D., Blum, W. P., Dieterle, J. M., Cawley, J. D., Baxter, J. G.: Chemistry of vitamin A. XXV. Geometical isomers of vitamin A aldehyde and an isomer of its α-ionone analog. J. Amer. chem. Soc. **77**, 4120—4215 (1955).

Roelofson, B., DeGier, J., Van Deenen, L. K. M.: Binding of lipids in the red cell membrane. J. Cell. comp. Physiol. **63**, 233—243 (1964).

Schmidt, W. J.: Polarisationsoptische Analyse eines Eiweiß-Lipoid-Systems, erläutert am Außenglied der Sehzellen. Kolloid-Z. **85**, 137—148 (1938).

Schneider, E. E., Goodeve, C. F., Lythgoe, R. J.: The spectral variation of the photo-sensitivity of visual purple. Proc. roy. Soc. A **170**, 102—112 (1939).

Shichi, H., Lewis, M. S., Irreverre, F., Stone, A. L.: Biochemistry of visual pigments. 1. Purification and properties of bovine rhodopsin. J. biol. Chem. **244**, 529—536 (1969).

Shields, J. E., Dinovo, E. C., Henriksen, R. A., Kimbel, R. L., Millar, P. G.: The purification of amino acid composition of bovine rhodopsin. Biochim. biophys. Acta **147**, 238—251 (1967).

Sjöstrand, F. S.: Ultrastructure of retinal receptors of the vertebrate eye. Ergeb. Biol. **21**, 128—160 (1959).

— Electron microscopy of the retina. In: The structure of the Eye. (Smelser, G. K., ed.) pp. 1—28. New York: Academic Press 1961.

Sperling, W., Rafferty, C. N.: Relationship between absorption spectrum and molecular conformations of 11-*cis* retinal. Nature (Lond.) **224**, 591—594 (1969).

Stam, C. H., MacGillavry, C. H.: The crystal structure of the triclinic modification of vitamin-A acid. Acta Cryst. **16**, 62—68 (1963).

Suzuki, H., Takizawa, N., Kato, T.: Adiabatic potentials for *cis-trans* isomerization of retinal, I. J. Phys. Soc. Japan. In press (1970).

Thompson, A. J.: Fluorescence spectra of some retinyl polyenes. J. chem. Phys. **51**, 4106—4116 (1969).

WALD, G.: Vitamin A in the retina. Nature (Lond.) **132**, 316—317 (1933).
— Visual purple system in freshwater fishes. Nature (Lond.) **139**, 1017—1018 (1937).
— On rhodopsin in solution. J. gen. Physiol. **21**, 795—832 (1938).
— The porphyropsin visual system. J. gen. Physiol. **22**, 775—794 (1939).
— The molecular basis of visual excitation. Nobel Lecture 1967. The Nobel Foundation 1968.
— BROWN, P. K.: The role of sulfhydryl groups in the bleaching and synthesis of rhodopsin. J. gen. Physiol. **35**, 797—821 (1952).
— — The molar extinction of rhodopsin. J. gen. Physiol. **37**, 189—200 (1953).
— — GIBBONS, I. R.: The problem of visual excitation. J. Opt. Soc. Amer. **53**, 20—35 (1963).
— — SMITH, P. H.: Iodopsin. J. gen. Physiol. **38**, 623—681 (1955).
WASSERMAN, P. M., MAJOR, J. P.: The reactivity of the sulfhydryl groups of lobster muscle glyceraldehyde 3-phosphate dehydrogenase. Biochemistry 8, 1076—1082 (1969).
WILLIAMS, T. P.: Rhodopsin bleaching: Relative effectiveness of high and low intensity flashes. Vision Res. **5**, 633—638 (1965).
— An isochromic change in the bleaching of rhodopsin. Vision Res. **10**, 525—533 (1970).
— MILBY, S. E.: The thermal decomposition of some visual pigments. Vision Res. 8, 359—367 (1968).
WIESENFELD, J. R., ABRAHAMSON, E. W.: Visual pigments: their spectra and isomerizations. Photochem. and Photobiol. 8, 487—493 (1968).
— — Unpublished observations (1969).
— LEWIS, A., ABRAHAMSON, E. W.: Unpublished observations (1970).
WOLKEN, J.: Studies of photoreceptor structures. Ann. N. Y. Acad. Sci. **74**, 164—181 (1958).
WULFF, V. J., ADAMS, R. G., LINSCHITZ, H., ABRAHAMSON, E. W.: Effect of flash illumination on rhodopsin in solution. Ann. N. Y. Acad. Sci. **74**, 281—290 (1958).
YAMAMOTA, T., TASAKI, K., SUGAWARA, Y., TONOSAKI, A.: Fine structure of the octopus retina. J. Cell. Biol. **25**, 345—359 (1965).
YOSHIZAWA, T., KITÔ, Y.: Chemistry of the rhodopsin cycle. Nature (Lond.) **182**, 1604—1605 (1958).
— WALD, G.: Pre-lumirhodopsin and the bleaching of visual pigments. Nature (Lond.) **197**, 1279—1286 (1963).
— — Transformations of squid rhodopsin at low temperatures. Nature (Lond.) **201**, 340—345 (1964).
ZONANA, H. V.: Fine structure of the squid retina. Bull. Johns Hopk. Hosp. **109**, 185—205 (1961).

Chapter 4

Photosensitivity

By

H. J. A. Dartnall, Falmer, Brighton (Great Britain)

With 8 Figures

Contents

I. Introduction

In photochemical reactions, light can be regarded as one of the reactants, the other being the absorbing molecules. An important property of these reactions is the *quantum efficiency*, which is defined as the ratio of the number of molecules changed to the number of photons absorbed.

In one sense the quantum efficiency is always unity, for a photon excites the molecule that absorbs it. But the overall quantum efficiency, as measured by some permanent change, depends on the consequences of the excitation.

In some cases all the excited molecules may return to the ground state by radiationless transfers of their energies, the net result being no permanent change but only a rise in temperature of the system. For such molecules (photostable pigments) the overall efficiency is zero. Alternatively a part of the acquired energy may be re-radiated (at a longer wavelength than that of the exciting radiation) as fluorescence or phosphorescence. Again there is no permanent change to the system and the quantum efficiency is still zero, though one could measure the quantum efficiency of fluorescence (or phosphorescence) as the ratio of the number of photons emitted (of wavelength λ_2) to the number of those absorbed from the incident light (λ_1).

Sometimes the absorbing molecule, though not itself permanently affected, may pass its energy to another molecular species which, as a result, is changed. This is photosensitization, and the appropriate measure of quantum efficiency would be the ratio of the number of molecules changed to the number of photons absorbed by the unaffected species.

In yet other cases excitation may be followed by a permanent change to the molecule that absorbs the photon. This might occur either directly (e.g. because the molecule dissociates) or indirectly because during its brief life in the excited state the molecule meets another (of the same or different species) with which it can react. Such are the photosensitive molecules for which the quantum efficiency may range from values as low as 0.01 (where deactivating processes are dominant) to several thousands, where energy or molecular chain reactions are initiated.

In some photochemical experiments it is possible to arrange the concentration of the reactant to be so high that — throughout the experiment — all incident light is absorbed. In this event the total photon dose received by the system is simply the product of the average incident intensity (in photons per second) and the duration of the exposure. The number of molecules changed is ascertained by chemical analysis, and the quantum efficiency can then be calculated.

Such a course is not generally open for the study of the visual pigments. These are normally obtained as a few millilitres of extract, about 10^{-5}M in pigment, and with an optical density at the absorbance maximum that rarely exceeds unity in the thin optical cells (e.g. 0.5 cm) commonly used. Thus even at the beginning of an experiment only 90% of the incident light would be absorbed and, as the extract bleached, this percentage would become progressively less, approaching zero for a fully-bleached solution. Moreover, even if it were practicable to prepare an extract of very high density (and this can be done in some cases) and to irradiate it for a limited period so that the part-bleached extract still had a sufficiently high density at the end to absorb practically all the incident light, there would remain the problem of assessing how much of the pigment had been bleached. There are no chemical methods of assaying the visual pigments and the spectrophotometric method (except at very long wavelengths, where extinctions are low and not reliably known) is not applicable — one could hardly distinguish between, for example, an original pigment density of 5 (99.999% absorption) and a final density of 3 (99.9% absorption) even though 40% of the pigment had bleached.

These difficulties are avoided by the *method of photometric curves* (DARTNALL, GOODEVE and LYTHGOE, 1936) which, though especially devised for the visual pigments, can be applied to any photochemical system that undergoes measurable changes in transmissivity when irradiated.

In the method, which is described in some detail later on, the transmissivity of the photosensitive solution is recorded at convenient intervals during its exposure to a steady light. The data, when plotted as a certain function of the transmissivity against time, yield a straight line of slope equal to $\alpha\gamma I_i$, where α is the extinction (absorbance) coefficient of the pigment for the wavelength of the bleaching light, γ is the quantum efficiency, and I_i is the intensity of the inciden light. Since the slope and the intensity are measured the value of $\alpha\gamma$ can be ob tained.

The product $\alpha\gamma$ consists of two efficiency terms. One, α, the extinction absorbance, is a measure of the efficiency with which the bleaching light is absorbed the other, γ, the efficiency with which the absorbed light causes the change tha is measured. The method cannot separate these factors but it does allow the product to be measured with precision — in spite of the accumulation of absorbin products, and moreover, in preparations of unknown concentration. It is the of particular value for the visual pigments and has the additional general ac vantage of requiring only a knowledge of the intensity of the *incident* light — in those instances when arrangements can be made for all the incident light to l absorbed.

The method focused attention on the product $\alpha\gamma$ and in 1938 Goodeve an Wood proposed that a special name be given to it — "photosensitivity". It ha a similar role in the reaction kinetics of photochemical processes to that of tl "velocity constant" of thermal reactions. Since the quantum efficiency, γ, is ratio it is dimensionless. Hence photosensitivity has the same dimensions absorbance, i.e. $[L]^2$.

II. The Coefficient of Extinction (Absorbance)

A. Significance and Physical Dimensions

The loss of intensity that a beam of light suffers as it passes through an abso bent material can be interpreted in two ways. In the wave theory the loss is due a progressive reduction in amplitude as the energy of the wave motion is transferre to the absorbent material. On this basis every ray in the beam is attenuated, but never wholly extinguished no matter how thick the absorbent. Alternatively, i the quantum theory the light beam (as regards its interactions with matte behaves as a stream of energy "particles" called photons. Each photon, in i passage, either "collides" with an absorption centre — and suffers extinction, else it misses every such centre — and emerges unscathed.

Both theories lead to the same expected relation between incident and tran mitted intensities, and it is only in special cases that philosophical distinctior arise. To take an extreme example, the wave theory suggests that every ray sunlight that strikes the Earth is represented (though reduced to an infinitesim fraction) in a seam cf the deepest coal mine; the quantum theory, on the oth hand, suggests that in this situation there are long periods of utter darknes punctuated every 10^x years on average by the arrival of a lucky photon or tw that shot through without losing anything. On either theory, however, the energ transmitted — steadily on the wave theory, or intermittently on the quantu theory — is the same when integrated over a sufficiently long time.

The relation between the incident and transmitted light intensities, and th properties of the absorbing medium can be easily derived. In the present contex it is relevant to consider the absorptive properties of a solution (e.g. an extract visual pigment) but the following treatment is equally valid for solids and gase

Consider, then, a sample of an extract in a transparent optical cell that is bounded by plane parallel faces, and coaxial with a beam of parallel monochromatic light (Fig. 1). We require to find the relation between I_i, the light that enters the first surface AA, and I_t, the light that reaches the second surface BB. The extract, of thickness l, can be regarded as a pile of very thin identical plates dl. Then, if the intensity of light incident on one of these plates is I, a portion dI will be absorbed, the remainder being transmitted to the next plate. The fraction of

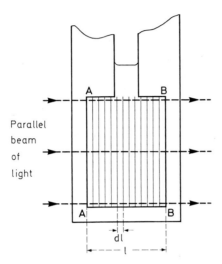

Fig. 1. Cross section of optical cell and contents as arranged for the measurement of optical densities. The solution, of thickness l, can be regarded as a pile of an infinite number of discs of thickness dl (DARTNALL, 1957)

light absorbed, dI/I, is independent of the intensity I and depends only on the plate thickness dl, the pigment concentration c, and a coefficient α_λ peculiar to the absorptive power of the pigment and the wavelength of the light. Thus we may write

$$ - dI/I = \alpha_\lambda \cdot c \cdot dl$$

(the minus sign arising because absorption is a decrement in I). By integrating this between the limits $I = I_i$ and $I = I_t$ we obtain

$$\log_e (I_i/I_t) = \alpha_\lambda \cdot c \cdot l. \tag{1}$$

The quantity $\log_e (I_i/I_t)$ is the optical density[1], and α_λ is the *extinction (absorbance)*

---

[1] The quantities I_i and I_t as defined above cannot be directly measured because of the reflexions that occur at the two cell/air interfaces and the two cell/liquid interfaces. This practical difficulty can be solved in the case of solutions by having, as a control or reference point, a second identical cell filled with solvent alone. The two cells are moved successively into the light beam and readings taken of the light intensities leaving the rear surface of the reference cell (I_r) and of the sample cell (I_s) respectively. It can be shown (taking first order reflexions into account but omitting the negligible effect of second and higher order reflexions) that the density of the solute (pigment) is given by

$$D_\rho = \log_e I_r/I_s$$

coefficient — a characteristic of the pigment and the wavelength of the light. When the concentration c is in number, n, of molecules per cubic centimetre, and the path length, l, is in centimetres, Eq. (1) becomes

$$\log_e (I_i/I_t) = \alpha_\lambda \cdot n/A$$

where A is the area exposed to light. Since the left hand side of this equation (optical density) is a numeric, the right hand side must also be dimensionless. From this it follows that α_λ has the dimensions of an area, and is expressed in square centimetres.

In the measurement of an extinction coefficient we are performing an operation that is analogous to firing bullets from random positions at right angles to a vertical plane (AA) that encloses a number of identical and impenetrable targets. We take note of the number of rounds fired (the incident intensity I_i) and of those that miss the targets and consequently hit the butts behind (the transmitted intensity I_t). From these numbers we can deduce the area of the targets (the absorption centres in molecules). Thus when all the targets lie in one plane, the ratio of $(I_i - I_t)$ to I_i, i.e. $\Delta I/I$, gives the fraction of the total shooting area that is occupied by the targets. When, on the other hand, the targets are distributed randomly in three dimensions (as are solute molecules in solution) the appropriate measure of target area is $\int dI/I$ which, as we have seen, is $\log_e (I_i/I_t)$, an expression that takes care of the screening effects of targets on each other.

In the concentration units mentioned above α_λ is the *molecular* (or, more precisely, the *chromophoric*) extinction coefficient, and is related to the effective physical area of a single absorption site (the chromophore) multiplied by the probability that a photon arriving within this area shall be absorbed. The change with wavelength of α_λ — the absorbance spectrum — can thus be construed as the variation of the probability term within its limits of zero and unity.

According to Braude (1945) the maximum area of a chromophore is likely to lie between the orders 10^{-16} and 10^{-15} cm^2, which led him to suggest that there is a theoretical limit of this order for the extinction coefficient of a chromophore, assuming the probability term is unity at the absorbance maximum. Rhodopsin has an α_{max} of 1.56×10^{-16} cm^2 per chromophore. In 1936 Dartnall, Goodeve and Lythgoe reported that a partial search of the literature on substances having continuous simple spectra in the visible or near ultra-violet had failed to reveal any with α_{max} in excess of 1.2×10^{-16} cm^2. One substance overlooked by them in this search is astacene, a carotenoid which, untypically, has a simple absorption band, and one of a shape and spectral position almost identical with that of rhodopsin. The α_{max} of astacene is 3.3×10^{-16} cm^2, which is in keeping with the fact that its conjugated chain is about twice the length of the prosthetic group of rhodopsin.

Thus the maximum values of α_{max} are consistent with Braude's hypothesis. Moreover the values cited relate to measurements in solution, in which the molecules are randomly oriented in space. It is shown below that when a molecule is oriented so that its dipole lies in the plane of the electric vector of the light, its extinction coefficient is three times as great as the average value for an unoriented molecule. Thus the appropriate value in Braude's sense for the α_{max} of rhodopsin is 4.68×10^{-16} cm^2, and for astacene is 9.9×10^{-16} cm^2. These are in good agreement with his hypothesis, and suggest that for these substances the probability term approaches unity at α_{max}.

The units in which the extinction coefficient has so far been expressed are not the usual ones. Usually the *molar absorbance*, ε_λ, is quoted, a quantity that is defined by the equation

$$\log_{10} (I_i/I_t) = \varepsilon_\lambda \cdot c \cdot l$$

where the concentration, c, is in moles (gramme-molecular weight) per litre, the path length, l, is in centimetres (as before), and the optical density is in decadic (not napierian) logarithms. In these units the value of ε_{max} for rhodopsin in solution is 4.06×10^4 litre per cm mole (WALD and BROWN, 1953). Since these units are not homogeneous, however, the figure does not give the area occupied by a mole of chromophores. This area can be obtained by adjusting the figure to the base of napierian logarithms (multiply by 2.303) and to concentration in moles/cm^3 instead of moles/litre (multiply by $c. 1000$). The result is 9.35×10^7 cm^2 per mole and this is the effective area occupied by a mole of randomly oriented rhodopsin chromophores for, on dividing it by Avogadro's Number (6.02×10^{23}) — the number in a mole — we obtain 1.56×10^{-16} cm^2, as before, for the chromophoric extinction coefficient.

B. Directional Properties (Dichroism)

The absorptive properties of the visual pigment molecule are highly directional. Only that component of the electric vector of light that is parallel to the long axis of the chromophoric group is absorbed in the principal band. If the electric vector of a particular ray of light makes an angle θ with this axis, then the effective amplitude of the vector is $\cos \theta$ and its intensity is the square of this. Thus if α' is the extinction coefficient of a molecule that is parallel to the electric vector, then the effective extinction coefficient for one that makes an angle θ with the vector is $\alpha' \cos^2 \theta$.

In an extract of visual pigment the molecules are random; in the retina they are partly organised. Thus in the photoreceptors the molecules lie within a series of planes (the lamellae) that are at right angles to the axis of the photoreceptor[2]. Within each plane, however, the molecules are randomly disposed. Consider, first, a beam of plane polarized light falling axially on the photoreceptor. The electric vectors in this beam are all parallel and at right angles to the photoreceptor axis. They consequently lie in the planes and make all angles with the molecules. If we consider a quadrant it is clear (since all angles are equally likely) that for every molecule that makes an angle θ with an electric vector there exists, on average, another molecule that makes the angle $(90° - \theta)$. Thus the effective extinction coefficient of *two* such molecules is given by

$$\alpha' (\cos^2\theta + \cos^2 (90° - \theta))$$
$$= \alpha' (\cos^2\theta + \sin^2\theta)$$
$$= \alpha'$$

Since all the molecules can be paired in this way it follows that the effective extinction coefficient for an assemblage of molecules randomly disposed in a series of planes at right angles to the direction of a light beam is $\alpha'/2$. Since ordinary light

---

[2] The dichroism so caused is not complete, however, the average orientation of the electric dipole responsible for the absorption having axial and transverse components in the ratio 1:9. (For discussion see Chapter 7, Section I B).

can be regarded as a mixture of polarized light of all angles of polarization (to each of which the above argument can be applied) it follows that the effective extinction coefficient is $\alpha'/2$ for unpolarized light also.

It can be similarly shown that in a random assemblage of molecules (e.g. as in an extract of visual pigment or a suspension of photoreceptor outer limbs) the effective extinction coefficient, whether for polarized or for unpolarized light, is $\alpha'/3$. Thus in the partially organized arrangement of molecules in photoreceptors the extinction is 50% greater than in a random assemblage (DENTON, 1959) (see also Chapter 7).

C. Variation with Wavelength

This section is intended only as a guide to the interpretation of the absorbance spectra of some conjugated polyenes. For a more rigorous treatment of some of the problems involved the reader is referred to Chapters 1 and 3.

In the structural formulae of chemistry each single-valency bond represents two electrons, more or less equally shared between the two atoms forming the bond. Similarly a double bond represents four shared electrons. When the molecule is conjugated, i.e. has a chain of alternate single and double bonds, a special situation can arise. For example, the formula for the conjugated fragment

can equally well be written

provided the terminal groups of the chain permit this rearrangement of valencies. In such cases most of the molecules can be regarded as existing in an intermediate condition that we can represent by the formula

in which the black dots are unpaired electrons.

The "π" electrons that remain (five in the present example), after allocation of a single bond linkage between adjacent atoms, are not limited to the spaces between atoms. Instead they occupy a series of molecular orbitals that embrace the whole length of the conjugated chain. By PAULI's exclusion principle each orbit can only accommodate one electron (of given spin). Consequently the more electrons there are (i.e. the longer the chain of conjugation) the more ground-state orbits have to be filled, and less energy (i.e. a photon of lower frequency) is needed to raise the "nearest" electron to an excited-state orbit.

As the length of the conjugated chain increases, therefore, the spectral location of the absorption band advances to longer wavelengths (where the quantal energy is less). Thus in the diphenylpolyenes, $C_6H_5-(CH=CH)_n-C_6H_5$, the simplest members ($n = 1$ and 2) absorb in the ultraviolet, and are colourless. When $n = 3$ the polyene is pale yellow; when $n = 5$ it is orange; when $n = 11$ it is violet, and when $n = 15$ it is green — the absorption bands being respectively centred in the violet, blue, green, and red regions of the spectrum.

The most familiar conjugated substances are the carotenoids, which exist in many varieties and are widely dispersed in nature. They contain forty carbon atoms per molecule, and can be regarded as formed from eight isoprene ($CH_2=CH$ $-C(CH_3)=CH_2$) units.

As exemplified by β-carotene (Fig. 2) the carotenoids absorb light in three spectral regions. The main band lies in the visible (centred usually between 400 and 500 nm), a subsidiary band is found in the near ultraviolet (centred at 340 nm) — the region of *cis* peaks, and another in the far ultraviolet (centred at 275 nm). The following interpretation of these spectra is based on the ideas of LEWIS and CALVIN (1939), PAULING (1939) and ZECHMEISTER (1944).

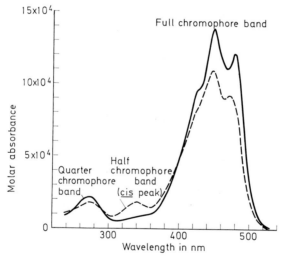

Fig. 2. Absorbance spectra of two molecular conformations of β-carotene. The continuous curve gives the spectral absorbance of *trans-β*-carotene, the dashed curve that of *cis-β*-carotene

The oscillating electric vector of light induces π-electrons to surge backwards and forwards along the conjugated chain. When the light is of a frequency to correspond with the rhythm of these movements it is strongly absorbed. This gives rise to the fundamental band in the visible. The intensity (absorbance) of the band is proportional to the square of the regularly alternating dipole moment of the molecule, and hence to the square of the length of the conjugated chain.

The *cis*-peak (at 340 nm) is attributed to induced oscillations of π-electrons from the two ends towards the middle of the conjugated chain, and back. The dipoles of these "half" oscillations are opposed. Consequently in "straight" (all-

trans) isomers absorption is negligible in this spectral region. In *cis*-isomers, however, the molecule is bent, and consequently has a resultant dipole due to these half-oscillations at right angles to the main axis of the chain. This dipole gives rise to a moderately intense absorption in the *cis*-, or "half-chromophore" band (Fig. 2).

In *cis*-isomers the intensity of absorption in the fundamental band is less than that for the all-*trans* isomer. A *cis* bond has its greatest effect in this respect when it is located in the middle of the chain, for it then reduces the chromophore length by the factor cos 30°, and hence decreases the intensity of the "full-chromophore" band to $\cos^2 30° = 0.75$ times that for the *trans* isomer (Fig. 2).

The band at 275 nm in the ultraviolet is attributed to induced concentrations of π-electrons alternately in the first and third and in the second and fourth quarters of the chain. These quarter oscillations confer an overall dipole moment on the molecule that is maximal for the all-*trans* isomer and less for any *cis* form (Fig. 2).

The maxima of these three bands in carotenoids (450 nm, 340 nm and 275 nm for β-carotene) are separated by roughly equal frequency intervals (about 7,100 wave numbers).

The spectra of the vitamins A, i.e. the retinols and 3-dehydroretinols, and of their corresponding aldehydes the retinals and 3-dehydroretinals can be similarly interpreted. Since these substances have conjugated chains only half as long as those of the carotenoids, however, their main absorption bands are in the near ultraviolet, and (when present) their *cis* peaks and "quarter oscillation" bands are displaced to the further ultraviolet (see Chapter 2).

The visual pigment molecule consists of a protein (in the "opsin" series) in combination with a single prosthetic group (Hubbard, 1954) that is based either on vitamin A_1 or on vitamin A_2. Apparently the prosthetic group is always in the 11-*cis* conformation (Wald, 1958). Because of the close association between opsin and prosthetic group the main absorption band of the visible pigment is displaced to longer waves by comparison with that for the detached prosthetic group (retinal or 3-dehydroretinal). No entirely satisfactory explanation of this bathochromic shift has been advanced (for a discussion see Chapter 3, Section III C, p. 91). Thus in the A_1 series the spectral location of maximum absorbance ("λ_{max}") ranges from 433 nm for the green-rod pigment of the frog (Dartnall, 1967) to 575 nm for the cone iodopsin of the frog (Liebman and Entine, 1968). Fewer pigments are known in the A_2 series but the λ_{max} ranges from 438 nm for the green-rod pigment of the frog tadpole to 620 nm for the cone cyanopsin of the same species (Liebman and Entine, 1968).

Within these ranges several pigments have been characterized. There is evidence from surveys of nearly 200 animal species that the λ_{max} of visual pigments are not randomly distributed but tend to occur at certain points in the spectrum, one set of positions for the A_1 pigments (Dartnall and Lythgoe, 1965a, b) and another for the A_2 pigments (Bridges, 1964, 1965).

The absorbance spectrum of a typical visual pigment, bovine rhodopsin, is shown in Fig. 3. In addition to the principal band (at 498 nm in this case) there is a secondary ("*cis*") band at about 340 nm and considerable absorption, largely due to the opsin moiety, in the ultraviolet. On bleaching there is little change in this region. Hubbard (1969) reports that the absorbance of rhodopsin at 280 nm decreases by only about 3% when it is bleached by light and, from this and other evidence considers that the prosthetic group chromophore contributes but little to the absorbance of rhodopsin in this far-ultraviolet region.

The *cis* band has λ_{max} ranging from about 340 to 380 nm in different pigments, being separated by about 1000 wave numbers from the main band λ_{max}. The fact that the photosensitivity spectrum of frog rhodopsin (Fig. 3) also possesses a *cis* peak is evidence that it belongs to the same chromophore as the main band

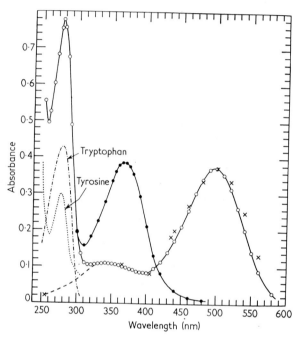

Fig. 3. Absorbance and photosensitivity spectra of typical visual pigments. The curve through the plain circles gives the absorbance spectrum of an extract of bovine rhodopsin (pigment 498_1) at pH 9.2; curve through filled circles, the same after bleaching. Note that the main band at 498 nm and the *cis* band at 340 nm are replaced by a photoproduct band at 370 nm but that the "protein band" at 278 nm is little affected by the bleaching. The protein band is due largely to tyrosine and tryptophan. The crosses are photosensitivity data from SCHNEIDER, GOODEVE and LYTHGOE (1939) and GOODEVE, LYTHGOE and SCHNEIDER (1942) for frog rhodopsin (pigment 502_1) scaled to agree with the bovine rhodopsin absorbance curve at 500 nm. (Modified from COLLINS, LOVE and MORTON, 1952)

(GOODEVE, LYTHGOE and SCHNEIDER, 1942). HELLER (1968a, b), however, has recently published a spectrum of purified bovine rhodopsin that lacks the *cis* peak and has an A_{280}/A_{500} ratio of 1.55—1.68 instead of the usual 2.2. HELLER suggested that the *cis* peak is an artifact due to photoproduct contamination. This view is difficult to accept, however, not only because of the photosensitivity data but also because frog rhodopsin shows in this region a very marked circular dichroic absorption (see Chapter 6) that disappears when the pigment is bleached (CRESCITELLI, MOMMAERTS and SHAW, 1966). Possibly the stringent purification methods used by HELLER resulted in some "surgery" to the visual pigment molecule without causing it to lose its photosensitivity and the other properties that we associate with visual pigments. In any case HELLER's important observations and methods should be extended.

III. The Bleaching Kinetics of Visual Pigments

When exposed to a continuous beam of light a visual pigment preparation "bleaches", i.e. its transmissivity of most wavelengths increases until a final value for the fully-bleached condition is reached. Some typical transmission/time curves for room-temperature bleachings of extracts are shown in Fig. 4 for various visual pigments and bleaching wavelengths.[3]

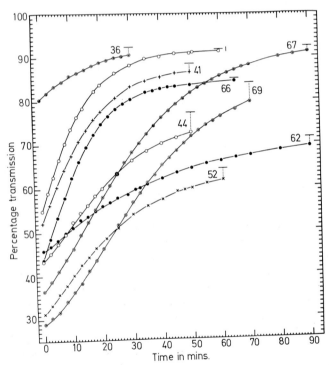

Fig. 4. Transmission/time curves for the bleaching of visual pigment extracts from various species. Plain circles are for frog extracts (502_1), diagonal crosses for a gurnard extract (492_1), centred circles for conger eel extracts (486_1), upright crosses for a carp extract (523_2) and filled circles for tench extracts (530_2). The short horizontal lines, connected by dots to the last readings, indicate the final transmissions, I_f, after prolonged exposure. Temperature $25°$ C, pH 8—9, no hydroxylamine present. Various bleaching wavelengths were used, as follows: Experiment 44; 460 nm: Experiments 52, 62 and 69; 480 nm: Experiments 36, 67; 510 nm: Experiment 1 and 66; 540 nm: Experiment 41; 560 nm. (DARTNALL, 1958)

---

[3] When bleaching is carried out by light of less than the isosbestic wavelength the preparation becomes less transmitting as it "bleaches", and $I_f - I_t$ on the left hand side of Eq. (2) must be replaced by $I_t - I_f$ (GOODEVE, LYTHGOE, and SCHNEIDER, 1942).

A. Method of Photometric Curves

It has been shown (DARTNALL, GOODEVE and LYTHGOE, 1936, 1938; DARTNALL, 1958, 1968) that the equation

$$\log_e \frac{I_t}{I_f - I_t} = \phi \cdot \alpha_\lambda \cdot \gamma \cdot I_i \cdot t + \text{constant} \tag{2}$$

describes the bleaching kinetics of all visual pigments tested, under all conditions — provided certain requirements are met.

In Eq. (2) the symbols have the following meanings.

I_i, the intensity (in number of quanta per sec. per cm^2) of a constant, uniform beam of parallel monochromatic light incident on the front surface of an extract contained in an optical cell having plane parallel faces at right angles to the light.

I_t, the intensity of light (in any convenient units) transmitted through the rear surface of the bleaching extract at the time t.

I_f, the intensity of light (in the same convenient units) finally transmitted through the fully-bleached extract.

t, the time (in seconds) from the initial exposure to light.

γ, the quantum efficiency of the photochemical change, a ratio defined as

$$\frac{\text{number of chromophores destroyed}}{\text{quanta absorbed by the chromophores}}$$

α_λ, the extinction coefficient (cm^2) of a single chromophore for the bleaching light of wavelength λ, as defined by the equation

$$\log_e \frac{I_i}{I_t} = \alpha_\lambda \cdot c \cdot l$$

where c is the chromophore concentration (number per cm^3) and l is the length (cm) of light path through the extract.

The validity of equation (2) is not affected by the presence of other light-absorbing species (e.g. impurities that may have accompanied the visual pigment into the extract) provided they are stable and do not act as catalysts or photosensitizers. This follows from the derivation of the equation (DARTNALL, GOODEVE and LYTHGOE, 1936, 1938) and has also been shown by practical tests (DARTNALL, unpublished observations) in which the presence or absence of added inert pigment has made no difference to the value obtained for the photosensitivity, $\alpha_\lambda \gamma$, of the visual pigment. The light absorbed by impurities is generally small, for modern methods of extraction yield preparations of high spectrophotometric purity. But when the bleachings are carried out with shortwave light, the absorption in the protein band (Fig. 3) of the visual pigment itself can be appreciable. However, to the extent that no energy transfer to the prosthetic group chromophore occurs, this absorption by the opsin moiety has the same effect as though a stable impurity were present, and is similarly compensated by the factor ϕ (see below).

More surprising, perhaps, is the fact that neither the setting up of a concentration gradient in the unstirred extract as bleaching proceeds, nor the formation of light-absorbing photoproduct seriously disturbs the validity of Eq. (2). For a consideration of these points the reader is referred to the literature (DARTNALL, 1936, 1957; DARTNALL, GOODEVE and LYTHGOE, 1936, 1938; GOODEVE, LYTHGOE and SCHNEIDER, 1942; SCHNEIDER, GOODEVE and LYTHGOE, 1939).

The presence of inert impurities, and the accumulation, as bleaching proceeds, of stable photoproduct result, of course, in a slower rate of visual-pigment bleaching than would otherwise be the case, for these other pigments compete for the light. But the reduction in rate from either or both these causes is precisely allowed for by the slope-compensating factor, ϕ, in Eq. (2).

The function ϕ is given by

$$\phi = \frac{I_f}{I_f - I_t} \cdot \frac{I_i - I_t}{I_i} \cdot \frac{\log I_f/I_t}{\log I_i/I_t}$$

and hence, since it contains I_t, is a variable. However the value of ϕ in any one experiment alters only very slowly as I_t changes from its initial value of I_i to its final value of I_f. In the majority of actual experiments the total change in ϕ is less than 1%, and mean values can be used without introducing significant error[4].

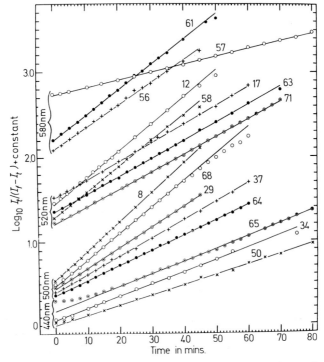

Fig. 5. Examples of the linear plots obtained in the bleaching experiments by the method of photometric curves. The visual pigment extracts were from various species (frog, gurnard, conger eel, carp and tench as symbolized in Fig. 4), and the bleachings were carried out at 25° C and pH 8—9 by monochromatic lights of various wavelengths, as indicated (Dartnall, 1958)

---

[4] In practice a correction must be made to I_i to allow for the light reflected back into the visual pigment extract from the rear surfaces of the optical cell (usually about 5%). This reflected light increases as the extract becomes more transmitting, thus acting in the opposite sense to the decrease in ϕ that occurs in these conditions. The two effects are also opposed when the extract becomes less transmitting as it bleaches, i.e. when bleached with light shorter than the isosbestic wavelength.

Since ϕ is effectively constant in any one experiment it follows from Eq. (2) that the values of the function $\log I_t/(I_f-I_t)$ should lie on a straight line when plotted against the time. This found to be so, provided certain conditions are met, and Fig. 5 illustrates the acceptably linear plots that can be obtained.

From Eq. (2) the slopes, S, of such lines are given by

$$S = \phi \cdot \alpha_\lambda \gamma \cdot I_i$$

and hence, since ϕ and the intensity I_i are known, it is possible to calculate the value of $\alpha_\lambda \gamma$, the photosensitivity of the visual pigment at λ, the bleaching wavelength.

B. Applicability of the Method

Eq. (2) was derived for the simple photochemical reaction,

$$A \xrightarrow{\;h\nu\;} B$$

in which a photosensitive substance A is converted to a photoproduct B that is both thermally and photochemically stable. The equation would also apply if the immediate photoproduct B were very unstable and decomposed by an extremely rapid thermal process to a stable product C, for in this event the amount of C present at any time would be a strict measure of the total amount of B that had been formed, and of the total amount of A that had been photolysed. The number of unstable intermediate stages before a stable end product is reached is clearly immaterial, and Eq. (2) applies to the general case

$$A \xrightarrow{\;h\nu\;} B \longrightarrow C \longrightarrow D \longrightarrow \ldots X$$

unstable intermediates   Stable
end product

provided that the amounts of the unstable intermediates are vanishingly small at all times during the bleaching. This requires that all the intermediates shall be very unstable, and also that the rate of production of B, the first of them, shall be low. This, in turn, means that the intensity of the bleaching light must be relatively low. In summary we may say that Eq. (2) will apply provided the rate-limiting factor of the total reaction is the initiating photolytic process.

The bleaching of a visual pigment is just such a complex process — initiated by light and followed by a sequence of purely thermal reactions. The complexities of this sequence are the subject of some controversy (for discussion see Chapter 3, Section IVB) but for our purpose the scheme of Ostroy, Erhardt and Abrahamson (1966) for rhodopsin, as set out in Fig. 6, will suffice.

Many satisfactory experiments by the method of photometric curves have been carried out at room temperatures and above under mildly alkaline conditions (and with bleaching light intensities of $10^{13}-10^{14}$ quanta sec^{-1}cm^{-2})[5]. In these circumstances the "final" product is the alkaline form of N-retinylidene opsin, which is only moderately stable and slowly hydrolyses to retinal (Fig. 6). Fortunately, however, the spectra of these two substances are not very dissimilar, and the "end point" is sufficiently sharp for Eq. (2) to apply, particularly at the longer

---

[5] In these orders of intensity, photoreversal (see Chapter 5, Sections V and VI) is calculated to be negligible.

wavelengths where the absorbances of N-retinylidene opsin and retinal are low
It is better, however, to carry out the bleachings in the presence of 0.02—0.06 M
hydroxylamine (DARTNALL, 1968) for then the final product is the stable retina
oxime, irrespective of pH, and there is the additional advantage that hydroxylamine, by capturing prosthetic-group retinal as oxime, shortens the lifetimes of
the intermediates (BRIDGES, 1962).

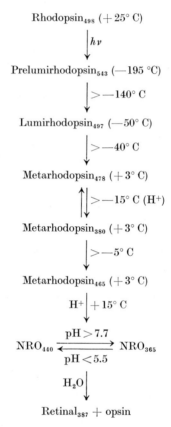

Fig. 6. Thermal reactions following photolysis of bovine rhodopsin according to OSTROY,
ERHARDT and ABRAHAMSON (1966). (Compare with Fig. 14 in Chapter 3). The subscript figures
give λ_{max} of the various intermediates at the temperatures given in brackets. The metarhodopsins 478, 380 and 465 are also called metarhodopsin I, II and III respectively, and the last is
also known as pararhodopsin. NRO denotes N-retinylidene opsin. Prelumirhodopsin is also
known as bathorhodopsin to distinguish it from hypsorhodopsin (see YOSHIZAWA, Chapter 5,
Fig. 1)

Although linear plots of log $I_t/(I_f - I_t)$ against time are generally obtained in
the absence of hydroxylamine it had been noticed in a few cases (particularly with
short-wave bleachings of the 486_1 pigment of the conger eel) that there was an
appreciable divergence from linearity in the early part of the experiment, as
though "the bleaching took some time to get under way" (DARTNALL, 1958).
A clear example of this is given by experiment 65 in Fig. 5.

In a later investigation (DARTNALL, 1968) it was found that the addition of hydroxylamine removed this anomalous behaviour, and perfect straight lines for the whole period of the experiment were obtained with all the visual pigments examined. Another effect of the presence of hydroxylamine was to increase the slopes of the straight lines, i.e. to increase the values of the photosensitivities. The magnitude of this increase was found to vary with different visual pigments (though it was always the same for any one pigment). Thus in the presence of hydroxylamine the photosensitivity of the 520_1 pigment of the freshwater fish gwyniad is raised by 4%, that of the 502_1 pigment of the common frog by 16% and that of the conger 486_1 pigment by no less than 31%.

More significant is the fact that the maximum photosensitivities of all the retinal-based pigments examined were found to be the same, within experimental error, when measured in hydroxylamine whereas without it they showed some variation (Fig. 8).

At the time it was thought probable that the effect of hydroxylamine was due to inhibition of visual pigment regeneration, but a subsequent investigation (DARTNALL, unpublished observations) showed that it was due simply to its property of drastically shortening the lifetimes of the intermediates (and thus validating the assumptions made in deriving Eq. (2)). This result was obtained in the following way. A series of bleaching experiments was carried out at 25° C on frog rhodopsin extracts without hydroxylamine but, instead of exposing the extracts continuously to the light, they were exposed for periods of two minutes only, followed by ten minutes in darkness. They were then re-exposed for another two minutes followed again by ten minutes in the dark. The experiments were continued in this way until bleaching was complete. It was found that there was appreciable loss of optical density in the dark periods. From such experiments carried out with bleaching lights of various wavelengths between 440 and 560 nm it was possible to construct the difference spectrum of the substance that was fading in the dark periods. It had λ_{max} at about 480 nm and was, presumably, principally due to the fading of metarhodopsin III (Fig. 6). It had not been anticipated that this intermediate would interfere with the applicability of Eq. (2) at a temperature as high as 25° C.

When the functions $\log I_t(I_f - I_t)$ were plotted against time for these discontinuous-exposure experiments (ignoring the ten minute dark periods) the *same* slopes were obtained as in continuous-exposure experiments carried out in the presence of hydroxylamine. This indicates that the effect of hydroxylamine is simply to hasten the decomposition of interfering intermediates, and explains the varying of this effect from pigment to pigment as due to variations in the thermal stability of the metarhodopsins. It also suggests that thermal regeneration of visual pigment from intermediates (BRIDGES, 1960) is negligible under these experimental conditions.

By bleaching extracts in discontinuous bursts, viz. by short exposures to light followed by lengthy periods in darkness to allow unstable intermediates to be cleared from the extract, the applicability of the method of photometric curves can be extended to quite low temperatures. With the technique[6] Mr E. D.

---

[6] This technique was first used by BAUMANN (1965) in his photochemical study of the rate of bleaching of the perfused frog-retina.

FOLLAND and I (unpublished observations in 1968) have obtained satisfactorily linear plots at temperatures down to $-15°$ C using extract/glycerol mixtures to prevent freezing. In some of these experiments only two 2-minute light exposures were made each day, the intervening darkness periods having to be very long (alternately 6 hours and an "overnight" 18 hours) to allow the very slow thermal changes following exposure to be completed before the next exposure was made. Such experiments took well over a week to complete, yet yielded results as precise as the fast ones at room temperature.

IV. Photosensitivities of the Visual Pigments

A. Extracts

1. In the Visible

In the first use of the method of photometric curves (DARTNALL, GOODEVE and LYTHGOE, 1936, 1938) measurements were made on frog rhodopsin at a wavelength close (506 nm) to the absorbance maximum, and the value 9.1×10^{-17} cm^2 was obtained for the photosensitivity, $\alpha_{506}\gamma$, in absolute units. This corresponds to an $\varepsilon_{max}\gamma$ of 2.39×10^4 litre per cm mole, where ε_{max} is the molar absorbance at the maximum (502 nm). This result was confirmed by SCHNEIDER, GOODEVE and

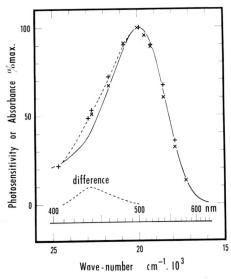

Fig. 7. Comparison between the absorbance spectrum of pure frog rhodopsin (full-line curve) and the photosensitivity spectrum as determined (in the absence of hydroxylamine) on retinal extracts. The upright crosses are SCHNEIDER, GOODEVE and LYTHGOE's (1939) data (436—560 nm) and the value at 405 nm is from GOODEVE, LYTHGOE and SCHNEIDER (1942). The diagonal crosses are derived from DARTNALL's (1958) data. Note the discrepancy (dashed portion of curve) between absorbance and photosensitivity, maximal at 430—440 nm, and separately plotted as a difference. This is probably due to the presence of green-rod pigment, $\lambda_{max} = 433$ nm, in the hydroxylamine-free extracts used for the photosensitivity measurements (DARTNALL, 1968)

LYTHGOE (1939) who in addition measured the photosensitivity to lights between 436 and 560 nm, and found that it varied with wavelength in practically the same way as did the absorbance. This indicated that γ, the quantum efficiency, is independent of wavelength. A comparison of their results with a modern absorbance spectrum for pure frog rhodopsin is made in Fig. 7. This confirms the correspondence between the wavelength variations of photosensitivity and of absorbance on the long-wave side of the maximum but there is a clear discrepancy on the short-wave side, maximal at 430—440 nm. This is due to the presence in the rhodopsin extracts of the 433_1 pigment, the pigment of the green rods. Frog extracts contain about 91% rhodopsin and 9% green-rod pigment (DARTNALL, 1967) and the unsuspected presence of the latter would lead to spuriously high values for the photosensitivity of rhodopsin at wavelengths below 500 nm. There seem no grounds, therefore, for doubting that the wavelength variation of the photosensitivity of pure rhodopsin exactly matches that of its absorbance, and hence that γ, the quantum efficiency is invariant, at least for wavelengths > 436 nm.

In 1958 DARTNALL reported the results of photosensitivity measurements at various wavelengths on some other visual pigments using frog rhodopsin for comparison. The pigments used were the 486_1 pigment of the conger eel, the 493_1 pigment of the gurnard and, in the A_2 series, the 523_2 pigment of the common carp and the 530_2 pigment of the tench. These four pigments were all found to have photosensitivities comparable to that of frog rhodopsin, the values at their respective maxima ranging from 66 to 104% of that for the frog pigment.

A more precise comparison between the photosensitivities of different visual pigments was made possible by carrying out the experiments in the presence of hydroxylamine. In this investigation (DARTNALL, 1968), already mentioned above (p. 137), the use of hydroxylamine revealed a dichotomy of photosensitivity corresponding to the A_1/A_2 dichotomy of the prosthetic group. Thus all seven A_1 (retinaldehyde-based) pigments examined had maximum photosensitivities within the range $2.63—2.85 \times 10^4$ litre per cm mole; the five A_2 (3-dehydroretinal-based) pigments values between 1.89 and 1.95×10^4 litre per cm mole, i.e. about 70% of the A_1 values (see Fig. 8 and Table 1). These results are linked to the value of 2.78×10^4 litre per cm mole for frog rhodopsin, obtained on increasing by 16% the previous figure of 2.39×10^4 litre per cm mole (DARTNALL, GOODEVE and LYTHGOE, 1938; SCHNEIDER, GOODEVE and LYTHGOE, 1939) (see p. 137). KROPF (1967) measured the photosensitivity of frog rhodopsin *(Rana pipiens)* to light of 436 nm by a different method in which potassium ferrioxalate was used as an actinometer (HATCHARD and PARKER, 1956). This was done in the presence of 0.1 M hydroxylamine so the result is directly comparable with those just quoted. He obtained the value 1.14×10^4 litre per cm mole for the photosensitivity at 436 nm. To relate this with the value for the photosensitivity at λ_{max} we need the value of the ratio $\varepsilon_{502}/\varepsilon_{436}$. Unfortunately this is not known very precisely but KROPF (1967) takes ε_{436} for rhodopsin as 1.76×10^4 litre per cm mole. Since ε_{502} is 4.06×10^4 litre per cm mole (WALD and BROWN, 1953) the ratio $\varepsilon_{502}/\varepsilon_{436}$ is 2.31 on this reckoning. The writer, on the other hand, (DARTNALL, 1968) has estimated this ratio to be 2.58. If we use the mean, 2.44, and multiply KROPF's photosensitivity value by it we obtain 2.78×10^4 litre per cm mole as the photosensitivity at λ_{max}. This is the same figure as was obtained in the photometric curves experiments when hydroxylamine was present (DARTNALL, 1968) and reinforces SCHNEIDER, GOODEVE and LYTHGOE's conclusion that the quantum efficiency is independent of wavelength in the visible spectrum.

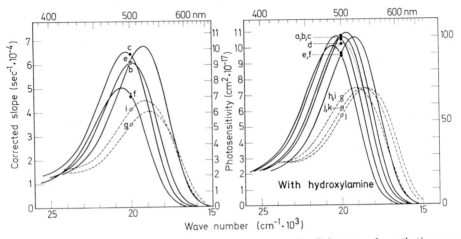

Fig. 8. The dichotomy of photosensitivity corresponding to the dichotomy of prosthetic group in the visual pigments. Measurements at 25° C in the absence and presence of hydroxylamine, as indicated. Left ordinate scale, slopes of the straight lines obtained by photometric curve analyses: centre ordinate scale, photosensitivities ($\alpha\gamma$) in absolute units: right ordinate scale, photosensitivities as percentages of that for *Rana temporaria* at λ_{max}. Filled circles give the photosensitivity values at 500 nm (20,000 wave-numbers) of A_1-based pigments; plain circles those of A_2-based pigments. The curves, full-line for A_1 pigments (dotted-line in one case to avoid confusion) and dashed-line for A_2 pigments are absorbance spectra scaled to pass through these values. The data on the left (filled and plain circles) were obtained in the 1958 work and agree with those of the 1968 work (crosses) that were also obtained without hydroxylamine. The data on the right were obtained in the presence of hydroxylamine (1968 work), and fall into two classes having maximum photosensitivities of either $10.1 - 10.9 \times 10^{-17}$ cm² per chromophore (A_1 pigments) or 7.4×10^{-17} cm² per chromophore (A_2 pigments). Key to letters as follows: a *Salvelinus alpinus* (508_1); b *Rana temporaria* (502_1); c *Trigla cuculus* (493_1); d *Rana cancrivora* and *Galago crassicaudatus agisymbanus* (502_2 and 501_1 respectively); e *Coregonus clupeoides pennantii* (520_1); f *Conger conger* (486_1); g *Tinca tinca* (530_2); h *Carassius carassius* (523_2); i *Cyprinus carpio* (523_2); j *Coregonus clupeoides clupeoides* (536_2); k *Rutilus rutilus* (536_2); l *Osmerus eperlanus* (543_2) (DARTNALL, 1968)

2. In the Ultraviolet

GOODEVE, LYTHGOE and SCHNEIDER (1942) extended the method of photometric curves to the violet and ultraviolet by making measurements of the photosensitivity of rhodopsin at 405, 365 and 254 nm. Their values at 405 and 365 nm were in line with what we know to be the variation of absorbance with wavelength in this region (Fig. 3) and indicate that absorption in the β-band of rhodopsin is just as effective as in the α-band in promoting bleaching, i.e. that the quantum yield is invariant down to 365 nm at least. Their value at 254 nm however was very low (Fig. 3) though absorption in this region — the γ-band of rhodopsin — is very high indeed. This suggested that energy absorbed by the "protein moiety" of the molecule was not available to the chromophore in the prosthetic group.

Recently, however, KROPF (1967) has measured the photosensitivity of frog rhodopsin in the ultraviolet (at 254 and 280 nm) and has obtained evidence that there is a substantial intramolecular transfer of energy absorbed in the protein part of the molecule to the prosthetic part carrying the retinal-based chromophore. KROPF established that bleaching by irradiation with ultraviolet light was "normal", i.e. that the prosthetic group product of bleaching, as with visible light, was in the all-trans form (HUBBARD and WALD, 1952) and that the free opsin was capable of regenerating rhodopsin, a criterion for native opsin (HUBBARD, 1958).

KROPF's values for the photosensitivities to 254 and 280 nm radiation are $1.10 \pm 0.40 \times 10^4$ and $2.30 \pm 0.50 \times 10^4$ litre per cm mole respectively, (compare with 2.78×10^4 litre per cm mole for the photosensitivity at λ_{max}).

In this work KROPF tacitly assumed that the rhodopsin chromophore has no absorption in the 254—280 nm region, i.e. that all the ultraviolet is absorbed by the opsin moiety. HUBBARD (1969) considers that the contribution from the chromophore must be small for the "absorption of rhodopsin at 280 nm decreases[7] by only about 3% when it is bleached by light to all-*trans* retinal and opsin, and the molar absorbance of all-*trans* retinal is only about 4% that of rhodopsin at 280 nm".

B. In Situ

In 1954 HAGINS reported measurements of the photosensitivity of mammalian rhodopsin *in situ*. By following the time course of the rise in retinal reflectivity of the excised eye (of a dark-adapted albino rabbit) as it bleached in light of known intensity and wavelength (516 nm) he was able to determine the photosensitivity as a rate constant. He calculated his result to the λ_{max} for rabbit rhodopsin (498 nm) and reported $\varepsilon_{max}\gamma$ as 2.7×10^4 litre/cm mole (corresponding to $\alpha_{max}\gamma = 10.3 \times 10^{-17}$ cm²/mole). Digitonin extracts of rabbit rhodopsin, solidified as agar gels and treated in the same way gave a distinctly lower result, 1.7×10^4 litre/cm mole (corresponding to $\alpha_{max}\gamma = 6.5 \times 10^{-17}$ cm²/mole). The difference between these results is nicely accounted for by the 50% enhancement of absorbance that one would expect from orientation of the *in situ* pigment. It is less easy, however, to relate these results to the values found in extracts by conventional methods (Table 1), mainly because of the uncertainties in the light losses by pre-retinal absorption and reflection.

Soon afterwards the photosensitivity of rhodopsin in the living human eye was measured by RUSHTON (1956) who calculated from his results a value for the photosensitivity at 507 nm that was 1.7 times that reported by DARTNALL, GOODEVE and LYTHGOE (1938) for extracted frog rhodopsin at 506 nm. This was after allowances for the effect of orientation, and for the pre-retinal light losses (LUDVIGH and McCARTHY, 1938; WEALE, 1954). This can be regarded as tolerable agreement considering that the bleaching was done by white light (the calculations consequently involving the use of the scotopic luminosity function and the appropriate relative spectral energy distribution for the colour temperature (2750° K) of the white light), and the assumption of the value of 44% for light losses in his subject's

---

[7] KROPF's (1967) spectra show a slight *increase* in absorbance at 280 nm on bleaching. The A_{280}/A_{500} ratio for his rhodopsin extracts was about 4.3, considerably more than the 2.2 for a pure specimen (WALD, 1949).

eye. Nevertheless, Rushton drew attention to the possibility that the discrepancy might arise from an approximately $2:1$ concentration of light intensity incident on the pigment in the outer segments by the funnelling action of the inner segments.

Most of the uncertainties inherent in the above measurements were avoided by Baumann (1965) in his study of the rate of bleaching of the perfused isolated retina of the edible frog, *Rana esculenta*. He used light of wavelength 504 nm and intensity 2.57×10^{14} quanta per second per cm^2 of retina and measured the transmissivity of the retina at various times. In order to avoid the complication that would otherwise be caused by the relatively slower thermal decomposition *in situ* of the intermediate products he invented the discontinuous exposure technique that was described in Section III B, employing $15-30$ sec exposures followed by $20-30$ min in darkness. He analysed his results by the method of photometric curves, using the stable values for the transmissivities at the end of the dark periods, and found a photosensitivity at 504 nm for rhodopsin of 14.6 ± 1.8 (S. D.) $\times 10^{-17}$ cm^2 per chromophore (equivalent to an $\varepsilon_{max}\gamma$ of $3.81 \pm 0.47 \times 10^4$ litre per cm mole).

The value for unoriented frog pigment in the extracted condition is 10.4×10^{-17} cm^2 per chromophore. The absorbance spectra of extracted and *in situ* rhodopsin are identical (Dartnall, 1961) and hence if their only difference is in the partial organisation of the latter (Section II B) one would expected an $\alpha_{max}\gamma$ for *in situ* pigment of 15.6×10^{-17} and this, in fact, is well within one standard deviation of Baumann's value.

V. Quantum Efficiency of Bleaching

The parameter photosensitivity is the product of the extinction coefficient (α or ε) and the quantum efficiency γ, and the measurements of it described in the previous pages can only give indirect information about its component factors. Thus in the original and early papers it was concluded (from the constancy of photosensitivity over ranges of temperature, concentration and pH, and from certain photochemical considerations) that the quantum efficiency for the bleaching of frog rhodopsin "is equal to or not much less than unity" (Dartnall, Goodeve and Lythgoe, 1936, 1938) and again "not less than 0.6" (Schneider, Goodeve and Lythgoe, 1939). No more precise statements from these results seem possible.

We are delivered from this uncertainty, however, by the measurements of extinction coefficients that have been independently made, both for A_1- and A_2-based pigments. Thus cattle rhodopsin ($\lambda_{max} = 498$ nm) has an absorbance of 4.06×10^4 litre per cm mole (Wald and Brown, 1953) assuming one retinal equivalent per molecule (Hubbard, 1954), and chicken iodopsin ($\lambda_{max} = 562$ nm) practically the same value (Wald, Brown and Smith, 1955). The only published information on A_2-based pigments is the statement in Brown, Gibbons and Wald (1963) that "the molar extinction of porphyropsin is about 30,000[8] (Wald, Brown

---

[8] This measurement was made on a digitonin extract (to which hydroxylamine had been added) of the yellow perch, *Perca flavescens*, and the molarity of the pigment was computed, as in the case of rhodopsin, by reference to the spectrum of the oxime formed on bleaching (private communication from Prof. Wald).

and BROWN, unpublished observations)". In none of these species has the pigment photosensitivity been measured but it is clear from the many published spectra that the α-band intensities of the visual pigments stand in nearly constant relation to those of their retinal (or dehydroretinal) oximes after bleaching. Thus the ε_{max} values of 4.06 and 3.00 $\times$ 10^4 litre per cm mole are applicable (at least approximately) to all A_1- and A_2-based pigments respectively. The quantum efficiencies can be obtained, therefore, by dividing the values of $\varepsilon_{max}\gamma$ by the appropriate figure. The results of doing this are set out in Table 1, which shows that the quantum efficiency is practically the same (2/3) for all visual pigments, A_1- and A_2-based alike.

Table 1. *The photosensitivities of the visual pigments and the quantum efficiencies of their bleaching at 25° C in the presence of hydroxylamine* (DARTNALL, 1968)

Species	Pigment	Photosensitivity			Quantum efficiency γ
		% frog pigment	$\alpha_{max}\,\gamma^a$	$\varepsilon_{max}\,\gamma^b$	
Conger conger	486_1	94·7	10·1	2·63	0·65
Trigla cuculus	493_1	100·6	10·7	2·80	0·69
Galago crassicaudatus agisymbanus	501_1	96·4	10·2	2·68	0·66
Rana temporaria	502_1	100·0	10·6	2·78	0·68
R. cancrivora	502_1	96·4	10·2	2·68	0·66
Salvelinus alpinus	508_1	102·6	10·9	2·85	0·70
Coregonus clupeoides pennantii	520_1	100·0	10·6	2·78	0·68
Mean for A_1-based pigments			10·5	2·74	0·67
Cyprinus carpio	523_2	67·9	7·2	1·89	0·63
Carassius carassius	523_2	69·8	7·4	1·94	0·65
Rutilus rutilus	536_2	69·4	7·4	1·93	0.64
Coregonus clupeoides clupeoides	536_2	70·3	7·5	1·95	0·65
Osmerus eperlanus	543_2	69·7	7·4	1·94	0·65
Mean for A_2-based pigments			7·4	1·93	0·64

[a] in $cm^2 \times 10^{-17}$ per chromophore (napierian base).
[b] in litre $cm^{-1} \times 10^4$ per mole of chromophore (decadic base).

Recently a much lower value for ε_{500}, namely 2.31 $\pm$ 0.80 $\times$ 10^4 litre per cm mole has been reported by HELLER (1968a) for bovine rhodopsin. This value, were it confirmed for all A_1-based pigments, would suggest a γ of near unity but, as mentioned above (Section IIC, p. 131) HELLER's absorbance spectrum lacked a *cis* peak, and there is doubt as to the relevance of his preparation to the present purpose. In any case, three groups of workers have since confirmed WALD and BROWN's (1953) original measurement. Thus SHICHI, LEWIS, IRREVERRE and STONE (1969) have reported 4.2 $\times$ 10^4 litre per cm mole for the maximum absorbance of bovine rhodopsin, BRIDGES (1970) the value of 4.19 $\times$ 10^4 for frog rhodopsin and DAEMEN, BORGGREVEN and BONTING (1970) the value 4.30 $\pm$ 0.70 $\times$ 10^4 for bovine rhodopsin.

Thus there seems little doubt about the molar absorbances of the visual pigments and consequently a strong suggestion from the photosensitivity values (Table 1) that the quantum efficiency of bleaching both in extracts and *in situ* is distinctly below unity. GUZZO and POOL (1968) have reported that the quantum efficiency of fluorescence of rhodopsin is only 0.005, so the one in three absorbed quanta that do not lead to bleaching cannot be accounted for in this way.

References

BAUMANN, CH.: Die Photosensitivität des Sehpurpurs in der isolierten Netzhaut. Vision Res. 5, 425—434 (1965).

BRAUDE, E. A.: Intensities of light absorption. Nature (Lond.) 155, 753—754 (1945).

BRIDGES, C. D. B.: Regeneration of visual pigments from their low-temperature photoproducts. Nature (Lond.) 186, 292—294 (1960).

— Studies on the flash-photolysis of visual pigments — IV. Dark reactions following the flash-irradiation of frog rhodopsin in suspensions of isolated photoreceptors. Vision Res. 2, 215—232 (1962).

— Periodicity of absorption properties in pigments based on vitamin A_2 from fish retinae. Nature (Lond.) 203, 303—304 (1964).

— The grouping of fish visual pigments about preferred positions in the spectrum. Vision Res. 5, 223—238 (1965).

— Molar absorbance of rhodopsin. Nature (Lond.) 227, 1258—1259 (1970).

BROWN, P. K., GIBBONS, I. R., WALD, G.: The visual cells and visual pigment of the mudpuppy, *Necturus*. J. Cell Biol. 19, 79—106 (1963).

COLLINS, F. D., LOVE, R. M., MORTON, R. A.: Studies in rhodopsin, 4: Preparation of rhodopsin. Biochem. J. 51, 292—298 (1952).

CRESCITELLI, F., MOMMAERTS, W. H. F. M., SHAW, T. I.: Circular dichroism of visual pigments in the visible and ultraviolet spectral regions. Proc. nat. Acad. Sci. (Wash.) 56, 1729—1734 (1966).

DAEMEN, F. J. M., BORGGREVEN, J. M. P. M., BONTING, S. L.: Molar absorbance of rhodopsin. Nature (Lond.) 227, 1259—1260 (1970).

DARTNALL, H. J. A.: The photochemistry of visual processes. Ph. D. Thesis. Univ. of London (1936).

— The visual pigments. London: Methuen & Co., Ltd.; New York: John Wiley & Sons. Inc. (1957).

— The spectral variation of the relative photosensitivities of some visual pigments. *In:* "Visual Problems of Colour", National Physical Laboratory Symposium No. 8, pp. 121—148. London, H.M.S.O. (1958).

— Visual pigments before and after extraction from visual cells. Proc. roy. Soc. B 154, 250—266 (1961).

— The visual pigment of the green rods. Vision Res. 7, 1—16 (1967).

— The photosensitivities of visual pigments in the presence of hydroxylamine. Vision Res. 8, 339—358 (1968).

— GOODEVE, C. F., LYTHGOE, R. J.: The quantitative analysis of the photochemical bleaching of visual purple solutions in monochromatic light. Proc. roy. Soc. A 156, 158—170 (1936).

— — — The effect of temperature on the photochemical bleaching of visual purple solutions in monochromatic light. Proc. roy. Soc. A 164, 216—230 (1938).

— LYTHGOE, J. N.: The clustering of fish visual pigments around discrete spectral positions, and its bearing on chemical structure. Ciba Foundation Symposium on Physiology and Experimental Psychology (Editors G. E. W. WOLSTENHOLME and JULIE KNIGHT). pp. 3—21 J. and A. Churchill Ltd., London: (1965a).

— — The spectral clustering of visual pigments. Vision Res. 5, 81—100 (1965b).

DENTON, E. J.: The contributions of the oriented photosensitive and other molecules to the absorption of whole retina. Proc. roy. Soc. B. 150, 78—94 (1959).

GOODEVE, C. F., LYTHGOE, R. J., SCHNEIDER, E. E.: The photosensitivity of visual purple solutions and the scotopic sensitivity of the eye in the ultraviolet. Proc. roy. Soc. B. **130**, 380—395 (1942).
— WOOD, L. J.: The photosensitivity of diphenylamine *p*-diazonium sulphate by the method of photometric curves. Proc. roy. Soc. A. **166**, 342—353 (1938).
GUZZO, A. V., POOL, G. L.: Visual pigment fluorescence. Science **159**, 312—314 (1968).
HAGINS, W. A.: The photosensitivity of mammalian rhodopsin *in situ*. J. Physiol. (Lond.) **129**, 22P (1954).
HATCHARD, C. G., PARKER, C. A.: A new sensitive chemical actinometer. II. Potassium ferrioxalate as a standard chemical actinometer. Proc. roy. Soc. A **235**, 518—536 (1956).
HELLER, J.: Structure of visual pigments. I. Purification, molecular weight and composition of bovine visual pigment$_{500}$. Biochemistry **7**, 2906—2913 (1968a).
— Structure of visual pigments. II. Binding of retinal and conformational changes on light exposure in bovine visual pigment$_{500}$. Biochemistry **7**, 2914—2920 (1968b).
HUBBARD, R.: The molecular weight of rhodopsin and the nature of the rhodopsin-digitonin complex. J. gen. Physiol. **37**, 381—399 (1954).
— The thermal stability of rhodopsin and opsin. J. gen. Physiol **42**, 259—280 (1958).
— Absorption spectrum of rhodopsin: 280 nm absorption band. Nature (Lond.) **221**, 435—437 (1969).
— WALD, G.: *Cis-trans* isomers of vitamin A and retinene in the rhodopsin system. J. gen. Physiol **36**, 269—315 (1952).
KROPF, A.: Intramolecular energy transfer in rhodopsin. Vision Res. **7**, 811—818 (1967).
LEWIS, G. N., CALVIN, M.: The colour of organic substances. Chem. Rev. **25**, 273—328 (1939).
LIEBMAN, P. A., ENTINE, G.: Visual pigments of frog and tadpole, *(Rana pipiens)*. Vision Res. **8**, 761—775 (1968).
LUDVIGH, E., McCARTHY, E. F.: Absorption of visible light by refractive media of the human eye. Arch. Ophthal., **20**, 37—51 (1938).
OSTROY, S. E., ERHARDT, F., ABRAHAMSON, E. W.: Protein configuration changes in the photolysis of rhodopsin. II. The sequence of intermediates in the thermal decay of cattle rhodopsin *in vitro*. Biochim. biophys. Acta (Amst.) **112**, 265—277 (1966).
PAULING, L.: Recent work on the configuration and electronic structure of molecules, with some applications to natural products. Fortschr. Chem. org. Naturstoffe **3**, 203—235 (1939).
RUSHTON, W. A. H.: The difference spectrum and the photosensitivity of rhodopsin in the living human eye. J. Physiol. **134**, 11—29 (1956).
SCHNEIDER, E. E., GOODEVE, C. F. LYTHGOE, R. J.: The spectral variation of the photosensitivity of visual purple. Proc. roy. Soc. A **170**, 102—112 (1939).
SHICHI, H., LEWIS, M. S., IRREVERRE, F., STONE, A. L.: Biochemistry of visual pigments. I. Purification and properties of bovine rhodopsin. J. biol. Chem. **244**, 529—536 (1969).
WALD, G.: The photochemistry of vision. Docum. ophthal. (Den Haag) **3**, 94—134 (1949).
— Retinal chemistry and the physiology of vision. In "Visual Problems of Colour", National Physical Laboratory Symposium No. 8, pp. 7—61. H. M. S. O. London (1958).
— BROWN, P. K.: The molar extinction of rhodopsin. J. gen. Physiol. **37**, 189—200 (1953).
— — SMITH, P. H.: Iodopsin. J. gen. Physiol. **38**, 623—681 (1955).
WEALE, R. A.: Light absorption by the lens of the human eye. Optica Acta **1**, 107—110 (1954).
ZECHMEISTER, L.: *Cis-trans* isomerization and stereochemistry of carotenoids and diphenylpolyenes. Chem. Rev. **34**, 267—344 (1944).

Chapter 5

The Behaviour of Visual Pigments at Low Temperatures

By

T. Yoshizawa, Toyonaka, Osaka (Japan)

With 19 Figures

Contents

I. Historical Introduction

One of the most fascinating problems in vision is the identification of the chemical process that triggers the excitation of the photoreceptor. To elucidate the molecular basis of this event, many workers have studied the sequence of intermediate products that are formed after a visual pigment molecule has captured a photon. Since the intermediates have short lives, these studies have been helped by working at low temperatures.

The first measurements at low temperatures were those of LYTHGOE and QUILLIAM (1938), who found that irradiation of frog rhodopsin at near 0° C yielded an orange-coloured intermediate ($\lambda_{max} =$ ca. 470 nm), which they called "transient orange". On warming to room temperature the transient orange was transformed into "indicator yellow", a pH-sensitive product that is pale yellow in alkaline solution and deep yellow ($\lambda_{max} =$ 440 nm) in acid (LYTHGOE, 1937). Then the introduction by BRODA and GOODEVE (1941) of a non-freezing solvent consisting of 75% glycerol and 25% water made it possible to measure the spectral absorbances of visual pigments well below 0° C. The photoproduct of frog rhodopsin obtained at dry-ice temperature ($-73°$ C) was considered by them to be identical with LYTHGOE's transient orange. Later, COLLINS and MORTON (1950) reported that when the photoproduct, formed by irradiating frog rhodopsin at $-70°$ C, was allowed to warm up to room temperature in the dark, half the original amount of photopigment was regenerated, though its λ_{max} was situated some 8 nm towards shorter wavelengths than rhodopsin. This was the first mention of *isorhodopsin*, a name later appropriated for the 9-*cis* isomer of rhodopsin (HUBBARD and WALD, 1952). (It is probable that COLLINS and MORTON's isorhodopsin was a mixture of rhodopsin (11-*cis*) and isorhodopsin (9-*cis*)).

WALD, DURELL and ST. GEORGE (1950) also measured the spectra of rhodopsin and its photoproducts at low temperatures (between $-30°$ C and $-100°$ C) but observed, on irradiating cattle rhodopsin in a 2:1 glycerol/water mixture, that the absorbance maximum shifted only about 5 nm towards the blue (and increased about 5% in height). Since the photoproduct thus obtained differed from LYTHGOE's transient orange, it was given another name, "lumirhodopsin". On warming this to about $-20°$ C in the dark, the maximum shifted a further 7—9 nm towards the blue, owing to the formation of a second intermediate, which was called "metarhodopsin". On further warming to room temperature in the dark metarhodopsin was converted to a final product that consisted of about equal amounts of photopigment and retinal + opsin.

It had been thought for a number of years that photoproducts reverted to rhodopsin or isorhodopsin by thermal processes. Then HUBBARD and ST. GEORGE (1958) obtained conclusive evidence that squid metarhodopsin, which, unlike vertebrate metarhodopsin, is stable below 15° C and pH sensitive, could be converted to rhodopsin by light. Similarly, HUBBARD and KROPF (1958) showed that cattle "metarhodopsin" is not, as had been supposed, a single substance, but a mixture (in photochemical equilibrium) of rhodopsin, isorhodopsin and a thermolabile fraction that hydrolyzes to all-*trans* retinal and opsin above about $-15°$ C in the dark. They, therefore, redefined the terms lumi- and metarhodopsin as the thermally labile fractions.

At the same time, YOSHIZAWA and KITÔ (1958a, b) began to find evidence that the irradiation of cattle rhodopsin at liquid-air ($-186°$ C) or liquid-nitrogen ($-196°$ C) temperatures yielded an even earlier intermediate than lumirhodopsin, the colour of the preparation changing from an orange-red to a pinkish red as the original rhodopsin was replaced by an equilibrium mixture of rhodopsin, isorhodop-

sin and intermediate. It was also shown that at these very low temperatures lumi-
and metarhodopsins partly revert to rhodopsin on irradiation (Yoshizawa and
Kitô, 1958 b; Kitô and Yoshizawa, 1960). The new intermediate, which is stable
below − 140° C (Yoshizawa, Kitô, and Ishigami, 1960; Yoshizawa, 1962), is
formed maximally when rhodopsin at − 195° C is irradiated by short-wave light
(440 nm), and is almost completely photoreversed to rhodopsin or isorhodopsin
by long-wave light (612 nm) (Kitô, Ishigami, and Yoshizawa, 1961; Yoshizawa,
1962). This suggested that the absorbance spectrum of the new intermediate must
lie well towards the red compared with rhodopsin.

In 1963, Yoshizawa and Wald, using a specially-designed Dewar vessel and
an opal glass technique, worked with extract-glycerol mixtures (1 : 2) at liquid-
nitrogen temperature. They confirmed the previous observations and also measured the absorbance spectrum of the new intermediate ($\lambda_{max} = 543$ nm) which
was given the name "pre-lumirhodopsin".

More recently, Horiuchi and I (unpublished) have developed a technique
for spectrophotometry at liquid-helium temperature, in order to examine whether
or not there exists an even earlier photoproduct than pre-lumirhodopsin. It was
found that irradiation of cattle rhodopsin under these conditions can result in two
different kinds of photoproducts. Irradiation with light of wavelengths greater
than 520 nm shifts the spectrum towards the blue because of the formation of a
photoproduct called "hypsorhodopsin", while irradiation with short-wave light
(437 nm) causes a bathochromic shift, owing to the conversion of rhodopsin to
"bathorhodopsin" (which is the same as pre-lumirhodopsin). On warming hypsorhodopsin above − 250° C in the dark, it changes into bathorhodopsin. In this
chapter the name, bathorhodopsin, is used in preference to pre-lumirhodopsin.

Thus continuing developments in the techniques of low-temperature spectrophotometry have been followed by the disclosure of an increasing number of
ntermediate stages in the bleaching process. It should be noted that the "true"
nitial photoproduct is the excited state itself.

II. The Bleaching Sequence

On exposure to light, visual pigment "bleaches" via a series of intermediates
to the final products, all-*trans* retinal and opsin. The various products and their
interrelationships are summarized in Fig. 1 for cattle rhodopsin, the most extensively studied of all the visual pigments.

Irradiation of cattle rhodopsin at liquid-helium temperature yields two different kinds of all-*trans* chromoproteins, hypsorhodopsin ($\lambda_{max} = $ ca. 430 nm) and
bathorhodopsin ($\lambda_{max} = 548$ nm) (Yoshizawa and Horiuchi, unpub.). On absorption of light, hypsorhodopsin is largely converted into bathorhodopsin, though
a small fraction may possibly revert to rhodopsin. Hypsorhodopsin is also changed
into bathorhodopsin in the dark when the temperature rises above − 250° C. It
seems probable, therefore, that hypsorhodopsin is an earlier product than bathorhodopsin. It is, in fact, uncertain whether rhodopsin, on irradiation, can change
directly to bathorhodopsin or whether bathorhodopsin is all formed via hypsorhodopsin. When bathorhodopsin, which is stable below − 140° C, is irradiated

at liquid-helium or -nitrogen temperatures, it reverts completely to rhodopsin. These conversions at liquid-helium temperature probably involve changes in side chain interactions between prosthetic group and opsin, presumably owing to conformational changes (*cis-trans* isomerization) of the former.

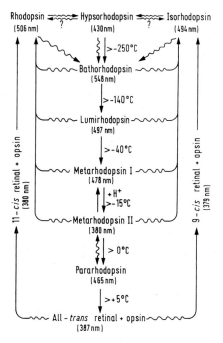

Fig. 1. Stages in the bleaching of cattle rhodopsin. Photoreactions are symbolized by wavy lines, thermal reactions by straight ones. λ_{max} for rhodopsin, hypsorhodopsin, isorhodopsin and bathorhodopsin at —268° C; lumirhodopsin and metarhodopsin I at —65° C; other pigments at near 0° C

When warmed above — 140° C in the dark, bathorhodopsin changes into lumirhodopsin, which is stable up to about — 40° C. Above this temperature lumirhodopsin is converted to metarhodopsin I. The thermal conversion of bathorhodopsin through lumirhodopsin to metarhodopsin I is interpreted as changes of interaction between the prosthetic group and opsin, arising from the stepwise changes of opsin structure (HUBBARD and KROPF, 1959a; YOSHIZAWA and WALD, 1963).

Metarhodopsin I is stable up to about — 15° C. Above this temperature it comes into tautomeric equilibrium with metarhodopsin II (MATTHEWS, HUBBARD, BROWN and WALD, 1964). On warming above about 0° C, metarhodopsin II changes to pararhodopsin (metarhodopsin III) (WALD, 1967b). These last two intermediates are also interconvertible by light. Finally, pararhodopsin hydrolyzes to all-*trans* retinal and opsin on warming above 5° C in the dark.

As already stated, most of these intermediates have been discovered at low temperatures where the rates of thermal reactions are reduced without affecting the rates of photoreactions. In general, if irradiation of a photosensitive pigment at low temperature results in the same final product as obtained at room temperature, it is usually concluded that any intermediates disclosed at the low temperature are also part of the process at room temperature. Indeed, a study of rhodopsin in a dried-gelatine film has indicated that lumi- and metarhodopsins appear in the bleaching process of the rhodopsin at room temperature (WALD, DURELL, and ST. GEORGE, 1950). Again in flash-photolysis studies of rhodopsin in solution and in a suspension of rod particles, metarhodopsin I has been detected at temperatures above 0° C (WULFF, ADAMS, LINSCHITZ, and ABRAHAMSON, 1958), and batho- and lumirhodopsins at and below − 25° C (GRELLMANN, LIVINGSTON, and PRATT, 1962; PRATT, LIVINGSTON, and GRELLMANN, 1964). It seems reasonable, therefore, to regard these products as intermediates in the normal bleaching process of rhodopsin rather than as low-temperature artifacts.

On the other hand, isorhodopsin, which is thermostable at normal temperatures, is regarded as an artifact for it has never been observed in an intact retina. However, isorhodopsin transforms to the same intermediates, when irradiated, as does rhodopsin. The photosensitivity of isorhodopsin is somewhat lower than that of rhodopsin (HUBBARD and KROPF, 1958).

III. Spectrophotometry at Low Temperatures

In the measurement of spectral absorbances at low temperature, the main problems are the selection of a solvent that remains optically clear, and the construction of a cryostat with windows that do not fog.

A. Solvents

Retinals and carotenoids are soluble in many organic solvents, several of which are suitable for spectrophotometric work above dry-ice temperature (− 78° C). At liquid-nitrogen temperature (− 196° C), however, most solvents freeze with crazing. To avoid this the carotenoid may be dissolved in a mixture of ether, isopentane (or isohexane) and alcohol (5 : 5 : 2), called EPA or EHA; or of ether, isohexane and triethylamine (5 : 5 : 2), called EH amine (JURKOWITZ, 1959). These mixtures remain clear at liquid-nitrogen temperature, though they become highly viscous, and contract in volume by about 23%.

Visual pigments, on the other hand, are not only insoluble in organic solvents, but are also denatured by some of them. Usually visual pigment is extracted by the aid of an aqueous solution of detergent such as digitonin. The extract when mixed with twice its volume of glycerol will congeal to a glass without cracking at temperatures above − 100° C. Below this temperature, however, some crazing occurs. This causes scattering of light with distortion of the apparent spectral absorbance. To eliminate the distorting effect of the scattering, the use of an opal glass (see Fig. 3) is recommended (YOSHIZAWA and WALD, 1963). When the glycerol-extract mixture is rapidly cooled, it freezes to a glass without cracking. The contraction in volume has been estimated at 7.7% in 67% glycerol and at 6.5% in 50% glycerol.

B. Cryostats for Spectrophotometry

In order to measure spectral absorbances at low temperatures, a cryostat must be designed for attachment to the spectrophotometer. The manufacturers of some spectrophotometers will provide a suitable cryostat. The cryostats here described were designed for use with the Hitachi recording spectrophotometer (EPS-3T).

1. Dry-Ice Temperature (—70° C)

As shown in Fig. 2, a cryostat suitable for work down to − 70° C consists of two separable parts, a copper cell holder and a container for the coolant (dry-ice/acetone). These parts are surrounded by blocks of polyurethane to insulate against the inflow of radiant heat from outside. Standard absorption cells can be fitted into the two outer compartments of the cell holder by the aid of copper jackets. Light from the spectrophotometer passes through the optical vacuum windows cemented on to the ends of the horizontal holes through the poly-urethane block, and thus reaches the absorption cells. The "cold finger" of the coolant container is inserted into the middle compartment of the cell holder. Light, for irradiation of the sample, passes through a vertical hole bored in the polyurethane block and impinges on the sample cell from above. The temperature is directly measured by inserting a thermocouple into the sample cell. The cryo-stat will maintain a constant temperature of about − 70° C without causing fogging of the windows.

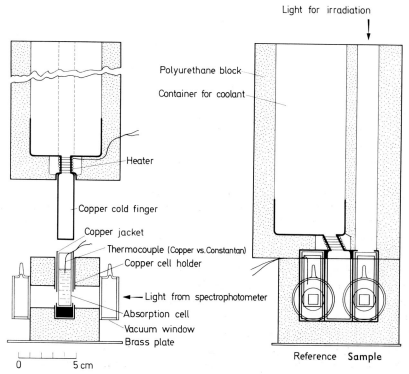

Fig. 2. Diagram of absorption vessel for measurement of spectral absorbance at above dry-ice tem-peratures. Left, side view; right, front view (YOSHIZAWA and HORIUCHI, hitherto unpublished)

2. Liquid-Nitrogen Temperature (—190° C)

This cryostat (Fig. 3) was based on one described by Cunningham and Tomp-kins (1959). The sample is put into a compartment consisting of a silicone-rubber ring (0.8—2.0 mm thick) and a front quartz plate and back opal glass. This compartment is fixed by means of a screw-on ring into a sample holder made of copper. The holder is fitted to a copper tube at the bottom of the cold finger and the whole is enclosed within a glass jacket. The space between the cold finger and the jacket is then evacuated by a rotary pump. The preparation is then cooled by pouring

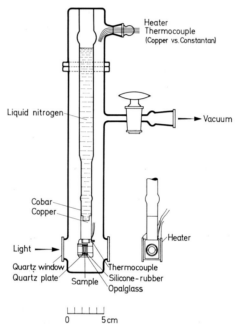

Fig. 3. Diagram of absorption vessel for the measurement of spectral absorbances at liquid-nitrogen temperature (Yoshizawa and Horiuchi, hitherto unpublished)

liquid nitrogen into the cold finger. The cryostat is positioned in the cell compartment of the spectrophotometer, a similar plate of opal glass being placed in the comparison beam. With this device the temperature of the preparation is brought to about − 190° C, according to measurements made with a copper-constantan thermocouple inserted into the sample holder. Since the volume of the cold finger is rather small, the liquid nitrogen evaporates in 30 min or so. However, when used in conjunction with an automatic supply of liquid nitrogen, it is easy to keep the preparation at the low temperature as long as required. If dry-ice/acetone is used instead of liquid nitrogen, the preparation can be kept at about − 73° C.

3. Liquid-Helium Temperature (—268 °C)

In constructing a cryostat for working at liquid-helium temperature the greatest care must be taken to insulate against the inflow of radiant heat from outside, because liquid helium, having a small heat of evaporation (0.65 cal/cm³), is easily lost. The cryostat is usually designed so that the container for liquid helium is surrounded by another, containing liquid nitrogen.

The metal cryostat (Fig. 4a) was constructed for use with a double-beam spectrophotometer. The copper holder, the sample and reference cells are connected to a copper block at the base of the liquid-helium container and are protected by a copper radiation shield (4.2° K) screwed to the bottom of the container. The procedure for loading the preparation is similar to that described above for the liquid-nitrogen cryostat. The 4.2° K radiation shield and the liquid-helium container are surrounded by a second radiation shield (77° K), welded to the bottom of the liquid-nitrogen container. The lower part of this outer shield is separable from the upper part at the level of the base of the liquid-helium container. The whole apparatus is enclosed in a jacket, the upper part of which surrounds the coolant containers, and the lower part the sample holder. The lower part is fitted with two pairs of quartz optical windows in alignment with the sample and reference cells. To bring the cryostat into commission the space between jacket and containers is first evacuated to about 10^{-5} mm Hg by a diffusion pump. The liquid-nitrogen container is then filled to pre-cool the apparatus and finally the liquid-helium container is filled.

In the double-vacuum glass cryostat (Fig. 4b), only the sample (with opal glass) is set in the holder (cf. the liquid-nitrogen cryostat). In the comparison beam, a similar plate of opal glass is placed. The copper sample holder is supported

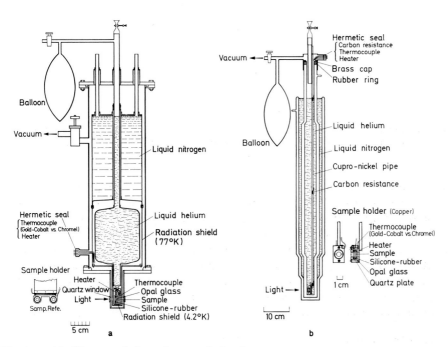

Fig. 4a and b. Diagram of absorption vessels for the measurement of spectral absorbances at liquid-helium temperature. a) metal cryostat for double beam spectrophotometer, b) double vacuum glass cryostat (YOSHIZAWA and HORIUCHI, hitherto unpublished)

by a cupro-nickel tube soldered to a brass cap. The inner vacuum vessel containing the liquid helium is surrounded by an outer vacuum vessel containing liquid nitrogen, except at the base where it is enclosed only by the outer wall of the outer vessel. Thus the outer wall of the inner vessel serves as a radiation shield. All glass parts of the cryostat are silvered, except for the windows. The sample holder is directly immersed into the liquid helium of the inner vessel. Thus light from the spectrophotometer passes directly through the triple glass wall and liquid helium to the sample, without crossing any liquid nitrogen. The spectrum can be measured at 4.2° K without any interference from bubbling of the liquid helium. When the inner vessel is brought to a reduced pressure (by a rotary pump), the bubbling of the liquid helium ceases altogether and the absorbance spectrum of the sample can be measured below 4.2° K.

In both the cryostats shown in Fig. 4 the temperature of the preparation is measured continuously by a gold-cobalt vs. chromel thermocouple inserted into the holder.

IV. The Spectral Absorbance of Visual Pigments and Retinal at Low Temperatures

A. Retinal and Related Substances

The spectra of carotenoids at liquid-nitrogen temperature have been extensively studied by Jurkowitz (1959) and by Loeb, Brown, and Wald (1959), and a theoretical interpretation of the results has been given by Wald (1959).

When all-*trans* retinal is cooled to liquid-nitrogen temperature, the $\lambda_{\max}$ of its spectrum moves by 14 nm to longer wavelengths, and $\varepsilon_{\max}$ rises about 10% (Fig. 5).

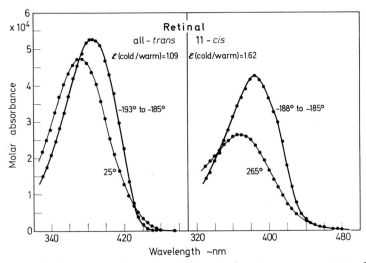

Fig. 5. Spectral absorbances of all-*trans* and 11-*cis* retinals, at room temperature and at liquid-nitrogen temperature (Jurkowitz, 1959)

In addition, the long-wave tail of the absorbance band is abbreviated (JURKOWITZ, 1959). Similar changes have been found not only in other retinal, retinol and carotenoid isomers (see Table 1), but also in the diphenyl-polyenes (HAUSSER, KUHN, and SEITZ, 1935).

At liquid-nitrogen temperature almost all molecules are in the lowest vibrational level of the ground state, from which transition to the first electronically-excited state takes place on absorption of a photon. At room temperature, on the other hand, some of the molecules are in higher vibrational levels of the ground state. Transitions from these higher levels to the excited state involve smaller energies, which can thus be provided by photons of longer wavelength. Thus the long-wave tail of the absorbance band, present at room temperature, is lost at low temperature (WALD, 1959). For the same reason, however, the general shift of the spectrum to longer waves on cooling is opposite in direction to that expected. Indeed, it is opposite to that observed in porphyrin derivatives (ESTABROOK, 1956),

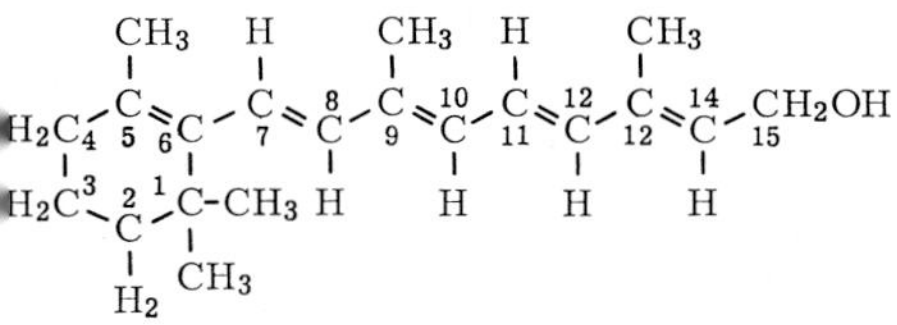

all-trans retinol ($C_{19}H_{27}CH_2OH$)

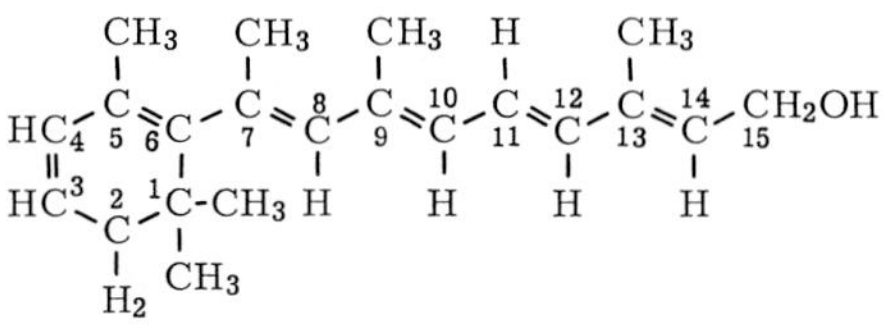

all-trans dehydroretinol ($C_{19}H_{25}CH_2OH$)

retinal

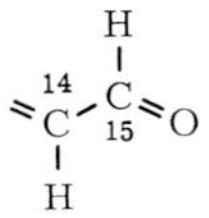

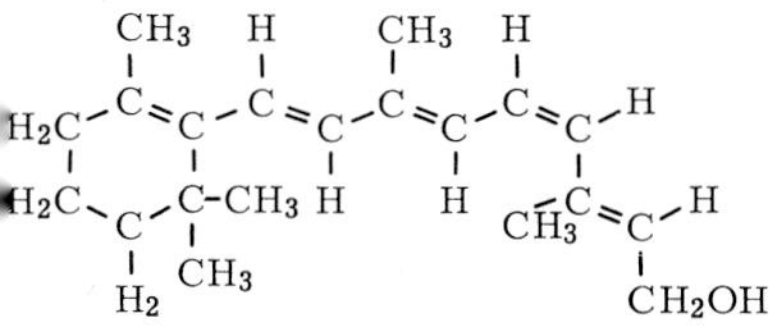

11-cis retinol

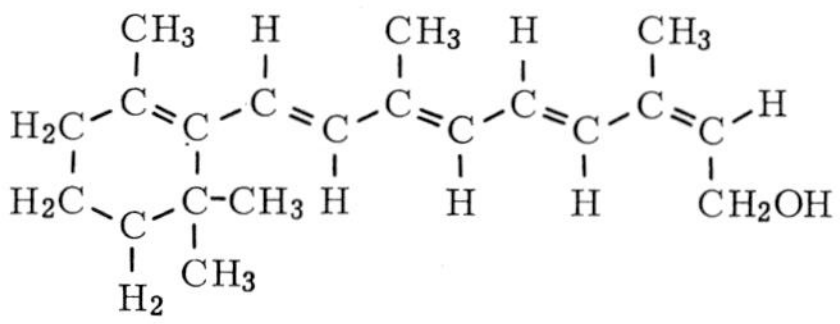

13-cis retinol

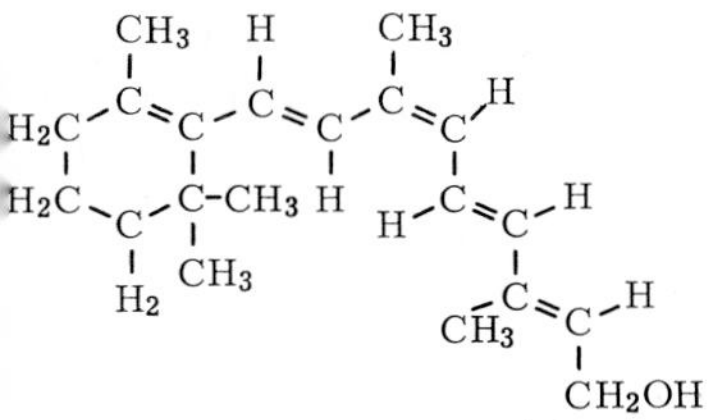

9-cis retinol

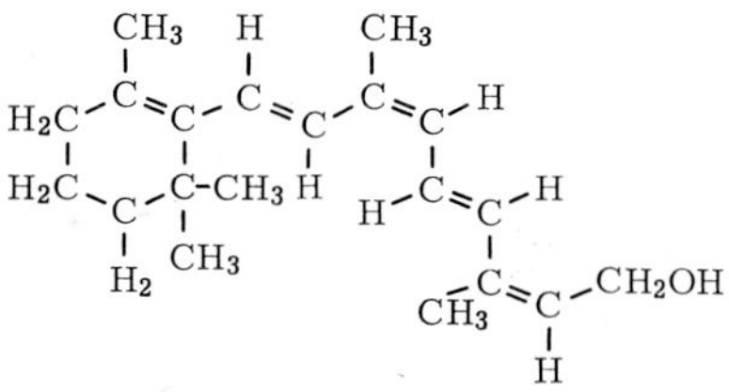

9.13-dicis retinol

Fig. 6. Structural formulae of some geometric isomers of retinol, dehydroretinol and retinal: the all-*trans* isomers, the two unhindered mono-*cis* isomers (9-*cis* and 13-*cis*), the unhindered *dicis* isomer (9, 13-*dicis*) and the sterically hindered mono-*cis* isomer (11-*cis*)

which have a rigid ring structure. Retinals and carotenoids, however, possess conjugated systems of alternate single and double bonds in linear array, so that they readily undergo conformational changes; bending and twisting to some extent because of molecular motion in the warm. In the cold, however, the molecule is subject to less deformation, with the result that it tends to an extended and planar conformation. Now the λ_{max} is proportional to the square of the distance between the ends of the conjugated system (Mulliken, 1939) and consequently cooling, which favours an increase in this length, will shift the spectrum towards the red (Wald, 1959).

Table 1. *Effects of cooling upon carotenoid spectra* (Loeb, Brown, and Wald, 1959)

Geometric isomer	Room temperature		$-185°$ to $-195°$		Ratio of ε_{max} (cold/warm)	Shift of λ_{max} (cold—warm) (nm)
	ε_{max} ($\times 10^{-3}$)	λ_{max} (nm)	ε_{max} ($\times 10^{-3}$)	λ_{max} (nm)		
Retinal						
All-*trans*[a]	47 · 6	373	51 · 7	387	1 · 09	14
9-*cis*	39 · 7	366	44 · 1	379	1 · 11	13
13-*cis*	38 · 8	366	43 · 5	380	1 · 12	14
9, 13-*dicis*	35 · 6	360	39 · 9	371	1 · 11	11
(Dehydroretinal, all-*trans*)	42 · 0	392	45 · 5	409	1 · 09	17
11-*cis* (hindered)[b]	26 · 4	369	43 · 0	384 · 5	1 · 63	15 · 5
β-Carotene						
All-*trans*[c]	137 · 5[d]	451 · 5	184	469	1 · 34	17 · 5
15-*monocis*	98 · 3	447	140	465	1 · 42	18
(Lycopene, all-*trans*)[c]	186	472	272	484	1 · 46	12
11, 11'-*dicis*	46 · 2	403	134	452 · 5	2 · 90	49 · 5
Vitamin A						
All-*trans*	52 · 1	324	54 · 2	333 · 5	1 · 04	9 · 5
(Vitamin A_2 acetate, all-*trans*)	39 · 5	349	45 · 0	360	1 · 14	11
11-*cis*	34 · 3	318	48 · 7	332 · 5	1 · 42	14 · 5

[a] Averages from three sets of measurements.
[b] Averages from four.
[c] Averages from two.
[d] For carotene and lycopene, ε_{max} and λ_{max} are of the 'middle' maximum, that of next-to-longest wave-length.

When 11-*cis* retinal is cooled to liquid-nitrogen temperature, ε_{max} increases to about 1.62 times its room temperature value. This remarkable rise in absorbance, characteristic also of hindered *cis* carotenoids, is thought to be due to a reduction in the steric hindrance between a hydrogen atom at carbon 10 and a methyl group at carbon 13, presumably because of contraction of the effective van der Waals' radii of the methyl group (Wald, 1959).

Another interesting low-temperature phenomenon is the appearance or accentuation of fine structure in the spectral absorbance curves of β-carotene and lycopene (Figs. 7 and 8; Loeb, Brown, and Wald, 1959). At room temperature all-*trans* β-carotene exhibits three maxima in the visible region. On cooling to liquid-nitrogen temperature, the spectrum shifts to longer wavelengths and the fine structure is greatly accentuated, five maxima now being distinguishable (Fig. 7). Unhindered *cis* isomers display a similar effect on cooling, while the hindered *cis* isomer behaves very differently. But 11, 11′-*dicis* β-carotene, which contains *two* hindered *cis* linkages shows a single broad maximum at room temperature, while in the cold, five distinct maxima appear (Fig. 7) as if it were an unhindered *cis* β-carotene. Thus cooling relieves steric hindrance in this instance as in 11-*cis* retinal (WALD, 1959).

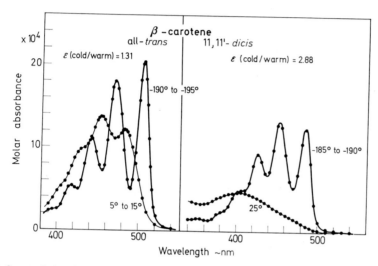

Fig. 7. Spectral absorbances of all-*trans* and 11, 11′-*dicis* β-carotene in EPA at room temperature and at liquid-nitrogen temperature (LOEB, BROWN, and WALD, 1959)

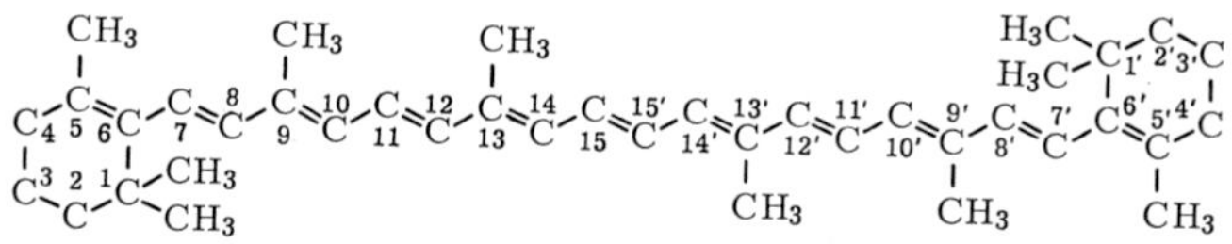

β-carotene, $C_{40}H_{56}$ (all-trans)

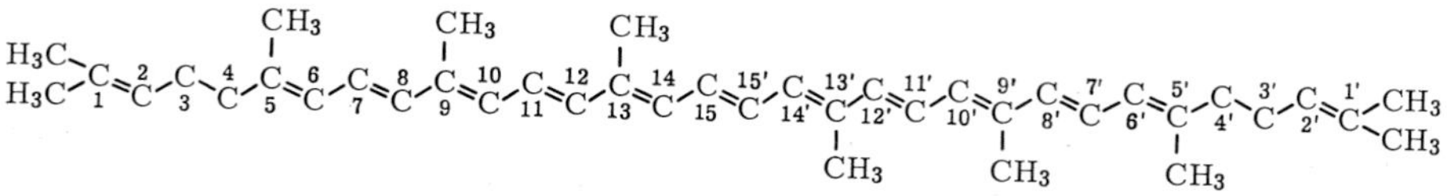

lycopene, $C_{40}H_{56}$ (all-trans)

Fig. 8. Structures of all-*trans* β-carotene and lycopene

B. Visual Pigments

In order to measure the spectra of visual pigments and their derivatives at low temperatures, extracts of these substances are usually mixed with glycerol, as mentioned earlier. These glycerol-water mixtures, when cooled to liquid-nitrogen temperature, form a rigid and amorphous glass containing numerous cracks. Since the cracks give rise to multiple reflections, the effective light path is increased with consequent intensification of the spectral absorbance. When a 45—55% glycerol is used, and a microcrystalline state is induced by warming from liquid-nitrogen temperature, the spectral absorbance of the solute can be intensified more than ten fold. This intensification is purely optical, the micro-crystals causing a massive degree of multiple reflection. This effect was discovered by KEILIN and HARTREE (1949, 1950), who applied the technique to the investigation of a variety of haemoproteins.

A typical example of the results of this technique with cattle rhodopsin is shown in Fig. 9 (YOSHIZAWA and WALD, 1966). It should be noted that before recording each of the spectra in Fig. 9, the apparent absorbance was adjusted to zero at 700 nm, where the absorbance of rhodopsin is negligible. On cooling the preparation from room temperature (curve 1) to liquid-nitrogen temperature (curve 2), the maximum absorbance increases about 1.8 times and there is a bathochromic shift of λ_{max} from 498 nm to 505 nm. The intensification is due partly

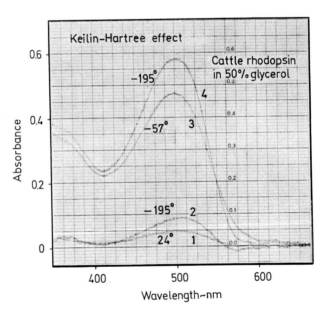

Fig. 9. Intensification of the spectral absorbance of cattle rhodopsin (curve 2 → 3) due to the formation of micro-crystals in the medium (1 : 1 glycerol/water mixture) on warming to about —57° C from liquid-nitrogen temperature (YOSHIZAWA and WALD, 1966)

to contraction, partly to cracking of the vitreous solvent and partly to the effect of cooling *per se*. On increasing the temperature from —195° C to —120° C, a gradual decrease in absorbance is observed, a further decrease occurring at about —120° C when the cracks in the solvent begin to disappear. At about —80° C microcrystals start to form, and the absorbance then increases, reaching a maximum at -57 to $-55°$ C (curve 3, Fig. 9). At $-57°$ C the maximum absorbance is about 9.7 times that at room temperature, and λ_{max} is 499 nm. Further warming would cause the microcrystals to melt, so at this point the preparation is re-cooled to liquid-nitrogen temperature. At $-195°$ C the maximum absorbance is 11.9 times the original value, and λ_{max} is 501 nm (curve 4, Fig. 9).

Thus, because of the Keilin-Hartree effect, it is possible to obtain a considerable intensification of the spectrum with little displacement or distortion. The same procedure should be particularly useful in the identification and study of any visual pigment that is obtained only in very low concentration (e.g. a cone pigment). The photochemistry of iodopsin at liquid-nitrogen temperature has been studied by this method (YOSHIZAWA and WALD, 1967).

In order to determine the effect of cooling *per se* on a visual pigment, the solvent must be frozen to an amorphous glass, free from cracks and microcrystals. Rapid cooling of glycerol-water mixtures (2 : 1) to liquid-nitrogen temperature sometimes results in a clear glass. This can be checked by measuring the apparent absorbance at a wavelength where the absorbance of the visual pigment is negligible (in the red). Spectra of cattle rhodopsin in such relatively clear media at low temperatures are shown in Fig. 10. These show that the absorbance maximum moves from 498 nm at room temperature to 505 nm at liquid-nitrogen temperature and to 506 nm at liquid-helium temperature.

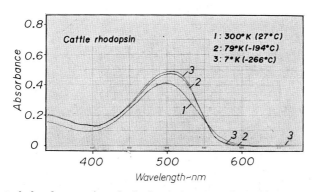

Fig. 10. Spectral absorbances of cattle rhodopsin in a 2 : 1 glycerol/water mixture containing 0.05 M hydroxylamine at pH 6.4. The spectra were recorded at 27° C (curve 1), then —194° C (curve 2) and finally at —266° C (curve 3) (YOSHIZAWA and HORIUCHI, to be published)

Similar effects are observed on cooling carp porphyropsin (YOSHIZAWA and HORIUCHI, 1969). It is interesting to note that the spectrum of porphyropsin at low temperature has a small shoulder near 560 nm (Fig. 12). Since such a shoulder has never been observed in A_1-based visual pigments, it must be attributed to the A_2-prosthetic group, namely, dehydroretinal. Similar shoulders have been observed in the spectra of the intermediates of porphyropsin and isoporphyropsin (Figs. 12 and 13).

V. Reversible Photochemical Reactions

A. Mixtures in Photochemical Equilibrium

When an isomer of free retinal is irradiated at room temperature, the product is not a single isomer, but an equilibrium mixture of all possible isomers. In ethyl alcohol about 25% of this mixture is 11-*cis*, about 25% is composed of other *cis* isomers, and about 50% is all-*trans* (Brown and Wald, 1956). Similar isomerizations can occur when the retinal is attached as prosthetic group to opsin. Thus when a visual pigment molecule absorbs a photon the prosthetic group is isomerized from the 11-*cis* to the all-*trans* form. If, now, the all-*trans* intermediate absorbs a second photon, the prosthetic group is further isomerized to a mono-*cis* form. Prolonged irradiation at low temperature (when the intermediate is stable) continues to isomerize and re-isomerize the prosthetic group, resulting in an equilibrium mixture composed of visual pigment (11-*cis* form), isopigment (9-*cis* form) and intermediates (all-*trans* and other isomeric forms). The possible reactions may be summarized as follows:

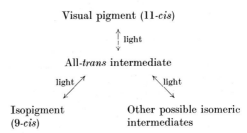

As yet there is no positive proof of the formation of isomeric intermediates other than the all-*trans* form. Flash photolytic studies, however, have indicated that there are three concurrent first order reactions in the thermal decay of batho-rhodopsin, presumably because there are three different species of bathorhodopsin having similar spectral absorbances (Grellmann, Livingston, and Pratt, 1962; Pratt, Livingston, and Grellmann, 1964).

The photochemical interconversions at liquid-nitrogen temperature between visual pigment, batho-intermediate and isopigment are illustrated for carp porphyropsin in Fig. 11 (Yoshizawa and Horiuchi, 1969). As shown in Fig. 11a, irradiation with 506 nm of the original (11-*cis*) porphyropsin (curve 1) results in a progressive shift of the spectrum to longer wavelengths (curves 2—5), owing to the formation of bathoporphyropsin (all-*trans*). On further irradiation with the same light (Fig. 11b) the spectrum returns to shorter wavelengths (curves 6—9) because of the formation of isoporphyropsin (9-*cis*). The final position of the spectrum (curve 9, Fig. 11b) represents the equilibrium mixture of porphyropsin, isoporphyropsin and bathoporphyropsin. On the other hand, as shown in Fig. 11c, when porphyropsin is irradiated with light exceeding 580 nm in wavelength (which isoporphyropsin hardly absorbs) mainly isoporphyropsin is formed, probably via bathoporphyropsin (curves 2—7, Fig. 11c), the final spectrum (curve 7) representing a mixture of 95% isoporphyropsin and 5% porphyropsin. Further irradiation of this mixture (curve 7, Fig. 11d) with 463 nm finally converts it to an equilibrium

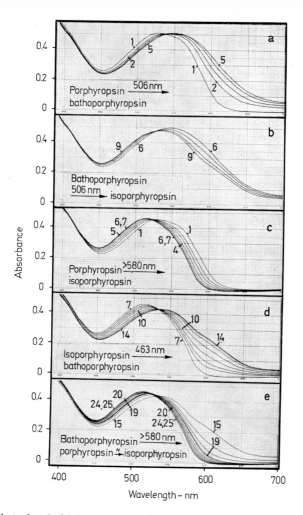

Fig. 11a—e. Photochemical interconversions between porphyropsin, bathoporphyropsin and isoporphyropsin at liquid-nitrogen temperature. a) and b) The course of the photoconversion of porphyropsin to an equilibrium mixture of porphyropsin, bathoporphyropsin and isoporphyropsin. Curve 1a: Carp porphyropsin in a 2:1 glycerol/water mixture. Curves 2a to 9b: Products of irradiation by 506 nm after successive exposure periods of 1, 1, 2, 4, 8, 16, 32, and 64 min. The final spectrum (curve 9b) represents an equilibrium mixture of porphyropsin, bathoporphyropsin and isoporphyropsin. c) The course of photoconversion of porphyropsin to isoporphyropsin. Curve 1c: Porphyropsin in a 2:1 glycerol/water mixture. Curves 2c—7c: Products of irradiation by wavelengths longer than 580 nm after successive exposure periods of 1, 1, 2, 4.5, 8, and 16 min. The final spectrum (curve 7) is due to isoporphyropsin (95 per cent) with a small admixture of porphyropsin (5 per cent). d) The course of the photoconversion of isoporphyropsin to an equilibrium mixture. Curve 7d: The same as curve 7c. Curves 8d—14d: Products of irradiation by 463 nm after successive exposure periods of 0.5, 0.5, 1, 2, 4, 8, and 16 min. The final spectrum (curve 14d) represents the equilibrium mixture of porphyropsin, bathoporphyropsin and isoporphyropsin. e) The course of the photoconversion of bathoporphyropsin to porphyropsin and then to isoporphyropsin. Curve 15e: The equilibrium mixture of 14d irradiated for a further 5 min by 463 nm. Curves 16e—25e: Products of irradiation by wavelengths longer than 580 nm after successive exposure periods of 1, 1, 2, 4 sec and 1, 1, 2, 4, 8, and 16 min. The final spectrum (curve 25e) is due to isoporphyropsin (95 per cent) with a small admixture of porphyropsin (5 per cent) (YOSHIZAWA and HORIUCHI, hitherto unpublished)

mixture (curve 14, Fig. 11 d) of porphyropsin, isoporphyropsin and batho-porphyropsin, just as in the case of porphyropsin (curve 9, Fig. 11 b). When, now, the mixture (curve 15, Fig. 11 e) is irradiated with light of wavelengths exceeding 580 nm, the bathoporphyropsin in the mixture rapidly changes to porphyropsin (curves 15—19), which then converts slowly to isoporphyropsin (curves 20—25). These experiments clearly demonstrate that porphyropsin, iso-porphyropsin and bathoporphyropsin are freely interconvertible by light at liquid-nitrogen temperature. Similar photoisomerizations at liquid-nitrogen temperature have also been observed in A_1-based visual pigments, namely, cattle and squid rhodopsins, and chicken iodopsin; and also at the level of lumi, meta I and meta II intermediates.

B. Calculation of the Spectra of Intermediates

Since the irradiation of visual pigment at low temperature yields an equilibrium mixture of visual pigment, isopigment and intermediate, the spectrum of the intermediate can be calculated by subtracting the spectra of visual pigment and of isopigment from the spectrum of the mixture.

In the case of experiments carried out above $-100°$ C, when lumi- and/or meta-intermediates are present in the equilibrium mixture, the mixture is warmed to room temperature. The visual pigment and isopigment remain unchanged but the intermediates bleach to the final products (opsin and retinal oxime in the presence of hydroxylamine). The preparation is then re-cooled to the original temperature and its spectrum measured. Subtraction of this spectrum from that

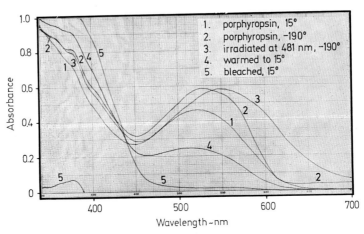

Fig. 12. The photoconversion of carp porphyropsin to bathoporphyropsin at liquid-nitrogen temperature. Curve 1: Carp porphyropsin in a 2 : 1 glycerol/water mixture containing 0.05 M hydroxylamine, at pH 6.4 and 15° C. Curve 2: After cooling to —190° C. Irradiation by 481-nm light for 2 min converted this to an equilibrium mixture of porphyropsin, bathoporphyropsin and isoporphyropsin (curve 3). On warming to 15° C in the dark the bathoporphyropsin in the mixture bleached to all-*trans* dehydroretinal oxime ($\lambda_{max} = 378$ nm), leaving a residual mixture of porphyropsin and isoporphyropsin (curve 4). Finally the preparation was completely bleached by orange light at 15° C to a mixture of all-*trans* dehydroretinal oxime and opsin (curve 5) (YOSHIZAWA and HORIUCHI, hitherto unpublished)

of the equilibrium mixture gives the difference spectrum of the intermediate. In this way, the spectra of lumi- and meta-intermediates have been estimated (KROPF and HUBBARD, 1958; HUBBARD and KROPF, 1958; HUBBARD, BROWN, and KROPF, 1959; HUBBARD and KROPF, 1959a and b).

In experiments carried out below $-120°$ C, however, the second cooling results in a different pattern of cracking in the glycerol-water mixture, which would introduce some error. In these cases, therefore, it is necessary to determine the proportions of each component in the equilibrium mixture. As an example, we may consider an experiment designed to determine the spectral absorbance curve of bathoporphyropsin (YOSHIZAWA and HORIUCHI, 1969). Carp porphyropsin in a 2 : 1 glycerol-water mixture, M/20 in hydroxylamine (curve 1, Fig. 12) was cooled to liquid-nitrogen temperature (curve 2). The preparation was then irradiated with 481-nm light which produced an equilibrium mixture (rich in bathoporphyropsin) of porphyropsin, isoporphyropsin and bathoporphyropsin (curve 3). On warming the preparation to room temperature in the dark, the porphyropsin and isoporphyropsin remained intact, while the bathoporphyropsin bleached to all-*trans* dehydroretinal oxime + opsin (curve 4, Fig. 12). Finally, the preparation was completely bleached, at room temperature, to all-*trans* dehydroretinal oxime by irradiating it with orange light (>500 nm). This orange light does not isomerize all-*trans* dehydroretinal oxime, for the oxime hardly absorbs at wavelengths above 470 nm. That part of curve 5 in Fig. 12 above 470 nm thus represents the absorbance of impurity. By subtracting curve 5 from the other "room temperature" curves (curves 1 and 4 in Fig. 12), therefore, the "true" spectra (in the range above 470 nm) are obtained. We may denote these as curves 1′ and 4′.

Since porphyropsin and isoporphyropsin have the same absorbance at 515 nm, the difference in absorbance between curves 1′ and 4′ at this wavelength is a measure of the amount of bathoporphyropsin, the percentage of which (B) is given by:

$$B = \frac{E^{1'}_{515} - E^{4'}_{515}}{E^{1'}_{515}} \times 100 . \tag{1}$$

The proportions of porphyropsin and isoporphyropsin in the equilibrium mixture (curve 3, Fig. 12) can be estimated from curve 4′ by HUBBARD's procedure (1956). Thus the absorbance in curve 4′ at 480 nm ($E^{4'}_{480}$) is equal to the sum of absorbances of porphyropsin ($E^{P4'}_{480}$) and isoporphyropsin ($E^{I4'}_{480}$), i.e.

$$E^{4'}_{480} = E^{P4'}_{480} + E^{I4'}_{480} . \tag{2}$$

Similarly, for 550 nm

$$E^{4'}_{550} = E^{P4'}_{550} + E^{I4'}_{550} . \tag{2'}$$

In the case of pure porphyropsin (curve 1′), the ratios of the absorbances at 480 nm and at 550 nm to that at the maximum (522 nm), namely, (E^{P}_{480}/E^{P}_{522}) and (E^{P}_{550}/E^{P}_{522}) are 0.726 and 0.879 respectively. The corresponding ratios for pure isoporphyropsin ($\lambda_{max} = 506$ nm) are 0.872 (E^{I}_{480}/E^{I}_{506}) and 0.668 (E^{I}_{550}/E^{I}_{506}). Thus, from equations (2) and (2′):

$$E^{4'}_{480} = 0.726 \times E^{P4'}_{522} + 0.872 \times E^{I4'}_{506} , \tag{3}$$

$$E^{4'}_{550} = 0.879 \times E^{P4'}_{522} + 0.668 \times E^{I4'}_{506} , \tag{3'}$$

in which $E_{522}^{P4'}$ and $E_{506}^{I4'}$ are the absorbances at the $\lambda_{\max}$ of the porphyropsin and isoporphyropsin contained in curve 4'. From the Eqs. (3) and (3'), one can derive $E_{522}^{P4'}$ and $E_{522}^{I4'}$ as functions of the absorbances of the mixture (curve 4') at the wavelengths 480 nm and 550 nm. Thus, for porphyropsin,

$$E_{522}^{P4'} = -2.38 \times E_{480}^{4'} + 3.12 \times E_{550}^{4'}, \tag{4}$$

and for isoporphyropsin,

$$E_{506}^{I4'} = 2.95 \times E_{480}^{4'} - 2.44 \times E_{550}^{4'}. \tag{4'}$$

The percentages of porphyropsin (P), isoporphyropsin (I) and bathoporphyropsin (B) in the equilibrium mixture can now be calculated from Eq. (1) together with Eqs. (5) and (6):

$$P = \frac{E_{522}^{P4'}}{E_{522}^{V}} \times 100, \tag{5}$$

$$P + I + B = 100. \tag{6}$$

By subtracting the spectra of porphyropsin and isoporphyropsin (at liquid-nitrogen temperature) in amounts corresponding to these values from the spectrum of the equilibrium mixture, one can then obtain the spectral absorbance curve of bathoporphyropsin. In Fig. 13 are shown the spectral absorbance curves of equivalent amounts of porphyropsin, isoporphyropsin and bathoporphyropsin. By a similar procedure the spectral absorbance curves of hypsorhodopsin (curve 3,

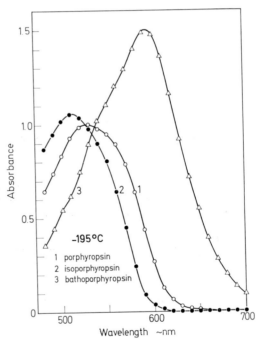

Fig. 13. The spectral absorbances of carp porphyropsin (curve 1), isoporphyropsin (curve 2) and bathoporphyropsin (curve 3) at liquid-nitrogen temperature. The maximum absorbance of the porphyropsin is normalized at 1.0 and the other curves are plotted in quantitative relation (YOSHIZAWA and HORIUCHI, to be published)

Fig. 15) and of the bathorhodopsins of cattle (YOSHIZAWA and WALD, 1963) and of squid (YOSHIZAWA and WALD, 1964) have been calculated.

C. Calculation of Relative Quantum Efficiencies

The equilibrium mixtures produced by irradiation of visual pigment at low temperature can be formulated as:

$$\text{Visual pigment} \rightleftarrows \text{Intermediate} \rightleftarrows \text{Isopigment.} \qquad (7)$$

The proportion of each isomer in an equilibrium mixture obviously depends on the wavelength of the radiation used, for the isomer that absorbs minimally will accumulate. This was illustrated in Fig. 11 in which it was shown that irradiation of porphyropsin by green light (506 nm), which is preferentially absorbed by porphyropsin, favors the formation of bathoporphyropsin; whereas orange light (>580 nm), which isoporphyropsin hardly absorbs, favors the formation of that pigment.

The rate of any photochemical reaction at a time t is given by the product of the quantum efficiency (γ) and the intensity of light flux absorbed at that time (J_t) by the sensitive species. Quantum efficiency is defined as the ratio of the number of molecules reacting to the number of quanta absorbed. The intensity of light absorbed is approximately proportional to the product of the molar extinction ε_λ at the wavelength, λ, of the light used and the concentration, c_t, of the photosensitive pigment. Thus, using the superscripts a, b and c to denote visual pigment, intermediate and isopigment respectively, and the subscript e to indicate equilibrium concentrations, we can write,

$$\varepsilon_\lambda^a \cdot \gamma^{a \rightarrow b} \cdot C_e^a = \varepsilon_\lambda^b \cdot \gamma^{b \rightarrow a} \cdot C_e^b, \qquad (8)$$

$$\varepsilon_\lambda^b \cdot \gamma^{b \rightarrow c} \cdot C_e^b = \varepsilon_\lambda^c \cdot \gamma^{c \rightarrow b} \cdot C_e^c. \qquad (9)$$

If, as a convention, the quantum efficiency of the change $a \rightarrow b$, i.e. visual pigment $\rightarrow$ intermediate, is taken as unity, the quantum efficiencies of the other photochemical changes can be evaluated from a consideration of the proportions of the pigments in an equilibrium mixture and their ε values at the wavelength of irradiation. Thus from the compositions of the various equilibrium mixtures obtained by irradiating rhodopsin at $-20°$ C by lights of 450, 500 and 550 nm, and from a direct comparison of the bleaching rates of rhodopsin and isorhodopsin at $25°$ C, KROPF and HUBBARD (1958) deduced the following *relative* quantum efficiencies:

$$\text{Rhodopsin} \underset{0.5}{\overset{1}{\rightleftarrows}} \text{Metarhodopsin} \underset{0.3}{\overset{0.1}{\rightleftarrows}} \text{Isorhodopsin.}$$

VI. Properties and Relationships of the Intermediates

A. The Hypso-Intermediate

Hypsorhodopsin is preferentially formed when rhodopsin is irradiated at low temperatures by long-wave light. Thus when cattle rhodopsin at the temperature of liquid helium ($-269°$ C) is exposed to light of wavelengths exceeding 540 nm, the spectral absorbance curve shifts progressively towards the "blue" (Fig. 14a) owing to conversion of the rhodopsin to a mixture consisting primarily of hypsorhodopsin but containing also some rhodopsin and isorhodopsin. The spectrum of pure hypsorhodopsin is shown in Fig. 15 in relation to that of rhodopsin at the same temperature. The $\lambda_{\max}$ of hypsorhodopsin is ca. 430 nm and its maximum absorbance is about 0.9 times that of the parent rhodopsin. With the exception

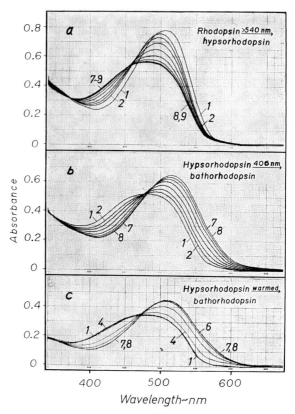

Fig. 14a—c. The photochemical formation of hypsorhodopsin and its photochemical and thermal conversions. a) The course of photoconversion of rhodopsin to hypsorhodopsin at liquid-helium temperature. Curve 1a: Cattle rhodopsin in a 2:1 glycerol/water mixture. Curves 2a—9a: The products of irradiation by wavelengths longer than 540 nm after successive exposure periods of 1, 1, 2, 4, 8, 16, 32, and 64 min. The final spectrum (curve 9a), measured at a slightly higher than liquid-helium temperature, is due to a mixture of rhodopsin, isorhodopsin and hypsorhodopsin. b) The course of the photoconversion of hypsorhodopsin to bathorhodopsin at liquid-helium temperature. Curve 1b: The mixture of rhodopsin, isorhodopsin and hypsorhodopsin formed by irradiation of rhodopsin by wavelengths longer than 540 nm. Curves 2b—8b: The products of irradiation by 406 nm after successive exposure periods of 5, 5, 10, 20, 40, 80, and 160 sec. The final spectrum (curve 8b) is due to a mixture of rhodopsin, isorhodopsin and bathorhodopsin. c) The thermal conversion of hypsorhodopsin to bathorhodopsin. Curve 1c: The equilibrium mixture of rhodopsin, isorhodopsin and hypsorhodopsin similar to curves 9a and 1b. Curves 2c—8c: The products formed by warming in the dark to —259°, —250°, —239°, —229°, —221°, —210°, and —194° C respectively. The final spectrum (curve 8c) is due to a mixture of rhodopsin, isorhodopsin and bathorhodopsin (Yoshizawa and Horiuchi, hitherto unpublished)

of metarhodopsin II ($\lambda_{max} = 380$ nm), hypsorhodopsin thus has the shortest λ_{max} of the intermediates.

When exposed to short-wave light hypsorhodopsin is converted to batho-rhodopsin (Fig. 14b). Thus in Fig. 14b curve 1 represents the equilibrium mixture, consisting mainly of hypsorhodopsin, that was formed by exposure to long-wave light (curve 9, Fig. 14a). When this mixture is further irradiated with 406 nm

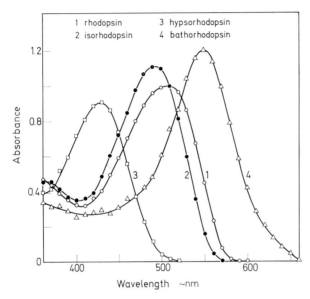

Fig. 15. The spectral absorbances of cattle rhodopsin (curve 1), isorhodopsin (curve 2), hypso-rhodopsin (curve 3) and bathorhodopsin (curve 4) at liquid-helium temperature. The maximum absorbance of rhodopsin ($\lambda_{max} = 506$ nm) is plotted arbitrarily at 1.0, and the other curves stand in quantitative relation. Isorhodopsin ($\lambda_{max} = 494$ nm), hypsorhodopsin ($\lambda_{max} = $ ca. 430 nm and bathorhodopsin ($\lambda_{max} = $ ca. 548 nm) of equivalent concentration thus possess maximum absorbances about 1.12, 0.91 and 1.21 times that of rhodopsin (YOSHIZAWA and HORIUCHI, to be published)

light there is an opposite shift of spectrum to the "red". During the early period of this irradiation (curves 1—4 in Fig. 14b) the curves have an isosbestic point at 476 nm due to the conversion of hypsorhodopsin to bathorhodopsin. In the later part of the irradiation, however, the curve-intersection point moves from 476 nm towards longer wavelengths. This is probably because of the production of batho-rhodopsin from the rhodopsin and isorhodopsin already present in the mixture at the outset. Thus cattle rhodopsin when irradiated at liquid-helium temperature with 437 nm light converts to a mixture of rhodopsin, isorhodopsin and (mainly) bathorhodopsin (Fig. 16a) while further irradiation with orange light (> 600 nm) brings the mixture back, i.e., mainly to rhodopsin with, possibly, a little isorhodop-sin (Fig. 16b).

It should be noted that there is no evidence for the photochemical transfor-mation of bathorhodopsin into hypsorhodopsin. On the other hand, conversion of hypsorhodopsin into bathorhodopsin can occur, not only photochemically but also in darkness by simply raising the temperature above − 250° C (Fig. 14c). These facts suggest that hypsorhodopsin is an earlier intermediate than bathorhodopsin in the photolysis of rhodopsin, though this is not certain for the following reasons. In the first place the conversion of rhodopsin to hypsorhodopsin is not a simple process (Fig. 14a), isorhodopsin being formed as well. When isorhodopsin

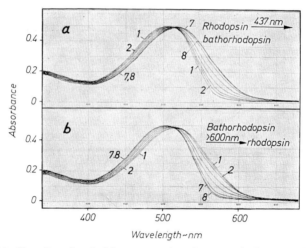

Fig. 16a and b. The photochemical interconversions between rhodopsin and bathorhodopsin at liquid-helium temperature. a) The course of photoconversion of rhodopsin to an equilibrium mixture, mainly of rhodopsin and bathorhodopsin but with a little isorhodopsin. Curve 1a: Cattle rhodopsin in a 2 : 1 glycerol/water mixture at 7 °K. Curves 2a—8a: The products of irradiation by 437 nm after successive exposure periods of 1, 1, 2, 4, 8, 16, and 32 min. The final spectrum (curve 8a) is due to an equilibrium mixture of rhodopsin, bathorhodopsin and isorhodopsin. b) The course of photoreversion of bathorhodopsin to (mainly) rhodopsin. Curve 1b: The equilibrium mixture of rhodopsin, bathorhodopsin and (some) isorhodopsin (cf. curve 8a). Curves 2b—8b: The products of irradiation by wavelengths longer than 600 nm after successive exposure periods of 0.5, 0.5, 1, 2, 4, 8, and 16 sec. The final spectrum (curve 8b) is due to rhodopsin with a small amount of isorhodopsin (Yoshizawa and Horiuchi, to be published)

is similarly illuminated it converts to rhodopsin with some formation of hypsorhodopsin in the early part of the irradiation. Second, the irradiation of rhodopsin with 579-nm light (which both hypsorhodopsin and isorhodopsin hardly absorb) results mainly in the production of isorhodopsin and only a little hypsorhodopsin. Third, the kinetics of the formation of bathorhodopsin by irradiation of rhodopsin with 437-nm light fits the simpler scheme:

$$\text{Rhodopsin} \underset{hv}{\overset{hv}{\rightleftarrows}} \text{Bathorhodopsin}$$

better than the alternative:

$$\text{Rhodopsin} \xrightarrow{hv} \text{Hypsorhodopsin} \xrightarrow{hv} \text{Bathorhodopsin}$$

These considerations suggest that it is premature to conclude that hypsorhodopsin is the first photoproduct in the photolysis of rhodopsin. All that can be said with certainty is that at the temperature of liquid helium, any of the chromo-proteins rhodopsin, isorhodopsin, hypsorhodopsin and bathorhodopsin can be converted into any other, either directly or indirectly, by suitable radiation.

B. The Batho-Intermediate

The batho-intermediates so far discovered are, in general, characterized by the possession of a longer λ_{max} and a greater ε_{max} than either their parent pigment or any other of their intermediate forms (Table 2). The only exception is squid bathorhodopsin ($\lambda_{max} = 543$ nm) which has a lower ε_{max} than the alkaline form of squid metarhodopsin ($\lambda_{max} = 380$ nm). The thermostability of the batho-intermediates varies from species to species but all are stable at the temperature of liquid nitrogen (Table 3). The batho-intermediates are formed by irradiation

Table 2. *Absorption properties of visual pigments and their intermediates*

	Measured at (°C)	Absorption property	Cattle rhodopsin	Squid rhodopsin	Chicken iodopsin	Carp porphyropsin
isual pigment (11-*cis*)	R.T.	λ_{max} (nm)	498[e]	493[c]	562[f]	522[h]
		ε_{max}	40,600[e]	40,600[c]	40,600[f]	30,000[g]
	—195	λ_{max}	505[j]	498[k]	575[l]	528[h]
		$\varepsilon_{-195}/\varepsilon_{R.T.}$	1.14[i]	1.15[k]	—	1.06[h]
so (9-*cis*)	R.T.	λ_{max} (nm)	485[j]	473[k]	510[l]	506[h]
		ε_{max}	43,000[j]	47,700[k]	—	30,100[h]
	—195	λ_{max} (nm)	491[j]	481[k]	550[l]	514[h]
		$\varepsilon_{-195}/\varepsilon_{R.T.}$	1.13[i]	1.12[k]	—	1.10[h]
ypso (ll-*trans*)	—269	λ_{max} (nm)	430[i]	—	—	—
		$\varepsilon_{H}/\varepsilon_{R}$	0.91[i]	—	—	—
atho (ll-*trans*)	—195	λ_{max} (nm)	543[j]	543[k]	640[l]	592[h]
		$\varepsilon_{B}/\varepsilon_{R}$	1.13[j]	1.39[k]	1.50[l]	1.48[h]
umi (ll-*trans*)	—65	λ_{max} (nm)	497[b]	530[k,1]	518[l]	542[h,1]
		$\varepsilon_{L}/\varepsilon_{R}$	1.15[b]	1.03[k,1]	—	1.16[h,1]
eta I (ll-*trans*)	—65	λ_{max} (nm)	481[b]	500[b,α]	495[b,2]	509[h,1]
		$\varepsilon_{MI}/\varepsilon_{R}$	1.06[b]	1.36[b,α]	—	1.07[h,1]
eta II (ll-*trans*)	above 0	λ_{max} (nm)	380[d]	380[b,β]	380[l]	408[a]
		$\varepsilon_{MII}/\varepsilon_{R}$	1.00[d]	1.50[b,β]	—	1.11[a]

Notes: $\varepsilon_{-195}/\varepsilon_{R.T.}$: Ratio of maximum absorbance of the pigment at —195° C to that at room temperature. $\varepsilon_{H}/\varepsilon_{R}$, $\varepsilon_{B}/\varepsilon_{R}$, $\varepsilon_{L}/\varepsilon_{R}$, $\varepsilon_{MI}/\varepsilon_{R}$ and $\varepsilon_{MII}/\varepsilon_{R}$ are the ratios of the maximum absorbances of hypso, batho, lumi, metarhodopsin I and II, respectively, to that of rhodopsin at the temperature shown in the second column.
[α] Acid metarhodopsin, [β] Alkaline metarhodopsin, [1] Measured at about —190° C, [2] at — 38° C. Data are from following sources: [a] Bridges (1967), [b] Hubbard and Kropf (1959a), [c] Hubbard and St. George (1958), [d] Matthews, Hubbard, Brown, and Wald, (1964), [e] Wald and Brown (1953), [f] Wald, Brown, and Smith, (1955), [g] Wald, Brown, and Brown, (1963), [h] Yoshizawa and Horiuchi (1969), [i] Yoshizawa and Horiuchi (to be published), [j] Yoshizawa and Wald (1963), [k] Yoshizawa and Wald (1964), [l] Yoshizawa and Wald (1967).

of visual pigment at this temperature. Normally an equilibrium mixture of visual pigment, isopigment and batho-intermediate results. On irradiation with light of wavelength 30—50 nm shorter than the visual pigment λ_{max}, the proportion of bathorhodopsin in the mixture is maximal (Yoshizawa and Wald, 1963, 1964, 1967; Yoshizawa and Horiuchi, 1969).

Table 3. *Temperatures at which intermediates begin to transform to the next intermediates*

Visual pigment	Batho	Lumi	Meta I	Meta II
Cattle rhodopsin	—140°	—40°	—15°	0°
Squid rhodopsin	—170°	—60°	+20° (a)	+20° (b)
Chicken iodopsin	—180°	—45°	—30°	0°
Carp porphyropsin	—180°	—60°	—10°	0°

(a) acid metarhodopsin; (b) alkaline metarhodopsin.

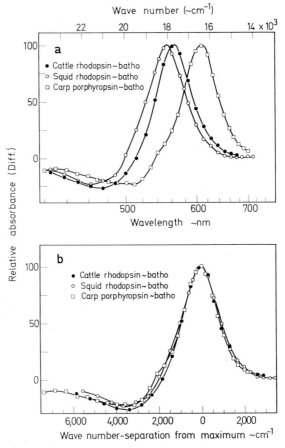

Fig. 17a and b. Comparison of the spectral differences between the visual pigment and its batho-intermediate among different species. a) The spectral differences for cattle, squid and carp are plotted against a regular wave-number scale. b) The same as a, but with the curves translated along the horizontal axis so that their maxima coincide

It has already been noted that the spectral absorbance curve of bathoporphy-ropsin has a shoulder (at 540 nm), a feature not found in the batho-intermediates of A_1-based pigments (Figs. 13 and 15). Nevertheless, the spectral difference curve between visual pigment and batho-intermediate is the same shape for both A_1- and A_2-based systems when the curves are plotted on a regular frequency (as distinct from wavelength) scale (Fig. 17) — even though the spectra of the parent pigments are so different at low temperature (Figs. 10 and 11). This suggests that the conversion of visual pigment to batho-intermediate is independent of the β-ionone ring part of the prosthetic group and depends only on the photoisomeri-zation (from 11-*cis* to all-*trans*) of the polyene chain part.

It has been reported that the opsin moiety of iodopsin behaves differently from that of other visual pigments in several respects, e.g. stability to alum, hydroxylamine, *p*-chloromercuribenzole, etc.; and in reaction velocity constant of regeneration, which is about 500 times that of the rhodopsin case (WALD, BROWN, and SMITH, 1955). In spite of this the photochemical behaviour of iodopsin at liquid-nitrogen temperature resembles that of rhodopsin, and in Fig. 18 (left hand side) the conversion of iodopsin, when irradiated with 546-nm light, to an equi-librium mixture of iodopsin and bathoiodopsin is shown. On the other hand there is a striking difference between the behaviour of bathoiodopsin and the batho-intermediates of other pigments when warmed in the dark; bathorhodopsin and

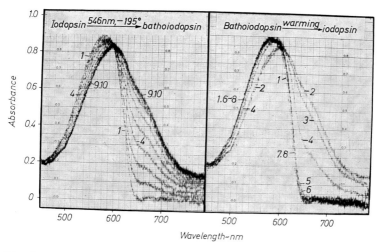

Fig. 18. The photoconversion of iodopsin to bathoiodopsin (left) and the thermal reversion of bathoiodopsin to iodopsin (right). *Left:* Curve 1: Chicken iodopsin in a 1 : 1 glycerol/water mixture at —195° C (λ_{max} = 575 nm) after intensification by the Keilin-Hartree procedure. Curves 2—10: The products of irradiation by 546 nm after successive exposure periods of 1, 1, 2, 4, 8, 16, 32, 64, and 128 sec. The final spectrum (curve 10, left) is due to an equilibrium mixture of iodopsin and bathoiodopsin. *Right:* Curve 1: Iodopsin at —195° C (identical with curve 1, left). Curve 2: The equilibrium mixture of iodopsin and bathoiodopsin (identical with curve 10, left). Curves 3—8: The products formed by warming in the dark to —180°, —160°, —140°, —120°, —100°, and —80° C respectively and re-cooling each time to —195° C to record the spectrum (YOSHIZAWA and WALD, 1967)

bathoporphyropsin are converted to their respective lumi-intermediates, whereas bathoiodopsin reverts to iodopsin (Fig. 18, right hand side). Yoshizawa and Wald (1967) have interpreted these results as follows. When light isomerises the chromophoric group of a visual pigment from the 11-*cis* to the all-*trans* form, the molecule is in a highly strained condition (batho-intermediate). The strain can be thermally relieved in two ways — by re-isomerization of the chromophoric group back to 11-*cis*, or by a change in the opsin. In the bathorhodopsin and batho-porphyropsin case relief is obtained by an opsin change with formation of the lumi-intermediate; in bathoiodopsin the chromophoric group isomerizes to 11-*cis* with reversion to the parent pigment.

C. The Lumi-Intermediate

Although, with the exception of bathoiodopsin, the lumi-intermediate can be formed by warming the corresponding batho-intermediate, the most convenient way of producing lumi-intermediates is by irradiating the visual pigments at dry-ice temperature. The λ_{max} of a lumi-intermediate is shorter than that of its batho-intermediate, but may be either shorter or longer than that of its parent visual pigment (Table 2). Thus the λ_{max} of squid lumirhodopsin is about 30 nm longer than that of squid rhodopsin (Yoshizawa and Wald, 1964) while the λ_{max} of chicken lumi-iodopsin is about 40 nm shorter than that of its parent pigment (Yoshizawa and Wald, 1967). The ε_{max} of the lumi-intermediates are usually greater than those of the originating visual pigments, but lower values have been reported in the cases of the octopus and bullfrog (Hubbard and Kropf, 1959a; Hubbard, Brown, and Kropf, 1959). In spite of these species differences, how-ever, the spectral absorbance curves of the lumi-intermediates are all much the same shape (on a frequency basis).

As shown in Table 3, the transition temperature for the change from batho- to lumi-intermediate varies with species, owing, presumably, to species differences in the opsin structures. This may mean that the thermal conversion of batho- to lumi-intermediate involves some changes in the opsin structure. These confor-mational changes can be reversed by irradiation of the lumi-intermediate at liquid-nitrogen temperature, when the parent visual pigment or isopigment are first formed, and then the batho-intermediate. This photochemical conversion of lumi- to batho-intermediate has been shown to occur perfectly in the squid rhodopsin system (Yoshizawa and Wald, 1964), but is not complete in the case of cattle rhodopsin (Yoshizawa, 1962; Yoshizawa and Wald, 1963). The mecha-nism of the conversion is probably as follows: the first photon absorbed by the lumi-intermediate molecule isomerizes the chromophoric group from the all-*trans* configuration to the 11-*cis* one, and the residual energy from the absorbed photon induces the re-arrangements of opsin needed to form visual pigment or isopigment. Then the absorption of another photon further isomerizes the chromophoric group back to all-*trans*, to form the batho-intermediate (Yoshizawa and Wald, 1963).

The behaviour of iodopsin at dry-ice temperature differs from that of other visual pigments in that lumi-iodopsin is not generally formed (but see below). This is because of the thermal reversion of bathoiodopsin to iodopsin. Thus Hubbard and Kropf (1959b) reported that the photosensitivity of iodopsin decreases markedly on lowering the temperature, and irradiation of iodopsin at dry-ice temperature with green light (546 nm) causes no change of spectrum. Apparently, the green light photoisomerizes iodopsin to bathoiodopsin, which then reverts thermally to iodopsin so rapidly that no change is observed. When isoiodopsin is irradiated under the same conditions, it is converted to iodopsin (Fig. 19). This transformation apparently involves the photoisomerization of iso-iodopsin to bathoiodopsin, which is then thermally converted to iodopsin. Never-theless, on irradiation of iodopsin at dry-ice temperature with intense orange-red light, which lumi-iodopsin hardly absorbs, the latter is slowly trapped as a photo-product (Fig. 19). Re-irradiation of the lumi-iodopsin formed with the green light converts it to iodopsin for, in spite of the fact that the green light is absorbed more effectively by iodopsin than by lumi-iodopsin, the iodopsin is effectively inert because of the rapid thermal reversion from bathoiodopsin mentioned above.

This unique behaviour of iodopsin at low temperature can be attributed to the two competing thermal pathways open to bathoiodopsin; one to lumi-iodopsin, the other back to iodopsin. Which of them takes precedence depends on the tem-perature of irradiation. At lower temperatures bathoiodopsin preferentially reverts to iodopsin, while at higher temperatures the forward reaction to lumi-iodopsin is predominant (YOSHIZAWA and WALD, 1967).

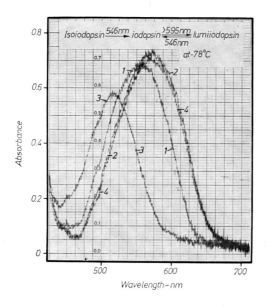

Fig. 19. The photochemical interconversions between isoiodopsin, iodopsin and lumiiodopsin at dry-ice temperature. Curve 1: Isoiodopsin, synthesized from 9-*cis* retinal and chicken cone opsin, in a 1 : 1 glycerol/water mixture at — 78° C, after intensification by the Keilin-Hartree procedure. Irradiation by 546 nm for 10 min converted this almost entirely to iodopsin (curve 2). Irradiation at —78° C for 128 min by wavelengths longer than 595 nm then converted the iodopsin almost wholly to lumiiodopsin (curve 3). Re-irradiation at 546 nm for 40 min brought it back to iodopsin (curve 4) (YOSHIZAWA and WALD, 1967)

D. The Meta-Intermediates

When a "vertebrate" lumi-intermediate is warmed in the dark, it is converted to the meta-intermediate I, and there is a hypsochromic shift in the spectral absorbance. Meta-intermediate I also can be produced by irradiating the visual pigment at about $-20°$ C in solution or at room temperature in the dry state. Irradiation of vertebrate visual pigment under these conditions yields an equilibrium mixture of visual pigment, isopigment and meta-intermediate I, these components being perfectly interconvertible by light. However, irradiation at $-65°$ C or $-195°$ C does not convert meta-intermediate I to visual pigment or isopigment (HUBBARD, BROWN, and KROPF, 1959; YOSHIZAWA and WALD, 1963). This indicates that the structural changes in opsin corresponding to the transformation of lumi- to meta-intermediate are too large to permit the reverse reaction at these low temperatures. In general the λ_{max} of meta-intermediate I lies at a shorter wavelength than that of its parent visual pigment (Table 2). According to HUBBARD, BROWN, and KROPF (1959), the shapes of the spectra of the metarhodopsins I exhibit little species variation when presented on a frequency scale. The meta-intermediates I from different species do vary, however, in their thermostabilities (Table 3).

An apparently exceptional metarhodopsin I is that derived from the cusk. Cusk metarhodopsin I has λ_{max} at 507 nm, a longer wavelength than that of its parent rhodopsin (500 nm), and also of the metarhodopsins I from other species (482 to 489 nm); the shape of its spectrum is also different from that of other metarhodopsins I (HUBBARD, BROWN, and KROPF, 1959). These peculiar properties of spectral absorbance are attributable to the thermostability of cusk metarhodopsin I, which decomposes more readily than those of the others. Thus, before the conversion of cusk lumirhodopsin to metarhodopsin I is complete, some metarhodopsin I begins to transform to the next product (probably metarhodopsin II). It is therefore likely that the λ_{max} of cusk "metarhodopsin" represents a mixture of lumirhodopsin and metarhodopsin I.

When warmed in the dark, meta-intermediate I enters into a tautomeric equilibrium with meta-intermediate II. In the case of the cattle rhodopsin system, this involves the large displacement of λ_{max} from 478 nm to 380 nm. This conversion is accompanied by the net uptake of a proton by a group with pK 6.4 (possibly an imidazole group of a histidine residue on opsin) and by some re-arrangement of opsin structure. In contrast to the preceding reactions, the conversion of metarhodopsin I to II is reversible. Increase in temperature, in acidity or in ionic strength, and the replacement of water by glycerol or methanol, all shift the equilibrium towards metarhodopsin II (MATTHEWS, HUBBARD, BROWN, and WALD, 1964). Chicken metaiodopsin and carp metaporphyropsin appear to behave in a similar way to cattle metarhodopsin (HUBBARD, BOWNDS, and YOSHIZAWA, 1965; BRIDGES, 1967).

"Invertebrate" metarhodopsins differ in thermostability from the "vertebrate" metarhodopsins; cephalopod metarhodopsins, such as those of the squid, octopus and cuttlefish, are quite stable even at room temperature (HUBBARD and ST. GEORGE, 1958; BROWN and BROWN, 1958; KROPF, BROWN, and HUBBARD, 1959; HARA and HARA, 1965, 1967; HARA, HARA, and TAKEUCHI, 1967), and arthropod metarhodopsins, such as those of lobsters, crabs, crayfishes, appear to decay very slowly at room temperature (WALD and HUBBARD, 1957; GOLDSMITH and FERNANDEZ, 1966; HUBBARD and WALD, 1960; WALD, 1967a). Cephalopod and possibly other invertebrate metarhodopsins also behave as pH indicators, but the fundamental difference between vertebrate and cephalopod rhodopsins is the fact that the equilibrium between two forms of metarhodopsins is affected by pH in completely opposite ways. Thus cephalopod metarhodopsins are red ($\lambda_{max} = 475-500$ nm) in neutral and mildly acid solution (acid metarhodopsin) and yellow (378−380 nm) in alkaline solution, there being some species differences in λ_{max}. The pK of cephalopod metarhodopsin varies from 7.3 (*Octopus ocellatus*) to 9.1 (*Ommastrephes sloani pacificus*) (TAKEUCHI, 1966).

In addition to the hydrolysis of meta-intermediate II to all-*trans* retinal, or dehydroretinal, and opsin this intermediate exhibits another reaction on warming above 0° C (MATTHEWS, HUBBARD, BROWN, and WALD, 1964). Thus, in the dark at 3° C, metarhodopsin II is slowly converted to pararhodopsin ($\lambda_{max} = 465$ nm) (WALD, 1967b). All those conditions that favour the conversion of metarhodopsin I to metarhodopsin II favour also the formation of pararhodopsin. When warmed above 5° C, pararhodopsin hydrolyzes to retinal and opsin. The conversion of metarhodopsin II to pararhodopsin is reversible in the light but not in the dark. Irradiation of metarhodopsin II with ultraviolet light yields pararhodopsin, and subsequent irradiation with visible light reverses the process. From a consideration of the photoreversibility of pararhodopsin MATTHEWS, HUBBARD, BROWN, and WALD (1964) suggested that its chromophoric group may be a *cis*-isomer of retinal other than 9- or 11-*cis* (i.e. presumably 13-*cis*). They considered pararhodopsin to be an artifact that does not ordinarily enter into the bleaching sequence. On the other hand, OSTROY, ERHARDT, and ABRAHAMSON (1966), from studies on the kinetics of thermal decay of intermediates, concluded that the conversion of metarhodopsin II to pararhodopsin (meta 465) was a refolding process of the opsin, and the thermal decay of pararhodopsin a folding one. Furthermore they believe that pararhodopsin (meta 465) is a genuine intermediate in the bleaching process of rhodopsin. This opinion seems to be supported by measurements of the early receptor potential of the retina or excised eye (WALD, 1967b; CONE, 1967; EBREY, 1968).

VII. Mechanism of the Bleaching Process

We have seen that the bleaching of a visual pigment is characterized by the appearance of a succession of coloured intermediates, all with their characteristic spectral properties. Before attempting to interpret the properties of these intermediates, one must consider the relationship between the chromophoric group and the opsin in the original visual pigment molecule. This consideration is here confined to a qualitative explanation, and the reader is referred to Chapter 3 for a more quantitative treatment.

It is generally accepted that in the visual pigment molecule a chromophoric group based on 11-*cis* retinal (or dehydroretinal) is bound to opsin in a Schiff-base linkage formed by the condensation of the aldehyde group of retinal with an amino group of opsin (COLLINS, 1953; MORTON and PITT, 1955). This amino group has recently been identified in cattle rhodopsin as the ε-NH$_2$ group of lysine (BOWNDS, 1967). The Schiff-base linkage shifts the absorbance maximum of 11-*cis* retinal from 380 nm to about 367 nm. Acidification causes a bathochromic shift to about 440 nm, owing to the formation of the protonated Schiff base (COLLINS, 1953; MORTON and PITT, 1955). In order to account for the shift to the position of rhodopsin's λ_{max}, DARTNALL (1957), HUBBARD (1958), and KROPF and HUBBARD (1958) assumed that the chromophoric group closely fits the surface structure of opsin, so as to result in a strong interaction between the two parts. HUBBARD and KROPF (*loc. cit.*) considered that this interaction was principally between a negative charge on opsin, such as COO$^-$, and a positive charge of the nitrogen atom on the binding site. Recently, KITO, SUZUKI, AZUMA, and SEKO-GUTI (1968) reported that cattle rhodopsin that has been denatured with trichloro-acetic acid, so that its λ_{max} falls to 440 nm, displays a bathochromic shift to 495 nm when cooled to liquid-nitrogen temperature. They considered that this shift may be due to the second linkage between a carboxyl group of opsin and the chromophoric group in an acidic and proton-rich environment. At the same time ERICKSON and BLATZ (1968) showed that a protonated Schiff base displays a bathochromic shift ($\lambda_{max} = 490$ nm) in a nonpolar solvent (1,2-dichloroethane) with perchloric acid. Thus they suggested that the λ_{max} of visual pigment may simply be dependent upon the dielectric constant of the local environment about the chromophoric group, and upon the association between the cation and its counter-ion. In any event it seems reasonable to suppose that the bathochromic shift depends upon the strength of the interaction between chromophoric group and opsin. KROPF (1962) stated some years ago that changing the configuration of the chromophore would result in a shift in λ_{max} and that, likewise, conform-ational changes in the opsin would also cause other shifts.

Cooling to liquid-helium temperature has almost no effect on the interaction between the secondary linkages and the environment around the chromophoric group, as judged by the spectral absorbance at this temperature (Fig. 10). Photo-isomerization of the 11-*cis* chromophoric group, however, involves breakdown of some of the secondary linkages, and a re-interaction of the resulting all-*trans* chromophoric group to the opsin. The formation of hypso- and bathorhodopsins by irradiation at liquid-helium temperature may fairly be attributed to a con-figurational change in the chromophoric group, for the opsin is hardly likely to change at this temperature. Judged from its spectroscopic properties, hypso-rhodopsin may possess little or no interaction between its chromophoric group and opsin, while bathorhodopsin may possess a strong interaction between them. If hypsorhodopsin is an earlier intermediate than bathorhodopsin, the process of photoisomerization of rhodopsin can be accounted for as follows: In the excited state, the chromophoric group, because of the breakdown of the secondary link-ages, is potentially free to undergo simultaneous rotations about the (originally) single or double bonds in the polyene chain. The particular pathway of such con-formational changes, however, would be governed by the surface structure of opsin surrounding the chromophoric group. Thus, rotation about the 11—12 double bond (Fig. 6), for example, might be preceded by rotation about any single bond (from s-*trans* to s-*cis* or vice versa) in order to avoid interference with the opsin structure. Such an isomerization would result in little or no interaction between the chromophoric group and opsin, and could be the model to account for the spectroscopic properties and thermostability of hypsorhodopsin. Upon the absorption of a further photon, or on warming above $23°$ K in the dark, however, the chromophoric group might again undergo a rotation about the same (or other) single bond, with the consequent establishment of a new side chain that interfered strongly with opsin to give a highly strained and distorted molecule (bathorhodopsin). The strained condition of such a molecule, in which the potential energy of the ground state would be high, could account both for the instability and the bathochromic shift (YOSHIZAWA and WALD, 1963).

The first thermal re-arrangement of opsin, which appears in the change from batho- to lumi-intermediate, would allow the relaxation of this strained condition, resulting in an all-*trans* chromophoric group of normal geometry. Thus interaction between the chromophoric group and opsin would become weaker, the energy-level of the ground state would fall and the spectrum would shift to shorter wavelengths. According to flash photolytic studies on cattle rhodopsin (GRELLMANN, LIVINGSTON, and PRATT, 1962; PRATT, LIVINGSTON, and GRELLMANN, 1964), the activation energy for this conversion is 10 kcal per mole, and the entropy of activation is zero, or close to it. These kinetic parameters suggest that the transition from batho- to lumi-intermediate involves only minor conformational changes.

According to HUBBARD, BOWNDS, and YOSHIZAWA (1965), the first large changes in kinetic parameters occur in the next step in the bleaching sequence, i.e. from lumirhodopsin to metarhodopsin I, indicating a large conformational change in the opsin structure. ERHARDT, OSTROY, and ABRAHAMSON (1966) reported quite different kinetic parameters for this conversion and suggested it was a charge orientation process. For further details the reader is referred to Chapter 3.

The chromophoric group (11-*cis* retinal or dehydroretinal) of a visual pigment is the veritable trigger of visual excitation. It is not stereotyped; it is, *per contra*, so adoptable that, by suitable changes of its geometry, it can accommodate to the key site of any particular opsin, and thus, when pulled, can induce that conformational change in protein by which visual excitation is initiated.

Acknowledgments

The recent work described in this Chapter was supported by The National Institute of Neurological Diseases and Blindness of The National Institutes of Health (No. NB-06204). I express my sincere thanks to Mr. S. HORIUCHI and Miss H. SAKASHITA for generous assistance. I am also grateful to Dr. H. J. A. DARTNALL for his considerable help in the preparation of the manuscript.

References

BOWNDS, D.: Site of attachment of retinal in rhodopsin. Nature (Lond.) **216**, 1178—1181 (1967).
BRIDGES, C. D. B.: Spectroscopic properties of porphyropsins. Vision Res. **7**, 349—369 (1967).
BRODA, E. E., GOODEVE, C. F.: The behaviour of visual purple at low temperature. Proc. roy. Soc. A **179**, 151—159 (1941).
BROWN, P. K., BROWN, P. S.: Visual pigments of the octopus and cuttlefish. Nature (Lond.) **182**, 1288—1290 (1958).
— WALD, G.: The neo-b isomer of vitamin A and retinene. J. biol. Chem. **222**, 865—877 (1956).

Collins, F. D.: Rhodopsin and indicator yellow. Nature (Lond.) **171**, 469—471 (1953).
— Morton, R. A.: Studies in rhodopsin 3: Rhodopsin and transient orange. Biochem. J. **47**, 18—24 (1950).
Cone, R. A.: Early receptor potential: Photoreversible charge displacement in rhodopsin. Science **155**, 1128—1130 (1967).
Cunningham, J., Tompkins, F. C.: Spectra of sodium and potassium azide crystals coloured by ultraviolet and X-ray radiation. Proc. roy. Soc. A **251**, 27—40 (1959).
Dartnall, H. J. A.: The visual pigments. London, Methuen & Co: New York, John Wiley & Sons, Inc. (1957).
Ebrey, T. G.: The thermal decay of the intermediates of rhodopsin in situ. Vision Res. **8**, 965—982 (1968).
Erhardt, F., Ostroy, S. E., Abrahamson, E. W.: Protein configuration changes in the photolysis of rhodopsin. 1. The thermal decay of cattle lumirhodopsin in vitro. Biochim. biophys. Acta (Amst.) **112**, 256—264 (1966).
Erickson, J. O., Blatz, P. E.: N-retinylidene-1-amino-2-propanol: A Schiff base analog for rhodopsin. Vision Res. **8**, 1367—1375 (1968).
Estabrook, R. W.: The low temperature spectra of hemoproteins. I. Apparatus and its application to a study of cytochrome C. J. biol. Chem. **223**, 781—794 (1956).
Goldsmith, T. H., Fernandez, H. R.: Some photochemical and physiological aspects of visual excitation in compound eyes. In: The functional organization of the compound eye. London: Pergamon Press (1966).
Grellmann, K.-H., Livingston, R., Pratt, D.: A flash-photolytic investigation of rhodopsin at low temperatures: Nature (Lond.) **193**, 1258—1260 (1962).
Hara, T., Hara, R.: New photosensitive pigment found in the retina of the squid Ommastrephes. Nature (Lond.) **206**, 1331—1334 (1965).
— — Vision in octopus and squid. Rhodopsin and retinochrome in the squid retina. Nature (Lond.) **214**, 573—575 (1967).
— — Takeuchi, J.: Vision in octopus and squid. Rhodopsin and retinochrome in the octopus retina. Nature (Lond.) **214**, 572—573 (1967).
Hausser, K. W., Kuhn, R., Seitz, G.: Lichtabsorption und Doppelbindung. V. Über die Absorption von Verbindungen mit Konjugierten. Kohlenstoffdoppelbindungen bei tiefer Temperatur. Z. phys. Chem. **29**, 391—416 (1935).
Hubbard, R.: Retinene isomerase. J. gen. Physiol. **39**, 935—962 (1956).
— On the chromophores of the visual pigments. In: Visual problems of colour, No. 8, pp. 153 to 169. London: H. M. Stationary Office (1958).
— Bownds, D., Yoshizawa, T.: The chemistry of visual photoreception. Cold Spr. Harb. Symp. quant. Biol. **30**, 301—315 (1965).
— Brown, P. K., Kropf, A.: Action of light on visual pigments. Vertebrate lumi- and meta-rhodopsins. Nature (Lond.) **183**, 442—446 (1959).
— St. George, R. C. C.: The rhodopsin system of the squid. J. gen. Physiol. **41**, 501—528 (1958).
— Kropf, A.: The action of light on rhodopsin. Proc. natl. Acad. Sci. **44**, 130—139 (1958).
— — Molecular aspects of visual excitation. Ann. N. Y. Acad. Sci. **81**, 388—398 (1959a).
— — Action of light on visual pigments. Chicken lumi- and meta-iodopsin. Nature (Lond.) **183**, 448—450 (1959b).
— Wald, G.: Cis-trans isomers of vitamin A and retinene in the rhodopsin system. J. gen. Physiol. **36**, 269—315 (1952).
— — Visual pigment of the horseshoe crab, Limulus polyphemus. Nature (Lond.) **186**, 212—215 (1960).
Jurkowitz, L.: Photochemical and stereochemical properties of carotenoids at low temperatures. (1) Photochemical behaviour of retinene. Nature (Lond.) **184**, 614—617 (1959).
Keilin, D. F. R. S., Hartree, E. F.: Effect of low temperature on the absorption spectra of haemoproteins; with observations on the absorption spectrum of oxygen. Nature (Lond.) **164**, 254—259 (1949).
— — Further observations on absorption spectra at low temperatures. Nature (Lond.) **165**, 504—505 (1950).
Kitô, Y., Ishigami, M., Yoshizawa, T.: On the labile intermediate of rhodopsin as demonstrated by low temperature illumination. Biochim. biophys. Acta (Amst.) **48**, 287—298 (1961).

KITÔ, Y., SUZUKI, T., AZUMA, M., SEKOGUTI, Y.: Absorption spectrum of rhodopsin denatured with acid. Nature (Lond.) **218**, 955—956 (1968).
— YOSHIZAWA, T.: Photochemical properties of rhodopsin at low temperature. Ann. Zool. Jap. **33**, 7—13 (1960).
KROPF, A.: The role of geometrical isomerism in the visual process. Symp. Reversible Photochemical Processes, at Durham, preprint 592—609 (1962).
— BROWN, P. K., HUBBARD, R.: Action of light on visual pigments. Lumi- and metarhodopsins of squid and octopus. Nature (Lond.) **183**, 446—448 (1959).
— HUBBARD, R.: The mechanism of bleaching rhodopsin. Ann. N. Y. Acad. Sci. **74**, 266—280 (1958).
LOEB, J. N., BROWN, P. K., WALD, G.: Photochemical and stereochemical properties of carotenoids at low temperatures. (2) Cis-trans isomerism and steric hindrance. Nature (Lond.) **184**, 617—620 (1959).
LYTHGOE, R. J.: The absorption spectra of visual purple and of indicator yellow. J. Physiol. (Lond.) **89**, 331—358 (1937).
— QUILLIAM, J. P.: The relation of transient orange to visual purple and indicator yellow. J. Physiol. (Lond.) **94**, 399—410 (1938).
MATTHEWS, R. G., HUBBARD, R., BROWN, P. K., WALD, G.: Tautomeric forms of metarhodopsin. J. gen. Physiol. **47**, 215—240 (1963—1964).
MORTON, R. A., PITT, G. A. J.: Studies on rhodopsin. 9: pH and the hydrolysis of indicator yellow. Biochem. J. **59**, 128—134 (1955).
MULLIKEN, R. S.: Intensities of electronic transitions in molecular spectra III. Organic molecules with double bonds. Conjugated dienes. J. chem. Phys. **7**, 121—135 (1939).
OSTROY, S. E., ERHARDT, F., ABRAHAMSON, E. W.: Protein configuration changes in the photolysis of rhodopsin. II. The sequence of intermediates in thermal decay of cattle metarhodopsin *in vitro*. Biochim. biophys. Acta (Amst.) **112**, 265—277 (1966).
PRATT, D. C., LIVINGSTON, R., GRELLMANN, K.-H.: Flash Photolysis of rod particle suspensions. Photochem. and Photobiol. **3**, 121—127 (1964).
TAKEUCHI, J.: Photosensitive pigments in the cephalopod retinas. J. Nara med. Ass. (in Japanese) **17**, 433—448 (1966).
WALD, G.: Photochemical and stereochemical properties of carotenoids at low temperatures: (3) Discussion. Nature (Lond.) **184**, 620—624 (1959).
— Visual pigments of crayfish. Nature (Lond.) **215**, 1131—1133 (1967a).
— The molecular basis of visual excitation. Nobel lecture, preprint 1—21 (1967b).
— BROWN, P. K.: The molar extinction of rhodopsin. J. gen. Physiol. **37**, 189—200 (1953).
— — BROWN, P. S.: Quoted by BROWN, P. K., GIBBONS, I. R., WALD, G. (1963): The visual cells and visual pigment of the mudpuppy, *Necturus*. J. Cell Biol. **19**, 79—106 (1963).
— — SMITH, P. H.: Iodopsin. J. gen. Physiol. **38**, 623—681 (1955).
— DURELL, J., ST. GEORGE, R. C. C.: The light reaction in the bleaching of rhodopsin. Science **111**, 179—181 (1950).
— HUBBARD, R.: Visual pigment of a decapod crustacean. The lobster. Nature (Lond.) **180**, 278—280 (1957).
WULFF, V. J., ADAMS, R., LINSCHITZ, H., ABRAHAMSON, E. W.: Effect of flash illumination on rhodopsin in solution. Ann. N. Y. Acad. Sci. **74**, 281—290 (1958).
YOSHIZAWA, T.: Further studies on labile intermediates of rhodopsin. Ann. Rep. Sci. Works, Fac. Sci., Osaka Univ. **10**, 1—12 (1962).
— HORIUCHI, S.: Intermediates in the photolytic process of porphyropsin. Exptl. Eye. Res. **8**, 243—244 (1969).
— — Conversion of cattle rhodopsin at extremely low temperature. In preparation.
— KITÔ, Y.: Studies on rhodopsin illuminated at low temperature. Ann. Rep. Sci. Works, Fac. Sci., Osaka Univ. **6**, 27—41 (1958a).
— — Chemistry of the rhodopsin cycle. Nature (Lond.) **182**, 1604—1605 (1958b).
— — ISHIGAMI, M.: Studies on the metastable states in the rhodopsin cycle. Biochim. biophys. Acta (Amst.) **43**, 329—334 (1960).
— WALD, G.: Pre-lumirhodopsin and the bleaching of visual pigments. Nature (Lond.) **197**, 1279—1286 (1963).
— — Transformations of squid rhodopsin at low temperatures. Nature (Lond.) **201**, 340—345 (1964).
— — Visual pigments and the Keilin-Hartree effect. Nature (Lond.) **212**, 483—485 (1966).
— — Photochemistry of iodopsin. Nature (Lond.) **214**, 566—571 (1967).

Chapter 6

The Circular Dichroism and Optical Rotatory Dispersion of Visual Pigments

By

Trevor I. SHAW, London (Great Britain)

With 6 Figures

Contents

I. Introduction

A. Circular Dichroism

The phenomenon of circular dichroism is well illustrated in an experiment first performed by the French physicist COTTON (1896). One looks through a strong solution of potassium chromium tartrate, prepared from optically active tartaric acid, introducing pieces of right and left circularly polarizing material between the light and the solution. It is seen that the fields presented by the two polarizers are not identical, differing in brightness if the light is monochromatic, and in hue if white light is used. The solution preferentially absorbs one of the two forms of circularly polarized light and is said to be circularly dichroic. HAIDINGER (1847) had previously reported differences in absorption of the components of circularly polarized light by crystals of amethyst quartz but COTTON's extensive quantitative studies on solutions of coloured tartrates revealed the principal features of the phenomenon.

At this point it might be well to remind the reader of the nature of polarized light and of conventions associated with it. The electromagnetic wave theory of light associates it with both an electric and a magnetic vector, which oscillate and which are perpendicular to each other and at right angles to the direction of propagation. In unpolarized light, the electric vector has no preferred plane, while in plane polarized light its oscillations occur in a single plane. Unfortunately, the term 'plane of polarization' was used before the development of electromagnetic theory and it is now known that the 'plane of polarization' is in fact a plane at right angles to the electric vector and is therefore in the plane of the magnetic vector.

It is perhaps a little more difficult to form a mental picture of circularly polarized light than it is of plane polarized light. The following representation may help. The sinusoidal displacements of a spot in the X-axis of a cathode ray oscilloscope may be imagined as representing the electric vector found at any point traversed by a ray of plane-polarized monochromatic light. If the same sinusoidal wave form were also applied in the Y-axis then the beam would, of course, be displaced in both directions. Provided the deflections along both axes had the same maximal amplitudes but were a quarter of a wavelength out of phase then the spot would follow a circular course. In an optical mount that uses a doubly refracting material it is easily possible to delay one component of monochromatic plane polarized light by a quarter of a wavelength so that the emergent beam has an electric vector, the limit of which moves progressively round a circle: such light is called circularly polarized.

Returning to the oscilloscope representation of the electric vector of light — if the oscillations of the spot in the X- and Y-axes are not equal or, indeed, if the phase delay between the deflections in the two directions is not exactly a quarter of a wave then the beam will in general move in an ellipse. Correspondingly, a misalignment of the birefringent plate in an optical mount intended to give circularly polarized light, or a birefringent plate that gives greater or less retardation than a quarter of a wavelength will yield emergent beams that in general are elliptically polarized.

In the oscilloscope representation of the light's electric vector the spot can move either in a clockwise or in an anti-clockwise sense: so too circularly or elliptically polarized light must have a sense associated with it. When the electric vector at any point moves in a clockwise sense — when seen by an observer looking into the light beam — then the light is said to be right circularly polarized and *per contra* the anticlockwise beam is said to be left circularly polarized.

So far, the time course of the direction of the electric vector at one point in space has been considered but one can also consider the directions taken up by the electric vector as a function of distance at any particular time. If the beam is circularly polarized and is traversing a homogeneous medium the vector limit will be represented by a helix, the sense of which is determined by whether the light is right or left circularly polarized.

The right or left sense attributed to circularly or elliptically polarized light must be noted carefully because it must be consistent with the nomenclature used in another phenomenon; optically active materials rotate the plane of plane polarized light, and if this rotation is clockwise as seen by an observer looking into the light then the rotation is said to be right (dextro- or positive), while it is said to be left (laevo- or negative) if the rotation is in the opposite sense. These conventions, though now widely used have not always been employed and even relatively recent texts (for example Ditchburn, 1952, p. 380) have described positive rotations of plane polarized light as being clockwise when seen by an observer looking in the direction in which the light is travelling.

From Cotton's studies and subsequent work by Mitchell (1933), Kuhn (1933), Lowry (1935), Velluz, Legrand, and Grosjean (1965) and Crabbé (1965), several of whom used circular dichroism to elucidate organic chemical problems, it was established that optically active compounds in general discriminate between right and left circularly polarized light, absorbing one form more than the other. The effect is restricted to wavelengths where there are normal absorption bands for the material, but not all absorption bands in an optically active material necessarily show circular dichroism. This latter point is illustrated by the failure of sucrose solutions, coloured by magenta dye, to show circular dichroism in the visible region of the spectrum. Indeed the normal absorption at a particular wavelength gives no indication as to how powerful a circular dichroism is to be found at that wavelength, and when the circular dichroism is studied at wavelengths covering several normal absorption bands it can be found that one form of circularly polarized light is preferentially absorbed in one absorption band, and the opposite form in another band.

The usual way of expressing the effect quantitatively is by the difference between the molar extinction coefficients of the substance for left and right circularly polarized light. This difference, $(\varepsilon_L - \varepsilon_R)_\lambda$, is called the circular dichroic extinction, $\Delta\varepsilon_\lambda$, and can be either positive or negative; for example, the values of $\Delta\varepsilon_\lambda$, for enantiomorphs are opposite in sign at all wavelengths. To evaluate $\Delta\varepsilon_\lambda$, the molecular weight of the pigment must be known. Measurements are made of the optical densities $(D_L)_\lambda$ and $(D_R)_\lambda$ (or directly of their differences, $(D_L - D_R)_\lambda = \Delta D_\lambda$), and $\Delta\varepsilon_\lambda$ is calculated from the relation $\Delta\varepsilon_\lambda = \Delta D_\lambda/c.l$ where c is the concentration of the material in moles per litre and l is the path length of light through that material in centimetres. The relation between the molar extinction coefficients for unpolarized light, $(\varepsilon_N)_\lambda$ and for circularly polarized lights is taken as

$$(\varepsilon_N)_\lambda = \frac{(\varepsilon_L + \varepsilon_R)_\lambda}{2} \ .$$

A secondary phenomenon associated with circular dichroism gives an alternative method of expressing it quantitatively. Plane polarized light can be regarded as composed of equal parts of right and left circularly polarized forms, and, therefore, on traversing a circularly dichroic material, in which one form is preferentially absorbed, the beam becomes elliptically polarized. The extent to which this occurs can be measured and is expressed in terms of an angle ϕ, called the ellipticity. The angle ϕ is given by

$$\mathrm{Tan}\ \phi = \frac{a_R - a_L}{a_R + a_L},$$

a_R and a_L being the amplitudes of the right and left circular components respectively. The ellipticity, ϕ, in degrees, is related to ΔD_λ, by the equation

$$\Delta D_\lambda = \frac{\phi}{180} \cdot 4\pi \log_{10} e.$$

An approximation in deriving this relationship assumes ϕ to be small, as is found in practice. Early experimental studies on circular dichroism gave ellipticities as an angle directly observed and even some recent workers, (e.g. HOLZWARTH and DOTY, 1965) have presented results in terms related to ϕ rather than as $\Delta\varepsilon_\lambda$.

B. Optical Rotatory Dispersion

The phenomenon of circular dichroism, occurring as it does in optically active materials, suggests there might be a relationship with another phenomenon found in such materials namely the rotation of the plane of plane polarized light which, when studied as a function of wavelength, is called optical rotatory dispersion. The relationship between the two effects can be understood by regarding the beam of plane polarized light as the resultant of two equal beams of circularly polarized light, one right and one left-handed: rotation of the plane of polarization arises when the *refractive index* of the medium differs for the two circular components, for the phase relationship between the two beams then changes progressively as the light traverses the medium. FRESNEL (1825) demonstrated the validity of this concept by using prisms constructed of right and left-handed quartz to separate a single beam of plane polarized light into two beams, one having left, the other right circular polarization. A measurement of ϱ, the optical rotation by any material gives the difference between its refractive indices n_L and n_R for left and right circularly polarized light according to the equation

$$\varrho = \pi (n_L - n_R) \cdot \frac{l}{\lambda}$$

where l is the path length of light through the optically active medium and λ is the wavelength of the light used. If the measurement is made in a circularly dichroic absorption band then, although the incident ray is plane polarized, the emergent ray is elliptically polarized, and ϱ then represents the angular rotation of the major axis of the ellipse.

C. Cotton Effects

In general the rotatory power of material varies with wavelength, even in spectral regions free from absorption bands. By analogy with studies upon coloured materials with unpolarized light, which commonly show a variation of refractive index with wavelength known as dispersion, the term rotatory dispersion has come to denote a variation of optical rotatory power with wavelength. As COTTON (1896) first showed, the rotatory dispersion in absorption bands of an optically active compound can be 'anomalous' in that the curve relating rotation to wavelength has an S-form with a maximum and minimum. To illustrate this a plain rotatory dispersion curve, together with an anomalous curve are shown in figure 6. Anomalous rotatory dispersion occurs only in absorption bands that also show circular dichroism, such bands being said to show a COTTON effect. Indeed the close relationship between optical rotatory dispersion and circular dichroism is evinced by Natanson's rule for isolated absorption bands which has been stated in the form "On the red side of the absorption band, the ray which is less absorbed is propagated with the greater velocity; on the violet side the reverse is the case" (cf. Lowry, 1935).

D. Theory

The Kronig-Kramers theorem establishes the quantitative relationship between circular dichroism and optical rotatory dispersion. This theorem allows the calculation of optical rotation, ϱ_{λ_1} at any wavelength λ_1 in terms of the ellipticity ϕ_λ, a function of which is integrated over the whole spectrum. The equation (Djerassi, 1960) is

$$\varrho_{\lambda_1} = \frac{2}{\pi} \int_0^\infty \frac{\phi_\lambda \lambda}{\lambda_1^2 - \lambda^2} \cdot d\lambda.$$

If ϕ_λ can be expressed as the sum of a series of gaussian curves or as the sum of a series of curves closely related to gaussian curves then the integral is readily evaluated from tables such as those given by Lowry (1935).

From the theorem and the equation given above it is clear that optical activity and circular dichroism must have a common theoretical background. Early efforts to provide a theoretical basis for optical activity have been rejected as erroneous or implausible, and current theory is based upon the realisation that dispersion electrons (i.e. electrons contributing to refractivity) vibrating in a potential well of the form $V = \frac{1}{2}ax^2 + \frac{1}{2}by^2 + \frac{1}{2}cz^2 + Axyz$, would rotate the plane of polarized light, the term in A giving the necessary dissymmetry. The theory has been extended by Moffit and Moscowitz (1959) to a form more easily manageable with respect to circular dichroism and in terms of the electric and magnetic moments involved in the electronic transitions giving rise to each absorption band. The essential feature required in a chromophore for it to show circular dichroism is that either the chromophore or its immediate environment are not superimposable on their mirror images. Changes in circular dichroism and optical rotatory dispersion are sensitive indicators of changes in conformation of a chromophore or its immediate environment although, in complex molecules, it has only rarely been possible to deduce the nature of the particular conformation or its changes.

E. Techniques

With few exceptions the values of $(\Delta\varepsilon)_\lambda$ that have been measured are small compared with the normal molar extinction coefficient $(\varepsilon_N)_\lambda$. It therefore requires a sensitive apparatus to detect the differences in absorption of right and left circularly polarized light. One exception to this rule is potassium chromium tartrate, which Cotton originally studied, and for that compound the circular dichroism is readily measured by inserting a piece of polaroid and a quarter wave plate in the light beam of a conventional spectrophotometer. The quarter wave plate is rotated through 90° so that the emerging circularly polarized light falling on the sample is changed from right to left handedness or *vice versa*; the change in optical density then brought about, is directly given by the spectrophotometer. (Many photocells are sensitive to polarized light and blank readings must be taken into account.) With a 20-fold scale expansion applied to a conventional spectrophotometer the circular dichroism of visual pigments can be detected in this way, though the measurements are not of high accuracy (CRESCITELLI and SHAW, 1964). Allowance has to be made for the failure of a quarter wave plate to give true circularly polarized light at more than a single wavelength, and another difficulty associated with the method is that bleaching can occur during a single measurement, changing the true optical density by an amount that may be significant with respect to $(\varDelta D)_\lambda$.

A much more sensitive method was described by GROSJEAN and LEGRAND (1960), and is now applied to commercially available instruments. The method depends upon what is known as the POCKELS effect, which occurs in certain crystals. These crystals, sectioned in a selected plane so that they are non birefringent (when seen through that plane) become so when a potential difference is applied across the section. The optical retardation depends upon the applied voltage, and reversing the voltage reverses the fast and slow axes of the crystal. Plane polarized light traversing a suitably oriented crystal (excited with the appropriate voltage) becomes circularly polarized, and by simply reversing the voltage the sense of polarization of the emergent light is reversed. Thus without any mechanical interference a sample can be presented in rapid succession with right and left circularly polarized light. In the apparatus described by GROSJEAN and LEGRAND light from a monochromator is plane polarized by a quartz prism. After traversing the crystal the light then passes through the sample and falls on an end-windowed photomultiplier, selected for its insensitivity to changes in the form of polarized light. An alternating potential difference is applied to the faces of the POCKELS-effect crystal and the sample and photomultiplier are thus presented successively with right and left circularly polarized lights that are of equal intensity. If a circularly dichroic material is interposed in the beam the output of the photomultiplier oscillates and then it does so only with a frequency identical to that of the alternating voltage applied to the crystal. The sense of dichroism in the sample will determine whether the oscillating output from the photomultiplier is in phase or antiphase with the voltage applied to the crystal. The procedure allows of an ingenious method for increasing the signal-to-noise ratio of measurements; the output from the photomultiplier is led into an a.c.-coupled amplifier where the signal can be filtered to exclude virtually all frequencies other than that employed to excite the crystal. The amplifier output is phase-sensitively rectified by mechanical switches operated in phase with the alternating voltage applied to the crystal, and then gives rise to a steady potential. This steady potential is not itself a direct measure of $\varDelta D_\lambda$ of the sample. Thus a high intensity light falling on the photomultiplier after traversing a given sample would produce a large oscillating output from the photomultiplier, giving rise to a large steady potential after phase-sensitive rectification. A low intensity light falling on the same sample, however, would yield only a small steady potential after phase-sensitive rectification. To obtain a measure of $\varDelta D_\lambda$ the output of the phase sensitive rectifier is divided by the photomultiplier output. With such a technique values of $\varDelta D_\lambda$ of 10^{-5} can be measured.

One advantage of basing the optical retardation upon a POCKELS-effect crystal is that by adjustment of the applied voltage a true quarter-wave action can be obtained for any wavelength. The adjustment of voltage is simple because for these crystals a substantially linear relationship holds for retardation as a function of wavelength. The commercial instruments available for circular dichroimetry record automatically over the ultraviolet and visible regions of the spectrum. A sensitive manually-operated instrument can be constructed, however, from commercially available spectrophotometers, provided that a suitable photomultiplier is installed, a quartz Rochon prism and Pockels-effect crystal being inserted in the light beam. In constructing such an apparatus care must be taken to have a parallel light beam incident on the crystal (which has a very limited acceptance angle); moreover it is important to establish how far into the ultraviolet the apparatus can operate without error arising from the stray light that can be present in a single prism monochromator.

Certain precautions must be taken when using any instrument for measuring circular dichroism. In particular the cells used to hold the sample should be strain-free, otherwise they will distort the circularly polarized light to an elliptical form. The most convenient test of cells is to use them for measurements on a substance showing a strong circular dichroism, and for which the measurement has already been carefully recorded (Velluz, Legrand, and Grosjean, 1965). The crystal must also be oriented with respect to the plane of polarization of the incident light, and placed so that the light beam falls normally. Finally, in using a dichroimeter it should be remembered that generally a sine and not a square wave of voltage is applied to the crystal so that between peak voltages linearly polarized light falls on the sample. In principle a linearly dichroic material in the light beam should not give a reading. However, any slight error of operation of the mechanical switches in the phase sensitive rectifier, or misalignment of the crystal, can give false measurements. Moreover, a linearly dichroic material generally possesses linear birefringence, which will distort the circularly polarized light. These factors should be considered when a material such as a whole retina is examined.

II. Circular Dichroism and Optical Rotatory Dispersion of Extracted Visual Pigments

A. Circular Dichroism in the A-Band

A preliminary study of the circular dichroism of visual pigments was first made by Crescitelli and Shaw (1964), who reported that the A-band of rhodopsin, extracted with digitonin from the retinae of *Rana pipiens*, showed positive circular dichroism. Further work by Crescitelli, Mommaerts, and Shaw (1966) showed that a positive circular dichroism was associated, not only with the A-band of *Rana pipiens* rhodopsin (Fig. 1) but also with the A-bands of other visual pigments. Thus the rhodopsins of the ox, the frog (*R. catesbeiana*) and, as we now know, the conger eel show positively dichroic A-bands, and so does the porphyropsin of the carp, *Cyprinus carpio* (Crescitelli and Shaw, 1964; Crescitelli, Mommaerts, and Shaw, 1967). With such studies on visual pigments a problem arises from the use of digitonin as an extractant, for this substance is optically active and could conceivably impose a dissymmetry on an otherwise symmetric chromophore in the visual pigment, when aggregated in micelles with the extractant. However, when the non-ionic detergent Triton X100 was used as an extractant for the rhodopsin from bullfrog retinas it gave results identical with those obtained with digitonin.

The form and magnitude of circular dichroism associated with the A-band is of interest; a rhodopsin solution from *R. pipiens* having a unit optical density at the maximum of its A-band when measured with unpolarized light, gave a maximum optical density difference between left and right circularly polarized lights of about 5×10^{-4}. According to WALD and BROWN (1953) and HUBBARD (1954)

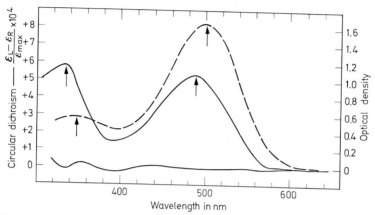

Fig. 1. Optical density spectrum (interrupted curve) and circular dichroism of unbleached (upper continuous curve) and bleached (lower continuous curve) frog rhodopsin. Arrows indicate peaks. The circular dichroism is given in terms of a rhodopsin solution having unit density at 502 nm. (After CRESCITELLI, MOMMAERTS, and SHAW, 1966)

the molar extinction coefficient for rhodopsin is 40,600 so that the molar circular dichroic extinction $\Delta\varepsilon_{max}$ amounts in this material to 20 cm^2 millimole^{-1}. This is almost twice the maximum value found for $\Delta\varepsilon_{max}$ in some 400 compounds listed by VELLUZ, LEGRAND, and GROSJEAN (1965), most of which contained a carbonyl chromophore. Another surprising result was that the peak circular dichroism associated with the A-band occurred at a slightly shorter wavelength than the wavelength of peak absorption for ordinary light. The shift was of the order of 10 nm both for frog rhodopsin and carp porphyropsin, and a similar shift has been found by KITO, AZUMA, and MAEDA (1968) for squid rhodopsin. A small shift may be expected if the *dissymmetry factor* g_λ defined as $\left(\dfrac{\varepsilon_L - \varepsilon_R}{\varepsilon_N}\right)_\lambda$ (cf. LOWRY, 1935) varies slightly with frequency; VELLUZ, LEGRAND, and GROSJEAN (1965) p. 16, point out there can be a direct proportionality but the observed shift for rhodopsin is larger than can be accounted for in this way. It may be that the electronic transition giving rise to the A-band has higher frequency components due to associated vibrational transitions and that these latter are dissymetric.

B. Circular Dichroism in the B-Band

The B-band (*cis* peak) of frog rhodopsin has also been explored for circular dichroism and found to show dissymmetry. Although the normal absorbance of the

B-band is very much less than that of the A-band its circular dichroic absorbance has about the same maximum value as that found in the A-band. In terms of the dissymmetry factor g_λ, therefore, it is more powerful. However, the circular dichroism of the B-band does not appear to be universal since carp porphyropsin, explored to wavelengths down to 380 nm failed to show signs of it (Fig. 2). Judging by the absorbance spectrum of yellow perch (Wald, 1959) we can expect the B-band to peak at 377 nm, beginning to rise at 422 nm, so that any strong circular dichroism associated with it should have been detected. It may be that a circularly dichroic B-band is only to be found in rhodopsins, and is absent from porphyropsins; but only an extensive survey would establish such a generalisation.

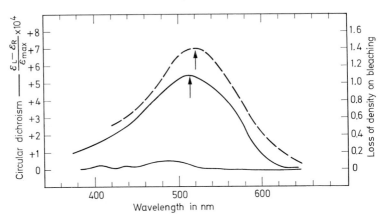

Fig. 2. Difference spectrum on bleaching (interrupted curve and optical density scale) and circular dichroism of unbleached (upper continuous curve) and bleached (lower continuous curve) of carp porphyropsin. Arrows indicate peaks. The circular dichroism is given in terms of a porphyropsin solution having unit loss of density (at maximum) on bleaching. (After Crescitelli, Mommaerts, and Shaw, 1966)

C. Circular Dichroism after Bleaching by Light and Heat

After the bleaching of visual pigments by light the circular dichroism of both the A- and B-bands is lost, the spectral region from 650 nm down, in the case of frog rhodopsin, to 320 nm being virtually free from circular dichroism. This loss of dichroism occurs whether hydroxylamine is present or not, which is a point of some interest for in its absence the retinal can be expected to have remained in association with opsin while in those solutions to which hydroxylamine had been added the retinal would have been detached from the opsin and formed into an oxime. The dichroism was lost whether digitonin or Triton X100 had been used as the solubilising agent for the visual pigment.

In light-induced bleaching of the visual pigments the prosthetic group changes from the 11-*cis* to give the *all trans* retinal configuration (Wald, 1959), and the question arises whether this transformation is the change primarily associated with the loss of dissymmetry on bleaching. There is some evidence relevant to this question arising from Hubbard's (1958) observation that during thermally induced bleaching of rhodopsin the retinal formed retains the 11-*cis* configuration.

Experiments in which frog rhodopsin was bleached by heat (30 min at 66° C) showed that the thermally bleached product was not circularly dichroic in the visible and near ultraviolet regions of the spectrum. TAKEZAKI and KITO (1967) have confirmed the effects of light and heat on the circular dichroism of cattle rhodopsin. A subsequent paper by KITO, AZUMA, and MAEDA (1968) describes results of studies upon squid rhodopsin. The circular dichroic extinction for the A-band of squid rhodopsin is more than twice that found in cattle rhodopsin though that for their B-bands is about the same. Of particular interest is their finding that the relatively stable squid metarhodopsin produced by light has little circular dichroism such dichroism as was associated with the exposed sample being attributable to unaltered rhodopsin (a photoequilibrium being set up). Indeed neither the acid nor alkaline metarhodopsin gave indications of circular dichroism. This is the first indication that the Cotton effects associated with the A- and B-bands are lost at a relatively early stage in the thermal reactions succeeding the photochemical event.

D. Optical Rotatory Dispersion

From the close relationship between circular dichroism and optical rotatory dispersion one would expect that the A-band of rhodopsin would show anomalous rotatory dispersion (Cotton effect). KITO and TAKEZAKI (1966) found that unbleached cattle rhodopsin extracted with digitonin had a large negative rotation in the visible that decreased (became less negative) as the wavelength decreased. They did not detect any clear S-shaped anomaly associated with the A-band in the optical rotatory dispersion curve but they did observe that the curve changed as a result of bleaching; down to wavelengths of 330—340 nm the unbleached pigment was less laevorotatory than its light-bleached products, while at still shorter wavelengths it was more laevorotatory; at about 450 nm the bleached and unbleached pigments had nearly the same rotatory power. WILLIAMS (1966) constructed a difference curve for optical rotatory dispersion in the visible region of the spectrum, subtracting rotations obtained after light-bleaching from those obtained prior to the bleach (Fig. 3). He used pigment from *Rana pipiens*, extracted by Triton X100 as well as by digitonin, and found the changes on bleaching to be represented by an S-shaped curve characteristic of chromophore groupings showing a Cotton effect. The positive peak of the curve occurred at longer wavelengths, so that towards the red the refractive index for left circular rays was greater than for right and their velocity therefore less. Applying Natanson's rule to WILLIAMS' (1966) data leads to the prediction that left circularly polarized rays would be preferentially absorbed, which is in accord with the results of circular dichroism. The Kronig-Kramers theorem can be applied to the circular dichroism measurements; although a detailed analysis has not been done. We can assume to a first approximation that the circular dichroic extinction curve of CRESCITELLI, MOMMAERTS, and SHAW (1966) for the A-band is gaussian in form. The gaussian curve is centred on 490 nm and has a width of 100 nm at half its maximum height, indicating that (under the conditions described by WILLIAMS) the anomaly in the optical rotatory dispersion curve should show a diphasic form with maximum and minimum at 545 nm and 435 nm, and a difference in rotation between the peak and trough amounting to 0.0014°. The observed maximum and minimum occur at 542 and 454 nm while the difference in rotation between the peak and trough amounts to 0.007°. The fact that the circular dichroism is only approximated by an isolated gaussian curve accounts for at least some of this discrepancy; for the B-band will contribute to the rotations by raising the difference curve above the zero line, as WILLIAMS observed, and by tending to reduce the difference between the peak and trough of the recorded anomaly.

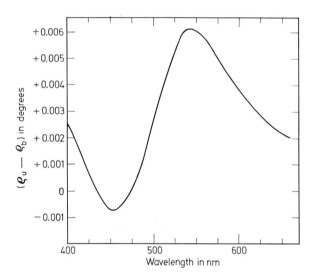

Fig. 3. Optical rotatory dispersion changes that occur when rhodopsin is bleached. ϱ_u and ϱ_b are the optical rotations before and after bleaching. The solution contained 1.76×10^{-5} moles per litre of rhodopsin and had a 1.0 cm path length. (After WILLIAMS, 1966)

WILLIAMS' observations go further than simply providing optical rotatory dispersion curves for normal rhodopsin. By flashing rhodopsin during bleaching he reisomerised some *all-trans* retinal to its 11-*cis* form thus regenerating rhodopsin by photoreversal. The regenerated rhodopsin was as optically active as fresh rhodopsin. Apparently the Cotton effect of the A-band of rhodopsin is not only associated with the pigment as generated in the retina, where dissymmetric enzymes might be involved in its formation. The point is of some importance for as TAKEZAKI and KITO (1967) and CRESCITELLI (1969) have stressed, 11-*cis* retinal is not only bent but twisted also, there being steric interference between adjacent hydrogen and methyl groups that resist a planar configuration. Enzymically formed 11-*cis* retinal might have a right or left handedness, although the free forms probably racemise rapidly. Nevertheless, it is possible that retinal could be twisted in one sense only when in combination with opsin to form a visual pigment, and one might then expect that the steric interaction between the hydrogen and methyl groups would be essential for the Cotton effect in the A-band. TAKEZAKI and KITO (1967) disposed of this possibility by finding that iso-rhodopsin also showed Cotton effects associated with the A- and B-bands

(Fig. 4). The iso-pigment is based upon 9-*cis* retinal an isomer that, though bent, lacks the steric interference of 11-*cis* retinal and can freely exist with a plane of symmetry. Nevertheless the circular dichroism of the iso-pigment appears to be somewhat weaker than that of the pigment containing 11-*cis* retinal, and one cannot rule out the possibility that the Cotton effect is enhanced in the latter material by steric interference, even though it cannot be primarily due to this.

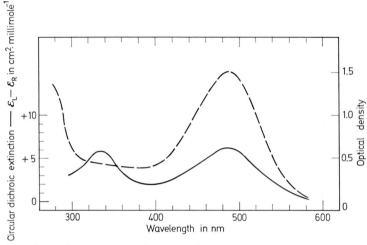

Fig. 4. Optical density spectrum (interrupted curve) and circular dichroic extinction (continuous curve) of isorhodopsin from cattle. (After TAKEZAKI and KITO, 1967)

III. Circular Dichroism and Optical Rotatory Dispersion of Pigments *in situ*

The Cotton effects in visual pigments discussed so far have been observed in pigments that have been extracted. It is natural to wonder whether the pigments show the same behaviour whilst they are still in the visual receptors. It is by no means self evident that the same effects should exist for there can be a drastic change in optical activity on solution, as, for example, when crystals of sodium chlorate, optically active in the solid state, completely lose their activity when dissolved. LOWRY (1935) nevertheless points out that all crystals yielding optically active solutions are themselves optically active. ARDEN (1954) showed it was possible to study the properties of the pigments in suspensions of isolated rod outer segments, and KITO and TAKEZAKI (1966) were the first to demonstrate that a change in the optical rotatory dispersion curve occurred between 546 and 600 nm when sonicated rod preparations from cattle were bleached; the change was in the same sense as that with extracted pigments. CRESCITELLI, FOSTER, and SHAW (1969) studied the circular dichroism of rod outer segments suspended in 40 % sucrose. (These suspensions had been stored for several days in a refrigerator.) Even in the bleached state there existed a large apparent circular dichroism associated with the rod outer segments and this dichroism increased relatively rapidly with decreasing wavelength. At least part of this apparent circular dichroism seems to be due to preferential scattering of one form of circularly polarized light, for when light scattered sideways from the sample was directed on to the photomultiplier this light was found to have the opposite sense of dichroism from that obtained from the sample directly. The question arises as to what dissymmetry in the rod outer segment suspension gives rise to this discrimination between the two forms of circularly polarized light; the wavelength dependence suggests that the dissymmetry probably occurs on a scale comparable with the wavelength of visible light, but there is as yet no indication what structural characteristic of the rod outer segments provides the necessary lack of symmetry. While there is evidence that circular dichroic scattering occurred in these bleached rod outer segment suspensions there is no assurance that the whole of the apparent circular dichroism arose in this manner, and a Cotton effect that persists after bleaching may contribute to the measurements. Unbleached rod outer segments show a wavelength-dependent circular dichroism very similar to that found in the bleached preparations. Careful measurements on rod suspensions, however, reveal a decrease in circular dichroism in the region of the A-band of rhodopsin and a curve of differences between bleached and unbleached can be obtained, though great accuracy cannot be expected from such measurements. The difference curve is similar in form to that obtained for unbleached rhodopsin extracts although, when referred to the amount of rhodopsin observed, it is some 30% larger. The enhancement of the Cotton effect may represent a difference in the configuration of rhodopsin when it occurs *in situ* or it may arise from a difference in the refractive index of the environment for the rhodopsin (Sidman, 1957, gives a figure of 1.41 for the refractive index of frog rod outer segments). However, there is an alternative explanation for the discrepancy. The rhodopsin in the rod outer segments was estimated from the decrease in optical density for unpolarized 500 nm light when the rods were light-bleached; Dartnall (1961) has investigated the optical properties of frog rod outer segments and found a light stable photoproduct of bleaching that absorbs at this wavelength. The presence of this photoproduct leads to an underestimate of the true quantity of rhodopsin present, an underestimate that would amount, according to Dartnall's data, to 27%. Indeed as Crescitelli, Foster, and Shaw (1969) pointed out, if correction for this photostable pigment is applied to their measurements then it seems that the circular dichroism associated with the A-band of rhodopsin is very similar whether the pigment is *in situ* or in detergent extracts (at least under the conditions in which they studied the outer segments). It would be interesting to explore the B-band spectral region for circular dichroism by rod outer segments but this has not yet been done.

IV. Studies in the Far Ultraviolet

A. Extracted Pigments

The spectral absorbance of visual pigment for unpolarized light becomes very great in the farther ultraviolet, and one might expect that measurements of optical rotatory dispersion and circular dichroism would be very difficult in that region.

However, KITO and TAKEZAKI (1966) were able to make measurements, and reported changes on bleaching in the optical rotatory dispersion curve for cattle rhodopsin at wavelengths down to 220 nm. A minimum in the optical rotatory dispersion curve occurred at 235 nm and they attributed the changes they found on bleaching to changes in the helical structure of the opsin. Using circular dichroism CRESCITELLI, MOMMAERTS, and SHAW (1966) found that measurable effects could be obtained with diluted digitonin extracts of frog rhodopsin almost down to 200 nm. That the circular dichroism is measurable at all in that region of the spectrum depends upon the large value of the dissymmetry factor (g_λ) at these wavelengths as compared with its value in the A-band region of the spectrum. Unbleached frog rhodopsin and carp porphyropsin both show a negative circular dichroism with two extrema, one at about 224 nm, the other at approximately 210 nm, and a shallow intervening trough. The pattern is very similar to that found in several proteins and in solutions of polypeptides which, on other grounds, are believed to be in an α-helical configuration. These latter materials show yet a third and positive peak at 190 nm, a wavelength not yet accessible with visual pigment extracts. While the circular dichroism between 260 and 200 nm for both rhodopsin and porphyropsin extracts resembles that found in α-helical polypeptides and proteins it must be realised that such extracts probably contain protein other than visual pigment opsin. Contaminating proteins are probably extracted from the rods, and may well contribute to the circular dichroism seen in this spectral region. Indeed carp porphyropsin showed almost twice the circular dichroism found in frog rhodopsin when scaled to unit optical density as measured in ordinary light at the A-band peak. This could well have been because of the greater impurity of the carp extract.

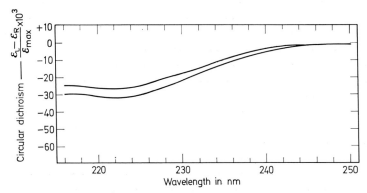

Fig. 5. Circular dichroism of frog rhodopsin in the far ultra-violet, before (lower curve) and after (upper curve) bleaching by white light. Data scaled to refer to a rhodopsin solution with unit optical density at 502 nm. (After CRESCITELLI, MOMMAERTS, and SHAW, 1966)

Nevertheless some of the dichroism in the far ultraviolet is certainly due to the visual pigments, for light-bleaching caused a significant decrease in circular dichroism, as can be seen in Fig. 5. In the case of the frog pigment illustrated, approximately $\frac{1}{6}$ of the dichroism in the far ultra-violet was lost on bleaching by light, while a much larger decrease occurred (presumably due to a much larger disorganization of the protein in the extract) when heat was used to bleach the pigment. Whereas studies in the A- and B-band spectral regions were carried out with both digitonin and Triton X100 extracts, the ultraviolet absorption of the latter material prevented its use at very short wavelengths. Fortunately digitonin does not have a strongly dichroic band in that spectral region, and blank measurements made upon the extractant alone can readily be subtracted from the data for the pigment. Using cattle rhodopsin Takezaki and Kito (1967) obtained similar curves for the circular dichroism in the far ultraviolet, their magnitude being about 60% and the decrease on bleaching about 25% of that found with frog pigment.

From the studies of Kito, Azuma, and Maeda (1968) it appears that the simple isomerisation of prosthetic group that follows irradiation is not alone sufficient to yield the decrease in circular dichroism seen in the ultraviolet after exposure to light. Specifically these authors showed that squid rhodopsin that had been exposed to light at pH 8.5 underwent no decrease of circular dichroism at wavelengths between 220 and 260 nm although a substantial fraction of the rhodopsin had been converted to alkaline metarhodopsin. Subsequent heating, however, did cause a major decrease in the ultraviolet circular dichroism of the pigment.

B. Pigments *in situ*

Suspensions of frog rod outer segments in 40% sucrose have also been examined for circular dichroism in the far ultraviolet (Crescitelli, Foster, and Shaw, 1969); in the unbleached state they show a wavelength dependence of circular dichroism (between 220 and 250 nm) that is rather similar in form and magnitude to that of the extracted pigment. It is surprising that true circular dichroism (at these short wavelengths) seems to be much more marked than scattering circular dichroism. Although a detailed wavelength curve of circular dichroism, showing the effects of light bleaching, has not been obtained for frog rod outer segments it has been found that, as with the extracted pigment, there is a decrease of the dichroism at 220 nm on bleaching, and this decrease is of the same size as that found in extracts. At 250 nm neither suspensions nor pigment extracts undergo a significant change of circular dichroism with bleaching. There is therefore some evidence that similar dissymmetry changes can occur, whether rhodopsin is bleached *in situ* or in extracts.

Shichi, Lewis, Irreverre, and Stone (1969) studied suspensions of rod outer segments from cattle retinas and likewise detected circular dichroism in the far ultraviolet. But no change in circular dichroism at 220 nm could be detected on bleaching the suspension, though extracted pigment showed a significant decrease in this region when bleached. These observations, which contrast with those of Crescitelli, Foster and Shaw on the frog, may be attributable to species difference, or to the effect of storage.

V. Cotton Effects in Relation to the Conformation of Visual Pigments

Ideally the results for the circular dichroism and optical rotatory dispersion of visual pigments given above should be compared with those for a detailed model of the molecule for which the Cotton effects had been calculated from theory. Since the theoretical treatment is difficult for even simple and well understood compounds this ideal is probably to be regarded as a distant hope. Nevertheless indirect arguments can be employed and comparisons made, though, at present, such interpretations must be regarded as very tentative. In the first instance, there is the surprising finding that the A-band of the visual pigments shows a Cotton effect at all. It may not be right to regard retinal as synonymous with the whole chromophore for that band, but it undoubtedly approximates closely to it. Recent evidence by POINCELOT, MILLAR, KIMBEL, and ABRAHAMSON (1969) and by BOWNDS (1967) shows that the attachment is originally to an amino group of phosphatidyl ethanolamine while, at the metarhodopsin II stage of bleaching, transfer occurs to an ε-amino group of lysine. Neither of these attachments closely involves an asymmetric carbon atom. After bleaching, the retinal, which has been detached from opsin, shows no dichroism in the region of its absorption band at 385 nm. Indeed in the *all trans* form there is no reason why retinal should be dissymmetric for it has a plane of symmetry, but heat-bleached pigment, which liberates *11-cis* retinal with its sterically imposed twist, also seems inactive, and presumably racemises very readily. However, situations are known where a symmetric chromophore develops a Cotton effect from the dissymmetry of its environment. Such Cotton effects are called extrinsic, and examples are to be found among carbonyl groups, which have been extensively studied (VELLUZ, LEGRAND, and GROSJEAN, 1965). Another and possibly more relevant example has been investigated by STRYER and BLOUT (1961). These authors found that the dye acridine orange, which itself is optically inactive, gives a pronounced Cotton effect in its visible absorption band if adsorbed on to poly-L-glutamate when that material is in the α-helical configuration (Fig. 6). Among naturally occurring compounds giving an extrinsic Cotton effect is the enzyme phosphorylase b, which has pyridoxal-5-phosphate as a prosthetic group (TORCHINSKII, LIVANOVA, and PIKHELGAS, 1967). At neutrality a positively dichroic absorption band is found at 333 nm, which corresponds to an absorption band of pyridoxal-5-phosphate; neither protein nor prosthetic group are separately active at this wavelength. CRESCITELLI (1969) gives other examples. STRYER and BLOUT (1961) in their original observations on the Cotton effect given by acridine orange adsorbed on polyglutamate noted that the effect was lost when, by raising the pH, the polyglutamate was changed from a α-helical into a random-coil configuration. It seems from their observations that a loss of α-helix by the adsorbing material can be sufficient to destroy the extrinsic Cotton effect given by an associated dye. Sufficient though such a change may be it seems that the loss of α-helix does not necessarily destroy an extrinsic Cotton effect, for MYHR and FOSS (1966) have found that if the dye is adsorbed after the polyglutamate has taken up a random coil configuration then an extrinsic Cotton effect develops, though it is not identical with that developed with the α-helical polypeptide. It is clear at least that conformational changes in a polypeptide to which a dye is attached can influence the extrinsic Cotton effect shown by the dye.

In contrast with the extrinsic Cotton effects, which are induced by the environment on otherwise symmetrical chromophores, there are intrinsic Cotton effects, which arise from the dissymmetry of the chromophore itself. An example of

13*

a chromophore showing an intrinsic effect is hexahelicene in which six benzene rings are arranged in a helical array and the conjugated double bonds co-operate to give a single chromophore.

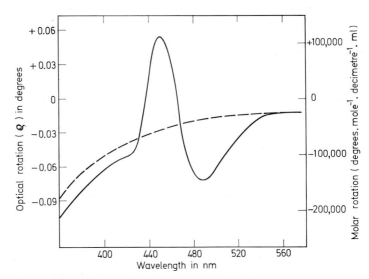

Fig. 6. Optical rotatory dispersion of a complex of acridine orange and poly-L-glutamic acid in the helical conformation (continuous curve) and of helical poly-L-glutamic acid alone (interrupted curve). (After STRYER and BLOUT, 1961)

The circular dichroism seen in the far ultraviolet in visual pigment extracts compares so closely with that observed with proteins and polypeptides that it would appear to be due to protein. Not all polypeptides show the same circular dichroism in the ultra-violet and its dependence upon wavelength is determined by the configuration taken up by the molecule. As SARKAR and DOTY (1966) showed poly-L-lysine occurring in the β-configuration and studied at wavelengths greater than 200 nm has a single negative peak of circular dichroism at 218 nm; poly-L-lysine together with other poly-L-peptides when they occur as α-helices, however, possess a double negatively-peaked curve of circular dichroism with extrema at about 222 and 206 nm, while at still shorter wavelengths (below 200 nm) the curve becomes positive (HOLZWARTH and DOTY, 1965). Another configuration that has been studied is the random coil form, which gives its own characteristic curve of circular dichroism as a function of wavelength; a large positive peak occurs at about 200 nm but there is only weak negative dichroism at wavelengths between 235 and 210 nm. The probable electronic transitions associated with the various peaks have been allocated by HOLZWARTH and DOTY (1965) — the positive and the shorter wavelength negative peak in α-helical L-polypeptides have been attributed to the $\pi \to \pi^*$ transition of amide groups, and the longer wavelength negative peak to the $n \to \pi^*$ transition occurring in the helical peptide structure. These two negative peaks, seen in visual pigment extracts, would seem to be intrinsic COTTON effects.

All three polypeptides so far studied in their α-helical form have circular dichroic extinctions per amino acid residue of similar values, namely 12 cm^2 per residue millimole (HOLZWARTH and DOTY, 1965; MOMMAERTS, 1966). It is clear that the decrease in circular dichroism in the ultra-violet that occurs when visual pigments are bleached can be accounted for by supposing that there is a net loss of right handed α-helix from the opsin and that this occurs whether the pigment is present in the rods or in extracts. As SIMMONS, COHEN, SZENT-GYÖRGYI, WETLAUFER, and BLOUT (1961) have pointed out, the COTTON effect shown by polypeptides and proteins in the far ultra-violet may be used to provide an estimate of α-helical content. From the rather limited data as yet available on polypeptides and the molecular absorbance of rhodopsin (WALD and BROWN, 1953; HUBBARD, 1954) it appears that a loss of some 17—19 amino acid residues from the α-helical configuration could account for the observed change of intrinsic COTTON effect arising in the bleaching of frog rhodopsin (SHAW, 1968). Indeed if the intrinsic circular dichroism seen in frog rhodopsin extracts is entirely due to opsin and not to other protein impurities a similar calculation leads to the view that perhaps one third of the amino acid residues (average molecular weight 150) in unbleached rhodopsin occur in α-helical portions of the protein. In cattle pigment, studied by TAKEZAKI and KITO (1967), the smaller effect would suggest the involvement of fewer amino acids. Such calculations must be regarded at the moment with considerable caution, partly in view of the limited number of polypeptides studied, but also because, as SARKAR and DOTY (1966) observed, the nature of other materials present can alter the magnitude of the circular dichroism seen in polypeptides. Indeed the theoretical treatment of circular dichroism indicates that the band strength should depend upon the refractive index of the material within which the chromophore is located (VELLUZ, LEGRAND, and GROSJEAN, 1965; p. 196).

CRESCITELLI (1969) has reviewed the experimental results for the COTTON effects in visual pigments with reference to studies that various authors have made upon enzymes with prosthetic groups. He points out that there may be a distortion of the protein molecule on combination with the prosthetic group and this conformational change he likens to a "cocking" process. Certainly the results so far observed on visual pigments can be interpreted in those terms; a portion of the opsin close to either *11-cis* or *9-cis* prosthetic group takes up the α-helical configuration and loses that configuration at some stage after the group has been isomerized to the *all trans* form. Judging from the results of KITO, AZUMA, and MAEDA (1968) on squid rhodopsin the loss of α-helix must occur after the stage of metarhodopsin. The recent paper by SHICHI, LEWIS, IRREVERRE, and STONE (1969) on very carefully purified bovine rhodopsin, showed a circular dichroism in the far ultra-violet that indicated an apparent helical content of 60%. One fifth of this was lost on bleaching the pigment extract; none on bleaching rod suspensions.

The role, if any, that the changes shown up by circular dichroism of visual pigments play in stimulation of the rods is a matter of pure conjecture. CRESCITELLI (1969), pointing out that rhodopsin is almost certainly associated with the extensive membranes in the rod outer segments, suggests that conformational changes of the pigment may alter the properties of those membranes extensively. From the studies by KITO, AZUMA, and MAEDA (1968) it seems that the conformational change shown up by the loss of circular dichroism associated with the A- and B-bands of rhodopsin occurs, at least in the squid, prior to the formation of metarhodopsin. It may, therefore, be involved in the stimulation of the rods, though changes associated with the dichroism in the far ultra-violet seem to occur too late in the sequence of thermal reactions that follow the initial photochemical event to be so involved (Wald, Brown, and Gibbons, 1963). The latter changes could nevertheless be concerned with the alternations of visual threshold, attendant upon the bleaching of rhodopsin, that have been given quantitative expression by Rushton (1965). Clarification of the stage at which the conformational changes shown up by the circular dichroism occur in vertebrate rhodopsin — whether, for example, some occur during the generation of prelumirhodopsin (Yoshizawa and Wald, 1963), or in the formation of lumi- or metarhodopsin I (Matthews, Hubbard, Brown, and Wald, 1963) — awaits low temperature studies in which the intermediate compounds of bleaching can be stabilised. Moreover, studies on the circular dichroism of visual pigments should be extended to intact retinae where artefacts arising from the linear dichroism of the rods will have to be carefully excluded.

References

Arden, G. B.: Light sensitive pigment in the visual cells of the frog. J. Physiol. (Lond.) **123**, 377—385 (1954).

Bownds, D.: Site of attachment of retinal in rhodopsin. Nature (Lond.) **216**, 1178—1181 (1967).

Cotton, A.: Recherches sur l'absorption et la dispersion de la lumière par les milieux doués du pouvoir rotatoire. Ann. Chim. Phys. 8, 347—432 (1896).

Crabbé, P.: Optical rotatory dispersion and circular dichroism in organic chemistry. San Francisco: Holden Day 1965.

Crescitelli, F.: The role of photopigments in vision. In: The Control of behaviour: Proceedings of the centennial year conference of the University of California, Univ. Calif., Irvine. London: Academic Press 1969 (in the press).

— Foster, R. F., Shaw, T. I.: The circular dichroism of suspensions of frog rod outer segments. J. Physiol. (Lond.) **202**, 189—195 (1969).

— Mommaerts, W. F. H. M., Shaw, T. I.: Circular dichroism of visual pigments in the visible and ultra- violet spectral regions. Proc. natl. Acad. Sci. (Wash.) **56**, 1729—1734 (1966).

— — Shaw, T. I.: The circular dichroism of visual pigments, particularly in the ultra-violet. J. Physiol. (Lond.) **189**, 74—75P (1967).

— Shaw, T. I.: The circular dichroism of some visual pigments. J. Physiol. (Lond.) **175**, 43—45P (1964).

Dartnall, H. J. A.: Visual pigments before and after extraction from visual cells. Proc. roy. Soc. B, **154**, 250—266 (1961).

Ditchburn, R. W.: Light. London: Blackie 1952.

Djerassi, C.: Optical rotatory dispersion. New York: McGraw-Hill 1960.

Fresnel, A. T.: Extrait d'un mémoire sur la double refraction particuliere que présente le cristal de roche dans la direction de son axe. Ann. Chim. Phys. **28**. 147—161 (1825).

Grosjean, M., Legrand, M.: Appareil de mesure du dichroisme circulaire dans le visible et l'ultraviolet. C. r. hebd. Séanc. Acad. Sci. (Paris) (1960).

Haidinger, W.: Über den Pleochroismus des Amethysts. Ann. Phys. Chem. 70, 531—544 (1847).

Holzwarth, G., Doty, P.: The ultra-violet circular dichroism of polypeptides. J. Amer. chem. Soc. 87, 218—228 (1965).

Hubbard, R.: The molecular weight of rhodopsin and the nature of the rhodopsin-digitonin complex. J. gen. Physiol. 37, 381—399 (1954).

— Bleaching of rhodopsin by light and by heat. Nature (Lond.) 181, 1126 (1958).

Kito, Y., Azuma, M., Maeda, Y.: Circular dichroism of squid rhodopsin. Biochim. biophys. Acta (Amst.) **154**, 352—359 (1968).

— Takezaki, M.: Optical rotation of irradiated rhodopsin solutions. Nature (Lond.) **211**, 197—198 (1966).

KUHN, W.: In: Stereochemie (K. FREUDENBERG, Ed.) Leipzig: Deuticke 1933.

LOWRY, T. M.: Optical rotatory power. London: Longmans, Green 1935. Reprint. New York, Dover.

MATTHEWS, R. G., HUBBARD, R., BROWN, P. K., WALD, G.: Tautomeric forms of metarhodopsin. J. gen. Physiol. 47, 215—240 (1963).

MITCHELL, S.: The Cotton effect. London: Bell 1933.

MOFFIT, W., MOSCOWITZ, A.: Optical activity in absorbing media. J. Chim. Phys. 30, 648—660 (1959).

MOMMAERTS, W. F. H. M.: Ultra-violet circular dichroism of myosin. J. molec. Biol. 15, 377—380 (1966).

MYHR, B. C., FOSS, J. G.: Polyglutamic acid-acridine orange complexes. Cotton effects in the random coil region. Biopolymers 4, 949—952 (1966).

POINCELOT, R. P., MILLAR, P. G., KIMBEL, R. L., ABRAHAMSON, E. W.: Lipid to protein transfer in the photolysis of visual pigments. Nature (Lond.) 221, 256—257 (1969).

RUSHTON, W. A. H.: Bleached rhodopsin and visual adaptation. J. Physiol. (Lond.) 181, 645—655 (1965).

SARKAR, P. K., DOTY, P.: The optical rotatory properties of the β configuration in polypeptides and proteins. Proc. nat. Acad. Sci. (Wash.) 55, 981—989 (1966).

SHAW, T. I.: Some aspects of the effects of light on visual pigments. Symp. zool. Soc. (Lond.) 23, 63—74 (1968).

SHICHI, H., LEWIS, M. S., IRREVERRE, F. STONE, A. L.: Biochemistry of visual pigments 1. Purification and properties of bovine rhodopsin. J. biol. Chem. 244, 529—536 (1969).

SIDMAN, C. L.: The structure and concentration of solids in photoreceptor cells studied by refractometry and interference microscopy. J. Biophys. biochem. Cytol. 3, 15—30 (1957).

SIMMONS, N. S., COHEN, C., SZENT-GYÖRGYI, A. G., WETLAUFER, D. B., BLOUT, E. R.: A conformation-dependent Cotton effect in α-helical polypeptides and proteins. J. Amer. chem. Soc. 83, 4766-4769 (1961).

STRYER, L., BLOUT, E. R.: Optical rotatory dispersion of dyes bound to macromolecules. Cationic dyes: poly-glutamic acid complexes. J. Amer. chem. Soc. 83, 1411—1418 (1961).

TAKEZAKI, M., KITO, Y.: Circular dichroism of rhodopsin and isorhodopsin. Nature (Lond.) 215, 1197—1199 (1967).

TORCHINSKII, Y. M., LIVANOVA, N. B., PIKHELGAS, V. Y.: Circular dichroism and optical rotatory dispersion of muscle phosphorylase b. Mol. Biol. 1, 23—28 (1967).

VELLUZ, L., LEGRAND, M., GROSJEAN, M.: Optical circular dichroism. Principles, measurements and applications. London: Academic Press 1965.

WALD, G.: In: Handbook of Physiology Section 1, Vol. 1. Washington D. C.: Amer. Physiol. Soc. (1959).

— BROWN, P. K.: The molar extinction of rhodopsin. J. gen. Physiol. 37, 189—200 (1953).

— — GIBBONS, I.: The problem of visual excitation. J. Opt. Soc. Amer. 53, 20—35 (1963).

WILLIAMS, T. P.: Induced asymmetry in the prosthetic group of rhodopsin. Vision Res. 6, 293—300 (1966).

YOSHIZAWA, T., WALD, G.: Prelumirhodopsin and the bleaching of visual pigments. Nature (Lond.) 197, 1279—1286 (1963).

Chapter 7

Physical Changes Induced by Light in the Rod Outer Segment of Vertebrates

By

G. Falk and P. Fatt, London (Great Britain)

With 3 Figures

Contents

I. Relation of Visual Pigment to Rod Structure

Information on the distribution and physical state of the visual pigment within the rod outer segment is basic to the subject of this chapter. An understanding of the changes produced by light must include the manner in which a localized physico-chemical event initiated at the site of absorption of a photon by a pigment molecule is able to affect spatially separated regions. Visual excitation requires that all (or nearly all) pigment molecules be so situated that the photochemical conversion of any one of them should have a high probability of initiating an excitatory process capable of propagating to other cells in the visual pathway (PIRENNE, 1967; BRINDLEY, 1970).

A. Distribution of Pigment

The outer segments of frog and cattle rods contain rhodopsin in concentrations of about 2mM and 1mM respectively. These values are based on the amounts of visual pigment extractable by digitonin solution, and the information that the digitonin micelle of a particular size that is formed contains one molecule of rhodopsin, which has a single chromophoric group (11-*cis*-retinaldehyde) (BRODA, GOODEVE, and LYTHGOE, 1940; HUBBARD, 1954; PESKIN, 1957). Similar values can be derived from measurements of the optical density of rhodopsin *in situ* in frog and in man (DENTON and WYLLIE, 1955; RUSHTON, 1956; LIEBMAN, 1962), when use is made of the extinction coefficient of 40,600 litre/cm mole, as determined for digitonin-solubilized cattle rhodopsin (WALD and BROWN, 1953), and molecular orientation with respect to the rod axis is taken into account. From the protein content of the micelles formed on solubilization of cattle rhodopsin, the molecular weight of the pigment is estimated to be in the region of 28,000 (SHIELDS, DINOVO, HENRIKSEN, KIMBEL, and MILLAR, 1967; HELLER, 1968; SHICHI, LEWIS, IRREVERRE, and STONE, 1969) to 40,000 (HUBBARD, 1954). In terms of mass per volume of fresh rod, rhodopsin is present to the extent of about $0.08g/cm^3$ in frog and $0.035g/cm^3$ in cattle (HUBBARD, 1954).

From these findings one may reasonably infer that the amount of solid matter comprising the pigment is too great for more than a very small proportion of it to be attached to the surface of the rod (considered as a cylinder without extensive infolding of its surface). Supporting evidence is provided by observations on rods separated from the retina and immersed in aqueous solutions of different refractive indices, which show that, on the scale of the minimum distance resolvable with visible light, the solid matter is uniformly distributed through the cross-section (SIDMAN, 1957).

B. Dichroism due to Rhodopsin

Evidence that the major part of the visual pigment is fixed to the solid structure of the rod is provided by optical observation of the dichroism of rhodopsin in the outer segment. The dichroism is such that absorption is maximal when the impinging light is linearly (plane) polarized with its electric vector perpendicular to the rod axis, (SCHMIDT, 1938; DENTON, 1959; LIEBMAN, 1962; WALD, BROWN, and GIBBONS, 1962), i.e. when the electric vector lies in the plane of the transverse lamellae occupying the rod interior. The dichroism is not complete, however, the absorption when the rod is illuminated from the side being (for the same optical path length) 22% of that when illuminated from the end. When account is taken of the random orientation of molecules in directions perpendicular to the rod axis, consistent with axial symmetry, this indicates an average orientation of the electric dipole responsible for absorption such that its components in the axial and transverse directions are in the ratio of 1 to 9.

The deviation from complete dichroism may be explained in several ways. One possibility is that the electric dipoles of the chromophores are directed at a constant small angle out of the plane of the transverse lamellae, but with projections on the plane of variable orientation from molecule to molecule. Another is that there is a limited freedom of rotation of the molecule so that the electric dipole of the chromophore is not confined strictly to the plane of the lamellae, but can vary from instant to instant. Yet another is that there is a constant small fraction of visual pigment that is in a different situation from the rest; it might, for example, consist of molecules that are attached to the surface membrane rather than to the transverse lamellae.

Some information is provided by the failure to induce any measurable dichroism (i.e., persisting beyond a minimum resolution time of about 0.1 sec) in rods illuminated from their end, by bleaching away an oriented component of rhodopsin with an intense flash of linearly polarized light (Hagins and Jennings, 1959). This absence of photodichroism has been interpreted to mean that the rhodopsin molecule is free to rotate about an axis normal to the lamellae, so that any preferred orientation of molecules remaining after partial bleaching is rapidly lost by thermal motion. It is possible that such freedom of rotation about one spatial direction may be accompanied by some restricted degree of rotation about other spatial directions.

It has been shown recently that long-lasting photodichroism may be induced in the retina after restricting the rotational freedom of rhodopsin by glutaraldehyde fixation (Brown, 1971) or by cooling to $-196°$ C (Strackee, 1970). The failure to detect photodichroism in the earlier work was due to the limited time resolution. The rotational relaxation time, τ, of a spherical molecule will be given by

$$\tau = 4\,\pi\,\eta\,r^3/kT$$

where η is the viscosity in poise, r is the radius, k is Boltzmann's constant and T is the absolute temperature. The rotational relaxation time of N-retinyl-opsin in digitonin solution has been determined (Tao, 1971). The value of 0.15 μsec was obtained, consistent with the size of the N-retinyl-opsin-detergent micelle. Cone (1971) has constructed an instrument for detecting transient photodichroism with a time resolution of 40 nsec. Two relaxation times for rhodopsin in fresh frog retinas at 10° C were found: 4 and 50 μsec. The latter is what might be expected for a spherical molecule of radius 20 Å in a medium having the viscosity of castor oil.

The relaxation time of rhodopsin is within the lifetime of the transient product, lumirhodopsin. Cone observed that there was no photodichroism if measurements were made at a wavelength of 520 nm. at which lumirhodopsin is isosbestic with rhodopsin. It would appear that lumirhodopsin and rhodopsin have the same relaxation times and the electric dipoles of their chromophores are similarly oriented.

The question whether there was any change in the dichroism after photochemical alteration of rhodopsin had previously been examined only with a time resolution of about one minute. The yellow product that appears during this time (presumably metarhodopsin II) is dichroic in the same sense as rhodopsin (Schmidt, 1938; Denton, 1959). Using linearly polarized light and the edge-fold retinal preparation, Denton found a reversal of the dichroism in the near ultra-violet region of the spectrum which occurred within about 15 min after bleaching of rhodopsin. He interpreted this result to mean that the final product of bleaching, vitamin A, had its electric dipole oriented parallel to the axis of the rod. This conclusion was strongly supported by DENTON's further observations on the fluorescence of the bleached, colourless retina. The green fluorescence of the bleached rod outer segments, first described by EWALD and KÜHNE (1878a), was brightest when the exciting light (near ultra-violet) was polarized with its electric vector parallel to the rod axis. DENTON found that the fluorescence likewise was partially linearly polarized, the emission and the absorption having the same direction of polarization. The fluorescence observed was that which would be expected from the emission spectrum for vitamin A (HAGINS and JENNINGS, 1959). HAGINS and JENNINGS (1959) described a yellow fluorescence of rod outer segments that was partially linearly polarized (such that its intensity was greatest parallel to the axis of the rods) and that became evident upon the appearance of a yellow photoproduct of rhodopsin.

WALD, BROWN and GIBBONS (1962) have reached the opposite conclusion as to the orientation of vitamin A in the rods. They measured the spectral absorbance of a frog's retina with unpolarized light passing along the axes of the rods in the dark-adapted state, and also after bleaching the rhodopsin, when the final product had been formed. The difference spectrum was compared with that occurring in solution. Since the difference spectra, suitably scaled, were found to be similar, they concluded that vitamin A and rhodopsin had the same orientation in the retina. It may be noted, however, that these measurements, which extended into the ultra-violet, would be strongly affected by any systematic changes in the light scattering of the retina during the period required to obtain the difference spectrum.

C. Birefringence

The existence of other oriented molecules (which may well be associated with the visual pigment) is inferred from the intrinsic birefringence of the rod outer segment. This takes the form that the refractive index is greater for light having its electric vector parallel to the rod axis than perpendicular to it (corresponding to uniaxial positive birefringence) (SCHMIDT, 1938). This component of birefringence is nearly compensated in the fresh rod by form birefringence attributable to a difference in isotropic refractive index between the transverse lamellae of the rod interior and the intervening aqueous spaces. That the intrinsic birefringence is not due to the chromophoric group of the rhodopsin molecule is indicated by the sign of the effect, which requires that the electric dipole responsible for the anisotropy of refractive index (which is equal to the square root of the dielectric constant at the frequency of the light) should lie normal to the plane of the lamellae. In addition the intrinsic birefringence is found to vanish rapidly on exposure of the dark-adapted rod to osmium tetroxide. This change occurs well in advance of any alteration in dichroism due to the pigment (SCHMIDT, 1935, 1938).

The total birefringence (form plus intrinsic birefringence) of rods in an aqueous milieu does not alter permanently with the bleaching of rhodopsin (SCHMIDT, 1951). A transient decrease in birefringence following flash illumination has been detected by means of an infrared polarizing microscope (JAGGER and LIEBMAN, 1970). The time constant of this birefringence change (of the order of milliseconds) and the effect of temperature are consistent with the change occurring during the conversion of metarhodopsin I to metarhodopsin II.

D. Electron Microscopy

Electron microscopic studies (Sjöstrand, 1949, 1953; Fernández-Morán, 1954; de Robertis and Lasansky, 1961; Moody and Robertson, 1960; Cohen, 1961; Nilsson, 1965; Dowling, 1965) reveal that the interior of the rod is occupied by closely spaced, transversely oriented lamellae, paired to form discs. These are apparently composed of unsaturated phospholipid (as indicated by combination with osmium tetroxide and uranyl ions) together with protein (as indicated by combination with basic lead ions or phosphotungstate). In the case of the frog rod, 6 μm in diameter, these lamellae, pairs of which occur at a repeat interval of 0.03 μm exceed the surface membrane in area by a factor of 100. Since the presence of these lamellae and the high concentration of mainly protein pigment are the characteristic features of the visual receptor, one is strongly inclined to associate the two, and to suppose that the visual pigment is attached to, or forms an essential structural component of the lamellae. The structure of the lamellae and the location of rhodopsin in the lamellae have been the subjects of recent X-ray diffraction studies (Blaurock and Wilkins, 1969; Gras and Worthington, 1969; Blaisie, Worthington and Dewey, 1969; Blaisie and Worthington, 1969).

In the rod the transverse lamellae are arranged with the two members of each pair in contact along their circumference (thus forming a loop, as seen in longitudinal section). The discs (or membranous sacs) so formed have deep incisures around their circumference, the incisures of adjacent discs being in alignment.

One indication that the lamellae of rods have a composition distinct from that of other membranes is that they disintegrate when treated first with osmium tetroxide and then with tris-(hydroxymethyl)-aminomethane or pyridine (Falk and Fatt, 1969). Neither the surface membrane of the rods nor any other membranous structures in the receptor cell region of the retina (including the lamellae of the cones and the mitochondrial membranes of the inner segments) are as susceptible. The edges of the rod discs remain intact under this treatment, and therefore one presumes that they also are materially different from the lamellae, as has been surmised by Sjöstrand (1949, 1961). The specific action on the rod lamellae may indicate that they have a mosaic macromolecular structure, with consequent weakening of cohesive forces by comparison with those existing in other membranes that include a continuous bimolecular layer of lipid.

There is no indication, at least for the great majority of discs within the rod, of continuity between the membranes comprising the discs and the surface membrane. The incisures do not seem to hold any special significance in this respect, since the surface membrane that envelops the disc stack maintains a fairly constant distance from the disc edges and does not penetrate the incisures. The possibility of continuity between adjacent discs has also been carefully investigated, since such an occurrence could permit all of the transverse lamellae in a rod to function as a single continuous membrane. The conclusion reached is that there is no continuity between the discs themselves nor between the discs and the surface membrane, except for a very limited region at the proximal end of the rod (near the inner segment), where a few pairs of lamellae are continuous with the surface membrane along a part of their circumferences, and appear as infoldings of the surface membrane (Moody and Robertson, 1960; Cohen, 1961, 1963, 1968; Nilsson, 1965).

From studies on the incorporation and subsequent disposition of labelled amino acid in rod outer segments, the conclusion has been reached that the transverse lamellae are formed continuously at the proximal end of the rod, and are then progressively displaced distally (DROZ, 1963; YOUNG, 1968; YOUNG and DROZ, 1968; HALL, BOK, and BACHARACH, 1969). One may thus suppose that the few pairs of lamellae at the proximal end of the rod that are connected with the surface membrane are ones that have recently been formed by an expansion and infolding of the surface membrane. After being formed in this way the paired lamellae are presumably pinched off from the surface and displaced distally by further growth at the proximal end. The continuity between the proximal lamellae and the surface membrane can thus be regarded as a feature of vertebrate rod outer segments consistent with the continuous replacement of lamellae.

The situation in cones is different, and is more variable from species to species. In amphibia (NILSSON, 1965; DE ROBERTIS and LASANSKY, 1961; BROWN, GIBBONS, and WALD, 1963), fishes (SJÖSTRAND, 1959) and reptiles (YAMADA, 1961), most, if not all, the transverse lamellae that occupy the cone interior are continuous with the surface membrane along about one-third of the circumference of the receptor. The infoldings of the surface membrane that give rise to the lamellar pairs are here very clearly revealed. In mammals (COHEN, 1961; DOWLING, 1965; COHEN, 1970) and birds (COHEN, 1963) the majority of lamellae are in the form of discs that are isolated from the surface membrane similarly as in rods. Over much of the length of the cone, however, there do occur occasional pairs of lamellae that differ from their neighbours in being continuous with the surface membrane.

E. The Early Receptor Potential

Additional information about the physical state of the visual pigment in relation to the structure of the receptor can be obtained from the early receptor potential. This is a fast transient potential change recorded from the retina on flash illumination (BROWN and MURAKAMI, 1964; CONE, 1964a; PAK and CONE, 1964; BRINDLEY and GARDNER-MEDWIN, 1966). This type of potential change can be reasonably attributed to a change in either the orientation or magnitude (or possibly both) of the electric dipole of the pigment molecule. (It should be noted that this electric dipole — determined largely by the presence of ionized groups — is not related to the dipole that resides in the chromophore. This latter is set into oscillation by the electric field of the light and through its resonance is responsible for light absorption). The dependence of the early receptor potential on changes occurring in the pigment molecule is strongly suggested by the fact that the potential can be divided into a number of components, each of which can be related to a change in the absorbance spectrum of the molecule (ARDEN, IKEDA, and SIEGEL, 1966; CONE, 1967; PAK and BOES, 1967; HAGINS and McGAUGHY, 1967; CONE and COBBS, 1969). For a potential change of the observed time course and magnitude to appear between electrodes in contact with opposite sides of the retina, it would seem essential that the change in electric dipole should take place within the thickness of a high-resistance membrane separating the interior of the rod from the external space. In this situation a change in the dipole would be equivalent in action to a displacement of charge on the membrane capacitance. This would then result in the transient flow of current between the inner and outer segments; in one direction in the interior of the receptor cell, and in the opposite direction in the external medium (the potential drop here being recorded as the early receptor potential).

Lettvin (1965) and Brindley and Gardner-Medwin (1966) have discussed an alternative possibility for the origin of the early receptor potential — namely that it arises from an asymmetric arrangement of electric dipoles, as would occur if rhodopsin were attached only to one face of each of the discs within the rod. Apart from the improbability of such an arrangement (in view of the way in which the lamellae are formed) there are other grounds that make this unlikely. If the majority of the lamellae are not connected with the surface membrane, one would have to assume that the current path included a low-resistance membrane of the rod outer segment separating the internal and external conducting spaces. Impedance measurements on isolated rod outer segments of the frog (Falk and Fatt, 1968a) give no indication of such a low-resistance path involving most of the rod surface.

In the case of some invertebrate receptors (squid and horseshoe crab), there is strong evidence that the early receptor potential arises as a result of charge displacements in the rhodopsin molecules located in the surface membrane, the area of which is vastly expanded by the presence of microvilli (Hagins and McGaughy, 1968; Smith and Brown, 1966).

The recognition that in apparently all vertebrate receptors a small proportion of lamellae pairs are in the form of infoldings of the surface membrane (so that the space between the members of these pairs will have a low electric resistance to the external space) raises the possibility that the early receptor potential is accounted for entirely by the action of visual pigment in these few lamellae that are continuous with the surface membrane. In the case of the mammalian retina this implies that only a very small fraction (perhaps a few per cent) of the total visual pigment is concerned in the generation of the recorded potential. It should be noted that this possibility would not militate strongly against the production of an appreciable potential change in the space external to the receptor. For example, if 3% of the lamellae of a mammalian rod, 2.0 μm in diameter, were continuous with the surface membrane, the membrane containing the effective rhodopsin would equal in area all the rest of the surface membrane of the outer segment. The area of the surface of the inner segment, through which current flows to complete the circuit for production of the response, is probably about equal to that of the outer segment. Consequently, if there were much increase in the area of lamellae continuous with the surface of the outer segment, the amplitude of the recorded potential change would come to be limited by the inner segment (on the assumption that all membranes, those containing the active pigment as well as those responding passively, have the same capacitance per unit area).

Strong evidence that only the pigment located in lamellae continuous with the surface membrane is effective in generating the response is provided by the finding that in the frog retina, (where the proportion of such lamellae is much greater in the cones than in the rods), the early receptor potential can be shown to arise predominantly from the cones. This is deduced on the grounds that the action spectrum of the response, and the recovery from bleaching, corresponds to the cone rather than the rod pigments, even though the cone outer segments occupy a much smaller volume in the retina than do the rods (GOLDSTEIN, 1967). From a comparison of the responses recorded from the fovea and from the more peripheral regions of the mixed rod and cone retina of the macaque monkey, BROWN, WATA-NABE, and MURAKAMI (1965) had already suggested that the early receptor potential generated by cones might be larger than that generated by rods. Thus they were unable to record an early receptor potential from the nearly all-rod retina of the night monkey at light intensities that evoked an easily recorded signal (about 0.3 mV) from the cone-containing macaque retina.

The early receptor potential from single rods in the amphibian retina has been recorded with intracellular microelectrodes by MURAKAMI and PAK (1970). The intracellularly recorded potential is approximately 20 times greater in amplitude than the externally recorded potential, is of the opposite polarity and has a slower decay. These features of the early receptor potential are what would be expected for a potential generated by charge displacement across the membrane capacitance, with the decay of the potential across the membrane determined by the passive electrical properties of the receptor. An analysis of the early receptor potential of rat rods, based on measurements of the voltage gradients in the conducting spaces surrounding the receptors and considerations of the passive electrical properties of the receptors, has been made by HAGINS and RÜPPEL (1971). The conclusion drawn is that the early receptor potential can be accounted for by charge displacement within the thickness of the membrane generated by visual pigment molecules located in a small number of lamellae continuous with the surface membrane.

II. Morphological Changes on Illumination

Ever since the specialized structure of the visual receptor was recognized by light microscopists and correlated with the presence of a light-sensitive pigment, attempts have been made to detect structural changes related to the bleaching of the visual pigment.

A readily observed morphological change, produced by exposure to light of moderate intensity for a period of a few hours, is a shortening of the myoid of the cone cells of fishes, amphibians and birds (see GARTEN, 1907; WALLS, 1942). The myoid is the elongated portion of the inner segment, containing longitudinally oriented fibrils, that extends between the region of densely packed mitochondria (the ellipsoid) and the cell nucleus. Indeed, the term myoid ("like muscle") was introduced by ENGELMANN (1885) in recognition of the contraction of this portion of the visual cell on illumination of the retina. There is no information regarding the location and character of the light-absorbing material nor how the effect of light on the myoid is brought about.

In rod cells the changes in myoid length are less striking and less consistent, and are generally in the opposite sense to those in cones (AREY, 1916a, b). There is the possibility that the change generally observed − an elongation under the influence of light − may merely be a passive mechanical response to lateral compression by the adjacent cones.

According to EWALD and KÜHNE (1878b), prolonged and intense illumination of the isolated eyecup of the frog (containing the retina together with pigment epithelium and sclera) causes changes in the dimensions of the rod outer segments. An increase in cross-sectional area of the rods was detected by observing the diminution of the spaces between the rods when the retina was viewed from the distal ends of the rods after detachment of the sclera and pigment epithelium. An increase in diameter (up to 15%) of the rod outer segments has also been described on the basis of measurements on fixed and sectioned material, particularly in the case of the large diameter rods of the salamander (Angelucci, 1894; Garten, 1907). A shortening of the rod outer segment was also reported by Angelucci and Garten though the percentage decrease in length was less than the increase in diameter and was considerably more variable, suggesting that this effect might be a passive mechanical response to other morphological changes taking place in the eyecup. It is important to bear in mind that these changes in dimensions of the rod outer segment require much more intense and prolonged illumination than is required to bleach the pigment and to keep it bleached for the period during which the morphological change develops. The swelling of the rod outer segments has been found to be reversed in the dark, provided the retina is placed in contact with the pigment epithelium (Ewald and Kühne, 1878b). It seems possible that the changes in rod diameter seen in these studies is the result of an alteration in the chemical environment of the retina, e.g. a shift in pH, which might have a slowly developing effect on the osmotic properties of the rod through changing the amount of fixed charge in its interior. The structure in which light is absorbed to initiate a chemical change in this way cannot be ascribed on the reported findings, but it is entirely possible that the pigment epithelium, rather than the receptor cells, may be concerned.

Microscopic observations on individual isolated rod outer segments of the frog have been made in an attempt to detect any changes in dimensions that might follow rapidly on bleaching (Fatt, unpublished observations). Suspensions of isolated rod outer segments were prepared in dim red light by removing the dark adapted retina from the eyecup, placing it in Ringer solution (pH 7.0) and then agitating the solution. The degree of agitation was limited so that no appreciable fraction of the rod outer segments was carried into the air-water interface. The majority of the outer segments appeared soon after isolation as highly refractile, straight, apparently rigid circular cylinders mostly about 6 μm in diameter and 50 μm long. To the limit of resolution of the light microscope they were devoid of any fine internal structure, apart from longitudinally-running lines that presumably corresponded to refractive index changes at the incisures present in the disc stack. The lamellar composition of the rod interior would not have been be visible, for the repeat interval of the lamellae is well below the limit of resolution of the light microscope.

For the detection of any change in dimensions, the isolated rod outer segment was viewed under high magnification (employing an oil immersion objective) with deep red illumination (light from a tungsten-filament lamp filtered through 4-mm thicknesses each of Schott-RG 10 and Chance-HA 1 glasses, the transmittance of this filter combination being flat at 0.27 ± 0.03 between 725 and 765 nm but falling off steeply at shorter wavelengths to less than 10^{-4} at 600 nm and below). A comparison was made between the dimensions of the rod measured a few seconds before and a few seconds after exposing the rod to a one-second flash of white light. This was sufficient to bleach most of the visual pigment in the rod and to allow time for the thermal conversion of rhodopsin photoproducts to proceed to the stage of metarhodopsin II. Some observations were carried out on rods in suspensions that had been prepared with sodium chloride as the major solute, and others with potassium chloride. No change was found in either case, the accuracy of measurement being such that a change of 2% in length or of 5% in diameter would have been detectable. An upper limit of 0.1% for any change (a decrease) in the dimensions of the rod that might follow within 2 sec of bleaching is given by impedance measurements on isolated rod outer segments (described in detail in a later section, see p. 220). Clearly such a change could not be observed microscopically.

It has been claimed (WOLKEN, 1961) that bleaching of the visual pigment causes structural disorganization of the rod outer segments, namely a loss of rigidity and an appearance of cross-striations. The idea that such an alteration in structure is an immediate response to bleaching can be denied, however. In a suspension of freshly isolated rod outer segments of the frog, no obvious change in structure is observed to occur to a significant fraction of the population for up to one-half hour following complete bleaching. At room temperature changes in rod structure occur within a few hours after isolation, but these changes are not the result of bleaching, for they can be seen in rod suspensions (prepared as usual from dark-adapted animals) that have not been exposed to bleaching light. These changes in rod structure are of two kinds. In one kind the rods appear to lose their rigidity and high degree of refractility. They increase somewhat in length, become curved, and develop cross-striations at irregular intervals. Their surface, as seen under high power, puckers at irregular intervals and small refractile droplets frequently occur attached to it. On the further progress of this kind of change the interior appears granular between the increasingly prominent cross-striations. In the other kind of change the rod remains highly refractile and does not develop any conspicuous internal structural pattern. Instead, the rod swells at one end, or develops a sharp bend at one position along its length. It then proceeds to curl up into a tight spiral, which in its final form has the appearance of a highly refractile flattened sphere. It is uncertain, even, whether a significant difference in the relative numbers of rods undergoing morphological change exists between bleached and unbleached suspensions after storage for longer periods, for under both conditions the majority of rods appear altered. The structural changes are similar in appearance to those that take place when rods are put into hypotonic solutions. These changes have been well known to light microscopists for a long time (SCHULTZE, 1869, p. 380; KOLMER, 1936, p. 310; SCHMIDT, 1938). Indeed, observations on the appearance of cross-striations form the basis for the idea put forward by SCHULTZE that the fine structure of the outer segments consisted of discs with spacings below the resolution of the light microscope.

Nevertheless, it can be readily shown, by keeping outer segments for short periods at elevated temperatures, that the bleaching of the rhodopsin in rod outer segments does affect their structural stability (FALK and FATT, unpublished observations). Thus, when a suspension of rods, prepared by shaking a retina in Ringer solution, is divided into a number of aliquots, half of which are bleached and the others unbleached, and then warmed for periods of 10 min at different temperatures, the following morphological changes are observed. At temperatures up to 35° C the bleached and unbleached rods both appear normal under the light microscope; i.e. about 90% are straight, highly refractile, rigid cylinders, devoid of cross-striation, the remainder having either bulges or bends, or being curved with fine cross-striations. At 38° C the rods that had been unbleached at the time they were warmed continue to appear normal when subsequently examined at room temperature, while of the bleached rods only about 55% appear straight and free of cross-striation. At 41.5° C the proportion of straight, cross-striation-free rods among those that were unbleached is reduced to about 80%, but among the bleached rods the proportion in such condition is only about 1%, about 60% being curled, and 40% elongated with prominent cross-striations. Only when the temperature is raised to 48° C is the proportion of structurally unaltered rods in the unbleached population reduced to 50%, there being at this temperature no normal rods among the bleached population. The warming of a suspension of unbleached frog rods at a temperature of 52° C for 10 min causes virtually the entire rod population to lose its normal structure. It should be emphasized that this treatment does not produce any significant bleaching of the rods. Thermal bleaching of most of the rhodopsin of frog rods however, is produced by heating at 62° C for 10 min. A steep relation between temperature and thermal bleaching of rhodopsin is evident from the work of LYTHGOE and QUILLIAM (1938), HUBBARD (1958) and WILLIAMS and MILBY (1968) who measured the energy of activation of the process.

It is thus seen that photochemical bleaching of visual pigment lowers by about 10° C the temperature required to produce a morphological change in the rod over a period of 10 min. These findings are evidently related to HUBBARD's (1958) observations on the greater thermal stability of rhodopsin as compared with opsin. She showed that the thermal denaturation of opsin (judged by the loss of ability of the protein to regenerate rhodopsin on incubation with 11-*cis*-retinaldehyde) occurs at a temperature 15—20° C lower than that required to bleach and denature rhodopsin (the initial products of thermal bleaching being denatured opsin and 11-*cis*-retinaldehyde).

Since the structural changes in frog rods described above appear before there is any appreciable thermal bleaching of rhodopsin, it must be supposed that there is some change involving rhodopsin that precedes its thermal bleaching. A change in rod properties described by CONE and BROWN (1967) is the decrease of the early receptor potential in the isolated rat retina when warmed at 48—58° C for a few minutes. This degree of warming does not bleach the visual pigment to any significant extent, but it does abolish the dichroism of the rods. The interpretation placed on these observations is that the warming disorientates the visual pigment within the receptors. It seems quite possible that gross morphological changes may follow from a disorientation of rhodopsin (or opsin), which is probably a major constituent of the rod lamellae, and that stability of rod structure is conferred normally by the existence of oriented rhodopsin molecules. It is also noteworthy that the thermal stability of opsin and rhodopsin is greater when they form part of the organized solid structure of the rod than when in solution (HUBBARD, 1958).

Morphological changes involving irreversible destruction of rod cells have been described in rats maintained under illuminated conditions for 20 hrs or more (NOELL, WALKER, KANG, and BERMAN, 1966). The initial degenerative changes, observed with the light microscope in fixed and stained retinas, involve the inner segments, the nuclei of which appear shrunken. The dependence of these effects on the wavelength of illumination, and spectrometric analysis of the content of visual pigment both suggest that the changes are associated with the maintenance of a large fraction of the visual pigment in a bleached condition. The induction of the changes in structure is, moreover, facilitated by maintaining the animals at a raised body temperature. One wonders if the degeneration follows from the diminished thermal stability of opsin, and is related to the thermally-induced structural changes described in isolated rod outer segments. Although the outer segments of illuminated rat retinas were observed to degenerate within a few days, no early changes in the outer segments were noted at the time that changes had become apparent in the inner segment. It should be noted, however, that many of the conventional histological procedures used in light microscopy cause changes in rod outer segments (e.g. the appearance of gross cross-striations). Any such changes, if produced under the conditions of illumination, might have escaped detection, especially in view of the small diameter of rat rods (about 1.5 μm).

With the higher resolution of the electron microscope, KUWABARA and GORN (1968) have shown that the earliest changes that can be detected occur in the outer segments. Initially there is swelling of the discs which leads progressively to vesiculation of the discs, loss of alignment of the disc stack and irregular bending of the outer segments. They made the interesting observation that the changes begin at the distal end of the outer segment and extend gradually towards the proximal end. This result would be expected from the foregoing. The discs at the distal ends of the rods are the oldest. The probability that they would contain denatured or disoriented rhodopsin molecules is greater than for those discs at the proximal end containing newly synthesized rhodopsin.

III. Transfer and Conversion of Absorbed Energy

Visual excitation involves a process in which a photon absorbed by any one of some 10^9 rhodopsin molecules within a single rod has a high probability of producing a change that can be signalled to the nervous system. It is this property of the visual process that has led to consideration of the various forms of long-range energy transfer (over distances many times greater than molecular dimensions), such as exciton migration, resonance transfer and photoconduction, that might occur. A general account of energy transfer is given by REID (1957).

The diagram (Fig. 1) shows the quantum-mechanically allowed energy levels for a molecule in its ground- (D) and electronically-excited (D*) states. The more closely spaced levels correspond to different vibrational states. The transition from D to D* may be effected by absorption of a photon, with the particular vibrational level reached in the excited state depending on the positions of the atomic nuclei in the molecule at the instant of absorption. At room temperature this would be followed by a rapid vibrational relaxation to the lowest energy level of the excited state, as indicated by the wavy arrow. In the absence of a photo-

14*

chemical reaction, the excited state of the molecule is terminated by radiative or radiationless transitions to the ground state (which may involve other excited states whose energy level is less than D*). The energy may appear as fluorescence, phosphorescence or heat. Under certain conditions electronic excitation can be transferred to an acceptor molecule A before being lost to competing processes. It is emphasized that the processes of energy transfer to be considered do not depend on chemical reaction. Indeed to the extent that a chemical change occurs, it may reduce the efficiency of the transfer process. Phosphorescence of rhodopsin has not been observed, and, as will be discussed later (p. 216), the quantum yield of fluorescence of rhodopsin is extremely low (Guzzo and Pool, 1968).

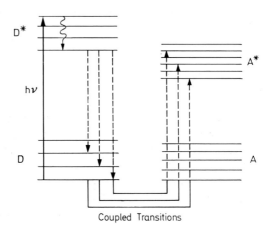

Coupled Transitions

Fig. 1. Energy levels of donor and acceptor molecules and their coupled transitions. Absorption of radiant energy hν raises the donor species into an upper vibrational level of an excited state D* which is followed by nuclear relaxation to the lowest vibrational level (shown by wavy arrow) of this excited state of the molecule, as thermal equilibrium takes place. The broken lines show the coupled transitions in which excitation energy from D* is transferred to the acceptor molecule A

A. Dissipation of Energy as Heat

Observations have been made on the heat dissipated following the absorption of light by rhodopsin. These have an important bearing on the possibility of long-range energy transfer in rods.

Conductance changes have been observed in suspensions of frog rod outer segments illuminated by a 1-msec flash from a xenon lamp (Falk and Fatt, 1968b). One component of conductance change (the heat component) has its origin in a rise in temperature that causes an increased mobility of ions initially present in the aqueous spaces of the suspension. As is consistent with this mode of origin, the amplitude of the heat component varies in proportion to the conductivity of the suspending medium. The development of the heat component is very rapid, (generally indistinguishable from the time integral of the light used to expose the rods). It then decays slowly along a time course that appears to be determined by the thermal properties of the conductivity cell used for the measurement. The amplitude of this component (when considered as a fractional increase in the real part of the admittance of the rod suspension), and its onset are nearly independent of the frequency of measurement over a wide range extending both above and below the region in which conductance changes in the interior of the rod come under observation.

This result requires that thermal equilibration should take place rapidly between the internal spaces of the rod, where heat is evolved by the visual pigment, and the external spaces. One may place an upper limit for equilibration at about 300 μsec, this being the time resolution for the observation of rapid conductance changes. One may note further that this applies even at the lowest temperatures at which observations have been made, namely in the region of $-2°$ C. Such behaviour is, in fact, consistent with the proposed mechanism of origin of the response. Thus in water the thermal diffusivity (which approximates numerically to the thermal conductivity expressed as cal/cm sec $°$ C) is 0.0012–0.0014 cm²/sec over the temperature range of interest. For the lipid portion of the rod one may expect a slightly smaller thermal diffusivity, i.e. in the region of 0.0008 cm²/sec (taken as that for olive oil). For a volume fraction occupied by the rods in the suspension of 0.80, and for an average thermal diffusivity of 0.0010 cm²/sec, the temperature in the external space is then calculated to reach 90% of its final level (corresponding to thermal equilibrium between inside and outside) in 6.6 μsec (CRANK, 1956 § 5.33). If the volume fraction were much less, so that practically complete transfer of heat would occur from the rod interior to the outside (where the temperature rise would be much less than in the previous case), the time to approach thermal equilibrium would be greater, but still very short (90% completion in 30 μsec).

Of the total conductance increase that is attributable to heating in rods when exposed to a 460–560 nm flash, about 82% depends on the absorption of light by rhodopsin. The remainder is due to absorption by other substances in the rod suspension as shown by the decline in the magnitude of the heat component as rhodopsin is removed by bleaching. This is so whether the rods are suspended in a normal solution or in one containing 0.1 M hydroxylamine, the latter being used to check on the effect of absorption by long-lived products of rhodopsin. The magnitude of the heat component is found to vary in proportion to the amount of rhodopsin bleached when fresh preparations (in which the rods contain one-half or more of their initial rhodopsin content) are exposed to flashes bleaching up to 20% of the initial rhodopsin.

The measurement of the heat component allows a quantitative estimate to be made of the amount of energy dissipated as heat per mole of rhodopsin bleached in the rods. For a flash that bleaches 1.75% of the initial rhodopsin content, the conductance increases by 0.0084%. Assuming a specific heat of 1.0 for the rod suspension, and a temperature coefficient of conductivity of 3.0%/° C (applicable to the sucrose-containing solution used in preparing the rod suspension), the conductance change is calculated to have arisen from a release of heat amounting to 2.8 mcal/cm³ of rod suspension. From the estimated amount of bleaching, and taking the rhodopsin concentration in the rod suspension to be 1.8 mM (corresponding to 2.2 mM rhodopsin in the rod outer segment), this corresponds to

89 kcal per mole of rhodopsin bleached[1]. This is equivalent to 1.6 einsteins at 500 nm (the peak of absorbance by rhodopsin). This result may be compared with the quantum efficiency for the photochemical bleaching of rhodopsin solubilized with digitonin, i.e. 1.5 photons absorbed for every rhodopsin molecule bleached (DARTNALL, 1968). There is evidence that the quantum efficiency for the bleaching of rhodopsin *in situ* is the same as in extracts (HAGINS, 1954; compare the results of BAUMANN, 1965, with DARTNALL, 1968). Furthermore, observations of the heat liberated in a concentrated rhodopsin solution when a measured quantity of light is absorbed (measurements being carried out with a thermocouple) indicate that at least 90% of the energy of the absorbed light is degraded into heat (HAGINS, reported in HAGINS and McGAUGHY, 1967). Thus three kinds of measurement (the amount of heat released per rhodopsin molecule bleached, the number of molecules bleached per photon absorbed, and the heat released per photon absorbed) are in reasonable agreement.

It can be concluded that all the radiant energy absorbed by rhodopsin in the rods is degraded into heat. Since this occurs within about 300 μsec (the limit of resolution of the method by which the heat component of conductance change was determined), one can eliminate from consideration any long-lasting energy-transfer mechanisms requiring the persistence (longer than 300 μsec) of states of higher energy. This is consistent with the fact that no long-lived excited state of rhodopsin has been observed and, if a triplet state of rhodopsin exists, it must have a lifetime of less that 10 μsec (ABRAHAMSON, ADAMS, and WULFF, 1959). However, 300 μsec is long compared with the expected lifetime of an excited state of rhodopsin (less than 0.1 μsec) so that long-range energy transfer is not ruled out by the heat measurements, though as will be shown below, it is extremely improbable on other grounds.

B. Transfer of Electronic Excitation Energy

In the case of exciton migration there is strong interaction between neighbouring molecules of a crystal so that transfer of electronic excitation energy may occur in a shorter time than molecular vibration (which requires $10^{-13} - 10^{-12}$ sec). The excitation, migrating in a time that is more nearly comparable to the time for transition to the excited state (about 10^{-15} sec), can be regarded as belonging to an assembly of molecules rather than as localized at any particular instant to a single molecule. A necessary condition is extensive overlap between orbitals of adjacent molecules, so that an excited electron is effectively delocalized. This condition may be realized in periodic structures (crystals) of high dielectric constant.

Even where the interaction between molecules is relatively weak, it is still possible to have transfer of electronic excitation energy by a mechanism known as reasonance transfer, involving dipole-dipole interaction. The theory in its most useful form has been given by FÖRSTER (1959).

Consider the transitions between the electronic states of the molecules D and A (Fig. 1): $D^* \rightarrow D$, $A \rightarrow A^*$, where the star designates the molecule in the state of

---

1 The earlier estimate (FALK and FATT, 1968b) of the heat release, namely 117 kcal per mole of rhodopsin bleached, was based on an assumed value of 1.7 mM rhodopsin in frog rod outer segments. Optical-density measurements (DENTON and WYLLIE, 1955; LIEBMAN, 1962) suggest that this is an underestimate of the rhodopsin content.

higher energy. These two transitions may be coupled when the transition dipoles have a common frequency, i.e. when the energies of the separate transitions are the same. A radiationless transfer of energy from D* to A can then occur, leading to D* + A → D + A*. Provided that the donor molecule is in thermal equilibrium with its surroundings before there is any energy transfer, the energy transferred will depend only on the frequency common to the emission spectrum of the donor and the absorbance spectrum of the acceptor. The probability of energy transfer will be proportional to the lifetime of the excited state of the donor (which can be estimated from the quantum yield of the donor emission in the absence of transfer) and to factors that depend on the overlap of the two spectra and the relative orientation of the transition dipoles in donor and acceptor; and will be inversely proportional to the sixth power of the distance between donor and acceptor. Thus the critical dependence of transfer on intermolecular distance makes transfer unlikely over distances greater than about 10 nm, even in most favourable circumstances, if the transfer is restricted to a single stage. However, the donor and acceptor need not be different molecular species but can be different electronic states of the same molecular species. The transfer act can then take place repeatedly if the concentration is high enough.

The possibility of migration of electronic excitation energy in frog rod outer segments has been examined by HAGINS and JENNINGS (1959). They sought for such energy transfer among the fluorescent molecules of a rhodopsin product after bleaching dark-adapted rods. They illuminated a small region (about 2 μm wide) of a bleached frog rod with the 405 or 436 nm Hg line and looked for any spread of the yellow fluorescence beyond the area illuminated. This was done both in the case when the rod axis lay perpendicular, and also when it was parallel to the exciting image. In neither case did the fluorescence extend beyond the region excited by the incident light (resolution 0.5 − 1.0 μm).

This negative result has no necessary relevance to the possibility of energy transfer among rhodopsin molecules. There is some question as to which of the rhodopsin photolytic products was under observation (see p. 203; GUZZO and POOL, 1968 and 1969; LIEBMAN and LEIGH, 1969); hence there is the possibility that the fluorescing species was present in significantly lower concentration than rhodopsin in dark-adapted rods. In that event the observations on the fluorescence would have no bearing on the question of energy transfer in dark-adapted rods, for, as has been noted, the probability of transfer decreases as a high power of the distance between donor and acceptor molecules.

More recently, LIEBMAN (1962) has made microspectrophotometric observations on single rod outer segments of the frog. He attempted to determine directly if the excitation energy of rhodopsin molecules could spread over distances comparable with the dimensions of the rod. Dark-adapted rods were illuminated locally with a beam of light of 3 μm diameter and of 500 nm wavelength, so that a large fraction of the rhodopsin in this region was bleached within about one minute. LIEBMAN then looked, in various regions of the rod, for optical density changes that might indicate bleaching beyond the region illuminated. None was observed at distances greater than 2 μm from the illuminated region. Any spread of bleaching over distances less than 2 μm would not have been detected owing to the limitations of the method. In any case, migration of electronic excitation energy over distances as large as 2 μm in the direction parallel with the rod axis would seem *a priori* to be improbable if there is no continuity among lamellae. Unfortunately, in order to detect any spread of bleaching in directions perpendicular to the rod axis, it was necessary to compress the rods so that the width was about twice the diameter of a normal rod. As LIEBMAN pointed out, there is some question whether continuity of structure within a disk is maintained under these conditions.

Thus radiationless migration of electronic excitation has not been detected experimentally, though it has not been excluded by these observations. It is worth considering if, in theory, one could expect excitation transfer in the rods. HAGINS and JENNINGS (1959) attempted to make such calculations using the theory of FÖRSTER outlined above. At the time, the fluorescence spectrum of rhodopsin had not been observed, and in order to obtain an estimate of the spectral overlap integral, they assumed that the emission and absorbance spectra of rhodopsin would show the same proportional red shift as in the case of vitamin A (absorbance maximum 327 nm; emission maximum 510 nm). HAGINS and JENNINGS calculated that even assuming a fluorescence yield of unity, the mean distance between rhodopsin molecules in the rod was 3—6 times (depending on how the rhodopsin was distributed in the rods) the critical transfer distance at which there would be an equal probability of excitation transfer and of spontaneous deactivation. Since the probability for radiationless transfer of excitation energy falls as the sixth power of the distance, the probability of transfer would be vanishingly small if there were no local clustering of rhodopsin molecules. The distance between clusters would then be such as to make the transfer of electronic excitation energy over distances comparable with rod dimensions even less likely.

The fluorescence spectrum and quantum yield of the fluorescence of cattle rhodopsin in digitonin extracts, and in freeze-dried rod outer segments has recently been determined by GUZZO and POOL (1968). The emission spectrum has a maximum at 575—600 nm so that the overlap between the emission spectrum and the absorbance spectrum of rhodopsin is very much greater than was assumed by HAGINS and JENNINGS. However, the fluorescence yield in digitonin solution is extremely low (only about 0.005) indicating a very short radiative lifetime. One if forced to conclude that the radiationless transfer of excitation energy in the rods is improbable.

C. Photoconduction

In the case of photoconductivity, as known in the solid state of matter, a mobile charge becomes available when the energy of an absorbed photon promotes an electron from a filled valence band of allowed energy states into an empty conduction band. The electron, having entered a previously empty conduction band, leaves behind a positively charged hole, which also may migrate under the influence of an electric field. Alternatively, the presence of impurities gives rise to other energy levels such that excitation of an electron from a donor level into the conduction band yields a mobile electron and a bound hole, while excitation of an electron from the valence band into an acceptor level yields a mobile hole and a bound electron.

The magnitude of photoconductivity depends on the number of charge carriers generated, their mobility and their lifetime. If photoconductivity is to have any role in vision (so that a single photon absorbed anywhere in a rod outer segment could have a high probability of being counted some distance away) it is necessary for the charge carriers to have either a high mobility or a long life or some combination of the two. The evidence, that all radiant energy absorbed by rhodopsin in the rods is rapidly degraded into heat, rules out the occurrence of any photoconductivity in rods that involves charge carriers with an average lifetime greater than about $300\mu sec$. In further measurements at frequencies up to 16 MHz (FALK and FATT, unpublished) with a time resolution of 50 μsec, no evidence for photoconduction was obtained, the initial transient rise in conductivity of the rod suspension being attributable to a change in ionic mobility in the aqueous spaces as a result of an increase in temperature (the heat component).

Using a d.c. voltage-current method with a time resolution only of the order of seconds, ROSENBERG, ORLANDO, and ORLANDO (1961) claimed to have observed photoconductivity in dried rod outer segments of sheep. The maximum increase in specific conductance that they observed on illumination was extremely small (less than 10^{-9} mho/cm). The fact that a photocurrent was observed only under conditions in which it was thought that the samples still contained water makes it likely that conduction was ionic (i.e. involved the migration of atomic nuclei) rather than electronic. Moreover, if the observed phenomenon were due to photoconductivity, the lifetime of the electronic charge carriers would have to be several seconds long − a possibility that appears to be ruled out by observations on the rapid heat dissipation already discussed. It seems possible that what was measured corresponds, in fact, to the heat component. That the generation of electronic charge carriers by direct optical excitation might compete effectively with photoisomerization of rhodopsin (ROSENBERG, 1966) is unlikely in view of the apparent absence of a significant photoconductivity and the high quantum efficiency of bleaching of rhodopsin both in solution and in the rods.

IV. Uptake of Hydrogen Ions

One component of the conductance change observed upon illumination of a packed suspension of frog rod outer segments (FALK and FATT, 1968b) arises through the uptake of hydrogen ion in the dark reaction in which metarhodopsin I is converted to metarhodopsin II (MATTHEWS, HUBBARD, BROWN, and WALD, 1963; OSTROY, ERHARDT, and ABRAHAMSON, 1966). A conductance change having the same origin is seen also in solutions of rhodopsin solubilized with digitonin (T. HARA, 1958; R. HARA, 1963). An uptake of hydrogen ions was first recognized to occur at an early stage in the conversion of rhodopsin photoproducts by using a pH-sensitive glass electrode, though this technique of recording was too slow to permit the resolution of changes occuring in less than about 10 sec (RADDING and WALD, 1956). By a back-titration method, the uptake was found to amount to one H^+ per molecule of rhodopsin bleached. The apparent pK of the acid-binding group was estimated to be 6.5. In contrast to these findings on solubilized cattle rhodopsin, potentiometric measurements of pH changes in a suspension of frog rod outer segments have indicated a pK of roughly 7.9 (FALK and FATT, 1966). A maximum H^+ uptake of 1.7 mM − estimated from the change in pH, a knowledge of the buffering capacity of the suspending medium and of the rods (at pH 6.8) and a pK of 7.9 – is somewhat less than the rhodopsin content of the rods (about 2.2 mM). It would appear that a better estimate of the pK would be 7.3, which would be consistent with a H^+ uptake equal on a mole basis to the amount of rhodopsin bleached.

It seems possible that the difference in pK for H^+ uptake between the solubilized cattle rhodopsin and the suspension of frog rods is due to the difference in the environment of the pigment, which in the former case is contained in digitonin micelles, and in the latter is fixed in the rod lamellae. However, the data of McCONNELL, RAFFERTY, and DILLEY (1968) on the H^+ taken up by fragments of cattle rod outer segments per mole of rhodopsin bleached would indicate a pK in the region of 6.4, this value being about the same as that obtained by RADDING and WALD (1956) and by MATTHEWS, HUBBARD, BROWN, and WALD (1963) for cattle rhodopsin in digitonin solution. The different values of pK may, therefore, be species related.

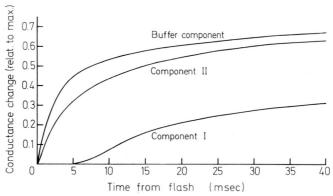

Fig. 2. Computed time courses for different components of conductance change observed in a suspension of frog rod outer segments at a temperature of 20° C. The curve for the buffer component is taken from measurements on the pH changes produced in solutions of rhodopsin following flash illumination. The curve for component II is taken from records of the change in absolute value of admittance at 100—300 kHz with the rods suspended in a low-conductivity medium, suitable corrections being made for heat and buffer components. The curve for component I is derived from records obtained with the rods suspended in high-conductivity media, containing 100—300 mM NaCl, on the assumption that in 100 mM NaCl the final level of response contained contributions from components I and II in the ratio 1:2.0, and in 300 mM NaCl in the ratio 1:1.1 (FALK and FATT, 1968b)

A time course of H^+ uptake (FALK and FATT, 1966) in close agreement with the reported time course of metarhodopsin II formation (WULFF, ADAMS, LINSCHITZ, and ABRAHAMSON, 1958; HAGINS, 1956; ABRAHAMSON, MARQUISEE, GAVUZZI, and ROUBIE, 1960) was obtained in potentiometric pH measurements on solubilized rhodopsin (using either digitonin or Triton X-100 as solubilizer). The time course of this response to a brief flash is not exponential (Fig. 2). It rises to 30% of its final level in 1.5 msec, to 50% in 5 msec and to 70% in 20 msec (at 20° C). Variations in the rate of metarhodopsin II formation, depending on whether the rhodopsin has been solubilized by digitonin or by a cationic detergent, have been reported by WILLIAMS and BREIL (1968).

On the other hand, the time course of the pH change recorded from the rod suspension indicates a lag of about 300 msec between the uptake of H^+ by rhodopsin and the subsequent removal of H^+ from the buffer in the suspending medium. It seems possible that this lag is determined by the passage, across the surface membrane of the rod, of low-molecular-weight molecules capable of serving as buffers.

The time lags inherent in the potentiometric method of measurement of H^+ uptake in suspensions of rods can be overcome in admittance (reciprocal of impedance) measurements when the frequency of measurement is sufficiently high (above the characteristic frequency) for a major fraction of the current flowing across the suspension to pass through the rod interior (FALK and FATT, 1968b). With the rods suspended in a low-conductivity, phosphate-buffered solution (the major ions present being usually 6 mM phosphate and 12 mM Na^+, together with 1% serum albumin) and packed into a conductivity cell to occupy a volume fraction of about 0.8, the measurement of admittance at 300 kHz shows a prominent component of conductance increase that follows rapidly on illumination. This can be attributed to an increase in conductivity of buffer in the interior of the rod as a result of H^+ uptake by rhodopsin. Thus, the removal of a hydrogen ion from the buffer would result in an increase in its state of ionization, with $H_2PO_4^-$ being converted to $HPO_4^=$, and hence an overall increase in conductivity. (This depends on the fact that the pigment molecule receiving the H^+ is immobile, so that a change in its charge has no effect on the conductivity).

A feature of this component of admittance change, distinguishing it from others observed on illumination of the rod suspension, is the possibility of reversing the sign of the change on replacing the anionic phosphate buffer by a cationic buffer such as imidazole. When the latter type of buffer is used, the effect of the uptake of H^+ by visual pigment is a diminution in the degree of ionization of buffer (imidazole being converted from the ionized, protonated form to the un-ionized form). As a consequence, there is a decrease in conductivity. From the known equivalent conductances for the various buffer ions concerned, it is possible to calculate the amount of H^+ removed from the buffer to produce the measured conductance change. This calculation indicates an uptake of one H^+ for each rhodopsin molecule bleached, in agreement with the results of pH measurements. Furthermore, by use of the reversal of the sign of the conductance on replacement of an anionic by a cationic buffer, the time course of the buffer component has been accurately determined, and is found to agree with the time course of H^+ uptake found by the potentiometric (pH) measurement on solubilized rhodopsin. It is further observed that this component of conductance change varies in proportion to the amount of rhodopsin bleached.

V. Changes in Electrical Properties that Depend on Rod Structure

The conductance changes so far described, i.e. the heat component and the buffer component of response, do not depend in any way on rod structure and can be observed in rhodopsin solutions. Two other components of conductance change that do depend on an intact rod structure have been identified (Falk and Fatt, 1968b). These are called components I and II. They are distinguished by their differing dependence on the frequency of measurement (within the frequency range investigated, extending, from 15 Hz to 16 MHz) as well as by their different time courses. Each component appears as an increase in admittance of the packed suspension of frog rod outer segments. This increase is maintained indefinitely (up to at least 8 min, the maximum time over which a change of the magnitude of the response can be followed, as limited by unpredictable drift in the measurements).

A. Component I

Component I is measured as an increase (ΔG) in the real part of admittance. This is independent of the frequency of measurement, from very low frequencies (presumably from zero frequency) up to the characteristic frequency for admittance, f_Y, this being defined as the frequency at which the real part of admittance of the suspension equals the algebraic mean of its limiting values reached above and below the frequency range over which the surface membrane of the rods is prominent in effecting a frequency-dependent behaviour. Roughly, f_Y may be taken to correspond to the frequency above which the voltage gradient in the external solution extends to the interior of the rod. The response for a given amount of rhodopsin bleached varies in direct proportion to the conductivity of the suspending medium, G_0, which can be controlled by the addition of electrolyte. The response is not dependent on the particular ion species used for this purpose. Since the specific conductance, G_1, of the suspension measured at frequencies much below the characteristic frequency also varies in proportion to G_0 (owing to the reproducibility of the volume fraction, p, occupied by the rods when suspended in media of different conductivities), the response regarded as a fractional increase in G_1 is nearly constant. That the response depends on the absorption of light by rhodopsin is shown by the agreement between the action spectrum of the conductance change and the absorbance spectrum of rhodopsin. It is likely that this component of response corresponds to the conductance increase observed by T. Hara (1958) in a suspension of cattle rods in 0.15 M NaCl measured at a frequency of 1 kHz.

The time course of component I (Fig. 2) has been determined by the application of a bleaching flash lasting less than 1 msec, and after subtraction of other, more rapidly developing, components of conductance change (heat component, buffer component and component II as described below). Following a latent period of about 5 msec the response at 20° C develops to reach 50% of its final amplitude in about 90 msec, and 90% in about 400 msec.

A saturation of the response mechanism severely limits the amplitude of conductance change obtainable with flashes that bleach more than 1% of the rhodopsin in the rods. At weaker flash intensities the response is proportional to the amount of rhodopsin bleached. Recovery from saturation occurs slowly, so that the response to a weak flash is affected by a preceding bright flash for intervals up to 10 min (at 20° C). The time course of the response to a brief flash is unaltered by saturation, as observed for flashes bleaching up to 15% of the rhodopsin. This indicates that the process that saturates is completed within the latent period of the response.

Two mechanisms can be envisaged for the production of component I. One is that it arises from an increase in permeability of the surface membrane of the rod, which increase is not specific to any particular ion in the suspending medium. Another is that it has its origin in a decrease in the volume occupied by the rods. A response arising from either of these processes would appear as a frequency-independent increase in the real part of the admittance so long as the measuring frequency were well below the characteristic frequency, f_Y, of the suspension. The two mechanisms can however be discriminated by observation of the behaviour of ΔG close to f_Y. On the assumption that the major dispersion of admittance for the rod suspension is determined by the capacitance of the rod surface membrane, one can make the following inferences: If the response observed at low frequencies arises from a change in surface membrane conductance, then as the frequency of measurement is raised to approach f_Y, ΔG will fall steeply toward zero, with the greater part of this fall taking place within one decade of frequency below f_Y. Alternatively, if the response arises from a change in the volume of the rods, ΔG will remain nearly constant until f_Y is reached. Only when this frequency is surpassed may ΔG be expected to decline, to an extent dependent on the geometry of the suspension (including variation in the cross-section of conducting paths through the external medium as described below) and on any difference in ionic mobility between inside and outside the rods.

Examination of the response in the required frequency region (0.3–10 MHz) shows component I to remain constant in amplitude with increasing frequency up to f_Y. At higher frequency the response declines, but then only partly and to a variable extent. This mode of behaviour rules out the possibility that component I might have its origin in an increase in conductance of the surface membrane of the rod. On the other hand, it is consistent with a light-induced decrease in the volume of the rod.

It is important to note that a change in rod volume (which may be indicated relative to the volume of the suspension as a change, Δp, in volume fraction) can lead to an admittance change of the kind observed even if only water, unaccompanied by ions, moved between the interior of the rod and the external medium. It is necessary to consider this possibility because component I, although slower than some other components of response seen in the rod suspension, is still sufficiently rapid to make it unlikely that those ions that determine the conductivity of the internal and external spaces would be able to move across the membrane in the course of the response. This view is taken on the assumption that a passive exchange of ions between the outside and inside would require several minutes and that the final level of the observed response (which reaches 90% completion in 0.4 sec) is indicative of the relaxation of the driving force producing the response. If only water moved out of the rod during the response, then a decrease in rod volume will result in a dilution of the constant quantity of ions present in the external space and hence a reduction in the conductivity G_0 within this space. There will nevertheless occur an increase in the low-frequency specific conductance G_1 for the suspension, the value of which is determined entirely by ionic conduction in the external space, provided that diffusion occurs in this space so that the concentration of ions within it remains nearly uniform. The reason for this sensitivity of G_1 to the movement of water is that, in a path through the external medium in the direction of current flow, there are variations in the width of the gap between neighbouring particles. The conductance of the suspension is affected by the narrow portions of the path to an extent greater than the proportion of external space included in them. Consequently a decrease in p that produces a fairly constant (not proportional) widening of the gaps between particles will produce a greater relative increase in G_1 than the relative increase in the external volume fraction, $1-p$.

For a suspension of randomly oriented cylinders, the dependence of G_1 on p and G_0 is

$$G_1 = (\sqrt{4 - 3p} - 1)^2 G_0$$

[FALK and FATT, 1968a, the expression being equivalent to the one given by Eq. (19)]. On the assumption that during the response the amount of electrolyte in the external space remains constant, G_0 will vary in inverse proportion to the external space, that is

$$G_0 = \frac{K}{1 - p}$$

where K is a constant. For a small change in rod volume one can write for a change in G_1

$$\Delta G_1 = \frac{dG_1}{dp} \cdot \Delta p \,,$$

when the above relations yield

$$\frac{\Delta G_1}{G_1} = \frac{-\Delta p}{(1 - p)\sqrt{4 - 3p}} \,.$$

The response is here represented as a fractional change in G_1 which would be independent of the conductivity, G_0, of the suspending medium in accordance with the observed proportional relations between component I (i.e. ΔG_1), G_0 and G_1.

Exposure of a packed suspension of rods to a flash that bleaches 1% of the initial rhodopsin produces a maintained increase in the low-frequency conductance (component I) that can be expressed as $\Delta G_1 = 7 \times 10^{-5} G_0$. This represents an upward revision by a factor of 3 of the value previously given (FALK and FATT, 1968b, Fig. 6). The response can be alternatively expressed as a fractional change in the low-frequency conductance, $\Delta G_1/G_1 = 10^{-3}$. Owing to saturation, the maximum response obtainable for flashes bleaching 10% or more of the initial rhodopsin is only about three times that for one bleaching 1%. For the rod suspensions studied, the volume fraction, p, was about 0.80. One can thus calculate that the maximum response to an intense flash is a relative change in rod volume of $\Delta p/p = 10^{-3}$. The change in linear dimensions of the rod required to produce such a volume change is well below the limits of resolution of direct microscopic observation.

A decrease in rod volume might result from a decrease in the concentration of osmotically effective solutes in the rod interior as this would cause water to leave the rod. Another possibility is a change in electrostatic forces acting within the lamellae. Thus, a change in the distribution of charge in the visual pigment molecule, by electrostatic interaction with neighbouring molecules that are also oriented and carry an asymmetric distribution of charge, could cause a reduction in forces acting to maintain the lamellae in planar configuration. Brownian motion would then produce a crumpling of the lamellae, thence leading to a diminution in cross-sectional area of the lamellae and of the rod as a whole.

B. Component II

Component II is distinguishable from component I by its frequency dependence, being detectable as an increase in the real part of admittance only when the measuring frequency is greater than 0.3–3 kHz. Above this cut-off frequency, which is fairly sharply defined, the response rises linearly with the logarithm of the frequency up to the characteristic frequency of admittance, f_Y. The position of f_Y can be made to vary over a wide range (0.3–3 MHz) by experimental variation of the conductivity of the suspending medium. When this is done, the amplitude of component II (measured as ΔG) is found to reach a limiting, maximum value at f_Y. At still higher frequencies ΔG remains constant up to the highest frequency at which measurements have been made (16.5 MHz). In addition to the upper frequency limit for the increase in component II, the low-frequency cut-off and the slope of the relation of response amplitude against log frequency also show a positive correlation with the conductivity of the solution used for suspending the rods. In accordance with these effects of conductivity, the frequency range over which ΔG increases logarithmically with frequency is seen to maintain a constant width of 3 decades, while the maximum amplitude of response varies linearly with the conductivity of the suspending medium. The form of this relation is similar to that found for the internal conductivity of the rods.

In an earlier report, component II was described as being independent of the conductivity of the suspending medium over a wide range of conductivities, corresponding to NaCl concentrations of 5–50 mM, with the response amplitude increasing at higher conductivities (FALK and FATT, 1968b). In the light of later measurements, carried out at higher frequencies, it is concluded that the apparent constancy of response amplitude with conductivity was a fortuitous result of comparing measurements of ΔG at a fixed frequency of 60 kHz (which was close to the upper limit of measurement for most of the early experiments). This frequency lay in the region of linear increase in ΔG with log frequency. In such circumstances the upward shift of the cut-off frequency with increasing conductivity compensated for the increased steepness of the response versus log frequency relation.

Since component II is not affected by the type of buffer used in preparing the suspension, that is whether anionic or cationic, a clear separation can be made between component II and the buffer component, which latter appears at high frequencies (above f_Y), and this allows an accurate comparison of the time course of the two components (Fig. 2). The time course of component II cannot be fitted by a single exponential curve. It rises with negligible latency to 30% of its final amplitude in 4 msec, to 50% in 15 msec and to 70% in about 50 msec (at 20° C). Completion of the final 30% of the response is slow (taking about 2 sec) in which respect it resembles the buffer component. Component II is observed to follow the buffer component with a delay that at the level of 30% of the final amplitude

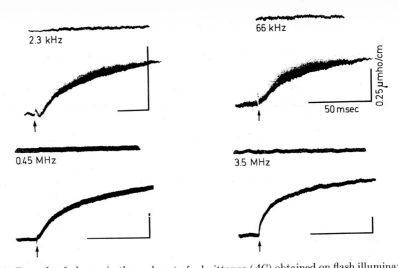

Fig. 3. Records of change in the real part of admittance (ΔG) obtained on flash illumination of a packed suspension of frog rod outer segments in a high-conductivity medium. The rod outer segments, after separation from dark-adapted retinas, were suspended in a solution consisting of 300 mM NaCl, 6 mM imidazole, 24 g sucrose/100 ml, 1 g bovine serum albumin/100 ml, pH 7.0. They were packed by centrifugation into the conductivity cell where they occupied a volume fraction of 0.82 (calculated from the limiting value of G at low frequencies and the conductivity of the suspending medium).— The records were obtained using a marginal oscillator. Each record at a given frequency consists of two sweeps. During the first sweep, at the time indicated by the arrow, the preparation was exposed to a flash of blue-green light lasting about 0.7 msec (a xenon arc filtered to pass a band of wavelengths between 465 and 610 nm). The second sweep, started 2 sec after the first, gives the approximate final level reached in the displacement of G produced by the flash. An upward deflexion corresponds to an increase in G. — The integrated intensity of the flash was sufficient to bleach 1.0% of the rhodopsin present in the rods at the time of flashing, except in the case of the record at 2.3 kHz when it was sufficient to bleach 2.0%. Owing to progressive bleaching of the rods due to repeated flashing, including flashes interpolated between those for which records are shown, the amount of rhodopsin present and hence the amount bleached per flash was not the same for each flash. The order of delivery of the flashes and the amount of rhodopsin present at the time of flashing (relative to the dark-adapted condition) for the responses illustrated was as follows: 66 kHz, 97%; 2.3 kHz, 96%; 0.45 MHz, 92%; 3.5 MHz, 86%. — The calibration bars given for each record represent horizontally 50 msec and vertically 0.25 μmho/cm, the latter having been calculated taking into account the cell constant of the conductivity cell. The calibrations in ΔG have been adjusted, so that each record corresponds to bleaching 1% of the initial rhodopsin content of the rods. The calibration for the record at 2.3 kHz has been additionally adjusted to allow for the fact that a 2%-bleaching flash was used. This has involved multiplying the calibration by a factor of 1/1.59 (the difference from 1/2 arising from non-linearity of the bleaching-response relation due to saturation). All flashes to which the preparation was exposed, each bleaching 1—2% of the rhodopsin content, were delivered at intervals greater than 10 min to allow for decay of the response saturation phenomenon. — The time resolution of the records, considered to represent the response to an impulse of light, was limited at 0.45 and 3.5 MHz by the flash duration. At 2.3 and 66 kHz there was an additional distortion of the records due to the narrow bandwidth of the tuned circuit in the marginal oscillator. This had the effect of imposing a lag corresponding to that of a single-RC circuit with a time constant of about 5 msec at 2.3 kHz and 0.5 msec at 66 kHz. A further effect of the delay in recording was a prolongation of the artefact due to operation of the flash lamp. Thus, in the record at 2.3 kHz the artefact, starting at the arrow and taking the form of an upward deflexion of the trace, greatly outlasted the flash. A less severe prolongation of the artefact occurred at 66 kHz, while at 0.45 MHz the artefact appeared as a rapid transient downward deflexion of the trace. — The fuzzy appearance of the records at 2.3 and 66 kHz arises from the fact that, unlike the records at the higher frequencies, the alternating voltage used for the measurement was not greatly attenuated by low-pass filtering and the records were obtained as a limit of the envelope formed by the alternating voltage. — The temperature was between 14.3 and 15.5° C. The conductivity of the suspending medium (G_0) was 10,100 μmho/cm. The characteristic frequency (f_r), at which G would be at the mean of its limiting values at high and low frequencies, was estimated to be about 2.9 MHz

(the two components of response being scaled to the same final amplitude) amounts to about 2 msec.

The response of frog rod outer segments, suspended in a high conductivity medium, to a flash of light is shown in Fig. 3, the records being obtained at different measuring frequencies as indicated. For the small fraction of rhodopsin bleached and the high conductivity of the suspending solution, the buffer contribution to the response would be negligibly small at all frequencies. The responses consist of a small initial step (the heat component) followed by the summed contributions of components I and II. The differences in the time course arise because component I is nearly independent of frequency while component II increases with frequency over the range represented. Since component II has the more rapid time course, the overall response develops more rapidly at the higher frequencies.

A finding that points to a dependence of component II on the maintained presence of metarhodopsin II is an alteration in response produced by treatment of the rods with 0.1 M hydroxylamine. In hydroxylamine component II is not maintained. Instead the conductance increase is transient; it develops to almost the normal amplitude with a time course similar to that in normal solution, but then decays in a few seconds. This behaviour resembles the slow reversal of H^+ uptake observed in potentiometric measurements on rod suspensions when treated with hydroxylamine (FALK and FATT, 1966). It is probably due to the instability of metarhodopsin II in the presence of hydroxylamine. Component I is not affected by hydroxylamine.

On increasing the flash intensity a saturation in component II is observed, qualitatively similar to that seen with component I. For flashes that bleach less than about 2% of the rhodopsin, the final amplitude of component II varies in proportion to the amount bleached. For more intense flashes the response increases less than in proportion to the amount bleached. The maximum (saturation) response amplitude is 10 times that given by a flash that bleaches 1% of the pigment. According to the theory of photoregeneration by the absorption of even numbers of photons per pigment molecule, no more than 50% bleaching can be achieved by a brief flash, no matter how intense (WILLIAMS, 1964). By repeated flashes, recovery from saturation is found to occur in about 5 min. The saturation of component II is thus found at a higher level of rhodopsin bleaching than for component I. Nevertheless, the general similarity of the phenomenon for the two components (which probably involve different stages in the conversion of the rhodopsin photoproduct, and originate at different sites in the suspension) suggests that non-linear depressant effects of some change in the rod lamellae is responsible for both.

It should be noted that the quantitative difference in the stimulus-response relation between components I and II described here is made somewhat uncertain by the occurrence of a light-induced negative change in G. Like component I, this negative-going response is frequency-independent below f_Y, but it differs in being proportional to the amount of rhodopsin bleached. Since component I is obtained from ΔG observed at low frequencies where there is no variation in total response amplitude with frequency whereas component II is obtained from the difference in ΔG between low and high frequencies, a failure to allow for the negative-going component will introduce an error in the estimation of component I, but not in that of component II. At low light intensities the magnitude of the negative component is about one-fifth that of component I. As the negative component is proportional to bleaching, the effect of its presence will be to subtract from the steepness of the proportional variation of component I at low levels of bleaching and hence to accentuate the apparent non-linearity of this component at higher levels of bleaching. The possibility cannot be excluded that the apparently greater deviation from proportionality that has been described for component I in comparison with component II is due to superposition of the negative component.

The finding that with increasing frequency of measurement component II first becomes detectable at about 1 kHz, increases logarithmically with frequency over a range of about 3 decades up to f_Y, and then remains constant at higher frequencies denies certain sites of conductance change from being concerned in production of the response. Thus, the progressive increase in ΔG over a range of frequencies below f_Y eliminates a change in membrane conductance or in rod volume, as considered in relation to component I. It also eliminates a change of conductance in the major portion of the internal space of the rods, such as was shown to account for the buffer component for which ΔG increased with frequency above f_Y. The low-frequency cut-off of component II some 3 decades below f_Y would appear to require some different site of conductance change that, because of either a high value of resistance within the conducting path or a high value of capacitance in series with it, will give the observed cut-off. One possibility which has been considered is that the response might arise from a change in surface charge on the rods, producing a change in surface conduction. By "surface conduction" is here meant variation in ionic conduction (over that occurring in the bulk of the aqueous solution) induced by the presence of a nearby solid surface. Since the influence of the surface normally extends for only a very short distance into the aqueous solution (0.1–1 nm depending on ionic strength), surface conduction will be effectively tangential to the surface; and for a suspension of particles it will be frequency-dependent with a low-frequency cut-off determined by the linear extent of the particle surface in the direction of the electric field used in the measurement. As an example of this type of mechanism, which might be invoked to explain component II, an increase in surface conduction could arise from the dissociation of some substance on the exposed surface of the rod, with the result that ions would be introduced into the external medium, and fixed charged groups would appear on the rod surface. The fixed charges, if of the same sign as charges already present on the surface, would act to restrict the movement of ions of opposite charge (counterions) by causing them to remain within the electrostatic field of the charged surface. The result would be an increase in ionic surface conduction having a frequency dependence of the kind observed (an increase in real part of admittance that would increase with frequency).

A difficulty with this proposal is that it predicts the occurrence of a frequency-independent as well as of a frequency-dependent part of the response, the relative amounts of these two parts varying with the ionic strength of the suspending medium. This is because the surface charge on the rod would be balanced by a depletion of ions of opposite sign to the fixed charge in addition to an augmentation of ions of the same sign. By assuming a reasonable figure for the initial surface density of fixed charge, one can calculate that for a suspending medium of ionic strength 6 mM (equal in value to the concentration of a univalent electrolyte) the fraction of the response that would be frequency-dependent would be 0.92; but for an ionic strength of 300 mM, this fraction would be only 0.32. This prediction conflicts with observation in that component II, identified by its relatively rapid time course (compared with component I) and by its sensitivity to treatment of the rods with hydroxylamine, is absent at low frequencies even when the conducti- vity of the solution is raised. Figure 3 illustrates an experiment carried out with a high-conductivity suspending medium. In the record of response taken at 2.3 kHz no measurable change in G is seen to occur up to 7 msec following the flash, by which time component II has developed to about 40% of its final level, as can be seen in the early rapid rise of response in the record at 3.5 MHz. In this particular experiment, owing to the high conductivity of the suspending medium, the low- frequency cut-off of component II was above 2.3 kHz while f_Y was slightly below 3.5 MHz. Additional characteristics of component II which cannot be explained by a process of surface conduction are variation in the position of the low-frequency cut-off with the conductivity of the medium and the consistently close agreement between the frequency at which the response reached a maximum value and f_Y. It would seem necessary therefore to seek an alternative mechanism for the pro- duction of component II, in particular one that would account for the levelling off of component II in the region of f_Y.

In the analysis of the admittance of a rod suspension whereby the surface membrane capacitance is found to have a value of about 0.8 $\mu F/cm^2$, it is assumed that the characteristic frequency f_Y is effectively determined by the passage of current across the surface membrane capacitance and across the internal conduct- ing space of rods oriented with their axes perpendicular to the alternating electric field used in the measurement. The reason for making this assumption is that, within a suspension of randomly oriented cylinders, symmetry considerations require that 70% of the cylinders lie with their axes within 45° of a plane perpen- dicular to the electric field and only 30% lie with their axes within 45% of the direction of the field. Such rods as do lie with their axes nearly parallel with the direction of the electric field might nevertheless account for the appearance of component II at frequencies well below f_Y. The interior of the rods may be ex- pected to be anisotropic in its electrical properties, owing to the transverse arrange- ment of lamellae, so that within the range of frequencies over which component II is observed to increase, the effective conductivity of the rod interior will be much lower in the axial direction than in the transverse direction. On the assumption that conduction in the longitudinal (axial) direction is restricted to the gap between the edges of the stacked discs and the surface membrane and to the incisures within the discs, the effective longitudinal conductivity may be estimated to be reduced by a factor of 1/40 relative to the conductivity of the solution filling the internal aqueous spaces. On the other hand, the effective transverse conductivity is expected to be reduced by a factor of 1/2 owing to the exclusion of current from the space occupied by the discs, which would be in parallel with the conducting path in the transverse direction.

One may now examine the possibility that component II arises from an increase in the longitudinal conductance of the rod interior. Rods oriented with their axes in the direction of the electric field will make the major contribution to the response seen at fairly low frequencies and will determine the low-frequency cut-off. One may apply cable theory to calculate the contribution to the measured admittance made by such rods. On the assumption that the resistance for unit length in the interior of the rods is high, relative to the resistance of other paths through the suspension, the contribution to the measured admittance made by those rods oriented parallel to the field will be

$$Y = \frac{n}{r_l}\left(1 - \frac{\tanh \sqrt{jf/f_{\mathrm{II}}}}{\sqrt{jf/f_{\mathrm{II}}}}\right)$$

where n is the number of rods per unit area in a plane through the suspension perpendicular to the direction of the applied field, r_l is the resistance of the rod interior per unit length, f is the measuring frequency, and f_{II} is a characteristic frequency dependent on the properties of the rods. For rods in the form of circular cylinders the following relations will apply:

$$\frac{1}{2\pi f_{\mathrm{II}}} = c_m r_l \left(\frac{l}{2}\right)^2 = \frac{C_m l^2}{G_l\, 2a}$$

where c_m is the surface membrane capacitance per unit length of rod, C_m is the same capacitance per unit area of membrane, G_l is the effective longitudinal conductivity of the interior, l is the length of the rod and a its radius. Differentiation of the above expression for Y with respect to G_l can be readily carried out to obtain ΔY corresponding to an increment in ΔG_l, as

$$\Delta Y = \frac{dY}{dG_l}\,\Delta G_l\,.$$

This leads to the prediction that ΔG, the real part of ΔY, will be absent at low frequencies, make its appearance at close to f_{II} and then increase with frequency over about one decade before levelling off. (Owing to the distributed, cable properties of the rod, this range of frequencies over which ΔG increases is about twice as wide on a logarithmic scale as that for a lumped resistance-capacitance network.) The much wider range of frequencies over which component II is observed to rise (about 3 decades) can be accounted for by a distribution in the orientation of rods relative to the field. A deviation from the assumed parallel orientation would have the effect of introducing an additional conductance (having its origin in the transverse conductance of the rod) in parallel with the longitudinally conducting elements, thus causing the response to appear at higher frequencies. The levelling-off of the response at f_Y is also consistent with this scheme, since above that frequency the capacitance at the surface of the rod would no longer restrict the passage of current into the interior for any orientation. Furthermore, one may note that the failure of the response amplitude to increase further above f_Y is a clear indication that the spaces between the discs, conduction within which determines the transverse conductivity of the rod interior, are not involved in the production of component II.

Taking into consideration the structure of the rod interior, one notes that there are two different kinds of structures, changes within which would affect the longitudinal conductance. There might occur a change in conduction in the gap between the surface membrane and the disc edge and in the incisures within the disc, or alternatively a change in membrane conductance of the lamellae forming the disc.

The response could conceivably depend on a change in the lamellae even though their conductance formed a relatively small fraction of the effective longitudinal conductivity, and hence would not influence significantly the position of the low-frequency cut-off. From the position of the low-frequency cut-off of component II, the effective longitudinal internal conductance G_l is estimated to be about 200 μmho/cm for rods suspended in a solution having the conductivity of Ringer solution. This value is in agreement with the fraction of unobstructed aqueous space seen by electron-microscopy in transverse sections of rods.

The change in internal conductivity, ΔG_l, can be derived from the limiting amplitude of component II, ΔG_{II}, recorded at high frequencies. From symmetry considerations (with the electric field existing in one of the three dimensions of space) the suspension of randomly oriented rods may be treated as if the response occurred in rods occupying a reduced volume fraction, $p' = 1/3\, p$, these rods being oriented with their axes parallel to the electric field. The remaining rods would act merely to increase the conductance, G_0', of the space external to them. Maxwell's theory for a dilute suspension of particles distributed through the three spatial dimensions may be applied, on the assumption that $G_l \ll G_0'$, to give the proportional relation

$$\Delta G_{II} = \frac{9\,p'}{(2 + p')^2}\, \Delta G_l \,.$$

A flash bleaching 1 % of the rhodopsin content of dark-adapted rods produced a response in which component II had a limiting value of about 1.0 μmho/cm. On the above theory this would correspond to a change in the rod interior of $\Delta G_l = 2.1$ μmho/cm. (The fact that, for rods oriented with their axes oblique to the applied field, the longitudinal component of internal conductance is shunted by a transverse component, the combination of the two being in series with the membrane capacitance, and that this greatly increases the frequency of measurement required to obtain the limiting value does not influence the present calculation.) For an intense flash yielding a response close to saturation, ΔG_l would be about 8 μmho/cm, corresponding to a 4 % increase of G_l. It is possible that this represents the maximum variation of G_l that can be sustained and that the observed recovery of responsiveness following a saturating response involves a slow, as yet undetected, reversal of ΔG_{II} in the dark.

It is not possible on the basis of the measurements thus far carried out to decide whether component II has its origin in a change in the unobstructed area of the rod cross-section (perhaps a widening of the incisures) or in a change of ionic permeability of the disc membranes. The difficulty of distinguishing between these possibilities is that the current paths involved appear electrically in parallel for the electric-field configuration in measurements on suspensions. It is nevertheless of some value to examine further in a quantitative way the possibility that the response may arise in the disc membranes, since an increase in disc-membrane permeability can be envisaged to constitute an essential step in the process of visual excitation. For a disc-repeat interval (including a pair of membranes) of 30 nm, the indicated change in G_l produced by bleaching 1% of the rhodopsin is calculated to correspond to a change in the conductance of these membranes amounting to 1.4 mho/cm². This is an extraordinarily high value, being several times greater than the maximum change occurring during the propagation of an action potential in a nerve fibre. It may be considered in relation to the number of rhodopsin molecules, as these have been regarded as fixed to the disc membrane and may form channels locally through it. For rhodopsin present in the frog rod in a concentration of 2.5 mM and for the indicated disc-repeat interval, the density of rhodopsin molecules in the disc membrane is calculated to be 2.2×10^{12} cm^{-2}. For the bleaching of 1 % of the rhodopsin to produce a membrane conductance increment of 1.4 mho/cm^2 requires that each rhodopsin molecule effects a conductance increase of 6.4×10^{-11} mho. The value which thus emerges is similar to that estimated for a single Na$^+$-carrying channel, capable of being blocked by a single tetrodotoxin molecule, in the case of the nerve fibre membrane exposed to Ringer solution. The separate, unidirectional fluxes of univalent ions that would take place through such a channel in the absence of an electrochemical potential difference across the membrane can be obtained by multiplying the conductance by RTN_0/F^2. For the present case this indicates a flux of 9×10^6 sec^{-1}. One is encouraged by this result to entertain the idea that in component II one is observing an early stage of amplification in the visual excitation process.

VI. Visual Excitation

Any changes produced by light in the properties of the surface membrane are of particular interest in view of the important role that this structure has in nerve excitation, and of general interest because it is a structure that continues over the entire cell and consequently may be concerned in the propagation of the response. The most obvious of such changes that one is led to seek is a change in ionic permeability.

Evidence for a permeability increase specific to Na$^+$ has been found in the squid visual receptor (HAGINS, 1965). Exploration of the potential fields in the neighbourhood of an illuminated region of the squid receptor (HAGINS, ZONANA, and ADAMS, 1962; HAGINS, 1965) shows the existence of an inward current into that region, consistent with the view that a sodium movement is activated by light, while the other ions move passively in response to the alteration in membrane potential (depolarization of the photoreceptor). A detailed analysis of the potential changes generated across the squid retina suggests that the alteration in membrane potential due to the influx of sodium would be adequate to account for visual excitation, the rate of sodium ion entry produced by the bleaching of a single molecule of visual pigment being sufficient to produce a change that would stand out significantly above the thermally-induced electrical noise. In the squid the surface membrane of the receptor is expanded by the presence of villi, which are analogous to the transverse lamellae of vertebrate receptors, and probably contain the visual pigment as a constituent of their membrane (ZONANA, 1961). Thus changes in molecular configuration of the visual pigment may, in the squid, control the local permeability of what is effectively a single continuous membrane separating the interior of the cell from the external solution. There appears to be no need to postulate any amplification process involving a multiplication in the number of molecules concerned in excitation, except insofar as the photochemical alteration of a single pigment molecule would permit a large number of sodium ions to pass across the membrane (see HARTLINE, WAGNER, and MacNICHOL, 1952; FUORTES, 1959; STIEVE, 1965; FULPIUS and BAUMANN, 1969; MILLECCHIA and MAURO, 1969; BROWN, HAGIWARA, KOIKE, and MEECH, 1970 for some other invertebrates).

A. Retinal Potential Changes

Intracellular electrical recording from receptor cells in the retinae of various vertebrates (teleost fish, amphibians and reptiles) has been accomplished by the use of fine pipette electrodes (BORTOFF and NORTON, 1967; TOMITA, KANEKO, MURAKAMI, and PAUTLER, 1967; TOYODA, NOSAKI, and TOMITA, 1969; WERBLIN and DOWLING, 1969; BAYLOR and FUORTES, 1970; TOYODA, HASHIMOTO, ANNO, and TOMITA, 1970). The intracellular position of the electrode is revealed by the recording of a resting membrane potential (with the preparation in the dark this has usually amounted to only -20 to -40 mV, the interior of the cell being negative with respect to extracellular fluid) and by marking with a dye ejected from the electrode. These studies have consistently failed to detect any light-induced depolarization or any regenerative action-potential type of electrical activity under any conditions. Instead, when the electrode tip is in a receptor cell (in the inner or outer segment or in the region of the nucleus), illumination produces hyperpolarization (an increase in internal negativity).

At low intensities the response is proportional to the stimulus, the rate of absorption of photons required to produce a maintained hyperpolarization of 1 mV being about 1000 photons/sec. With increasing light intensity, the response shows saturation, the maximum hyperpolarization obtainable being 20 mV. Recorded from the cone receptors of the carp, *Necturus* and turtle, the response to a weak flash rises and falls exponentially with a time constant of about 0.2 sec. As the stimulus-response relation becomes non-linear with increasing illumination, the response develops an early peak, owing to a sag of the hyperpolarization while the light is maintained. It is of interest that the peak amplitude of the response varies in a non-linear manner with light intensity over a very wide range of light intensity (about 1000-fold) before being limited by saturation.

In the case of rods the region of proportionality of the stimulus-response relation is limited sharply by saturation. Thus, whilst sensitivity to light as seen in the linear stimulus-response relation at low light levels is about the same in the rods as in the cones, a gradation in response amplitude with light intensity extends to much higher intensities in the latter. In addition to inducing saturation of response, high intensity stimulation results in a prolongation of the decay of the response on cessation of the stimulus. The time scale of the rod response, especially its decay, is greater than that of the cones (BROWN, WATANABE, and MURAKAMI, 1965; TOYODA, NOSAKI, and TOMITA, 1969; TOYODA, HASHIMOTO, ANNO, and TOMITA, 1970; TOMITA, 1970).

To enquire into the origin of the hyperpolarization in terms of a change in electrical properties of the surface membrane of the receptor cell, pulses of current have been applied through the intracellular electrode between the cell interior and the surrounding medium. It has been found that, coincident with the hyperpolarization produced by light, there is an increase in resistance between the interior of the cell and the outside. The resistance in the dark of all receptor cells that have been successfully impaled is in the range $10-20$ MΩ. On illumination, this is increased by a maximum amount of about 5 MΩ. Variation of the stimulus intensity and duration shows that the hyperpolarization and the resistance increase are directly proportional to each other and may be considered to be causally releated. This resistance increase, measured with small displacements of membrane potential, represents a change in the dynamic (slope) resistance of the cell in the region of membrane potential within which the hyperpolarizing response occurs.

Additional information is obtained by displacing the membrane potential with a steady current and observing the effect upon the transient potential change evoked by light. Hyperpolarization by inward current across the surface of the cell causes an increase in the hyperpolarizing response to light, while depolarization by outward current results in a decrease in the response. The relationship between response for a given light stimulus and the membrane potential on which it is superimposed is approximately linear. Close to zero membrane potential the potential change evoked by light is absent. With further displacement of membrane potential the response is inverted, appearing as an increase in the positivity of the interior of the cell with respect to the exterior.

On the basis of the above findings, the response of the receptor cell can be interpreted as a reduction in overall membrane conductance, with the channel of membrane conductance modulated by the light stimulus depending on the passage of ions, which are so distributed and have relative membrane permeabilities (assuming more than one ion species is involved) that, at zero membrane potential, there is no current through the channel. (For brevity this has often been termed "equilibrium potential", though with more than one species of ion involved, as is probably the situation for the photoreceptor cell response, the concept of an equilibrium would not be applicable.) The type of membrane change envisaged in the receptor cell, whereby the membrane potential is driven away from the level of zero potential, is a decrease in permeability towards Na^+ ions (and probably to some extent K^+ ions). The hyperpolarization evoked by light would be the result of a reduction in the inward passage of Na^+ through the active region of cell membrane.

Exploration of extracellular potential fields in a slice of the retina of the rat (the plane of the slice including the axial direction of the receptor cells) has shown that in the dark-adapted state there is a distally-directed steady current in the receptor region, with the source of current at the level of the inner segments and the sink at the level of the outer segments (PENN and HAGINS, 1969; HAGINS, PENN, and YOSHIKAMI, 1970). This current is dependent on metabolic processes, being rapidly abolished on treatment of the retina with CN^-. It is further found that illumination causes a reduction of this current (see also SVAETICHIN, NEGISHI, and FATEHCHAND, 1965). It is this transient reduction of the distally-directed steady current that underlies the major part of PIII of the electroretinogram (GRANIT, 1933, 1968; BROWN, 1968). Another part of PIII is probably brought about by activity in cells proximal to the receptors (MURAKAMI and KANEKO, 1966).

One may reasonably assume that the reduction in the steady, distally-directed current is a direct consequence of the resistance increase with associated hyperpolarization seen by intracellular recording. The steady current itself indicates that, in the dark-adapted state of the cell, the membrane potential (taken as the magnitude of internal negative potential with respect to external potential) is less in the outer segment than in the inner segment. This in turn would appear to depend on a relatively high permeability towards Na^+ of the outer-segment surface membrane. The consequent inward flux of Na^+ passively following the electro-chemical potential across the membrane would be balanced, to maintain a steady-state condition, by a metabolically driven sodium pump, extruding Na^+, probably in the region of the inner segment. A reduction by light of the Na^+ permeability of the outer segment would produce a reduction of current flow. Owing to the cable properties of the receptor cell, the inward flux of Na^+ across the membrane of the outer segment in the dark-adapted state would have the effect of depressing the membrane potential over the entire cell, the effect extending, with some atten-uation, to the pre-synaptic terminals of the receptor cell within the outer plexi-form layer of the retina. (The exact picture of membrane potential distribution along the cell would depend on whether and to what extent the metabolically driven ion pump, extruding Na^+ from the cell, is electrogenic. To the extent that the pump is electrogenic, i.e. entails a net transfer of charge across the membrane, its operation would affect the distribution of membrane potential. The change in membrane potential arising from a change in membrane conductance in part of the cell would, however, spread to distant parts of the cell in accordance with its cable properties, irrespective of the site of the sodium pump mechanism.)

It would be expected that inhibition of the sodium pump would reduce or abolish the light-induced receptor potential change because of dissipation of the ionic concentration gradients without interfering with the light-induced conduct-ance change. In agreement with this idea, SILLMAN, ITO, and TOMITA (1969) and ARDEN and ERNST (1970) have shown that receptor potential changes can still be obtained on illumination of a retina in which the sodium pump has been inhibited by ouabain, provided that the composition of the solution surrounding the recep-tors is manipulated so as to set up a sodium concentration gradient. As ARDEN and ERNST have demonstrated for cones, when the ionic concentration gradient is reversed, so is the light-induced potential change.

It should be noted that the mechanism of production of the ion-permeability decrease of the surface membrane of the outer segment underlying the usual hyperpolarization of the receptor cell has not been explained. In the case of verte-brate rods and mammalian cones, the surface membrane conductance change cannot be a direct and immediate effect of light, since most of the lamellae bearing the visual pigment are isolated from the surface membrane and from each other. One must postulate, therefore, at least one intermediate stage between the absorp-tion of light and the membrane conductance decrease, probably involving the release from the discs of some diffusible substance that acts on the surface membrane to decrease its permeability. Calcium ions would be a possible candidate for this role of intracellular transmitter. A light-induced change in properties of the rod interior, in the form of an increase in conductance in the longitudinal direction, has already been described (component II in Section V). On the basis of its rapid time course of development following a brief flash, this change in the rod interior can be envisaged to reflect a process concerned in the initiation of the surface membrane conductance decrease and consequent hyperpolarization. The fact that the surface membrane change saturates at a lower level of light intensity than does the internal change is not an obstacle to this view. One may presume that this saturation at low-stimulus intensity takes place locally in the surface membrane, where a chemical receptor controlling the ionic permeability may become fully occupied with increasing intensity while preceding stages, including the postulated intracellular transmitter, capable of reacting with the receptor continue to build up in concentration. An indication of such a process is the finding that with strong light flashes, in excess of that required to give a surface membrane conductance decrease of maximum peak amplitude, increasing flash intensity causes the response to develop a plateau of increasing duration, which in the rods may last for minutes (TOYODA, HASHIMOTO, ANNO, and TOMITA, 1970).

Although the potential change in the receptor is a hyperpolarization, it is not difficult to conceive of a scheme whereby this change is signalled to the optic nerve. Let us assume that the transmitter released from the pre-synaptic terminals of the receptor cell is an excitatory one, i.e. produces a non-specific increase in ionic permeability of the post-synaptic membrane. The absorption of light, by reducing the rate of transmitter release from its level in the dark-adapted state, will bring about a transient hyperpolarization of the post-synaptic cell. This inference is consistent with the intracellular recording of potential changes from bipolar and horizontal cells (SVAETICHIN and MACNICHOL, 1958; NAKA and RUSHTON, 1966; WERBLIN and DOWLING, 1969; STEINBERG, 1969; KANEKO, 1970). The responses of the horizontal cells designated luminosity(L)-type, slow(S)-potentials consist solely of a hyperpolarization that is graded with light intensity and may be recorded when the light falls anywhere within a radius of about 200 μm from the electrode. Evidence in support of the idea that the hyperpolarization results from a decrease in excitatory synaptic activity is provided by the demonstration of an increase in the resistance between the interior of the horizontal cell and the outside (TOYODA, NOSAKI, and TOMITA, 1969). Further, by applying current pulses across the retina so as to depolarize the pre-synaptic terminals of receptor cells, BYZOV and TRIFONOV (1968) have recorded transient potential changes in horizontal cells having the characteristics of excitatory post-synaptic potentials.

In contrast to horizontal cells, the potential change in bipolar cells produced by illumination of the centre of their receptive fields is reversed by illumination of the surround. Depolarization of bipolar cells produced by surround illumination might be explained if one were to suppose that horizontal cells pre-synaptic to bipolar cells release an inhibitory transmitter and that the release is diminished in the light. The same effect would be achieved if the horizontal cells made presynaptic contact with receptor cells. Illumination of a distant region of the retina causing a depolarization of the receptor cell, presumably through a reduction in the release of inhibitory transmitter from a contacting horizontal cell, has been observed in turtle cones (BAYLOR, FUORTES and O'BRYAN, 1971). This depolarization of the receptor, by causing an increase in the release of excitatory transmitter at its presynaptic contacts on bipolar cells, would thus produce a depolarization of the bipolar cell distant from the region of illumination.

One might suppose that hyperpolarization of a bipolar cell would reduce the release of transmitter from its pre-synaptic endings which, if the transmitter were an inhibitory one, would result in the depolarization of an amacrine or ganglion cell post-synaptic to the bipolar cell. Observations with intracellular electrodes show that amacrine cells generate action potentials but that they rapidly accommodate to depolarization (WERBLIN and DOWLING, 1969; KANEKO, 1970). Having post-synaptic contacts with bipolar cells and pre-synaptic contacts with ganglion cells, as well as being connected with one another, amacrine cells would exert a powerful excitatory action on ganglion cells (assuming that the transmitter released by it is an excitatory one) reinforcing the action of bipolar cells to give centre-on-responses. Both amacrine and ganglion cells may give off-responses (in the form of transient depolarization with superimposed action potentials). The interposition of a cell like the horizontal cell in the neuronal chain between receptor and bipolar cell could account for this effect.

B. Sensitivity of the Visual Mechanism

The results of intracellular recording from bipolar and horizontal cells described above strongly suggest that an excitatory transmitter is continually released from the presynaptic terminal of the receptor cell in the dark and produces a steady depolarization of the postsynaptic cell membrane. It is reasonable to assume, in conformity with observations on many types of vertebrate neurones, that the resting potential of the bipolar cell, occurring in the absence of synaptic activity, would be about -75 mV and that the excitatory transmitter would have the effect of introducing an additional conductance across the membrane with a series voltage source driving the membrane potential toward 0 mV. Even though membrane conductances are assumed to be independent of potential, synaptic potentials will fail to add linearly because of the reduction in driving force for their generation as the membrane is progressively depolarized. Quantitatively, the dependence of the depolarization of the postsynaptic membrane V_{post} on the transmitter-induced conductance increment Δg will be given for the steady state by the hyperbolic relation

$$V_{post} = \frac{V_r}{1 + \dfrac{g_m}{\Delta g}}$$

where V_r is the voltage source in series with the conductance increment (measured, like V_{post}, from the resting potential) and g_m is the conductance presented by the resting (i.e. non-synaptic) membrane. The relation of the postsynaptic to the presynaptic potential can be derived by combining this relation with the following ones which describe the release and postsynaptic action of transmitter (LILEY, 1956; KATZ and MILEDI, 1967): (1) The rate of transmitter release, T, is an exponential function of presynaptic membrane potential, V_{pre}, expressible as

$$T \propto e^{bV_{pre}}$$

where b is a constant which, for the experimental observation that a 10-fold variation in transmitter release rate is given by a 15 mV change in V_{pre}, amounts to 2.3/15 mV. (2) The conductance change produced in the postsynaptic membrane is proportional to the rate of transmitter release, i.e.

$$\Delta g \propto T$$

a behaviour that may depend on the transmitter's acting on different chemo-
receptive sites of the postsynaptic membrane. One thus obtains

$$V_{post} = V_r \left(1 + ce^{-bV_{pre}}\right)^{-1}$$

where c is a numerical constant which may be regarded as describing the synaptic
matching between pre- and postsynaptic structures, its value being determined
by the factors of proportionality for the relations in (1) and (2) and by g_m.

The sensitivity S for the synapse, describing the change in postsynaptic
potential produced by a small change in presynaptic potential, can then be obtained by

$$S \equiv \frac{dV_{post}}{dV_{pre}} = \frac{1}{4} V_r b \left[\cosh\left(\frac{1}{2} b V_{pre} - a\right)\right]^{-2}$$

where $a = \frac{1}{2} \ln c$.

Alternatively, the sensitivity may be expressed as a function of the postsynaptic
potential by the simple parabolic relation

$$S = bV_{post} \left(1 - \frac{V_{post}}{V_r}\right).$$

This last relation shows that the sensitivity will be maximum when the background
depolarisation of the postsynaptic cell is one-half maximum. It is consistent with
the observation that in the dark, where maximum sensitivity is demanded,
transmitter is released from the receptor at a rate sufficient to produce a large, but
partial depolarization of the bipolar cell. An additional point to be noticed is that
the maximum value of S is fixed at $\frac{1}{4} V_r b$, which for the values $V_r = 75$ mV and
$b = 0.15$ mV^{-1} yields a maximum sensitivity of 2.7.

Information on the absolute sensitivity of the complete visual mechanism has
been provided by subjective experiments (Hecht, Shlaer and Pirenne, 1942;
Pirenne, 1967) which have shown that a light stimulus involving the absorption
of only some 5 photons within a period of time of about 0.1 sec and distributed
over an area of retina containing about 500 rods gives rise to a visual sensation
with a probability of 60%. With variation of the flash intensity the probability
of seeing falls on a curve given by summation of a Poisson series, which describes
the probability of the number of absorbed photons in a large number of trials
being not less than the critical number. The spatial extent of the stimulus over
which there occurs nearly complete summation of the effectiveness of absorbed
photons in evoking a response has been considered to correspond to the receptive
field of a retinal ganglion cell. Further studies (Barlow, 1956) have suggested that
the critical number of absorbed photons required to evoke a visual sensation is
determined by the presence in the visual mechanism of continual random fluctuations in excitability equivalent in their action to the stimulus giving 60%, probability of seeing. Thus, assuming that the source of fluctuation is in the rod cells
and that the only effect of this fluctuation transmitted to the ganglion cell is one
equivalent to the absorption of a photon, then it would be predicted that spontaneous
fluctuations in the rod should reach a critical level for transmission at intervals
having an average value of $(500 \times 0.1)/5 = 10$ sec.

Thermal noise in the membrane potential of the presynaptic terminal of the rod
receptor, due to random fluctuations in the number of ions crossing the membrane

in any given time interval, has been considered by HAGINS, PENN and YOSHIKAMI (1970). They have been concerned to show that such noise would not exceed the potential change, produced by a single absorbed photon, more often than once in ten seconds on the average, as required by the above calculation. On the assumption that the terminal of the receptor behaves as a low-pass filter with a time constant (integration time) of 200 msec they calculate the root-mean-square (equal, for random fluctuations, to the standard deviation) of voltage fluctuation to amount to only 0.9 μV, while the response to a single photon would be about 3.6 μV. If, however, the integration time determined by the membrane capacitance were 20 msec, corresponding more closely to that found for other neuronal membranes, with the electrical properties being otherwise the same as used by HAGINS et al., the fluctuations would be calculated to be ± 2.8 μV while the response would amount to 6 μV. For the critical level for signal transmission to have a probability of occurrence within each period of 20 msec of only $0.02/10 = 0.002$ requires that the critical level, which must be surpassed by the graded response of the receptor, be 3 times the standard deviation of random fluctuations.

The above consideration of thermal noise represents a very fine point, however, in view of the probable occurrence of very much larger fluctuations in signal transmission, arising in the process of transmitter release from the presynaptic terminal of the receptor. By electron microscopy this terminal is observed to possess structural features typical of chemically transmitting synapses, including an accumulation of vesicles of about 30 nm in diameter, which have been generally regarded as constituting the minimum unit for release of transmitter (KATZ, 1962). Recordings of membrane potential from the postsynaptic region of a wide variety of cell types have shown the synaptic response to fluctuate in increments of discrete size, owing to the transmitter's being released from the presynaptic terminal in packets estimated to comprise a few thousand molecules of transmitter. When seen in isolation, i.e. in the absence of other synaptic activity, the response to a single packet of transmitter is designated a miniature synaptic potential, and is found at many synapses, where an excitatory transmitter is operative, to consist of a transient depolarization having a peak amplitude of about 0.5 mV, a rapid rising phase, and a slower approximately exponential decay with a time constant of about 20 msec (FATT and KATZ, 1952; BLACKMAN, GINSBORG, and RAY, 1962; KATZ and MILEDI, 1963).

Assuming now that in the dark the bipolar cell is depolarized from a resting potential of -75 mV to -25 mV as a result of the superposition of miniature synaptic potentials occurring in a random time sequence, one can calculate from the relation previously given between depolarization and conductance increment (the latter considered proportional to transmitter release rate) that transmitter would have to be released at a rate corresponding to what would produce a potential change of 150 mV if linear summation of synaptic potentials applied. The mean rate of release of packets of transmitter acting on the bipolar cell in the dark is thus calculated to be $150/(0.5 \times 0.02) = 15,000$/sec. For an integration time of the postsynaptic cell membrane of 20 msec, the mean number of packets of transmitter controlling the level of membrane potential at any instant will be effectively 300. (The foregoing calculation involves a certain simplification whereby the number of packets considered to be effective are those that together contribute 63% to the depolarization, on the basis of linear summation of synaptic potentials. Additionally, it is assumed in the statistical consideration that follows that these packets contribute equally.)

One may suppose, as has been found to hold at other types of synapse, that the release of packets of transmitter is a probabilistic occurrence, such that the number released within the time period under consideration will fluctuate about the mean according to a Poisson distribution for which the standard deviation equals the square-root of the mean (Fatt and Katz, 1952). For the present case this gives 300 ± 17, corresponding to a relative fluctuation about the mean of $\pm 5.8\%$. If the rate of release increased 10-fold for a 15 mV change in presynaptic membrane potential, the spontaneous fluctuation in release rate would be equivalent to that produced by fluctuations in the potential of the receptor terminal having a standard deviation of 0.39 mV. As mentioned previously, a light-induced potential change 3 times greater, i.e. in the region of 1 mV, would be the minimum signal required to give a response, on the criterion that random fluctuations in the dark should not reach the critical level for signal transmission from receptor to ganglion cell more often than once in 10 sec. The equivalent receptor noise set by the release of transmitter in packets is thus seen to be greater by a factor of 200 than thermal noise calculated on the basis of the electrical properties of the receptor. It is also much greater than the potential change that experimental studies have indicated would be evoked as the result of the absorption of a single photon.

In all the above considerations on the sensitivity of post- to presynaptic potentials and the fluctuation in synaptic activity, a major simplification has been to ignore the fact that the bipolar cell receives synaptic contacts from a number of rod cells, only one of which would have absorbed the photon (in absolute threshold determinations) whereas all would contribute to the background depolarization of the bipolar cell. (A similar convergence exists in the contact of bipolar cells with a ganglion cell, but the possibility of the local initiation of action potentials and the intervention of amacrine cells causes the present argument to apply with less stringency.) Histological studies on the primate retina (Dowling and Boycott, 1966) indicate that in the parafoveal region bipolar cells receive synaptic contact from about 15 rod cells, this number increasing to about 45 in regions more distant from the fovea. In the observed absence of action potentials or other regenerative electrical activity, it is presumed that synaptic activity on all the postsynaptic areas of the dendrites of a bipolar cell are summed, effectively as if these areas were contiguous to give a spatially uniform membrane potential. One may continue to use the model in which the bipolar cell in the dark is at any time depolarized by the action of 300 ± 17 packets of transmitter released from the terminals of all the receptor cells contacting it. Considering these to be released independently with equal probability from 15 receptor cells, each therefore contributing a mean number of 20 packets, one is forced to conclude that even the complete cessation of transmitter release from the single receptor absorbing a photon would be insufficient to produce a change in synaptic activity capable of standing out from random fluctuation in such activity.

A way out of this dilemma would be to suppose that rod cells do not respond independently at low light levels, but the absorption of a photon in one receptor causes a similar hyperpolarization to occur in a group of receptors including all those converging onto the bipolar cell. The situation would then be equivalent to the one analysed on the assumption of the bipolar cell's being contacted by a single receptor. Regions of specialization, indicative of synaptic contact, have been observed between adjacent cones and between rods and cones in the primate retina (COHEN, 1965; DOWLING and BOYCOTT, 1966; MISSOTTEN, APPELMANS, and MICHIELS, 1963). However, inter-rod contacts have not been found (DOWLING and BOYCOTT, 1966) or have been seen only occasionally (COHEN, 1965). Even if synaptic contacts did exist between rod cells in sufficient density to cause a nearly uniform spread of hyperpolarization among the group of rod cells converging onto a bipolar cell, then these contacts would themselves become a source of synaptic noise.

Some other mechanism for the transfer of potential changes between receptor cells, finer grained than the usual synaptic transmission mechanism, would appear to be required. It may be relevant to consider in this connection the generation of the b-wave. With a wide field of retinal illumination the b-wave recorded across the rat retina is observed to increase proportionally with flash intensity up to a mean number of 0.06 photons absorbed per rod, with a transretinal potential change of 10 μV being recorded at 0.01 photons per rod (CONE, 1964b). This may be compared with the receptor-generated a-wave for which a 100-fold increase in brightness is required for the same response amplitude. It is interesting to note that the proportional variation in b-wave amplitude with flash intensity holds only within the region in which for each group of rods converging onto a bipolar cell, only one rod receives a photon, or only a few do. Intracellular recording (MILLER and DOWLING, 1970) has revealed that the production of the b-wave involves a depolarization of the large glial cells of the retina (Müller cells), while the exploration of potential gradients with extracellular electrodes (ARDEN and BROWN, 1965) has shown the existence of a sink of current at a retinal depth corresponding to the synaptic contacts between receptor and bipolar cells with a limited source more distal and a larger, more extensive source more proximal. How the change in the Müller cells, which occupy the correct position to give rise to these gradients, is brought about has not been explained. It would appear to involve interactions between cells that are non-synaptic in character. A lateral spread of activity among receptor cell terminals would result if the relation between these terminals and the Müller cells were reciprocative.

Acknowledgement

Original work was supported by a grant from the Medical Research Council.

References

ABRAHAMSON, E. W., ADAMS, R. G., WULFF, V. J.: Reversible spectral changes in retinene solutions following flash illumination. J. phys. Chem. 63, 441—443 (1959).
— MARQUISEE, J., GAVUZZI, P., ROUBIE, J.: Flash photolysis of visual pigments. Z. Elektrochem. 64, 177—180 (1960).
ANGELUCCI, A.: Untersuchungen über die Sehtätigkeit der Netzhaut und des Gehirns. Untersuch. zur Naturlehre d. Menschen u. d. Thiere (Moleschott) 14, 231—357 (1894).
ARDEN, G. B., BROWN, K. T.: Some properties of components of the cat electroretinogram revealed by local recording under oil. J. Physiol. (Lond.) 176, 429—461 (1965).

— ERNST, W.: The effect of ions on the photoresponses of pigeon cones. J. Physiol. (Lond.) **211**, 311—339 (1970).

— IKEDA, H., SIEGEL, I. M.: New components of the mammalian receptor potential and their relation to visual photochemistry. Vision Res. **6**, 373—383 (1966).

AREY, L. B.: The movements in the visual cells and retinal pigment of the lower vertebrates. J. comp. Neurol. **26**, 121—201 (1916a).

— Changes in the rod-visual cells of the frog due to the action of light. J. comp. Neurol. **26**, 429—442 (1916b).

BARLOW, H. B.: Retinal noise and absolute threshold. J. opt. Soc. Amer. **46**, 634—639 (1956).

BAUMANN, C.: Die Photosensitivität des Sehpurpurs in der isolierten Netzhaut. Vision Res. **5**, 425—434 (1965).

BAYLOR, D. A., FUORTES, M. G. F.: Electrical responses of single cones in the retina of the turtle. J. Physiol. (Lond.) **207**, 77—92 (1970).

— — O'BRYAN, P. M.: Receptive fields of cones in the retina of the turtle. J. Physiol. (Lond.) **214**, 265—294 (1971).

BLACKMAN, J. G., GINSBORG, B. L., RAY, C.: Spontaneous synaptic activity in sympathetic ganglion cells of the frog. J. Physiol. (Lond.) **167**, 389—401 (1963).

BLAISIE, J. K., WORTHINGTON, C. R.: Planar liquid-like arrangement of photopigment molecules in frog retinal receptor disk membranes. J. mol. Biol. **39**, 417—439 (1969).

— — DEWEY, M. M.: Molecular localisation of frog retinal photopigment by electron microscopy and low-angle X-ray diffraction. J. mol. Biol. **39**, 407—416 (1969).

BLAUROCK, A. E., WILKINS, M. H. F.: Structure of frog photoreceptor membranes. Nature (Lond.) **223**, 906—909 (1969).

BORTOFF, A., NORTON, A. L.: An electrical model of the vertebrate photoreceptor cell. Vision Res. **7**, 253—263 (1967).

BRINDLEY, G. S.: Physiology of the retina and visual pathway, 2nd Ed. London: Edward Arnold 1970.

— GARDNER-MEDWIN, A. R.: The origin of the early receptor potential of the retina. J. Physiol. (Lond.) **182**, 185—194 (1966).

BRODA, E. E., GOODEVE, C. F., LYTHGOE, R. J.: The weight of the chromophore carrier in the visual purple molecule. J. Physiol. (Lond.) **98**, 397—404 (1940).

BROWN, H. MACK, HAGIWARA, S., KOIKE, H., MEECH, R. M.: Membrane properties of a barnacle photoreceptor examined by the voltage clamp technique. J. Physiol. (Lond.) **208**, 385—414 (1970).

BROWN, K. T.: The electroretinogram: its components and their origins. Vision Res. **8**, 633—677 (1968).

— MURAKAMI, M.: Biphasic form of the early receptor potential of the monkey retina. Nature (Lond.) **204**, 739—740 (1964).

— WATANABE, K., MURAKAMI, M.: The early and late receptor potentials of monkey cones and rods. Cold Spr. Harb. Symp. quant. Biol. **30**, 457—482 (1965).

BROWN, P. K.: Rhodopsin rotates in the visual receptor membrane. Biophys. Soc. Abstr. **1971**, 284a.

— GIBBONS, I. R., WALD, G.: The visual cells and visual pigment of the mudpuppy, *Necturus*. J. Cell. Biol. **19**, 79—106 (1963).

BYZOV, A. L., TRIFONOV, J. A.: The response to electric stimulation of horizontal cells in the carp retina. Vision Res. **8**, 817—822 (1968).

COHEN, A. I.: The fine structure of the extrafoveal receptors of the rhesus monkey. Exp. Eye Res. **1**, 128—136 (1961).

— The fine structure of the visual receptors of the pigeon. Exp. Eye Res. **2**, 88—97 (1963).

— Some electron microscopic observations on inter-receptor contacts in the human and macaque retinae. J. Anat. (Lond.) **99**, 595—610 (1965).

— New evidence supporting the linkage to extracellular space of outer segment saccules of frog cones but not rods. J. Cell Biol. **37**, 424—444 (1968).

— Further studies on the question of the patency of saccules in outer segments of vertebrate photoreceptors. Vision Res. **10**, 445—454 (1970).

CONE, R. A.: Early receptor potential of the vertebrate retina. Nature (Lond.) **204**, 736—739 (1964a).

— The rat electroretinogram I. Contrasting effects of adaptation on the amplitude and latency of the b-wave. J. gen. Physiol. **47**, 1089—1105 (1964b).
— Early receptor potential: photoreversible charge displacement in rhodopsin. Science **155**, 1128—1131 (1967).
— Relaxation times of rhodopsin detected by photodichroism. Biophys. Soc. Abstr. **1971**, 246a.
— BROWN, P. K.: Dependence of the early receptor potential on the orientation of rhodopsin. Science **156**, 536 (1967).
— COBBS W. H.: Rhodopsin cycle in the living eye of the rat. Nature (Lond.) **221**, 820—822 (1969).
CRANK, J.: The mathematics of diffusion. Oxford: Clarendon Press 1956.
DARTNALL, H. J. A.: The photosensitivities of visual pigments in the presence of hydroxylamine. Vision Res. **8**, 339—358 (1968).
DENTON, E. J.: The contributions of the oriented photosensitive and other molecules to the absorption of whole retina. Proc. roy. Soc. B, **150**, 78—94 (1959).
— WYLLIE, J. H.: Study of the photosensitive pigments in the pink and green rods of the frog. J. Physiol. (Lond.) **127**, 81—89 (1955).
DE ROBERTIS, E., LASANSKY, A.: Ultrastructure and chemical organization of photoreceptors. In: Structure of the eye. (Ed. G. K. Smelser) 29—49. New York: Academic Press 1961.
DOWLING, J. E.: Foveal receptors of the monkey retina: fine structure. Science **147**, 57—59 (1965).
— BOYCOTT, B. B.: Organization of the primate retina: electron microscopy. Proc. roy. Soc. B, **166**, 80—111 (1966).
DROZ, B.: Dynamic condition of proteins in the visual cells of rats and mice as shown by radioautography with labelled amino acid. Anat. Rec. **145**, 157—167 (1963).
ENGELMANN, T. W.: Über Bewegungen der Zapfen und Pigmentzellen der Netzhaut unter dem Einfluß des Lichtes und des Nervensystems. Pflügers Arch. ges. Physiol. **35**, 498—508 (1885).
EWALD, A., KÜHNE, W.: Untersuchungen über den Sehpurpur. I. Untersuch. physiol. Inst. Univ. Heidelberg **1**, 139—218 (1878a).
— — Untersuchungen über den Sehpurpur. III. Untersuch. physiol. Inst. Univ. Heidelberg **1**, 370—422 (1878b).
FALK, G., FATT, P.: Rapid hydrogen ion uptake of rod outer segments and rhodopsin solutions on illumination. J. Physiol. (Lond.) **183**, 211—224 (1966).
— — Passive electrical properties of rod outer segments. J. Physiol. (Lond.) **198**, 627—646 (1968a).
— — Conductance changes produced by light in rod outer segments. J. Physiol. (Lond.) **198**, 647—699 (1968b).
— — Distinctive properties of the lamellar and disk-edge structures of the rod outer segment. J. Ultrastruct. Res. **28**, 41—60 (1969).
FATT, P., KATZ, B.: Spontaneous subthreshold activity at motor nerve endings. J. Physiol. (Lond.) **117**, 109—128 (1952).
FERNÁNDEZ-MORÁN, H.: The submicroscopic structure of nerve fibres. Progr. Biophys. **4**, 112—147 (1954).
FÖRSTER, T.: Transfer mechanism of electronic excitation. Discussions Faraday Soc. **27**, 7 —17 (1959).
FULPIUS, B., BAUMANN, F.: Effects of sodium, potassium and calcium ions on slow and spike potentials in single photoreceptor cells. J. gen. Physiol. **53**, 541—561 (1969).
FUORTES, M. G. F.: Initiation of impulses in visual cells of *Limulus*. J. Physiol. **148**, 14—28 (1959).
GARTEN, S.: Die Veränderungen der Netzhaut durch Licht. Graefe-Saemisch, Handbuch der gesamten Augenheilkunde, Aufl. 2, Bd. 3, Kap. 12, Anhang, 1—130, Leipzig 1907.
GOLDSTEIN, E. B.: Early receptor potential of the isolated frog *(Rana pipiens)* retina. Vision Res. **7**, 837—848 (1967).
GRANIT, R.: The components of the retinal action potential in mammals and their relation to the discharge in the optic nerve. J. Physiol. (Lond.) **77**, 207—239 (1933).

— The development of retinal neurophysiology. In: Les Prix Nobel en 1967. pp. 232—241. Stockholm: Nobel Foundation 1968.

Gras, W. J., Worthington, C. R.: X-ray analysis of retinal photoreceptors. Proc. nat. Acad. Sci. (Wash.) **63**, 233—238 (1969).

Guzzo, A. V., Pool, G. L.: Visual pigment fluorescence. Science **159**, 312—314 (1968).

— — Fluorescence spectra of the intermediates of rhodopsin bleaching. Photochem. Photobiol. **9**, 565—570 (1969).

Hagins, W. A.:The photosensitivity of mammalian rhodopsin in situ. J. Physiol. (Lond.) **126**, 37P (1954).

— Electrical signs of information flow in photoreceptors. Cold Spr. Harb. Symp. quant. Biol. **30**, 403—418 (1965).

— Jennings, W. H.: Radiationless migration of electronic excitation in retinal rods. Discussions Faraday Soc. **27**, 180—190 (1959).

— McGaughy, R. E.: Molecular and thermal origins of fast photoelectric effects in the squid retina. Science **157**, 813—816 (1967).

— — Membrane origin of the fast photovoltage of squid retina. Science **159**, 213—215 (1968).

— Penn, R. D., Yoshikami, S.: Dark current and photocurrent in retinal rods. Biophys. J. **10**, 380—412 (1970).

— Rüppel, H.: Fast photoelectric effects and the properties of vertebrate photoreceptors as electric cables. Federation Proc. **30**, 64—78 (1971).

— Zonana, H. V., Adams, R. G.: Local membrane current in the outer segments of squid photoreceptors. Nature (Lond.) **194**, 844—847 (1962).

Hall, M. O., Bok, D., Bacharach, A. D. E.: Biosynthesis and assembly of the rod outer segment membrane system. Formation and fate of visual pigment in the frog retina. J. mol. Biol. **45**, 397—406 (1969).

Hara, R.: Changes in electrical conductance of rhodopsin on photolysis. J. gen. Physiol. **47**, 241—264 (1963).

Hara, T.: The effect of illumination on the electrical conductance of rhodopsin solutions. J. gen. Physiol. **41**, 857—877 (1958).

Hartline, H. K., Wagner, H. G., MacNichol, E. F.: The peripheral origin of nervous activity in the visual system. Cold Spr. Harb. Symp. quant. Biol. **17**, 125—141 (1952).

Hecht, S., Shlaer, S., Pirenne, M.: Energy, quanta, and vision. J. gen. Physiol. **25**, 819—840 (1942).

Heller, J.: Structure of visual pigments. I. Purification, molecular weight and composition of bovine visual pigment 500. Biochemistry 7, 2906—2913 (1968).

Hubbard, R.: The molecular weight of rhodopsin and the nature of the rhodopsin-digitonin complex. J. gen. Physiol. **37**, 381—399 (1954).

— The thermal stability of rhodopsin and opsin. J. gen. Physiol. **42**, 259—280 (1958).

Jagger, W. S., Liebman, P. A.: Birefringence transients in photoreceptor outer segments. Biophys. Soc. Abstr. **1970**, 59 a.

Kaneko, A.: Physiological and morphological identification of horizontal, bipolar and amacrine cells in goldfish retina. J. Physiol. (Lond.) **207**, 623—634 (1970).

Katz, B.: The transmission of impulses from nerve to muscle, and the subcellular unit of synaptic action. Proc. roy. Soc. B, **155**, 455—477 (1962).

— Miledi, R.: A study of spontaneous miniature potentials in spinal motoneurones. J. Physiol. (Lond.) **168**, 389—422 (1963).

— — A study of synaptic transmission in the absence of nerve impulses. J. Physiol. (Lond.) **192**, 407—436 (1967).

Kolmer, W.: Die Netzhaut. In: Handb. mikros. Anat. d. Menschen. (Möllendorff). Bd. 3, Teil 2: Auge. Berlin: Julius Springer 1936.

Kuwabara, T., Gorn, R. A.: Retinal damage by visible light. Arch. Ophthal. (N. Y.) **79**, 69—78 (1968).

Lettvin, J. Y.: General discussion: early receptor potential. Cold. Spr. Harb. Symp. quant. Biol. **30**, 501—502 (1965).

Liebman, P. A.: In situ microspectrophotometric studies on the pigments of single retinal rods. Biophys. J. **2**, 161—178 (1962).

— Leigh, R. A.: Autofluorescence of visual receptors. Nature (Lond.) **221**, 1249—1251 (1969).

LILEY, A. W.: The effects of presynaptic polarization on the spontaneous activity of the mammalian neuromuscular junction. J. Physiol. (Lond.) **134**, 427—443 (1956).

LYTHGOE, R. J., QUILLIAM, J. P.: The thermal decomposition of visual purple. J. Physiol. (Lond.) **93**, 24—38 (1938).

MATTHEWS, R. G., HUBBARD, R., BROWN, P. K., WALD, G.: Tautomeric forms of metarhodopsin. J. gen. Physiol. **47**, 215—240 (1963).

McCONNELL, D. G., RAFFERTY, C. N., DILLEY, R. A.: The light-induced proton uptake in bovine retinal outer segment fragments. J. biol. Chem. **243**, 5820—5826 (1968).

MILLECCHIA, R., MAURO, A.: The ventral photoreceptor cells of *Limulus* III. A voltage-clamp study. J. gen. Physiol. **54**, 331—351 (1969).

MILLER, R. F., DOWLING, J. E.: Intracellular responses of the Müller (glial) cells of the mudpuppy retina: their relation to b-wave of the electro-retinogram. J. Neurophysiol. **33**, 323—341 (1970).

MISSOTTEN, L., APPELMANS, M., MICHIELS, J.: L'ultrastructure des synapses des cellules visuelles de la rétine humaine. Bull. Mém. Soc. Franç. Ophtal. **76**, 59—82 (1963).

MOODY, J. F., ROBERTSON, J. D.: The fine structure of some retinal photoreceptors. J. biophys. biochem. Cytol. **7**, 87—92 (1960).

MURAKAMI, M., KANEKO, A.: Differentiation of PIII subcomponents in cold-blooded vertebrate retinas. Vision Res. **6**, 627—636 (1966).

— PAK, W. L.: Intracellularly recorded early receptor potential of the vertebrate photoreceptors. Vision Res. **10**, 965—976 (1970).

NAKA, K. I., RUSHTON, W. A. H.: S-potentials from luminosity units in the retina of fish (Cyprinidae). J. Physiol. (Lond.) **185**, 587—599 (1966).

NILSSON, S. E. G.: The ultrastructure of the receptor outer segments in the retina of the leopard frog *(Rana pipiens)*. J. Ultrastruct. Res. **12**, 207—231 (1965).

NOELL, W. K., WALKER, V. S., KANG, B. S., BERMAN, S.: Retinal damage by light in rats. Invest. Ophthal. **5**, 450—472 (1966).

OSTROY, S. E., ERHARDT, F., ABRAHAMSON, E. W.: Protein configuration changes in the photolysis of rhodopsin. II. The sequence of intermediates in thermal decay of cattle metarhodopsin *in vitro*. Biochim. biophys. Acta (Amst.) **112**, 265—277 (1966).

PAK, W. L., BOES, R. J.: Rhodopsin: Responses from transient intermediates formed during its bleaching. Science **155**, 1131—1133 (1967).

— CONE, R. A.: Isolation and identification of the initial peak of the early receptor potential. Nature (Lond.) **204**, 836—838 (1964).

PENN, R. D., HAGINS, W. A.: Signal transmission along retinal rods and the origin of the electroretinographic a-wave. Nature (Lond.) **223**, 201—205 (1969).

PESKIN, J. C.: Concentration of visual purple in a retinal rod of *Rana pipiens*. Science **125**, 68—69 (1957).

PIRENNE, M. H.: Vision and the eye, 2nd ed. London: Chapman & Hall 1967.

RADDING, C. M., WALD, G.: Acid-base properties of rhodopsin and opsin. J. gen. Physiol. **39**, 909—922 (1956).

REID, C.: Excited states in chemistry and biology. London: Butterworth 1957.

ROSENBERG, B.: A physical approach to the visual receptor process. Adv. Radiat. Biol. **2**, 193—241 (1966).

— ORLANDO, R. A., ORLANDO, J. M.: Photoconduction and semiconduction in dried receptors of sheep eyes. Arch. Biochem. **93**, 395—398 (1961).

RUSHTON, W. A. H.: The rhodopsin density in the human rods. J. Physiol. (Lond.) **134**, 30 —46 (1956).

SCHMIDT, W. J.: Doppelbrechung, Dichroismus und Feinbau des Außengliedes der Sehzellen vom Frosch. Z. Zellforsch. **22**, 485—522 (1935).

— Polarisationsoptische Analyse eines Eiweiß-Lipoid-Systems, erläutert am Außenglied der Sehzellen. Kolloid-Z. **85**, 137—148 (1938).

— Polarisationsoptische Analyse der Verknüpfung von Protein- und Lipoidmolekeln, erläutert am Außenglied der Sehzellen der Wirbeltiere. Pubbl. Staz. Zool. Napoli **23**, Suppl. 158—184 (1951).

SCHULTZE, M.: Ueber die Nervendigung in der Netzhaut des Auges bei Menschen und bei Thieren. Arch. mikr. Anat. **5**, 379—403 (1869).

Shichi, H., Lewis, M. S., Irreverre, F., Stone, A. L.: Biochemistry of visual pigments I. Purification and properties of bovine rhodopsin. J. biol. Chem. **244**, 529—536 (1969).

Shields, J. E., Dinovo, E. C., Henriksen, R. A., Kimbel, R. L., Millar, P. G.: The purification and amino-acid composition of bovine rhodopsin. Biochem. biophys. Acta (Amst.) **147**, 238—251 (1967).

Sidman, R. L.: The structure and concentration of solids in photoreceptor cells studied by refractometry and interference microscopy. J. biophys. biochem. Cytol. **3**, 15—30 (1957).

Sillman, A. J., Ito, H., Tomita, T.: Studies on the mass receptor potential of the isolated frog retina II. On the basis of the ionic mechanism. Vision Res. **9**, 1443—1451 (1969).

Sjöstrand, F. S.: An electron microscope study of the retinal rod of the guinea pig eye. J. cell. comp. Physiol. **33**, 383—403 (1949).

— The ultrastructure of the outer segment of rods and cones of the eye as revealed by the electron microscope. J. cell. comp. Physiol. **42**, 15—44 (1953).

— Ultrastructure of retinal receptors of vertebrate eye. Ergebn. Biol. **21**, 128—160 (1959).

— Electron microscopy of the retina. In: The structure of the eye. (Ed. G. K. Smelser) pp. 1—28. New York: Academic Press 1961.

Smith, T. G., Brown, J. E.: A photoelectric potential in invertebrate cells. Nature (Lond.) **212**, 1217—1219 (1966).

Steinberg, R. H.: Rod and cone contributions to S-potentials from the cat retina. Vision Res. **9**, 1331—1344 (1969).

Stieve, H.: Interpretation of the generator potential in terms of ionic processes. Cold Spr. Harb. Symp. quant. Biol. **30**, 451—456 (1965).

Strackee, L.: Dichroism in the retina at —196° C. Vision Res. **10**, 925—938 (1970).

Svaetichin, G., MacNichol, E. F.: Retinal mechanism for chromatic and achromatic vision. Ann. N. Y. Acad. Sci. **74**, 385—404 (1958).

— Negishi, K., Fatehchand, R.: Cellular mechanisms of a Young-Hering visual system. In: Ciba Foundation symposium on colour vision: physiology and experimental psychology. (Ed. A. V. S. de Reuck & J. Knight). pp. 178—203. London: Churchill 1965.

Tao, T.: Rotational mobility of a fluorescent rhodopsin derivative in the rod outer-segment membrane. Biochem. J. **122**, 54P (1971).

Tomita, T.: Electrical activity of vertebrate photoreceptors. Quart. Rev. Biophys. **3**, 179—222 (1970).

— Kaneko, A., Murakami, M., Pautler, E. L.: Spectral response curves of single cones in the carp. Vision Res. **7**, 519—531 (1967).

Toyoda, J., Hashimoto, H., Anno, H., Tomita, T.: The rod response in the frog as studied by intracellular recording. Vision. Res. **10**, 1093—1100 (1970).

— Nosaki, H., Tomita, T.: Light induced resistance changes in single receptors of Necturus and Gekko. Vision Res. **9**, 453—463 (1969).

Wald, G., Brown, P. K.: The molar extinction of rhodopsin. J. gen. Physiol. **37**, 189—200 (1953).

— — Gibbons, I. R.: Visual excitation: A chemo-anatomical study. Symp. Soc. exp. Biol. **16**, 32—57 (1962).

Walls, G. L.: The vertebrate eye. Bloomfield Hills: Cranbrook Institute of Science 1942.

Werblin, F. S., Dowling, J. E.: Organization of retina of the mudpuppy, Necturus maculosus. II. Intracellular recording. J. Neurophysiol. **32**, 339—355 (1969).

Williams, T. P.: Photoreversal of rhodopsin bleaching. J. gen. Physiol. **47**, 679—689 (1964).

— Breil, S. J.: Kinetic measurements on rhodopsin solutions during intense flashes. Vision Res. **8**, 777—786 (1968).

— Milby, S. E.: The thermal decomposition of some visual pigments. Vision Res. **8**, 359—367 (1968).

Wolken, J. J.: A structural model for a retinal rod. In: The structure of the eye. (Ed. G. K. Smelser) pp. 173—191. New York: Academic Press 1961.

Wulff, V. J., Adams, R. G., Linschitz, H., Abrahamson, E. W.: Effects of flash illumination on rhodopsin in solution. Ann. N. Y. Acad. Sci. **74**, 281—290 (1958).

Yamada, E.: Observations on the fine structure of photoreceptive elements in the vertebrate eye. J. Electron-microscopy (Tokyo) **9**, 1—14 (1960).

Young, R. W.: Passage of newly formed protein through the connecting cilium of retinal rods in the frog. J. Ultrastruct. Res. **23**, 462—473 (1968).

— Droz, B.: The renewal of protein in retinal rods and cones. J. cell. Biol. **39**, 169—184 (1968).

Zonana, H. V.: Fine structure of the squid retina. Bull. Johns Hopk. Hosp. **109**, 185—205 (1961).

Chapter 8

The Visual Cells and Visual Pigments of the Vertebrate Eye

By

FREDERICK CRESCITELLI*

Los Angeles, California (USA)

With 30 Figures

Contents

* The original work reported in this chapter was aided by a grant from the Division of Research Grants and Fellowships, National Institutes of Health, US Public Health Service.

I. Introduction

Information about the environment is received by animals *via* a number of sensory structures, each specialized to respond optimally to a particular physical or chemical change in the environment. Of these structures, photoreceptors are of common occurrence, and mediate information that is of primary significance to the life of the organism and the species. Photoreceptors function by means of pigments that absorb light in the near ultraviolet and visible regions of the spectrum, i.e., roughly 300 to 800nm. The lateral eyes of vertebrates possess such photopigments located intracellularly in specialized segments of the retinal receptors. In these outer segments light quanta are absorbed, and after a transduction and amplification process — about which little is known — excitation of the retinal neurones occurs, leading to impulses that proceed out of the retina to the visual centers of the brain. This chapter is concerned with the vertebrate visual cells and the photopigments contained therein. It deals with the manifold types of visual receptors throughout the various vertebrate groups, and the possible biological significance of this multiplicity. It deals similarly with the visual pigments within these receptors and attempts to sort out some ecological and phylogenetic relations suggested by the properties and distribution of these photopigments. Because of the manner in which this volume is organized, this chapter has a limited scope, being concerned mainly with those pigments that have been extracted out of the retina by appropriate solvents, chiefly digitonin solution. For this reason it will deal almost exclusively with the photopigments of the rods or rod-like cells. Other chapters will examine the cone pigments and the results obtained using methods of study other than the technique of extraction.

A. Historical Introduction to the Visual Cells

The specialized receptors of the vertebrate retina are derived embryologically from the ependymal cells of the neural tube and in their ultrastructure they reveal their relation to these cells. With respect to various detailed morphological characters the vertebrate visual cells are divided into two categories: rods and cones. The finding of retinas with many rods in nocturnal or crepuscular animals, and with many cones in diurnal forms, led SCHULTZE (1866, 1867) to conclude that the cone is the functional receptor in bright light while the rod functions in dim light. SCHULTZE also associated the cone with a role in the detection of color. Thus was established the duplex nature of the vertebrate retina and of retinal function, which later received impressive support from physiology, and led to what has become known as the Duplicity Theory of Vision.

SCHULTZE employed several morphological characters to distinguish rods and cones (Fig. 1). Some of these were; the longer, cylindrical outer segments of the rods in some animals compared to the shorter, tapered outer segments of the cones; the stouter, flask-shaped inner segments of the cones compared with the slenderer rod inner segments; the more internal (vitread) location of the tips of the cones in certain animals; the presence of oil-droplets in the inner segments of some cones, and their absence in typical rods; and certain differences in the appearance and location of the nuclei of rods and cones.

Schultze admitted having difficulty in distinguishing rods from cones under some circumstances. He pictured the visual cells of the human fovea as being slender and rod-like and without the characteristic flask-shaped inner segments of the peripheral cones. He observed a similar change in shape of the visual cells in passing from the periphery to the center of the retina in several other animals. In the guinea pig and rabbit retinas Schultze was unable to distinguish rods and cones on the basis of the inner segment but the outer segment's shape made a distinction possible. In the pigeon and falcon it was not easy to pick out the cones because the outer segments were slender and rod-shaped, but the presence of oil-droplets — absent in the rods — was useful in making a distinction. Oil-droplets in visual cells had been discovered previously by Hannover (1840) but Schultze added to Hannover's description. He observed that some oil-droplets were colored and he argued on the basis of these that hue discrimination is a property associated with cones. Schultze examined the oil-droplets in the developing chicken retina and noted a chronological order in appearance of the differently colored droplets, the order being colorless, red, yellow. This sequence has been confirmed for the chicken retina in a recent study (Meyer, Cooper, and Gernez, 1965). Schultze was aware of the presence of oil-droplets in the cones of the turtle and of certain amphibians, as well as their absence in teleost fishes and placental mammals. The presence of strikingly colored droplets in the cones of certain vertebrates eventually led to speculations about the possible role of such droplets in color vision. This idea, first proposed by Krause (1863), assumed the existence of cones with but a single photopigment, the wavelength specificity arising from the optical filter action of the colored oil droplets. On the basis of the occurrence and lack of occurrence of colored droplets, or specifically colored droplets, in certain species and in specific retinal regions, Walls (1942b) rejected Krause's suggestion. Walls was not successful in dispelling the idea, and it periodically reappears in connection with specific investigations. This, in spite of the fact that visual pigment research has advanced to the stage of showing that no single photo-pigment exists that effectively spans the visible spectrum, and of showing that multiple cone pigments probably occur in diurnal vertebrates. King-Smith (1969) recently resurrected the theory of Krause in a study of the spectral transmittance of the droplets in the pigeon retina. Three spectrally different types of droplets were described for the yellow and red retinal fields of this bird. King-Smith viewed these droplets as short-wave cut-off filters with one type serving to remove light below about 590 nm, a second type removing light below about 540 nm and the third absorbing below about 460 nm. King-Smith cited Bridges' finding of only one pigment, i.e. $P544_1$ — in addition to rhodopsin — in extracts of the pigeon retina. Knowledge of cone visual pigments in birds is noticeably deficient and even Bridges' result has not been confirmed. The situation is somewhat better for the turtle retina which also contains colored oil droplets: red, orange and yellow. In both the freshwater turtle *(Pseudemys scripta)* and the marine turtle *(Chelonia mydas)* three different cone pigments were detected by means of single-cell micro-spectrophotometry (Liebman and Granda, 1971). Liebman and Granda rejected, for the turtle, Krause's single cone pigment hypothesis. As possible functions for the colored oil droplets we are left with the idea that they serve to improve visual acuity by reducing light scattering and/or chromatic aberration.

SCHULTZE also reported the presence, in the inner segment of both rods and cones, of a light-refracting organelle, which he called the lenticular body (SCHULTZE, 1873) and which KRAUSE previously had seen and called the optic ellipsoid (cited by SCHULTZE, 1873). This organelle is apparently the mitochondrion-rich structure that we now call the ellipsoid. SCHULTZE also described the double cones, which he referred to as Zwillingszapfen and which had been already seen by HANNOVER (SCHULTZE, 1867). He recognized that these were present in the retinas of birds, reptiles, amphibians and fishes but not in placental mammals. It is clear that he recognized the two classes of Zwillingszapfen that we now call twin cones and double cones. The twin cones were seen by SCHULTZE as consisting of a pair of similar cones attached to each other at the inner segments. We now recognize twin cones as characteristic components in the retinas of some teleost fishes, although their special role in vision in these fishes is not known. The second type — the double cone — was found by SCHULTZE in the retinas of amphibia, reptiles and birds. These were described as being a pair of dissimilar cones, one of which, the chief or principal member (Hauptzapfen), was pictured as different in shape and in relative position from the accessory member (Nebenzapfen). An oil-droplet was shown as a characteristic organelle of the chief member whereas no trace of such a structure was seen in the accessory member of the frog and tortoise double cones. In the retina of the lizard *(Lacerta agilis)* the accessory member showed no structured oil-droplet but instead a diffuse yellow pigment in the inner segment at the comparable location of the oil-droplet in the chief member. In chicken double cones SCHULTZE noted a yellow droplet in the accessory member. The thoroughness of SCHULTZE's observations is revealed by recent confirmations of the oil-droplet in the accessory members of the chicken double cones. Missed by several retinologists, this was seen as a small droplet by MEYER and COOPER (1966) and as a granular vesicle by MORRIS and SHOREY (1967), who employed electron microscopy. SCHULTZE also was able to detect slight differences in the shapes of the outer segments of the two members of the double cones. In the frog retina, for example, he described the outer segment of the chief member as thick and clearly conical, whereas the outer limb of the accessory member was seen to be less tapered. Another difference between the two members of the double cones was pictured by SCHULTZE in the swelling of the accessory cell in the region of the myoid. This structure, now known as the paraboloid, is a glycogen-containing organelle (see SAXÉN, 1955). Many of these features described in this section are illustrated by Fig. 1, which includes drawings taken from SCHULTZE's publications.

In his studies SCHULTZE made a rather good sampling of animals from the several vertebrate classes and came to some general formulations about the nature and distribution of rods and cones in vertebrates. As to cyclostomes, SCHULTZE examined the retina of Lampetra fluviatilis and concluded, very tentatively, that it was a cone-free retina. Examination of other species was not made. According to SCHULTZE (1873) cones were also absent from the retinas of elasmobranchs such as sharks and rays. I shall have occasion to remark later that these conclusions about the cyclostome and elasmobranch retinas are probably not correct. For the chondrosteans, only the sturgeon retina was explored, and SCHULTZE, on the basis of a somewhat uncertain drawing of the visual cells of *Acipenser* made by LEYDIG (1853), concluded that no cones were present. In contrast, WALLS (1942a)

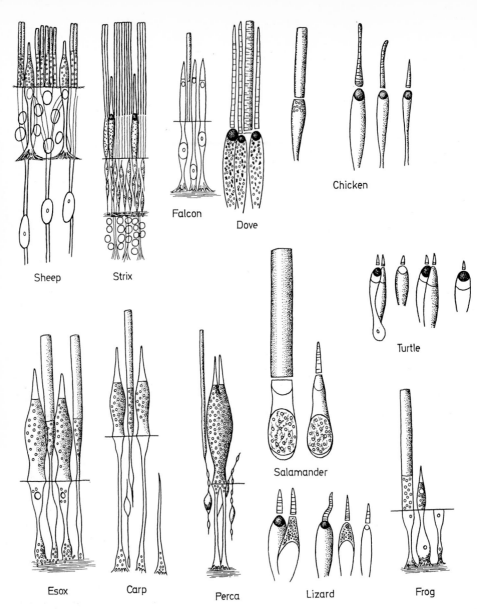

Fig. 1. Selected sketches to illustrate SCHULTZE's concepts of the visual cells in various vertebrates. Sheep: 2 cones and 9 rods; rods were incompletely shown. Owl *(Strix)*: 12 rods and 2 cones; the cones were shown as having light-yellow oil-droplets. Falcon: 3 cones and 1 rod, the nucleus of the rod was not shown, cones have oil-droplets. Dove: 3 cones with red oil-droplets and the outer segment of a rod. Chicken: rod without nucleus and 3 cones, the larger cone with a yellow oil-droplet, the 2 smaller cones with red oil-droplets. Fish *(Esox)* 2 cones and 2 rods. Fish *(Carp)*: 2 cones and 1 rod. Fish *(Perca)*: 1 rod and 1 double cone. Salamander: 1 rod and 1 cone. Lizard *(Lacerta)*: 1 double cone with yellow oil-droplet in one member and 3 types of single cones, one with an orange oil-droplet, the second with a diffuse yellow pigment in the ellipsoid and the third with a small colorless oil-droplet. Turtle *(Emys)*: 2 double cones, with orange-yellow oil-droplets in one member of each double, a single cone with colorless oil-droplet and a single cone with red oil-droplet. SCHULTZE found no **rods** in the turtle retina. Frog: 1 rod and 1 cone

pictured for *Acipenser fulvescens* a cone with colorless oil-droplet and paraboloid, as well as an easily distinguishable rod. SCHULTZE (1867) considered that enough was known about the distribution of rods and cones in vertebrates to permit him to state that rods are phylogenetically ancestral to cones. The presence of the colorless oil-droplet in the sturgeon visual cells (LEYDIG, 1853) suggested to SCHULTZE that these elements probably represent evolutionary transitional forms between rods and cones. The difficulty with SCHULTZE's hypothesis of the rod as the ancestral cell is that recent work has not confirmed the pure-rod nature of the sub-teleost retina, although no oil-droplets and no double cells have been reported for the cyclostomes and elasmobranchs.

The teleost fishes were considered by SCHULTZE to possess duplex retinas although he conceded the occurrence, as in the eel, of cone-free systems. In amphibia, SCHULTZE had no difficulty in distinguishing rods and cones since he observed between numerous colossal rods, as he called them, a few small cones (Fig. 1). It is surprising, perhaps, that SCHULTZE, thorough observer though he was, failed to see the green rods of amphibians. These were seen later by SCHWALBE (1874), by BOLL (1877) and by KÜHNE (1877, 1878). These green or SCHWALBE rods occupy only about 8 percent of the total retinal area in the frog (DENTON and WYLLIE, 1955) a fact that may account for SCHULTZE's failure to observe them. In his sample of reptiles SCHULTZE looked at the retinas of lizards, the tortoise and some alcohol-preserved snakes. Disagreeing with HULKE (1867), SCHULTZE considered that lizards, such as *Anguis fragilis* and *Lacerta agilis*, have retinas that are rod-free. He noted the presence of colorless and yellow oil-droplets in the lizard cones and the presence of red and orange oil-droplets in the tortoise visual cells. SCHULTZE might have adopted a broader view of the reptilian system if he had extended his sample somewhat. If he had looked at the alligator retina, and the retina of some fresh water turtles, he might have seen rods as well as cones (WALLS, 1942a). If he had examined the retinas of certain nocturnal lizards, including geckos, he would have discovered pure rod retinas in lizards (ROCHON-DUVIGNEAUD, 1917; DETWILER, 1923; WALLS, 1934). He also would have discovered, in geckos, retinas with double, as well as single, rods (DETWILER, 1923; WALLS, 1934; UNDERWOOD, 1951) and eventually, if he had continued his studies of geckos, he would have discovered the presence of oil-droplets in rods (UNDERWOOD, 1951). One wonders how he would have responded to these findings, which to a considerable extent blur the distinctions between rods and cones. And yet, if he had examined enough geckos, he might have found great support for his duplexity concept of the vertebrate retina, for eventually he would have come upon diurnal, round-pupiled geckos, with retinas whose visual cells he would have named cones. He would have contrasted these with nocturnal geckos whose pupils close down to a vertical slit and whose visual cells, by the usual morphological criteria, he would have classified as rods (TANSLEY, 1964).

For his study of the bird visual cells SCHULTZE employed the chicken, the pigeon, the falcon, the crow (two species) and three species of owls. In all these, he was able to recognize both rods and cones, the cones, in turn, having red, yellow and colorless oil-droplets. He reported seeing changes in visual cell morphology correlated with retinal location, the peripheral rods being thicker, and becoming thinner toward the fovea and being lost (in the falcon) from the fovea. The falcon fovea showed only yellow oil-droplets in the cones and at the foveal edge, whereas toward the periphery red and yellow droplets were observed. In the crow the fovea was seen to have rods (though thin ones) in addition to cones; and to retain in the latter both red and yellow oil-droplets. In the retinas of the owls the rods were found to be numerous and long; the cones were seen to be relatively short, having pale yellow droplets that were colorless at the ora.

The retinas of several common mammals were studied by Schultze including those from man, monkey (Macacus cynomolgus), sheep, cattle, pig, horse, dog, bat, hedgehog, mole, mouse, guinea pig, rabbit, cat, and rat. He believed cones to be absent in the bat, the hedgehog, the mole and the mouse; these animals being classed as nocturnal forms. A sort of intermediate condition was assigned to the retinas of the rabbit, the cat and the rat in whose systems rods were believed to predominate, with the cones being relatively thin. Most of the remaining species were viewed as having typically duplex retinas with the visual cells changing in morphology and relative numbers over the retinal surface in somewhat the same manner as the rods and cones of the human retina, which Schultze studied in some detail. The progressive change in shape of cones in going from more peripheral regions to the central fovea is now considered to have functional significance in terms of the Stiles-Crawford directional sensitivity phenomenon. According to Westheimer (1967), the rod-like cones of the central fovea, compared with the more conical cones of the parafovea, exhibit a significantly smaller Stiles-Crawford effect. Westheimer considered this evidence sufficient to support the idea that the Stiles-Crawford effect is associated with the shape of the retinal receptors. The occurrence of a significant directional sensitivity away from the fovea emphasizes the importance of optimizing the orientation of cones with respect to the direction of the incident light rays. It is significant, therefore, that the retina, in its development, possesses mechanisms for achieving such optimal orientation. Employing special techniques to preserve the normal receptor orientation, Laties (1969) demonstrated a graded deviation of receptor axis angle over the retinal surface so as to achieve optimal acceptance of light incident upon the retina at different retinal regions (Laties, Liebman and Campbell 1968). The deviation with respect to the normal to the retinal surface was as much as 40° at the extreme periphery.

B. Historical Introduction to the Visual Pigments

A number of pioneer investigators are on record as having seen the reddish coloration associated with the retinas of invertebrates and vertebrates (see Kühne, 1877). It is certain that Schultze himself observed a red satiny appearance of the long rods in the rat, the owl and the frog. None of these early investigators associated the red color with light or with photochemical events in the visual cells. The discoverer of this important relationship was Franz Boll (1876) who presented to the November 23, 1876 meeting of the Berlin Academy a short communication describing the purple-red color of a freshly-removed frog retina, and its bleaching out in the presence of light. Boll associated the red color with rods and noted that rod-rich retinas such as those of amphibia, elasmobranchs, teleost fishes and certain mammals, showed the color especially well. The colored oil-droplets of the bird and reptile retinas made it difficult for him to detect the purple-red color but BOLL eventually was able to observe it in the center of the pigeon retina. The purple-red color, Sehrot (as he named it), was shown to regenerate in the dark. He was uncertain of the nature of Sehrot, whether it was a physical or chemical color, but he correctly interpreted the color changes as being related to the act of vision. BOLL erroneously associated the color with the living state of the retina and he attributed the failure of previous investigators to see Sehrot as the result of having the retinas in a poor physiological condition.

Stimulated by BOLL's discovery, FRIEDRICH WILHELM KÜHNE, director of the Physiological Institute at Heidelberg, began his classic observations and analyses, which established the foundations and structure of modern retinal photochemistry. KÜHNE (1877) quickly confirmed BOLL's discovery and proved that the living state was not required in order to preserve the red color. He was able to extract the color into a solution of bile salts and thus to show that the color was not the result of physical interference but of a chemical substance, which he named Sehpurpur and then Rhodopsin (KÜHNE, 1879). Later, digitonin was introduced and proved to be an effective extractant for visual pigments (TANSLEY, 1931). KÜHNE examined many physical and chemical properties of Sehpurpur, which led eventually to its formal recognition as a protein (WALD, 1935). KÜHNE obtained a crude absorption spectrum for Sehpurpur and studied the bleaching effectiveness of light of various wavelengths. He examined the products of bleaching and observed the regeneration of Sehpurpur from these products, noting especially the role of the pigment epithelium in promoting regeneration.

KÜHNE's comparative studies were influenced by the work of SCHULTZE, and he selected a number of animals on the basis of SCHULTZE's descriptions of the visual cell composition. He noted a faint coloration in the retina of the lamprey, *Lampetra fluviatilis*, that disappeared on exposure of the retina to light. He confirmed BOLL's finding of Sehpurpur in elasmobranchs and teleosts, seeing it in a shark, the eel, the loach and the carp. With amphibia, KÜHNE studied especially the Sehpurpur of the frog but he also observed its presence in newts and salamanders. KÜHNE was well aware of SCHULTZE's association of rods and cones with the nocturnal and diurnal habits of life, respectively, and he attempted to find a parallel correlation with the presence and absence of Sehpurpur. In the retinas of snakes (*Tropidonotus natrix, Coronella laevis*) he found no trace of red color and he concluded that in such diurnal animals there was no Sehpurpur. In the retina of a lizard (*Anguis fragilis*) the yellow oil-droplets were sufficiently far apart as not to interfere with the observations of the retina between the droplets and in such regions KÜHNE was unable to detect Sehpurpur. He concluded that Sehpurpur was absent in retinas without rods. In the retinas of owls, however, KÜHNE confirmed SCHULTZE's claim of many rods with large outer segments; in these he noted the presence of Sehpurpur. KÜHNE examined the retinas of the tower falcon, the pigeon and the fowl. Unlike BOLL, he was unable to see the red color in the pigeon retina. We know now that rhodopsin is indeed present in the pigeon retina and can be extracted therefrom (BRIDGES, 1962). KÜHNE failed to see Sehpurpur in the chicken retina but this animal, too, is now known to possess rhodopsin (Bliss, 1946). The rods in the tower falcon were seen to have a definite purple coloration but this was not found for all rods since those rods intermingled between cones with colored oil-droplets were seen as colorless. Kühne introduced the concept of rods without Sehpurpur and he considered that such rods existed in the tower falcon, the pigeon and the chicken. This, in turn, suggested the concept of vision without Sehpurpur and he believed that Sehpurpur was deficient in a retina that had other means of absorbing light, e.g., the colored oil-droplets. Kühne was unable to see Sehpurpur in the retina of a bat whose rods were not surrounded by cones, and he was forced to the conclusion that vision is absent or deficient in the bat. Here again, Kühne's failure to see the red pigment is unreliable, and bats have been shown to yield rhodopsin to digitonin extraction, as I have demonstrated with several species.

Kühne also accepted the idea of cones without Sehpurpur, i.e., without visual pigment. This idea was gained from his failures to see the characteristic color in the retinas of diurnal snakes and of *Anguis*. It was reinforced by the absence of color in the fovea and macula of the human and monkey retinas. Together with rods without Sehpurpur, the existence of cones without Sehpurpur, led Kühne to postulate the concept of vision without visual pigment (*Sehen ohne Sehpurpur*). We now know that this concept is incorrect. Rods have been shown to contain photopigments other than the traditional red-appearing Sehpurpur, and cones have been found to house characteristic photolabile pigments. A common photochemical basis underlies all vision whether it is mediated by Sehpurpur or other visual pigments.

Kühne apparently employed the term Sehpurpur in the generic sense rather than to indicate one specific substance. He was aware that the retinal photo-pigments of different species varied as do the hemoglobins. In the lamprey retina, though the color was faint, it appeared to be different, showing a violet or blue appearance. The carp retina, like that of the eel, was described as being, not purple-red, but of a "bläulich-purpurfarben". Kühne did not explore further these differences in different species but such a study was made subsequently by Köttgen and Abelsdorff (1896) who prepared solutions of visual pigments by the method of Kühne and analyzed these solutions by the technique of direct difference spectrophotometry. Based on the difference spectra, a categorization of pigments into two distinct spectral classes was suggested: one class, comprising the data for the extracts from four mammals, one bird (owl) and three amphibia, showed an absorbance maximum at 500 nm; the second class, containing the data for eight species of teleosts, was characterized by a maximum at 540 nm. While this study could be criticized on the basis of unjustified employment of difference spectra, there probably is no reason to doubt the general conclusion that a difference in color of photopigments was indeed present in the extracts from fishes as compared with the solutions derived from the other vertebrates. In fact, a basic duality of visual pigments was eventually demonstrated to be present as a result of the investigations of Wald (1936a, 1936b, 1937a, 1939). While details of these studies will be found in other chapters of this volume, it is necessary here to point out certain salient features that are relevant to the purposes of this chapter.

(1) Rhodopsin was shown to be a conjugated protein with a protein, called opsin, complexed to a colored prosthetic group (WALD, 1953). In the formation of this complex the absorbance maximum was shown to shift from 385 nm (in chloroform), the spectral maximum for the prosthetic group, to about 500 nm, the corresponding maximum for rhodopsin in digitonin solution.

(2) The prosthetic group, originally called retinene, was found to be related to the then known vitamin A and to be converted to this vitamin after bleaching a retina with light and allowing it to decolorize completely (WALD, 1935). Vitamin A is now called vitamin A_1 or retinol.

(3) As a result of the important work of MORTON and his colleagues (MORTON, 1944; MORTON and GOODWIN, 1944; BALL, GOODWIN and MORTON, 1948) retinene was identified as the aldehyde of vitamin A_1. This aldehyde, formerly called retinene$_1$ and later retinal$_1$, is now referred to simply as retinal or retinaldehyde. Retinal is believed to be covalently bonded to a free amino group of the opsin, probably the $\varepsilon\text{-}NH_2$ of lysine (BOWNDS, 1967), although recently (POINCELOT, MILLAR, KIMBEL, and ABRAHAMSON, 1969) a Schiff-base binding to the lipid moiety has been suggested.

(4) A second system of visual pigments was extracted from the retinas of certain freshwater fishes (WALD, 1939). These pigments, called porphyropsins by WALD, were considered to be conjugated proteins with the opsin bound to retinene$_2$, the aldehyde of vitamin A_2, the vitamin found in the livers of many freshwater fishes. Vitamin A_2 is now called 3-dehydroretinol while retinene$_2$ is referred to as 3-dehydroretinal. The latter plays the same role in the porphyropsin system that retinal plays in the rhodopsin system. The chemistry of these two chromophores of the visual pigments is discussed in other chapters of this volume.

(5) According to WALD (1939), the porphyropsins absorb maximally at about 522 nm whereas the 3-dehydroretinal prosthetic group has a spectral maximum at 405 nm (in chloroform). The discovery of the porphyropsin system clarified the report of KÖTTGEN and ABELSDORFF (1896) of a unique system in fishes. Apparently, these investigators employed freshwater teleosts in their study although their maximum at 540 nm is not in agreement with the porphyropsin maximum at 522 nm.

(6) According to WALD, marine fishes, with possible exceptions in the family Labridae (the wrasses), have rhodopsin; freshwater fishes have porphyropsin (WALD, 1960). In WALD's writings, the spectral maximum for porphyropsin was given variously. In 1937 this location was given as 522—525 (WALD, 1937a); in 1939 it was given as 522 ± 2 nm (WALD, 1939); in 1960 it was placed at 523 ± 3 nm with the added information that certain labrids showed porphyropsins at 513 and 510 nm (WALD, 1960). This variation is pointed out merely to show that as more fishes have been examined and as methods of analyzing the visual pigment composition of an extract have improved, including the testing of homogeneity, the spectral definition of porphyropsin has broadened. As will be shown later, the same has happened to rhodopsin. One way out of this dilemma is to ignore etymology, as WALD (1960) proposed, and to define rhodopsin as the 11-*cis* retinal-opsin complex, and porphyropsin as the 11-*cis* 3-dehydroretinal-opsin complex. In this chapter I propose to follow, where possible, the lead of

LIEBMAN and ENTINE (1968) and to use the designations: Pn_1 or Pn_2, where n is the wavelength for maximal absorbance and the numbers refer to retinal or 3-dehydroretinal.

(7) On the basis of an examination of the visual system of certain fishes that are able to withstand marked changes in osmotic pressure, WALD (1941) concluded that an association exists between the nature of the visual system and this tolerance to changes in osmotic pressure. The retinas of certain salmonid fishes (brook trout, rainbow trout, chinook salmon) showed the presence of both vitamins A_1 and A_2, with the latter predominating. The photopigment absorbance curves revealed maxima, not at 522 nm, nor at 500 nm, but at the intermediate region of 510—515 nm, which was taken to mean the presence of a mixture of rhodopsin and porphyropsin. In the American eel, *Anguilla rostrata*, which spawns in the sea, WALD concluded that retinal vitamin A_1 predominates in quantity over the vitamin A_2 and that the visual pigment system, extracts of which gave spectral absorbance maxima at 498 and 502 nm, consisted of a mixture with rhodopsin in great preponderance. In the case of the killifish *(Fundulus heteroclitus)* which he classified as catadromous, WALD found a visual pigment much as in the eel. In contrast, the anadromous white perch *(Morone americana)* was interpreted as having only vitamin A_2 and porphyropsin in the retina. WALD assumed that phylogenetic considerations, rather than environment *per se* were involved in determining this visual pigment pattern and he used the expression "primacy of the spawning environment" to suggest that the visual pigment system that predominates in the retina is that appropriate to the spawning environment as defined by item 6 above. The association of porphyropsin with fresh water led WALD (1942 b) to suggest that this system may represent the ancestral vertebrate system, an idea that seemed to be supported by the finding of vitamin A_2 in the retina of the lamprey, *Petromyzon marinus*.

(8) WALD also considered the rhodopsin system to be characteristic of terrestrial vertebrates, but amphibia were thought of as transitional animals in the sense that porphyropsin, characteristic of the aquatic phase, as in bullfrog tadpoles, was replaced by rhodopsin in the terrestrial phase, as in bullfrog adults. These fundamental explorations by WALD and his colleagues, supplemented by the chemical findings of the Liverpool group under MORTON firmly established the duality of vertebrate visual pigments on the basis of the two aldehydes: retinal and 3-dehydroretinal.

(9) WALD's work also demonstrated that the nature of the opsin was relevant in determining the color and other properties of the visual pigment. From the chicken retina, for example, a second photopigment, in addition to rhodopsin, was extracted (WALD, BROWN, and SMITH, 1955). This pigment, named iodopsin, absorbed maximally at about 562 nm but possessed the same prosthetic group as rhodopsin, i.e., retinal. Iodopsin was shown to be less stable in solution than rhodopsin and was shown to regenerate faster than rhodopsin from its specific opsin and 11-*cis* retinal. In other words, the chicken retina was shown to yield two separate photopigments both with the same prosthetic group but based on different opsins. Nature has devised two separate and independent methods to achieve multiplicity and diversity of visual pigments in vertebrates: (i) a duality based on the two A vitamins and (ii) a multiplicity related to a number of specific

opsins. An opsin may combine with either one of these aldehydes, according to availability, and either of these aldehydes may complex with any one of a number of opsins. In the remainder of this chapter I shall explore how different vertebrates have utilized these two methods to evolve their unique visual pigments and to produce modifications adaptively related to the environment, or significant within a phylogenetic context.

II. A Paradigm: The Receptors and Visual Pigments of an Anuran

An important aim of vision research is the complete accounting of the visual cell types within a given retina, including the identification of the visual pigments housed within these cells. With modern techniques of electron microscopy and microspectrophotometry this aim appears to be within reach. In fact, this has been almost, if not completely, realized already for an anuran amphibian, i.e., *Rana pipiens*. The visual cells of this frog were recently examined with the electron microscope (NILSSON, 1964a). They are shown in Fig. 2. The following cells, already known before NILSSON's study, are pictured: red rods, green rods, single cones and double cones. The distribution of these different cell types was not uniform over the entire retina, but NILSSON enumerated for the posterior pole a count of 204 receptors which included 50% red rods, 15% green rods, 20% single cones and 15% double cones. No pattern or mosaic arrangement of cell types was noted. These different cell types were distinguished from each other by a number of identifying features some of which are illustrated in Fig. 2. These features included the sizes and shapes of the outer segments; the sizes and shapes of the inner segments; the size of the ellipsoids; the size and packing of the mitochondria within the ellipsoids; the length and thickness of the myoids; the shape, density and position of the nuclei; the size, shape and density pattern of the synaptic bodies; and the locations of the different organelles relative to the external limiting membrane and to the basement membrane. The double cone deserves special mention even though its functional significance is unknown. The principal member was like the single cone except for the longer and thinner myoid. In contrast, the accessory member lacked the oil-droplet, and the mitochondria were larger and denser than in the principal member. In addition, the accessory member showed a prominent paraboloid internal to the ellipsoid and closely packed against the principal member. Each member was seen to have its own nucleus and its own synaptic body but the two members were in intimate contact, except for the outer segments. Neither pigment-cell processes nor MÜLLER cells were observed to intervene between the two members at the surfaces of contact, so that a minimum of resistance to possible cross-talk exists between the members of the double cones. NILSSON pictured the outer segments of the two members to be similar, but on this point there appears to be a difference with some previous statements. As already mentioned, SCHULTZE described the outer segment of the frog accessory member as less tapered than that of the chief member. KRAUSE (1892) pictured the double cones of *Rana fusca* showing the chief member's outer segment as longer and thicker than the outer segment of its mate. The most recent indication of asymmetry for these two outer segments is found in a paper by Saxén (1953) who showed in *Rana temporaria* that the outer segment was conical for the chief member and rod-shaped for the accessory member. In addition, a difference in staining properties for these two outer segments was indicated. Using Heidenhain's azocarmine, Saxén recorded the chief outer segment to be light red, as were also the outer limbs of the single cones, while the outer limbs of the accessory cones and rods stained blue. Saxén interpreted this finding to mean that double cones originate through a fusion of already differentiated visual cells, in this case a rod and a cone. This would mean that the name double cone is inaccurate since the double entity would then represent a rod-cone coupling.

Nilsson's study is also relevant in relation to the old problem of whether rods and cones are ontogenetically independent. This independence was questioned by Bernard (1900) and by Cameron (1905) who believed they saw a graded series of developmental stages in the frog visual cells from early cone-shaped cells to fully developed rods. The Bernard-Cameron view was that cones were developmental stages in the formation of mature visual cells and that there is no such thing as Schultzian duplexity. This idea was resurrected recently by Muntz (1964a) who determined the spectral sensitivities of tadpoles of *Rana temporaria*, using the b-wave of the ERG as the index of response. At an early stage (stage 6 of Saxén, 1954) no Purkinje shift was found and the sensitivity was maximal at about 570nm. With further development (stages 8 and 9 of Saxén) the scotopic sensitivity curve shifted stage-wise to shorter wavelengths until in the adult the typical rhodopsin-based function was obtained. Because of sensitivity considerations, Muntz eliminated an explanation based on mixed responses of both rods and cones and adopted the view that the change in sensitivity was the result of developing rods which in the early stages contained a cone pigment that was gradually replaced by rhodopsin or some intermediate photopigment as development took place. The difficulty with Muntz's hypothesis is that it is based on indirect evidence, i.e., on the b-wave which does not simply or directly reflect the activity in receptor cells. The b-wave of the frog appears to originate, not in the visual cells, but at retinal levels internal to these (Nilsson and Crescitelli, 1969). Such a b-wave probably is the result of complex interacting activity from numerous converging pathways. Deductions about the receptors from such a processed signal are likely to be insecure. In any case there is some evidence against the Bernard-Cameron interpretation. Nilsson (1964b) suggested that rods and cones could be easily identified at the stage when the double-membraned discs appeared. By following development through to the stage when rods and cones were easily identified, Nilsson associated the cones with closely-packed double membranes, and rods with double membranes having a light interspace of 5—10nm. On this basis Nilsson concluded that rods and cones are independent cells from very early stages of development. Furthermore, the photopigment situation of tadpoles, to be presented next, offers direct evidence against the idea of ontogenetic gradualism.

The morphological description of the visual receptors in *Rana pipiens* has been complemented by an account of the photopigments within these receptors (Liebman and Entine, 1968). By use of a sensitive and stable microspectro-

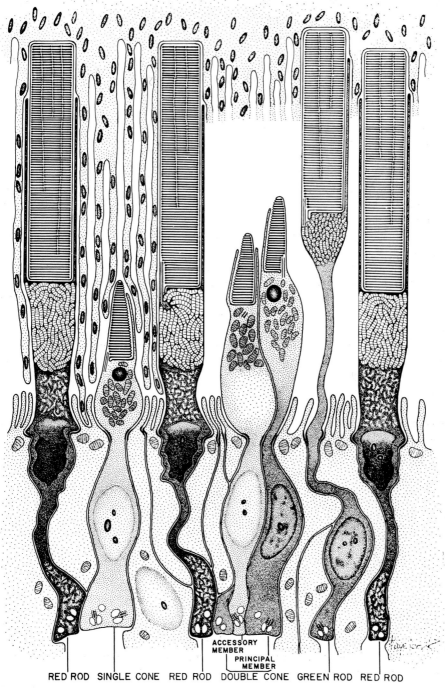

RED ROD   SINGLE CONE   RED ROD   DOUBLE CONE   GREEN ROD   RED ROD

ACCESSORY MEMBER

PRINCIPAL MEMBER

Fig. 2. Schematic drawing of visual receptors in *Rana pipiens* as shown by NILSSON and reproduced with permission of Dr. S. E. G. NILSSON. Some of the pigment epithelium processes have been omitted. Explanation in text

photometric technique, the *in situ* pigment composition of the rods and cones of the adult frog and of the tadpole was ascertained. The results, which in some respects are novel, may be summarized as follows:

Pigments of the adult: all vitamin A_1-based.

1. Red rods: $P502_1$; this is in agreement with the pigment extracted from the retina of adult *Rana pipiens* (Crescitelli, 1958a).

2. Single cones: $P575_1$; no such pigment has been extracted from the frog retina although Chase (1938) reported the presence of one or more red-sensitive components in retinal extracts of the frog (species not named). This work of Chase has not been confirmed. Although some variability (from 565 to 580nm) was noted for the pigment in single cones, Liebmann and Entine concluded that the $P 575_1$ was spectrally distinct from the iodopsin ($P 562_1$) of chicken.

3. Double cones

(a) Chief member: $P575_1$; the chief member was found to be similar to the single cone in certain morphological characteristics and in the nature of its visual pigment.

(b) Accessory member: $P502_1$; this finding was a surprise for here is a cell which, on the criteria of Schultze, would be called a cone and is called a cone, and yet houses rhodopsin. Is it a rod or a cone? Biochemically, this finding offers some support to Saxén's thesis that the anuran double cone is a rod-cone doublet.

4. Green rods: $P432_1$; I have detected evidence of a blue-absorbing photopigment in retinal extracts of adult *Rana pipiens* but the definitive study of the green rod pigment was made by Dartnall (1967) who extracted the retinas of the crab-eating frog *(Rana cancrivora)*. Dartnall determined the maximum for the spectral absorbance to be at 433nm, in excellent accord with the *in situ* measurements of Liebman and Entine made with *Rana pipiens*. Another study of the green rod pigment was made by Reuter (1966) who employed *Rana temporaria*. He placed the spectral maximum at 440nm. Reuter discovered the green rod pigment to be especially liable to destruction by hydroxylamine, a characteristic of certain other visual pigments, and Dartnall put this property to use in the analysis of the pigment from the crab-eating frog. The green rods of the frog are green, as Boll (1877) pictured in drawings and as Denton and Wyllie (1955) proved by photographs. No orange-red absorbing pigment that would account for the photo-stable green appearance was extracted by Dartnall, and no such pigment was detected in the outer segments by the microspectrophotometric probings of Liebman and Entine. The green color of the green rods is still unexplained.

Pigments of the tadpole: all vitamin A_2-based.

1. Red rods: $P527_2$; the name red rods is employed for the larval single rods although the photopigment is not the rose-colored rhodopsin of the adult red rods. I have recently found a classical porphyropsin in extracts of larval *Rana pipiens* similar to that I earlier found in tadpoles of the bullfrog, *R. catesbeiana* (Crescitelli, 1958a).

2. Single cones: $P620_2$; this is an interesting result for it established the natural occurrence of a retinal photopigment first discovered in a test tube synthesis. This synthesis was accomplished by mixing the opsin derived from chicken iodopsin with 3-dehydroretinal. A photopigment, named cyanopsin, was generated (Wald, Brown and Smith, 1953).

3. Double cones

(a) Chief member: $P620_2$; here, as in the adult, the visual pigment is like that of the comparable single cone.

(b) Accessory member: $P527_2$; the situation is parallel to that of the adult; biochemically the accessory member is like the single red rod.

4. Green rods: $P438_2$; the green rod pigment of the tadpole is only 6nm displaced from the $P432_1$ of the adult green rods. This contrasts with the 25nm displacement for the red rods and accessory members and the 45nm displacement for the single cones and chief members. The replacement of retinal by 3-dehydroretinal in combination with a specific opsin apparently does not lead to a constant spectral displacement in absorbance but to a shift that is related to the spectral location of the absorbance curve. The chemical meaning of this relation is not known.

These data demonstrated in a convincing manner the metamorphic transition of the visual pigment system in *Rana pipiens* and the fact that all the visual cells participated in this transition. This transition apparently involved a molecular change occurring within each cell while the morphological integrity of the cell was maintained. This was suggested by the finding that in tadpoles at an advanced stage of metamorphosis the red rods contained *both* $P527_2$ and $P502_1$. All rods at this stage yielded the same result suggesting a simultaneous, rather than a sequential, transition. The cones at this stage were not examined so that no information was obtained on the relative rates at which this transition occurred in rods and cones. Finally, LIEBMAN, and ENTINE's results obtained with tadpoles at various stages of development showed no evidence for MUNTZ's idea that rods at an early stage possess a cone pigment that is replaced, as development proceeds by rhodopsin or by intermediate-type photopigments (MUNTZ, 1964a). Replacement occurred, true enough, but only within the context of an A_2 to A_1 transition.

In contrast to the situation for other vertebrates, this relatively tidy state of knowledge about the visual cells and visual pigments of *Rana pipiens* offers to the physiologist one preparation where a minimum of guessing is required in the interpretation of results requiring knowledge of the retinal receptor systems.

III. Introduction to the Phylogenetic Sections

A. The Origin of Vertebrates from Invertebrates

For some 150 years, speculations have been made as to the specific invertebrate line that may have given rise to vertebrates. At various times, insects, annelids, arachnids, nemerteans, and echinoderms have been awarded this honor. The retina and eye offer little help in regard to the problem of vertebrate ancestry. There are some similarities, it is true, between vertebrate visual cells and invertebrate photoreceptors. The association of both groups of receptors with ciliated cells is well recognized. EAKIN (1965) differentiated two categories with respect to the evolution of photoreceptors: (a) the ciliary type derived from a cell with a cilium or flagellum and (b) the rhabdomeric type, thought to be an off-shoot of the ciliary type, which is not associated with a cilium or flagellum. Vertebrates, along with certain specific invertebrates, were classed as having the ciliary type while the remaining invertebrates were assigned to the rhabdomeric classification. The folding of the cell membrane into villi, tubules, lamellae has occurred in the visual cells of many invertebrates and these foldings appear to be functionally comparable to the outer segment rod and cone discs (EAKIN, 1965). The invertebrate visual pigments, insofar as they have been examined, are all based on vitamin A_1. There are differences, however. Nothing like the duplex rod-cone system seems to have developed in invertebrates. Moreover, there appears to be some fundamental difference in the mechanism of excitation by light of vertebrate and invertebrate visual cells, at least in the few cases that have been studied. This difference relates to the fact that the action of light on the invertebrate receptor involves a graded depolarization associated with a conductance increase, whereas on the vertebrate receptors it involves a hyperpolarization accompanied by a decrease in conductance (Toyoda, Nosaki, and Tomita, 1969).

B. Vertebrates and the Deuterostomia

The Deuterostomia designates an assemblage of animals including Echinodermata, Pogonophora, Hemichordata, Protochordata (Urochordata, Cephalochordata) that possesses a number of vertebrate affinities. For this reason the vertebrates are included within this assembly (Barrington, 1965). Though most zoologists probably agree that these affinities indicate evolutionary relationships between the various members of this assemblage, few agree as to the exact nature of these relationships. For those readers who may be interested I give here references to some recently expressed views on this subject: Berrill (1955), Carter (1957), Whitear (1957), Bone (1958). The primary difficulty, as both Berrill (1955) and Bone (1958) indicated, is the absence of fossil evidence to help us reduce the number of possible explanations of chordate ancestry that have been proposed. The finding of the ostracoderm, *Jamoytius kerwoodi*, from the Silurian shale of Lanarkshire, Scotland, aroused great interest because it was considered to be the earliest known fossil in the vertebrate line. Berrill (1955) attached great significance to *Jamoytius*, considering it to be an ancient naked form dating from the Ordovician period, and more primitive than the ostracoderms with which it was contemporary. He assigned to *Jamoytius* a relationship close to the basic chordate stock leading to the gnathostomes. Even *Jamoytius* is controversial, however, and recently Ritchie (1968), on the basis of the lamprey-like branchial apparatus, concluded that *Jamoytius*, instead of having the significance given to it by Berrill, was, in fact, only an anaspid-like ostracoderm on, or near, the line leading to the living cyclostomes.

Do the photoreceptors of living deuterostomes help us in tracing out relationships within this strategic assembly of animals? Little is known about light sensitivity and photoreceptors in the lower deuterostomes but one or two points can be made. Echinoderms, like vertebrates, appear to have photoreceptors of the ciliary type. Eakin (1963) portrayed the photoreceptor in the ocellus of sea stars as a cell with a cilium containing the characteristic fibrillar apparatus and with numerous tubules, which were assumed to contain the photosensitive pigment. No such pigment has been reported for echinoderms but the presence of a simple cornea-negative electrical response to a flash of light was reported for the ocellus of the starfish (Hartline, Wagner, and MacNichol, 1952). The hemichordates (Pterobranchia and Enteropneusta) show clear-cut affinities to the echinoderms, most striking being the tornaria larva of the enteropneust, which was originally mistakenly identified as the larva of an aberrant starfish. Virtually nothing is known about photoreception in hemichordates. Knight-Jones (1952) described a number of cells in the epidermis of the enteropneust, *Saccoglossus cambrensis*, which he interpreted to be sensory in nature. The ability of *Dolichoglossus kowalevskyi* to respond to light was demonstrated by Hess (1938) who believed that this photosensitivity was due to cells in the epidermis comparable to the visual cells of vertebrates. No one seems to have seriously followed up this suggestion and Hess's case was based on little more than a statement that the receptor cells were more numerous and larger in the more photosensitive regions of the animal.

The urochordates and cephalochordates are generally conceded to be so much more advanced toward the vertebrate condition than are hemichordates that they have been assigned a special grouping, along with the vertebrates, in the phylum Chordata. This is the most one can say, however, and the relationships between these two, and between both of them and vertebrates, are far from understood. It would be interesting to determine whether or not the photoreceptors can contribute anything towards the elucidation of these relationships. The urochordates (tunicates) are especially interesting in this regard. Adult tunicates seem to be sensitive to light but, the receptors responsible have not been recognized. For the larval tunicate, however, a relatively simple, but well organized, ocellus has been described (DILLY, 1961, 1964). This ocellus from the larva of *Ciona intestinalis* is situated within the wall of the posterior portion of the cerebral vesicle. Made up of about 10 cells, the structure was described as a lens cell composed of 3 vesicles, a large pigment cell containing numerous pigment granules and 4 to 9 retinal cells each with a process imbedded within the pigment cell. DILLY described the retinal cell as consisting of three parts: a photoreceptor end made up of a pile of membrane discs, a connecting cilium and a cell body. The discs were stated to be 15—20 nm thick and up to 2.5 μm in diameter. The discs made up a segment several micrometres long. Connected to this photoreceptor end, and passing through the pigment cell, was a tubular, membrane-bound portion within which were found some 50—100 filaments each about 15 nm in diameter. These filaments, believed to be solid and unstriated, ran the length of the tubular process but were not observed to extend into the cytoplasm of the cell body. Even though the filament structure was unlike that of the typical cilium, DILLY speculated that the ascidian retinal cell is probably comparable to the vertebrate visual cell. In one respect, however, the photoreceptor cells of *Ciona* differ from vertebrate rods and cones, and that is in the apparent absence of synaptic structures. How these cells communicate their state of excitation to effector cells or to neighboring neurons remains an intriguing problem for the future. Because of the lack of centrioles, the large number of filaments, and the lack of precise organization in pattern of these filaments, EAKIN (1963) initially questioned the homology of the ascidian larval receptor cells with vertebrate visual cells. More recently EAKIN and KUDA (1971) added some valuable information about the structure of the larval ascidian ocellus. Their description established beyond doubt the ciliary character of the tunicate photoreceptor, thus relating it to the vertebrate visual cell. The ocellus was described as consisting of a 3-celled lens, a group of 15—20 sensory cells and a pigmented, cup-shaped supportive cell. Each receptor cell contained (a) an outer segment made up of an aggregation of regularly oriented lamellae with axes parallel to the outer-segment inner-segment axis, (b) an inner segment bearing the basal body of the modified cilium, but, unlike the inner segment of the vertebrate visual cell, lacking the mass of mitochondria, (c) a narrow shaft with many microtubules connecting the inner segment with the soma, and (d) the broader soma containing the nucleus, mitochondria, ribosomes and other organelles. Recently, electrical responses to light were reported to occur in the larval photoreceptors of another tunicate, *Amaroucium constellatum*

(Gorman, McReynolds ,and Barnes, 1971). The responses, thought to be intracellular, were hyperpolarizations of the membrane associated with a conductance decrease, actions similar to those of the vertebrate visual cell. From another tunicate *(Salpa democratica)* hyperpolarizing potentials to light were also recorded, but these were associated with a membrane conductance increase. The *Salpa* photoreceptors were said to be of the microvillous type. Finally, there is the interpretation of Berrill (1955) that the ascidian eye has been lost in evolution and that the vertebrate eye is a new addition.

The photoreceptor cells of the ascidian larva show some apparent similarities to vertebrate visual elements but the same cannot so easily be said of the cephalochordates. There is no good evidence that the anterior pigment spot of amphioxus is photoreceptive, or even sensory in function (Walls, 1942 b). On the other hand, Walls (1942 b) considered the ciliated columnar cells of the misnamed infundibular organ in the floor of the cerebral vesicle of amphioxus to be light-sensitive, and to be the most primitive homologues of the vertebrate visual cells. This statement, of course, was made before Dilly's study of the ocellus of the ascidian larva. Eakin and Westfall (1962) examined the cells of the infundibular organ and reported them to be cilia-like with a string of vesicles at the base of the cilia. The possibility was mentioned that these vesicles contain a photopigment but I know of no experiments intending to test this possibility and, in fact, there is no compelling reason to believe that this organ is sensitive to light. In fact, there are reasons for believing that the cells of the infundibular organ have a secretory function (Barrington, 1965). Except for the ascidian larva, therefore, we seem to be left with the theory mentioned by Walls (1942 b), and ascribed to Froriep, that the vertebrate eye evolved suddenly like "the birth of Athena, full-grown and fully armed, from the brow of Zeus". Fortunately, I believe, the ascidian larva spares us from this implausible theory.

C. The Vertebrates

Whatever the origin of the vertebrate eye, it seems clear that the duplex retina evolved early in vertebrate evolution and has been retained in its basic form throughout the millions of years of this evolution. During these millions of years vertebrates have become adapted to a variety of environments, and the eye and retina faithfully reflect these adaptations. In the sections that follow I propose to describe some of these adaptations insofar as the visual cells and visual pigments are concerned. To assist the reader in this account I have prepared a palaeontological time chart (Fig. 3), which illustrates some of the ideas of vertebrate phylogeny.

Ancestral chordates are assumed to have been part of the fauna of the Cambrian period but because of the absence of hard parts, no fossil remains exist of these forms. Primitive Agnatha (jawless vertebrates) apparently appeared some time during the Ordovician and led eventually to the heavily armored ostracoderm agnathans of the Silurian and Devonian. Some writers have expressed the view that the earliest agnathans were naked, and consequently not represented in the fossil record (Berrill, 1955). One group of ostracoderms, now extinct, was the Heterostraci, believed to have been active forms with eyes placed laterally on the head. According to some palaeontologists, modern hagfishes have evolved

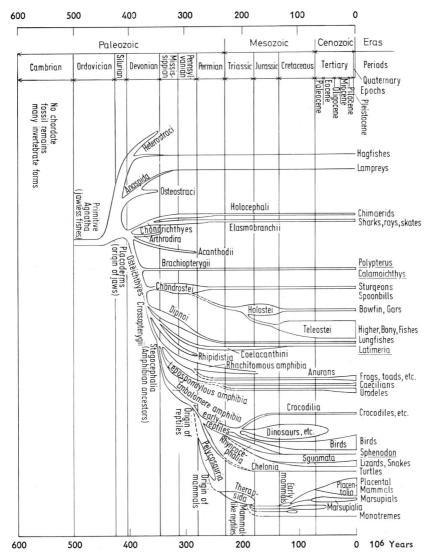

Fig. 3. Palaeontological chart illustrating modern views on vertebrate phylogeny

from them. An important line of ostracoderms was the Anaspida, fish-like forms with a light dermal armor composed of small plates of bony tissue, aspidine. The Osteostraci probably originated from the Anaspida. Modern cyclostomes are believed to have evolved either from the Osteostraci or directly from the Anaspida.

The next great step in vertebrate evolution was the origin of jaws and the rise of the gnathostomes, with the consequent change in food to nektonic organisms. The most primitive of these gnathostomes, the placoderms, formed the ancestral stock for several lines, among which were the Arthrodira and the Acanthodii. The Arthrodira line appears to be related to the ancestors of the existing cartilaginous fishes, the Holocephali and the Elasmobranchii. The higher bony fishes were probably derived from a primitive stock close to the Acanthodii. This stock of Osteichthyes appeared in the Devonian period during which it diverged into several lines. Some retained many primitive features and these features are preserved in living forms like Polypterus and Calamoichthys whose exact taxonomic position is still a matter of doubt. Another osteichthyan development was the evolution of the Chondrostei, which persist today as the sturgeons and spoonbills. Late in the Permian period there appeared a different line of fishes, the Holostei, which were so successful that they became the dominant aquatic vertebrate fauna of the Triassic and Jurassic periods. Their numbers decreased throughout the Cretaceous period and they were replaced by their descendants, the teleosts, which are the dominant fishes today. Holostei are now represented by living remnants, the bow-fin and gars. The very significant line of crossopterygian fishes arose in the Devonian period. The lung-fishes (Dipnoi) probably branched off earlier. They evolved rapidly for the first 100 million years and then slowed down until today there are only three genera of living Dipnoi. The primitive character of lung-fishes is suggested by the presence, in living forms, of a permanent notochord. The Coelacanthini, another crossopterygian line, were common throughout most of the Mesozoic era but died out except for one living representative. Some palaeontologists have suggested that the Rhipidistia, not now represented by living forms, may have been close to the ancestral stock that gave rise to the Amphibia and the tetrapod condition.

The amphibian ancestry dates back to the late Devonian period with the first appearance of the Stegocephalia. These early tetrapods, which were quite different from modern amphibia, possessed a number of crossopterygian-like features. A number of stegocephalian lines evolved during the Paleozoic era and these included both aquatic and terrestrial forms. Most of these died out by the early Mesozoic era. The origin of modern amphibians from these stegocephalian forms is somewhat uncertain although it is believed that the different lines of living amphibia arose in various ways. Anurans are considered to have arisen from small rhachitomous Stegocephalia during the Permian or lower Triassic. In the lower Carboniferous (Mississippian) there occurred a group of palaeontologically enigmatic lepospondylous Stegocephalia which may have been the ancestral stock, perhaps by separate branches, for the modern Apoda (caecilians) and Urodela.

During the Carboniferous period there existed a stegocephalian group of amphibia, the Embolomeri, which may have been close to the ancestral stock that evolved the seymourians, believed by some to have been the first reptile-like amphibians. From these, or similar cotylosaurian forms arose, not only modern reptiles, but many extinct reptiles, too numerous to mention here. The rise of the active, predacious reptiles probably was the cause of the end for the stegocephalian amphibia. The ancestors of modern amphibia probably peristed because they were small, secretive, or nocturnal forms, or else lived where reptiles could not survive.

Modern birds have a number of characteristics that reveal their reptilian origin. Already in the Triassic period evidence has been found of lizards that employed their hind legs in running, the forelegs being significantly shortened. First evidence of true birds appeared in the Jurassic period, as is indicated by the presence of feathers in *Archaeopteryx*. The further evolution of birds is not well known but in the Cretaceous period, apparently, birds comparable to modern birds appeared, i.e., birds without teeth.

Mammals appear to have had a reptilian origin dating back to the late Carboniferous and early Permian periods. These carnivorous reptiles, the Pelycosauria, were replaced by their descendants, the Therapsida, quadruped forms that evolved into the herbivorous dicynodonts and the carnivorous theriodonts. The theriodonts evolved into several lines of mammal-like reptiles during the Triassic period but by the end of the Triassic they had almost entirely disappeared. All these synapsid reptiles occurred before the early Jurassic, some 170 million years ago. For the next 90 million years mammal-like animals were present as small, insectivorous forms, some of which gave rise to the modern mammals. Monotremes may have evolved from the Mesozoic Docodonta; monotremes still show some of the primitive features of these Mesozoic forms. The origin of the Marsupialia is in doubt although they probably had a common origin with the placental mammals, and evolved in a parallel manner in the Australasian region.

With this sketch of some 500—600 million years of zoological history, I can now proceed to the account of vertebrate visual cells and visual pigments.

IV. The Cyclostomes

Cyclostomes are ancient vertebrates belonging to the subphylum Agnatha and related to the extinct ostracoderms of the Silurian and Devonian periods. One idea (SCHMALHAUSEN, 1968) is that the cyclostomes arose directly from a primitive group of ostracoderms, the Anaspida, which are conceived as being free-swimming, fish-like Agnatha with a light dermal armour made up of plates of bony tissue (aspidine). The living cyclostomes comprise two subclasses: the hagfishes (Myxini) and the lampreys (Petromyzones). The relation of these two subclasses has been the subject of some dispute, STENSIÖ suggesting a diphyletic origin for these two, and others believing in a more common origin for hagfishes and lampreys (see SCHMALHAUSEN, 1968). Recently, some illumination of this problem was obtained by the discovery of six fossil impressions in the Pennsylvanian shale deposits of northeastern Illinois (U.S.A.) that were quite clearly of an extinct lamprey, which was assigned the name *Mayomyzon pieckoensis*. *Mayomyzon* had many basic similarities to living lampreys but no resemblances to living hagfishes. The evidence suggested to the discoverers of this interesting fossil (BARDACK and ZANGERL, 1968) that hagfishes and lampreys probably arose from separate phyletic lines at least before the Pennsylvanian. The hagfishes, fundamentally marine and parasitic, have eyes in various stages of degeneracy (WALLS, 1942b; ROCHON-DUVIGNEAUD, 1943; DUKE-ELDER, 1958). In some hagfishes, apparently, functional eyes are present. KOBAYASHI (1964) described the rudimentary eye of *Myxine garmani* beneath the skin of the head as containing a colorless lens, a vitreous body, a layered retina and definite visual cells. Apparently, the neuronal layers of the retina were not differentiated to the degree of the typical vertebrate eye. From the prolongation of the reaction time to light that occurred after removal of the eyes, KOBAYASHI concluded that the eyes were photosensitive and that conduction of optic nerve impulses to the central nervous system occurred in this hagfish. The idea of functional eyes was supported by the recording of electro-retinograms, made up of a- and b-waves, from the isolated eyes of the hagfish. The electrical responses were employed to obtain a spectral sensitivity curve, which showed a peak at about 500 nm for both the dark- and light-adapted state. Another hagfish, *Myxine glutinosa* was shown to have eyes without lens, without vitreous body and with a poorly differentiated retina (Holmberg, 1970). While the visual receptors were found to lack the characteristic outer-segment-inner-segment structure of the vertebrate photoreceptor, electron microscopy revealed the presence of bodies containing parallel arrays of membranes some of which consisted of discs closed at both ends, like rods. In addition, the receptors possessed a connecting piece with 9 microtubule pairs and a basal body, all features of the ciliate type photoreceptor. This species of hagfish was studied by Newth and Ross (1955) who concluded, by observing the light-induced motor activity, that skin receptors mediated this activity and that destruction of the eyes did not abolish it.

Lampreys, in one order and one family of 8 genera (5 of which are found throughout the N. hemisphere) have well-developed eyes and visual cells bearing photopigments. Ecologically, lampreys show considerable diversity (Gage, 1928). Some, like the brook lampreys, remain throughout life in fresh water, spawning in tributaries upstream, growing and metamorphosing in the stream system, and then migrating upstream to spawn at sexual maturity. The brook lamprey has no parasitic phase but lives in a non-feeding phase until maturity. An example is the Michigan brook lamprey, *Ichthyomyzon fossor*. Another strictly freshwater group consists of the lake lampreys which spawn in tributaries to the lake, grow, metamorphose to young adults after which they swim to the lake where they parasitize fishes, and then return to the stream, as sexually mature adults, to spawn and then to die. The silver lamprey, *Ichthyomyzon unicuspis*, of the Great Lakes (U.S.A.) is an example. Somewhat similar to the lake lampreys are the river lampreys, such as *Ichthyomyzon castaneous* of the Mississippi basin. These spend the parasitic, feeding phase of their adult life in large rivers and return to spawn in tributary creeks. A different ecological grouping is seen in the marine lampreys. In these the fertilized eggs develop on the sandy or gravelly bottom of freshwater streams far from the sea. The young larvae, ammocoetes as they are called, live in the mud and are plankton feeders for 4 to 5 years. They metamorphose to young adults and then migrate to the sea where they parasitize fishes, often going to depths of 500 meters or more (Nicol'skii, 1961). During this period of ingesting blood and tissues of the host fishes they grow rapidly. Eventually, they stop feeding, migrate back into fresh water, mature sexually, and then after a long journey to the spawning grounds far inland, deposit and fertilize the eggs and then, apparently, die. Examples of marine lampreys are the European *Lampetra fluviatilis*, and the Pacific form, *Entosphenus tridentatus*. The common marine lamprey of the North Atlantic, *Petromyzon marinus*, is especially interesting here because in North America this species is found in three distinct ecological populations which I shall refer to as the sea-run (SR), the Finger Lakes (FL) and the Great Lakes (GL) populations. SR is the normal marine form which spawns in freshwater streams and then migrates to the sea. The FL population is a landlocked lamprey probably derived from SR originally but separated from its parent stock since the Pleistocene. The GL population probably originated from SR lampreys that entered Lake Ontario and its tributaries, but it was not until after the Welland Canal between Lake Ontario and Lake Erie was opened in 1829 that access to the upper Lakes was possible for these lampreys. In 1921 the first specimen of *Petromyzon marinus* was recovered from Lake Erie, and in the next 17 to 20 years the lamprey spread throughout the whole of Lakes Erie, Huron, Superior and Michigan.

1. The Visual Cells of Lampreys

Because cyclostomes are living representatives of an ancient vertebrate stock the visual cells of lampreys are of special significance. Unfortunately, however, the nature of the lamprey visual receptors has been a matter of disagreement in the literature for almost 100 years. Some of the earlier literature was unavailable to me and for this I have had to rely on a review by WALLS (1935). In 1856 MÜLLER noted the retina of *Lampetra fluviatilis* to contain long and short visual cells in approximately equal numbers. He called them cones but later, after examining the retina of *Petromyzon marinus*, MÜLLER concluded that the short elements might be rods (cited by WALLS, 1935). SCHULTZE, too, went through a period of uncertainty regarding the nature of the lamprey receptors but eventually he settled on the conclusion that *Lampetra fluviatilis* had a pure-rod retina (SCHULTZE, 1867). This conclusion, along with his belief that sharks and rays also had only rods, led him to the generalization that rods were the simpler receptors, functionally, and the older receptors, phylogenetically, and that cones were evolved gradually from rods (SCHULTZE, 1867; 1873). In 1873 LANGERHANS studied the retina of *Lampetra planeri* and described the long cells as rods and the short cells as cones (cited by KRAUSE, 1876), a view adopted by KRAUSE (1876) in his later work. As WALLS (1935) explained, uncertainty and disagreement continued, with some investigators confirming the presence of rods, others supporting the idea of an all-cone retina and still others suggesting that the visual cells were neither rods nor cones but undifferentiated elements. In a later paper FRANZ (1932) resurrected SCHULTZE's notion of an all-rod retina for *Lampetra fluviatilis*, showing cylindrical forms for all outer segments and explaining the staggered arrangement of visual cells on the basis of an accommodation for the interference of adjacent bulky ellipsoids. WALLS (1935) was critical of much of this early work claiming that the use of improper fixatives might have resulted in the production of artifactual outer segment shapes. Using special fixatives, WALLS made preparations from eight species and, like MÜLLER, concluded that the lamprey retina was typically duplex, the long cells being identified as cones and the short cells as rods. WALLS based his conclusion on outer segment shapes, on the presence of rhodopsin, which he observed visually, on the extent of summation, and on certain ecological characteristics of lampreys. Disagreeing with FRANZ (1932), WALLS suggested that lampreys are not strictly nocturnal animals and that, indeed, the possession of a yellowish lens suggested a diurnal mode of life. Reading all this vague literature, I am forced to the admission that in the case of lampreys the designations rods and cones are neither very appropriate, nor very easy to apply (Fig. 4A). The situation emphasizes the difficulties, which

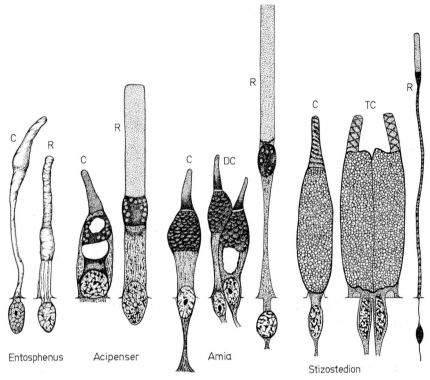

Fig. 4a

Fig. 4a and 4b. Visual cells of selected vertebrates to illustrate phylogenetic relationships and other properties of vertebrate visual receptors. a) Cone and rod of lamprey (*Entosphenus tridentatus*); cone and rod of sturgeon (*Acipenser fulvescens*), the oil-droplet is colorless; single cone, double cone and rod of bowfin (*Amia calva*); single cone, twin cone and rod of teleost (*Stizostedion vitreum*). These drawings are taken from Walls (1935, 1942a). b) Visual cells of selected reptiles. *Sphenodon punctatum:* 1. from nasal periphery, 2. from central fovea. Cells of periphery include large single rod, small single rod and double rod. These rods are enigmatic and are called cones by some writers. The small single cone is very rare and is absent from the fovea. *Alligator mississippiensis:* 1. from ventral periphery, 2. from tapetal region. In the ventral retina one sees a single cone, a double cone and a single rod. From the tapetal region, according to Walls, one sees evidence of partial transmutation to rods. *Aristelliger praesignis:* this illustrates the typical gecko visual cells, i.e., single (type A), double (type B) and double (type C). In this case the cells may be called rods on the basis of the outer segments but colorless oil-droplets are present in the cells shown with circles in the ellipsoid regions. *Chelydra serpentina:* standard single cone, small single cone, double cone and rod. Colored oil-droplets in cones but not in rod, the rod has a paraboloid. *Anolis lineatopus:* single cone (A_1) with yellow oil-droplet, smaller single cone (A_2) with colorless oil-droplet and double cone (B) with yellow oil-droplet in the chief member. Note that the chief member is the smaller of the two members. A few triple cones are present but are not shown here. *Lialis burtonis*, a crepuscular pygopodid: types A_1 and A_2 singles and type B double are shown. No type C double is present. The quadriplex snake pattern (VII) from *Vipera berus:* type A single cone, type B double cone, type C small cone and the single rod (type D of Underwood or type C′ of Walls). Note the ophidian paranuclear body in the accessory member of the type B double cone. Also note, that unlike *Anolis*, the chief member is the large member. Information for making this figure was obtained from the many drawings and descriptions of reptilian visual cells given by Underwood and Walls as given in the text. Vertical scale lines are 20 μm

several investigators have admitted to, in sometimes distinguishing rods and cones on the basis of light microscopy (ROZEMEYER and STOLTE, 1931). Neither the techniques of electron microscopy nor of physiology have been yet applied to the lamprey visual system.

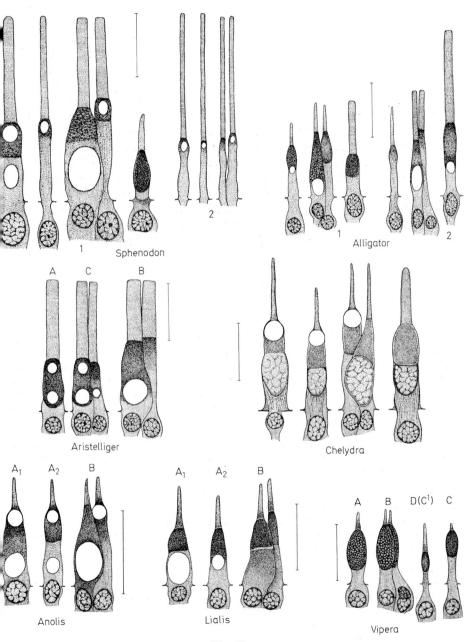

Fig. 4b

2. The Visual Pigments of Lampreys

If there is doubt about the nature of the lamprey visual cells there is no such uncertainty about the visual pigments that have been extracted from the lamprey retina. These ancestral vertebrates possess *both* the retinal and 3-dehydroretinal pigment systems.

KÜHNE (1878) described the pigment in the fresh retina of *Lampetra fluviatilis* as of a bluish-violet hue. From observations of the retinas of *Petromyzon marinus* WALLS (1935), however, believed the pigment to be purple in color and to be present in the short cells. The possession of rhodopsin was one characteristic that WALLS associated with rods. The retinal vitamin A content of upstream migrants from the SR population of *Petromyzon marinus* was analyzed by WALD (1942 a) who found both A vitamins in a ratio, A_2/A_1, of 89/11 in the bleached retinas. No extracts of the visual pigment were prepared but on the basis of the vitamin A composition and the unusual colors reported for the lamprey retinas by KÜHNE and by WALLS, the suggestion was made that porphyropsin, the 3-dehydroretinal pigment, was the dominant pigment of the lamprey retina. Integrating this information with previous findings on teleost visual pigments, WALD (1942 b) reached two conclusions: (i) the A_2-system is associated genetically with the freshwater spawning environment and (ii) porphyropsin is the ancestral pigment of vertebrates. The first direct analysis of cyclostome visual pigments was made by CRESCITELLI (1956a) who worked on (a) downstream migrants of the GL population of *Petromyzon marinus* and (b) upstream and downstream migrants of the Pacific lamprey, *Entosphenus tridentatus*. Using the technique of partial bleaching, CRESCITELLI obtained evidence in both lampreys, not of porphyropsin, but of a single vitamin A_1-based photopigment, a typical rhodopsin (Fig. 5). This result was especially interesting for it demonstrated the presence of a rhodopsin in lampreys going upstream to spawn, and also going downstream to Lake Michigan and to the sea for the adult feeding phase of life. At the time this appeared to contradict WALD's suggestion of the presence of porphyropsin but actually it was not applicable to WALD's conclusion since WALD used only upstream migrants, and not of *Entosphenus*, but of *Petromyzon*. Later, WALD (1957) reopened this problem, first confirming CRESCITELLI's finding of rhodopsin in downstream migrants of the GL population of *Petromyzon*. He then returned to his original animals, upstream migrants of the SR population of *Petromyzon*, and found in these a P 518_2 which he called porphyropsin. This finding confirmed his original deduction based on vitamin A analysis. Lumping together the results from the SR and GL populations, WALD concluded that the sea lamprey possessed a metamorphic transition of visual pigments with rhodopsin and porphyropsin associated with downstream and upstream migrations, respectively. CRESCITELLI's finding of rhodopsin did not deter WALD from expressing the view that the porphyropsin system was the ancestral vertebrate visual system for, as he stated, the change to porphyropsin "is part of the second metamorphosis, marking the return to the original environment." I am reluctant to accept this interpretation for it ignores the contrary findings with *Entosphenus tridentatus*. In this sea lamprey, rhodopsin was found in animals going upstream to spawn, as well as in downstream migrants on their way to the sea (Fig. 5). Using WALD's argument based on a second metamorphosis, rhodopsin becomes the ancestral visual pigment. WALD also supported his thesis that porphyropsin represents the ancestral vertebrate visual system by citing the views of SMITH (1932) and ROMER and GROVE (1935) that vertebrates originated in freshwater. The freshwater origin of early vertebrates is not accepted by all paleontologists, and DENISON (1956), who made a thorough analysis of this question, rejected this view. He concluded that known Ordovician vertebrates were near-shore, marine forms. In the Silurian, furthermore, certain

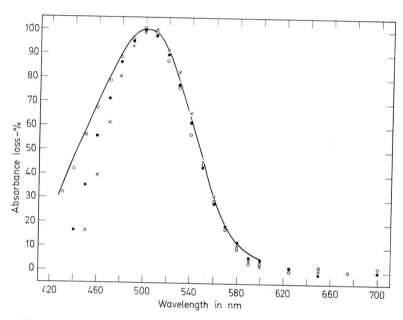

Fig. 5. Normalized difference spectra (density loss) for 3 lamprey extracts. *Plain circles*: recently transformed downstream migrants of *E. tridentatus*, taken from Minter Creek, Washington State, USA. *Filled circles*: upstream migrants of *E. tridentatus*, taken from Columbia River basin, Oregon, USA. *Crosses*: land-locked downstream migrants of Great Lakes population of *P. marinus*, taken from Carp Lake River, Michigan, USA. *Full line*: curve based on the DARTNALL nomogram for an A_1-pigment with maximum at 501 nm. The data for downstream migrants of *E. tridentatus* (*plain circles*) were obtained with an extract to which had been added NH_2OH, which explains the better accord of these data at shorter wavelengths with the DARTNALL nomogram. A classical rhodopsin was found in all 3 lampreys

forms (Cyathaspinae, Euphanerida, Acanthodii, and certain Coelolepida) were considered to be marine while the Osteostraci and Anaspida became established in brackish and fresh waters. Accordingly, cyclostomes may have had a fresh-water history since the Silurian, but before that in the Ordovician a marine ancestry is indicated by DENISON's study.

It is quite clear that the lamprey story is an unfinished one. An examination of brook, river, lake and sea lampreys needs to be made, and care should be taken to compare the upstream and downstream migrants of the same species and the same ecological population.

V. The Chondrichthyes — Cartilaginous Fishes

A. The Elasmobranchs

Sharks, dogfishes, skates and rays are cartilaginous fishes, which are believed to be descendants of Devonian forms that evolved from placoderm-like ancestors. The cartilaginous skeleton is not primitive but probably derived secondarily since the jawed ancestors of elasmobranchs possessed bony plates. There are at present some 150 to 200 species of living elasmobranchs. These are mainly marine forms, living in the sea from the shallow coastal zone to great depths, *Raja abyssicola* being found at about 3,000 meters in the Bay of Bengal according to Nikol'-skii (1961). A few species inhabit large rivers in the tropical and subtropical zones.

1. Visual Cells

Though rods predominate, cones are not always absent, as Schultze (1873) believed, and cones that are present may not be unimportant in the retinal responses to light. Krause (1889) reported the presence of cones, along with rods, and even described double cells, which he thought were like reptilian double cells except for the absence of oil-droplets. He also suggested that the accessory member of these double cells was like the amphibian green rod. These latter observations have never been confirmed, and neither double cells, nor green rods, are believed to be present in the elasmobranch retina. A recent study of the Lemon Shark *(Negaprion brevirostris)* presented unmistakable evidence for the occurrence of cones (Gruber, Hamasaki, and Bridges, 1963). The cones were characterized by the presence of short, tapering outer segments; pyramidal inner segments containing both ellipsoids and paraboloids; and with nuclei that were similar to the rod nuclei. At the posterior pole the ratio of rods to cones was 12:1. The visual cells were all free of oil-droplets. Similar cones were seen in *Negaprion* and in three other species of sharks. The ERG in these sharks was shown to be markedly different according to the state of adaptation. For the light-adapted eye the ERG consisted of a typically cornea-negative PIII response with a prominent, positive off-effect; for the fully dark-adapted eye the ERG consisted of a- and b-waves but with no off-response (Hamasaki and Bridges, 1965). Unlike lampreys, there seems to be less difficulty in distinguishing rods and cones in the elasmobranch retina, even though some of the characteristics of the cones of higher forms, such as oil-droplets and double cells, are missing. The retinas of some elasmobranchs lack cones, and Dowling and Ripps (1970) made use of this by studying the course of dark adaptation in *Raja erinacea* and *Raja ocellata*, two skates whose retinas were considered to be of the all-rod classification. After demonstrating that the b-wave and the single ganglion cell discharge behaved in a kinetically similar fashion during dark adaptation, Dowling and Ripps established the point that during the slow dark adaptation, following an initial rapid period of recovery, the rhodopsin regeneration was such as to indicate a relation in which rhodopsin concentration was a function of log threshold. Such a relation had already been noted for the eyes of humans and of the rat.

2. Visual Pigments

In his original discovery BOLL (1876) mentioned seeing Sehrot in the retinas of elasmobranchs, and KRAUSE (1889) saw Sehpurpur in the rod outer segments of a ray. The first study of retinal extracts was made by BAYLISS, LYTHGOE, and TANSLEY, (1936) who placed the absorbance maxima for the pigments of the dog-

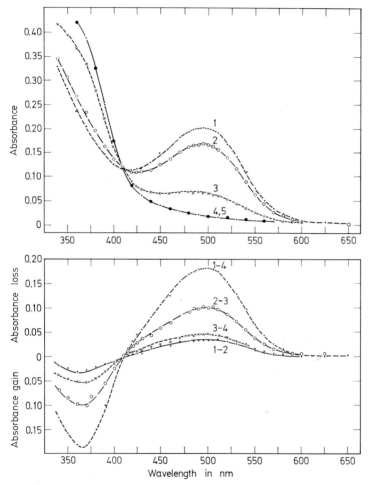

Fig. 6. Elasmobranch rhodopsin. Retinal extract of shovel-nosed guitarfish (*R. productus*). Analysis carried out in presence of added NH_2OH. *Upper frame*: bleaching sequence showing absorbance of unbleached extract (*1*); after exposure to light at 650 nm from a monochromator (*2*); after exposure to light at 645 nm (*3*), after exposure to light at 600 nm (*4*). Completion of bleaching and absence of any other photopigment is shown by lack of effect of an exposure to light at 500 nm (*5, filled circles*). Lower frame: difference spectra derived from this bleaching sequence. First bleach (*1—2*), second bleach (*2—3*), third bleach (*3—4*), and total of all bleachings (*1—4*). The results indicate the photic removal of a single pigment with maximum at 497 nm and the formation of a product at 366 nm, i.e., retinal oxime. A similar result was obtained with an extract of the retinas of the gray smooth hound shark (*M. californicus*). This figure serves to illustrate the technique of partial bleaching as applied to the analysis of visual pigments in extracts

fish, *Scyllium canicula*, and the ray, *Raia clavata*, at 505 and 510 nm, respectively Their method of determining the spectral absorbance by measuring the differences in optical density between bleached and unbleached samples of the extract is not always reliable because of the color of the bleached solution. Consequently, their data cannot be accepted without reservation. Wald (1939) next showed that light-exposed, completely faded retinas of the smooth dogfish *(Galeorhinus laevis)* contained vitamin A_1 and that the extracted photopigment of the spiny dogfish *(Squalus acanthias)* had a spectral absorbance typical of rhodopsin. The photo- pigment *in situ* was studied in *Squalus acanthias* and *Scyliorhinus canicula* by Denton and Nicol (1964) who placed the absorbance maximum at about 500 nm Recently, I had occasion to prepare extracts of the retinas of the gray smooth houndshark *(Mustelus californicus)* and of the shovel-nosed guitarfish *(Rhinobatus productus)*. The extracts were analyzed by the method of partial bleaching, and only one photopigment was present in each extract. The prosthetic group was identified from the oxime formed after bleaching the extract in the presence of hydroxylamine. For both species the visual pigment was found to be a typical rhodopsin, a $P497_1$ (Fig. 6). This result confirms precisely the results of Beatty (1969a) with *Squalus suckleyi* and *Raja binoculata*.

It must not be concluded that there is no diversity in spectral absorbance for the elasmobranch pigments obtained by the method of extraction. Deep-sea elas- mobranchs appear to have developed pigments absorbing at shorter wavelengths This was demonstrated by Denton and Shaw (1963), for the sharks, *Centroscymnus coelolepis*, *Centrophorus squamosus* and *Deania calcea*. These were caught at night from a depth of about 1150 meters. The retinas which looked neither red nor purple but golden, were extracted with digitonin and analyzed spectrophotometrically Neither partial bleaching, to test the homogeneity of the extracts, nor chemical identification of the prosthetic group was carried out, but the results, as far as they go, suggest the presence of photopigments, not at about 500 nm, the posi- tion of rhodopsin, but at significantly shorter wavelengths, i.e., 472 and 484 nm This result is of more than passing interest for it confirms in elasmobranchs what we had learned earlier in teleosts, i.e., that the deep-sea habit is associated with the evolution of retinal pigment absorbing at shorter wavelengths than rhodopsin the pigment of surface-inhabiting teleosts and elasmobranchs. A remarkable example of parallel evolution in dissimilar groups is indicated. I shall return to this deep-sea photopigment system later in this chapter.

B. The Holocephali

The shark-like chimaerid fishes (order Chimaeriformes) are believed to have arisen from early elasmobranchs. These fishes are of some interest here because some of them go to great depths in the sea. *Chimaera monstrosa*, for example, has been reported as going down to 1800 meters (Dean, 1906). Denton and Nicol (1964) measured the spectral absorbance of the visual pigment *in situ* for *Hydro- lagus affinis*. They established the fact that the maximum was at 477 nm, another example, apparently, of the deep-sea type of pigment. Following this report, the retinal photopigments of two other chimaerid species were examined by the method of extraction. In *Hydrolagus colliei* (Beatty, 1969a; Crescitelli, 1969) a single photopigment, P484$_1$, was found; in *Callorhynchus callorhynchus* (McFARLAND, 1970) another single pigment, P499$_1$, was identified. In these three species — the deep sea form, *Hydrolagus affinis*, the vertical migrator, *Hydrolagus colliei*, which has been caught at moderate depths as well as near the surface, and the shallow water form, *Callorhynchus* — three different spectral locations (477, 484, and 499 nm) have been noted for the respective visual pigments obtained by extraction. A correlation between habitat depth and spectral location of the visual pigment thus appears in these three chimaerid fishes.

VI. The Osteichthyes — Bony Fishes

Evidence of Osteichthyes is found in early Devonian deposits. These early fishes had a number of similarities to the Acanthodii which are the oldest forms known of jawed vertebrates. The early Osteichthyes evolved into a number of forms two of which have living representatives today. These are the Dipnoi and the Crossopterygii. One line of Crossopterygians now extinct, the Rhipidistia, is believed to have led to the evolution of the amphibia.

A. The Dipnoi — Lungfishes

Living lungfishes consist of three genera found separately in Australia, South America and Africa. They are all freshwater fishes that are able to obtain oxygen either by means of gills or by means of the highly vascularized, physostomous swim bladder acting as a lung. The Dipnoi are believed to have arisen in the Lower Devonian from an ancestor common both to the lungfishes and the Crossopterygii.

The visual cells of lungfishes are of biological interest because they reveal features not seen in the retinas of cyclostomes and elasmobranchs. Double cones are present as well as oil-droplets in *both* rods and cones. SCHIEFFERDECKER (1886) reported the presence in *Neoceratodus* and *Protopterus* of single rods and single cones. Oil-droplets were reported to occur in the cones. KERR (1903) studied the development of visual cells in *Lepidosiren* and saw the large oil-droplet in the inner segments. According to KERR only rods were present and he considered SCHIEFFERDECKER's cones to be young rods that had not yet developed their mature form. Apparently, KERR subscribed to the BERNARD-CAMERON concept of the ontogenetic origin of rods. According to MUNK (1969), however, the visual cells of *Lepidosiren paradoxa* should be classified as cones. WALLS (1942a) pictured the *Protopterus* visual cells as consisting of (a) single, droplet-bearing cones; (b) double cones with only one member having an oil-droplet; and (c) rods with large, cylindrical outer segments, oil-droplets and paraboloids. The rod nucleus was described as like that of the cones. The cone-like features of the *Protopterus* rods led WALLS to speculate on the phylogenetic derivation of such rods from cones.

Nothing is known, unfortunately, about the visual pigments of the lungfish although the droplet-bearing rods offer an interesting challenge. WALD (1942b) mentioned a preliminary examination of a single specimen of *Protopterus* that suggested to him the possession by this lungfish of a porphyropsin system. He interpreted this to mean that the freshwater habitat had once again determined the nature of the visual pigment. WALD assumed that the lungfish has a long freshwater ancestry back to earliest vertebrate forms. On the other hand, Denison (1956) pointed to fossil remains from the Early Devonian that suggested a marine origin for the Dipnoi although he admitted that later Dipnoi from the Middle and Late Devonian occupied a freshwater habitat.

B. The Crossopterygii — Lobe-Fin Fishes

Although the Dipnoi have characteristics in common with Amphibia, it is generally agreed that they were not the forms that eventually led to the tetrapod vertebrates. This honor has been conferred on the Crossopterygii, a primitive group of fishes that appear to be linked to the oldest Dipnoi, on the one hand, and, through many transitions, to the original terrestrial vertebrates, on the other. Fossil remains of Crossopterygii from the Devonian belong to two separate lines: the Rhipidistia and the Coelacanthini. The Rhipidistia, which are considered to have given rise to the early Amphibia, became extinct before the termination of the Paleozoic. The Coelacanthini flourished, but by the late Mesozoic almost vanished and at one time it was believed they had so disappeared. In 1938, however, a coelacanth was captured in a trawl at a depth of 80 meters off the east coast of South Africa. This living relic of the past was named *Latimeria chalumnae*. In 1952 a second specimen was caught off the coast of the Comoro Archipelago in the Indian Ocean, and by now some 35 or so of these living crossopterygians have been captured. The retina of *Latimeria* was examined in a preliminary way by Millot and Carasso, (1955) who reported the presence in it of numerous long and thin rods and some cones with colorless oil-droplets. There is no report yet on the nature of the photopigment or of the vitamin A of the *Latimeria* retina.

C. The Brachiopterygii (Polypteri)

There are two genera of living fishes formerly classed with the Crossopterygii but now placed in the superorder Brachiopterygii or Polypteri (Nikol'skii, 1961). In some characters these fishes show relationships to the Dipnoi. The two genera consist of *Polypterus*, having several species, and *Calamoichthys*, with a single species, *calabaricus*. The species of Polypterus are rather large fishes inhabiting the rivers and lakes of Africa. *Calamoichthys* is an anguilla-shaped fish living in the delta of the Niger. The retina of *Polypterus congicus* was pictured by Rochon-Duvigneaud (1943) as duplex with bulky rods resembling those of urodeles and salamanders. In contrast, the visual cells of *Calamoichthys* were pictured as all cones. Munk's description of the retina of *Calamoichthys calabaricus* differed from that of Rochon-Duvigneaud, however, in suggesting the presence of single cones, double cones and rods (Munk, 1964). An oil droplet was said to be present in both single cones as well as in the principal members of the double cones. Nothing is known about the visual pigments of these fishes whose systematic position is still debatable and whose ancestry dates back to the Middle Devonian.

D. The Chondrostei — Spoonbills and Sturgeons

These fishes, whose ancestral bony skeleton has been largely lost and replaced by cartilage, include two living families; the sturgeons and the spoonbills. The visual cells of some sturgeons have been studied and LEYDIG (1853) reported the presence of rods with oil-droplets but WALLS (1942b) listed only single rods without oil-droplets, and single cones with colorless oil-droplets in the retina of *Acipenser fulvescens* (see Fig. 4a). The paddlefish *(Polyodon spathula)* apparently has a similar complement of visual cells (MUNK, 1969).

I know of no publications on the retinal photopigments of these fishes although such studies would be of interest in the light of the ecology of this group. Spoonbills are freshwater inhabitants but many sturgeons are migratory and anadromous. Like the sea lamprey they travel long distances upstream to spawn but, unlike the lamprey, they return to the sea after spawning. During their lifetime, which may be very long for some sturgeons (the beluga may live more than 100 years according to NIKOL'SKII, 1961) they make this round trip many times. What happens to the visual pigment in these periodic journeys ? Does it remain constant or does it shuttle back and forth between a porphyropsin and a rhodopsin ? It would be interesting to know.

E. The Holostei — The Bowfin and Gars

These fishes, closely related to the teleosts, appeared first in the Permian, flourished in the Jurassic, began to decline in the Cretaceous, and are represented now only by the bowfin *(Amia calva)* and several species of gars. The bowfin and gars are all North American freshwater inhabitants. WALLS (1942a) pictured the visual cells of *Amia* as consisting of single cones without oil-droplets, and double cones without oil-droplets but with a paraboloid in each accessory member (Fig. 4a). In addition he showed single rods that, as in many teleosts, possessed extensible myoids. The holostean visual cells were also studied by MUNK (1968) whose description agreed with that of WALLS except for the detail that every visual cell type possesses a paraboloid. The visual pigments of two holosteans, *Amia calva* and *Lepisosteus platyrhincus* (the Florida spotted gar) were studied by BRIDGES (1964a) who found two pigments, P 525_2 and P 523_2, respectively, in retinal extracts, thus conforming to WALD's association of A_2-based pigment with the freshwater habit.

F. The Teleostei

About 95% of all living fishes are members of the superorder Teleostei or higher bony fishes. Arising from holostean stock in the Triassic, evolving widely during the Cretaceous, these fishes virtually established themselves to their present status by the Eocene. At present there are over twenty thousand species of teleosts so that any statements about the visual pigment situation in these fishes must be tempered by the fact that only a minuscule sample has been studied. From this sample, however, it appears that ecology, rather than taxonomy, is associated with the nature of the visual pigments in the teleosts. For this reason I will follow an ecological organization in presenting the information on their retinal photopigments.

Of all the vertebrate groups that have been examined none shows such a multiplicity and diversity of photopigments as does the teleost group. This may be associated with the fact that the higher bony fishes inhabit a variety of environments, and have successfully adapted themselves to almost every niche in the hydrosphere. Fishes live in marine, brackish and fresh water; some inhabit clear, others, muddy or turbid waters. Some fishes are pelagic, others occupy the coastal zones. Some have invaded the great depths of the sea where no surface light penetrates, others are inhabitants of the twilight zone, still others occupy the photic zone near the surface. Teleosts are found in the arctic and antarctic regions, the temperate regions of both hemispheres and the tropics. Cave fishes have adapted themselves to an absence of light by a degeneration of the eyes and the visual system. Some teleosts require a continuous supply of well-oxygenated water, others are able to survive in somewhat stagnant water; some are bottom dwellers. A number of teleosts have evolved structures for obtaining oxygen from the air and some, like *Periophthalmus*, are able to leave the water and "walk" on land. Many teleosts are capable of migrating from one environment to another and in so doing of withstanding marked changes in salinity, temperature, light, etc. Some of these migrations involve long journeys to the spawning grounds; the Atlantic eel going to sea to spawn deep in the Sargasso Sea and some salmon, in contrast, ascending rivers and streams to spawn in fresh water. These migrations are often accompanied by striking morphological, physiological and biochemical alterations in the migrating fishes.

1. Visual Cells

No short account such as this can hope to review adequately the large literature on the teleost visual receptors. A good account of some of this literature was made by Kolmer (1936) and by Engström (1963a). The visual cells of teleosts are different in a number of features from the receptors of lower fishes. Typically, both rods and cones are present and the two receptors are easily distinguishable on the basis of the shapes of the outer and inner segments; the sizes, locations and internal structure of the nuclei; the width and length of the myoids; and the opposing photomechanical movements to light. I know of no teleost with a rod-free retina but there are some that are considered to be cone-free. The deep-sea fish, *Bathytroctes*, was reported by Brauer (cited by Wunder, 1926a) to have an all-rod retina, and this was confirmed for *Argyropelecus* by Contino (1939) and for *Bathylagus* by Vilter (1953). These rods were described as having long, cylindrical, and closely-packed outer segments, thus providing a large surface for the capture of light quanta. Vilter (1953, 1954a, b, c) reported an arrangement of the rods in regular layers. A fovea was reported to be present in the temporal region, and in this foveal area six layers of rods were noted. Vilter considered the *Bathylagus* retina to have mechanisms for binocular fixation and for increased visual acuity.

Perhaps this is the place to describe certain adaptations of the eyes and retinas of teleosts inhabiting the twilight and aphotic zones of the deep sea where light from the surface is absent or greatly attenuated. In such teleosts the eyes have either degenerated or evolved structures to maximize vision in this dim environment. In those species in which ocular degeneration has occurred one finds eyes in various stages of atrophy (Munk, 1966a). There are species in which all that is left of the eye is a capsule containing a mass of pigmented cells. In other species the lens, though present, is rudimentary and the retina has degenerated, with visual cells that are swollen and fragmented. In those species in which the eye persists and vision is present a number of specializations have evolved (MUNK, 1966a, b). The eye is enlarged, relatively speaking, in some species and sometimes has assumed unusual shapes such as the tubular eye, and the eye of *Bathylychnops exilis* which has a rostro-ventral protuberance forming a smaller secondary globe. This secondary globe has a scleral lens and a retina that appears to be a diverticulum-like extension of the retina in the eye ball. The lens of the deep-sea eye is typically spherical, relatively large, and close to the cornea — features designed to achieve a large aperture. The retinas of these fishes also show specializations, some of them unique. In tubular eyes a common feature is the division of the retina into two distinct moieties: a main retina at the bottom or ventral portion of the tube, and an accessory retina along the median wall. In some species light may reach the accessory retina by pathways other than the corneal-lens aperture, i.e., through the skin or the roof of the mouth. In such cases the eyeball has developed a pigment-free "window". The visual cells of these deep-water fishes have been considered to be rods, all in possession of long outer segments packed closely together and forming, in some species, a series of layers sometimes 6 tiers in depth. One has difficulty in assessing the conclusion by MUNK (1965) that *Omosudis lowei* has an almost all-cone retina. Perhaps, this emphasizes, once again, the subjective nature of the morphological criteria employed to distinguish rods and cones in some species. In any case, even MUNK (1965, 1966a) recognized the uncertain nature of *Omosudis* by invoking the transmutation theory of WALLS, which is discussed later in this chapter. The presence of long outer segments, especially arranged in tiers, poses some problems as LOCKET (1970) recognized. In retinas of this character the processes of the pigment epithelium are retracted away from many of the outer segments. If the epithelium is involved in the transfer of retinol between the visual cell and the epithelium, as many believe, how is this accomplished in the special situation of these tiered retinas? Additionally, how is the process of phagocytizing the apical tips of the outer segments accomplished as the rods add new discs from their basal ends and the apical discs are discarded? A feature reported for the retinas of some deep-sea teleosts, but not limited to deep-sea forms, is the presence of visual cells in groups or bundles. A good description of these was given by LOCKET (1970) who reported them as occurring in the posterior portion of the main retina of *Scopelarchus guentheri*. Each bundle consists of some 23 rods ensheathed within a casing made of the processes of the pigment epithelial cells, which contain a reflecting layer made up of oriented crystals of what LOCKET thinks to be guanine. Perhaps the most remarkable feature of these photoreceptor bundles is the existence of membrane-to-membrane tight junctions between adjacent receptors at the level of the inner segments. The presence of such junctions suggests, of course, the possibility of functional cross-talk between receptors. LOCKET, in fact, described these bundles as macro-receptors, realizing the possibility of functional linkage by way of the tight junctions and, optically, through the multiple reflections of the tapetal layer.

There are a few reports claiming the absence of cones in teleosts other than deep-sea forms. Such claims exist for the catfish, *Clarias batrachus* (VERRIER, 1927), for the mooneye, *Hiodon tergisus* (MOORE, 1944) and for the goldeye, *Amphiodon alosoides* (MOORE and McDOUGAL, 1949). These last two closely-related clupeoid fishes were reported to have a guanine tapetum lucidum and to be adapted to vision in dim light. In assessing all such claims one must keep aware that a master histologist, such as was Schultze (1873), considered the eel retina to have no cones, although investigators soon after him (Krause, 1881; Denissenko, 1882) noted the presence of these receptors. Cones are not always uniformly distributed over the retina. Vilter (1951a) for example, reported the retina of the freshwater eel to have a high density of rods in the dorsal portion and only few cones. This is the reverse of the distribution in the eel elver in which the ventral region of the retina was seen to have a high density of rods.

Despite these exceptional cases, the visual cells of most teleosts consist of single rods, single cones, and double cones. Not all single cones are the same and some investigators, especially Engström (1960, 1963b), reported the presence, in the same retina, of both long single cones and short single cones. As Fig. 7 shows, the morphological characteristics of the long and short single cones are sufficiently different to suggest that these two forms are genuinely different cells, rather than one cell type with either a contracted or an elongated myoid. Multiple cells such as triple and quadruple elements have been detected in the teleost retina (Lyall, 1956; Engström, 1960, 1961, 1963a), and Engström (1963a) credited Vrabec as first seeing triple cones in the retinas of the chub, the tench and the carp. In some retinas these cells were found to be so abundant that they could not be treated as aberrant structures (Lyall, 1956). Engström (1963a) pointed out that the triple cones in the cyprinids that he examined were all of the linear type, i.e., with the three members in a row, whereas in gadids and certain other fishes they were arranged in a triangular array. Engström (1963a) also reported the quadruple cones to be in the form of a square in some species and in the form of a triangle with one member in the center, in other species. The significance of these multiple cells, which occur also in the retinas of frogs and geckos, is not known.

One striking feature of the visual cells of many teleosts is the action of light and darkness in inducing opposite movements, inward and outward, for the rods and the cones. In fact, this photomechanical action differentiates rods and cones about as well as many of the morphological characteristics that have been mentioned. In the presence of light the cone myoids contract, bringing the outer segments closer to the external limiting membrane and out of the region of extended pigment granules in the processes of the epithelial cells. Simultaneously, the rod myoids elongate thus burying the rod outer segments within the protective enclosure of the pigment. In darkness these movements all reverse: the pigment retracts, the cone myoids elongate and the rod myoids contract. The whole system behaves as if to protect the rods in bright light while permitting adequate exposure of the cones. These photomechanical responses are most prominent in teleosts, although they also occur in some amphibia and in some birds. They are said to be absent in the visual cells of placental mammals and are of minor occurrence in the reptilian retina. It is perhaps significant that they are so well developed in teleosts in which pupillary movements are either absent or small, whereas the visual cell movements are insignificant in lizards, which characteristically possess rapid and effective pupillary control of light. The mechanism of these photomechanical responses and the reason why rods and cones behave in opposite ways are completely unknown. One great obstacle to exploration of this phenomenon is that the responses cannot be observed directly in isolated pre-

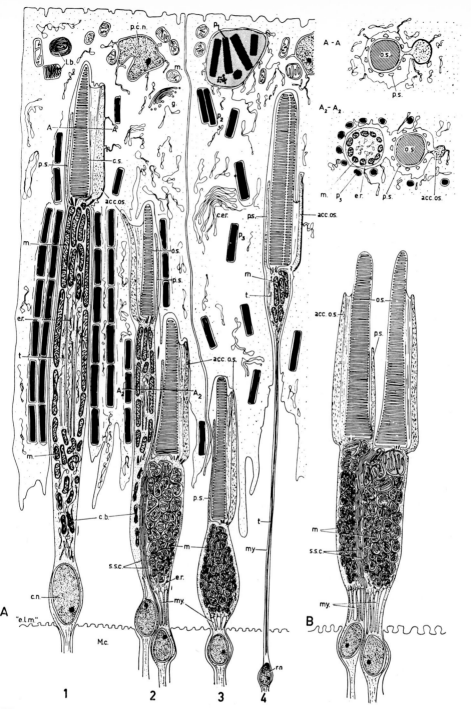

Fig. 7. Schematic drawing of selected teleost visual cells as pictured by ENGSTRÖM (1963b). On the left (A) is shown ENGSTRÖM's *Crenilabrus* type in which the double cones are grossly dissimilar in length and structure. Shown here are the long single cone (*1*), the short single cone (*3*), the unequal double cone (*2*) and the rod (*4*). On the right (B) is a double cone of the *Ctenolabrus* type. Though not a twin cone, the two members are rather similar. This figure is reproduced through the courtesy of Dr. K. ENGSTRÖM

parations but require that the retina be removed *after* the exposure to light or darkness and then prepared for microscopic observation. It is no wonder that the literature in this field contains contradictions and uncertainties. For the reader who is interested I can recommend the following references: Arey (1916), Wunder (1926b), Engström and Rosstorp (1963), O'Connell (1963), Nicol (1965), Blaxter and Jones (1967).

At present it is not possible to make secure biological generalizations regarding the visual cells in teleosts. This is so for several reasons. In the first place a broad spectrum of fishes from diverse ecological categories has not been examined with a specific aim and with adequate and identical histological technique. The little work that has appeared has had limited aims with respect to specific taxonomic groups or specific ecological situations. In the second place a systematic sampling of different retinal regions has not been made in a sufficient number of species to discover meaningful biological relations. I have already referred to Vilter's claim of some regional segregation of rods in the retina of the eel (Vilter, 1951a). In the benthic fish, *Callionymus lyra*, Vilter (1947) reported the presence of a dorsal retinal region containing cones, a ventral area where rods were found in large numbers and cones rarely, and an intermediate central band having high cone density. O'Connell (1963) reported the occurrence of some rather striking regional differences in the distribution of rods, single cones and double cones in the retinas of six species of pelagic marine teleosts. Such regional segregations have been noted for the retinas of other vertebrates. They probably represent specializations for specific visual tasks in different regions of the retina in cases where the visual fields are markedly different. In some fishes there is a region of specialization in the form of a horizontal band of thickened retina located near the center of the fundus. Munk (1970) described the single band in the mudskippers (*Boleophthalmus* and *Periophthalmus*) and the double band in the freshwater *Aplocheilus lineatus* and *Epiplatys grahami*. Munk concluded that the horizontal band in the amphibious mudskipper is an area of improved movement perception along the horizontal at or near ground level, where objects of visual interest occur while the fish is on land. The freshwater fishes with the double band swim just below the surface of the water and catch insects that are on, or just above, this horizontal surface. In both cases the horizontal bands may serve to fixate the eyes along the horizontal region of interest. This was also the interpretation given by Brown (1969) for the role of the linear central area that he observed in the turtle retina. It is also the interpretation applicable to the function of the ribbon-shaped area found in the retinas of some birds that are active in open country (Duijm, 1958; Pumphrey, 1948). Anyone who has tried to keep in fixation a high flying plane knows what advantage a horizontal area of high acuity would be in the human retina. Bifurcation of vision is well developed in the four-eyed fish, *Anableps*, which is a genus of cyprinodonts living in South America, Central America and the southern portion of Mexico. This remarkable fish skims the surface of the water with one half of each eye above water, the lower half in the water. The cornea, pupil and lens are dualized so as to permit both aerial and aquatic vision. I know of no detailed studies of the retina of this interesting fish but Schwassmann and Kruger (1965) mentioned some significant differences in the ventral retina, which perceives the aerial field, and the dorsal retina, which views the aquatic field. The ventral retina was found to have about twice as many smaller cones as the dorsal retina, the inner nuclear layer in the ventral region was shown to be thicker, as well as to have more bipolar cells. In addition, the inferior retina was found to contain more ganglion cells. Correlated with these histological observations were the electrophysiological findings of a magnified tectal projection for the aerial field, and of a lower size-threshold for movement in the aerial visual field. Insects floating on the surface of the water or moving just above it seem to be part of the food of *Anableps*, and for the catching of this food the aerial retina with its better acuity seems to have evolved.

One investigator who attempted to make a correlation between the numbers and characteristics of rods and cones, on the one hand, and the photic habitat, on the other, is WUNDER (1926b). Studying twenty-four species of fishes from different environments WUNDER made detailed measurements of sizes and numbers of visual cells. He found in an 80 μm stretch of retina that the mean number of rods for the twenty-four species was 66.3, with a range of 11 to 260 in the different species; that the mean number of cones was 7.9 with a range of 3 to 16. With regard to length of outer segment, WUNDER found for the rods a mean length of 25 μm with a range of 8 to 42 μm and for the cones a mean length of 9.4 μm with a range of 4 to 17 μm. One relationship that WUNDER observed was that not always was a large, bulky rod outer-segment associated with dim-light vision, for he noted the presence in some dim-light species of numerous rods containing fine and short outer segments. In some species, in fact, the rod outer segments were smaller than the corresponding cone outer segments. If these observations are correct they suggest, for teleosts at least, that sensitivity to dim light may be achieved either by increasing the volume of the rod outer segments or by increasing the density of rods.

Unlike the cones of chondrosteans, dipnoans and *Latimeria* the cones of teleosts possess no oil-droplets, and the occasional vesicles that have been reported in the ellipsoids do not have the properties of oil-droplets (BUTCHER, 1938). In place of colored oil-droplets, however, the corneas of many diurnal teleosts have developed a yellow pigmentation that serves the same purpose as other intraocular filters, i.e., to absorb light of shorter wavelength, and to reduce intraocular scatter and chromatic aberration, thus improving visual acuity (WALLS and JUDD, 1933; MORELAND and LYTHGOE, 1968).

The so-called double cone is a prominent feature of the teleost retina. Skepticism is advisable in the case of those reports claiming the absence of such elements in a teleost retina. ENGSTRÖM, for example, was able to demonstrate double cones in retinas in which WUNDER (1926b) saw only single cones (ENGSTRÖM, 1963a). Such negative findings are likely to be uncertain if based on transverse sections alone. Double cones, as well as triple and quadruple cones, are better recognized by means of tangential sections which have not always been employed. Double cones were first described by HANNOVER (1840), later further described and pictured by SCHULTZE (1867), and then classified by DOBROWOLSKY (1871) who thought he saw some double cones with a single nucleus, some double cones with a dividing nucleus, and some double cones with two nuclei. DOBROWOLSKY apparently held the view that double cones arose by the division of single cones. The erroneous idea of a single nucleus associated with the two members has persisted and sometimes is found even in the more recent literature. A distinction has been made between twin cones and double cones but this distinction may not be as clear as hitherto believed. Walls (1942b) considered the typical double element of the teleost retina to be a twin cone, i.e., having two identical members, although he did admit to the possible existence of double cones, i.e., with two members different in size and structure. Since the holostean double element is also an unequal double cell, Walls conceived the presence of such unequal double elements in teleosts to support the origin of such doubles from the holostean counterparts. He considered that twin cells evolved later in the higher teleosts. Unfortunately, however, Walls himself, and later, Engström (1963a) pointed out the occurrence of unequal double cells in advanced teleosts. In point of fact if we broaden the definition of twin cones to include identity in size, position, structure and biochemistry of the two members it is a question whether or not many twin cones remain. Engström (1960) studied the visual cells in thirteen cyprinids and found, on the basis of morphology alone, that all the doubles were unequal double cones. In ten species of gadid fishes, Engström (1961) found double cones that were characteristically different from the double cones of cyprinids. In *Gadus callarias* the two members were so nearly alike in structure, size and location that they were called twin cones but in other species there were slight differences between the two members, although not so pronounced as for the cyprinids. A study of five labrid species (Engström, 1963b) revealed the presence of a highly differentiated visual cell system containing long single cones, short single cones and double cones that were highly unequal in some species and slightly unequal in others (Fig. 7). Engström and Ahlbert (1963) also examined the retinas of four species of flatfishes and observed the presence of double cones that varied from equal members to slightly unequal ones. Engström mentioned that even in the so-called twins there were differences in staining of the two members which to him suggested the possibility that the two members "are not physiologically equal." Lyall (1957a) earlier had reported that for the so-called twin cones of the trout (*Salmo trutta*), the two members did not stain similarly with haematoxylin or Mallory. All these studies weaken the concept of a double element with biochemically and physiologically identical members even though gross morphology may be identical. The functional role of double cones in teleosts is unknown although some guesses have been made on the basis of the distribution of double cones in different ecological forms. Wunder (1926b) and Walls (1942b) associated the presence of double cones with vision in bright light; Lyall (1957a) with vision in deep water.

One of the most remarkable features of the teleost retina is the orderly arrangement of the different visual cell types in mosaic patterns. Though such patterns occur in the retinas of other vertebrates, they are nowhere better developed than in the retinas of these bony fishes. The nature of these patterns varies with the species, with the region of the retina and with the age of the animal. First observed by Hannover (1840), denied by Nunneley (1858), they were later confirmed by a number of investigators who described in varying detail the nature of the mosaic patterns. Using young fish of *Salmo salar*, Ryder (1894) described a mosaic whose fundamental repeat unit was a quadrangular arrangement of single and double cells with four single cells each at a corner, one single cell in the center and four double cells each at one side in between the corner singles. Believing these units, each of thirteen cells, to have some homology to the ommatidia of the compound eye, RYDER named them retinidia, a term that has not survived. A modification of this pattern was noted by EIGENMANN (1899) in the cyprinodont, *Zygonectes notatus*. It was next pointed out (EIGENMANN and SHAFER, 1900) that a number of variations in pattern existed in different species. The fact that some variations occurred in different retinal regions of the same species was indicated by SHAFER (1900) for the large mouthed black bass, *Micropterus salmoides*. In addition, SHAFER indicated that as the eye increased in size with age no new elements were added to the pattern but instead the size of the elements and the area of the pattern increased in proportion to the increase in retinal area. While admitting to an enlargement of the pattern unit as the trout retina grew, LYALL (1957a, b) conceived of a change in pattern by loss of the single cones at the corners of the quadrangular mosaic. This loss was thought to be a conversion of single cones to rods, associated with growth of the eye. This idea, similar to the BERNARD-CAMERON hypothesis of ontogenetic transmutation in the frog, is not supported by any evidence and NILSSON, as was earlier pointed out, gave reasons for believing that rods and cones were separate entities with no transmutation of one to the other occurring during development. DETWILER and LAURENS (1921) had earlier denied an ontogenetic transmutation for the developing cells in *Amblystoma* while admitting that all visual cells looked cone-like in the early stages of outer segment formation. In addition, they observed double cones very early in development of the visual receptors, and even at this stage each of the two members had its own nucleus indicating the origin of double cones by fusion of two single members rather than as a result of division of a primordial cell. As SAXÉN (1953) pointed out, a process of fusion better explains the occurrence of triple cells. ENGSTRÖM recently made a study of the visual cell patterns in a number of teleosts. In cyprinids the pattern was fundamentally the same but showed varying degrees of development in different species (ENGSTRÖM, 1960). No pattern was observed in the retina of the carp (*Cyprinus carpio*) but a very regular one was seen in *Leuciscus rutilus*, the dace. In the latter fish, in the horizontal, equatorial region of the retina a most remarkable arrangement of single cones and unequal double cones was found, and is illustrated in Fig. 8. Arranged in rows running radially in the retina, the double cones were found to alternate with rows of single cones. In each row of double cones the two members of the doubles were seen to alternate in position as shown in Fig. 8. Each row of single cones contained both short and long singles that alternated regularly along the row. A somewhat similar pattern was found in gadids (ENGSTRÖM, 1961) although here again some species differences in the degree of development was noted. In *Gadus minutus* rows of twin cones, running radially, were found but the single cones were not arranged regularly, being scattered among the twin cones. The cone mosaic in flatfishes was shown to consist of quadrangular units with a single central cone surrounded by four double cones. In some flatfishes ENGSTRÖM and AHLBERT (1963) noted the irregular appearance of single cones at the corners of the units. A full quadrangular unit was also reported to occur in labrid fishes with a long single cone in the center, short single cones at the four corners and double cones forming the sides of the square (ENGSTRÖM, 1963b). This was the appearance in tangential sections at the level of the ellipsoids. At the level of the outer segments the unit appeared to be two double cones and one single cone (the long single). The short single cones were not apparent or only revealed by the tips of the outer segments. A very unusual arrangement of visual cells was found by McEwan (1938) in two species of mormyrid fishes from South Africa. These fishes inhabit fresh, muddy water and avoid bright light. McEwan found both rods and cones to be present and these were found in bundles, each bundle being enclosed in a sheath of pigment epithelial cells. There were some nineteen to forty-four cones in each bundle with each cone probably surrounded by eight slender rods. Moore (1944) studied the pure rod retina of *Hyodon tergisus* and found the rods also to be grouped into bundles. Thus

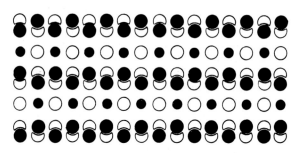

Fig. 8. The idealized cone mosaic pattern of *Leuciscus rutilus* illustrating the very regular arrangement of double cones in rows each row alternating with a row of single cones. The rows of single cones comprise both the long and short single cones of Fig. 7. In each row of doubles the two members alternate in zig-zag fashion. Taken from Engström (1960)

a variety of mosaic patterns exists in teleosts, some of which appear to be modifications or degenerations of some basic arrangement; others appear to be quite independent. For the reader who is interested further the general summary by Engström (1963a) is recommended. In spite of all this descriptive work on the visual cell patterns no one knows the role in vision of these beautiful arrays of receptors. Statements such as a role in bright light vision or a role in movement perception have appeared in the literature but no direct attacks on the functional significance of the mosaics have been made.

A differentiation of teleost rods and cones also can be made on the basis of the rod and cone nuclei. One of the most thorough studies of this point was made by Menner (1929) who pointed out that teleost retinas were especially useful for this purpose since the two types of cells could be identified readily on the basis of their form. In the common savetta, *Chondrostoma nasus*, Menner noted some marked differences between the cone and the rod nuclei. The cone nuclei formed a row of relatively large, slightly elliptical bodies, which showed a loose network of chromatin substance. This row was located just external to the external limiting membrane. In contrast, the rod nuclei consisted of several layers of smaller, elongated bodies with dense, coarse granulations of the chromatin. These were all located internally to the external limiting membrane. No intermediate cells were seen, suggesting to Menner that these nuclei were of fully-formed mature cells of two distinct types. A somewhat similar differentiation was made for the nuclei of the three-spined stickleback, *Gasterosteus aculeatus*. The rod and cone nuclei of the burbot, *Lota lota*, could also be differentiated by MENNER on the basis of their positions, their sizes, shapes and chromatin structure.

MENNER extended his study to include representatives from the other vertebrate classes. Excepting the amphibia for the moment, he always observed two types of nuclei in the external nuclear layer in the case of duplex retinas, and the numbers of these two types corresponded to the numbers of rods and cones. In retinas having many rods and few cones the rod nuclei predominated as, for example, in the case of the deer, *Capreolus capreolus*. In retinas considered to be of the pure rod classification, he noted the presence of only one class of nuclei in the external layer, and these nuclei resembled, cytologically, the nuclei associated with rods of the duplex retina. This situation was found in the badger, the domestic cat, the bat, the owl and certain elasmobranchs. The retinas in some of these animals are probably not entirely free of cones but the rods undoubtedly are in great abundance. For the retinas of certain diurnal reptiles and for the swift *(Cypselus apus)*, which MENNER considered to be pure-cone in nature, only one type of nucleus was identified in the external nuclear layer and this was characterized as a cone nucleus. An interesting category studied by MENNER was those retinas in which the visual cells could not be clearly identified on the basis of form but in which the external nuclear layer showed evidence of duplexity. The tree squirrel is of special interest here for its visual cells are somewhat enigmatic and sometimes have been classified as all cones (ARDEN and TANSLEY, 1955a). Despite this, MENNER reported the presence of two separate layers of nuclei in the external nuclear layer; one, more external, consisted of larger elements, presumably cone nuclei; the second, more internal, comprised smaller bodies with different chromatin structure, presumably rod nuclei. On the basis of MENNER's findings, what was considered a simplex, or at most an enigmatic retina, turned out to be classically duplex. A somewhat similar situation was noted for the retinas of certain birds and mammals whose bacillary layer appeared uniform but whose external nuclear layer, when studied carefully, was found to be duplex.

The amphibian retina was shown to be paradoxical. Though an unmistakable difference was noted between the inner and outer segments of the rods and cones, the nuclei of these two classes of cells were shown to be so similar in size, in form and in chromatin structure that they could not be differentiated. This is a curious contrast to the apparent duplexity of the external nuclear layer in the other vertebrate classes. Even at the ultrastructural level a clear rod-cone duplexity was not evident in the nuclei of *Rana pipiens* (NILSSON, 1964a). As Fig. 2 shows, while the nuclei of the red rods appear to be different, the nuclei of the green rods are like those of the chief cone member and the nuclei of the single cones and accessory cone members form a third grouping. No explanation is available for the apparently special morphology of the amphibian visual cell nuclei.

2. Visual Pigments

As already indicated in the historical section of this chapter, the study of the teleost retina led to the important conclusion that there are two separate photo-pigment systems: one utilizing retinal, the other utilizing 3-dehydroretinal, as the prosthetic group. This conclusion now has been amply confirmed in investigations involving some 230 species of teleosts. What has not been confirmed is that there are two classes of colored pigments: one purple, i.e., porphyropsin, the other red, i.e., rhodopsin. Instead, it has been discovered that the retinal photopigments of teleosts are diverse in color ranging in their spectral absorbance all the way from pigments with absorbance peaks at about 470 nm to pigments with peaks at about 520 nm for the A_1-system; and from about 513 nm to about 543 nm for the A_2-system. This diversity is apparently due to the effect of specific opsins in different species, which leads to shifts in absorbance of the chromophoric group to different regions of the visible spectrum and which thus offers a fine adjustment in the working range of the photopigment. In addition, it has been discovered that a significant number of teleosts employ both A_1- *and* A_2-based pigments in the retina at the same time, and in some of these fishes the ratio of the two pigments may change according to season or according to the light schedule to which the fish is subjected. A relationship of the photopigment composition to the photic environment has been revealed by the finding that the color or range of absorbance of a pigment is related to the spectral quality of the photic habitat of the fish. In the next section I elaborate on some of these matters (see also Chapters 11 and 14).

VII. The Multiplicity of Teleost Visual Pigments and the Bases for it

To DARTNALL, I believe, should go the credit for initiating and stimulating the investigations that have led to the present broadened knowledge. DARTNALL emphasized two matters that are critical in assaying the visual pigment composition of a retinal extract: (a) the homogeneity of an extract may not be assumed, it must be tested; and he devised the method of partial bleaching for doing this (DARTNALL, 1957) and (b) the spectral absorbance maximum cannot be always ascertained from the absorbance curve of the extract since this curve may be distorted by the presence of colored impurities. This means that the judicious use of difference spectra coupled with the method of partial bleaching is often the preferred procedure in the analysis of photopigment composition. This is the procedure employed by most investigators at the present time. Using this method, DARTNALL (1957) soon demonstrated two points: (a) a spectral distribution of pigments in fishes was found that was shown to be broader than was indicated by the rhodopsin-porphyropsin terminology and (b) extracts often were found with more than one photopigment. In the twenty years since DARTNALL began to examine the fish retina a considerable body of information has appeared about teleost visual pigments. A summary of most of these data is given in Fig. 9. This summary illustrates several points: (a) Either A_1- or A_2-based pigments occur over a considerable range of the visible spectrum. This is especially so for the pigments of marine teleosts whose absorbance maxima range from 478 nm (ignoring the single case at 468 nm) to 528 nm. (b) More pigments at shorter wavelengths have been noted in retinal extracts of marine, than of freshwater, fishes. (c) Although there is some spectral overlap between the A_1- and A_2-pigments in the marine teleosts, the distribution of the two systems is clearly separate in freshwater teleosts with the A_2-pigments inhabiting the longer wavelength region. (d) The pigments of freshwater teleosts extend further toward the red. (e) There is some indication of grouping around certain preferred spectral locations. DARTNALL and LYTHGOE (1965) made a special study of this clustering phenomenon and concluded, for one hundred and two A_1-pigments from eighty-three species, that preferred locations were at 486.5, 494, 500.5, 506, and 511.5 nm with two possible additional positions at 478 and 519 nm. These groupings are also indicated by the data that are reproduced in Fig. 9 except for an additional peak at about 503 nm which is due to the fact that I have included new data by SCHWANZARA (1967) on tropical freshwater fishes that were not available to DARTNALL and LYTHGOE. The clustering hypothesis was also applied to the distribution of A_2-based pigments by

BRIDGES (1965a) who assembled data from thirty four species including two holosteans. BRIDGES gave the preferred positions for his data at 511.5, 523.5, 534 and 543 nm. The data of Fig. 9 show, in addition to these, a prominent representation at 527 nm and this is due to the fact that here too I have included newer data. The clustering hypothesis has important implications regarding the chemical structure of visual pigments as DARTNALL and LYTHGOE (1965) pointed out. They suggested that in the interaction of prosthetic group and opsin, wherein the specific color is determined, there occur only certain permitted interaction forms. The future will determine the fate of the clustering hypothesis. The data of Fig. 9 include only about 0.01 % of the earth's teleost species.

Fig. 9 pools all acceptable data without reference to the ecology of the fishes from which the data were gathered. I shall now proceed to dissect these data in terms of ecological considerations.

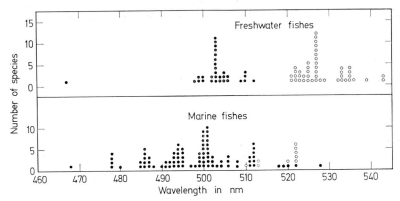

Fig. 9. Distribution of visual pigments in marine and freshwater teleosts. Each point represents the wavelength for maximal absorbance for a single species. *Filled circles.* A$_1$-photopigments. *Plain circles*; A$_2$-photopigments. These data were all obtained using partial bleaching analyses of extracts. The data were obtained from the publications of BRIDGES (1965a), CRESCI-TELLI and DARTNALL (1954), DARTNALL and LYTHGOE (1965), MUNZ (1956, 1957a, b, 1958a,b,c, 1965), MUNZ and BEATTY (1965), SCHWANZARA (1967)

A. The Marine versus the Freshwater Environment

WALD's well-known thesis that A$_1$-pigments are associated with the freshwater habitat and A$_2$-pigments are associated with the marine environment was derived from an analysis of the retinal vitamin A and of visual pigment extracts of marine teleosts and of freshwater teleosts (WALD, 1936a, 1937a, 1939, 1941, 1942b). Migratory fishes were found to have both vitamins in the retina and both classes of visual pigments, the dominant system being that associated with the spawning environment of the fish. WALD did not test homogeneity of his extracts, depending, instead, on the vitamin A composition of the retina and the spectral maximum of the photopigment absorbance curves.

Some apparent exceptions to this view have appeared. WALD (1960) mentioned the presence, in several marine labrids, of an A$_2$-system. MUNZ (1957a) found in the marine puffer, *Sphoeroides annulatus* (family Tetraodontidae), two pigments,

P 500$_1$ and P 522$_2$ in almost equal amounts (optical densities). Several reports have indicated the presence, in retinal extracts, of both A$_1$- and A$_2$-pigments in freshwater fishes. One report was that on the rudd (*Scardinius erythrophthalmus* family Cyprinidae) published by Dartnall, Lander and Munz (1961). Another report was that of Bridges (1964a) listing five species of freshwater fishes in which were found both classes of photopigments. In the case of such apparent exceptions refuge can sometimes be taken in expressions of doubt about the primary habitat of the fish. In the case of the marine puffer, for example, one can read (Nikol'skii 1961) that in the order Tetraodontiformes some species (not *Sphoeroides annulatus*) have become adapted to fresh water. Despite these apparent exceptions there are still some good examples of related fishes that have an A$_1$-system in marine representatives and an A$_2$-system in the freshwater species. One such example is cited by Beatty (1969b) for the fishes of the family Gadidae. Three Pacific marine gadids were found to have typical rhodopsins, P 498$_1$ and P 499$_1$. In contrast, the freshwater *Lota lota* was found to have a pigment pair: P 503$_1$ and P 527$_2$. These two pigments were not constant over the year but varied in proportion, with P 527$_2$ tending to decrease during spring and early summer. A discussion of this seasonal effect is given later in this section.

A thorough examination was recently made by Schwanzara (1967) who selected fifty-five species of tropical freshwater fishes taken from forty-eight genera and twenty families. The data were segregated according to whether the families belonged to one of three salinity tolerance groups: primary, secondary or peripheral. Primary families were those known to be strictly confined to fresh water; secondary families were those known to be capable of tolerating some salinity beyond that of fresh water but known to be chiefly in fresh water and peripheral families included those that were recognized as inhabiting fresh and brackish water and that were known to enter the sea sporadically or as part of a life cycle. Schwanzara also included data, similarly classified, from forty-eight species of temperate zone freshwater species. Her summary (Table 1) suggests the following conclusions about the occurrence of A$_1$- and A$_2$-pigments in freshwater fishes. (a) Out of a grand total of one hundred and three species just as many showed A$_1$-pigments as A$_2$-pigments. Of the fifty-nine species of strictly freshwater fishes, thirty-five or 59% had A$_1$-pigments alone or had both classes. Of these fifty-nine species, fifty-one or 86% had A$_2$-pigments alone or had both. These figures indicate that in these fifty-nine species of strictly freshwater species the A$_2$-system predominated. (b) When the tropical and temperate zone fishes were looked at separately a somewhat different picture emerged. Of the thirty-four species from the primary group of tropical fishes, twenty-seven or 79% had A$_1$-pigments alone or had the mixture. The same figures apply for the A$_2$-pigments alone or the mixture. Apparently, in tropical freshwater fishes there is no preference for either of the two pigment systems. In contrast, the temperate zone primary fishes showed a definite preference for the A$_2$-system. Out of twenty-five species, twenty-four or 96% had the A$_2$-pigment alone or had the mixture. (c) The data in Table I also suggest that possession of a mixture was not an exclusive property of euryhaline or migratory teleosts. Out of a total of fifty-nine strictly freshwater species, twenty-seven or 45% possessed the mixture although eighteen out of twenty-three or 78% of the peripheral species also showed a mixture. Again, the excess was related to a predominance of the purely vitamin A_2-system in the temperate zone fishes. Of the thirty-four species of tropical primary fishes, twenty or 59% possessed a mixture but in the twenty-five temperate zone primary fishes only seven or 28% had the mixture. This interesting survey by SCHWANZARA suggests that the hypothesis of a vitamin A_2-pigment association with the freshwater habitat probably arose as the result of the study, by investigators, of temperate zone fishes.

Table 1. *Retinal (A_1) and 3-dehydroretinal (A_2) Visual Pigments in Freshwater Fishes*

Family category	Number of families	Number of genera	Number of species			
			A_1	A_2	A_1+A_2	total
IA. Tropical Zone Fishes						
Primary	11	31	7	7	20	34
Secondary	4	12	8	0	8	16
Peripheral	5	5	4	0	1	5
Total	20	48	19	7	29	55
IB. Temperate Zone Fishes						
Primary	7	22	1	17	7	25
Secondary	3	5	2	1	2	5
Peripheral	4	7	1	0	17	18
Total	14	34	4	18	26	48
IC. Tropical + Temperate Zone Fishes						
Primary	17	53	8	24	27	59
Secondary	5	16	10	1	10	21
Peripheral	9	12	5	0	18	23
Grand Total	31	81	23	25	55	103

Data from SCHWANZARA (1967).

B. The Seasonal Cycle

The presence in a retina of a mixture of A_1- and A_2-photopigments is neither an incidental nor an atypical characteristic. In SCHWANZARA's compilation (Table 1) over 50% of the species contained such a mixture. The proportion of the two pigments was, of course, not the same for all species and SCHWANZARA cited examples showing the A_1-pigment predominating, the A_2-pigment predominating or the two equally represented. Actually, the proportion of the two may not remain constant at all times. An example of a fish with a seasonal variation is the rudd *(Scardinius erythrophthalmus)*, a non-migratory cyprinid freshwater teleost. Retinal extracts revealed the presence of two photopigments: an A_2-pigment with maximum density loss on bleaching at 543 nm and an A_1-pigment with maximum loss at 510 nm (DARTNALL, LANDER, and MUNZ, 1961). Although the total density of photopigment in the extracts remained constant, the proportion of the two components changed with the season in such a way as to indicate an association of the A_1-system with the coming of summer and of the A_2-system with the coming of winter. The possible role of light in this cyclic change was indicated in an experiment in which placing the rudd in constant darkness prevented the normal increase of the A_1-pigment, whereas exposing the fish to daylight increased the A_1-pigment at the expense of its A_2-partner. The retinal composition of the A vitamins was correspondingly changed but the liver vitamin A (predominantly A_1) was not affected. This work with the rudd was carried out in London (lat 52°N but a similar investigation was made by Bridges (1964b, 1965a, 1965b) at Miami Florida (lat 25°N) with two other species: a cyprinid, *Notemigonus crysoleucas* and a poecilid, *Belonesox belizanus*. Though individual variations in the proportions of the A_2-A_1 mixture were encountered from fish to fish, these were not enough to hide the seasonal effect, which was similar to that of the rudd. The photic envi ronment also was altered: darkness prevented the increase of the A_1-pigment while light had the reverse effect. In the results from London and from Miami the total density of pigment in the extracts remained about the same, only the proportion of the two pigments changed. This suggested that the same opsin was employed in the two systems, only the prosthetic group varied with the season i.e., the light. Dartnall (1962) has expressed the view that this "rudd effect' as he called it, may not be an aberrant or atypical phenomenon but may turn out to be a widespread and biologically useful adaptation. Its adaptive significance can only be guessed at but one guess is that the winter shift to the longer-wavelength A_2-system is associated with a change in transmission properties toward longer wavelengths of the water in which the fishes live.

Further studies of this seasonal effect have provided a number of new facts but it is doubtful whether any real understanding of this phenomenon has yet been achieved. Bridges and Yoshikami (1970a, b) established the identity of the two extractable pigments of the rudd retina to be $P535_2$ and $P507_1$. They then con firmed the seasonal effect and showed the summer increase in $P507_1$ to be less in older fish. The conversion of $P535_2$ to $P507_1$, produced by light, did not occur, or was retarded, in eyes capped with an opaque covering, although it did take place in the uncapped second eye of the same fish or in the second eye capped with a transparent covering. The light effect thus appears to be a local ocular effect rather than a systemic action by way of the endocrine or nervous systems. An analysis of the pigment epithelium revealed that changes involving the retinol and 3-dehydroretinol content were associated with light and darkness in parallel with the changes in $P507_1$ and $P535_2$, respectively. This suggested the occurrence, even in darkness, of a continuous turnover of the visual pigment chromophoric group and an exchange with the retinol and 3-dehydroretinol of the pigment epithelium Bridges and Yoshikami postulated the occurrence, in the epithelium, of a 3,4-dehydrogenation/hydrogenation enzyme reaction under photic control that serves to regulate the ratio of vitamins A_1 and A_2 for any light level, and thus to control the ratio of $P507_1$ to $P535_2$ in the outer segments. An alternative suggestion was that the regulation resides in the stereo-specific nature of an enzyme that acts more effectively on the all-*trans* isomer released by light bleaching than on the 11-*cis* chromophore liberated during the dark turnover of the visual pigment. In support of the turnover hypothesis is the finding of a constant replacement of outer segment discs known to occur in adult rods. While the older discs at the apical ends of the rods are eroded off and phagocytised by the pigment epithelium new discs containing new visual pigment are added at the base (Young, 1967 Young and Droz, 1968; Young, 1969). Thus a continuous turnover of visual pigment, even in the dark though at a reduced rate, was demonstrated, as required by the hypothesis of BRIDGES and YOSHIKAMI. There are several observations, however, that do not accord easily with this hypothesis. The developing tadpole eye of the frog *(Rana pipiens)* is known to have an A_1-A_2 pigment pair (CRESCI-TELLI, 1958a). When tadpoles are allowed to develop in the dark there is a shift in the proportions of these pigments the reverse of that found for the rudd. BRIDGES himself reported this (BRIDGES, 1970) and I have obtained the same result. In addition, a fundamental difference between rods and cones has been reported by YOUNG (1971) with respect to the renewal of outer segment discs. Whereas rods were noted to produce new discs throughout adult life, the replacement of discs in cones ceased after completion of growth. YOUNG considered this difference to be the basis for the difference in shape of the cone and rod outer segments in the frog. However, in spite of the fact that the cone outer segments of the tadpole are the same in size and shape as the outer segments of the adult (indicating, presumably, that no new discs have been added) an A_1-pigment in all the adult cones never-theless replaces the A_2-pigment of the tadpole cones (LIEBMAN and ENTINE, 1968). These facts appear to require a different turnover mechanism for the cone visual pigments. Even more troublesome to a general understanding of the seasonal effect and the mechanism of visual pigment turnover are the new facts revealed by ALLEN in a paper I read in galley proof (ALLEN, 1971). ALLEN extracted the pigment pair $P531_2-P506_1$ from the retina of the redside shiner, *Richardsonius balteatus balteatus*. He found a seasonal change similar to that of the rudd, i.e., $P531_2$ increased its proportion in winter, decreased it in summer. Significantly, however, the effects of light and darkness were the converse of those reported for the rudd. Light was reported to induce a percentage increase of $P531_2$ or else a retardation of the decrease associated with the season. Darkness, on the other hand, tended to increase the proportion of $P506_1$. Unlike the rudd, the total amount of extractable photopigment was not constant with season or with varying photic conditions. Instead, the amount was correlated with changes in $P531_2$. The cytological or ultrastructural basis for these changes in total pigment is unknown. Though light intensity and total quantity of light were factors in controlling the pigment composition of the shiner retina, ALLEN observed that the distribution of light in time was also an important parameter. In two separate experiments a 12/12 daily light/dark distribution was found to be more effective than either a 6/18 or 18/6 period when the light half-periods were equated in respect to intensity or to total quantity of light. A photoperiodism is suggested, indicating a control of visual pigment composition by extra-ocular systemic mechanisms. In fact, ALLEN demonstrated a dramatic increase in the proportion of the A_2-pigment as a result of adding thyroxine to the water containing shiners with a low $P531_2$. So far as this writer is aware, no experiments have been performed to test the effect of capping one eye of the shiner as was done with the rudd.

A complicating factor in these experiments with the rudd, unrecognized at the time of these studies, is the fact that the visual pigment composition is not uniform over the retina. MUNTZ and NORTHMORE (1971) observed that extracts of the superior half of the rudd retina contained a greater proportion of $P507_1$ than did extracts of the lower half. Such a non-uniform distribution has also been detected in the bullfrog retina, where the A_2-system was found to predominate in the upper half of the retina (Reuter, White, and Wald, in press). In the summer months at least, porphyropsin was found to comprise 30—40 % of the total extracted photopigment of the adult retina. The porphyropsin was found exclusively in the superior half of the retina, the portion that views the lower visual field below the water surface. The ventral retinal half yielded rhodopsin, and its concentration was significantly less than the concentration of porphyropsin. The proportions of retinol and 3-dehydroretinol in the underlying pigment epithelium paralleled the distribution of rhodopsin and porphyropsin. This segregation of the vitamins A permitted the authors to carry out a Kühne-type experiment. A light-adapted or bleached dorsal retina when placed on the ventral pigment epithelium led to the regeneration of rhodopsin. Contrariwise, the bleached ventral retina after lying on the dorsal epithelium regenerated porphyropsin. In both cases the regenerated pigment was determined by the composition of the epithelium; presumably the opsin was the same. The authors have suggested a segregation of the presumptive enzyme, 3,4-dehydrogenase, in the dorsal epithelium where it is able to produce 3-dehydroretinol which, in turn, leads to the formation of porphyropsin in the dorsal retinal half. It is a notable fact that in *Rana pipiens*, another frog that has been studied extensively, the adult retina apparently contains no porphyropsin, even though a metamorphic shift from porphyropsin to rhodopsin occurs as in the bullfrog. No one yet has examined the visual pigment composition of *Anableps*, the four-eyed fish, which views the upper visual field with the inferior retina and the lower aquatic field with the superior retina.

C. The Deep-Sea Environment

The point raised in the preceding paragraph about the photic environment has been investigated by an examination of the visual pigments of deep water marine teleosts. These fishes live in an environment that is biologically unique. Here temperatures are low, reaching almost to 0°C at about 3000 meters. The pressures are high, and light from the surface continually decreases with depth until at about 1000 meters all surface light is absent and the only light is that arising from bioluminescence. As light is absorbed down to the twilight zone, the selective removal of longer wavelengths leads to a remnant illumination that is predominantly blue or blue-green. This has been established by measurements of the spectral transmittance of ocean waters at various depths, one of the most recent of these measurements being that of Boden, Kampa, and Snodgrass (1960). These measurements, made in the Bay of Biscay, involved readings starting at 50 meters and continuing down to 400 meters at 50 meter intervals. The spectral transmittance curves showed the continual change in optic environment from the broad solar band at the surface to the ever-narrowing band, maximal at 475—480 nm, as depth increased.

In addition, light of biological origin at these depths is colored, that being emitted by luminescent fishes being blue-green. Nicol (1960) analyzed the spectral composition of light from the photophores of the lantern fish, *Myctophum punctatum*, and found the range of emission to be 410 to 600 nm with the maximum at about 470 nm. It is generally assumed that such light is biologically useful, serving such functions as species or sex recognition, as lures to entice prey, or as

defensive screens to confuse or evade predators. The eyes of many deep-sea fishes
are well developed with large corneas, pupils and lenses and with retinas provided
with numerous, closely-packed rods that have long, cylindrical outer segments
(CONTINO, 1939). Knowing the ecological situation, CLARKE (1936) suggested that
deep-sea fishes might be expected to have a spectral sensitivity shifted toward
shorter wavelengths as an adaptation to the quality of light in the deep-sea
environment. A similar idea was in the minds of BAYLISS, LYTHGOE, and TANSLEY
(1936) in their examination of visual pigments of several fishes. Their method of
measuring spectral absorbance by recording the difference in absorbance between
bleached and unbleached extracts, was not suited, as we know now, to give reliable
data for all conditions of the extracts. Moreover, they were under the impression,
obtained from some observations by SAWYER and by BEEBE (cited by BAYLISS,
LYTHGOE, and TANSLEY, 1936) that light at wavelengths above 510 nm is transmitted maximally in deep water.

CLARKE's suggestion was eventually revealed to be prophetic, for it was found
that bathypelagic teleosts have special photopigments that absorb maximally, not
at 500 nm, but at wavelengths some 20 nm below this value. DENTON and WARREN
(1956, 1957) used isolated retinas and measured the spectral density change after
bleaching, for nineteen different species of deep-sea fishes belonging to twelve
different families. All of them revealed the presence of a golden-colored pigment
system, named chrysopsin (visual gold), whose spectral absorbance was shifted
some 15−20 nm toward shorter wavelengths away from the position of classical
rhodopsin. The *in situ* density of the pigment was often relatively high, in some
species so high as to indicate the absorption of 95% of the blue-green light incident
on the retina. The varied taxonomic positions of these fishes eliminated
systematics as a factor in the evolution of the chrysopsin system; instead the
deep-sea environment appeared to be the common factor in all of these. At about
the same time that DENTON and WARREN were making their measurements,
MUNZ (1957b, 1958a) was preparing extracts from retinas of fishes caught at night
from depths of 510 to 870 meters in the Pacific Ocean off Guadalupe Island, Baja
California. In six species MUNZ obtained evidence for the presence of pigments
absorbing maximally at 478, 485, 488 and 490 nm. The extracts were analyzed by
the technique of partial bleaching and all, except one species, showed but a single
photopigment. *Bathylagus wesethi* revealed the presence of a major component
absorbing maximally at 478 nm and another component, which made up about
20−25% of the density loss on bleaching, with a maximum at 500 nm. MUNZ
identified the prosthetic group of all these pigments by means of the spectrum of
the oxime formed in the presence of hydroxylamine. They were all identified as
A_1-based photopigments. A summary of some published data on the pigments
of deep-sea fishes is given in Fig. 10. Considerable variability exists for the pigments
from different species but all of them absorb at wavelengths significantly lower
than that characteristic for the pigments of surface marine fishes. The photopigments of deep-sea teleosts are apparently chemically similar to other visual
pigments. They are able to regenerate, for example, from the specific opsin and
added 11-*cis* retinal (WALD, BROWN, and BROWN, 1957). It is the nature of the
opsin apparently that confers on the chromoprotein the special property of
absorbing at shorter wavelengths. The evolution of a special deep-water visual

pigment system has occurred not only in teleosts, but, as was noted earlier, also in elasmobranchs and in the Holocephali. Ecological considerations have determined the visual pigment situation irrespective of taxonomic relations.

It is interesting to compare the adaptations to dim light that have evolved in the retinas of deep-water elasmobranchs and teleosts (Denton and Nicol, 1964). The teleosts have no reflecting tapeta except in special cases such as that described by Locket (1970), but have rods that are about twice as long and a retinal photo-pigment density that is about twice as great as in elasmobranchs, which have evolved an efficiently reflecting tapetum. The fraction of light incident on the retina that is absorbed is therefore the same for the teleosts and the elasmobranchs, though the latter are able to achieve this with about half the pigment. Denton and Nicol speculated that this could be of advantage to the elasmobranch in that it could lead to an improved signal-to-noise ratio or to a faster dark adaptation without sacrifice of sensitivity.

D. The Coastal Zone

If the quality of the photic environment is implicated in the evolution of a visual pigment then marine fishes that inhabit shallow coastal waters, which are sandy, muddy, turbid, or which have a growth of algae, should have evolved a system absorbing at longer wavelengths. This is because such waters tend to transmit maximally yellow or yellow-green light, for red light is lost by absorption and light of shorter wavelengths is lost by scattering and by absorption. It is perhaps significant, therefore, that the longjaw goby (*Gillichthys mirabilis*), which is found in tidal mudflats and salt marshes of the Gulf of California and along the Pacific Coast from northern California to Baja California, was found to have a

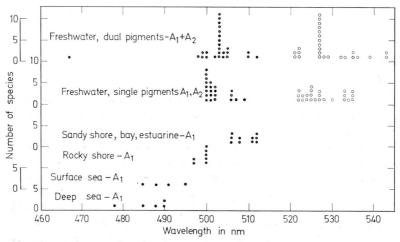

Fig. 10. Distribution of visual pigments according to the habitat of the fishes. *Filled circles*: A₁-pigments; *plain circles*: A₂-pigments. The data for the freshwater fishes have been segregated into two groups: those fishes with only one pigment in the extract, and those with a dual A₁-A₂-system. These data were all obtained by partial bleaching analyses of retinal extracts. Sources: same as for Fig. 9

P512₁ (MUNZ, 1956). This is not an isolated occurrence for MUNZ (1958b) obtained evidence for the existence of A_1-based pigments absorbing maximally at 504 to 512 nm in a number of fishes inhabiting sandy shores, bays and estuaries (Fig. 10).

In contrast to the open sea, freshwater lakes, rivers, ponds, etc. tend to have optical properties more like bays, marshes, mud flats and estuaries. Moreover, the optical properties tend to vary much more with the seasons due to varying quantities of silt washed in by rains and to varying amounts of plant life. Several investigators (MUNZ, 1965; BRIDGES, 1965a; SCHWANZARA, 1967) have expressed the view that the evolution of the A_2-system could have come about in response to the yellowish optical environment of fresh water. BRIDGES (1965a) suggested that the possession of a dual system of mixed pigments, found in so many freshwater fishes, would confer a broader spectral sensitivity in the face of a labile photic environment. Finally, evolutionary adaptability is not limited to vertebrates. GOLDSMITH and FERNANDEZ (1968) pointed out, for example, that ultraviolet light receptors, common in insects, are rare in crustacea, possibly because ultraviolet light, present in the terrestrial environment, is absent in the aquatic habitat.

E. The Migratory Habit

In association with the search for food, or the reproductive cycle, or environmental changes, etc. certain fishes make long migrations. The migrations that concern us here are those that take place between the sea and fresh water in connection with the reproductive cycle. These migrations are known to be accompanied by a number of morphological, physiological and biochemical alterations. The visual system is involved in this complex of changes, which is the reason for considering this subject here. I will be concerned chiefly with the catadromous migrations of the eel and the anadromous migrations of the salmon. Nothing can be said about the monadromous spawning migrations such as occur in the cod, *Gadus callarias* (TROUT, 1957; WOODHEAD, 1959) since no studies have appeared on the visual pigments of this fish.

1. The Eel

The family Anguillidae consists of one genus, *Anguilla*, with several species inhabiting the Atlantic, Indian and Pacific Oceans. The European eel, *Anguilla anguilla*, is found along the coast and in rivers of Europe from the White Sea to the Black Sea. This eel is catadromous, that is it travels to the sea to spawn. By following the distribution of the leptocephalus larva as it decreased in size, the Danish oceanographer JOHANNES SCHMIDT (1923) traced the smallest larvae to the Sargasso Sea, the region of the Atlantic between 22° and 30° N. lat. and 48° and 65° W. long. This is presumed to be the deep-sea spawning area for the eel. The young larvae, released seasonally between the end of winter and the middle of summer, drift for about three years in the Atlantic currents, eventually reaching the European coast. Here the larvae metamorphose into young adult yellow eels, which proceed to swim upstream into the rivers, sometimes even going overland to reach inland fresh water. They feed at first on certain invertebrates; later, when larger, they may capture small fishes. After 9 to 12 years in fresh water the eels begin their spawning migration back to the sea. During this journey metamorphic changes occur: the swim bladder decreases in size, the eyes enlarge and the body color changes from a greenish-yellow to a darker hue. The eel, now known as the silver eel, eventually reaches sexual maturity on its way back to the Sargasso Sea where it spawns and presumably ends its life. During its catadromous journey in the sea the eel is said not to feed, but there is some uncertainty on this point. The American eel, *Anguilla rostrata*, is said to spawn in an area of the Atlantic somewhat west of that used by the European eel. It is said to develop more rapidly than its European counterpart, its journey to the American coast is much shorter, and a number of characteristic morphological differences exist in the two species. Schmidt, for example, cites the European eel as having, on average, 7.5 more vertebrae than the American eel (Schmidt, 1923).

Although further studies are required, it appears that changes in retinal photopigments accompany the metamorphic transitions of the eel life cycle. Nothing is known about the visual pigments of the leptocephalous larva nor about changes in the visual system during development to the yellow eel. Kühne (1877) noted the intense purple color of the eel retina. He did not state what stage of life his specimen represented but it was probably a river eel. Measurements of the visual pigment of the European river eel were first made by Bayliss, Lythgoe, and Tansley (1936) who found in the fresh water form a "high yield of visual purple" with maximum absorbance at 505 nm. A somewhat different result was reported later by Wald (1941), who employed the American eel and who noted the presence of both vitamins A_1 and A_2 in the retina, with A_1 in excess. The retinal extract was found to absorb maximally at 498—502 nm. Wald interpreted these results to mean the presence of both rhodopsin and porphyropsin in the eel retina with the former predominating, in conformity with the marine spawning habit of the eel. The first attempt to analyze separately the visual pigments of the yellow eel and the silver eel was made by Carlisle and Denton (1959). Using the *in situ* density loss on bleaching they found a pigment, with maximum loss at about 515 nm for the yellow eel, and another pigment with a maximum some 33 nm less for the silver eel. Though no identification of the prosthetic groups was made, Carlisle and Denton considered this transformation to be analogous to the porphyropsin-rhodopsin transition in the bullfrog and lamprey. Actually, it is not strictly analogous, for the transition in the eel is to a deep-sea type of visual pigment, a chrysopsin, as Carlisle and Denton fully appreciated. Biologically, this transformation in photopigment appears to be adaptive in nature. Not only does the visual pigment change to a spectral form better suited for the blue-green environment of its spawning fields, but the *in situ* density increases in transforming to the silver eel. Carlisle and Denton gave figures of 0.34 and 0.21 for the maximum density loss in two yellow eels whereas values of 0.58 and 0.52 were given for two silver eels while still in fresh water. This important paper of Carlisle and Denton was incomplete in two respects: (a) the nature of the prosthetic groups was not examined and (b) partial bleaching was not employed to prove that a dual pigment system is all that is involved in the yellow eel — silver eel transition. Wald (1960) clarified this situation by mentioning some work of his colleagues (Brown and Brown) showing the yellow eel retina to contain both $P 523_2$ and $P 501_1$ and the silver eel to have only vitamin A_1 in the retina. Details of this work have never appeared in published form but if they are true it would appear to indicate a double change in preparing the eel for the deep-sea spawning environment: first, a shift from the A_2-system to the A_1-system and second, a shift from an opsin giving an absorbance maximum at 501 nm to one giving λ_{max} at about 487 nm. This does not appear to be analogous to the metamorphic transition in the bullfrog. Clearly, however, more investigation of the eel visual system is required before the matter is entirely clarified.

An interesting problem in ichthyology is the nature of the relationship between the American and European eels. Normally, these are considered to be separate species, as SCHMIDT (1923) proposed. A different view was published by TUCKER (1959a,b) who proposed the theory that European eels derive from the American, and not from the European stock. The latter, according to TUCKER, never reach the spawning area, dying before they arrive at this distant portion of the Atlantic. According to TUCKER, the differences in the American and European eels are the result of environmental differences, possibly the temperature, to which the larvae are exposed in the eastward and westward migrations. TUCKER's proposal set off a lively exchange (JONES, 1959; D'ANCONA, 1959; DEELDER, 1960) in which various reasons, none decisive, were adduced for rejecting the single species theory. In an attempt to obtain objective evidence the hemoglobin types in the American and European eels were assayed by means of electrophoresis. After first finding no differences in the two hemoglobins (SICK, WESTERGAARD, and FRYDENBERG, 1962), a larger experimental sample was employed which revealed the American eel hemoglobin to have three electrophoretic bands clearly differentiated from the pattern of the European eel (SICK, BAHN, FRYDENBERG, NIELSEN, and VON WETTSTEIN, 1967).

The total visual pigment analysis of *Anguilla anguilla* and *Anguilla rostrata* might be useful in deciding between the one or two-species concepts. From the data given in the preceding paragraphs it appears that at least three visual pigments are a part of the yellow eel-silver eel cycle. Because spectrophotometrically-similar visual pigments do occur in different species, the finding of a similar trio of pigments in the American and European eels would not be decisive, but the finding of different pigments would support the two-species idea.

2. Salmonids

Many salmonid fishes perform an anadromous migration going upstream to spawn in fresh water. The newly hatched fish gradually make their way back to the sea for the feeding, growing stage. The old question as to whether or not a photopigment transition is associated with this migration has not been answered with certainty. The brown trout (*Salmo trutta*) was one of the fishes employed by KÖTTGEN and ABELSDORFF (1896) in their pioneer study in which it was concluded that the photopigments of fishes absorb maximally at a wavelength some 40 nm higher than the rhodopsin of amphibia, birds and mammals. This result was confirmed by BAYLISS, LYTHGOE, and TANSLEY (1936) who, like KÖTTGEN and ABELSDORFF, employed the method of directly measured difference spectra. The presence of a mixture of vitamins A_1 and A_2 in the retinas of salmonids was shown by WALD (1941) who, in addition, extracted the photopigments and found results that he interpreted as indicating the presence of both rhodopsin and porphyropsin. The occurrence of a dual system in extracts of the retinas of rainbow trout was verified by BRIDGES (1956) who found one pigment with maximum at 507 nm and a second one with maximum at 533 nm. He concluded, without positive evidence, that these two were A_1- and A_2-based pigments respectively. The most careful and comprehensive study of salmonid visual pigments so far published is that of MUNZ and BEATTY (1965) who analyzed over 1,000 extracts, most of them prepared from individual fish so that some measure of specimen variability could be obtained. They employed five species of the genus *Oncorhynchus* and four species of *Salmo*. They used partial bleaching analysis and employed hydroxylamine to identify the nature of the prosthetic group. One of the species that they included was the rainbow trout (*Salmo gairdneri*) used previously by WALD (1941) and by BRIDGES (1956). Their results confirmed WALD's expectation of a dual mixture but, unlike the data of BRIDGES, the positions of maximum absorbance were at 503 and 527 nm. This pair of photopigments ($P503_1$ and $P527_2$) was found in all species of salmonids that they examined. A significant finding of this study was that the proportions of the two pigments varied considerably in individual fish ranging all the way from 0 to 100% $P527_2$. It is not possible at present to assign a reason for this extensive variability. MUNZ and BEATTY obtained their fishes either wild or from a hatchery. One obvious factor is the stage in the migration of the fish but this factor remains to be explored systematically. A further study of salmonid fishes, of several genera, has indicated the occurrence of photopigments at spectral locations other than 503 and 527 nm (BRIDGES and YOSHIKAMI, 1970c). In some fishes a pair of A_1-A_2-pigments was detected in the extracts; in other fishes the A_1- or A_2-pigment was found singly.

F. Genetics

The structure and properties of the opsin are basic to the spectral absorbance and other properties of a visual pigment. One would expect the nature of the opsin in a given species to be under genetic control in the same way that hemoglobin and other proteins are controlled. In the case of the retinal photopigments tracing out genetic relations may be facilitated because color is specifically related to the nature of the opsin. This fact was employed recently in some studies of the inheritance of visual pigments in hybrid fishes (MUNZ and McFARLAND, 1965; McFARLAND and MUNZ, 1965). In this study advantage was taken of the fact that the speckled or brook char (*Salvelinus fontinalis*) and the lake char (*Salvelinus namaycush*) were found to have two separate pairs of visual pigments: $P503_1-P527_2$ and $P512_1-P545_2$, respectively. Moreover, the artificially fertilized hybrid of these two species (the splake) was found to inherit both pairs. The analysis of four photopigments in an extract is an arduous and somewhat uncertain task, so in order to simplify the procedure they resorted to an analysis of the opsins, of which there were only two in the splake, one for each pair of visual pigments. This analysis was accomplished by adding 11-*cis* retinal to the bleached extract, thus regenerating two A_1-photopigments which could then be analyzed by the method of partial bleaching. In this way the opsin composition was determined in the F_1 splake, the F_2 splake and the backcross ($F_1 \times$ brook

char). Individual fish were examined and the genetic segregation of the two
opsins, as indicated by the $P503_1-512_1$ distribution (see Table 4 in Chapter 11,
p. 444), was followed. It will be seen that the regenerated pigments were the two
native A_1-pigments of the parent species. The data indicate a single factor
inheritance of the codominant type. This follows from the $1:2:1$ segregation of
the F_2 hybrids and the $1:1$ segregation of the backcross. The authors of this
important study suggested the possibility that the two opsins in the two species
of chars may differ by one amino acid in the primary structure. McFarland and
Munz found no evidence of sex linkage in the inheritance of the two opsins.

G. Double and Twin Cones

The double and twin cones of the higher bony fishes are so prominent a feature
of the retina that one tends intuitively to assign a special role in vision to these
receptors. There are reports of fishes in which single cones are said to be entirely
absent (O'Connell, 1963). One type of information that would be useful in
thinking of a role for these elements is the visual pigment composition. Do both
members contain the same or different photopigments? If different, how many
kinds of pairs are there? In the case of retinas that have triple cones, as in the
minnow, what is the photopigment composition of the three members? Obviously,
such questions cannot be answered by the method of extraction even if different
cone pigments were present and could be analyzed in extracts. There are some
indications that the two members of even twin cones are not alike biochemically.
Lyall (1957a) reported that the two members stained differently with
haematoxylin or Mallory. In the minnow retina the twin cones were found to be
aligned regularly in rows and in each row the positions of the two members
alternated from one twin to the next. A similar alternation of the two members
of double cones was found by Engström (1963a). Microspectrophotometry is the
only technique at present that gives hope of answering some of the questions
posed earlier in this paragraph. Marks (1965) has made a beginning in this
direction. Using the goldfish visual cells, Marks determined that there were three
types of single cones: one absorbing maximally at about 625 nm; a second, at
about 530 nm; and a third, at about 455 nm. These occurred in the ratios, $2:4:1$,
respectively, in the sample examined. Analyses made on 30 twin cones indicated
that 29 were red-green pairs and one was a blue-green pair. This is but a beginning
in the assignment of visual pigments to specific cell types but this, along with the
work of Liebman and Entine (1968), which has already been mentioned, gives
some reason to hope that a meaning may eventually be found for the orderly
mosaics so common in the retinas of teleosts and certain other vertebrates.

VIII. Amphibians

The amphibian stock is believed to have arisen from the Devonian rhipidistian
Crossopterygii. Modern amphibians are derived from aquatic tetrapods of the
Carboniferous and Triassic periods and are very different from the original fish-like
Devonian ancestors, yet in many characteristics they reveal their relationship to

their aquatic past. There are some 2,000 living species of amphibians in about 250 genera. These are grouped under three subclasses or orders as follows: (a) caecilians, (b) urodeles, (c) anurans.

A. The Caecilians

These are legless, burrowing, tropical and subtropical forms with small eyes. The visual cells have been identified as rods without oil-droplets (Walls, 1942b). No information exists about their visual pigments.

B. The Urodeles (Caudata) — Newts and Salamanders

These are the newts and salamanders, which in the adult stage retain the tailed, elongated, fish-like larval form. Varying degrees of terrestriality occur in urodeles though most live in or close to water or in a moist environment. Certain structures of the larval stage appear to be anachronistic, the tetrapod condition being one such. There is one large family, the Plethodontidae, that is characterized by complete lunglessness. Some urodeles omit the aquatic larval stage and pass on directly to the terrestrial form. Others, like the North American

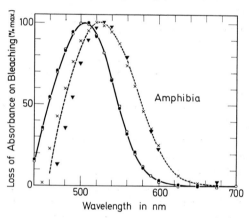

Fig. 11. Amphibian visual pigments. Spectral density losses following bleaching with red light (above 600 nm). Partial bleaching revealed the presence of only one photopigment, that shown by the curves, in each extract. Data are segregated into two groups: *Aquatic forms*; *Necturus maculosus* (interrupted line), *Diemictylus viridescens* adults (filled triangles), *Xenopus laevis* (crosses); *Terrestrial forms*; *Rana muscosa* (full line), *Bufo canorus* (plain circles), *Hyla cinerea* (filled circles). The curves for *Taricha torosa* and other terrestrial amphibia are not included in this figure to avoid confusion, but they agree with the rhodopsin assembly

Necturus and the European *Proteus*, are in the permanently aquatic and larval state. Terrestrial habitats are variable: cold and barren highlands; heavily forested tropical areas; arboreal, fossorial or semi-fossorial modes of life. There are salamanders that live in lightless caverns and appear to be almost blind as adults. Nearly all urodeles shun direct sunlight and are seldom found on a surface without ground cover.

The visual cells of urodeles, insofar as they have been studied, appear to be similar to the cells of anurans. Red rods are present, as are also single and double cones. Green rods have been described for some species. No oil-droplets are found in urodele visual cells although WALLS (1942b) mentioned the presence of paraboloids in the rods of *Necturus*. The *Necturus* visual cells, like those of other salamanders, are unique because of their relatively large diameters (HOWARD, 1908), a fact that explains their current use in electrophysiological studies.

No systematic investigation of the visual pigments of urodeles has been made. The limited information available suggests that both A_1- and A_2-based photopigments occur. The pigment of the neotenic *Necturus maculosus* (family Proteida) was examined by CRESCITELLI (1958a) who found, in retinal extracts, only one photosensitive component: a $P522_2$ (Fig. 11). In contrast with these results were the findings with the California newt, *Taricha torosa* (family Salamandridae). This newt lives in ponds and streams in the coastal region between Mendocino county and San Diego county. When the ponds dry up in summer it can, and does, survive on land. Adults of this newt were collected and extracts of the retinas were prepared and analyzed by the method of partial bleaching (CRESCITELLI, 1958a). A single photopigment, $P502_1$, was found in the extracts. Thus in these selected urodeles an A_2-based pigment was extracted from the retinas of the aquatic, larval-type *Necturus*, and an A_1-based pigment was similarly recovered from the more terrestrial, adult newt.

C. The Anurans (Salientia) — Frogs, Toads, etc.

This is a highly successful group comprising the frogs, toads and their relatives. These amphibians have lost the tail and have developed legs to become jumpers. They are found throughout temperate and tropical regions but are absent from snow-capped mountains, deserts and some islands of the Pacific. In general, anurans undergo a more extensive metamorphosis than do urodeles. The aquatic larvae change into adults, which in the various species show varying degrees of terrestriality. The true frogs (family Ranidae) have been especially valuable animals in studies of the retina. Various members of this family have served well in the pioneer studies of SCHULTZE, BOLL, KÜHNE, KRAUSE, LYTHGOE, WALD and others. The visual cells of frogs were discussed in section II, to which the reader is referred.

Of all amphibians, the visual pigments of adult anurans have received the most attention. In contrast to the spectroscopic diversity found in teleost fishes, the photopigments of adult anurans are remarkably constant. But for certain exceptions, all are A_1-based and all show a spectral absorbance maximal at 502 to 504 nm. The data of Figs. 11 and 20 summarize the present position with respect to these pigments. These rhodopsins, as they may be accurately called, have been found in the following anuran families: Discoglossidae (fire-bellies and midwives), Pelobatidae (the spade foots), Bufonidae (toads), Hylidae (tree frogs), Microhylidae (narrow-mouthed toads) and Ranidae (true frogs). An exception is the visual pigment extracted from the retina of the platanna (*Xenopus laevis*) which is an anuran in the family Pipidae (tongueless frogs). *Xenopus*, a native of South Africa, is aquatic even in the adult stage. The retina of *Xenopus* has been found to yield to extraction only a small amount of $P502_1$, the major pigment being one that absorbs maximally at 523 nm (Dartnall, 1954; Dartnall, 1956). I have shown this pigment to be a typical porphyropsin (Fig. 11). Wald (1955) demonstrated the presence of vitamin A_2 with a small amount of A_1 in the *Xenopus* retina. Thus in anurans, as in urodeles, the vitamin A_2 system is associated with the aquatic habitat. The adult form of *Xenopus* is somewhat enigmatic, for it is possible that the aquatic habit of the adult evolved secondarily *after* the evolution of a terrestrial form. This is the tentative view reached by Weisz (1945) on the basis of the early development of the lungs. This interpretation could mean that the porphyropsin of adult *Xenopus* was adopted secondarily and that the trace of $P502_1$ found by Dartnall could be a vestigial remnant of an ancestral condition. Perhaps it is wise to add a word of caution about the visual pigment situation in the genus *Xenopus*. Currently, I am exploring the retinal photopigments in extracts of *Xenopus mülleri*. The results suggest, provisionally at least, that the second pigment (λ_{max} about 500 nm) is not an A_1- but an A_2-pigment.

In addition to the red rods, anurans have a second type of rod (Fig. 2) known as the green or Schwalbe rod. This visual cell originally described by Schwalbe (1874) was further studied by Boll (1877) who observed that a minority of the frog rods was green, that these rods were bleached by light like the red rods, and that in the bleached state all rods looked the same. He questioned whether green and red rods were separate cell categories or whether they were different stages of the same cell. Kühne (1877; 1878) also observed these grass-green rods in the frog retina and found them to be, in certain respects, different from the red rods. Denton and Wyllie (1955) found the green rods of *Rana temporaria* to constitute 6—14% of the rods and to be bleached by blue light but not by green or red light; in other words, they behaved like blue-sensitive receptors. An important point was established by Donner and Rushton (1959) who determined that the green rods of the frog retina, like the red rods, and unlike the cones, showed little directional sensitivity (Stiles-Crawford effect). Finally, as shown in Fig. 2, Nilsson (1964a) pictured a number of morphological differences between the green rods and the other visual cells of the frog retina. Green rods appear to be characteristic of the amphibian retina. Boll (1877) attempted, without success, to find them in the retinas of certain mammals. I have not seen them described in any of the literature on vertebrate visual receptors except for amphibia. This does not mean, of course, that there are no blue-sensitive rods in other vertebrates, for, in fact, there may be. It simply means that the specific grass-green rods are an amphibian invention. The origin of the green color in these rods is still unexplained. Dartnall (1967) was unable to extract a red-absorbing pigment even though the photographs of Denton and Wyllie revealed the green color to be an objective phenomenon. The evidence so far merely indicates the presence somewhere in the green rods, other than the outer segments, of a pigment or physical structure that absorbs red-orange light. The outer segments are eliminated since Liebman and Entine (1968) obtained no evidence of such absorption in their microspectrophotometric study of the frog visual cells.

Several investigators (Dartnall, 1957; Donner and Reuter, 1962; Reuter, 1966) reported the presence, in frog retinal extracts, of a blue-sensitive component with maximum absorbance in the region 430—440 nm. These earlier reports are subject to several uncertainties among which is the possible isomerizing action of the second light treatment on the products formed after the rhodopsin was bleached out by the inital exposure to light. DARTNALL (1967) was aware of these uncertainties when he undertook the analysis of the green-rod photopigment of the crab-eating frog (*Rana cancrivora*). He made use of the fact, discovered by REUTER (1966), that the green-rod pigment, like certain other visual pigments, is specially sensitive to hydroxylamine, and bleaches in its presence to form the oxime. Frog rhodopsin, as is well known, is not so bleached by the usual concentrations of hydroxylamine employed in these analyses. In this way DARTNALL was able to effect a clear separation of the green-rod pigment from the rhodopsin and, along with the results of photobleaching in the absence of isomerization, to place the spectral absorbance maximum of the green-rod pigment at 433 nm. When account was taken of the *in situ* density of $P433_1$ the spectral absorption of this pigment was shown to account for the spectral sensitivity curve of DONNER and REUTER (1962). The final touch about this green-rod pigment was applied by LIEBMAN and ENTINE (1968) who found a $P432_1$ in the green rods of *Rana pipiens*. They showed that the *in situ* density per unit length of outer segment was the same as for rhodopsin, that the pigment *in situ*, like rhodopsin, was linearly dichroic, and that the photosensitivities were about the same for $P432_1$ and $P502_1$.

The role of the green rods in amphibian vision is unknown. MUNTZ (1962, 1964b) suggested that amphibia with green rods use them in a hue-discriminating capacity. First, he reported that the optic nerve fibres to the dorsal thalamus mediate blue-specific on-responses. Next, he demonstrated the presence of blue-specific, positive phototactic behavior in *Rana temporaria*. MUNTZ considered these reactions to blue to be of ecological significance in terms of directing the frog to water when it is disturbed at the edge of a pond or pool. A similar biologically adaptive positive response to blue was adduced to explain the seaward movements of green turtles and loggerhead turtles after hatching (HOOKER, 1911; CARR, 1965). The idea that green rods mediate information about hue weakens one of the tenets of the duplexity theory upheld since the time of SCHULTZE. To my knowledge no one yet has reported the presence of blue-absorbing cones in the amphibian retina. In their study of the visual cells of *Rana pipiens* LIEBMAN and ENTINE (1968) made no mention of such cones. It will be pointed out in a later section that geckos probably have rods with a blue-absorbing photopigment.

D. Visual Pigments and Metamorphosis

Amphibia have a complicated life cycle in which an aquatic larva is transformed to an adult, more or less adapted to the terrestrial habitat. The most complete form of metamorphosis is displayed in anurans in which a fish-like larval animal is progressively altered in morphology by resorption of the tail, emergence and growth of limbs, widening of the mouth, reconstruction of the gut, alterations of the skin and respiratory system, and other changes; all leading to the adult terrestrial form. Underlying these obvious morphological transformations are many biochemical and molecular alterations, which include the transition of larval to adult hemoglobin, the synthesis of such serum proteins as albumen, ceruloplasmin, etc., the formation of enzyme systems, and the transition from a ureotelic to an ammonotelic type of nitrogen excretion (FRIEDEN, 1967; COHEN, 1966). Meta-morphosis in urodeles is of shorter duration and is less complete than in anurans. The tail is not lost and the anachronistic limbs of the larva suffer no major alter-ations; instead metamorphosis is largely restricted to certain skin changes and to reduction of the external gills and the tail fin. ETKIN (1964) expressed the view that the urodele type of metamorphosis is perhaps the more primitive. In fact, some urodeles do not metamorphose and reproduction is neotenic, as in the genus *Necturus* and its European relative, *Proteus*. Some writers (NOBLE, 1931) have interpreted metamorphosis as reflecting in living forms what took place when the first vertebrates adapted themselves to the terrestrial mode of life. In fact, SCHMALHAUSEN (1968) noted the similarity in larval development of urodeles to that of the extinct Stegocephalia as shown by the fossil remains of larval stages of such forms as the branchiosaurian, *Tungussogyrinus*.

For these reasons knowledge of the visual pigments during metamorphosis in various amphibian groups would be of biological interest, although only a begin-ning in this direction has been made. It was first suggested by WALD (1945) that the bullfrog (*Rana catesbeiana*) undergoes a porphyropsin to rhodopsin transition in metamorphosis. This conclusion was based on the finding of a predominant vitamin A_2 content in the tadpole retina and a predominant vitamin A_1 content for the retina of the newly transformed adult. In addition, the extract of the tad-pole retina had a spectral absorbance maximal at 516 nm, intermediate in position to rhodopsin and porphyropsin. Using the method of partial bleaching, CRESCI-TELLI (1958a) carried out a complete pigment analysis of the bullfrog retina during metamorphosis. From the retina of the adult a single A_1-based, light-sensitive component with maximum at 503 was found (Fig. 12). A similar analysis of extracts of tadpole retinas showed the presence of a red-sensitive A_2-based pigment with maximum at about 525 nm and a smaller amount of the P 503_1. The ratio of densities (P 525_2: P 503_1) was 7.3:1. WALD's conclusion was therefore confirmed. A similar pigment transition was found to occur in the tree frog, *Hyla regilla* during metamorphosis. Adult tree frogs, two years after metamorphosis, were shown to possess only rhodopsin: P 504_1 (Fig. 13). *Hyla* tadpoles, however, were found to have a dual system, P 523_2 and P 504_1, the ratio of the two pigments varying with larval development. Animals in the stage before limb emergence (in prometamorphosis) yielded extracts that contained only P 523_2. Animals with hind limbs in various stages of development (still prometamorphosis) yielded results showing, on an optical-density basis, 83% porphyropsin and 17% rhodop-sin. When all four limbs had formed but with the tail still present, retinal extracts had increased their rhodopsin content to 25—40% of the total photopigment density. Finally, tadpoles with the tail completely, or almost completely resorbed, were revealed to have a composition consisting of 62 % P 504_1 and 38 % P 523_2. The trend is clear: metamorphosis in these amphibians is associated with a change-over of visual pigment class, from a larval A_2-based system, to an adult A_1-based pigment. LIEBMAN and ENTINE (1968) demonstrated that this change-over takes place in all the visual cells, cones as well as rods, of *Rana pipiens*. This view of a pigment change during metamorphosis has not gone uncontested. Using tadpoles and adults of *Rana temporaria* and *Rana esculenta*, COLLINS, LOVE, and MORTON (1953) concluded that rhodopsin was a constituent of both tadpoles and adults.

This conclusion was based on the spectral absorbance curves and no analyses by partial bleaching were carried out to test the homogeneity of the composition. DARTNALL (1962) expressed the opinion that the conclusion of COLLINS, LOVE, and MORTON was not justified on the basis of the absorbance curves that were published. A later study with *Rana temporaria* by MUNTZ and REUTER (1966) revealed the tadpole of this species to have a dual system: $P523_2$ and $P502_1$. Both pigments were reported to be present in very young tadpoles but during the metamorphic climax $P502_1$ rapidly replaced $P523_2$. It is doubtful, therefore, whether the conclusion of COLLINS, LOVE, and MORTON (1953) has seriously weakened the genera-

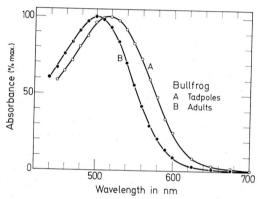

Fig. 12. Visual pigments during metamorphosis of the bullfrog, *R. catesbeiana*. These are spectral absorbance curves of retinal extracts for the tadpoles (*A*) and for the adults (*B*). Partial bleaching analyses revealed the presence in the extracts of only one photopigment, $P\,503_1$, for the adults and of two pigments, $P\,525_2$ and $P\,503_1$, in the ratio of 7.3 to 1 (on a density basis), for the tadpoles

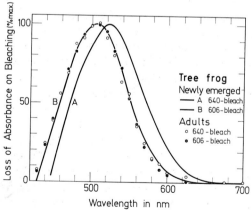

Fig. 13. Visual pigments during metamorphosis of the tree frog, *Hyla regilla*. Curve *A* (*full line*); normalized spectral density loss for a retinal extract of just metamorphosed (newly emerged) tree frogs after a bleaching with light at 640 nm. Curve *B* (*full line*); normalized spectral density loss in same extract after bleaching with light at 606 nm following the exposure to 640 nm. The filled and plain circles are similar results obtained with an extract from adult tree frogs. The filled circles represent the density loss for an initial bleaching with light at 640 nm, the plain circles show the result for the 606-bleaching that followed

lization of an A_2-to A_1-metamorphic change-over in the Ranidae, at least under the normal conditions of temperature, food, etc. to which these frogs are usually exposed.

The case is apparently different for the Bufonidae. Only rhodopsin was reported to be present in tadpoles and adults of *Bufo vulgaris* by Collins, Love, and Morton (1953), but they employed the same type of evidence as in the case of *Rana temporaria* and this, as indicated above, is inadequate to reveal the true composition of the extracts. In the event, however, their conclusion was confirmed for *Bufo boreas halophilus* (Crescitelli, 1958a) and for *Bufo bufo* (Muntz

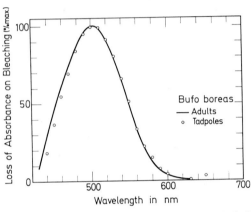

Fig. 14. Visual pigments during metamorphosis of the toad, *Bufo boreas*. Spectral density loss curves as a result of bleaching a retinal extract from adults (*full line*) and one from tadpoles (*plain circles*). Only rhodopsin (502_1) was found in both adults and tadpoles. This result can be contrasted with the data from the tree frog (Fig. 13) because both species of tadpoles were collected from the same pond at the same time

and Reuter, 1966) in analyses that cannot be as easily disputed. Crescitelli (1958a) obtained tadpoles of *Bufo boreas halophilus* from the same pond that had served as the source of the aforementioned tree frogs. The two species were at about the same stage of development when collected and were subject to identical conditions and food supply before being brought to the laboratory. After separating the two species, which was not difficult because their body movements were quite different, the toads were segregated into two major categories: (a) early larvae with no limbs and (b) larvae with tails and with hind limbs in various stages of growth. Extracts of the eyes revealed, even in the early tadpoles, only one pigment and that P 502_1 (Fig. 14). This result was especially convincing because the companion tree frogs treated and analyzed in the same manner displayed the presence of the A_2-system (Fig. 13). A similar conclusion was reached by Muntz and Reuter (1966) with another bufonid, *Bufo bufo*. Only a rash investigator would make a generalization on the basis of this limited evidence but the question is useful in terms of future inquiries: are the bufonid anurans unique in lacking the A_2-A_1 metamorphic transition found in the Ranidae and the Hylidae? Reuter (1969) has expressed the view that the presence of porphyropsin in tadpoles of *Rana temporaria* is, as in freshwater fishes, an adaptation to the photic environment. This may be, but there is still the straightforward observation that bufonid tadpoles lack porphyropsin. In my analyses (CRESCITELLI, 1958a) the tree-frog tadpoles and the toad tadpoles were derived from the same pond at the same time. Yet the toad tadpoles had $P 502_1$ while the tadpoles of the tree frog yielded $P 523_2$. REUTER (1969) cited a possible difference in microenvironment to explain this discrepancy between ranid and bufonid larvae but such an explanation requires, certainly, a level of quantitative information about the habits and habitats of frog and toad tadpoles that we presently do not possess.

The visual pigment situation in urodeles during metamorphosis is virtually unexplored even though these amphibians may have, as already indicated, a special significance in terms of phylogeny. The newt, *Diemyctylus viridescens*, has a type of metamorphosis in which, under some conditions, an aquatic larva passes into a red eft which is the adult terrestrial form. Following this the newt reenters the water as an adult aquatic form. The retinal vitamin A was examined by WALD (1958a) who concluded that vitamin A_1 was the major component of the eft and A_2 predominated in the aquatic adult, another example, according to WALD, of a terrestrial-A_1 and aquatic-A_2 association. I have extracted the visual pigment from the adult aquatic newt (Fig. 11) but attempts to extract the photopigment from the red eft have been unsatisfactory.

IX. Reptiles

Characteristically, reptiles have evolved a terrestrial mode of life, going further in this direction than the most terrestrial of amphibia. Reptiles probably have an amphibian ancestry; a fossil form, *Seymouria*, a cotylosaur found in the lower Permian of Texas suggests something of this ancestry. This animal, in its osteology, was so similar to the early stegocephalian amphibians that it has been a problem to make a true distinction. Whatever their specific origins, reptiles evolved rapidly throughout the Permian, Triassic, Jurassic and Cretaceous periods flowering eventually into the Dinosaurs of the Jurassic and Cretaceous. It is supposed that between the end of the Cretaceous and the Eocene there occurred a climatic change unfavorable to the then-existing forms. Whatever the specific nature of this change, the Dinosaurs and certain other reptiles gradually died out and disappeared. Living reptiles comprise but four of the twelve or so lines of reptiles that have existed on earth. They are the sole remnants of a once highly diversified and dominant form of life. Modern reptiles stem from four distinct evolutionary lines: (a) the Squamata or lizards and snakes, (b) *Sphenodon*, the tuatara of New Zealand, which is the single survivor of an order, the Rhyncocephalia that has existed since the Triassic, (c) the crocodiles, related to the archaic stock from which modern birds evolved, and (d) the Chelonia, turtles and tortoises which, retain a number of ancestral reptilian characteristics.

In general, reptiles inhabit the warmer regions of the planet. All are basically terrestrial, although the water habitat has been adopted in part by some turtles, crocodiles and some snakes. Reptiles tend to be active, diurnal animals often seeking the open sun and bright light, although crepuscular and nocturnal species do occur and will form an important portion of this section. Reptiles are found in hot, dry regions that are inimical to other form of life. They have done well in the tropics and in the lush forests of the tropics.

It is not surprising that the reptilian eye should present so many features related to diurnal vision. In the lacertilian eye, for example, the striated ciliary muscle, the scleral ossicles, the ringwulst of the lens, all represent adaptations for an efficient method of accommodation required in a diurnal, warm environment where rapid invasive and evasive responses are matters of life and death. The rapid pupillary movement is a similar adaptation. The snake eye, including the retina, is an enigma, and not all investigators agree on the origin of this unique ophidian organ. It is generally agreed that snakes have a lacertilian ancestry, possibly by way of the monitor lizards. Yet the snake eye displays features quite unlike those of the lizard eye. Missing are the scleral ossicles, the ringwulst, and the powerful ciliary muscle of lizards. The eye is spherical, the iris is apparently involved in accommodation, the cones have neither oil droplets nor paraboloids, a yellow lens is sometimes present in diurnal snakes, and there are several other differences listed by WALLS (1942b). One hypothesis that attempts to account for this non-lacertilian eye in snakes is that of WALLS (1942b) which states that the ophidian ancestral forms, related to lizards, became fossorial and this led to a degeneration of the eye. Modern snakes evolved from these fossorial forms, which eventually left the underground environment for the surface. The eye then became reconstituted but along a novel ophidian line that led to the unique eye of modern snakes. According to WALLS, the ophidian eye is not like the eye of a legless lizard, and neither is the retina. The two reptilian forms are phylogenetically distinct, and the visual cells, as will be shown, support this thesis.

A. Rhyncocephalia — Sphenodon

This single surviving member of the order Rhyncocephalia is another living fossil, its ancestry going back to the Mesozoic. The tuatara (*Sphenodon punctatum*), is a slit-pupilled, nocturnal reptile whose retina and visual cells are somewhat enigmatic for an animal with nocturnal habit. There is a shallow fovea and the receptors, called rods by WALLS (1942b) and cones by VILTER (1951b, c, d), include a standard single element, a fine single element, and a double element (Fig. 4b). Colorless oil-droplets are present both in single rods and in one member of the double rods. The true identity of these cells is therefore obscure. They possess oil-droplets, a characteristic of cones, but the outer segments are enlarged and cylindrical in form. WALLS (1942b) interpreted these *Sphenodon* visual cells as being derived from ancestral cones. WALLS also reported the presence, in the retina of the tuatara, of a droplet-free dwarf cone. These cells, which were very few in number, were considered by VILTER (1951b) to be receptors in process of growth. The retina of *Sphenodon* is so interesting it is unfortunate no information is available yet on the visual pigment content.

B. Chelonia — Turtles and Tortoises

The turtle and tortoise retinas have often been assumed to be rod-free, and physiologists sometimes have interpreted their results on this assumption. This idea appears to stem from SCHULTZE (1873) who considered that the retinas of all reptiles were "exclusively composed of cones" and who doubted the claims of HULKE (1863 — 65) who believed that both rods and cones occurred in *Testudo graeca* and *Chelonia mydas*. More recently, DETWILER (1916) concluded that the retinas of the tortoises, *Clemmys insculptus*, *Clemmys guttata* and *Chrysemys picta* contained no rods, confirming earlier workers who had made similar claims. These claims of rod-free chelonian retinas may be true for certain diurnal species but in several photophobic species rods have been reported to occur (WALLS, 1942b, DETWILER, 1943). UNDERWOOD (1970) gives a figure of 40% of the single cells as rods in *Chelydra serpentina* and 25% in *Emydoidea blandingii*. The visual cell composition of *Chelydra serpentina* includes a standard single cone, a fine single cone, a double cone and a cell, called a rod by WALLS (1942b), that has a paraboloid but whose outer segment is rod-like (Fig. 4B). The single cones and one member of the double cones show oil-droplets: colorless or colored (red, orange or yellow).

Several attempts have been made to extract photopigments out of the retinas of turtles or tortoises but the results have been either negative (KÖTTGEN and ABELSDORF, 1896; WALD, BROWN, and SMITH, 1953) or inconclusive. There is the claim by von STUDNITZ (1937) of the successful extraction of a cone photopigment from the retina of *Testudo graeca* but, as BLISS (1946) pointed out, this claim rests on unconvincing evidence because of the minuteness of the effect in relation to the sensitivity of the method that was employed. Several spectral peaks of density loss after bleaching were reported to occur in visual cell extracts prepared from the tortoise (HOSOYA, OKITA, and AKUNE, 1938; KIMURA and HOSOYA, 1956). No evidence for rhodopsin was obtained and the density losses after bleaching were related to possible cone pigments. As KIMURA and HOSOYA (1956) pointed out, however, the peaks were inconstant and the solutions unstable, making the prospect of identifying photopigments an uncertain one. I have repeatedly encountered this difficulty with extracts of turtle or tortoise retinas. For the demonstration of the chelonian rod pigment it well may be that the appropriate species has yet to be found.

Nevertheless, there are some data, preliminary though they may be, that suggest that both A_1- and A_2-photopigments exist in chelonia. The presence of vitamin A_2 was indicated for the retinas of *Pseudemys scripta* and *Pseudemys mobilensis* (WALD, BROWN, SMITH, 1953). Coupled with this is the recent reference to some unpublished data (LIEBMAN and ENTINE, 1967) suggesting the presence in the retina of the swamp turtle, *Pseudemys scripta*, of cones with a P 620_2. In the sea turtle, *Chelonia mydas*, however, an A_1-based pigment was found, i.e., P562_1. LIEBMAN and GRANDA (1971) have published what is presently the most comprehensive study of visual pigments in Chelonia. Some of their results, tentative at present, await chemical verification. Using single cell microspectrophotometry, LIEBMAN and GRANDA came to the following conclusions: (a) The marine turtle, *Chelonia mydas*, has an A_1-system while the freshwater *Pseudemys scripta* has an A_2-system of retinal photopigments. Thus WALD's generalization about the freshwater-A_2 association and the marine-A_1 association has been extended beyond the fishes and amphibia to the reptiles. (b) The pigments of *Chelonia* include the rod pigment P502_1 and the cone pigments, P440_1, P502_1 and P562_1. The pigments of *Pseudemys* consist of P518_2 in rods, and P450_2, P518_2 and P620_2 in cones. The striking feature in these data is that the classical rod pigments, rhodopsin and porphyropsin, were also found in cones. This repeats the situation previously reported for *Rana pipiens* (LIEBMAN and ENTINE, 1968). Additionally, it may be said that iodopsin occurs in *Chelonia* and cyanopsin occurs in *Pseudemys*. The occurrence in chelonia of several pigment systems, is supported by several studies of the spectral sensitivity of the turtle and tortoise eyes. These studies are deficient in some respects, one being the failure to account for the light absorption by the colored oil-droplets. Nevertheless, in a general way they indicate the types of spectral mechanisms that may occur in these animals. Using *Pseudemys scripta*, ARMINGTON (1954) obtained evidence for at least two possible spectral mechanisms: (a) a scotopic mechanism with a maximum at about 525 nm, revealed by means of a behavior response and (b) another in the red, detected by means of the ERG. With other freshwater turtles, including *Pseudemys*, the ERG technique was employed, and results were obtained that were interpreted to indicate a mechanism in the red, 640 to 650 nm, and three other less well-defined mechanisms at 605 to 640 nm, 560 to 590 nm and in the blue-green region (DEANE, ENROTH-CUGEL, GONGAWARE, NEYLAND, and FORBES, 1958). Confirmation of this result was provided later by GRANDA (1962) and GRANDA and STIRLING (1966) who claimed the possible existence of mechanisms at 640—650 nm, at about 575 nm and again in the blue-green. The possible presence of a system in the red and another at 420 to 500 nm was suggested for *Chrysemys picta picta* by SOKOL and MUNTZ (1966) who employed a behavioral response on the part of the turtle. Probably the most convincing study demonstrating a red-sensitive system is that of GRANIT (1955) who obtained the dominator sensitivity curve of the tortoise, *Testudo graeca*, and found it to be in good agreement with the cyanopsin (P 620_2) curve of WALD, BROWN, and SMITH (1953). In addition, there is the possibility of a second system at 540 nm in the Greek tortoise (GRANIT, 1941). The chelonian retina is certainly worthy of further study, especially with respect to accounting for the effects of the oil-droplets.

C. Lizards

1. Diurnal Lizards

The retinas of diurnal lizards conform to the expectations of the duplexity theory. A fovea is present and this is often of the deep, convexiclivate type. Cones are numerous or exclusively present (ROCHON-DUVIGNEAUD, 1917; DETWILER and LAURENS, 1920) and in these, yellow oil-droplets are common. The visual cells of *Anolis lineatopus* (Fig. 4b) may serve as examples to characterize the situation in the retinas of diurnal lizards. There is seen a standard single cone with yellow oil-droplet and a paraboloid, a small single cone with colorless oil-droplet and a paraboloid, a double cone with unequal members, one member having the yellow oil-droplet, the second member without oil-droplet but with a prominent paraboloid. The outer segments are all slender. Occasionally triple cells are seen. The double cells, as seen in tangential section, are arranged in horizontal rows with the two dissimilar members located alternately one above the other in zig-zag fashion. Both a central and a temporal fovea occur. This account of the *Anolis* receptors is applicable to other diurnal lizards, although the small single cones have not been seen in all retinas, in fact they are missing in WALLS' comprehensive accounts (WALLS, 1942a 1942b). There are no rods reported for the retina of *Anolis* and for the retinas of other diurnal lizards.

It is not surprising, therefore, that no success has been achieved in extracting the visual pigments of these reptiles. Although he saw the yellow color of the oil-droplets, KÜHNE (1877) was unable to see Sehpurpur in the retinas of the lizards that he examined. He used this apparent absence to support his concept of "Sehen ohne Sehpurpur", which he associated with cones. BLISS (1946) tried, without success, to extract photopigments out of 50 retinas of the fence lizard, *Sceloporus*. During the past ten years I have been equally unsuccessful in attempts to extract the visual pigments of a number of species of diurnal lizards. To my knowledge the microspectrophotometric technique has not been applied to lizard cones; these cells are rather slender and not favorable for such measurements.

Lizard spectral sensitivity curves have been derived from measurements with the ERG and these curves suggest the presence of multiple spectral systems in the retinas of these animals. As in turtles these curves are complex and uncertain for several reasons, especially with respect to the effect of the colored oil-droplets. The spectral sensitivity of two species of *Sceloporus* and of the collared lizard, *Crotaphytus collaris* was found to be double-peaked with one maximum at 560—565 nm and the second at about 580 nm (FORBES, FOX, MILBURN, and DEANE, 1960). A resemblance to the spectral absorbance of iodopsin was believed to exist. The sensitivity for the horned toad, *Phrynosoma* sp., was somewhat similar except for a greater sensitivity at shorter wavelengths, i.e., in the region of blue-green. A rather different result was obtained by HAMASAKI (1968) with the green iguana, *Iguana iguana*. HAMASAKI showed evidence for the presence in the retina of two mechanisms, which were partially isolated by selective adaptation. One system, with maximal sensitivity at about 600 nm, was isolated by adaptation to white or to green light, the curve so isolated being in reasonable agreement, except at 480—500 nm, with the DARTNALL nomogram-derived curve for a 600-pigment. The second mechanism, with maximum at about 530 nm, was more difficult to isolate and when so isolated, by the technique of adaptation to light at 630 nm, showed poor agreement with either 530- or 540-curves derived from the nomogram. It is of more than passing interest to note that the spectral mechanisms are apparently different for the parietal and lateral eyes of lizards. HAMASAKI (1969) noted such a difference for the green iguana and a difference was previously found for *Lacerta sicula campestris* (DODT and SCHERER, 1967, 1968).

2. Nocturnal Lizards

Apparently, SCHULTZE did not examine the visual cells of nocturnal lizards but had he done so he certainly would have discovered their prominent rod-like visual cells. Of nocturnal lizards the gekkonid forms have become especially important for reasons that will become apparent. Many geckos, but not all, are either nocturnal or crepuscular in habit and require a retina with high sensitivity. HULKE (1863—65) published drawings of gecko visual cells that are obviously inaccurate in terms of present knowledge but clearly portrayed the large cylindrical outer segments. HEINEMANN (1877) noticed the regular arrangement of what he thought to be thick and thin cells in two species of geckos. The outer segments were pictured as rod-shaped, and he was unable to distinguish rods and cones. The visual receptors of *Hemidactylus* were considered by Krause (1893) to consist of rods, with long, cylindrical outer segments, alternating with double cones. He observed the deep extension of the pigment epithelium in between the outer segments, and most interesting was his description of the Sehpurpur which he characterized as being violet-red rather than just red. A more accurate description of the visual cells of a nocturnal gecko was given by Rochon-Duvigneaud (1917) who characterized the retina as being pure-rod in composition, with single rods alternating with double rods, all the cells being of the same length. Detwiler added further information by describing the visual cells of *Gekko swinhonis* from China as made up of single rods alternating with double rods in a pattern in which a row of doubles alternated with a row of singles (Detwiler, 1923). Detwiler

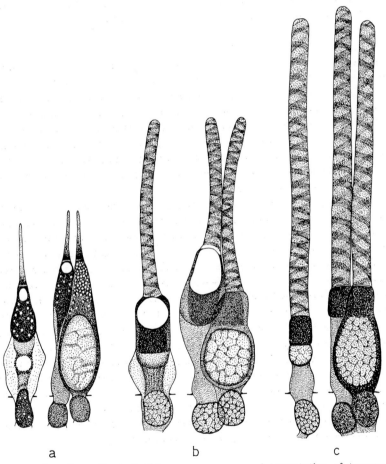

a   b   c

Fig. 15. The *Crotaphytus-Xantusia-Coleonyx* sequence, an interpretation of transmutation (Walls, 1942a). (a) *Crotaphytus collaris*: single and double cones with yellow oil-droplets and very small outer segments, no visual pigment extracted out of this retina. (b) *Xantusia riversiana*, a nocturnal lizard; outer segments are larger and oil-droplets are colorless, no visual pigment extracted. (c) *Coleonyx variegatus*, a nocturnal gecko; very large outer segments, no oil-droplets, visual pigment is not rhodopsin but P516$_1$

described the single rod outer segments as longer and slenderer than the outer segments of the double rods. He made the error of interpreting the double cells as single cells each with two outer segments. Nothing like this occurs in geckos, nor in any other vertebrate. DETWILER also mentioned the presence of a pink photolabile pigment, and noted the inward migration of the epithelial pigment after light adaptation.

A complete description of the gecko visual cells was made by WALLS (1934) who used the nocturnal, banded gecko, *Coleonyx variegatus* for his study. Once more the presence of single and double rods was confirmed (Fig. 15). The outer segments were seen to be long and cylindrical, a paraboloid was noted to be present in the single rod and in one member of the double rods. The double rods were clearly pictured as two complete cells fused together over part of their length. WALLS made two statements that have proved to be incorrect. He believed gecko visual cells to lack oil-droplets and to possess rhodopsin.

3. Uroplatidae and Pygopodidae

There are two groups of lizards that, though differing in some respects from geckos, have strong affinities to the gekkonid lizards. The uroplatids, which comprise one genus (*Uroplatus*) with three species, look like geckos, have a *Gekko* type pupil, and share many characteristics in common with geckos (UNDERWOOD, 1954). They differ, however, with respect to certain osteological details of the skull. I know of no published work on the visual cells of uroplatids and I have not succeeded yet in securing living animals for a visual pigment analysis. The presence of *Gekko*-type visual cells and visual pigments would argue in favour of including them within the gekkonid lizards.

The pygopodids are the legless lizards of the Australian region comprising eight genera and fourteen species. These lizards, without forelimbs and with only a trace of hind limbs, are nocturnal and most of them are fossorial. The pupil is vertical, a spectacle covers the cornea, and in other respects the pygopodid eye is lacertilian in character (UNDERWOOD, 1957). The visual cells of three species have been examined (O'DAY, 1940; UNDERWOOD, 1968) and the results appear to indicate a reptilian retina with some gekkonid characteristics. No oil-droplets have been seen in any of the cells which include, as do the cells of *Anolis*, *Chelydra* and *Sphenodon*, a standard single cell, a smaller single cell and a type B double cell. No type C double cell, as in geckos, was found. The outer segments were found to be intermediate between the slender, cone-shaped outer segments of *Anolis*, and the bulky, cylindrical outer segments of the nocturnal geckos. The similarity to the gekkonid retina is in the pattern of visual cells in rows, in which the type B double cells alternate with rows of single cells, and in which the two members of each type B double cell alternate in zig-zag fashion along each row of doubles. The nature of the visual pigment in pygopodids is not known.

D. Lizards and the Transmutation Theory of Walls

1. Visuals Cells and Transmutation

The most novel outcome of WALLS' studies was the interpretation of an homologous relationship of the *Coleonyx* single and double rods to the respective single and double cones of the diurnal lizard (*Crotaphytus collaris*), and to the single and double cells of the nocturnal *Xantusia riversiana*. This homology of visual cells in three species (Fig. 15) suggested to WALLS a systematic evolutionary relationship, a phylogenetic transmutation of visual cell types. According to this hypothesis the cones of *Crotaphytus*, the intermediate cells of *Xantusia* and the rods of *Coleonyx* form a series in three extant species that illustrate the stages in phylogenetic evolution through which a rod may have gone in evolving from a cone of its diurnal ancestral form. In this evolution the outer segments were conceived by WALLS to have become elongated, thickened and increased in volume, thus increasing the quantum-capturing capacity. The oil-droplets, originally yellow, as in diurnal lizards, lost the color and then disappeared entirely. The double rod was not formed *de novo* but arose through an evolution of the ancestral double cone, a cell type so common in living diurnal reptiles. The paraboloid still remains (in *Coleonyx*) where it serves as an indicator of phylogenetic history. This, in brief, is the speculation by WALLS known as the transmutation theory. This theory does not deny nor conflict with the duplexity theory; it attempts to explain the phylogenetic origin of the rods and cones. In some cases, as we shall see, it saves the duplexity theory from apparently contradictory positions.

WALLS expressed some disappointment that geckos, whose rods he considered to be prime examples of transmutation, should in their visual cells lack oil-droplets, as if this lack weakened his case for transmutation. He need not have been concerned, for in due time UNDERWOOD (1951) discovered, oil-droplet-bearing visual cells in several species of geckos, (Fig. 16). Pale yellow droplets were seen in the pure cone retina of *Gonatodes fuscus*. Colorless droplets were found in the rod-shaped cells of *Aristelliger praesignis*. No oil-droplets were observed in *Sphaerodactylus argus* (which has short outer segments), *Sphaerodactylus parkeri* (which has longer outer segments) and *Phyllodactylus tuberculosis* (which has long cylindrical outer segments). Another apparent sign of diurnal ancestry in geckos was discovered by UNDERWOOD (1951) in *Gonatodes fuscus*, *Sphaerodactylus argus*, and *Sphaerodactylus parkeri*. This was the presence of a temporal fovea; this would represent in *S. parkeri* another example of a fovea in a cone-free retina. Examining sections of the gecko retina, especially tangential sections, UNDERWOOD made another discovery, that of another type of double cell. This was a unique gecko-type double, which he named the type C double. It is illustrated for *Aristelliger* in Fig. 16. Using UNDERWOOD's designations, one sees the type A single rod, the type B double rod, with two highly asymmetric members, and the new type C double rod containing nearly equally-sized members, each having a paraboloid. The visual cells form a beautiful pattern (Figs., 17 and 18) in which a horizontal row of type B doubles alternates with a row containing both type A singles and type C doubles. In each row of type B doubles the chief and accessory members regularly alternate in position to form a zig-zag array, much as was discussed in connection with the linear arrays in the teleost retina. UNDERWOOD estimated the nasal portion of the *Aristelliger* retina to contain 50% type B doubles, 30% type A singles and 20% type C doubles. The type C doubles are not occasional cell types, and UNDERWOOD recorded their presence in all species of geckos that he examined. In addition to these three prominent cell types, twin cells, triple cells and other multiple cells have been reported to occur in the retinas of various geckos (UNDERWOOD, 1951; DUNN, 1965).

The transmutation theory of WALLS (1934) not only proposed the phylogenetic transformation of cones to rods in animal forms that were forced to adopt the nocturnal habit, but, additionally, it suggested the occurrence of a reverse trans-

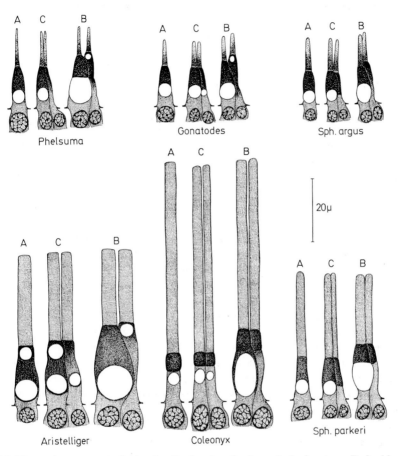

Fig. 16. The gecko sequence of visual cells showing the type A singles, type B doubles and type C doubles as pictured by UNDERWOOD. *Phelsuma cepediana*: diurnal gecko with all-cone retina; the oil-droplet is lacking in the type A and type C cones but is present in one member of the type B doubles. *Gonatodes albogularis*: visual cells are all cones and only one member of the type B doubles has a typical oil-droplet which is colorless. *Sphaerodactylus argus*: visual cells are still cone-like but larger than the cells of *Phelsuma*, there is no oil-droplet, and no photopigment was found in retinal extracts. *Aristelliger praesignis*: outer segments are rods but a colorless oil-droplet is found in the type A and in one member of the type B and type C doubles. An A_1-photopigment with maximum at about 530 nm was found in retinal extracts but the cell in which this occurs is not known. *Coleonyx variegatus*: typical rods with long, cylindrical outer segments, no oil droplets, although a paraboloid (granular or membranous) is found in the type A, both members of type C and one member of type B doubles. A $P 516_1$ was extracted from this retina but the cell of origin is not known. *Sphaerodytylus parkeri*: outer segments are tall and cylindrical, typically rod-like and no oil-droplets are present. An A_1-photopigment with maximum absorbance at about 528 nm was found in retinal extracts, also evidence for a second pigment absorbing at shorter wavelengths. Information for this figure and legend was obtained from the writings of WALLS, UNDERWOOD, DUNN, TANSLEY, and CRESCITELLI as cited previously

mutation of rods back to cones, a tertiary change as Walls termed it, apparently considering the evolution of the cones as the primary process. Walls named certain round-pupilled, diurnal geckos, e.g., *Phelsuma* and *Lygodactylus*, as having gone through such a tertiary change. The *Phelsuma* retina was recently examined by Tansley (1964) who found a pure cone retina with outer segments that were

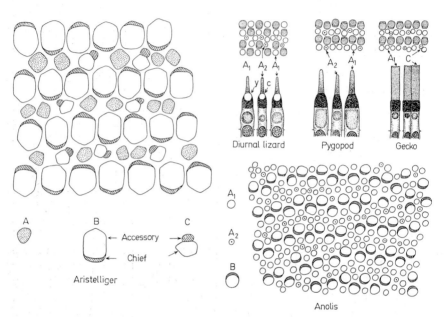

Fig. 17. Mosaic arrangements of visual cells in lizards. Left side illustrates the typical gecko array with rows of type B doubles alternating with rows constituted of type A singles and type C doubles. In each row of type B doubles the chief and accessory members alternate with each other in zig-zag fashion. In the pygopodid retina (*Lialis*) the two members of the type B rows alternate in the same manner but the rows in between the type B rows consist only of type A_1 and A_2 singles since there are no type C doubles in *Lialis*. The visual cells of diurnal lizards (*Anolis*) are arrayed somewhat differently for in each row of type B doubles the chief and accessory members do not zig-zag, gecko fashion, but each member is placed on the same side. But when one row of type B doubles is compared with its two neighboring rows on both sides, the two members are seen to be arrayed alternately, in other words an inter-row, rather than an intra-row, zig-zag alignment. The basis for this figure was in the drawings and descriptions of Underwood as cited in the text

observed to be very fine. Compared to the retina of the more nocturnal *Hemi-dactylus*, the bipolar and ganglion cell numbers were more like those of a diurnal retina. The lens was reported to be pale yellow, in contrast to the colorless lenses of nocturnal geckos. A typical complement was found of gecko visual cell types: type A singles, type B doubles and type C doubles. Tansley confirmed Under-wood's observation of an oil-droplet (colorless) in the chief member of the type B doubles but no such organelle was seen in either the type A singles or the type C doubles (Fig. 16). Taken together, all these characteristics were interpreted as

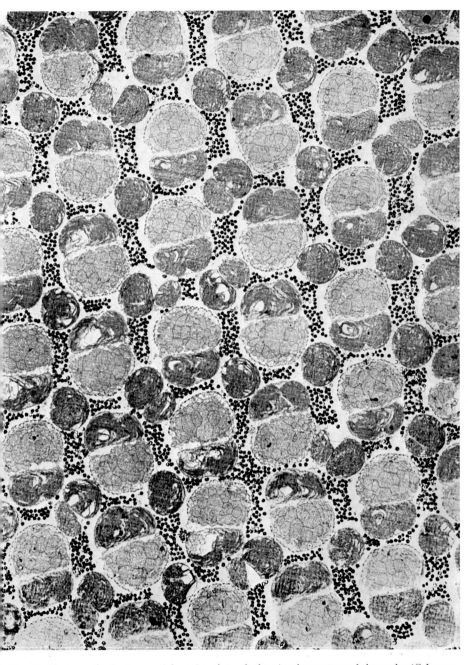

Fig. 18. Photograph of a tangential section through the visual receptors of the gecko *(Coleonyx variegatus)*. Note the rows of type B double cells alternating with rows that contain type A singles and type C doubles. In the rows of type B doubles the chief and accessory members are seen to alternate in zig-zag fashion. This figure was kindly presented by Dr. R. DUNN (DUNN, 1965). The retina was fixed in cold 40% osmium tetroxide in carbon tetrachloride; the section was stained with uranyl acetate and lead citrate; 3615 ×

supporting WALLS' concept of a tertiary evolution. Another study of the fine structure of the *Phelsuma* retina confirmed these features of the *Phelsuma* visual cells, as well as adding additional information about the ultrastructure (PEDLER and TANSLEY, 1963).

In summary, the transmutation theory was based on the interpretation of two separate series of apparent morphological relationships: (a) the intralacertilian homologous sequence as found in the collared lizard, the Rivers' night lizard and the banded gecko (Fig. 15) and (b) the intragekkonid sequence of intermediate cell types (Fig. 16). We shall turn next to other, and possibly more quantitative, characteristics of the gecko retina to evaluate the transmutation theory.

2. Visual Pigments and Transmutation

On the basis of information prior to 1953 there was little reason to believe that geckos would not have rhodopsin as an important constituent of the retina. Rhodopsin was considered to be the basic scotopic pigment of terrestrial animals; and, of all the vertebrates, reptiles, and especially lizards, are prime examples of the terrestrial habit. Despite his unique interpretation of the gecko rod, WALLS (1934) considered that these nocturnal lizards had evolved abundant rhodopsin, though it is not clear in what sense he employed this word — the general sense, or the specific sense that I employ, namely an A_1-based pigment with a spectral absorbance maximal at about 500 nm, i.e., a rose-red pigment, True, there was the statement by KRAUSE (1893) that the gecko pigment was violet-red, but this could always be brushed away as a limitation of the observational method. It was surprising, therefore, when the scotopic spectral sensitivity of *Gekko gekko* was reported to be maximal in a position, not as expected for a rhodopsin system, but some 20 nm further toward the red (DENTON, 1953). *Gekko gekko* is a nocturnal lizard with a typical gecko retina, and with no oil-droplets in the rods. The lens is not colored so there was no reason to believe that selective intraocular absorption was responsible for this unusual sensitivity function. The explanation soon appeared (CRESCITELLI, 1956b, 1958a, 1958b, 1963a, 1963b) when it was discovered that the photopigments extracted out of the retinas of various geckos, including *Gekko gekko*, absorbed at wavelengths longer than did the rhodopsins, although the maxima differed somewhat for the different species (Figs. 19 to 23). The interpretation of this pigment system, so typically associated with geckos, was made in terms of the transmutation theory. Accompanying the cytological transmutation, a photopigment transmutation from some ancestral cone pigment absorbing at longer wavelengths was assumed to have occurred. In this evolution various intermediate stages of visual pigment transformation might be seen in various gekkonid species, just as UNDERWOOD found various intermediate stages of visual cell transformation. The results of a comparative survey were briefly the following: (a) No photopigment was detected in a retinal extract made from four specimens of the diurnal *Lygodactylus capensis* obtained from Natal, South Africa. (b) Only a trace of a light-sensitive component was detected in an extract of fifteen specimens of *Sphaerodactylus argus* from Jamaica, B.W.I. (c) From *Sphaerodactylus parkeri*, whose visual cells have larger and longer outer segments than in the case of *S. argus*, a photopigment with maximum at 528 nm was extracted. (d) An extract of one specimen of *Aristelliger praesignis* showed a pigment with maximum at 530 nm. (e) The genus *Oedura* gave specially interesting results. Three species from New South Wales were examined: *O. monilis*, *O. lesueuri* and *O. robusta*. From *O. monilis* a very stable extract was prepared and this contained a photopigment with maximum at 518 nm. From *O. lesueuri* a pigment at 522 nm

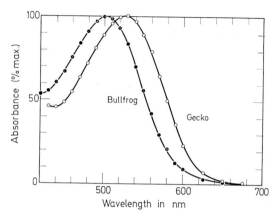

Fig. 19. Spectral absorbance curves to illustrate the displacement of the gecko visual pigment away from the position of classical rhodopsin. The gecko extract was obtained from *Tarentola mauritanica*; the rhodopsin source was the bullfrog

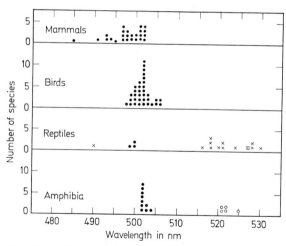

Fig. 20. Distribution of visual pigments obtained in retinal extracts of *amphibia, reptiles, birds,* and *mammals*. The A_1-pigments are indicated by filled circles and by the crosses (geckos) and the square (Nile crocodile). The A_2-pigments are shown by the plain circles. The second group of gecko pigments absorbing at lower wavelengths are not shown. These data were taken from BRIDGES (1959, 1962), CRESCITELLI (1956a, 1956b, 1958a, 1963a), CRESCITELLI and DARTNALL (1953), CRESCITELLI, WILSON, and LILYBLADE (1964), DARTNALL (1954, 1956, 1960, 1967), DARTNALL and LYTHGOE (1965), DARTNALL, ARDEN, IKEDA, LUCK, ROSENBERG, PEDLER and TANSLEY (1965), SILLMAN (1968) and LYTHGOE and DARTNALL (1971). I have also included here the pigments detected by microspectrophotometric examination by LIEBMAN and ENTINE (1968).

was extracted, while the extract from *O. robusta* showed the presence of but one light-sensitive component but with its maximum in the unusual location of 490 nm. (f) The banded gecko, *Coleonyx variegatus*, yielded a pigment with maximum at 516 nm, clearly not a typical rhodopsin. This gecko is a member of the family Eublapharidae, lizards without spectacles but with true eyelids. Some herpetologists do not consider the eublapharids to be true geckos. In terms of the visual pigment type, however, *Coleonyx* appears to fit nicely in with the spectacled geckos. A

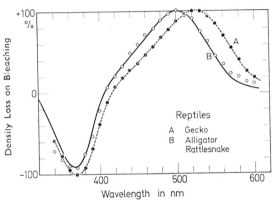

Fig. 21. The comparison of difference spectra for the photopigments from a gecko *(Phyllurus milii)*, the alligator *(Alligator mississippiensis)*, and the rattlesnake *(Crotalus viridis helleri)*. The bleaching was done in the presence of NH_2OH so the product maximum at 366 nm indicates an A_1-basis for all three pigments. Yet the gecko pigment is colored like classical porphyropsin, an effect of the different opsin

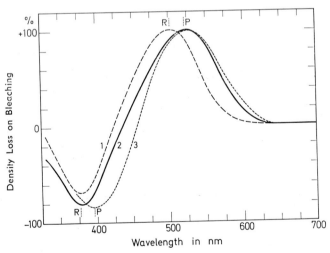

Fig. 22. Difference spectra obtained as the result of bleaching extracts each containing but one photosensitive component. The curves compare a classical rhodopsin *(1)*, from the alligator, a classical porphyropsin *(3)*, from the carp, and the unusual gecko pigment *(2)*, from *Phyllurus*. The figure illustrates that the same spectral shift may be accomplished either by substituting the opsin or the prosthetic group

summary of this information, and documentation of some of these statements are given in Fig. 20.

Insofar as analyses have been made, they indicate that the gecko pigments are all A_1-based pigments (Fig. 21). The shift in absorbance to longer wavelengths is due, therefore, not to the occurrence of 3-dehydroretinal as the prosthetic group, but to the specific nature of the gecko opsins. If transmutation is responsible for these unique pigments it has been a transmutation of the protein molecule. The

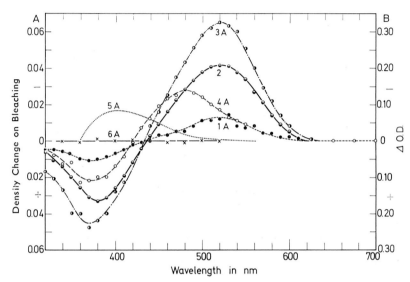

Fig. 23. The dual pigment system in *Gekko gekko*. Difference spectra obtained from a partial bleaching analysis of a retinal extract. Two different ordinate scales (A and B) are employed, the former applying to curves *1A*, *3A*, *4A*, *5A* and *6A*, and the latter to curve *2*. *1A*: bleaching by light of 709 and 691 nm. *2*: second bleaching by light of 660 nm. *3A*: third exhaustive bleaching by light of 660 nm. These 3 bleachings removed but a single photopigment with maximum at 521 nm. *4A*: the result of a fourth bleaching with light of 540 nm. This led to maximum density loss at 478 nm but a maximum gain position similar to that of the previous 3 bleachings. Control *5A* shows the effect of taking an extract from which all photopigment had been removed as in the previous 4 bleachings, and exposing it to white light. This caused an isomerization of the products of bleaching leading to *5A*. It will be seen that *5A*, an isomerization artifact, differs from *4A* which is interpreted as evidence of a photopigment. This interpretation is strengthened by the fact that curve *5A* was not obtained in the presence of NH₂OH; instead, there was no change (*6A*). Curve *4A* (478 pigment), was still obtained however, in the presence of NH₂OH (CRESCITELLI, 1963a)

gecko pigments illustrate the difficulty with the continued use of the rhodopsin-porphyropsin terminology. The gecko pigments cannot be called rhodopsins; they are not "red-appearing". Many of them have the appearance of porphyropsins from certain fishes, but they do not have 3-dehydroretinal as the prosthetic group (Fig. 22). It is for this reason that I prefer, when possible, to use the designations Pn_1 or Pn_2, as explained previously.

The gecko retina, as we have seen, is not uniform with respect to morphological visual cell types. It would be no surprise, therefore, if more than one photopigment were present in the gecko retina. This, in fact, is the case (Crescitelli, 1958b, 1963b). An example is the system of the Tokay gecko, *Gekko gekko* (Crescitelli, 1963a). Partial bleaching of a retinal extract revealed the presence of a $P 521_1$ (Fig. 23) which was entirely removed by exposure to light of longer wavelengths. Following this, the extract was exposed to light of shorter wavelengths. This resulted in the bleaching-out of another component with maximum at about 478 nm. The nature of the product formed in the presence of NH_2OH indicated that the 478-pigment was an A_1-based pigment (Crescitelli, 1963a). I have a private communication from Dr. Paul Liebman that he has

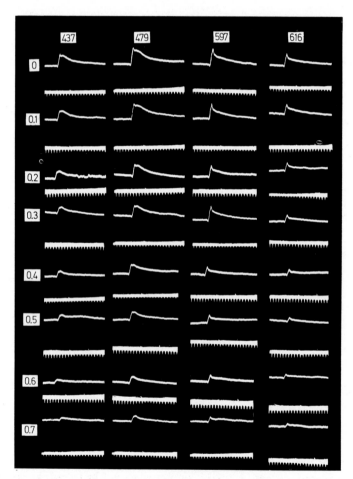

Fig. 24. Fast and slow components in the ERG of *Gekko gekko*. The recordings were made with flashes of light of different intensities and of 4 wavelengths (437, 479, 597, 616 nm) while the eye was adapted to light at 630 nm. This adaptation depressed the fast, more red-sensitive component and brought out the slower, more blue-sensitive wave. Note that in records of about the same magnitude the responses to 437 nm consist chiefly of the slow wave while the comparable responses to 616 nm are mainly fast potentials. A wavelength specificity for these two components is indicated and this suggests that the two waves are electrical signs of activity in two different spectral systems. Fig. 25 supports this interpretation

detected a blue-absorbing light-sensitive substance in some visual cells of *Gekko gekko*. I shall leave the description of this to him. The presence of an additional pigment absorbing at shorter wavelengths is not, apparently, an incidental phenomenon for I have obtained data similar to that shown for *Gekko gekko* with *Oedura monilis*, *Gehyra mutilata*, *Hemidactylus frenatus* and *Oedura robusta*.

3. Spectral Sensitivity and Transmutation

The spectral sensitivity curves for several species of geckos have been shown to be in general accord with the data on visual pigments. DENTON (1956) employed the efficient responses of the pupil of *Gekko gekko* to determine the spectral sensitivity, and he established the fact that this curve was in good agreement with the data of the visual pigment extracted by CRESCITELLI (1956b) from another gecko, *Phyllurus milii*. Later, CRESCITELLI (1963a) refined this comparison by making use of the pigment data from *Gekko gekko* itself. The discovery of two visual pigments in retinal extracts of *Gekko gekko* led to a further examination of the spectral sensitivity curve (CRESCITELLI, 1965). It was first found that the ERG of this lizard was compound, consisting of at least two separate and spectrally-specific components: the first one being faster, and red-sensitive; the second being

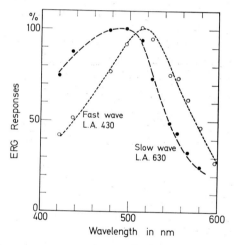

Fig. 25. The spectral sensitivities based on the fast wave and the partially-resolved slow wave of the *Gekko* ERG. The fast wave responses were recorded while the eye was adapted to light of 430 nm; the slow wave responses were obtained with the eye adapted to light of 630 nm

slower in time course and having a higher sensitivity to blue-green light (Fig. 24). An attempt was made to fractionate the ERG, using selective light adaptation, and to obtain the spectral sensitivity curves for these two components separately. The fast wave, isolated by adaptation to blue light (430 nm), showed a sensitivity curve maximal at about 520 nm, in good agreement with $P521_1$ (Fig. 25). The slow wave, more difficult to isolate because of residual fast wave activity that was difficult to remove (Fig. 24), was at least made more conspicuous by adaptation to red light (630 nm). Its spectral sensitivity function

(Fig. 25) was shifted to shorter wavelengths and had a maximum, not at 478 nm, but at 490 nm. I interpret this result to mean that the slow wave was not purged completely of fast wave activity and that the curve was contaminated by a contribution from the $P521_1$-system.

Compound sensitivity curves have been recorded from other species of geckos. Curves too broad to be easily attributed to a single photopigment were recorded from *Tarentola mauritanica* and *Hemidactylus turcicus* by Dodt and Walther (1959). The sensitivity function of the diurnal gecko, *Phelsuma inunguis*, was fractionated by selective adaptation to show a mechanism at 560 nm and another at about 460 nm (Arden and Tansley, 1962). It seems that geckos, whether diurnal or nocturnal in habit, have at least two spectral receptor systems. The role of such dual systems in nocturnal geckos is problematical. Perhaps the idea of Walls (1934) is relevant here, i.e., that cones in transmuting to scotopic receptors did not relinquish the capacity for hue discrimination.

4. Visual Responses and Transmutation

The equivocal nature of gecko visual cells is illustrated by some apparently anomalous physiological responses of the gecko retina. The first of such responses was reported by Crozier and Wolf, (1939) who demonstrated that the flicker response curve of the gecko, *Sphaerodactylus inaquae*, was simple in form, and agreed in all features with the comparable curve taken from the presumed pure-cone turtle, *Pseudemys scripta*. This similarity led Crozier and Wolf to question some of the implications of the duplicity theory of vision. Crozier and Wolf assumed that *S. inaquae* is nocturnal and that the retina is of the pure rod type. The Sphaerodactylidae, in general, are not strictly nocturnal and Goin and Goin, (1962) stated that this family of geckos tends to be more active during the day than are most geckos. The cells of *S. argus* (Fig. 16) might be called cones, and Underwood (1951) described a temporal fovea in *S. argus* and *S. parkeri*. It is unfortunate that Crozier and Wolf did not justify, with histological evidence, the assertion of a pure-rod retina in their gecko, or else use a more genuinely nocturnal genera of geckos. This criticism does not apply to the work of Dodt and Jessen (1961) who employed *Hemidactylus turcicus* and *Tarentola mauritanica*. The visual cells of these geckos were studied by Tansley (1959) who found typical gecko rods with large outer segments, paraboloids, no oil-droplets and the type A singles, type B doubles and type C doubles. Despite the absence of obvious cones, Dodt and Jessen demonstrated the occurrence of both scotopic and photopic fusion-frequency functions, and the presence of a duplex dark adaptation curve with an initial rapid kinetics, a break, and then a second, slower rate of recovery. The range of dark adaptation covered 6 log units. Duplex response from a pure-rod retina is embarrassing for the duplicity theory, but the concept of phylogenetic transmutation salvages the situation. All that is needed is to assume that some features of the photopic condition, quite independently of the morphology of the visual cells, have been retained. In this sense the duplex responses of Dodt and Jessen are indicators of a past ancestral condition. Tansley (1959) pointed out that the retinas of these nocturnal geckos showed relatively little summation as revealed by the numbers of visual cells and ganglion cells. She expressed the view that these geckos probably have better visual acuity than is usually associated with the pure rod condition. I know of no experiments to test this point.

E. Snakes and the Transmutation Theory

Here I do not wish to discuss the thorny problem of the origin of snakes, and the specific lacertilian group from which they may have been derived. Opinions differ on this question and the interested reader may be referred to recent articles by BELLAIRS and UNDERWOOD, (1951); McDOWELL and BOGERT, (1954); UNDERWOOD, (1967a,b). All I propose here is to present some of the unique features of ophidian visual cells, to show some characteristic cell types that are found in various groups of snakes and to relate the visual cells to the transmutation theory. My discussion is based mainly on the pioneer studies of WALLS (1934,1942a, 1942b) and on the accounts given by UNDERWOOD (1951, 1966, 1967a, 1970). The visual cells of snakes differ in certain characteristics from those of lizards. The oil-droplet is absent and so is the paraboloid. The curious double cells, both rods and cones, are unique, being found in no other vertebrate. Each double cell consists of a chief member, which contains a very large ellipsoid, like that of the large single cell, and of a thin accessory member. Adjacent to the nucleus of the accessory member is the unique ophidian organelle, the paranuclear body, discovered by WALLS, (1934). There is no such structure in the lacertilian visual cells. Moreover, in the latter, the large member of the double cells is the accessory member; in snakes the large member is the chief member. This follows if we define the chief member as that member similar to the comparable single cell. In snakes the comparable single cell is the large single cell (Fig. 4b). In addition, there is a small or thin single cell (Fig. 4b) and this, like the large single and the double, may be a rod or a cone, as explained in the next section.

The simplest snake retina is found in *Typhlops* and *Leptotyphlops*, the worm-like burrowing forms whose eyes are small and possibly degenerate. Herpetologists differ as to the taxonomic position of the two families, Typhlopidae and Leptotyphlopidae, and some have even questioned the classification of the Typhlopidae as snakes. In any case the retinas of these two species contain only single rods (UNDERWOOD, 1967a). It is questionable, however, whether these rods should be regarded as ancestral to the visual cells in other snakes because these burrowing forms, even if true snakes, may be aberrant, rather than primitive. If so, these rods may represent a secondary evolution from the duplex boid retina.

The primitive snakes of the family, Boidae, have a retina with well differentiated rods and cones, both singles. The cones house a bulky ellipsoid located just external to the external limiting membrane; the rods are longer, slenderer and their ellipsoids are still more external (WALLS, 1942a). This duplex retina, consisting only of single cells, is not entirely limited to the Boidae for it has been found in *Xenopeltis*, family Xenopeltidae, which UNDERWOOD considers a primitive and taxonomically isolated group, and in *Pareas*, a colubrid-type snake.

All snakes above the Boidae, except *Pareas* and other exceptions that may turn up in the future, have a more complicated visual cell composition. This includes the ophidian double cell as well as the large and small single cells mentioned previously. To clarify the visual cell types found in snakes I have grouped them into the following seven categories (Fig. 26). Next to each category I have given the descriptive terms used by Walls and by Underwood.

I. Single Rod Type. This is the Scolecophidian pattern of Underwood. It is found in Typhlops and in Leptotyphlops.

II. Duplex Mixed Type. This is the Boid pattern of Walls and of Underwood. It has been found in boids, pythons, *Xenopeltis* and *Pareas*. This consists of single rods and single cones.

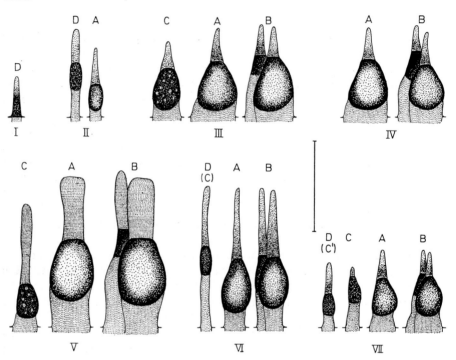

Fig. 26. Ophidian visual cell phylogeny to illustrate the views of Walls and of Underwood. The visual cell types are those given by Underwood (1967a) but in parentheses I have given Walls' designations (*C, C′*) for the single rods of categories *VI* and *VII*. The other designations are as used by both Walls and Underwood. Vertical scale = 20 μm. Further explanation in text

III. Triplex Cone Type. This is the colubrid pattern of Walls and the coluber pattern of Underwood. It has been found in some Colubridae but not in all that have been examined, and in some Natricidae and Elapidae. This category consists of a large (type A) single cone, a smaller (type C) single cone and a double cone (type B). These letter designations are ophidian descriptions and should not be confused with the letter designations of geckos.

IV. Duplex Cone Type. This is the *Malpolon* pattern of Underwood. This has been found in a few species of Colubridae and Elapidae. Only Type A single cones and type B double cones are present. Walls associated this category with the possession of high visual acuity: *Malpolon* has an area centralis and *Dryophis*, a fovea.

V. Triplex Rod Type. This is the *Hypsiglena* pattern of Walls and the *Phyllorhynchus* pattern of Underwood. Walls found this in the nocturnal snakes, *Hypsiglena ochrorhynchus* and *Phyllorhynchus decurtatus*. These snakes have vertical, slit pupils and colorless lenses. The retina consists of type A, type C and type B cells, all rods.

VI. Triplex Mixed Type. This is the Crotaline pattern of Underwood and of Walls. Type A single cones are present, as are type B double cones. The third cell is a single rod, which has replaced the type C single cone. This is called a type C rod by WALLS but a type D rod by UNDERWOOD, a designation that I prefer because of the next category. There are several variants of this category depending on the detailed morphology of the type A and type B cones. At our present state of knowledge I do not find it useful to subdivide this category further, though I recognize the possibility of several evolutionary stages within this category.

VII. Quadriplex Mixed Type. This is the Viperine pattern of WALLS and UNDERWOOD. This consists of the three types of category III with an additional element, the type D single rod, which WALLS designated type C'. UNDERWOOD found this category rather widespread in some of the Viperinae, the Lycodontinae, the Elapidae and a few Colubridae. One of the few reports giving figures for the relative abundance of these different cell types is that of UNDERWOOD (1966) who listed in *Enhydris pakistanica*, an Homalopsinae, the figures of type A (16%), type B (2.5%), type C (0.5%) and type D (81%) in a count of 945 cells.

In interpreting the phylogenetic relationships between these various categories both WALLS and UNDERWOOD agreed that the Boid pattern (category II) was probably ancestral to all the others, but beyond this they did not agree. WALLS believed the triplex cone type (category III) to be the central scheme from which the other categories evolved by (a) the loss of type C cones (III to IV), (b) by converting type C cones to type D rods while the other cells, though undergoing changes, remained as cones (III to VI), (c) by converting all cones to homologous rods (III to V), and (d) by converting some type C cones to type D rods while retaining some of the type C cones (III to VII). In this scheme the type C cone was visualized as the most plastic element in the process of evolutionary transmutation. The reader may find these hypothesized transmutations summarized in Fig. 26.

UNDERWOOD's view, on the other hand, placed the quadriplex mixed category (VII) as the central pattern from which the others evolved. This view was based upon the wide distribution of the quadriplex pattern. Loss of type C cones would then lead to the triplex mixed category (VII to VI), and loss of type D rods would give the triplex cone type (VII to III). UNDERWOOD agreed that categories IV and V could originate from category III as postulated by WALLS. On the basis of the observations that have been made it is not possible to critically evaluate these two schemes of ophidian visual cell evolution. There is a certain amount of subjectivism in identifying rods and cones here, and perhaps some other criteria should be employed to study the interrelationships. Knowledge of the visual pigments might be one such criterion.

It is clear from what has been said that snakes, in addition to geckos, provided WALLS with information relevant to his transmutation theory. The transition of category III to V was, in fact, one of WALLS' strongest arguments for transmutation. This case was documented by WALLS by citing the cones of the diurnal Indigo Snake, *Drymarchon corais couperi*, and the homologous rods of the nocturnal Spotted Night Snake, *Hypsiglena ochrorhynchus*. One possible explanation of this homology is that parallel and independent evolution occurred in separate lines ending, in one line, with the rods; in the other, with cones. Such a coincidence in evolution was rejected by WALLS who chose, instead, an explanation based on the transmutation of the three types of cones, as exemplified in *Drymarchon*, to the three types of rods as in *Hypsiglena*. This explanation was also favored by WALLS, (1934) because of the finding of what he interpreted to be visual cell types intermediate between cones and rods, as if transmutation had progressed only "part-way", as he put it. It is clear that

Walls based his theory of transmutation on observations of the visual cells of animals other than geckos. These observations led Walls to one of his formal conclusions, i.e., that "transmutations have occurred many times, independently of each other, so that unrelated forms have convergently attained similar final conditions".

It is unfortunate that we have no available information on ophidian visual pigments comparable with the elaborate knowledge of the visual cells. To my knowledge there is only one published paper on the visual pigments of snakes, and that is a report on the pigment of the Pacific rattlesnake, *Crotalus viridis helleri* (Crescitelli, 1956b). This report (Fig. 21) revealed the presence in the extract of but a single, light-sensitive pigment, peaking at 500 nm and containing retinal as the prosthetic group. The possession of rhodopsin by this crotaline snake is of interest in connection with the Walls and the Underwood concepts of the origin of the type D crotaline rod in category VI (Fig. 26). If the ancestral boid rod pigment was rhodopsin, and this was the belief of Walls (1942a), then a direct retention of the photopigment in the type D viperine rod (category VII), as suggested by Underwood, is a possibility. On the other hand, if the crotaline type D rod was the result of transmutation of the type C cone of category III, as Walls postulated, then a transmuted pigment, as in geckos, might be expected. The results offer no evidence for such a transmutation. The chemical identification of the visual pigments in the nocturnal, presumably-transmuted rods of *Hypsiglena* and *Phyllorhynchus* would be of great interest in this connection. Walls (1934) stated that rhodopsin was absent in the retinas of these snakes, presumably basing this conclusion on visual observation.

F. Crocodilia

The order Crocodilia includes some 25 species of large reptiles: the alligators and caimans, crocodiles and false gavial and the gavial. All are amphibious but lay their eggs on land; all inhabit fresh water except for the marine *Crocodylus porosus*.

The alligator retina has been the subject for most of the studies in this group of reptiles. This retina has had a special interest because of its regional specialization with a tapetum in the superior half which, according to Abelsdorff (1898), serves to increase the retinal sensitivity for light coming from the river bottom. The inferior half of the retina is free of this reflecting tapetum. In the approximate central region there is found, according to Walls (1942b), a horizontal *area centralis* containing slenderer and more closely packed visual cells. It is generally agreed that both rods and cones are present although the tapetal and non-tapetal regions differ with respect to visual cell composition and morphology. Laurens and Detwiler (1921) stated that the tapetal region contained about 85% rods and 15% cones, the majority of the latter being double cones. Within the non-tapetal region cones outnumbered the rods, and the majority of the cones were singles. The alligator retina suggests, as in the case of other retinas that have been discussed, a functional specialization into scotopic and photopic regions according to the visual field that is perceived. Walls (1942a) reported the presence of single cones, double cones and single rods, all without oil-droplets, the cones being from the lower, non-tapetal half of the retina. From the center of the tapetal region he described single and double cells that had enlarged, cylindrical outer segments as if "a local partial transmutation of cones into rods" had occurred within the same retina (Fig. 4b).

A light-sensitive pigment was seen by ABELSDORFF (1898) over both halves of the alligator retina. On the basis of visual observations, WALLS (1942a) believed the alligator pigment to be rhodopsin. The finding of a P500_1 in *Alligator mississippiensis* (Fig. 21) was first reported by CRESCITELLI (1956b) and confirmed by WALD, BROWN, and KENNEDY (1957) who, additionally, showed that regeneration of alligator rhodopsin occurred *in vitro* after the addition of 11-*cis* retinal to the bleached solution. No evidence was obtained by either of these groups of investigators for the presence, in the alligator retina, of gecko-type transmuted pigments. In one respect, however, alligator rhodopsin was shown to be interesting, and this was in its relatively high rate of regeneration. This rate, which was 10—20 seconds for half-completion at 25° C, was much higher than for the rhodopsins of frog, cattle or chicken, which showed figures of 4—6 minutes. Along with the rapid rate of regeneration of alligator rhodopsin *in vitro* was the relatively rapid rate of dark adaptation of the alligator retina, as measured by means of the ERG. Such adaptation was complete in 5—7 minutes whereas in the frog eye the comparable figure was 30 minutes or more. Clearly, the alligator system is unique, for after exposure to light the rhodopsin and the rods complete recovery more like a cone system, e.g., iodopsin. In this respect, therefore, the alligator rhodopsin system appears to show intermediate properties, behaving like rod rhodopsin in some respects, like the pigment of a cone in other respects. The situation is made intriguing, indeed, by the finding of a P527_1 in the Nile crocodile, *Crocodylus niloticus* (DARTNALL and LYTHGOE, 1965). This is reminiscent of the gecko-type visual pigments.

X. Birds

Certain skeletal characteristics, as well as other similarities, suggest that birds have a reptilian origin. The earliest known fossil with avian features is that of *Archaeopteryx* found in upper Jurassic beds in what is now Solnhofen, Bavaria. Though highly reptilian in osteology, the presence of a feather impression was regarded as conclusive for the avian classification of *Archaeopteryx*. Linked to this ancestry, it is not surprising that the avian eye displays so many features in common with the eyes of reptiles.

About 8,600 species of living birds are known, arranged in 28 orders and about 170 families. Birds utilize a wide variety of environments: marine, fresh water, terrestrial, temperate, tropical, arctic, alpine, etc.

1. Visual Cells

Most birds are highly active, diurnal animals and their retinas are characterized by the presence of many cones, both single and double, while rods may be relatively few. Oil-droplets are very common and such droplets may be colorless or colored yellow, orange, red (ROCHON-DUVIGNEAUD, 1943). Central and temporal foveas are common in diurnal birds and in these specialized regions the visual cells tend to be different in types and in morphology, as SCHULTZE (1866, 1867) long ago pointed out. It is, perhaps, instructive at this point to note that vision in typical diurnal birds is different in some important respects from photopic human vision and that this is the result of structural differences in the bird and human retinas. All this was considered some time ago by PUMPHREY (1948) in an essay of more than passing interest. PUMPHREY pointed out that the human retina with its shallow fovea, its localized central area, and its rapidly decreasing extra-foveal cone density is associated with a binocular mechanism of central fixation along a line. This implies the need for an efficient system of congruent eye movements. In contrast, the diurnal bird retina with its laterally-placed geometry, its central, steep-sided fovea, and its relatively high extra-foveal acuity serves the requirements of accurate monocular detection of movements over an area. Accurate fixation on a fixed point in the visual field is not as critical in birds that rely on dynamic rather than on static visual acuity. PUMPHREY described this as a "two-dimensional but virtually boundless" visual field for the bird and as a "three-dimensional but restricted" field for the human. I cannot resist the temptation of citing PUMPHREY's illustration of this difference; a man with a bird's eyes would be unable to thread a needle, and a bird with human eyes would have difficulty in detecting a cat approaching in directions other than the frontal one. Another adaptation in some birds is the horizontal retinal band of higher visual acuity (DUIJM, 1958) which apparently serves to concentrate visual attention on objects along a horizontal field for birds active in open areas. All this suggests that birds have retained, and even improved, a retinal system for movement detection that was present in their reptilian ancestors, and is found even today in living reptiles. It does not mean, however, that development of visual functions has not gone beyond this stage. PUMPHREY, in fact, recognized that the shallower temporal fovea of some birds is a structure designed for the binocular judgment of distance and of relative speed. Noctural birds, as SCHULTZE also noticed, had in their retinas a greater proportion of rods than did diurnal birds, and the oil-droplets were seen to be colorless or only weakly colored. In some birds the outer segments of rods and cones are not greatly different in length or thickness, and the two types of cells cannot be easily distinguished except on the basis of the oil-droplets. MEYER and COOPER (1966) described the visual cells of the chicken, observed with phase contrast microscopy, as consisting of rods, single cones with red oil-droplets, and double cones. In the latter the chief member was said to house a yellow droplet, and the accessory member a smaller yellow-green droplet. No colorless droplets were seen. A recent electron microscope study of the chicken visual cells (MORRIS and SHOREY, 1967) revealed the presence of the following types (Fig. 27): (a) a single rod with closely packed mitochondria, no oil-droplet and a paraboloid, (b) a double cone whose chief member included an oil-droplet and whose accessory member showed a large paraboloid and small granular vesicle in the ellipsoid, and (c) two kinds of single cones: type I, without paraboloid but with a heavy stain of lead in the droplet region; type II, without paraboloid and with a light-staining droplet region. The outer segments of the cones were seen as somewhat conical, and slenderer than the rods, but the length was not markedly different. MORRIS and SHOREY counted 286 receptors and found 15% rods, 36% double cones, 25% type I single cones, 11% type II single cones and 13%

unidentified. MORRIS (1970) has recently expanded this study of the chicken visual cells and reported the presence of a third type of single cone based on the electron density of the oil droplet. In addition she pointed out that the visual cells are organized in the form of an hexagonal pattern. If it is just a matter of the quantity of visual pigment that determines whether or not that pigment may be successfully extracted, as LIEBMAN and ENTINE (1968) have suggested, then the chicken retina, with its large and numerous cones, should be a favorable source for such a pigment.

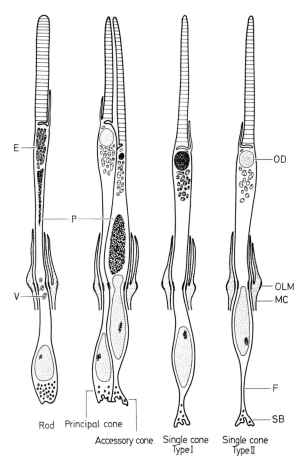

Fig. 27. Schematic drawing of chicken visual cells based on an electron microscope study by MORRIS and SHOREY (1967). *Single rod:* There are closely packed, elongated mitochondria in the ellipsoid (*E*). A paraboloid (*P*) is present as well as prominent vesicles (*V*) in the rod cytoplasma at the level of the outer limiting membrane (*OLM*). The nucleus is close to the synaptic body, which contains many synaptic vesicles. MEYER and COOPER (1966) refer to the glycogen-containing paraboloid as the hyperboloid of KRAUSE. *Double cone:* The chief member has a large yellow oil-droplet, the accessory member a small, yellow-green oil-droplet. The glycogen-containing paraboloid is seen in the accessory member. No MÜLLER cells (*MC*) intervene between the two members at their level of contact. Note the differences in oil-droplets, mitochondria and nuclei. The cellular origin of iodopsin is not yet known. This figure and legend are based on information by MORRIS and SHOREY (1967) and MEYER and COOPER (1966). The figure is reproduced through the courtesy of Dr. MORRIS

This has proved to be the case for chicken iodopsin was in fact the first presumptive, cone pigment to be brought into solution (Wald, 1937 b).

2. Visual Pigments

a) The Rhodopsin System. Nothing new or unusual has been revealed so far about the rhodopsins of birds. Retinal extracts have been shown to have A_1-based photopigments with maximum absorbance in the region of 500 nm. These rhodopsins have been detected in the retinas of nocturnal and diurnal birds, in diving birds, and in birds whose diets vary from seeds, fish, insects and small mammals. Data for the birds that have been examined are given in Fig. 20.

b) Cone pigments. Of all the vertebrates, birds are of special interest here because only from these animals has acceptable evidence been secured to indicate the successful extraction of cone pigments. This started when Wald (1937 b) published a brief note which showed, through the technique of difference spectro-photometry and selective bleaching with red light, that a digitonin extract of chicken retinas contained, in addition to rhodopsin, a light-sensitive component absorbing maximally at longer wavelengths. This component, called iodopsin from its presumed violet color, was considered to be a pigment of the chicken cones because of the resemblance of the photopic sensitivity curve of chickens, obtained by Honigmann (1921), to the difference spectrum of the iodopsin. Wald suggested that this iodopsin, in conjunction with three sets of oil-droplet filters (Wald and Zussman, 1937), might form the basis for a color vision system in chickens. Bliss (1946) confirmed the presence of iodopsin in extracts of the chicken retina and placed its spectral maximum at about 563 nm. Bliss observed, as Wald also had done, that iodopsin was different from rhodopsin in certain properties: it was not extracted from retinas previously kept below pH 4.4 for one hour; extraction at pH 8.5 yielded little iodopsin, neither glycocholate nor salicin extracted it; and it was destroyed by desoxycholate, formalin or acetone. Iodopsin was thus revealed as a more labile substance than rhodopsin.

Nevertheless, iodopsin was eventually shown to be a typical visual pigment (Wald, Brown, and Smith, 1955) with a spectral absorbance maximal at 562 nm, and based on 11-*cis* retinal as the prosthetic group. One distinguishing difference between iodopsin and chicken rhodopsin, other than the color, was the faster regeneration kinetics for iodopsin. This accords with the well-known fact that cone systems dark adapt faster than do rod systems. Plotted in a form showing log sensitivity (which is directly related to the concentration of visual pigment) as a function of time in the dark, the human cone dark-adaptation curve was found to be roughly similar to the regeneration curve of iodopsin. All these facts were considered to justify the conclusion that iodopsin was indeed a cone pigment. The fundamental similarity of iodopsin to the other visual pigments was also demonstrated by the finding of products of bleaching comparable to those already known for rhodopsin (Hubbard and Kropf, 1959; Yoshizawa and Wald, 1967). The difference between chicken rhodopsin and chicken iodopsin appears to reside entirely in the nature of the opsins. It is significant, in this connection, that just as opsin from various rhodopsins will combine with 3-dehydroretinal (probably the 11-*cis* isomer) to yield analogue photopigments absorbing maximally at 17 to 25 nm longer wavelength than the original rhodopsins, so it is that opsin from chicken iodopsin combines with this same isomer to form a photopigment, cyanopsin, absorbing at 620 nm, some 58 nm higher than iodopsin (WALD, BROWN, and SMITH, 1953). Until recently, cyanopsin was known only as a product of test tube chemistry, though the prediction was made that it might be present in the cones of freshwater fishes and the tortoise (WALD, BROWN, and SMITH, 1953). With the technique of single cell microspectrophotometry, cyanopsin now has been recognized in cones of the tadpole of *Rana pipiens* and the freshwater turtle (LIEBMAN and ENTINE, 1967, 1968).

The finding of a presumptive cone pigment in the chicken retina raises the question of its possible presence in the retinas of other birds. The turkey, another Gallinaceous bird, is one from whose retina iodopsin has also been extracted (CRESCITELLI, WILSON, and LILYBLADE, 1964). In one of his reviews, WALD (1958b) stated that iodopsin had been extracted from the pigeon retina but no data have appeared in print to support this statement. In fact, BRIDGES (1962) made a careful analysis of retinal extracts from the pigeon and obtained evidence, not for a pigment at 562 nm, but for one at 544 nm, a $P544_1$. The situation is somewhat enigmatic for there are some rather good spectral sensitivity curves for the pigeon eye that appear to support the existence of a mechanism at about 560 nm, rather than 544 nm. The electrophysiological measurements of GRANIT (1942) indicated the presence of a photopic dominator with maximum sensitivity at about 580 nm. GRANIT suggested that the true maximum was at shorter wavelengths, perhaps about 560 nm, if one corrected for the oil-droplet filtering effects. BLOUGH's careful measurements (BLOUGH, 1957) revealed a photopic curve that agreed approximately, except at wavelengths below 500 nm, with the iodopsin spectral absorbance. The scotopic sensitivity curve agreed well with the rhodopsin absorbance. There is no need at present to conclude that there is any conflict between WALD's claim for iodopsin and BRIDGES' finding of a $P544_1$, rather than a $P562_1$. Perhaps the pigeon retina has both these photopigments and, for reasons unknown, the WALD group found the latter, BRIDGES, the former. BLOUGH (1957) pointed out, in fact, that the pigeon spectral sensitivity function, like that of the human, may be compounded of several mechanisms. After all, there is more than one type of cone in the bird retina (Fig. 27) and color vision has been reported to be present in the pigeon (HAMILTON and COLEMAN, 1933). Perhaps the pigeon cone pigments are not grossly different in spectral location from the human cone pigments (see RUSHTON, next chapter).

XI. Mammals

It is generally agreed that mammals arose from reptiles, the early ancestral mammals being small, wary creatures that were very much at the mercy of the carnivorous reptiles. As the giant reptiles disappeared toward the end of the Mesozoic, the modern mammals evolved to their present dominant status. Mammals are active, adaptable and warm-blooded animals, and these characteristics have permitted them to spread over much of the solid earth and portions of the waters, and to achieve phylogenetic diversification not seen in the other vertebrate classes. Living mammals are divided into 19 orders comprising some 4,200 species.

A. Monotremes

These curious, primitive mammals, which inhabit Australia, Tasmania, New Guinea and nearby islands, have several reptilian characteristics, including yolked eggs with a tough, leathery shell, a cloaca, and a reptilian type osteology for the sternum. They have hair, suckle their young and are warm-blooded, though their thermoregulatory mechanism is thought to be inefficient. The visual cells of monotremes have been but little studied. Gunn (1884) examined two eyes of the duck-billed platypus (*Ornithorhynchus paradoxus*). These eyes had been sent to him preserved in whiskey. He reported the retina to be well fixed and to show both rods and cones, the latter cells having oil-droplets. Studying preparations and descriptions of O'Day (1938), Walls (1942b) saw the receptors of *Ornithorhynchus* as comprising single rods, single cones with oil-droplets, and double cones with one member having oil-droplets. The retina of the Echidna, *Tachyglossus* was described as being cone-free. Walls considered the monotreme retina to have retained certain sauropsidian characters. I know of no reports of the visual pigments of monotremes.

B. Marsupials

The marsupials are non-placental, pouch-bearing mammals that characteristically give birth to premature young, which continue development in a skin pouch. Marsupials now inhabit fairly restricted areas of the earth: Australia, Tasmania, New Guinea, Timor, Celebes, South America, Central America and the southern portion of North America. They are believed to be ancient mammals, perhaps survivors of some of the early mammals that lived alongside the now extinct reptiles. Marsupials in the past inhabited much of the earth's surface but are now limited to the regions named above. These pouched mammals have diversified into many forms, comparable to those of the placental mammals, so that we now recognize marsupial wolves, cats, badgers, squirrels, bears, otters, moles, anteaters, rats, mice, rabbits, etc. In Australia the marsupials have apparently filled the niches that were available owing to the absence of placental mammals.

As with monotremes, little has been published with respect to the marsupial retina. Hoffman (cited by O'Day, 1936) observed the presence of oil-droplets in the cones of *Macropus giganteus* and *Wallabia bennetti*. O'Day (1936) examined the retina of *Dasyurus viverrinus*, a small marsupial whose habits are mainly nocturnal. The pupil, when closed, formed a vertical ovoid slit, and a tapetum was found in the upper half of the retina. In spite of such strongly nocturnal signs, O'Day reported the presence of cones as well as of rods. The cones were both single and double, and oil-droplets were seen in them. O'Day stated that both members of each double cone had an oil-droplet; neither member had a paraboloid, and the two members were so nearly alike that they could be called twin cones. In the American opossum, Walls (1939) reported the presence of an oil-droplet only in the chief member. Walls (1942b) considered the visual cells of marsupials, as well as of monotremes, to be phylogenetically related to reptilian visual receptors.

There is only one marsupial for which information about the visual pigment is available and this is the American opossum, *Didelphis marsupialis virginiana*. This is a nocturnal animal and I obtained a living specimen, dark-adapted it and then prepared a digitonin extract of the retinas. The extract was relatively pure and a partial bleaching analysis in the presence of hydroxylamine showed the presence of only one photopigment, $P494_1$.

C. Placental Mammals

The dominant groups of mammals are the orders that have evolved the placental connection to the mother, the foetus remaining so connected until development is well advanced. In general, placental mammals have highly developed central nervous systems so that in their various niches they have become masters of their environment.

1. Visual Cells

The visual cells of placental mammals are different from the receptors of monotremes and marsupials in a number of features. The cones are all single, without paraboloids and without oil droplets. Though claims of photomechanical responses have been made for these visual cells, there is no good evidence of either pigment migration or of myoid contractility (DETWILER, 1924). Most placental mammals have evolved duplex retinas and many of these have specialized regions, such as an *area centralis* or a fovea to increase resolving power and to permit fixation. There are but few strictly diurnal mammals that possess retinas with only cones. One such group comprises the ground squirrels whose eyes are uniquely adapted to vision in bright light and whose retinas almost certainly are devoid of rods (ARDEN and TANSLEY, 1955b; TANSLEY, COPENHAVER, and GUNKEL, 1961; DOWLING, 1964; HOLLENBERG and BERNSTEIN, 1966). The common tree shrew (*Tupaia glis*) also was claimed to be of the all-cone variety (CASTENHOLZ, 1965) and in accord with this, the electrical responses to light were shown to be characteristic of a rod-free system (TIGGES, BROOKS, and KLEE, 1967). Contrasting these diurnal forms, a number of nocturnal mammals have been classified as possessing all-rod retinas. This claim has been made for the Douroucouli or Owl Monkey (*Aotes trivirgatus*), which is the only true monkey that is nocturnal; for the Slender Loris (*Loris tardigradus*); for the bush baby (*Galago crassicaudatus*); and for the Eastern Tarsier (*Tarsius spectrum*) (WOOLLARD, 1925; KOLMER, 1930; DETWILER, 1939; WOOLLARD, 1927; DETWILER, 1941; CASTENHOLZ, 1965; JONES, 1965; DARTNALL, ARDEN, IKEDA, LUCK, ROSENBERG, PEDLER, and TANSLEY, 1965). There are occasional statements in the literature to the effect that other nocturnal mammals such as bats, guinea pigs, mice, etc. have cone-free retinas (DETWILER, 1924; GRANIT, 1944) but some of these statements have been based, apparently, on incomplete evidence. O'DAY (1947), for example, confirmed KOLMER's finding (KOLMER, 1936) of a significant number of cones in the guinea-pig retina. SIDMAN (1958) cited evidence for the presence of cones in the retinas of the mouse, the rat and the guinea pig. Even the owl monkey has now been shown to have cones (HAMASAKI, 1967; FERRAZ DE OLIVEIRA and RIPPS, 1968) and these are in sufficient number to be revealed by duality behavior in the dark-adaptation curve, the critical fusion frequency function, and the electroretinographic b-wave (HAMASAKI, 1967). These examples suggest the caution that is required when interpreting physiological studies purporting to be based on a pure-rod retina.

2. Rod Pigments

There are almost 4000 species of placental mammals but the visual pigments of only about two dozen species have been extracted, and of these about half are rodents. On the basis of this sample it is presumptuous to generalize about the nature of mammalian rod pigments. All that can be said at this time is that the information so far available indicates an A_1-based group of pigments whose spectral absorbances are maximal in the region of 492 to 502 nm (Fig. 20). In these characteristics (nature of prosthetic group, color) these mammalian rhodopsins are similar to the rhodopsins of the marsupial opossum, the birds, the alligator, the rattlesnake, certain adult amphibia, certain larval amphibia, certain teleosts, many elasmobranchs, and the lampreys. A thread of generality seems to run through all these vertebrate classes suggesting that nature hit upon the right molecule early in vertebrate evolution; it has worked, and it has been retained all the way to the human animal. This tenacious retention of a particular type of molecule, not uncommon in biochemistry, makes all the more interesting the appearance of unusual visual pigments such as those of the deep-sea fishes, the geckos, and certain others that have been listed in this review. This situation illustrates the conservatism of nature in retaining a useful mechanism and, at the same time, the phylogenetic plasticity in modifying this mechanism to respond to ecological pressures.

3. Specific Problems

a) **Ground Squirrels.** The ground squirrels (genus *Citellus*, family Sciuridae) are a unique group of rodents for students of the visual system. This fact, now generally recognized, was appreciated by Walls who, some 20 years ago, put out a privately-circulated issue of the "Journalette of Sciurid Vision" intended for the purpose of keeping persons interested in squirrel vision informed on the latest developments. The Journalette died, due to lack of interest, before a second issue appeared. Ground squirrels are strictly diurnal, very active animals with large eyes, yellow-to-orange lenses, round pupils and an optic head that is not circular, but has the form of an horizontally-oriented, eccentric stripe. The retina is unquestionably free of rods and there is no fovea since no such specialization is required in a retina organized to have high resolving power over much of its area, a case of universal macularity, as Walls (1942b) named it. In many respects the ground squirrel retina reacts as would be expected from an all-cone retina. The ERG has a fast a-wave, a fast b-wave, no c-wave and a prominent d-wave (Crescitelli, 1961). The absolute visual threshold is high, the rate of dark-adaptation is rapid and the critical fusion frequency is high (Dowling, 1964). The morphology and physiology indicate the presence of an excellent diurnal visual system. The ground squirrel probably has the ability to discriminate on the basis of wavelength. It has been already shown that blue can be so discriminated from other colors, from black, and from various levels of white light (Crescitelli and Pollack, 1965, 1966). A study now in progress suggests that yellow can be similarly picked out. On the other hand, green, orange or red spectral lights were not so selected. Jacobs and Yolton (1969) trained ground squirrels *(Citellus tridecemlineatus, Citellus mexicanus)* to view three illuminated windows of equal brightness and to select which colored window could or could not be discriminated from white. A neutral point was indeed found, at 505 nm, which is at somewhat longer wavelengths than the neutral point (492—498 nm) of the human protanope. JACOBS and YOLTON concluded that both species of ground squirrels are dichromats comparable to the human protanope. Earlier, it was shown (CRESCITELLI, 1962) that wavelength-specific cortical evoked responses could be recorded from the ground squirrel, *Citellus leucurus*. The responses to flashes at 424 and 454 nm consisted of large on-waves and much smaller (1/6th or less) off-waves. Flashes between 469 and 590 nm elicited responses that had about equal on- and off-waves and no adjustment of stimulus intensity over 2 log units was able to match these responses with those obtained at the shorter wave-lengths. Flashes at still longer wavelengths (590 to 631 nm) often elicited a double off-wave, a response that was never seen with flashes below 590 nm. All these results suggest the existence of an opponent hue-discriminating mechanism for the antelope ground squirrel. In another ground squirrel, *Citellus tridecemlineatus*, DOWLING (1964) reported the presence of only one visual pigment with maximum at 523 nm. The spectral sensitivity curve, obtained by means of the ERG, was in accord with this 523-pigment. MICHAEL (1968a, b) ascertained that a spectral sensitivity function with maximum at about 525 nm was characteristic of the contrast-sensitive and the directionally-sensitive units of *Citellus mexicanus*. Neither of these units possessed color-specific properties. Presumably, cones with DOWLING's 523-pigment were responsible for activating these units. Because of the finding of only one pigment, DOWLING expressed doubt about the presence of color vision in the ground squirrel. I question DOWLING's result because the sensitivity curve of the antelope ground squirrel is bimodal, with one peak at 523 to 528 nm and a second peak — less precisely located — in the blue region (CRESCITELLI and POLLACK, 1966). This, in fact, confirmed previous reports with other species of ground squirrels (TANSLEY, COPENHAVER, and GUNKEL, 1961). Moreover, there is the study by JACOBS and YOLTON (1969) that indicated an ability on the part of *Citellus tridecemlineatus*, the species used by DOWLING, to discriminate colors. MICHAEL (1966, 1968c) also provided electrophysiological evidence for the presence, in *Citellus mexicanus*, of color-coded on-off units. As part of this evidence data were given that were collected from 99 units, out of the 410 optic nerve fibers studied, that showed antagonistic on-off, color-specific properties. Of these 99 a group of 49 was excited by green and inhibited by blue, i.e., green-on, blue-off units. The remaining 50 fibers were excited by blue and inhibited by green, i.e., blue-on, green-off units. Both groups were associated with a bimodal sensitivity curve with one peak in the blue, at about 460 nm, the other peak at about 560 nm. An apparent neutral point where excitation was antagonized by inhibition was found at about 500 nm. Some resolution of the two chromatic mechanisms was achieved through the use of selective color adaptation. In one blue-on, green-off unit, which was adapted to light at 440 nm, the on-response was abolished and the off-response, which persisted, showed a spectral maximum at about 525 nm. When the same unit was adapted to light at 600 nm the off-response dropped out leaving the on-response which was characterized by a spectral maximum at 460 nm. Green-on, blue-off units displayed the same properties except, of course, for the reversal of the impulse discharge at the "on" and "off" of the colored light flash. These results are in accord with the other investigations reviewed in this section in suggesting the presence of a dichromatic opponent system for hue discrimination in the ground squirrel, an obviously simpler system than occurs normally in man and, apparently, in fishes. This raises questions of biological interest. Has the third or "red" mechanism been lost in the course of evolution and been reinvented in primates, or has color vision evolved separately and independently several times during vertebrate phylogeny ? In this connection I make a note of the claim that the tree shrew *(Tupaia glis)* is a dichromat (Snyder, Killackey, and Diamond, 1969). This diurnal animal is said to have an all-cone retina and is an insectivore. This order of mammals is thought by many zoologists to be the ancestral form leading to the primates. The studies of Michael are of interest in still another connection. They suggest that the 523-cone system participates, not only in hue discrimination, but also in other, and achromatic, visual functions such as contrast discrimination and movement sensitivity.

It is a serious deficiency in knowledge that the photochemical basis for ground squirrel vision is not better established. The finding of a 523-pigment reported by Dowling (1964) was obtained by means of a microspectrophotometric study of a small retinal area. No photopigments have been reported yet in retinal extracts of these squirrels. Several years ago I made such extracts from the retinas of the antelope ground squirrel and the much larger Beechy ground squirrel *(Citellus beechyi)*. No rhodopsin was found, as expected, but no other photopigment was detected either. This failure may be due to several reasons one being the small amount of available pigment as suggested by Liebman and Entine, (1968). Dowling (1964) gave dimensions for the cone outer segments as $1.25 \, \mu$m wide and $6-7 \, \mu$m long. This would give a volume for the outer segments about 25 % of that of frog cones, and I have made extractions of as many as 48 retinas of bullfrogs without finding anything except $P502_1$. The only method that appears feasible at present is the method employed by Dowling, in which a small patch of retina is tested by means of a suitable microspectrophotometer.

b) Tree Squirrels. A successful extraction of photopigment was realized by using the retinas of the tree squirrel *Sciurus carolinensis leucotis* (Dartnall, 1960). In these extracts a $P\,502_1$ was found. Since the retina of this tree squirrel had been described as being of the all-cone variety, this finding seemed to indicate the presence of rhodopsin in cones, a result that was later obtained in the accessory members of the double cones in *Rana pipiens* (Liebman and Entine, 1968) and in cones, probably accessory members, of *Chelonia mydas* (Liebman and Granda, 1971). There are some reservations, however, about accepting this for the tree squirrel. Arden and Tansley (1955a) who described the tree squirrel as being free of rods, also described the visual cells as being arranged in two layers and as appearing neither like rods, nor like typical cones. Cohen (1964) stated the tree squirrel visual receptors were of two classes, based mainly on the form and location of the nuclei, and on the sizes and shapes of the outer segments. Cohen divided the visual cells into an R-class, with rod-like characteristics, and a C-class with cone-like properties, the ratio R/C being 4/5. There is no doubt of the duplex nature of the tree squirrel retina if one refers to the early work of Menner (1929) who employed the red variety of *Sciurus vulgaris*. The retina of this squirrel showed the clear separation of the outer nuclear layer into two zones, one more external and consisting of larger nuclei, the second more internal and having smaller nuclei with a different chromatin structure. Though the inner segments of the rods and cones were not very different, MENNER pictured the outer segments of the rods as being more massive than the cone outer segments. While all this does not entirely eliminate the possibility of the cones being the source of the rhodopsin in DARTNALL's extracts, it does indicate that the result was not as straightforward as it would have been in the case of a retina with an indisputably rod-free composition.

The data on the spectral sensitivity of *Sciurus carolinensis leucotis* also indicate the participation of a mechanism in addition to one based on rhodopsin. Using the ERG, ARDEN and TANSLEY (1955a) obtained a sensitivity curve, not in accord with a rhodopsin-mediated mechanism, but somewhat narrower and peaking at about 530 nm. The same curve was recorded for both the scotopic and photopic conditons indicating no Purkinje shift, in accord with the all-cone condition (as they thought) of the retina. The finding of rhodopsin suggests either that the ERG does not record the rhodopsin contribution, which would be surprising, or else that the sensitivity curve of the tree squirrel is determined by the interaction of more than one spectral mechanism. This, in fact, was the interpretation of DART-NALL (1960) who suggested that the physiological response was determined as a modulus of the difference between the spectral absorbance of P 502$_1$ and of a relatively stable 480-photoproduct of its bleaching. DARTNALL predicted that the type of sensitivity curve one would obtain would depend on the ratio 502/480 and that in the case of measurements at absolute threshold, where little or no 480-pigment would accumulate, the sensitivity curve would be that of a rhodopsin-based mechanism. Using a behavior response, ARDEN and SILVER (1962) determined such a sensitivity and found the curve to be that expected for a rhodopsin-mediated mechanism. Accordingly, spectral sensitivity measurements confirmed the presence of a rod-like mechanism in the tree squirrel retina.

c) **Human Rhodopsin.** In his pioneer studies KÜHNE (1877) was able to see evidence of Sehpurpur in the human retina and its apparent absence in the fovea and macula. Following the lead of KÜHNE, who showed that Sehpurpur could be extracted by use of bile salts, KÖNIG (1894) extracted the pigment from a freshly removed human retina. The solution was impure but KÖNIG obtained a difference spectrum and showed an agreement between it and the human scotopic sensitivity curve. This agreement proved directly and unequivocally the correctness of KÜHNE's hypothesis of Sehpurpur as the photochemical basis of vision. It is a curious fact that from 1894 to 1953 no one published any further information on human rhodopsin, although during this period the human scotopic sensitivity curve was being studied with increasing precision, and methods for the extraction and analysis of visual pigments were being developed and improved. The lack of data for the human pigment led to the comparison of human rod sensitivity with the absorbance curves for the pigments of lower vertebrates, an example being the study of HECHT and WILLIAMS (1922), who compared the human sensitivity curve with data on visual purple from rabbit and monkey as obtained by KÖTTGEN and ABELSDORFF (1896). HECHT and WILLIAMS, apparently, believed that the visual purples from various animals (monkey, cat, rabbit, frog) were very similar, if not identical, and they accepted KÖTTGEN and ABELSDORFF's figure of 500 nm as being the absorbance maximum for them all.

Eventually the rod pigment from the human retina was reexamined (CRESCI-TELLI and DARTNALL, 1953). In this reexamination the eye was first dark adapted and then removed, using red light as illumination. The extract was then prepared within two hours following the enucleation. Partial bleaching was carried out and only one photopigment, P 497$_1$, was detected in the extract. The spectral absorbance of the human pigment was shown to be significantly different from that of frog P 502$_1$ and was shown to accord well with the human scotopic curve (CRAWFORD, 1949) expressed in quantum terms and corrected for pre-retinal losses. The agreement between sensitivity and absorbance was so good that it revealed no evidence of a Kundt's rule shift as proposed by HECHT and WILLIAMS (1922) to explain the fact that their sensitivity curve was systematically shifted some 7—8 nm toward the red as compared with the monkey and rabbit visual purple data. In fact, HECHT and WILLIAMS' argument for a Kundt's rule shift was weakened by several defects in experimental design in addition to their use of non-human visual pigment. They expressed the sensitivity in terms of energy, rather than quanta, they failed to correct for pre-retinal absorption, and they employed KÖTTGEN and ABELSDORFF's somewhat uncertain difference spectra for absorbance curves. These defects were not present in a recent resurrection of the Kundt's rule idea (WALD and BROWN, 1958). In this work, human rhodopsin was extracted and found to be, not P497$_1$, as CRESCITELLI and DARTNALL had reported, but P 493$_1$. WALD and BROWN employed somewhat different methods, using not dark-adapted or fresh eyes, but retinas from eyes removed under ordinary surgery, the retinas being stored in the dark at $-10°C$ until used. Now the figure of 497, given by CRESCITELLI and DARTNALL, was stated to be within the limits of 497 ± 2 nm. The figure of 493, given by WALD and BROWN, probably has 1 or 2 nm uncertainty. This would make the difference between the results of the two groups of investigators a very small one, but WALD and BROWN's case for a Kundt's rule effect was actually based on the finding that an outer-segment suspension made from a fresh retina gave a spectral absorbance, not at 493 nm, but at 500 nm, a difference of 7 nm, which was the magnitude of the Kundt's rule shift claimed by HECHT and WILLIAMS. A difference of this magnitude cannot be ignored, for many of the comparisons of spectral sensitivity with pigment absorbance are made with the pigment in solution and not in the hydrophobic environment of the outer segment.

WALD and BROWN's results do not account for certain data in the literature that appear to contradict the operation of a significant Kundt's rule effect. The rhodopsin of red rods in *Rana pipiens*, for example, was found to absorb maximally at 502 nm for the pigment *in situ* (LIEBMAN and ENTINE, 1968). The same rhodopsin extracted into 2% digitonin, the solvent used by WALD and BROWN for human rhodopsin, absorbed maximally at 502 nm (CRESCITELLI, 1958a). DARTNALL (1961) made a special inquiry into this question and showed for the visual pigments of frog, conger eel and carp that the absorbance maxima at 502, 487 and 523 nm were the same for the pigments solubilized in digitonin or measured *in situ* with suspensions of outer segments, and using an opal glass technique to compute the effects of light scattering. Furthermore, the small difference of 2 nm found by DENTON and WALKER (1958) between the extracted pigment and the pigment *in situ* within the retina of the conger eel is well within the limits of error of their measurements. On the basis of these observations one cannot accept as final WALD and BROWN's thesis that a difference in absorbance exists for a visual pigment dissolved in digitonin solution and the same pigment located within the outer segment.

4. Replacement of Vitamin A_1 by Vitamin A_2

As already explained, there is good evidence that a given opsin may combine either with retinal or 3-dehydroretinal to give, respectively, an A_1 or A_2-photopigment. This is what happened when opsin from chicken iodopsin was mixed with retinal to regenerate iodopsin ($P\,562_1$) and was mixed with 3-dehydroretinal to form cyanopsin ($P\,620_2$) (WALD, BROWN, and SMITH, 1953). It is also believed that such transformations of visual pigment class occur naturally within the living retina. The anuran transformation of porphyropsin to rhodopsin during metamorphosis is apparently an example of this. The seasonal, light-dependent change of pigments in the rudd is another (DARTNALL, LANDER, and MUNZ, 1961). As far as present knowledge goes, the visual pigments of mammals are all A_1-based, and we know of no such changes in pigment type as occur in anurans and certain teleosts. Nevertheless, can an A_2-photopigment be induced to form under the pressure of a vitamin A_2 environment? This is the question for this section. It already has been demonstrated that this can occur in the test tube for cattle opsin, which was shown to combine with 3-dehydroretinal to form a synthetic $P517_2$ (WALD, 1953). Theoretically, the rhodopsin of a mammal might be changed to yield a photopigment absorbing at longer wavelengths thus shifting the scotopic sensitivity curve toward the red. In actual fact, however, there are several difficulties, one of these being that the vitamin A_1 reserves of the body are not easily depleted in order to pave the way for the exclusive vitamin A_2 environment that is required. Fortunately, this condition is possible to obtain in the laboratory rat, an animal in which the vitamin A may be depleted, leading eventually to a loss of visual sensitivity and to a degeneration of the outer segments (DOWLING and WALD, 1958). Both conditions may be repaired if vitamin A_1 is given in time.

What are the effects, in such depleted rats, of giving vitamin A_2? SHANTZ, EMBREE, HODGE, and WILLS (1946) first attempted to answer this question. They gave to depleted rats an extract of the tissues of wall-eyed pike. After twelve weeks of such supplementation they extracted the retinas and analyzed the visual pigment content by the method of difference spectrophotometry. The results appeared to indicate that the rhodopsin of the normal rat was replaced to the extent of about 80% by porphyropsin. The conclusion of SHANTZ, EMBREE, HODGE, and WILLS is subject to question on the basis of experimental design and technique. The spectral absorbance curve of the extract was not presented, partial bleaching was not carried out, and the nature of the prosthetic group in the so-called porphyropsin was not identified. For these reasons we have reopened this question and repeated the experiment (YOSHIKAMI, PEARLMAN, and CRESCITELLI, 1969). In this experiment the condition of the visual system was monitored by means of the ERG threshold and histological examination of the retina. The rats received retinoic acid to maintain normal tissue functions and, as a source of vitamin A, synthetic vitamin A_2 was employed. The result was not exactly the same as in the SHANTZ et al. experiment. Vitamin A_2 restored the impaired morphology of the visual cell layer

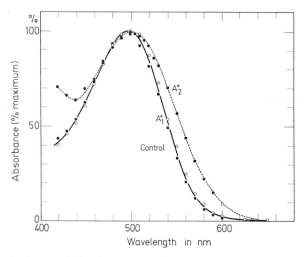

Fig. 28. Normalized spectral absorbance curves for photopigment from: control rats on Purina rat chow *(filled squares)*; vitamin A-deficient rats whose diet was supplemented with retinoic acid and crystalline all-*trans* vitamin A_1 *(plain circles)*; and vitamin A-deficient rats whose diet was supplemented with retinoic acid and crystalline all-*trans* vitamin A_2 *(filled circles)*. The results suggest the presence in the extract of the A_2-supplemented rats of an additional pigment absorbing at longer wavelengths

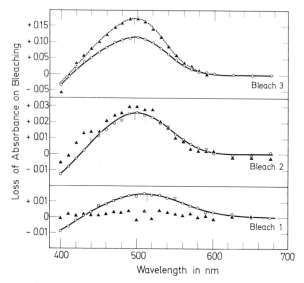

Fig. 29. Spectral density losses caused by three successive bleachings of retinal extracts from control rats *(filled triangles)* and from A_2-supplemented rats *(circles)*. The three exposures were: 3 hours to light of 650 nm *(bleach 1)*, 1 hour to light of 600 nm *(bleach 2)*, and exhaustive exposure to light of 550 nm *(bleach 3)*. Hydroxylamine was present during the bleachings. The results indicate that for the A_2-supplemented rats the photopigment in the extract consisted of about 90% (density-wise) of normal rat rhodopsin ($P 497_1$) but that about 10% was a $P 517_2$, as is proved by Fig. 30

and the lowered visual sensitivity. It was able to restore a photopigment in the retinas of the depleted rats, but this pigment was not porphyropsin but mainly rat rhodopsin ($P497_1$) along with a minor component ($P517_2$). Some details of this investigation are shown in Figs. 28, 29, 30. It appears that the rat retina is able to convert 3-dehydroretinol to retinal and thus to form normal rhodopsin, while a

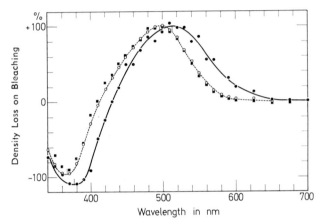

Fig. 30. Normalized difference spectra of Fig. 29. Continuous curve *(filled circles)* represents the 517-pigment removed by an initial bleaching with light of 650 nm of an extract from A_2-supplemented rats. Such a bleaching had no significant effect on an extract of control rats on a normal Purina rat chow diet (Fig. 29 bleach 1). Dotted curve *(plain circles)* is the result of further exhaustive bleaching with light at 550 nm to remove all rhodopsin. Dotted curve 2 *(filled squares)* shows the result of a total bleaching with light of 550 nm of an extract from control rats. This extract revealed the presence of no photopigment other than rhodopsin. The product peaks (oximes) indicate a vitamin A_2-base for the 517-pigment and vitamin A_1 for the remainder of the photopigment in the extract from the A_2-supplemented animals

small amount of 3-dehydroretinal is produced leading to the $P517_2$, the same pigment formed in the test tube with 3-dehydroretinal and cattle opsin from rhodopsin. In a second investigation of this problem no evidence was secured to implicate the thyroid hormone in this conversion (PEARLMAN and CRESCITELLI, 1971). Totally thyroidectomized rats depleted of their vitamin A stores responded similarly to the administration of 3-dehydroretinol as did depleted rats with thyroid glands intact.

XII. Summary

This chapter has been concerned with pointing out the wealth of morphological and biochemical diversity displayed by the vertebrate retina. This diversity has evolved, not through fortuitous factors in evolution but rather through the interaction of natural selection with diversity in the photic environment. Although we do not yet know the significance of all the structures that appear in the visual cells, most of them, when related to other properties of the eye, appear to have adaptive value in relation to the photic environment. In the body of this text

I have tried to show that such adaptations have involved the visual cell composition of the retina, the regional distribution of visual cell types, the detailed morphology of the rods and cones, and the nature of the photopigments housed within the visual cells. I have also indicated that while Schultze's concept of rod-cone duplexity has been extremely useful in helping us understand many functional attributes of the vertebrate retina, it cannot be applied too rigidly to the phylogenetic history of the visual cells.

Schultze's view that rods are the simpler of the two visual receptors cannot be easily defended. Indeed, as this review has indicated, rods have all the organelles and structures possessed by cones, and appear to perform visual functions that are fully as complex. In lower vertebrates at least there is no reason to reject a possible role of rods in hue discrimination. Schultze also suggested that rods were the ancestral cells from which cones eventually evolved. This idea arose out of his failure to find cones in the retinas of elasmobranchs and the lamprey. In the preceding pages I have pointed out that cones do indeed occur in the elasmobranch retina and that a duplex retina has been noted in lampreys. Schultze himself displayed vacillation on the question of cones in the lamprey retina.

In contrast to Schultze, Walls (1934) adopted the view that the cone is the ancestral cell. Walls supported this idea on the argument that visual cells have evolved from flagellated ependymal-like cells, the outer segment being derived by a modification of the flagellum. The original photoreceptors of the retina were conceived as filamentous, simple entities with low sensitivity to light, i.e., cone-like receptors. Walls invoked the biogenetic law of Haeckel in his support, stating that cones complete their ontogenetic development before rods, and rods, in their development, pass through a cone-like stage. It seems to be true that amphibian rods go through a stage of conically-shaped cells and that amphibian cones complete full development before rods, but both rods and cones appear to arise from one type of undifferentiated cell and at about the same time (Detwiler and Laurens, 1921; Saxén, 1954). Even if a clear duality in ontogenesis were present, it is not at all certain that this would reveal anything about the phylogeny of these two receptors. The law of recapitulation has received severe condemnation in recent years and de Beer (1954), who reviewed this subject, concluded that even if we knew all about the events of ontogeny, this alone would not elucidate phylogeny. He added that the concept of homology cannot be based on embryology but, instead, on comparative anatomy and palaeontology. This is the method I have employed in this review.

Because of the nature of palaeontological remains we shall never be able to answer the question of the visual cell ancestry. Willmer (1953, 1965) advanced the hypothesis of immutable phylogenetic duality of rods and cones starting from their ancestral origin in two types of cells of the surface epithelium. In my view, the data that have been summarized in this review do not support Willmer duplexity. Instead, these data suggest the occurrence of numerous and independent transmutations from one receptor type to the other in response to changes in the habitat of an evolving form. Though fully-evolved rods and cones are present in many vertebrates, the evidence of the whole phylogenetic series does not indicate a fixed and immutable duality. The occurrence of rods with organelles usually associated with cones, the finding of apparently intermediate cells whose identity as rods or cones is difficult to ascertain, and the presence in certain groups of an homologous series such as the *Crotaphytus-Xantusia-Coleonyx* sequences are all features of the visual cell biology that encourage an interpretation based on the lability and mutability of the visual receptors.

The appearance in printed form of WALLS' transmutation theory (WALLS, 1934) was followed shortly after by a severe denunciation of this theory by VERRIER (1935) who labelled it as imaginative, arbitrary and gratuitous. She selected for special criticism WALLS' interpretation of the visual cells of the Gila monster, *Heloderma suspectum*. The retina and eye of this lizard appeared to contradict both the duplexity theory and the transmutation theory. Believed to be nocturnal, *Heloderma* was described by WALLS as having a circular pupil and functional eyelids rather than spectacles. The visual cells, singles and doubles, were seen to have colorless oil-droplets but the outer segments were not described as being rod-like. VERRIER called them cones, and WALLS was placed in the position of calling them intermediate cells, "at the risk of seeming arbitrary". WALLS explained the *Heloderma* transmutation to nocturnal sensitivity by assuming the development of extensive summation in the neural layers. Actually, there was no necessity for WALLS to have invoked special transmutation in the case of *Heloderma* had he known more about the natural history of this lizard. A definitive study of the family Helodermatidae was made by BOGERT and MARTÍN DEL CAMPO (1956). In this study it was pointed out that the Gila monster is very probably not strictly nocturnal. Instead, chemoreception through the tongue — Jacobson's organ system — may play a more important role than vision in the finding of eggs, which form an important item in the diet of these lizards. BOGERT and MARTÍN DEL CAMPO described some observations in which Gila monsters were shown to be able to track down a buried egg over a trail laid down by drawing the egg over a circuitous path in the sand leading to the spot where the egg was buried. These eggs were traced and uncovered by the lizards even though they were unable to see an egg placed 15 cm away that had been placed on the sand without making a scent trail. Even if the Gila monster is more active at dusk, as it appears to be, this does not prove the presence of a nocturnal visual system. The sense of smell might easily be the dominant sense in dim light. It is obvious that a physiological study of the *Heloderma* retina might yield interesting results.

Of the two classes of visual pigments in vertebrates, we probably shall never know which represents the ancestral system. I have pointed out, however, that there is no reason to accept WALD's interpretation of porphyropsin, or an A_2-pigment, as the parent system. The known visual pigments in *Entosphenus* and in *Petromyzon* along with the real doubts that have been raised regarding the origin of vertebrates in fresh water, weaken WALD's case for porphyropsin as the ancestral photopigment. Moreover, a strict association of the A_2-system and the freshwater habit has not been confirmed to occur in all teleosts. Tropical freshwater fishes, according to SCHWANZARA, do not show, as do temperate zone fishes, a significant spezial association with the A_2-pigment system.

On the other hand, an apparent correlation between visual pigment and photic environment has been noted at least for those pigments appearing in retinal extracts. Of these, perhaps the most convincing is the finding, in deep-sea fishes, teleosts, elasmobranchs and chimaerids, of a pigment system whose absorptive properties are suited to the blue-green environment of the deep sea. These deep-sea forms display other adaptations of the visual system to the dim light of their environment. The teleosts have evolved retinas with all rods that have long and cylindrical outer segments and with a retinal photopigment density that is relatively high. The elasmobranchs possess an efficient *tapetum lucidum* while the rod outer segments are about half as long as those of the teleosts living in the same environment. The chimaerid fishes also have increased their sensitivity by developing a *tapetum*. The significance of the unique deep-sea photosystem is accentuated by the fact that marine teleosts that inhabit the yellow-green environment of sandy shores, bays and estuaries have retinal pigments with maximal absorbance at some 30 nm longer than in the case of the deep-sea pigments. The suggestion has been made that the A_2-system, with its absorbance at longer wavelengths, has evolved in close association with the redder environment of freshwater lakes, ponds, streams and swamps. Moreover, the presence of a dual A_1-A_2 visual system, which is known to occur in many freshwater species, might have developed in connection with life in a changing photic environment, where a greater spectral coverage would be advantageous. Such an advantage would be accentuated if the ratio of A_1 to A_2 pigments were to change according to the changing environment. This may be the meaning of the seasonal change in A_1/A_2 ratio found in the rudd and other fishes. All this is not to imply that light is the direct factor, or the only factor, involved in controlling the visual system. The effect of light might be mediated, for example, by way of the endocrine system.

It would be a mistake to interpret the spectroscopic nature of all visual pigments in terms of the nature of the photic environment. The presence of a porphyropsin-rhodopsin metamorphic transition in ranid and microhylid amphibians, but not in bufonids, indicates that a simple photic environment explanation is insufficient. The gecko visual pigments have presented a very special problem. In terms of their photic environment there is no reason to expect anything but a rhodopsin system of the classical type; yet they possess a scotopic pigment spectrally located 20 to 30 nm higher than rhodopsin. At present there is no better explanation for this gecko situation than in terms of the transmutation theory. An explanation based on an accident of evolution is unsatisfactory. The principal message of this chapter seems to be that nature has not left many, if any, random errors in evolving the visual system.

I have also presented in this chapter evidence indicating, as one would expect, that the visual pigments are genetically determined, insofar as the nature of the opsin is concerned. There are possibilities, however, that light might act through non-genetic channels to influence the visual cells and visual pigment composition of an animal. Several investigators have searched for such effects. KÜHNE (1877), it will be recalled, saw Sehpurpur in a 65 cm calf embryo whose eyes had never been exposed to light. Using tree frogs, which were allowed to develop from the gastrula stage through metamorphosis in total darkness, EAKIN (1965) found no effect on the development of the outer segment discs of rods and cones. These results suggest that light is not required for the development of the outer segments nor for the synthesis of rhodopsin. There are some effects of light that are understandable in terms of the greater thermal lability of opsin as compared to rhodopsin. DOWLING and SIDMAN (1962), for example, reported that dystrophic rats kept in the dark, beginning at 10 to 20 days after birth, showed a delay in the degenerative changes associated with the dystrophy. Compared with dystrophic rats kept in the lighted room, the rats in the dark showed considerable protection as indicated by the ERG, the histology, and the rhodopsin content. In respect to the effect of light the rhodopsin system of the rat differs from the photosynthetic apparatus of green plants and *Euglena*. When these are kept in darkness, the chlorophyll disappears and the chloroplast structure is altered. Under the influence of light, chlorophyll is synthesized, the normal structure is restored (KIRK and TILNEY-BASSETT, 1967), and a synthesis of plastid proteins occurs (DE DEKEN-GRENSON, 1954; POGO, BRAWERMAN and CHARGAFF, 1962). The photosynthetic system becomes unstable in the dark while the retinal rod system becomes unstable in the light. In both cases this may, in the end, be the same mechanism, i.e., the lability of the protein in the absence of the stabilizing prosthetic group.

The photic interconversion of the A_1- and A_2-photopigments that has been found in the rudd and other freshwater fishes appears to represent a mechanism in which the same opsin is employed but a replacement reaction between the two aldehydes takes place. DARTNALL (1964) postulated two possible types of replacement to account for the interconversion. In the light the A_2-pigment after bleaching was postulated to lose its 3-dehydroretinal which was then replaced by retinal, present in the blood in higher concentration. Thus long days would favor the A_1-system. In the dark, on the other hand, the retinal while still attached to the opsin was postulated to be dehydrogenated leading to the A_2-system. Thus short days, as in winter, would favor the A_2-system. (See also p. 469.)

An interesting and significant light-linked ophthalmological transformation has been noted, but not deeply explored, in certain cavernicolous forms such as cave fishes and the olm, *Proteus anguinus*. In the young or larval form after hatching, the eyes and retina develop up to a point and then degenerate, this degeneration involving the retina, cornea, lens and virtually all the structures of the eye. The eye then becomes imbedded within a fold of skin and the animal is said to be blind, although light-sensitive regions of the skin may be present (KOHL, 1891; EGGERT, 1931; KUHN and KÄHLING, 1954). The amount of degeneration and the final condition of the eye in the adult vary in different species of "blind fishes" (EIGENMANN, 1899). In the olm this degeneration of the eye has been shown to be preventable by keeping the animal in a lighted environment in which case the eye, not only does not degenerate, but proceeds to increase in size, to develop a normal lens and to form a retina with all layers and with differentiated rods and cones (KAMMERER, 1912). The mechanisms or reasons for this so-called "disuse effect" in the dark, and its reversal in the light, are entirely unknown but clearly some interesting possibilities for research in photobiology are offered by these cavernicolous forms.

References

ABELSDORFF, G.: Physiologische Beobachtungen am Auge der Krokodile. Arch. Anat. Physiol. (Physiol. Abt.) **1898**, 155—166.

ALLEN, D. M.: Photic control of the proportions of two visual pigments in a fish. Vision Res. **11**, 1077—1112 (1951).

ARDEN, G. B., SILVER, P. H. (née STRANGE): Visual thresholds and spectral sensitivities of the grey squirrel *(Sciurus carolinensis leucotis)*. J. Physiol. (Lond.) **163**, 540—557 (1962).

ARDEN, G. B., TANSLEY, K.: The spectral sensitivity of the pure-cone retina of the grey squirrel *(Sciurus carolinensis leucotis)*. J. Physiol. (Lond.) **127**, 592—602 (1955a).
— — The spectral sensitivity of the pure-cone retina of the souslik *(Citellus citellus)*. J. Physiol. (Lond.) **130**, 225—232 (1955b).
— — The electroretinogram of a diurnal gecko. J. gen. Physiol. **45**, 1145—1161 (1962).
AREY, L. B.: The movements in the visual cells and retinal pigments of the lower vertebrates. J. comp. Neurol. **26**, 121—200 (1916).
ARMINGTON, J. C.: Spectral sensitivity of the turtle, *Pseudemys*. J. comp. physiol. Psychol. **47**, 1—6 (1954).
BALL, S., GOODWIN, T. W., MORTON, R. A.: Studies on vitamin A. 5: The preparation of retinene$_1$ — vitamin A aldehyde. Biochem. J. **42**, 516—523 (1948).
BARDACK, D., ZANGERL, R.: First fossil lamprey: a record from the Pennsylvanian of Illinois. Science **162**, 1265—1267 (1968).
BARRINGTON, E. J. W.: The biology of Hemichordata and Protochordata. Edinburgh-London: Oliver and Boyd (1965).
BAYLISS, L. E., LYTHGOE, R. J., TANSLEY, K.: Some new forms of visual purple found in sea fishes with a note on the visual cells of origin. Proc. roy. Soc. B. **120**, 95—113 (1936).
BEATTY, D. D.: Visual pigments of three species of cartilaginous fishes. Nature (Lond.) **222**, 285 (1969a).
— Visual pigments of the burbot, *Lota lota*, and seasonal changes in their relative proportions. Vision Res. **9**, 1173—1183 (1969b).
BELLAIRS, A. D'A., UNDERWOOD, G.: The origin of snakes. Biol. Rev. **26**, 193—237 (1951).
BERNARD, H. M.: Studies in the retina; rods and cones in the frog and in some other amphibia. Quart. J. micr. Sci. **43**, 23—47 (1900).
BERRILL, N. J.: The origin of vertebrates. Oxford: Clarendon Press (1955).
BLAXTER, J. H. S., JONES, M. P.: The development of the retina and retinomotor responses in the herring. J. mar. biol. Ass. U. K. **47**, 677—697 (1967).
BLISS, A. F.: The chemistry of daylight vision. J. gen. Physiol. **29**, 277—297 (1946).
BLOUGH, D. S.: Spectral sensitivity in the pigeon. J. opt. Soc. Amer. **47**, 827—833 (1957).
BODEN, B. P., KAMPA, E. M., SNODGRASS, J. M.: Underwater daylight measurements in the Bay of Biscay. J. MARIN. biol. Ass. U. K. **39**, 227—238 (1960).
BOGERT, C. M., MARTÍN DEL CAMPO, R.: The Gila monster and its allies. Bull. amer. Mus. Nat. History **109**, 5—238 (1956).
BOLL, F.: Zur Anatomie und Physiologie der Retina. Mber. Berl. Akad. Wiss. **12**, 783—788 (1876).
— Zur Anatomie und Physiologie der Retina. Arch. Anat. Physiol. (Physiol. Abt.) **1877**, 4—35.
BONE, Q.: The origin of the chordates. J. Linn. Soc. Lond. (Zool.) **44**, 252—269 (1958).
BOWNDS, D.: Site of attachment of retinal in rhodopsin. Nature (Lond.) **216**, 1178—1181 (1967).
BRIDGES, C. D. B.: The visual pigments of the rainbow trout *(Salmo irideus)*. J. Physiol. (Lond.) **134**, 620—629 (1956).
— Visual pigments of some common laboratory mammals. Nature (Lond.) **184**, 1727—1728 (1959).
— Visual pigments of the pigeon *(Columba livia)*. Vision Res. **2**, 125—137 (1962).
— Periodicity of absorption properties in pigments based on vitamin A$_2$ from fish retinae. Nature (Lond.) **203**, 303—304 (1964a).
— Effect of season and environment on the retinal pigments of two fishes. Nature (Lond.), **203**, 191—192 (1964b).
— Absorption properties, interconversions, and environmental adaptation of pigments from fish photoreceptors. Cold Spr. Harb. Symp. quant. Biol. **30**, 317—334 (1965a).
— Visual pigments in a fish exposed to different light environments. Nature (Lond.) **206**, 1161—1162 (1965b).
— Reversible visual pigment changes in tadpoles exposed to light and darkness. Nature (Lond.) **227**, 956—957 (1970).
— YOSHIKAMI, S.: The rhodopsin-porphyropsin system in freshwater fishes. 1. Effects of age and photic environment. Vision Res. **10**, 1315—1332 (1970a).

BRIDGES, C. D. B., YOSHIKAMI, S.: The rhodopsin-porphyropsin system in freshwater fishes. 2. Turnover and interconversion of visual pigment prosthetic groups in light and darkness: role of the pigment epithelium. Vision Res. 10, 1333—1345 (1970b).
— — Distribution and evolution of visual pigments in salmonid fishes. Vision Res. 10, 609—626 (1970c).
BROWN, K. T.: A linear area centralis extending across the turtle retina and stabilized to the horizon by non-visual cues. Vision Res. 9, 1053—1062 (1969).
BUTCHER, E. O.: The structure of the retina of Fundulus heteroclitus and the regions of the retina associated with the different chromatophoric responses. J. exp. Zool. 79, 275—297 (1938).
CAMERON, J.: The development of the retina in amphibia: an embryological and cytological study. J. Anat. Physiol. 39, 135—153, 332—361, 471—488 (1905).
CARLISLE, D. B., DENTON, E. J.: On the metamorphosis of the visual pigments of Anguilla anguilla L. J. mar. biol. Ass. U. K. 38, 97—102 (1959).
CARR, A.: The navigation of the green turtle. Sci. Amer. 212, No. 5 (May), 78—86 (1965).
CARTER, G. S.: Chordate phylogeny (review of "The Origin of Vertebrates" by BERRILL, N. J.) Syst. Zool. 6, 187—192 (1957).
CASTENHOLZ, E.: Über die Struktur der Netzhautmitte bei Primaten. Z. Zellforsch. 64, 646—661 (1965).
CHASE, A. M.: Photosensitive pigments from the retina of the frog. Science 87, 238 (1938).
CLARKE, G. L.: On the depth at which fish can see. Ecology 17, 452—456 (1936).
COHEN, A. I.: Some observations on the fine structure of the retinal receptors of the American grey squirrel. Invest. Ophthal. 3, 198—216 (1964).
COHEN, P. P.: Biochemical aspects of metamorphosis: transition from ammonotelism to ureotelism. Harvey Lectures 60, 119—154 (1966).
COLLINS, F. D., LOVE, R. M., MORTON, R. A.: Studies in Vitamin A. 25. Visual pigments in tadpoles and adult frogs. Biochem. J. 53, 632—636 (1953).
CONTINO, F.: Das Auge des Argyropelecus hemigymnus. Morphologie, Bau, Entwicklung und Refraktion. von Graefe's Arch. Ophthal. 140, 390—441 (1939).
CRAWFORD, B. H.: The scotopic visibility function. Proc. phys. Soc. London B, 62, 321—334 (1949).
CRESCITELLI, F.: The nature of the lamprey visual pigment. J. gen. Physiol. 39, 423—435 (1956a).
— The nature of the gecko visual pigment. J. gen. Physiol. 40, 217—231 (1956b).
— The natural history of visual pigments. Proc. 19th Ann. Biol. Coll. Oregon State College, April, 1958, 30—51 (1958a).
— Evidence for a blue-sensitive component in the retina of the gecko, Oedura monilis. Science 127, 1442—1443 (1958b).
— The electroretinogram of the antelope ground squirrel. Vision Res. 1, 139—153 (1961).
— Some characteristics of on- and off-responses to flashes of colored light in ground squirrel visual system. J. Neurophysiol. 25, 141—151 (1962).
— The photosensitive retinal pigment system of Gekko gekko. J. gen. Physiol. 47, 33—52 (1963a).
— The duplicity theory: a phylogenetic view. In: General physiology of cell specialization (Ed. MAZIA, D., TYLER, A.) New York: McGraw-Hill 1963b.
— The spectral sensitivity and visual pigment content of the retina of Gekko gekko. In: Ciba Foundation Symp. Colour Vision. Physiology and Exper. Psychol. London: Churchill 1965.
— The visual pigment of a chimaeroid fish. Vision Res. 9, 1407—1414 (1969).
— DARTNALL, H. J. A.: Human visual purple. Nature (Lond.) 172, 195—196 (1953).
— — A photosensitive pigment of the carp retina. J. Physiol. 125, 607—627 (1954).
— POLLACK, J. D.: Color vision in the antelope ground squirrel. Science 150, 1316-1318 (1965).
— — Investigations into colour vision of the ground squirrel. In: Aspects of Comp. Ophthalm. (Ed. GRAHAM-JONES, O.). Oxford: Pergamon Press 1966.
— WILSON, B. W., LILYBLADE, A. L.: The visual pigments of birds I. the turkey. Vision Res. 4, 275—280 (1964).
CROZIER, W. J., WOLF, E.: The flicker response contour for the gecko (rod retina). J. gen. Physiol. 22, 555—566 (1939).
D'ANCONA, U.: Old and new solutions to the eel problem. Nature (Lond.) 183, 1405 (1959).

Dartnall, H. J. A.: A study of the visual pigments of the clawed toad. J. Physiol. **125**, 25—42 (1954).
— Further observations on the visual pigments of the clawed toad, *Xenopus laevis*. J. Physiol. **134**, 327—338 (1956).
— The visual pigments. London: Methuen & Co. Ltd. 1957
— Visual pigment from a pure-cone retina. Nature (Lond.) **188**, 475—479 (1960).
— Visual pigments before and after extraction from visual cells. Proc. roy. Soc. London B, **154**, 250—266 (1961).
— The photobiology of visual processes. In: The Eye. **2**, (Ed. Davson, H.). New York-London: Academic Press 1962.
— The visual pigments: a photobiological study. Ann. roy. Coll. Surg. Engl. **35**, 131—150 (1964).
— The visual pigment of the green rods. Vision Res. **7**, 1—16 (1967).
— Arden, G. B., Ikeda, H., Luck, C. P., Rosenberg, M. E., Pedler, C. M. H., Tansley, K.: Anatomical, electrophysiological and pigmentary aspects of vision in the bush baby: an interpretative study. Vision Res. **5**, 399—424 (1965).
— Lander, M. R., Munz, F. W.: Periodic changes in the visual pigment of a fish. Prog. in Photobiol., Proc. 3rd Internat. Photobiol. Congr. 203—213. Amsterdam: Elsevier 1961.
— Lythgoe, J. N.: The spectral clustering of visual pigments. Vision Res. **5**, 81—100 (1965).
Dean, B.: Chimaeroid fishes and their development. Carnegie Inst. Wash. **1906**, 3—186.
Deane, H. W., Enroth-Cugel, C., Gongaware, M. S., Neyland, M., Forbes, A.: Electroretinogram of fresh-water turtle: form and spectral sensitivity. J. Neurophysiol. **21**, 45—61 (1958).
De Beer, G.: Embryos and Ancestors. Oxford: Clarendon Press 1954.
De Deken-Grenson, M.: Grana formation and synthesis of chloroplastic proteins induced by light in portions of etiolated leaves. Biochim. biophysic. Acta (Amst.) **14**, 203—211 (1954).
Deelder, C. L.: The Atlantic eel problem. Nature (Lond.) **185**, 589—591 (1960).
Denison, R. H.: A review of the habitat of the earliest vertebrates. Fieldiana: Geology **11**, 359—457 (1956).
Denissenko, G.: Einiges über den Bau der Netzhaut des Aales. Arch. Mikroskop. Anat. **21**, 1—25 (1882).
Denton, E. J.: The spectral sensitivity of a nocturnal gecko. 19th Internat. Physiol. Congress. Abst. of Commun., 306 (1953).
— The responses of the pupil of *Gekko gekko* to external light stimulus. J. gen. Physiol. **40**, 201—215 (1956).
— Nicol, J. A. C.: The chorioidal tapeta of some cartilaginous fishes (chondrichthyes). J. mar. biol. Ass. U. K. **44**, 219—258 (1964).
— Shaw, T. I.: The visual pigments of some deep-sea elasmobranchs. J. mar. biol. Ass. U. K. **43**, 65—70 (1963).
— Walker, M. A.: The visual pigment of the conger eel. Proc. roy. Soc. (Lond.) B, **148**, 257—269 (1958).
— Warren, F. J.: Visual pigments of deep-sea fish. Nature (Lond.) **178**, 1059 (1956).
— — The photosensitive pigments in the retinae of deep-sea fish. J. mar. biol. Ass. U. K. **36**, 651—662 (1957).
— Wyllie, J. H.: Study of the photosensitive pigments in the pink and green rods of the frog. J. Physiol. **127**, 81—89 (1955).
Detwiler, S. R.: The effect of light on the retina of the tortoise and the lizard. J. exp. Zool. **20**, 165—189 (1916).
— Studies on the retina. An experimental study of the gecko retina. J. comp. Neurol. **36**, 125—141 (1923).
— Studies on the retina. Observations on the rods of nocturnal mammals. J. comp. Neurol. **37**, 481—489 (1924).
— Comparative studies upon the eyes of nocturnal lemuroids, monkeys and man. Anat. Rec. **74**, 129—145 (1939).
— The eye of the owl monkey *(Nyctipithecus)*. Anat. Rec. **80**, 233—241 (1941).
— Vertebrate Photoreceptors, New York: Macmillan 1943.

Detwiler, S. R., Laurens, H.: Studies on the retina. The structure of the retina of *Phrynosoma cornutum*. J. comp. Neurol. **32**, 347—356 (1920).

— — Studies on the retina. Histogenesis of the visual cells in *Amblystoma*. J. comp. Neurol. **33**, 493—508 (1921).

Dilly, N.: Electron microscope observations of the receptors in the sensory vesicle of the ascidian tadpole. Nature (Lond.) **191**, 786—787 (1961).

— Studies on the receptors in the cerebral vesicle of the ascidian tadpole. 2. The ocellus. Quart. J. micr. Sci. **105**, 13—20 (1964).

Dobrowolsky, W.: Die Doppelzapfen. Arch. Anat. Physiol. wiss. Med. **4**, 208—221 (1871).

Dodt, E., Jessen, K. H.: The duplex nature of the retina of the nocturnal gecko as reflected in the electroretinogram. J. gen. Physiol. **44**, 1143—1158 (1961).

— Scherer, E.: The electroretinogram of the third eye. II. Symp. Internat. Soc. clin. Electroret. (J.S.C.E.R.G.), Erfurt (1967).

— — Photic responses from the parietal eye of the lizard *Lacerta sicula campestris* (DeBetta). Vision Res. **8**, 61—72 (1968).

— Walther, J. B.: Über die spektrale Empfindlichkeit und die Schwelle von Gecko-Augen, Untersuchungen an *Hemidactylus turcicus* und *Tarentola mauritanica*. Pflügers Arch. ges. Physiol. **268**, 204—212 (1959).

Donner, K. O., Reuter, T.: The spectral sensitivity and photopigment of the green rods in the frog's retina. Vision Res. **2**, 357—372 (1962).

— Rushton, W. A. H.: Rod-cone interaction in the frog's retina analyzed by the Stiles-Crawford effect and by dark adaptation. J. Physiol. **149**, 303—317 (1959).

Dowling, J. E.: Structure and function in the all-cone retina of the ground squirrel. In: The Physiol. Basis for Form Discrimination, Symp., Brown Univ., Jan. 23—24, 1964.

— Ripps, H.: Visual adaptation in the retina of the skate. J. gen. Physiol. **56**, 491—520 (1970).

— Sidman, R. L.: Inherited retinal dystrophy in the rat. J. cell. Biol. **14**, 73—109 (1962).

— Wald, G.: Vitamin A deficiency and night blindness. Proc. nat. Acad. Sci. (Wash.) **44**, 648—661 (1958).

Duijm, M.: On the position of a ribbon-like central area in the eyes of some birds. Arch. néerl. Zool. **13**, 128—145 (1958).

Duke-Elder, S.: The eye in evolution. London: Henry Kimpton 1958.

Dunn, R. F.: Electron microscopy studies on the photoreceptor cells of the gecko, *Coleonyx variegatus*. Ph. D. Thesis, Univ. of Calif., Los Angeles (1965).

Eakin, R. M.: Lines of evolution of photoreceptors. In: General Physiology of Cell Specialization (Ed.: Mazia, D., Tyler, A.). New York: McGraw-Hill 1963.

— Differentiation of rods and cones in total darkness. J. cell. Biol. **25**, 162—165 (1965).

— Evolution of Photoreceptors. Cold Spr. Harb. Symp. quant. Biol. **30**, 363—370 (1965).

— Kuda, A.: Ultrastructure of sensory receptors in ascidian tadpoles. Z. Zellforsch. **112**, 287—312 (1971).

— Westfall, J. A.: Fine structure of photoreceptors in amphioxus. J. Ultra. Res. **6**, 531—539 (1962).

Eggert, B.: Der Bau des Auges und der Hautsinnesorgane bei den Gobiiformes *Amblyopus brachygaster* Gthr. u. *Trypauchen vagina* Bl. Schn. Z. Wissenschaft. Zool. **138**, 68—87 (1931).

Eigenmann, C. H.: The eyes of the blind vertebrates of North America. The eyes of the amblyopsidae. Arch. Entwicklungs. der Organismen **8**, 545—617 (1899).

— Shafer, G. D.: The mosaic of single and twin cones in the retina of fishes. The American Naturalist **34**, 109—118 (1900).

Engström, K.: Cone types and cone arrangement in the retina of some cyprinids. Acta Zool. **41**, 277—295 (1960).

— Cone types and cone arrangement in the retina of some gadids. Acta Zool. **42**, 227—243 (1961).

— Cone types and cone arrangements in teleost retinae. Acta Zool. **44**, 179—243 (1963a).

— Structure, organization and ultra-structure of the visual cells in the teleost family *Labridae*. Acta Zool. **44**, 1—41 (1963b).

— Ahlbert, I.-B.: Cone types and cone arrangement in the retina of some flatfishes. Acta Zool. **44**, 119—129 (1963).

Engström, K., Rosstorp, E.: Photomechanical responses in different cone types of *Leuciscus rutilus*. Acta Zool. **44**, 145—160 (1963).

Etkin, W.: Metamorphosis. In: Physiology of the Amphibia (Ed. Moore, J. A.) New York: Academic Press 1964.

Ferraz De Oliveira, L., Ripps, H.: The "area centralis" of the owl monkey *(Aotes trivirgatus)* Vision Res. **8**, 223—228 (1968).

Forbes, A., Fox, S., Milburn, N., Deane, H. W.: Electroretinograms and spectral sensitivities of some diurnal lizards. J. Neurophysiol. **23**, 62—73 (1960).

Franz, V.: Auge und Akkomodation von *Petromyzon (Lampetra) fluviatilis* L. Zool. Jahrbüch. Abteilung f. allgemeine Zoologie und Physiologie der Tiere. **52**, 144—178 (1932—33).

Frieden, E.: Thyroid hormones and the biochemistry of amphibian metamorphosis. Recent Progress in Hormone Res. **23**, 139—194 (1967).

Gage, S. H.: The lampreys of New York State. Life history and economics. In: A Biological Survey of the Oswego River system. Conservation Dept., State of N. Y., 158—191, Albany: J. B. Lyon Co., 1928.

Goin, C. J., Goin, O. B.: Introduction to Herpetology. San Francisco: W. H. Freeman & Co. 1962.

Goldsmith, T. H., Fernandez, H. R.: Comparative studies of crustacean spectral sensivity. Z. vergleich. Physiol. **60**, 156—175 (1968).

Gorman, A. L. F., McReynolds, J. S., Barnes, S. N.: Photoreceptors in primitive chordates: fine structure, hyperpolarizing receptor potentials, and evolution. Science **172**, 1052—1054 (1971).

Granda, A. M.: Electrical responses of the light- and dark-adapted turtle eye. Vision Res. **2**, 343—356 (1962).

— Stirling, C. E.: The spectral sensitivity of the turtle's eye to very dim lights. Vision Res. **6**, 143—152 (1966).

Granit, R.: A relation between rod and cone substances. Acta physiol. scand. **2**, 334—346 (1941).

— The photopic spectrum of the pigeon. Acta physiol. scand. **4**, 118—124 (1942).

— Stimulus intensity in relation to excitation and pre- and post-excitatory inhibition in isolated elements of mammalian retinae. J. Physiol. **103**, 103—118 (1944).

— Receptors and Sensory Perception. New Haven: Yale Univ. Press 1955.

Gruber, S. H., Hamasaki, D. H., Bridges, C. D. B.: Cones in the retina of the Lemon Shark *(Negaprion brevirostris)* Vision Res. **3**, 397—399 (1963).

Gunn, R. M.: On the eye of *Ornithorhynchus paradoxus*. J. Anat. Physiol. **18**, 400—405 (1884).

Hamasaki, D. I.: An anatomical and electrophysiological study of the retina of the owl monkey, *Aotes trivirgatus*. J. comp. Neurol. **130**, 163—169 (1967).

— The spectral sensitivity of the lateral eye of the green iguana. Vision Res. **8**, 1305—1314 (1968).

— Spectral sensitivity of the parietal eye of the green iguana. Vision Res. **9**, 515—523 (1969).

— Bridges, C. D. B.: Properties of the electroretinogram in three elasmobranch species. Vision Res. **5**, 483—496 (1965).

Hamilton, W. F., Coleman, T. B.: Trichromatic vision in the pigeon as illustrated by the spectral discrimination curve. J. comp. Psychol. **15**, 183—191 (1933).

Hannover, A.: Über die Netzhaut und ihre Gehirnsubstanz bei Wirbeltieren, mit Ausnahme des Menschen. Arch. Anat. Physiol. wiss. Med. 320—345 (1840).

Hartline, H. K., Wagner, H. G., MacNichol, E. F., Jnr.: The peripheral origin of nervous activity in the visual system. Cold Spr. Harb. Symp. quant. Biol. **17**, 125—141 (1952).

Hecht, S., Williams, R. E.: The visibility of monochromatic radiation and the absorption spectrum of visual purple. J. gen. Physiol. **5**, 1—33 (1922).

Heinemann, C.: Beiträge zur Anatomie der Retina. Arch. Mikroskop. Anat. **14**, 409—441 (1877).

Hess, W. N.: Reactions to light and the photoreceptors of *Dolichoglossus kowalevskyi*. J. exp. Zool. **79**, 1—11 (1938).

Hollenberg, M. J., Bernstein, M. H.: Fine structure of the photoreceptor cells of the ground squirrel *(Citellus tridecemlineatus)* Amer. J. Anat. **118**, 359—371 (1966).

HOLMBERG, K.: The hagfish retina: fine structure of retinal cells in *Myxine glutinosa*, L., with special reference to receptor and epithelial cells. Z. Zellforsch. **111**, 519—538 (1970).

HONIGMANN, H.: Untersuchungen über Lichtempfindlichkeit und Adaptierung des Vogelauges. Pflügers Arch. ges. Physiol. **189**, 1—72 (1921).

HOOKER, D.: Certain reactions to color in the young loggerhead turtle. Carnegie Inst. Wash. Papers from the Tortugas Laborat. **3**, 69—76 (1911).

HOSOYA, Y., OKITA, T., AKUNE, T.: Über die lichtempfindliche Substanz in der Zapfennetzhaut. Tohoku J. exp. Med. **32**, 447—459 (1938).

HOWARD, A. D.: The visual cells in vertebrates, chiefly in *Necturus maculosus*. J. Morphol. **19**, 567—629 (1908).

HUBBARD, R., KROPF, A.: Chicken lumi- and meta-iodopsin. Nature (Lond.) **183**, 448—450 (1959).

HULKE, J. W.: A contribution to the anatomy of the amphibian and reptilian retina. Roy. Lond. ophthal. Hosp. Rep. **4**, 243—314 (1863—65).

— On the retina of amphibia and reptiles. J. Anat. Physiol. **1**, 94—106 (1867).

JACOBS, G. H., YOLTON, R. L.: Dichromacy in the ground squirrel. Nature (Lond.) **223**, 414—415 (1969).

JONES, A. E.: The retinal structure of *Aotes trivirgatus*, the owl monkey. J. comp. Neurol. **125**, 19—27 (1965).

JONES, J. W.: Eel migration. Nature (Lond.), **184**, 1281 (1959).

KAMMERER, P.: Experimente über Fortpflanzung, Farbe, Augen und Körperreduction bei *Proteus anguinus* Laur. Arch. Entwicklungs. Organismen **33**, 349—461 (1912).

KERR, J. G.: The development of *Lepidosiren paradoxa*. Quart. J. microscop. Sci. **46**, 417—459 (1903).

KIMURA, E., HOSOYA, Y.: Further studies on cone substances. Jap. J. Physiol. **6**, 1—11 (1956).

KING-SMITH, P. E.: Absorption spectra and function of the coloured oil drops in the pigeon retina. Vision Res. **9**, 1391—1399 (1969).

KIRK, J. T. O., TILNEY-BASSETT, R. A. E.: The Plastids. London: W. H. Freeman & Co. 1967.

KNIGHT-JONES, E. W.: On the nervous system of *Saccoglossus cambrensis* (Enteropneusta). Phil. Trans. roy. Soc. London B., **236**, 315—354 (1952).

KOBAYASHI, H.: On the photo-perceptive function in the eye of the hagfish, *Myxine garmani* Jordan et Synder. J. Shimonoseki Univ. Fish. **13**, 141—157 (1964).

KÖNIG, A.: Über den menschlichen Sehpurpur und seine Bedeutung für das Sehen. Sitzungsberichte der Akademie der Wissenschaften zu Berlin. **1894**, 577—598.

KÖTTGEN, E., ABELSDORFF, G.: Absorption und Zersetzung des Sehpurpurs bei den Wirbeltieren. Z. Psychol. Physiol. Sinnesorg. **12**, 161—184 (1896).

KOHL, C.: Vorläufige Mittheilung über das Auge von *Proteus anguinus*. Zool. Anz. **14**, 93—96 (1891).

KOLMER, W.: Zur Kenntnis des Auges der Primaten. Z. Anat. Entwicklung. **93**, 679—722 (1930).

— Die Netzhaut. In: Handbuch der Mikroskop. Anatomie des Menschen. **3**, Auge. Berlin: Julius Springer 1936.

KRAUSE, W.: Über die Endigung der Muskelnerven. Z. rat. med. **20**, 1—18 (1863).

— Die Nerven-Endigung in der Retina. Arch. Mikroskop. Anat. **12**, 742—790 (1876).

— Über die Retinazapfen der nächtlichen Thiere. Arch. Mikroskop. Anat. **19**, 309—314 (1881).

— Die Retina. II. Die Retina der Fische. Monthly internat. J. Anat. and Physiol. **6**, 206—269 (1889).

— Die Retina. Monthly internat. J. Anat. and Physiol. **9**, 150—236 (1892).

— Die Retina. III. Die Retina der Amphibien. Monthly internat, J. Anat. and Physiol. **10**, 12—84 (1893).

KÜHNE, W.: Über den Sehpurpur. Untersuchungen aus dem Physiologischen Institut der Univ. Heidelberg **1**, 15—103 (1877).

— Nachträge zu den Abhandlungen über Sehpurpur. Untersuchungen aus dem Physiol. Institut der Univ. Heidelberg **1**, 455—470 (1878).

— Chemische Vorgänge in der Netzhaut. In: HERMANN, Handbuch der Physiologie der Sinnesorgane. Leipzig: F. C. W. Vogel 1879.

KUHN, O., KÄHLING, W. J.: Augenrückbildung und Lichtsinn bei *Anoptichthys jordani* Hubbs u. Innes. Experientia (Basel) **10**, 385—392 (1954).

Laties, A. M.: Histological techniques for study of photo-receptor orientation. Tissue Cell 1, 63—81 (1969).
— Liebman, P. A., Campbell, C. E. M.: Photoreceptor orientation in the primate eye. Nature (Lond.) 218, 172—173 (1968).
Laurens, H., Detwiler, S. R.: Studies on the retina. The structure of the retina. The structure of the retina of Alligator mississippiensis and its photomechanical changes. J. exp. Zool. 32, 207—234 (1921).
Leydig, F.: Anatomisch-Histologische Untersuchungen über Fische und Reptilien. Berlin: Georg Reimer 1853.
Liebman, P. A., Entine, G.: Cyanopsin, a visual pigment of retinal origin. Nature (Lond.) 216, 501—503 (1967).
— — Visual pigments of frog and tadpole (Rana pipiens). Vision Res. 8, 761—775 (1968).
— Granda, A. M.: Microspectrophotometric measurements of visual pigments in two species of turtle, Pseudemys scripta and Chelonia mydas. Vision Res. 11, 105—114 (1971).
Locket, N. A.: Deep-sea fish retinas. Brit. med. Bull. 26, 107—111 (1970).
Lyall, A. H.: Occurrence of triple and quadruple cones in the retina of the minnow (Phoxinus laevis). Nature (Lond.) 177, 1086—1087 (1956).
— The growth of the trout retina. Quart. J. microscop. Sci. 98, 101—110 (1957a).
— Cone arrangements in teleost retinae. Quart. J. microscop. Sci. 98, 189—201 (1957b).
Lythgoe, J. N., Dartnall, H. J. A.: A "deep-sea rhodopsin" in a mammal. Nature (Lond.) 227, 955—956 (1971).
Marks, W. B.: Visual pigments of single goldfish cones. J. Physiol. 178, 14—32 (1965).
McDowell, S. B., Jr., Bogert, C. M.: The systematic position of Lanthanotus and the affinities of the Anguino-morphan lizards. Bull. amer. Mus. nat. Hist. 105, 1—142 (1954).
McEwan, M. R.: A comparison of the retina of the mormyrids with that of various other teleosts. Acta zool. 19, 427—465 (1938).
McFarland, W. N.: Visual pigment of Callorhinchus callorynchus, a southern hemisphere chimaeroid fish. Vision Res. 10, 939—942 (1970).
— Munz, F. W.: Codominance of visual pigments in hybrid fishes. Science 150, 1055—1057 (1965).
Menner, E.: Untersuchungen über die Retina mit besonderer Berücksichtigung der Äußeren Körnerschicht. Ein Beitrag zur Duplizitätstheorie. Z. vergl. Physiol. 8, 761—826 (1929).
Meyer, D. B., Cooper, T. G.: The visual cells of the chicken as revealed by phase contrast microscopy. Amer. J. Anat. 118, 723—734 (1966).
— — Gernez, C.: Retinal oil droplets. In: The structure of the Eye. II. Symp. 8th Internat. Congr. Anatomists, Wiesbaden. Stuttgart: F. K. Schattauer 1965.
Michael, C. R.: Receptive fields of opponent color units in the optic nerve of the ground squirrel. Science 152, 1095—1097 (1966).
— Receptive fields of single optic nerve fibers in a mammal with an all-cone retina. I: Contrast-sensitive units. J. Neurophysiol. 31, 249—256 (1968a).
— Receptive fields of single optic nerve fibers in a mammal with an all-cone retina. II: Directionally selective units. J. Neurophysiol. 31, 257—267 (1968b).
— Receptive fields of single optic nerve fibers in a mammal with an all-cone retina. III. Opponent color units. J. Neurophysiol. 31, 268—282 (1968c).
Millot, J., Carasso, N.: Note préliminaire sur l'oeil de Latimeria chalumnae (Crossoptérygien coelacanthide). C. R. Acad. Sci. (Paris) 241, 576—577 (1955).
Moore, G. A.: The retinae of two North American teleosts, with special reference to their tapeta lucida. J. comp. Neurol. 80, 369—379 (1944).
— McDougal, R. C.: Similarity in the retinae of Amphiodon alosoides and Hiodon tergisus. Copeia 4, 298 (1949).
Moreland, J. D., Lythgoe, J. N.: Yellow corneas in fishes. Vision Res. 8, 1377—1380 (1968).
Morris, V. B.: Symmetry in a receptor mosaic demonstrated in the chick from the frequencies, spacing and arrangement of the types of retinal receptor. J. comp. Neurol. 140, 359—398 (1970).
— Shorey, C. D.: An electron microscope study of types of receptor in the chick retina. J. comp. Neurol. 129, 313—339 (1967).
Morton, R. A.: Chemical aspects of the visual process. Nature (Lond.) 153, 69—71 (1944).
— Goodwin, T. W.: Preparation of retinene in vitro. Nature (Lond.) 153, 405—406 (1944).

Munk, O.: The eye of *Calamoichthys calabaricus* Smith, 1865 (Polypteridae, Pisces). Vidensk. Medd. Dansk. Naturh. Foren. **127**, 113—126 (1964).
— *Omosudis lowei* Günther, 1887, a bathypelagic deep-sea fish with an almost pure-cone retina. Vidensk. Medd. Dansk. Naturh. Foren. **128**, 341—355 (1965).
— Ocular Anatomy of some deep-sea teleosts. Dana-Report **70**, 1—62 (1966a).
— On the retina of *Diretmus argenteus* Johnson 1863 (Diretmidae, Pisces). Vidensk. Medd. Dansk. Naturh. Foren. **129**, 73—80 (1966b).
— The eyes of *Amia* and *Lepisosteus* (Pisces, Holostei) compared with the branchiopterygian and teleostean eyes. Vidensk. Medd. Dansk. Naturh. Fornen. **131**, 109—127 (1968).
— On the visual cells of some primitive fishes with particular regard to the classification of rods and cones. Vidensk. Medd. Dansk. Naturh. Foren. **132**, 25—30 (1969).
— On the occurrence and significance of horizontal band-shaped retinal areae in teleosts. Vidensk. Medd. Dansk. Naturh. Foren. **133**, 85—120 (1970).
Muntz, W. R. A.: Effectiveness of different colours of light in releasing the positive phototactic behaviour of frogs, and a possible function of the retinal projection in the diencephalon. J. Neurophysiol. **25**, 712—720 (1962).
— The development of photopic and scotopic vision in the frog *(Rana temporaria)*. Vision Res. **4**, 241—250 (1964a).
— Vision in frogs. Sci. Amer. **210**, No. 3 (March.), 111—119 (1964b).
— Northmore, D. P. M.: Visual pigments from different parts of the retina in rudd and trout. Vision Res. **11**, 551—562 (1971).
— Reuter, T.: Visual pigments and spectral sensitivity in *Rana temporaria* and other european tadpoles. Vision Res. **6**, 601—618 (1966).
Munz, F. W.: A new photosensitive pigment of the euryhaline teleost, *Gillichthys mirabilis*. J. gen. Physiol. **40**, 233—249 (1956).
— The photosensitive retinal pigments of marine and euryhaline teleost fishes. Dissertation for the Ph. D degree, Univ. of Calif., Los Angeles (1957a).
— Photosensitive pigments from retinas of deep-sea fishes. Science **125**, 1142—1143 (1957b).
— Photosensitive pigments from the retinae of certain deep sea fishes. J. Physiol. **140**, 220—235 (1958a).
— The photosensitive retinal pigments of fishes from relatively turbid coastal waters. J. gen. Physiol. **42**, 445—459 (1958b).
— Retinal pigments of a labrid fish. Nature (Lond.) **181**, 1012—1013 (1958c).
— Adaptation of visual pigments to the photic environment. In: Ciba Foundation Symp. Colour Vision. Physiology and Exper. Psychol. London: J. & A. Churchill Ltd. 1965.
— Beatty, D. D.: A critical analysis of the visual pigments of salmon and trout. Vision Res. **5**, 1—17 (1965).
— McFarland, W. N.: A suggested hereditary mechanism for visual pigments of chars *(Salvelinus* spp.*)*. Nature (Lond.) **206**, 955—956 (1965).
Newth, D. R., Ross, D. M.: On the reaction to light of *Myxine glutinosa* L. J. exp. Biol. **32**, 4—21 (1955).
Nicol, J. A. C.: Spectral composition of the light of the lantern-fish, *Myctophum punctatum*. J. mar. biol. Ass. U. K. **39**, 27—32 (1960).
— Retinomotor changes in flatfishes. J. fish. Res. Bd. Canada **22**, 513—520 (1965).
Nikol'skii, G. V.: Special Ichthyology. Jerusalem: Israel Program for Scientific Translations, 1961.
Nilsson, S. E. G.: An electron microscopic classification of the retinal receptors of the leopard frog *(Rana pipiens)*. J. ultrastruct. Res. **10**, 390—416 (1964a).
— Receptor cell outer segment development and ultrastructure of the disk membranes in the retina of the tadpole *(Rana pipiens)*. J. ultrastruct. Res. **11**, 581—620 (1964b).
— Crescitelli, F.: Changes in ultrastructure and electroretinogram of bullfrog retina during development. J. ultrastruct. Res. **27**, 45—62 (1969).
Noble, G. K.: The Biology of the Amphibia. New York: McGraw-Hill 1931.
Nunneley, T.: On the structure of the retina. Quart. J. microscop. Science **6**, 217—241 (1858).
O'Connell, C. P.: The structure of the eye of *Sardinops caerulea, Engraulis mordax*, and four other pelagic marine teleosts. J. Morphol. **113**, 287—329 (1963).

O'DAY, K.: A preliminary note on the presence of double cones and oil-droplets in the retina of marsupials. J. Anat. **70**, 465—467 (1936).
— The visual cells of the platypus *(Ornithorhyncus)* Brit. J. Ophthalm. **22**, 321—328 (1938).
— The visual cells of Australian reptiles and mammals. Trans. Ophthal. Soc. Australia **1**, 12—20 (1940).
— Visual cells of the guinea pig. Nature (Lond.) **160**, 648 (1947).
PEARLMAN, J. T., CRESCITELLI, F.: Visual pigments of the vitamin A-deficient thyroidectomized rat following vitamin A_2 administration. Vision Res. **11**, 177—187 (1971).
PEDLER, C., TANSLEY, K.: The fine structure of the cone of a diurnal gecko *(Phelsuma inunguis)*. Exp. Eye Res. **2**, 39—47 (1963).
POGO, A. O., BRAWERMAN, G., CHARGAFF, E.: New ribonucleic acid species associated with the formation of the photosynthetic apparatus in *Euglena gracilis*. Biochemistry **1**, 128—131 (1962).
POINCELOT, R. P., MILLAR, P. G., KIMBEL, R. L., JR., ABRAHAMSON, E. W.: Lipid to protein chromophore transfer in the photolysis of visual pigments. Nature (Lond.) **221**, 256—257 (1969).
PUMPHREY, R. J.: The sense organs of birds. Ann. Rep. Smithson. Inst. **1948**, 305—330.
REUTER, T.: The synthesis of photosensitive pigments in the rods of the frog's retina. Vision Res. **6**, 15—38 (1966).
— Visual pigments and ganglion cell activity in the retinae of tadpoles and adult frogs *(Rana temporaria* L.). Acta Zool. Fenn. **122**, 1—64 (1969).
REUTER, T. E., WHITE, R. H., WALD, G.: Rhodopsin and porphyropsin fields in the adult bullfrog retina. J. gen. Physiol. (in press).
RITCHIE, A.: New evidence on *Jamoytius kerwoodi* White, an important ostracoderm from the Silurian of Lanarkshire, Scotland. Palaeontology, **11**, Part 1, 21—39 (1968).
ROCHON-DUVIGNEAUD, A.: Les fonctions des cones et des batonnets indications fournies par la physiologie comparée. Ann. D'Oculist. **154**, 633—648 (1917).
— Les Yeux et la Vision des Vertébrés. Paris: Masson et Cie, 1943.
ROMER, A. S., GROVE, B. H.: Environment of the early vertebrates. Am. midland Naturalist **16**, 805—856 (1935).
ROZEMEYER, H. C., STOLTE, J. B.: Die Netzhaut des Frosches in Golgi-Cox Präparaten. Z. mikroskop. Anat. Forschung. **23**, 98—118 (1931).
RYDER, J. A.: An arrangement of the retinal cells in the eyes of fishes partially simulating compound eyes. Proc. Acad. natural Sci. (Philad.) **47**, 161—166 (1894).
SAXÉN, L.: An atypical form of the double visual cell in the frog *(Rana temporaria* L.). Acta Anat. **19**, 190—196 (1953).
— The development of the visual cells. Ann. Acad. Sci. fenn. Series A. **23**, 1—93 (1954).
— The glycogen inclusion of the visual cells and its hypothetical role in the photomechanical responses. Acta anat. **25**, 319—330 (1955).
SCHIEFFERDECKER, P.: Studien zur vergleichenden Histologie der Retina. Arch. mikroskop. Anat. **28**, 305—396 (1886).
SCHMALHAUSEN, I. I.: The Origin of Terrestrial Vertebrates. New York-London: Academic Press, 1968.
SCHMIDT, J.: IV. The breeding places of the eel. Phil. Trans. roy. Soc. Lond., B. **211**, 179—208 (1923).
SCHULTZE, M.: Zur Anatomie und Physiologie der Retina. Arch. mikroskop. Anat. **2**, 175—286 (1866).
— Über Stäbchen und Zapfen der Retina. Arch. mikroskop. Anat. **3**, 215—247 (1867).
— The retina. In: Manual of Human and Comparative Histology (ed. Stricker) **3**, 218—298. London: New Sydenham Society 1873.
SCHWALBE, G.: Mikroskopische Anatomie des Sehnerven, der Netzhaut und des Glaskörpers. In: Handbuch der Gesamten Augenheilkunde (Ed. von Gräfe u. Saemisch), Bd. 1. Leipzig: Wilhelm Engelmann 1874.
SCHWANZARA, S. A.: The visual pigments of freshwater fishes. Vision Res. **7**, 121—148 (1967).
SCHWASSMANN, H. O., KRUGER, L.: Experimental analysis of the visual system of the four-eyed fish *Anableps microlepis*. Vision Res. **5**, 269—281 (1965).

SHAFER, G. D.: The mosaic of the single and twin cones in the retina of *Micropterus salmoides*. Arch. Entwicklungsmech. Org. **10**, 685—691 (1900).

SHANTZ, E. M., EMBREE, N. D., HODGE, H. C., WILLS, J. H., JR.: The replacement of vitamin A_1 by vitamin A_2 in the retina of the rat. J. biol. Chem. **163**, 455—464 (1946).

SICK, K., BAHN, E., FRYDENBERG, O., NIELSEN, J. T., WETTSTEIN, D. VON: Haemoglobin polymorphism of the American freshwater eel *Anguilla*. Nature (Lond.) **214**, 1141—1142 (1967).

— WESTERGAARD, M., FRYDENBERG, O.: Haemoglobin pattern and chromosome number of American, European, and Japanese eels *(Anguilla)*. Nature (Lond.) **193**, 1001—1002 (1962).

SIDMAN, R. L.: Histochemical studies on photoreceptor cells. Ann. N. Y. Acad. Sci. **74**, 182—195 (1958).

SILLMAN, A. J.: The visual pigment and oil droplet content of the retinas of several species of birds. Ph. D. Thesis, Univ. of Calif., Los Angeles (1968).

SMITH, H. W.: Water regulation and its evolution in the fishes. Quart. Rev. Biol. **7**, 1—26 (1932).

SNYDER, M., KILLACKEY, H., DIAMOND, I. T.: Color vision in the tree shrew after removal of posterior neocortex. J. Neurophysiol. **32**, 554—563 (1969).

SOKOL, S., MUNTZ, W. R. A.: The spectral sensitivity of the turtle *Chrysemys picta picta*. Vision Res. **6**, 285—292 (1966).

STUDNITZ, G. VON: Weitere Studien an der Zapfensubstanz. Pflüg. Arch. ges. Physiol. **239**, 515—525 (1937).

TANSLEY, K.: The regeneration of visual purple: its relation to dark adaptation and night blindness. J. Physiol. **71**, 442—458 (1931).

— The retina of two nocturnal geckos *Hemidactylus turcicus* and *Tarentola mauritanica*. Pflügers Arch. ges. Physiol. **268**, 213—220 (1959).

— The gecko retina. Vision Res. **4**, 33—37 (1964).

— COPENHAVER, R. M., GUNKEL, R. D.: Spectral sensitivity curves of diurnal squirrels. Vision Res. **1**, 154—165 (1961).

TIGGES, J., BROOKS, B. A., KLEE, M. R.: ERG recordings of a primate pure cone retina *(Tupaia glis)*. Vision Res. **7**, 553—563 (1967).

TOYODA, J., NOSAKI, H., TOMITA, T.: Light-induced resistance changes in single photoreceptors of *Necturus* and *Gekko*. Vision Res. **9**, 453—463 (1969).

TROUT, G. C.: The Bear Island cod: migrations and movements. Fish Invest. London, **21**, 1—57 (1957).

TUCKER, D. W.: A new solution to the Atlantic eel problem. Nature (Lond.) **183**, 495—501 (1959a).

— Eel migration. Nature (Lond.) **184**, 1281—1283 (1959b).

UNDERWOOD, G.: Reptilian retinas. Nature (Lond.) **167**, 183—185 (1951).

— On the classification and evolution of geckos. Proc. zool. Soc. London, **124**, 469—492 (1954).

— On lizards of the family Pygopodidae. A contribution to the morphology and phylogeny of the Squamata. J. Morph. **100**, 207—268 (1957).

— On the visual-cell pattern of a homalopsine snake. J. Anat. **100**, 571—575 (1966).

— A contribution to the classification of snakes. London, Trustees of the British Museum (Natural History) (1967a).

— A comprehensive approach to the classification of higher snakes. Herpetologica **23**, 161—168 (1967b).

— Some suggestions concerning vertebrate visual cells. Vision Res. **8**, 483—488 (1968).

— The Eye. In: GANS, C., PARSONS, T. S. (Ed.). Biology of the Reptilia. London-New York: Academic Press 1970.

VERRIER, M. L.: La structure de l'oeil de *Clarias batrachus* L. et d'*Ameiurus nebulosus* LeSueur, ses rapports avec l'habitat et le comportement biologique de ces deux silurides. Bull. Soc. Zool. France **52**, 581—588 (1927).

— Recherches sur l'histophysiologie de la rétine des vertébrés et les problèmes qu'elle soulève. Suppl. 20, Bull. biol. France Belg. 1—138 (1935).

VILTER, V.: Dissociation spatiale des champs photo-sensoriels à cônes et à bâtonnets chez un poisson marin, le *Callionymus lyra*. C. r. Soc. biol. **141**, 344—346 (1947).

Vilter, V.: Intervention probable de la lumière dans la naissance des structures rétiniennes révélée par l'étude comparée de la rétine chez les anguilles normales et cavernicoles. C. r. Soc. biol. **145**, 54—56 (1951 a).
— Valeur morphologique des photorecépteurs rétiniens chez la Hatterie *(Sphenodon punctatum)*. C. r. Soc. biol. **145**, 20—23 (1951 b).
— Organisation générale de la rétine nerveuse chez le *Sphenodon punctatum*. C. r. Soc. biol. **145**, 24—26 (1951 c).
— Recherches sur les structures fovéales dans la retine du *Sphenodon punctatum*. C. r. Soc. biol. **145**, 26—52 (1951 d).
— Existence d'une rétine a plusieurs mosaiques photoréceptrices chez un poisson abyssal bathypélagique, *Bathylagus benedicti*. C. r. Soc. biol. **147**, 1937—1939 (1953).
— Différentiation fovéale dans l'appareil visuel d'un poisson abyssal, le *Bathylagus benedicti*. C. r. Soc. biol. **148**, 59—63 (1954 a).
— Interpretation biologique des trames photoréceptrices superposées de la rétine du *Bathylagus benedicti*. C. r. Soc. biol. **148**, 327—330 (1954 b).
— Relations neuronales dans la fovea à bâtonnets du *Bathylagus benedicti*. C. r. Soc. biol. **148**, 466—469 (1954 c).
Wald, G.: Carotenoids and the visual cycle. J. gen. Physiol. **19**, 351—371 (1935).
— Pigments of the retina. I. The bull frog. J. gen. Physiol. **19**, 781—795 (1936 a).
— Pigments of the retina. II. Sea robin, sea bass, and scup. J. gen. Physiol. **20**, 45—56 (1936 b).
— Visual purple system in fresh-water fishes. Nature (Lond.) **139**, 1017—1018 (1937 a).
— Photo-labile pigments of the chicken retina. Nature (Lond.) **140**, 545—546 (1937 b).
— The porphyropsin visual system. J. gen. Physiol. **22**, 775—794 (1939).
— The visual systems of euryhaline fishes. J. gen. Physiol. **25**, 235—245 (1941).
— The visual system and vitamins A of the sea lamprey. J. gen. Physiol. **25**, 331—336 (1942 a).
— Visual systems and the vitamin A. In: Visual Mechanisms (Ed. Klüver, H.). Lancaster, Pa.: Jaques Cattell Press 1942 b.
— The chemical evolution of vision. Harvey Lectures **41**, 117—160 (1945).
— The biochemistry of vitamin A. In: Symp. on Nutrition (Ed. Herriott, R. M.). Baltimore: John Hopkins Press 1953.
— Visual pigments and vitamins A of the clawed toad, *Xenopus laevis*. Nature (Lond.) **175**, 390—394 (1955).
— The metamorphosis of visual systems in the sea lamprey. J. gen. Physiol. **40**, 901—914 (1957).
— The significance of vertebrate metamorphosis. Science **128**, 1481—1490 (1958 a).
— Retinal chemistry and the physiology of vision. Nat. phys. Lab. Symp. 8, **1**, 9—61 (1958 b).
— The distribution and evolution of visual systems. Comp. biochem. **1**, 311—345 (1960).
— Brown, P. K.: Human rhodopsin. Science **127**, 222—226 (1958).
— — Brown, P. S.: Visual pigments and depths of habitat of marine fishes. Nature (Lond.) **180**, 969—971 (1957).
— — Kennedy, D.: The visual system of the alligator. J. gen. Physiol. **40**, 703—713 (1957).
— — Smith, P. H.: Cyanopsin, a new pigment of cone vision. Science **119**, 505—508 (1953).
— — — Iodopsin. J. gen. Physiol. **38**, 623—681 (1955).
— Zussman, H.: Carotenoids of the chicken retina. Nature (Lond.) **140**, 197 (1937).
Walls, G. L.: The reptilian retina. Amer. J. Ophthal. **17**, 892—915 (1934).
— The visual cells of lampreys. Brit. J. Ophthal. **19**, 129—148 (1935).
— Notes on the retinae of two opossum genera. J. Morph. **64**, 67—87 (1939).
— The visual cells and their history. In: Visual Mechanisms (Ed. Klüver, H.). Lancaster, Pa.: Jacques Cattell Press (1942 a).
— The Vertebrate Eye and its Adaptive Radiation. Bloomfield Hills, Mich.: Cranbrook Institute of Science Bull. 19 (1942 b).
— Judd, H. D.: The intra-ocular colour-filters of vertebrates. Brit. J. Ophthal. **17**, 641—675; 705—725 (1933).
Weisz, P. B.: The development and morphology of the larva of the South African clawed toad, *Xenopus laevis*. J. Morphol. **77**, 163—191 (1945).
Westheimer, G.: Dependence of the magnitude of the Stiles-Crawford effect on retinal location. J. Physiol. **192**, 309—315 (1967).

WHITEAR, M.: Some remarks on the ascidian affinities of vertebrates. Ann. Mag. nat. Hist. **10**, 338—348 (1957).

WILLMER, E. N.: Determining factors in the evolution of the retina in vertebrates. Symp. Soc. exp. Biol. **7**, 377—394 (1953).

— Duality in the retina. In: Ciba Found. Symp., Colour Vision. Physiology & Exper. Psychol. London: J. A. Churchill Ltd. 1965.

WOODHEAD, A. D.: Variations in the activity of the thyroid gland of the cod, *Gadus callarias* L., in relation to its migrations in the Barents Sea. J. mar. biol. Ass. U. K. **38**, 407—415 (1959).

WOOLLARD, H. H.: The anatomy of *Tarsius spectrum*. Proc. zool. Soc. London 1071—1184 (1925).

— Differentiation of the retina in the primates. Proc. zool. Soc. London 1—17 (1927).

WUNDER, W.: Über den Bau der Netzhaut bei Süßwasserfischen, die in großer Tiefe leben (Corregonen, Tiefseesaibling). Z. vergl. Physiol. **4**, 22—36 (1926a).

— Physiologische und Vergleichend-Anatomische Untersuchungen an der Knochenfisch-Netzhaut. Z. vergl. Physiol. **3**, 1—61 (1926b).

YOSHIKAMI, S., PEARLMAN, J. T., CRESCITELLI, F.: Visual pigments of the vitamin A-deficient rat following vitamin A_2 administration. Vision Res. **9**, 633—646 (1969).

YOSHIZAWA, T., WALD, G.: Photochemistry of iodopsin. Nature (Lond.) **214**, 566—571 (1967).

YOUNG, R. W.: The renewal of photoreceptor cell outer segments. J. Cell Biol. **33**, 61—72 (1967).

— The organization of vertebrate photoreceptor cells. In: STRAATSMA, B. R., HALL, M. O., ALLEN, R. A., CRESCITELLI, F. (Eds.). The Retina: Morphology, Function and Clinical Characteristics. UCLA Forum Med. Sci. No. 8, Univ. of Calif. Press, Los Angeles 1969.

— An hypothesis to account for a basic distinction between rods and cones. Vision Res. **11**, 1—5 (1971).

— DROZ, B.: The renewal of protein in retinal rods and cones. J. Cell Biol. **39**, 169—184 (1968).

Chapter 9

Visual Pigments in Man

By

WILLIAM A. H. RUSHTON, Cambridge (Great Britain)

With 12 Figures

Contents

I. Introduction

The importance of being able to study the visual pigments in man lies in this; that visual performance depends upon the nature, amount and state of bleaching of the pigments in the rods and cones. There are two distinct ways in which visual pigments are related to vision. The first, (a), is easy to comprehend; roughly it is that receptors can only respond to the quanta they catch, and hence the spectral sensitivity of the receptor will correspond to the spectral absorption of the pigment it contains. The second, (b), is far more difficult to comprehend though the relation can easily be stated. Roughly it is that in recovery after bleaching, the logarithm of the visual threshold is raised by a quantity proportional to the fraction of pigment still in the bleached state.

Consider first (a). It is plain that quanta that are not absorbed cannot do anything, but it by no means follows that all quanta that *are* absorbed are equally effective, and (as we shall see) the evidence is that they are not. But it is impossible to measure directly the number of quanta caught in conditions where a visual response follows. We have to measure absorption accurately in very different conditions (e.g. rhodopsin in solution), and justify the use of this measurement, or its modification, in the living receptor.

A. Rhodopsin

1. Absorption Spectrum

The terms Density Spectrum (= Extinction or Absorbance Spectrum) and Absorption Spectrum are often used loosely as though they were synonymous. But they mean different things. If I_i is the light incident upon the trough of pigment and I_t is the light transmitted, the density D is defined as

$$D = \log (I_i/I_t) \text{ or } I_t/I_i = 10^{-D} = e^{-2 \cdot 3D}. \tag{1}$$

The absorption A is clearly the difference between I_i, the light entering the trough and I_t, the light leaving.

$$A = I_i - I_t = I_i (1 - I_t/I_i) = I_i (1 - 10^{-D}). \tag{2}$$

Therefore $A/I_i = 1 - e^{-2 \cdot 3D} = 2 \cdot 3D - (2 \cdot 3D)^2/2! + \cdots$

Thus when D is small compared with unity the absorption is nearly proportional to the density. At the molecular level we may regard D as the molecular quantum catching capacity. But molecules in solution look at the incident light through a coloured filter composed of other molecules: light of wavelength best caught will thus be that most sharply attenuated. Consequently this *self-screening* will flatten the peak of the absorption spectrum as compared with D the corresponding density spectrum. This is what is described quantitatively by Eq. (1) where D is the density at any wavelength.

2. In Solution

The most accurate measurements are made on rhodopsin in digitonin extract. Such extracts always contain some contaminants, and hence the density spectrum is the sum of that due to rhodopsin and that due to the contaminants. But the contaminants are not affected by exposure to a bleaching light. Consequently the *difference spectrum* (i.e. the change in density spectrum before and after bleaching) will eliminate them since their change is zero. Thus we are left with the change in uncontaminated rhodopsin — rhodopsin density *minus* photoproduct density. Now if hydroxylamine is added to the extract, it has no effect upon rhodopsin itself but converts the bleaching product into an oxime that is almost colourless. Since in this case the photoproduct density, in the visible is zero, the difference spectrum from bleaching rhodopsin in solution with hydroxylamine is nearly the same (in the visible) as the density spectrum of uncontaminated rhodopsin.

3. In the Rods

Rods are composed of a pile of discs normal to the rod axis, and rhodopsin molecules lie with their resonating axes in the planes of the discs and seem free to move in these planes, but not out of them. Density measurements of rhodopsin in the rods is less accurate than in solution, but the evidence is that the spectrum is the same.

In some animals the density of rhodopsin in rods may exceed 1.0 on single traverse (Denton and Warren, 1956; Denton and Walker, 1958) so here the density spectrum differs very considerably from the absorption spectrum upon which visual performance depends.

In man the density in rods is probably about 0.15, consequently self-screening is slight and the density spectrum hardly differs from the absorption spectrum.

4. Quantum Efficiency

Only about 60% of the quanta caught lead to the bleaching of rhodopsin; the remaining 40% have no known effect upon the molecule and are presumably degraded into heat. If monochromatic light of known wavelength falls steadily upon a trough of rhodopsin solution the incident light I_i, and also the transmitted light I_t may be sampled continuously. As we have seen in Eqs. (1) and (2) the difference of the energies give the light absorbed; the difference of the log energies, the pigment density. In this way Schneider, Goodeve, and Lythgoe (1939), Goodeve, Lythgoe, and Schneider (1942), measured the rate of density-loss as a function of light absorption for lights of various wavelengths. Knowing the molar extinction coefficient of rhodopsin (Wald and Brown, 1953; Hubbard, 1954) we can turn "density loss" into "molecules bleached". And expressing the light absorbed as "number of quanta caught" we can answer the question "How many quanta on average must be caught to bleach 1 molecule of rhodopsin". The result comes to about 1.7 quanta absorbed per molecule bleached, independent of wavelength. Hence the action spectrum is the same as the absorption spectrum for rhodopsin in solution, but about $1/3$ of the quanta caught at each wavelength appear to be degraded into heat, without any effect on bleaching.

5. Univariance

If rods are activated by the light absorbed by rhodopsin, and if every quantum so absorbed is equivalent in its contribution towards vision, an important and simple expectation follows: any two lights that are equally absorbed by rhodopsin will be equally seen by rods. Consequently the rhodopsin absorption spectrum should coincide with the twilight (scotopic) sensitivity function.

The first accurate comparison of these two kinds of measurement in man is shown in Fig. 1 (CRESCITELLI and DARTNALL, 1953). They measured the density spectrum of human rhodopsin extracted from a freshly excised human eye. The scotopic spectral sensitivity is taken from CRAWFORD (1949) with light energies expressed as quantum flux and corrected for absorption etc. in the pre-retinal eye media. It is plain that flashes that are equally absorbed are equally seen.

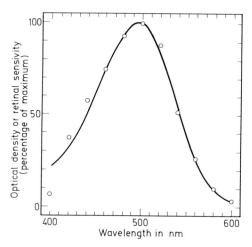

Fig. 1. Comparison between the density spectrum of human rhodopsin (curve) and CRAW-FORD's (1949) spectral sensitivity measurements for the dark adapted human eye. (After CRESCITELLI and DARTNALL, 1953)

Now we saw above (A.4) that flashes that were equally absorbed were equal in bleaching rhodopsin but for each wavelength it needed on average 1.7 quanta to bleach 1 molecule — as though 60% of the absorbed quanta caused bleaching and 40% did something else — or nothing. How is it with vision? Do only the 60% that bleach contribute to seeing, or do all absorbed quanta contribute — or could it be that the 40% that does "something else" is the very fraction that does whatever has to be done to make us see?

We have no measurements reliable enough to answer this question. I think that the 40% that cannot cause bleaching are also ineffective in promoting vision. For if they could so act, they would do so with such superior efficiency that this mechanism might be expected to supersede the other, and non-bleaching seeing would become the rule in the animal kingdom, which is certainly not the case.

One piece of experimental evidence bearing upon this arises from measurements of the absolute threshold of vision expressed as the minimum quantum catch from a flash. HECHT, SHLAER, and PIRENNE (1942) determined this quantum number in two ways — (a) by measuring photometrically the number of quanta entering the eye and then estimating the fraction absorbed by rhodopsin, (b) by presenting (in random order) flashes of various energies, and finding the frequency with which each flash was seen. Method (a) determines the number of quanta caught, (b) the number co-operating in the visual act. They found number (a) greater than (b) and so (though not so markedly) did Baumgardt (1960) who also made measurements by both methods. Unfortunately both methods rest upon estimates that are not very secure, but the result that more quanta are caught than are used for vision seems still to hold when more recent estimates are applied to their measurements.

B. Cone Pigments

1. Trichromacy

Thomas Young (1802) was the first to reconcile the continuous spectrum of Newton with the already accepted trichromacy of colour vision. As is well known, he did this by postulating that the input channels for colour information were "limited; for instance to three...." That is, the whole spectral range of light frequencies would set in motion just 3 resonators, but each frequency would produce a different set of relative amplitudes depending upon how nearly the light frequency coincided with the natural frequency of each resonator. Colour is judged by these relative amplitudes.

After Kühne's work on rhodopsin it became clear that Young's resonators were photosensitive chemicals, and his three input channels resulted from the quantum catches in three independent photosensitive pigments. Clerk Maxwell (1890) was the first to match all spectral colours with suitable mixtures of red, green and blue "primary" lights, and thus obtain trichromatic colour mixture functions. This work was repeated by Helmholtz and many others, and reached such perfection with Wright (1929, 1946) that the even more careful measurements of Stiles (1955) gave nearly identical results.

Knowing these colour matching functions, i.e. the energies of "primary" red, green and blue lights that when suitably mixed are identical to unity energy of the spectral light λ, it might have been hoped that we could deduce the spectral sensitivities of the three cone pigments erythrolabe, chlorolabe and cyanolabe. Unfortunately this is impossible, for it can be easily proved that if ε_λ, χ_λ, $\varkappa_\lambda$ are three pigment sensitivities that satisfy all matches, then replacing ε_λ by $(a_1 \varepsilon_\lambda + b_1 \chi_\lambda + c_1 \varkappa_\lambda)$, χ_λ by $(a_2 \varepsilon_\lambda + b_2 \chi_\lambda + c_2 \varkappa_\lambda)$, and $\varkappa_\lambda$ by $(a_3 \varepsilon_\lambda + b_3 \chi_\lambda + c_3 \varkappa_\lambda)$ will also satisfy. Since this holds for any values of the coefficients a_1 etc. there is a very large range of action spectra of the three pigments that could be made consistent with the colour matching functions.

Thus colour matches, exact as they are, cannot define the spectral sensitivity curves, but they do provide a very strict test that any proposed set of three curves must satisfy.

2. Colour Isolation by Adaptation

To determine the actual curves, then, something besides colour matching must be used. Many psycho-physical measurements have been pressed into this service — usually attempts by adaptation to suppress all but one of the colour sensitivities.

It is difficult to establish that all but one *have* been suppressed, and harder still to be sure that what remains is the result of quanta caught by only one pigment. Perhaps the best investigation is that of BRINDLEY (1953) in a paper of great analytical power, which has apparently proved too hard a biscuit for the loose teeth of most readers. He adapted to very bright lights of such a colour that the eye was left nearly monochromatic, so that the greater part of the spectrum appeared to be the same hue. One part could thus be matched exactly with another by varying intensity only, and such matches gave the spectral sensitivity when only red remains or when only green remains. When only blue remained the intensity discrimination was so poor that useful blue sensitivity curves could not be obtained.

The most extensive and accurate measurements on colour adaptation are those of STILES (1939, 1946, 1949, 1953, 1959) who measured the threshold for a flash of one colour upon a background of another, over the whole range of colours and intensities. He obtained three important generalizations: —

(i) for any test light λ on a background μ, the threshold intensity I_λ is related to the background intensity I_μ by Fechner's formula

$$I_\lambda = k(I_\mu + I_D)$$

where k is a constant (the Fechner fraction) and I_D the retinal noise ($= Eigengrau$).

(ii) If the test flash is altered in wavelength, but the background kept constant, then the energy I_λ must be changed to remain at threshold, and this energy as a function of wavelength λ gives the spectral sensitivity of the test flash mechanism. Similarly, we may measure the spectral sensitivity of the background I_μ by keeping λ fixed and changing the wavelength μ and also altering the energy I_μ so that I_λ remains still at threshold. STILES found that λ and μ have the same spectral sensitivities.

(iii) STILES discovered one rod and several cone mechanisms each acting independently and each satisfying conditions (i) and (ii). The actual threshold appearing in any condition was that which was most sensitive in that condition.

A simple and superficially plausible interpretation of these results is that of WALD (1964), namely that STILES had discovered a psycho-physical technique for measuring the sensitivity of the cone pigments. STILES himself, however, never claimed this, not only because reasons are weak for supposing it true, but because (as he had long established) they are strong for supposing it false. They are these:

a) On the fovea STILES has found five, not three independent spectral sensitivities at moderate luminosities.

b) At high luminosities another two appear.

c) The most likely three to correspond to pigment sensitivities do not quite satisfy the colour matching functions (though they are not far off).

d) The various colour mechanisms though nearly independent are not exactly so (BOYNTON, IKEDA, and STILES, 1964). Thus they cannot represent the activity of single pigments; they must involve a little nerve interaction.

The difficulties of arguing securely from excellent psycho-physical measurements back to visual pigments makes objective measurements of pigments in man of value, even though such measurements are rather limited in accuracy.

II. Principles of Retinal Densitometry in Man

A. Apparatuses and their Comparative Advantages

A parallel beam of light entering through the pupil of an eye focussed at infinity is brought to a focus at the retina and at the pigment epithelium in contact with it. Light is strongly absorbed by the black pigment and only about 1% incident on the retina is reflected, but much of this reflected light has passed twice through the rods and cones and hence bears the imprint of absorption by the visual pigments.

The reflected light may be separated from the in-going beam by an ophthalmscopic mirror device, and if we measure the reflected energy we may learn something about the visual pigments that have attenuated it. A single measurement cannot distinguish between absorption by the receptors or by the pigment epithelium (which is far greater). But receptor pigment will bleach and regenerate, whereas other light losses may be held nearly constant. In these conditions the *change* in light loss is entirely due to change in pigment absorption, and provides a measure of it.

A very small fraction of the light entering the pupil is reflected back from the ophthalmoscopic mirror for measurement. Reflexion at the fundus is diffuse so only 4% of the total 1% reflected there would emerge through a dilated pupil of diameter 8 mm if there were no transmission losses. But for the green light used for most of these measurements, the transmission loss each way is about 50% (Ludvigh and McCarthy; 1938) thus the emerging light is 10^{-4} of that entering.

The incident light must therefore be made as strong as possible in order to get a good signal, but since this light will bleach away the pigments to be measured, we are severely limited in the intensity admissable.

Rushton and Campbell (1954) constructed the first satisfactory human retinal densitometer; Weale (1959) built another good instrument upon a somewhat different principle, and virtually all the work on the living human eye has been performed on these instruments (and their modifications) by Rushton and Weale with their colleagues.

Weale's densitometer (Fig. 2) is designed to make measurements in rapid succession in light of 26 different wavelengths distributed through the spectrum. Full descriptions are given in Weale (1959) and the more recent modification (Fig. 2) in Ripps and Weale (1963). In principle the wheel W fitted with suitable interference filters is interposed in the beam of the powerful xenon arc S so that on rotation a rapid succession of coloured openings is presented, and a series of brief flashes of defined wavelengths delivered. The beam is divided by a biprism B so that it may fall on the fundus of the eye F_T and also on the orange fundus F_C of an artificial eye. Lights reflected from both eyes are deflected upwards and brought to fall upon a photomultiplier cell E.

Fig. 3 shows cathode ray traces of the photocell output. Each trace is the superposition of two responses, one in the dark adapted state, and one light adapted. Alternate waves come from the artificial eye, and the exact coincidence of these two waves (C) demonstrates the repeatability of the flashes. The other set of alternate waves shows a greater amplitude in the light adapted state (L) than in dark adaptation (D), since when the pigment is dense it absorbs more light. The "density", measured and plotted as "$\Delta D(2)$", was found by taking the logarithm of the ratio of amplitudes in each pair of superposed waves.

Rushton's densitometer (RUSHTON, 1956a) is designed to make measurements at one selected wavelength while bleaching at another. The feeble measuring light is flickered in alternation with the powerful bleaching light but only the reflected

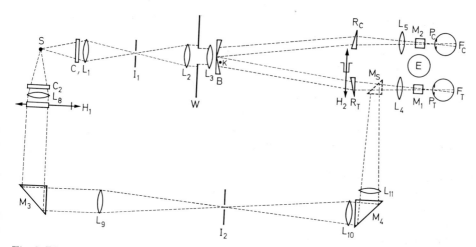

Fig. 2. Diagram of WEALE's retinal densitometer (for brief description, see text). F_T, subject's eye; F_C, artificial control eye. W, wheel bearing 26 interference filters which may be interposed in the measuring beam in rapid succession. (From RIPPS and WEALE, 1963)

Fig. 3. Typical pair of record sequences obtained with WEALE's densitometer, one from a dark adapted eye (D), the other (superimposed) from the same eye after bleaching (L). Alternate waves (from the control artificial eye C) show exact superposition. The intermediate waves (from the subject's eye) show a conspicuous change in amplitude resulting from the loss in pigment density after bleaching. The change is greatest at wave lengths most affected (example is for 552 nm) and hence allows a difference spectrum to be plotted from the log ratio of wave amplitudes. (From WEALE, 1961b)

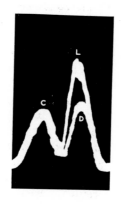

measuring light is permitted to reach the photocell. A phase-sensitive rectifier integrates signal/noise over 5 sec. or longer if necessary. The steadiness of output (when it occurs) is indication of reliable reading. This reliability could never be obtained with a separate control path to an artificial eye, for the continued tremor of the living eye changes the output from moment to moment in an irregular way. In order to eliminate this irregularity from tremor, a deep-red control light (700 nm) was sent along the same path as the measuring light instead of into an artificial eye. The measuring light was flickered against the deep red, which was adjusted in intensity to be equivalent at the photocell. The equivalence was hardly upset by eye tremor which affected the mixed beams equally, but change in pigment density changed the absorption of the (green) measuring light but not the deep red control. Thus bleaching of visual pigment upset the red-green balance in the photo-cell, which could be restored by withdrawing a photometric wedge from the red path. The balance was attained when as much wedge density had been removed from red as pigment density from green. Since light passes once through the wedge but there-and-back through the receptors, the wedge measures the "double density" ["$\Delta D(2)$"] of the pigment.

WEALE's instrument has the advantage that a whole range of spectral values can be measured at once, and hence it might be possible to record the difference spectrum of rapidly changing photoproducts. This is impossible in a single run with RUSHTON's densitometer. On the other hand in a situation limited by signal/noise it is clearly not possible to get such accurate results when, instead of concentrating upon measurement at one wavelength, we measure at 26 wavelengths all at once. In steady conditions with a good subject RUSHTON's measurements can have an accuracy of $\pm$ 3% of total pigment. It is questionable whether in Fig. 3, measurements can be made accurate to $\pm$ 3% of the maximum amplitude ratio of any pair.

The advantage of the control beam's having deep red mixed with the signal has been stated above. The disadvantage is that any change in retinal reflectivity that also affects equally the deep red signal will be missed, since there will be no differential change. Such a change was observed by WEALE (1961a) using the artificial eye control. It occurs after bleaching with very powerful lights, and is seen as a uniform increase in density throughout the spectrum — a "greying", which recovers in about 3 min. It may be due to heat oedema. The greying, however, appears not to be related to visual pigments, and the deep red control has the advantage of ridding the measurements of this as well as eye tremor and other unwanted perturbations.

In measurements by retinal densitometry it is hard to get consistent results and even when consistent it is hard to know whether perhaps they are simply consistent in their errors. It is, therefore, fortunate that many key measurements have been made on these two very different instruments with concordant results. I can certainly feel more confidence in my equipment when I find that it gives the same answer as WEALE's.

The measurement of pigment in single receptors, when satisfactorily performed, can answer important questions that cannot be touched by retinal densitometry in the living eye. These highly sophisticated measurements are treated in chapter 12 by DR. LIEBMAN.

B. Transmissivity, the Appropriate Measure for Retinal Mosaics

The most accurate measurements of visual pigments are made in solution, where the appropriate measure is density. Two solutions placed in troughs one behind the other in the measuring beam exhibit the same density reading as when mixed together and then replaced in the troughs. Densities are additive when each ray of the measuring light passes through both. They are like resistances: in series they add.

But in the living eye or in the excised retina we are not dealing with a homogenous mixture of pigments but with a mosaic. Light passes either through rods, or through cones either of one kind or another; or through interspaces; and there will be stray light in the living eye scattered in the lens etc., and somehow getting mixed with the signal. So here the densities are not in series; they are in parallel.

In parallel electric circuits it is not resistances but conductances that add, and obviously in the eye it is the lights transmitted through the various parallel channels that add at the photocell. If one pigment only is bleached there will be greater transmittance through that channel and no change in any other. If now a second pigment only is bleached, the increased transmittance in the new channel is added to the previous score. It is easy to obtain a general formula relating T, the light signal measured in the photo-cell, to the other quantities in the eye [on the lines of formula (1) in RUSHTON, 1965e].

The light T which is measured by the photocell comes partly from light superficially scattered in the eye, and partly from reflexion at the fundus. Some of the fundal light has passed through cones of one type or another, and some has passed between them. We assume here that light enters and returns through the same retinal channel, a) because it slightly simplifies the equations, b) because it is anatomically likely, c) because alternative paths give nearly identical results.

In the fully bleached eye, let $a\varrho$ be the amount of light reaching the photocell from between the cones, and $n_1\varrho$, $n_2\varrho$ .... be the amount passing through cones of type 1, 2, ... r.

Then the total light T_0 reaching the photocell will be

$$T_0 = b + \varrho \left(a + \sum^{r} n_r\right)$$

where b is the superficial stray light.

Now if cones r instead of being fully bleached contain pigment, this will reduce the light passing twice through these cones by a factor $(1 - \alpha_r)$, where α_r is the increased absorption (double passage) above the fully bleached value. Thus the contribution of these cones to the photocell light T will be reduced from ϱn_r to $(1 - \alpha_r)\,\varrho n_r$.

Consequently, the total increase of light on bleaching

$$T_0 - T = \varrho \sum^{r} \alpha_r n_r$$

and change in transmissivity

$$\frac{T_0 - T}{T'_0} = \frac{\sum^{r} \alpha_r n_r}{\sum^{r} n_r + a + b/\varrho}. \tag{3}$$

This formula applies to measurements at any given wavelength. Roman letters represent quantities independent of wavelength; Greek letter quantities are wavelength dependent. If b, the superficial stray light is zero, the denominator of Eq. (3) will be independent of wave length, and hence will simply scale down by a fixed fraction all the absorption spectra $\sum \alpha n$. If b is large, the scaling will depend upon ϱ, the spectral reflectivity of the fundus. In favourable conditions b/ϱ is only a few p.c. of the denominator, so that scaling is nearly the same at all wave lengths.

It is plain from equation (3) that each type of receptor r contributes to the transmissivity T/T_0 an amount proportional to the change in absorption α_r of its own pigment, and is independent of changes in other pigments.

If equivalent *density* were to be measured we should record

$$\log \left(\sum n_r \alpha_r \right)$$

from which the contributions of the various pigments can only be obtained by taking the antilog and going back to Eq. (3).

In what follows, therefore, we shall generally be concerned with transmissivities, for here the effects of various pigments are additive.

III. The Measurement of Rhodopsin

A. Validity of the Measurements

When anyone constructs an instrument intended to measure something much better than has hitherto been possible he is faced with the problem of how to test its performance. For there is then no better instrument in existence by which the new device may be calibrated.

If when CAMPBELL and I built our densitometer there had been no knowledge about visual pigments we should hardly have known how to test whether we could measure them. But a great deal was known about rhodopsin and its relation to twilight vision. Thus in our first full paper (CAMPBELL and RUSHTON, 1955) we were able to show that what we measured was rhodopsin because it satisfied certain expected criteria.

(1) *Bleaching and Regeneration.* In strong light the retinal density was diminished at a rate roughly proportional to the light intensity; in the dark it regenerated with a half-return time of some 5 min.

(2) *Local Effect.* The region of retina measured was a small patch (say 2°). When the *bleaching* light fell on this patch the density was diminished; when it fell elsewhere there was practically no change. Thus what is measured is the result of what the bleaching light does to the retina at the place where it falls, and is not due to any general effect upon the eye.

(3) *The Bunsen-Roscoe Law (It = k)* should hold for the bleaching of rhodopsin for times up to those where regeneration is significant. It was found when It had a value that bleached about 50% that the change in density was the same so long as the product It was constant and t not greater than 45 sec. But if It was increased or diminished the amount bleached was increased or diminished.

(4) *Action Spectrum.* Bleaching lights of different wavelengths matched to appear of the same brightness by scotopic vision should bleach rhodopsin equally. Lights, matched in twilight, were increased in luminance by a fixed amount (about 10^4 to produce a 50% bleach) and were then found all to bleach equally. But slightly mismatched intensities bleached unequally.

(5) *Retinal Distribution.* One would expect the density change measured to be zero when measurements were made upon a region of retina where there are no rods (optic disc or fovea) and to be greatest where the rod population is closest

packed. This was found to be so, in measurements right across the horizontal diameter of the retina.

All this is strong evidence that our densitometer in fact measured rhodopsin, for in various conditions where the rhodopsin level was expected to be the same, the densitometer readings were the same. These experiments give no information as to the relation between rhodopsin density and the readings of the densitometer. The measurements were mostly made far from the fovea (15°), where cones are comparatively scarce, with a pair of balanced wavelengths that practically excluded cones from the measurements.

WEALE (1961 b) tested his instrument in the same way six years later and obtained essentially the same results with rods in the periphery. He also made measurements nearer the fovea (8°) with conditions sensitive to cones as well as to rods, and obtained evidence of more than one pigment.

Two further measurements (RUSHTON, 1956a) show the densitometry measurements to be more or less proportional to the density of rhodopsin: a) the difference spectrum (obtained by measuring with lights of various wavelengths) and b) the photosensitivity curve (obtained by bleaching with brief flashes of various energies), both show what might be expected of rhodopsin. The early difference spectrum exhibits the presence of orange photoproducts, which later diminish in amount, and the bleaching rate was found to be more or less what would be predicted from bleaching of rhodopsin in solution (DARTNALL, GOODEVE, and LYTHGOE, 1936, 1938) after making corrections for light loss in the eye, molecular orientation in the rods etc. WEALE (1961 b) has confirmed these results also, 6.8 log td. sec. being the energy we both find necessary to bleach 50% of the rhodopsin within the Bunsen-Roscoe interval (45 sec). WEALE is able to record full difference spectra very quickly after bleaching and has demonstrated some conspicuous variations due to early photoproducts (WEALE, 1962).

B. Pigment Absorption and Transmissivity

Formula (3) gives the relation between the measured quantity transmissivity $(= T/T_0)$ and the pigment absorption α for double traverse. For a single type of receptor e.g. rods only

$$1 - \frac{T}{T_0} = \frac{n\,\alpha}{n + a + b/\varrho} \,. \tag{4}$$

If bleaching and regeneration are measured at some fixed wavelength

$$1 - \frac{T}{T_0} = c\,\alpha$$

where c is constant.

From estimates of various kinds (RUSHTON, 1956b) the full rhodopsin density is taken as about 0.15 (single passage), and for many purposes we may take the rhodopsin density as linear with transmissivity. But c, the constant of proportion is not easy to evaluate, it probably varies a great deal from eye to eye; and if this is due to the superficial stray light b (as is likely), then it may distort very greatly the difference spectra. For, transmissivity at various wavelengths will be attenuated by the size of the term b/ϱ, and ϱ the fundal reflectivity is strongly wavelength dependent.

C. Dark Adaptation and Regeneration

The quarter-century 1925—50 was the heyday of HECHT and WALD's photochemical theory. According to that doctrine, visual performance was in the main explicable in terms of the level of the visual pigment. A defect of the theory as applied to man (where it generally was applied) was that no one could measure the level of the visual pigment. The rhodopsin level in the rods was simply invented to support the theory. Where the invention was successful in explaining psychophysics (HECHT, 1937) it turned out to depart from fact by a factor of a million. This appeared at once when CAMPBELL and RUSHTON (1955) applied their retinal densitometer, but long before this the precise measurements of DARTNALL, GOODEVE, and LYTHGOE (1938) — results that were never mentioned by supporters of the Hecht-Wald theory — had shown that rhodopsin could not possibly be bleached away by the feeble lights in the short times required to change the level of rod performance in acuity, flicker etc. as the theory required.

KÜHNE (1878) had shown that strong lights bleached away rhodopsin which regenerated in the frog over a period of hours, and the photochemical theory had always claimed that the slow recovery of rod sensitivity after bleaching — the dark adaptation curve — was also closely connected with the regeneration of rhodopsin. But there was no settled view either as to the causal connexion or even what the empirical relation was.

Densitometry allows the regeneration after full bleaching to be measured objectively, and rhodopsin was seen to return along an exponential curve (RUSHTON, CAMPBELL, HAGINS, and BRINDLEY, 1955) running a course similar to the rod branch of the dark adaptation curve, at every stage taking about 5 min for further half return to full recovery. Measurements on the fovea (RUSHTON, 1957) showed a cone pigment that regenerated 4 times as fast, similar to the cone branch of the dark adaptation curve. WEALE (1959, 1962) has repeated these regeneration measurements and confirmed that rhodopsin regenerates much more slowly than cone pigments.

DOWLING (1960) was the first to establish that log rod threshold is rather accurately a linear function of the level of rhodopsin in the rods. But he did this not in man but in albino rats where the threshold measured was for the b-wave of the e.r.g. and the rhodopsin level was found by direct extraction of rhodopsin from excised retinas.

In man the difficulty is to measure the pigment and the threshold at the same stage of recovery, for after a full rhodopsin bleach it takes some 18 min before the rod threshold drops below that of the cones. Up till then rod threshold cannot be measured by ordinary techniques, but after that point rhodopsin will be more than 90% recovered so that little can be said about the correlation between rod dark adaptation and the 10% tail of rhodopsin regeneration.

The difficulty was overcome (RUSHTON, 1961) by using as subject a rod monochromat who had no functional cones to undersell the rods, so that the rod dark adaptation curve could be followed through a threshold range of over a millionfold. The results (replotted) are shown in Fig. 4. The dark adaptation curve of cones in a *normal* subject is indicated by the dotted curve; the wavy line starting after 6 min is the threshold plotted out by the rod monochromat starting at level

7 log units. The plain circles show the regeneration of rhodopsin in the normal; filled circles in the rod monochromat (scale on the right). It appears that the course

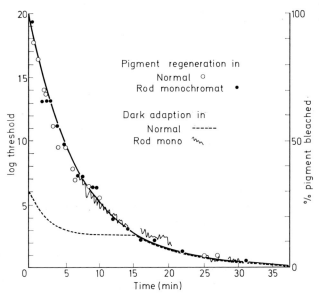

Fig. 4. Dark adaptation and rhodopsin regeneration in a rod monochromat. *Wavy line*, the trace of the subject's dark adaptation over a range of 6 log units (scale on left). *Dotted curve* indicates dark adaptation in the normal, showing only cone thresholds for 15 min after full bleach. *Filled and plain circles* plot the regeneration of rhodopsin in monochromat and normal (scale on right). (After RUSHTON, 1961)

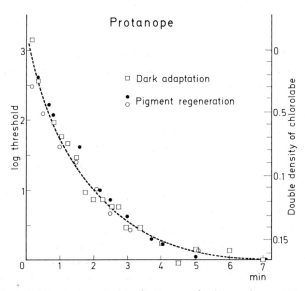

Fig. 5. Dark adaptation and pigment regeneration on the fovea of a protanope; scale of log threshold on left, of cone pigment chlorolabe on right. (After RUSHTON, 1963a)

of pigment regeneration is the same in both subjects and, when scaled so that full bleaching corresponds to 20 log units rise in threshold, the dark adaptation curve fits the rhodopsin regeneration curve. It follows that in man, each 5% of rhodopsin bleached raises the threshold 1 log unit.

Fig. 5 shows a similar measurement on the fovea of a protanope who also has only one measurable pigment, but here a cone pigment. The recovery time is 4 times as fast, and half bleaching raises the log threshold 1.5 instead of 10. But the dark adaptation and pigment regeneration curves still run together. Protanopes, deuteranopes and normals all have the same foveal dark adaptation curves.

The difficult question of adaptation is treated in a different place in this *Handbook* (Vol. VII/4, Chap. 1). It is mentioned here first because retinal densitometry has justified Hecht's original belief that dark adaptation was somehow closely related to the regeneration of visual pigment and has shown what in fact that relation is — namely that the log threshold is raised in proportion to the fraction of rhodopsin still bleached. Second it is further proof that what the densitometer measures is a *visual* pigment since the reflectivity change is so closely linked with the change in log threshold.

IV. The Measurement of Cone Pigments

Wald, Brown, and Smith (1955) proposed "that the ratio of the sensitivities of rod and cone vision in the intact animal is of the same order as the ratio of the absorption of visual pigments in the rods and cones". In man cone vision is 100 to 1,000 times less sensitive than rod vision, so the prospect of measuring cone pigments was not bright. However, while the above was being penned, cone pigments were in fact being measured on the human fovea (Rushton, 1955) where it was found that the density in the cones was about the same as that of rhodopsin in the rods and that protanopes lacked the normal red-sensitive pigment.

Clerk Maxwell had shown that in protanopes (the red-blind colour defectives), the red component of trichromacy was absent, and the lack of red-sensitive cones has always been a likely, and generally held explanation of this condition. When this was settled by densitometry it provided us with a fovea that contained only one measurable visual pigment, and hence a simple source of cone pigment where the hitherto unknown properties, kinetics etc., could be studied.

Nomenclature. Though it has long been recognized that there are no unique "primary" colours, trichromacy has generally been expressed in terms of red, green and blue inputs. Thus colour has been analysed in terms of R, G and B spectral sensitivity curves, R, G and B cones and R, G and B visual pigments. This is a better way of describing pigments than rhodopsin, iodopsin, cyanopsin etc. which name the visual pigments by the colours they do *not* absorb and to which their receptors are *in*sensitive. Human cone pigments have been named erythrolabe, chlorolabe, and cyanolabe (= red-, green-, blue-catching) to link them with the R, G and B of traditional psychophysics. These names imply nothing about the spectral regions where the maximum absorptions lie but are related simply to the $R:G:B$ cone excitations of psychophysics.

A. Foveal Measurements in the Protanope

The best evidence that the protanope contains only one foveal pigment in the red-green range is given by RUSHTON (1963a). The fovea was bleached by a red light and the transmissivities for lights throughout the spectrum measured, first dark adapted and then in equilibrium under this bleaching light. After recovery the experiment was repeated exactly as before except that the bleaching light was blue-green. The intensities used were such that when measured (say at 540 nm) the amounts bleached were half the total in each case. It was found, not only at 540 nm, but at every measured wavelength throughout the spectrum, that the transmissivity changes were the same in both experiments.

The triangles in Fig. 6 show the results of the two experiments (RUSHTON, 1965d). We are not concerned with the exact shape of the curve — that the point at 540 nm, for instance, lies low (as would happen if haemoglobin diminished the fundal reflectivity ϱ, formula (3), at this wavelength). What is relevant is the coincidence of triangles black and white, which show the differences after bleaching with red or blue-green light. For, if only one pigment were present only one kind of change could occur. But if two pigments were present only one kind of change could not occur: red light would bleach erythrolabe more, green would bleach chlorolabe more. That does not happen, thus there is only one measurable pigment on the fovea of the protanope. It is called chlorolabe.

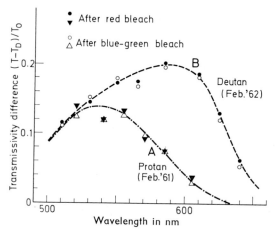

Fig. 6. The difference spectra obtained on the fovea of a protanope *(triangles)* or a deuteranope *(circles)*. *Filled symbols* show the difference after a 50% bleach by red light, *plain symbols* after 50% by blue-green light. The coincidence of filled and plain symbols means that no differential colour bleaching occurs. Thus protanopes and deuteranopes each have but one cone pigment in the foveal red-green range. (After RUSHTON, 1965d)

B. Foveal Measurements in the Deuteranope

The pigments in the deuteranope have long been disputed. Some teachers have held that only one pigment is present in the red-green range, so the condition is exactly analogous to that in the protanope. Others have held that both the normal red and green pigments are present but discrimination between the two inputs is ineffective because the pigments are mixed, or the signals are mixed, or the green signal is lacking though the green pigment is present.

The experiment of Fig. 6 performed now upon the deuteranope is decisive between these views. If there are two visual pigments in the deuteranope no matter how mixed are they or their signals, the changes after half bleaching by red or by blue-green will not be the same (as they certainly are not in normal eyes). But the filled and plain circles of Fig. 6 demonstrate that there is as good a coincidence in the results with deuteranopes (circles) as with protanopes (triangles). Thus protanopes and deuteranopes each have only one measurable cone pigment on the fovea. But they do not both have the same pigment. The deuteranope transmissivity spectrum absorbs much further into the red, corresponding to the fact that he can see much further into the red end of the spectrum than the protanope. His pigment is called erythrolabe.

C. Visual Pigments of Protanope and Deuteranope

If these photolabile pigments are *visual* pigments, then lights that appear equally bright to the fovea of the dichromat should bleach equally fast his pigment there. A densitometer that can measure the pigment in equilibrium during bleaching is well suited to compare these bleaching rates. We wish to compare two wavelengths λ_1, λ_2 to find the light energies I_1, I_2 that bleach *equally* the pigment on the fovea of a protanope (or deuteranope). Set λ_1 at a bleaching energy I_1 that at equilibrium bleaches about 50% of the pigment. Now suddenly change to light λ_2 of intensity I_2. In general this new light will bleach either more or less than does I_1 of λ_1, so the pigment level (measured always at some fixed convenient wavelength) will fall or rise. After a few trials a value of I_2 can be found that keeps the pigment level exactly unaltered. The relation between I_n and λ_n that keeps the pigment level always unchanged is the action spectrum for bleaching for the pigment. It can be measured correct to ± 0.06 log units with protanopes (Rushton, 1963a) and deuteranopes (Rushton, 1965a, b, c).

If these pigments are *visual* pigments then I_1 and I_2 that bleach equally should appear equally bright to that same dichromatic subject. This is an easy measurement to make since dichromats, being little confused by colour, can make excellent energy matches throughout the red-green spectral range. It was found that the subjective and objective measurements coincided to about ± 0.06 log units.

Thus the pigments measured are those that catch the quanta that result in the dichromat's foveal vision. The importance of this good correspondence is that it affords by far the best measure we have of the spectral sensitivity of cone pigments in the human eye. Dichromats have only one dimension of input in the red-green range and only one visual pigment is found there. Thus we should expect lights that appeared identical to bleach equally. This is found to be true correct to ± 0.06 log units. Thus we may believe that it is exactly true and accept the dichromat psycho-physical brightness match (that is certainly accurate to ± 0.01) as the action spectrum of the visual pigment.

It is known that the colour matching function is different at high intensities from that at low (Wright, 1936), a phenomenon analysed by Brindley

(1953, 1955) and attributed to variation in self-screening by the cone pigments. The action spectrum of the pigments therefore depends upon the bleaching level, and may be found by matching at that level. This method has the advantage over measurements of pigments in solution, excised retinas etc., that no spectral correction need be made for transmission losses in the eye media etc. when comparison is made with visual performance. The appropriate correction is automatically incorporated when bleaching is performed *in situ*.

The same applies to the Stiles-Crawford colour effect, the change in colour when light enters through different parts of the pupil. Now RIPPS and WEALE (1964) have shown that for different wavelengths the bleaching efficiency depends upon the point of pupil entry in the same way as does the efficiency for visual perception. Thus this effect also is compensated when bleaching rates and seeing are compared in identical conditions of light presentation.

All this, however, implies that pigments in the dichromat are the same as those in the normal eye.

D. Visual Pigments of the Normal Subject

It is well known that protanopes and deuteranopes each accept all normal colour matches. If normal eyes contain the chlorolabe of the protanope and the erythrolabe of the deuteranope this must follow. If they contain different pigments, those must each have an absorption spectrum that is the weighted mean of the absorption spectra of chlorolabe and erythrolabe. Biochemically this is unlikely. BAKER and RUSHTON (1965) showed that the red-sensitive pigment in a normal was identical with the erythrolabe of the deuteranope as judged by action spectrum, difference spectrum, photosensitivity, and regeneration rate. And RUSHTON (1964b) showed that the green-sensitive pigment in the normal was the same as chlorolabe in the protanope. RIPPS and WEALE (1963) have also studied the bleaching of mixed pigments on the normal fovea, but they have worked with densities, not transmissivities and the pigments remain mixed.

V. Cone Pigment Kinetics

A. Parameters

In the living eye cone pigments are under two main influences — bleaching by light and regeneration by chemical processes that are independent of light. The pigment level may be followed continuously with RUSHTON's densitometer throughout any light-dark manoeuvre that is not too rapid, and in this way the kinetics can be investigated. They turn out to be extremely simple to a first approximation, and may be expressed in these three statements.

(i) Pigment is bleached at a rate proportional to the quantum catch.

(ii) Regeneration proceeds at a rate proportional to the fraction of the pigment in the bleached state.

(iii) Processes (i) and (ii) are independent and hence are simply additive.

Let $I =$ strength of bleaching light (td),

   $t =$ time (sec),

   $p =$ fraction of pigment unbleached at t

   $Q_e =$ energy of flash (td. sec) that bleaches p from 1 to e^{-1},

   $t_0 =$ time constant of regeneration,

   $N =$ total number of pigment molecules/cm² of retina,

   $y =$ concentration of free 11-cis retinaldehyde,

   $k =$ velocity constant of the regeneration reaction.

Then expressing in symbols the three statements above we obtain

(i)   in bleaching, $-\dfrac{dp}{dt} = \dfrac{Ip}{Q_e}$ hence $ln\,\dfrac{1}{p} = \dfrac{It}{Q_e}$ if $p = 1$ when $t = 0$,   (5)

(ii)   in regeneration, $\dfrac{dp}{dt} = \dfrac{1-p}{t_0}$,   (6)

(iii)   in general, $-\dfrac{dp}{dt} = \dfrac{Ip}{Q_e} - \dfrac{1-p}{t_0}$.   (7)

   Relation (i) was established experimentally by bleaching with lights of various intensities exposed for 10 sec during which regeneration is negligible (when p starts from 1). This is too rapid a pigment change to be followed with the densitometer, but the total change produced could be measured at equilibrium as follows. At the end of the 10 sec exposure the bleaching light I_1 was not extinguished but suddenly reduced to a new value I_2, about 0.1 as strong, the precise value being found by trial to be that which held the pigment exactly in equilibrium. The pigment level was measured 15 sec after the 10 sec bleach and again at 60 sec. When I_2 was adjusted so that both readings were the same, it was found that measurement at all other times also gave the same reading and it was taken that this value of p was the level to which the pigment had been reduced by the 10 sec exposure to I_1, and that thereafter it remained in equilibrium under I_2.

   Fig. 7 (taken from Rushton, 1958) shows by filled circles the fraction p of pigment remaining after 10 sec of bleaching by intensity I_1 (scaled horizontally as log td. sec). The curve drawn through the points is derived from Eq. (5) which may be rewritten as

$$\log\left(ln\,\frac{1}{p}\right) = \log\,(It) - \log\,Q_e\,.   (8)$$

Changes in the value of Q_e will simply displace the curve sideways, and in Fig. 7 it has been displaced so as to fit the points. Q_e (the abscissa where $p = e^{-1}$) has the value 6.7 log td. sec.

   The plain circles of Fig. 7 plot p against I_2, the steady light that keeps the pigment in equilibrium at level p. Now from Eq. (5) the bleaching rate is $I_2 p/Q_e$, whose value can be found for each plain circle of Fig. 7, since its ordinate is p, its abscissa gives I_2, and Q_e is known from Eq. (8). But since plain circles represent equilibria where bleaching is exactly balanced by regeneration, this computed value is also the rate of regeneration under steady illumination, I_2. In Fig. 8 (plain circles) the regeneration rates so computed are plotted for various degrees of bleaching $(1 - p)$. They lie close to the straight line through the origin. Thus the regeneration rate under I_2 is proportional to $(1 - p)$ the amount bleached. This satisfies Eq. (6).

Now the regeneration rate in the dark may easily be found by plotting the regeneration curve (Fig. 5) and drawing a tangent at various times. When this was done for the subject of Fig. 8 the regeneration rate in the dark was found to give the values plotted as filled circles. Thus we establish the important fact, first that, both in the dark and at equilibrium under strong light, the rate of

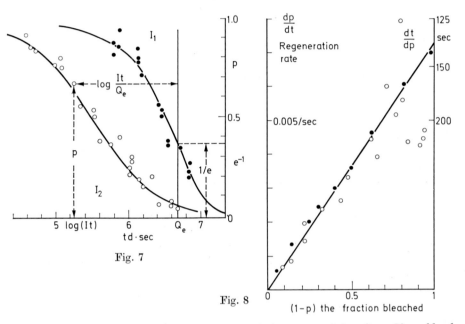

Fig. 7.

Fig. 8.

Fig. 7. *Filled circles* plot (vertically) the fraction p of pigment remaining after a 10 sec bleach of energy plotted horizontally in log td. sec. Curve through the points is that expected if bleaching is proportional to quantum catch Ip/Q_e. *Plain circles* plot the fraction p in equilibrium with steady light I_2, whose value × 10 sec is plotted as abscissa, Curve through the points is that expected if, in addition to the bleaching relation *(filled circles)* regeneration occurs at a rate proportional to (1—p), the fraction of pigment in the bleached state. (After RUSHTON, 1958)

Fig. 8. *Plain circles*, regeneration rate (under the bleaching light I_2) plotted against (1—p) from the plain circles of Fig. 7 (no arbitrary constants). *Filled circles*, regeneration rate in the dark, measured by drawing tangents to curves such as that of Fig. 5 at various stages of residual bleaching (1—p). Coincidence of filled and plain circles means that the regeneration rate is independent of concomitant bleaching. (After RUSHTON, 1958)

regeneration is proportional to the fraction of pigment in the bleached state. Second that the constant of proportion is identical in both cases since the slope of both lines is the same. The first establishes Eq. (6); the second, Eq. (7).

These results refer to mixed cone pigments on a normal fovea bleached by white light. In these circumstances erythrolabe and chlorolabe act nearly as a single pigment in their kinetics. The same results are seen more clearly with single pigments on the fovea of the protanope (RUSHTON, 1963b) and deuteranope (RUSHTON, 1965b), with some improvement in measurement after 6 years' practice.

B. The Equilibrium Condition

The equilibrium bleaching conditions are important in retinal densitomet because these states are simple, steady and reliable. In the circles of Fig. 7 t situation was complicated because there it was important that equilibrium shou be established from the start. But in general this is not required and any stea bleaching light will result in equilibrium in a few minutes. When this is establish the first member of Eq. (7) is zero and we obtain

$$\frac{It_o}{Q_e} = \frac{1-p}{p}.$$

This is the curve on the left of Fig. 7, through the circles. The curve has a fix shape and may be slid sideways to give the best fit to a set of experimental poir plotting p against $\log I$, as in Fig. 7. Calling I_0 the value of I where $p = 1/2$ we obta at once

$$I_0 t_0 = Q_e .$$

I_0 can be found accurately and rechecked at leisure in the equilibrium state and the time constant of regeneration, is also a reliable value, so probably the best wa to determine Q_e is from Eq. (10) (Rushton and Henry, 1968). The value of p most sensitive to changes in $\log I$ when $p = 1/2$; hence I_0 is the most accura bleaching power to use when comparisons are to be made.

One comparison has been mentioned earlier, the action spectrum in tl dichromat. Here I was changed in wavelength and also in energy in such a wa that the bleaching rate and hence the equilibrium value remained constant. $p = 0.5 \pm 0.03$, which is about what can be achieved in these steac conditions, it follows from Eq. (9) that $\log I = \log I_0 \pm 0.05$, so the actic spectrum can be obtained with good accuracy.

Glare and Scattered Light. Another application of equilibrium bleaching is the classical question of glare. When the fovea is surrounded by a very brig ring of light it becomes less sensitive just as though a veil of light fell upon the fov itself. Is this because a real veil of light is scattered from the bright ring and actual falls upon the fovea, or is it because of nerve interaction (lateral inhibition etc.

Many objective measurements have been made on light scatter in the retin they all measure the light seen to be scattered — seen either by eye or photocell. B the light *seen* as scattered from the fovea when surrounded by a bright annul clearly has not been absorbed by the foveal cones and hence could not hav contributed to the veiling light (though it could contribute to an estimate of it Obviously the relevant fraction of scattered light is that absorbed by the fove cones, and this can be measured by their bleaching. Rushton and Gubisch (196 showed that in fact the psycho-physical "equivalent veil" bleached the cones a much by direct light as the bright annulus did by scatter.

The retinal densitometer was set up to measure foveal bleaching in equilibriu and the direct foveal bleaching light intensity was 10^4 trolands which bleache about 50% of the cone pigment. This bleaching field could be suddenly exchange for a much brighter annulus, which did not fall upon the fovea but surrounded i The intensity of this was adjusted so that when the substitution was made n change in pigment level resulted at the fovea. This required the annulus to l 1.75 ± 0.05 log units brighter than the centre.

The psycho-physical measurements were made by projecting a test flash on to the fovea in the presence either of the luminous centre or the annular surround. The threshold was raised equally by centre and by surround when the surround was 1.7 log units brighter than the centre for all levels of the centre including 10^4 trolands.

Thus the psycho-physical veiling light is within $\pm\ 0.05$ of light that is scattered from the annulus and caught by the foveal cones, and lateral inhibition plays no part. And this result, measured directly at one high level applies to all, since the *proportion* of glare to equivalent veil was found experimentally to be independent of luminous level, and so also must be the *fraction* of the light scattered.

C. The Chemistry of Regeneration in Man

There is good evidence (HUBBARD and WALD, 1952) that the regeneration of rhodopsin is the combination of 11-*cis* retinaldehyde with rod opsin.

$$\text{free opsin} + 11\text{-}cis \text{ retinal} \to \text{rhodopsin} .$$
$$(1-p) \qquad\qquad y$$

Thus if $(1 - p)$ is the fraction of rhodopsin in the form of free opsin and y is the 11-*cis* concentration, then the rate of combination

$$\frac{dp}{dt} = ky\,(1 - p) \tag{11}$$

where k is the velocity constant. The fact that the regeneration curve for rods and cones is an exponential (equation 6)

$$\frac{dp}{dt} = \frac{(1-p)}{t_0}$$

means that, in these conditions, y, the 11-*cis* concentration is constant.

Recent measurements however (RUSHTON and HENRY, 1968) indicate that this is not always the case, nor would it be expected. We know from the work of v. JANCSÓ and v. JANCSÓ (1936) and DOWLING (1960) that after rhodopsin has been bleached, retinal leaves the retina and may be found in the pigment epithelium whence it returns, doubtless transformed from all-*trans* to 11-*cis*, ready to unite again with free opsin.

There is probably a small store of 11-*cis* in the human retina available for immediate regeneration — perhaps one retina's replacement. This implies that although, following a sudden full bleach, the 11-*cis* concentration would be high, it would rapidly fall as the small store was depleted faster than it could be replenished from the pigment epithelium. This is what was found by RUSHTON and HENRY (1968) on applying Eq. (11) to their densitometric results following full bleaches of short and long duration. From the regeneration curve, $(1 - p)$ is plotted as ordinate and dp/dt measured as tangent, so the value ky is easily found. Immediately after a sudden bleach, ky is about twice what it is after a long bleach that has exhausted the store.

There is quite a different condition that appears to affect the 11-*cis* material available for regeneration. Both rods and cones seem to require it and since cones regenerate 4 or 5 times as fast as rods do, they would be more effective in seizing it

if 11-*cis* were in short supply. Using the rod psycho-physical dark adaptation cur
as a measure of the rate of rhodopsin regeneration, Rushton (1968) showed th
rods regenerate more slowly when neighbouring cones are numerous and regenerati
fast. It is clear that rods and cones are in competition for some ingredient that l
in the retina outside the receptors, and a likely substance is 11-*cis* retinol.

The general kinetic Eq. (7) has proved rather satisfactory in predicting t
cone pigment level in a wide range of conditions. But it is doubtless much t
simple. It does not embrace changes in the 11-*cis* store nor the effects of fla
photolysis which are discussed in the next section.

VI. Photoisomerization

A. Balance between Photic and Thermal Processes

The bleaching of rhodopsin occurs in two main stages: (a) the photic stag
which Hubbard and Wald (1952) showed was essentially the change from t
11-*cis* to the all-*trans* configuration in the retinaldehyde component of the molecu
and (b) the thermal stage during which the retinaldehyde gets loose by steps a
finally comes away.

The thermal stage can be arrested by "bleaching" at low temperatures (e.
− 70° C) which does not affect the photic process. When Collins and Morton (195
studied the two stages separately, bleaching to excess in the cold and then allowi
the thermal reactions to take place at room temperature but in the dark, the
found two surprising facts. First, only about half the rhodopsin was bleached
matter how strong and prolonged the light exposure, second the "unbleached
residue was not exactly rhodopsin, it absorbed maximally at a slightly short
wavelength.

Hubbard and Kropf (1958) analysed what was happening. After bleachi
in the cold, where the all-*trans* retinaldehyde is held still strongly connected to t
protein, the absorbance spectrum remains very similar to that of rhodopsin itse
Thus the all-*trans* chromoproteins (lumirhodopsin etc.) will catch quanta from t
bleaching light and some of these quanta will re-isomerize the carotenoid. Abou
half these re-isomerizations restore the original 11-*cis* configuration, and abou
half generate 9-*cis*. Since this photo-reversal goes about as fast as the primar
bleaching process, at equilibrium some 50% is left in the all-*trans* state. Th
accounts for the observations of Collins and Morton (1950) though in detail t
situation may be a good deal more complex.

In the warm living eye some separation of the photic and thermal process
can be obtained by flash photolysis. The object of low temperature was to slo
down the thermal process relative to the photic. The same is achieved by speedin
the photic relative to the thermal by using extremely brief flashes, but stron
enough to provide incident quanta in excess.

Some effects of multiple quantum hits per molecule of cone pigment were studie
by Rushton on the fovea of Dr. H. D. Baker (Rushton, 1964a). Fig. 9 shows
the fraction of cone pigment remaining unbleached plotted against the energy
the bleaching light. Curve *A* is when the bleaching light was from a tungste

filament exposed for 10 sec. The relation is the same as the curve on the right of Fig. 7 but there the abscissa was log It and here it is It. The theoretical curves are the same, seen here as an exponential of constant $Q_e = 3.5 \times 10^6$ td. sec $= 6.55$ log td. sec (there $Q_e = 6.7$ log td. sec).

Curve B Fig. 9 shows the bleaching produced by the same range of energies when delivered in a 0.2 msec flash. One would expect that with very weak lights, when the probability of a double quantum hit per molecule is negligible, the pigment

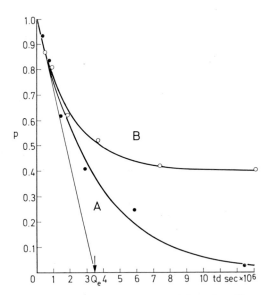

Fig. 9. *Filled circles*, fraction of cone pigment p remaining after 10 sec exposure of energy plotted horizontally in td. sec. *Plain circles* the fraction remaining when the energy was presented in a 0.2 msec flash. Even multiple quantum hits per molecule produce photoreversal. (After RUSHTON, 1964a)

molecules would not "know" whether their single quantum came from a steady light or an instantaneous flash. Thus for weak flashes curves A and B must run together. The flash energy needed for each molecule to catch effectively 1 quantum on average is Q_e. This can be formally established (RUSHTON and HENRY, 1968) but it is fairly obvious intuitively. As we have seen, for very weak bleaching lights double hits are negligible and each effective quantum hit bleaches a molecule. The tangent to the curve at $p = 1$, therefore, gives the rate of bleaching per troland seconds of retinal energy. Maintained at this rate, all would be bleached at 3.5×10^6 td. sec $= Q_e =$ the exponential constant of curve A.

On account of the random nature of individual quantum distributions the energy Q_e that on average hits each molecule once will actually leave some molecules unhit and will hit others twice, thereby changing them back to erythrolabe. Consequently we should expect curve B to lie above A, and in fact the points are seen to be close to the theoretical exponential curve which starts tangential to A and ends at about 50% bleached in photo-equilibrium (actually 60% bleached).

Since these results are exactly what was to be expected from Hubbard and Kropf's (1958) analysis of rhodopsin (bleaching at low temperatures) and the similar results of Williams (1964) with flash bleaching at room temperature, one might have supposed that the same would have been found with flash bleaching *rhodopsin* in living man. Fig. 10, however, shows the results of Ripps and Weale (1968) which show no sign of re-isomerization when the flash used had a time course (displayed in the left top corner) of only 0.5 msec.

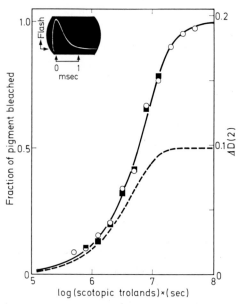

Fig. 10. Bleaching of rhodopsin in man. Ordinates show amount of pigment bleached by light energy (abscissa) plotted in log td. sec. *Circles* show results when the exposure lasted 30 sec, *squares* when it was about 0.5 msec, of time course shown by inset. *Dotted curve* is what would be expected if photoreversal occurred as it does in rhodopsin at room temperature. In the living eye there appears no sign of it. (From Ripps and Weale, 1968)

The curve drawn is the theoretical relation between pigment bleached and log bleaching energy ($Q_e = 6.9$ log td. sec), the same curve as on the right of Fig. 7 but inverted, since in Fig. 10 bleaching is plotted upwards. It is seen that when the energy is supplied by a 30 sec exposure, the circles constitute an excellent fit to the curve and 7.7 log td. sec bleaches some 95%. When the energy was nearly all delivered in 0.5 msec, if re-isomerization had occurred as it did in Fig. 9, the net amount of bleaching would consequently be less, and the experimental points should lie on a curve below that shown in Fig. 10, rising to only about half the full height at photo-equilibrium, as in the dashed curve. But in fact the results of flash bleaching (squares) lie precisely on the same curve as that for 30 sec bleaching. With so bright a flash it was not possible to obtain energy enough to bleach more than 75% of the pigment, but this is already more than the 50% Williams found at photo equilibrium. There seems no doubt that in Ripps and Weale's experiment photoreversal did not occur.

Now the brightest flash that they used was about 2 Q_e and hence each molecule on average received a double hit. It is, therefore, surprising that most of these double hits were incapable of inducing photoreversal. However, we know that when thermal decomposition has reached a certain stage, photoreversal is impossible. It is likely that this stage could be reached sooner in the warm human eye than at room temperature as in the experiments on solution (WILLIAMS, 1964) or on the excised rabbit's eye (HAGINS, 1955).

According to this explanation there is a short time after catching a quantum during which the all-*trans* isomer remains susceptible to photoisomerization by the catch of a second quantum. RUSHTON's 0.2 msec flash lay mainly within the susceptible period, (for cone pigments). RIPPS and WEALE's 0.5 msec flash lay largely outside it (for rhodopsin); but in the experiments (on rhodopsin) at room temperature, the susceptible period was somewhat prolonged, so that longer flashes might still fall within it.

The space between 0.2 and 0.5 msec seems rather narrow for this explanation to squeeze through, but current experiments by T. P. WILLIAMS (private communication) with rhodopsin solutions at different temperatures indicate that it may be on the right lines.

B. Double Quantum Hits and Dark Adaptation

If the result of double quantum hits per molecule is to restore the original visual pigment or to produce a new stable isomer (e.g. 9-*cis*) it might be expected to have some effects upon visual sensation. If, for instance, 9-*cis* has a different spectral absorption from 11-*cis* there should be a corresponding change in the spectral matching functions. None of the curious coloured phenomena associated with exposure to very bright bleaching lights has been proved to be due to a change from 11- to 9-*cis* and it is not likely that this change is the principal cause of the coloured effects.

We have seen (Fig. 5) that bleaching by steady light raises the log threshold in subsequent dark adaptation by an amount proportional to the amount of free opsin. But if the bleaching is produced by a very strong 0.2 msec flash, (curve B Fig. 9 instead of curve A) though most of the molecules have received more than one quantal hit, only about half the pigment remains bleached at the end of the flash; the rest has been re-isomerized. What happens to the dark adaptation curve, does it behave according to the 100% molecular hits or the 50% molecular bleachings?

As seen in Fig. 11 (lower curves) (from RUSHTON, 1964a) the foveal dark adaptation following a strong 0.2 msec bleaching flash does not run according to either expectation; the curve exhibits two branches, the second persisting for 15 min or more. The second branch (called the Θ effect) is not due to rods, for the test flashes fell upon the central fovea; moreover deep red, or green test flashes equated in intensity for cones had their thresholds raised equally at all stages of both branches of dark adaptation (Fig. 12 filled and plain triangles). This also shows that the kink is not a transition from red to green cone thresholds, nor the reverse.

Fig. 11 shows in the upper curves the usual effect of a 10 sec exposure upon the dark adaptation. With an exposure that delivered on average 1 quantum per molecule (filled circles) a fraction e^{-1} would be left unbleached; with 2, or 4 quanta/ mol the fraction would be e^{-2} or e^{-4}. Thus the three bleachings would be 63, 86, and 98%, and the upper curves appear to be roughly scaled in this proportion.

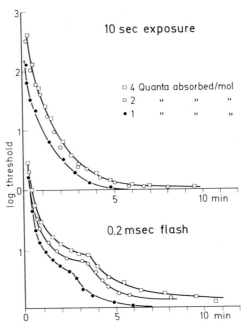

Fig. 11. Foveal dark adaptation curves following a bleaching exposure of 4, 2 or 1 quanta absorbed per molecule on average. Upper curves are when the exposure lasted 10 sec; lower when it lasted 0.2 msec. The kinks in the lower curves called 'the Θ effect' is the subject of this analysis. (After Rushton, 1964a)

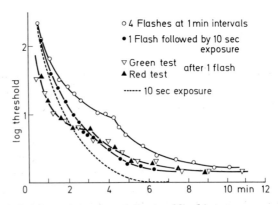

Fig. 12. Foveal dark adaptation curves following bleaching exposures of various kinds as indicated. The "flash" was always a 0.2 msec exposure of maximal strength that on average caused 4 quanta to be absorbed per molecule. (After Rushton, 1964a)

The lower curves show the same energy delivered in a 0.2 msec flash. The curves all show the kink and persistent tail of raised threshold characteristic of the Θ effect. It is greater the greater the average number of quantum hits per molecule. The curve (not shown) below this set i.e. with $\frac{1}{2}$ quantum absorbed/mol (on average) is the same whether the energy was delivered in 10 sec or in 0.2 msec. Thus it is plain from Fig. 11 that kinks begin at the intensity level where double quantum hits begin, and become prominent as double hits become frequent. It looks as though the first hit isomerizes 11-*cis* retinaldehyde to all-*trans* and the second hit changes this into — something new and strange, a pigment that lasts for 15 min and while it lasts keeps the threshold raised in some manner. But this is *not* the way of it.

If, immediately following the flash, we apply a full 10 sec exposure that would (and does) bleach away all pigments whether residual or new formed, it is found (Fig. 12 filled circles) that the Θ effect is *not* abolished. Thus multiple quantum hits can produce something that persists when all resulting pigments have been removed. This something is the result of the flash on cone pigments, not on other structures in the eye, for if the 10 sec full bleach instead of following the flash preceded it, then no Θ effect resulted. Clearly the flash must fall upon unbleached cone pigments to produce the something that then persists, despite further full bleachings. This suggests a procedure by which the Θ effect might be enhanced.

Apply a full flash that bleaches to photoequilibrium (60%) and generates the Θ effect. After 1 min delay (the charging time of our flasher) apply a second flash. This will fall upon cones that are about 70% regenerated and thus susceptible to receive the double hits that will generate a new Θ effect. But, as we have seen, the Θ effect produced by the first flash is not abolished by a second flash. It persists, and perhaps the second Θ adds to it. The plain circles of Fig. 12 show that this expectation is fulfilled. Four consecutive flashes were applied at 1 min intervals with the result that the Θ effect was increased several times. Now the energy of each flash used in that experiment was 4 Q_e (Fig. 9) which gives a double hit to 90% of the molecules. So if the condition for Θ was simply a double hit per molecule, Θ would be 90% maximal after the first flash and could not be further increased the several times shown by the empty circles of Fig. 12. Perhaps a more likely explanation is as follows.

1. A Speculation

Among the isomers produced by a double quantum hit is a *rare* kind so outrageous in shape that, at its birth, it deforms the protein nest and forthwith decomposes. The strained protein persists deformed for 15 min and further flash bleachings will increase the number of protein molecules so affected. The rare isomer will not be formed when the flash is given just after a full 10 sec bleach, for then there will be no pigment to absorb it; its Θ effect will not be abolished by a full bleach given just after the flash — for the rare isomer had already decomposed.

And how does deformation of protein raise the dark adapted threshold? Well, how does bleaching ever raise the threshold? Those who prefer the soaring kite of speculation to be stabilized by some weight of analysis in the tail, may find it in RUSHTON (1964a).

2. After-Images

One further correlation with the Θ effect is found in the foveal after-image. one half of the fovea is bleached with the full 0.2 msec flash and the other w the 10 sec exposure, (both bleaching to equilibrium), the brightnesses of the t images are not equal but show a sequence of time relations that follow closely t curves of Fig. 12, triangles and dotted, respectively. For the first 2 min after t bleach the 10 sec image is brighter; at 2 min they are about the same; the after the 0.2 msec flash image is brighter, and after 10 min can still be clearly se (on blinking in a fairly dim room) whereas the other half has long disappear entirely. If the whole fovea is exposed to the 10 sec bleach and then half is expos to the 0.2 msec flash, the latter has no effect, the fovea remaining uniform. If t whole fovea is exposed to the flash and then half to the 10 sec bleach, the latter h no cancelling effect (as with filled circles Fig. 12). Thus the long lasting aft image, like the Θ effect, persists despite the attempt to clear it by full bleachi

Ghosts, they say, appear to remind us of past injustice. Take heed, then, y photochemists how well you judge of pigments and visual performance, or yc darkness may be haunted by strange after-images.

References

Baker, H. D., Rushton, W. A. H.: The red-sensitive pigment in normal cones. J. Physi (Lond.) **176**, 56—72 (1965).

Baumgardt, E.: Mesure pyrométrique du seuil visuel absolu. Opt. Acta **7**, 305—316 (196

Boynton, R. M., Ikeda, M., Stiles, W. S.: Interactions among chromatic mechanisms ferred from positive and negative increment thresholds. Vision Res. **4**, 87—117 (1964)

Brindley, G. S.: The effects on colour vision of adaption to very bright lights. J. Physi (Lond.) **122**, 332—350 (1953).

— A photochemical reaction in the human retina. Proc. phys. Soc. (Lond.) B **68**, 860—8 (1955).

Campbell, F. W., Rushton, W. A. H.: Measurement of the scotopic pigment in the livi human eye. J. Physiol. (Lond.) **130**, 131—147 (1955).

Collins, F. D., Morton, R. A.: Studies on rhodopsin. 3. Rhodopsin and transient oran Biochem. J. **47**, 18—24 (1950).

Crawford, B. H.: The scotopic visibility function. Proc. phys. Soc. (London) B **62**, 321—3 (1949).

Crescitelli, F., Dartnall, H. J. A.: Human visual purple. Nature (Lond.) **172**, 195—1 (1953).

Dartnall, H. J. A., Goodeve, C. F., Lythgoe, R. J.: The quantitative analysis of the pho chemical bleaching of visual purple solutions in monochromatic light. Proc. roy. Soc. **156**, 158—170 (1936).

— — — The effect of temperature on the photochemical bleaching of visual purple solutio Proc. roy. Soc. A **164**, 216—230 (1938).

Denton, E. J., Walker, M. A.: The visual pigment of the conger eel. Proc. roy. Soc. B 1 257—269 (1958).

— Warren, F. J.: Visual pigments of deep-sea fish. Nature (Lond.) **178**, 1059 (1956).

Dowling, J. E.: The chemistry of visual adapation in the rat. Nature (Lond.) **188**, 114—1 (1960).

Goodeve, C. F., Lythgoe, R. J., Schneider, E. E.: The photosensitivity of visual pur solutions and the scotopic sensitivity of the eye in the ultra-violet. Proc. roy. Soc. B 1 380—395 (1942).

Hagins, W. A.: The quantum efficiency of bleaching rhodopsin *in situ*. J. Physiol. (Lon **129**, 22—23P (1955).

Hecht, S.: Rods, cones and the chemical basis of vision. Physiol. Rev. **17**, 239—290 (193

HECHT, S., SHLAER, S., PIRENNE, M. H.: Energy, quanta and vision. J. gen. Physiol. **25**, 819—840 (1942).

HUBBARD, R.: The molecular weight of rhodopsin and the nature of the rhodopsin-digitonin complex. J. gen. Physiol. **39**, 381—399 (1954).

— KROPF, A.: The action of light on rhodopsin. Proc. nat. Acad. Sci. (Wash.) **44**, 130—139 (1958).

— WALD, G.: Cis-trans isomers of vitamin A and retinene in the rhodopsin system. J. gen. Physiol. **36**, 269—315 (1952).

JANCSO, N. v., JANCSO, H. v.: Fluoreszenz, mikroskopisches Beobachten der reversiblen Vitamin A-Bildung in der Netzhaut während des Sehaktes. Biochem. Z. **287**, 289—290 (1936).

KÜHNE, W.: Zur Photochemie der Netzhaut. Untersuch. physiol. Inst. Univ. Heidelberg **1**, 1—14 (1878).

LUDVIGH, E., McCARTHY, E. F.: Absorption of visible light by the refractive media of the human eye. Arch. Ophthal. **20**, 37—51 (1938).

MAXWELL, J. C.: Scientific papers. Cambridge, Univ. Press. Vol. 1, 126—154 (1890).

RIPPS, H., WEALE, R. A.: Cone pigments in the normal human fovea. Vision Res. **3**, 531—543 (1963).

— — Photo-labile changes and the directional sensitivity of the human fovea. J. Physiol. (Lond.) **173**, 57—64 (1964).

— — Time exposures and flash photolysis of rhodopsin in the living human eye. J. Physiol. (Lond.) **196**, 67—68 P (1968).

RUSHTON, W. A. H.: Foveal photopigments in normal and colour-blind. J. Physiol. (Lond.) **129**, 41—42 P (1955).

— The difference spectrum and photosensitivity of rhodopsin in the living human eye. J. Physiol. (Lond.) **134**, 11—29 (1956 a).

— The rhodopsin density in human rods. J. Physiol. (Lond.) **134**, 30—46 (1956 b).

— Physical measurement of cone pigment in the living human eye. Nature (Lond.) **179**, 571—573 (1957).

— Kinetics of cone pigments measured objectively on the living human fovea. Ann. N.Y. Acad. Sci. **74**, 291—304 (1958).

— Rhodopsin measurement and dark-adaptation in a subject deficient in cone vision. J. Physiol. (Lond.) **156**, 193—205 (1961).

— A cone pigment in the protanope. J. Physiol. (Lond.) **168**, 345—359 (1963 a).

— Cone pigment kinetics in the protanope. J. Physiol. (Lond.) **168**, 374—388 (1963 b).

— Flash photolysis in human cones. Photochem. Photobiol. **3**, 561—577 (1964 a).

— Chlorolabe in the normal eye. J. Physiol. (Lond.) **170**, 10—11 P (1964 b).

— A foveal pigment in the deuteranope. J. Physiol. (Lond.) **176**, 24—37 (1965 a).

— Cone pigment kinetics in the deuteranope. J. Physiol. (Lond.) **176**, 38—45 (1965 b).

— The Ferrier Lecture: Visual adaptation. Proc. roy. Soc. B **162**, 20—46 (1965 c).

— The Newton Lecture: Chemical basis of colour vision and colour blindness. Nature (Lond.) **206**, 1087—1091 (1965 d).

— Stray light and the measurement of mixed pigments in the retina. J. Physiol. (Lond.) **176**, 46—55 (1965 e).

— Rod/cone rivalry in pigment regeneration. J. Physiol. (Lond.) **198**, 219—236 (1968).

— CAMPBELL, F. W.: Measurement of rhodopsin in the living eye. Nature (Lond.) **174**, 1096—1097 (1954).

— — HAGINS, W. A., BRINDLEY, G. S.: The bleaching and regeneration of rhodopsin in the living eye of the albino rabbit and of man. Opt. Acta **1**, 183—190 (1955).

— GUBISCH, R. W.: Glare: its measurement by cone thresholds and by the bleaching of cone pigments. J. opt. Soc. Amer. **56**, 104—110 (1966).

— HENRY, G. H.: Bleaching and regeneration of cone pigments in man. Vision Res. **8**, 617—631 (1968).

SCHNEIDER, E. S., GOODEVE, C. F., LYTHGOE, R. J.: The spectral variation of the photosensitivity of visual purple. Proc. roy. Soc. A **170**, 102—112 (1939).

STILES, W. S.: The directional sensitivity of the retina and the spectral sensitivities of the rods and cones. Proc. roy. Soc. B **127**, 64—105 (1939).

Stiles, W. S.: Separation of the "blue" and "green" mechanisms of foveal vision by mea urements of increment thresholds. Proc. roy. Soc. B **133**, 418—434 (1946).
— Increment thresholds and the mechanisms of colour vision. Docum. ophthal. ('s-Grav.) 138—163 (1949).
— Further studies of visual mechanisms by the two-colour threshold technique. Coloq. pro opt. vis. (Madrid) 65—103 (1953).
— The basic data of colour matching. Phys. Soc. Yearbook 1955, 44—65. Physical Societ London 1955.
— Colour vision: the approach through increment threshold sensitivity. Proc. nat. Acad. S (Wash.) **45**, 100—114 (1959).
Wald, G.: The receptors of human color vision. Science **145**, 1007—1017 (1964).
— Brown, P. K.: The molar extinction of rhodopsin. J. gen. Physiol. **37**, 189—200 (195:
— — Smith, P. H.: Iodopsin. J. gen. Physiol. **38**, 623—681 (1955).
Weale, R. A.: Photo-sensitive reactions in foveae of normal and cone-monochromatic o servers. Opt. Acta **6**, 158—174 (1959).
— Limits of human vision. Nature (Lond.) **191**, 471—473 (1961a).
— Further studies of photo-chemical reactions in living human eyes. Vision Res. 1, 354—3 (1961b).
— Photo-chemical changes in the dark-adapting human retina. Vision Res. **2**, 25—33 (196:
Williams, T. P.: Photoreversal of rhodopsin bleaching. J. gen. Physiol. **47**, 679—689 (196
Wright, W. D.: A re-determination of the trichromatic mixture data. Med. Res. Coun Spec. Rep. **139**, 1—38 (1929).
— The breakdown of colour match with high intensities of adaptation. J. Physiol. (Lond 87, 23—33 (1936).
— Researches on normal and defective colour vision. London: Henry Kimpton 1946.
Young, T.: On the theory of light and colours. Phil. Trans. roy. Soc. 12—48 (1802).

Chapter 10

The Regeneration and Renewal of Visual Pigment in Vertebrates

By

Ch. Baumann, Bad Nauheim (Germany)

With 5 Figures

Contents

I. Introduction

In the very first report on a visual pigment, Boll (1876) wrote: "Prolonged action of direct sunlight completely decolourizes the retina. In darkness, the intense purple colour is soon restored."[1] As is now known, the colour of the retina Boll referred to is due to a photolabile pigment, rhodopsin, situated in the rods. The action of light upon rhodopsin (as upon all other visual pigments) is to change its molecular configuration. Because of this, the pigment molecule becomes unstable and breaks down sequentially into a number of photoproducts. In the frog retina, which Boll worked with, the final breakdown products are retinol and opsin, a protein of unknown structure. Both these substances are colourless and consequently the retina loses its colour as their formation proceeds. The process underlying the restoration of colour is called regeneration and is the principal topic of this chapter.

In addition, however, and independently of whether or not the pigment is bleached, there is a continuous renewal of outer segment material, including the visual pigments contained therein.

Before the regenerative processes can be described in detail, it is desirable to summarize the essential steps involved in bleaching (for a complete description see Chapter 3 and 5). The visual pigment molecule consists of a protein to which a prosthetic group is attached. This prosthetic group can be either 11-*cis*-retinal (A_1-based pigments) or 11-*cis*-3-dehydroretinal (A_2-based pigments). When the molecule absorbs a photon, isomerization of the prosthetic group from the 11-*cis* into the all-*trans* configuration occurs. This change is accompanied by a marked loss in stability of the molecule, resulting in a progressive sequence of changes that terminate in stable end products. Nearly a dozen intermediate products are known, but for the present purposes they can be classified into two groups only: (1) the all-*trans*-chromoproteins (prelumi, lumi, meta I, II, III and retinylidene-opsin), the common feature of which is that the chromophore is still attached to the opsin moiety, and (2) photoproducts in which the two components (retinal and opsin) have parted company. Retinal is stable, but in the retina it disappears quickly because it is enzymatically reduced to retinol. Opsin is also stable, though less so than the original pigment. Thus, in the retina, retinol and opsin are the final products of bleaching. If, as is almost certain, the formation of new visual pigment after bleaching takes place from the decomposition products of the old, then the question arises: where does the regeneration start from? Is the pigment regenerated from the all-*trans*-chromoproteins or does the naked protein re-combine with retinol or retinal? As will be shown below, the latter is the physiological mode of regeneration of visual pigments (with a few possible exceptions in lower animals). It is nevertheless also of interest to consider the former mode of regeneration, which can be induced alike in both physiological and unnatural conditions.

II. Regeneration from all-*trans*-Chromoproteins

Regeneration from the all-*trans*-chromoproteins may occur either by thermal reactions or by photochemical ones.

A. Thermal Regeneration

Thermal regeneration from the pre-lumi intermediate has been observed in the case of iodopsin, the pigment of chicken cones. If, in the dark, a solution of pre-

---

[1] Längere Einwirkung direkten Sonnenlichtes entfärbt die Retina vollständig. In der Dunkelheit stellt sich die intensive Purpurfarbe alsbald wieder her.

lumiiodopsin that had previously been kept at —195° C is slightly warmed to above —180° C, this all-*trans*-chromoprotein reverts to the original pigment (YOSHIZAWA quoted by HUBBARD, BOWNDS, and YOSHIZAWA, 1965). A similar reversion does not occur in the case of rhodopsin. Thermal regeneration of visual pigment is likewise unknown from the later stages of breakdown (lumi, meta I, II, III or retinylidene-opsin) whether of iodopsin or rhodopsin, but thermal reversion of meta II to meta I does occur.

There is a possible exception to the general rule of no thermal regeneration from all-*trans*-chromoproteins in the case of certain lower animals, e.g. squid, octopus and cuttlefish. These animals possess a rhodopsin-like pigment that is transformed by light into a metarhodopsin that remains stable (HUBBARD and ST. GEORGE, 1958; BROWN and BROWN, 1958; HAMDORF, SCHWEMER, and TÄUBER 1968). This is true not only for solutions but also for visual cell suspensions, for isolated retinas, and hence probably also for the retina *in situ*. Thermal regeneration from this metapigment might therefore seem to be essential, but the situation in these animals is complicated by the presence of retinochrome in the retina (see Chapter 18).

Vertebrate metarhodopsin is unstable at temperatures above 0° C, and hydrolyses into all-*trans*-retinal and opsin. This hydrolysis, though fast, is not instantaneous. Consequently metarhodopsin may accumulate in the retina if it is formed quickly enough. This is the case, for instance, when intense photoflashes are used to bleach the visual pigment. In experiments of this kind (DOWLING and HUBBARD, 1963), the regeneration of rhodopsin in rat eyes was found to proceed rather slowly during an initial period of 20 to 30 mins in darkness. This delay does not appear to conform with the view that rhodopsin is effectively regenerated from metarhodopsin. The delay might be explained, however, if a competition between a slow hydrolysis of metarhodopsin and the re-formation of rhodopsin were assumed. This would mean that only those opsin molecules that had already lost by hydrolysis their "old" all-*trans*-chromophore could combine with "new" 11-*cis*-retinal to form rhodopsin.

Metarhodopsin, which can sometimes be present in the retina, will influence the form of the difference spectrum that should be used to characterize rhodopsin in the living human eye (see Chapter 9, p. 375). Thus, the bleaching difference spectrum of human rhodopsin has its maximum at wavelengths 5—10 nm longer than that of the extracted pigment (RUSHTON, 1956). This displacement is even more marked when the *in vivo* difference spectrum is taken after only a short exposure to light. RUSHTON supposes that metarhodopsin accounts for this effect. Thus if the presence of metarhodopsin is indicated by such displaced difference spectra, their analysis should yield evidence about the possible contribution of metarhodopsin to the regeneration of rhodopsin. In a recent study, WEALE (1967) has done this. He used a certain temporal pattern of dark periods followed by short bleaching periods, so obtaining a set of bleaching and regeneration spectra. In all of them interference from a breakdown product of rhodopsin, probably metarhodopsin III, was indicated. Mathematical analysis of these spectra led WEALE to conclude that rhodopsin is not even partly regenerated from metarhodopsin. (See also RIPPS and WEALE, 1969.)

B. Photoregeneration

A light quantum absorbed by a visual pigment causes photoisomerization of it prosthetic group. As long as the latter is still attached to protein, the absorption another quantum of light may again cause photoisomerization. The results of th two photochemical reactions are quite different, however. In the first case, th original pigment is converted into unstable photoproducts that, under most con ditions, result in bleaching. In the second case, the absorption of light results in regeneration of either the original pigment or in the formation of so-called iso pigment (in iso-pigments retinal has the 9-*cis*- instead of the normal 11-*cis*-con figuration). This is photoregeneration or photoreversal. Details of photoregenerativ reactions in pigment extracts are described by Yoshizawa in Chapter 5, p. 166 This section will be confined to photoregeneration *in situ*, i.e., to visual pigmen molecules situated in the photoreceptors.

In vertebrate rods the prelumi-, lumi- and metarhodopsins are very unstabl. Photoregeneration can only occur, therefore, if a sufficient fraction of these inter mediates can absorb light before they break down. This conditions can be fulfille by using intense short flashes to bleach the pigment; a method often called flas photolysis. In rat retinas that had been bleached by such intense flashes, Dowlin and Hubbard (1963) found a photoregenerated pigment consisting of a 5 : mixture of rhodopsin and isorhodopsin (see also Arden, Ikeda, and Siegel 1966a). Flash-irradiated suspensions of rod outer segments may likewise contain certain proportion of isorhodopsin (Bridges, 1962). In the frog retina, measurabl amounts of isorhodopsin are found, even under the conditions of continuou illumination (Reuter, 1964b, 1966). Reuter supposes that this is due to th greater stability of metarhodopsin *in situ* as compared with that in extracts. Whe isolated frog retinas are exposed to a high intensity flash of very short duratio indeed (2 nanoseconds; room temperature) the photoregenerated material is foun to be exclusively isorhodopsin (Baumann and Ernst, 1970).

Photoreversal, when achieved by the application of short flashes, is accompanied b electrical phenomena (Arden, Ikeda, and Siegel, 1966a, b; Cone, 1967; Pak and Boes 1967). These belong to a class of responses for which several terms are in use: fast photovoltages rapid photoresponses or early receptor potentials (for details see the chapter by Cone and Pa in volume I of this handbook). The existence of these phenomena is additional evidence for th view that photoreversal can occur in the retina.

III. Regeneration from Separated Components (Opsin plus Retinal or Retinol)

A. In Solution

1. Rhodopsin

Ewald and Kühne (1878) were the first to describe the regeneration of rho dopsin in solution. After bleaching their extracts and placing them in the dark they were able to detect visually some regeneration of colour after about 15 min and could detect no further deepening after about 1 hour. These early qualitativ observations were confirmed nearly 60 years later and placed on a quantitativ basis by the work of two groups (HECHT, CHASE, SHLAER, and HAIG, 1936; HOSOYA and SASAKI, 1938). The former group (CHASE, 1937; CHASE and SMITH, 1939) made the interesting additional observation that the colour of the bleaching light could influence the amount of rhodopsin regenerated on subsequent incubation in the dark. Thus regeneration was found to be nearly absent if the pigment had been bleached by yellow light while, after exposure to blue or violet light, solutions of rhodopsin frequently regenerated to the extent of 15 or 20 %. CHASE interpreted this in the sense that a photochemical process might be involved in regeneration. Later it was shown by HUBBARD and WALD (1952) that the process responsible for CHASE's observation was, in fact, an isomerization of retinal. Thus the blue light isomerizes a part of the all-*trans*-retinal, the stereoisomer released from opsin on bleaching, to the 11-*cis*-configuration, and in this latter form retinal can combine directly with opsin to regenerate rhodopsin.

The fact that only a specific isomer of retinal will condense with opsin to yield rhodopsin was established by HUBBARD and WALD (1952). These two authors had found that for the synthesis of rhodopsin in solution four well-defined components were required: these were opsin, the protein of rhodopsin; retinol, the precursor of the chromophore; and liver alcohol dehydrogenase and NAD (nicotinamide adenine dinucleotide), i.e. the enzyme and co-enzyme that oxidize retinol to retinal (HUBBARD and WALD, 1951)[2]. These experiments were first performed with fish liver oil concentrate as the source of retinol. When later, instead of liver oil concentrate, crystalline retinol was used, almost no rhodopsin was synthesized. This finding strongly indicated that stereoisomerism plays a decisive role in regeneration, for crystalline retinol is known to be a single isomer (all-*trans*) whereas liver oil contains a mixture of different stereoisomers of retinol. The site of this isomer specificity was found to be the coupling of retinal with opsin. In the oxidation of retinol to retinal there is little specificity.

HUBBARD and WALD (1952) studied five retinal isomers (all-*trans*, neo-a neo-b, iso-a, and iso-b) and tested their suitability for the synthesis of rhodopsin by incubating each of them with opsin in the dark. The result was very striking. All-*trans*-, neo-a- and iso-b-retinal were found to be inactive; the iso-a isomer yielded iso-rhodopsin, the photosensitive pigment that was mentioned above in connection with photoregeneration. Only neo-b-retinal yielded a visual pigment indistinguishable from the naturally occurring one. Fig. 1 shows that this synthesized pigment is spectrally identical to the native rhodopsin. OROSHNIK (1956) later synthesized neo-b-retinal by a route that established its configuration as 11-mono-*cis*.

It should be emphasized that when 11-*cis*-retinal and opsin condense to form rhodopsin the two components react directly without the intervention of an enzyme system. If neither of the two components is present in great excess, the synthesis follows a second order reaction (see Fig. 2). Regeneration according to the kinetics of a first order reaction has also been observed in cases where opsin was present in great excess (see for example CHASE and SMITH, 1939).

---

[2] What was synthesized by HUBBARD and WALD was, in fact, not rhodopsin but iso-rhodopsin (see HUBBARD, 1956, footnote on page 935). This in no way detracts, however, from the significance of the observation.

HUBBARD and WALD (1952) had to obtain their 11-*cis*-retinal from the all-*trans*-isomer by rather sophisticated chemical routes. This raises the question as to what system supplies the retinal receptors with the specific isomer they require.

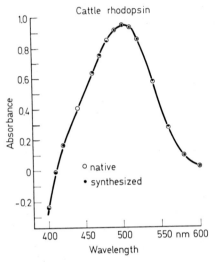

Fig. 1. Comparison between the difference spectra of cattle rhodopsin extracted from suspensions of dark-adapted rods (*plain circles*, average of four experiments), and of rhodopsin synthesized by incubating cattle opsin with 11-*cis*-retinal (*filled circles*, average of three experiments). (From HUBBARD and WALD, 1952)

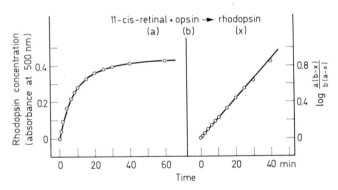

Fig. 2. The synthesis of rhodopsin in solution from 11-*cis*-retinal and cattle opsin. On the left is shown the rise in absorbance at 500 nm (a measure of the rhodopsin concentration). The straight line at the right shows that this reaction follows a bimolecular course. In this experiment opsin was only slightly in excess (23° C, pH 6.4). (From HUBBARD and WALD, 1952)

It is known that rhodopsin releases the all-*trans*-isomer when bleached. It is further known that retinal homogenates can regenerate rhodopsin from added all-*trans*-retinol (COLLINS, GREEN, and MORTON, 1953, 1954). Thus in addition to oxidation, isomerization must also occur. The latter reaction, however, cannot be attributed solely to the retinal tissue. There appears to be a contribution of the so-called pigment layers (pigment epithelium and chorioidea). KÜHNE wrote in his first paper on rhodopsin (1878) that contact of the retina with the pigment layer promotes regeneration, and EWALD and KÜHNE's (1878) solutions showed much more regeneration when retinas and pigment layers together were extracted than when the extracts were prepared from carefully isolated retinas. This finding was confirmed by HOSOYA and SASAKI (1938) who observed almost complete regeneration in bleached solutions of extracts from preparations containing a large excess of pigment layer. And when COLLINS, GREEN, and MORTON (1953) worked with frog and rat eyes, the homogenates were prepared from retinas *plus* chorioids and pigment epithelia. BLISS (1951b) and HUBBARD and WALD (1951) found in the pigment layers of the frog eye a heat-labile factor which had the properties of a protein and which clearly aided in the resynthesis of rhodopsin.

HUBBARD (1956) found a comparable factor present in cattle retinas, an enzyme that catalysed the isomerization of all-*trans*-retinal to 11-*cis*. This enzyme is not very effective, for, in the dark, it converts all-*trans*- and 11-*cis*-retinal to an equilibrium mixture containing only 5 % 11-*cis*, the rest being all-*trans*. If all-*trans*-retinal is irradiated, however, in the presence of the isomerase, the equilibrium shifts to 32 % 11-*cis*. The small amount of 11-*cis*-retinal, formed by the action of isomerase, can be trapped by any opsin that is present. Thus, although the isomerase can catalyse the synthesis of rhodopsin from all-*trans*-retinal, this reaction is too slow to account for rhodopsin regeneration rates *in vivo*. It seems to be worth emphasizing that HUBBARD used fairly long wavelength light for the irradiation of the enzyme-substrate complex (Tungsten light filtered through Corning No. 3484 transmitting wavelengths > 520 nm). Such light would, presumably, be only feebly absorbed by retinal. Several authors have investigated the effect of blue light (strongly absorbed by retinal) upon the yield of the 11-*cis* isomer, and hence upon the formation of rhodopsin. Experiments have been performed on living human eyes (RUSHTON, 1957), on the eyes of intact rats (LEWIS, 1957), on the excised eyes of frogs (REUTER, 1966) and on isolated frog retinas (BAUMANN, 1970). The results were negative except in the last instance, in which an intense short-wave beam from a xenon arc bulb impinged directly upon the retina.

2. Iodopsin

If retinas of Gallinaceous birds are carefully extracted, the extract may contain a substantial fraction of iodopsin, (WALD, 1937; BLISS, 1946; WALD, BROWN, and SMITH, 1955; CRESCITELLI, WILSON, and LILYBLADE, 1964), a pigment that, *in vivo*, is situated in the retinal cones (see LIEBMAN, Chapter 12). The spectral absorbance of this pigment peaks at 562 nm. Iodopsin possesses the same chromophore as rhodopsin, namely 11-*cis*-retinal, the pigments differing only in their opsin. The synthesis of iodopsin from its protein and 11-*cis*-retinal was shown by WALD, BROWN, and SMITH (1955) to be monomolecular, with a rate constant 527 times that of the comparable rhodopsin synthesis. In the living human retina the cone pigments are likewise more quickly regenerated than the rod pigment rhodopsin. But *in vivo* the two regeneration rates exhibit a ratio that hardly exceeds a value of 4 (cf. RUSHTON, Chapter 9, p. 385).

3. Porphyropsin

In the A_2-based pigments, frequently called the porphyropsins, the prosthetic group is based on 3-dehydroretinal. Little work has been done on the regeneration of these pigments. According to Wald, Brown, and Smith (Wald, 1953), a cis-isomer of dehydroretinal is required for the synthesis of porphyropsin in vitro. On the other hand, Crescitelli and Dartnall (1954) made an observation with carp porphyropsin that is hardly reconcilable with that view. They found that the λ_{max} of the light-absorbing photoproduct formed from this pigment at room temperature depended on the wavelength of the bleaching light. Thus with a short-wave (isomerising) bleach the λ_{max} of the photoproduct was shorter and its extinction was lower than with a long-wave (non-isomerising) bleach suggesting, as in the case of frog rhodopsin, that long-wave bleaching released 3-dehydroretinal in the all-trans-form. But, unlike the results obtained in similar experiments with frog rhodopsin, regeneration was most marked after a long-wave bleach and completely absent after a short-wave one. This finding of Crescitelli and Dartnall suggests that the carp pigment requires for its synthesis the unaltered all-trans-isomer and not a cis-isomer probably formed under the influence of isomerizing bleaching light.

The re-synthesis of porphyropsin in solution appears to be a rather rapid process (Wald, Brown, and Kennedy, 1957). This recalls the observations of Kühne and Sewall (1880) and of Abelsdorff (1897) who found in the retina of the living bream (Abramis brama) that regeneration is completed after less than one hour (Kühne gives the figure 40 min). This is much shorter than the regeneration time of other cold-blooded animals, e.g. frogs. According to Garten (1906), the spectral absorbance of the pigment extracted from bream retinas peaks at 536 nm, suggesting that the principal pigment of the bream retina is a porphyropsin (see also Köttgen and Abelsdorff, 1896).

B. *In situ*

For the purposes of this section the term in situ refers to the visual pigment molecules, rather than to the photoreceptor cells wherein these molecules are embedded. In other words, the subject of this section is not exclusively the regeneration in intact animals; studies in more or less isolated systems, e.g. excised eyes, isolated retinas, or even suspensions of visual cell outer segments, are included as well.

1. Suspensions of Rod Outer Segments

In fresh suspensions of frog photoreceptors, regeneration has been occasionally observed (Bridges, personal communication). The amount of pigment regenerated is small (about 5 %). If in the preparation of the suspensions the outer segments are first washed with pH 4.6 buffer, however, there is no longer any observable regeneration after bleaching (Bridges, 1962). This suggests that a substance promoting regeneration can be washed out of the preparation.

2. Isolated Retinas

There are several reports that regeneration following bleaching of isolated frog retinas is either absent or hardly detectable (Zewi, 1939; Baumann, 1965;

CRESCITELLI and SICKEL, 1968). Similarly, in the isolated perfused rat retina no regenerative properties have been observed (WEINSTEIN, HOBSON, and DOWLING, 1967).

On the other hand, EWALD and KÜHNE (1878) had reported that, even in retinas that had been carefully isolated from the pigment epithelium, there was a small amount of regeneration after bleaching. KÜHNE named this type of regeneration "autoregeneration" in order to emphasize that it referred to a retina in isolation rather than to one in its normal environment. WALD and HUBBARD (1950) estimated from their results that the isolated bleached retina of the frog could regenerate about 10 % of its potential content of rhodopsin. Recently, CONE and BROWN (1969) have observed up to 80 % regeneration in unperfused isolated rat retinas that had been sealed in very small chambers. This result suggests that the rat retina possesses an effective isomerizing system converting all-*trans*-retinol or all-*trans*-retinal back to the 11-*cis*-configuration. In other animals, such as frog and cattle, the retina probably receives the 11-*cis*-isomers mainly from the pigment layers, where substantial fractions of 11-*cis*-retinol esters are found (cf. p. 405 — 407). 11-*cis*-retinol is not present in the pigment epithelium of the rat eye (DOWLING, 1960). Some regeneration in bleached isolated frog retinas can also be induced by exposure of the retinas to short-wave light prior to incubation in darkness (FRANK, 1969; BAUMANN, 1970).

3. Living Animals[3]

When living animals are used to study regeneration, the general feature of the experiment is as follows: The animals are exposed to light intense enough to bleach most of the pigment within a reasonable time span. During the ensuing dark period, some animals are removed at intervals in order to estimate the pigment present in their retinas. The data obtained are usually plotted as a function of time in the dark. The experiment is continued until the pigment concentration has approached its maximum value.

Several methods of estimating or measuring the pigment content of the retina have been used; some are now of historical interest only. The first workers in the field simply inspected the isolated retina which was either still colourless or pale, or had regained its colour. KÜHNE sometimes used optograms to determine whether regeneration was complete. In the method of optography (KÜHNE, 1877) retinal images delineated by bleached rhodopsin fade as the rhodopsin is regenerated. GATTI (1901) on the other hand used a set of twelve papers all of the same red hue, but of different saturation. The colour of the retina was then compared with the colour of these standards, and in this way GATTI was able to measure approximately the time course of rhodopsin regeneration in frogs.

One modern method of studying regeneration rests upon the extraction of rhodopsin and the measurement of its optical density in a spectrophotometer (TANSLEY, 1931). Another depends upon the analysis of light reflected by the *fundus oculi* (RUSHTON, 1952; WEALE, 1953). For details of this method (fundus reflectometry or retinal densitometry) the reader is referred to Chapter 9 by RUSHTON, p. 364.

---

[3] For the regeneration of visual pigments in man, see Chapter 9 by RUSHTON, p. 376.

a) **Frog.** Most work on the regeneration of visual pigment in living eyes has been done on common laboratory animals such as frog, rat, rabbit and certain fishes, and the major part of this work refers to the regeneration of the scotopic pigments. KÜHNE (1879) has summarized his findings about regeneration of frog rhodopsin in an article in Hermann's Handbuch. KÜHNE emphasized that regeneration in the living eye is a very slow process. By optography, KÜHNE was able to detect the first trace of regenerated pigment only after 20 mins, and complete regeneration after 1—2 hours. Unfortunately, KÜHNE did not report the temperature of the eyes. The temperature dependence of regeneration was studied extensively by GATTI (1901) who used the colour standards mentioned above to measure approximately the time course of regeneration. He found a marked influence of temperature up to a limit of 25° C, above which the preparations deteriorated (cf. Table 1).

A considerable amount of data is available from more modern studies in frogs. Three species of this animal have been investigated. ZEWI (1939) made measurements with *Rana esculenta*, PESKIN (1942) with *R. pipiens*, and REUTER (1964a, 1966) with *R. temporaria*. PESKIN worked only with intact animals while the other authors used both these and excised eyes as well, their results with the latter confirming KÜHNE's (1878) observation that the isolated frog eye is well able to regenerate rhodopsin. The time course of regeneration in carefully treated excised eyes is nearly the same as in eyes of the intact animal (REUTER, 1966). Some of PESKIN's (1942) measurements are reproduced in Fig. 3.

The sigmoid curves that PESKIN drew through the averages of his measurements (Fig. 3) have been confirmed in full detail by REUTER (1964a, 1966). These curves characterize the regeneration of frog rhodopsin *in situ*. In solution, on the other hand, the synthesis of (cattle) rhodopsin from 11-*cis*-retinal and opsin follows the course of a second order reaction (HUBBARD and WALD, 1952). A first order kinetics may be found as well, if one of the reactants is present in excess in the solution (CHASE and SMITH, 1939). PESKIN (1942) explained the shape of the *in situ* curves in terms of a first order autocatalysed reaction, supposing that the regeneration of rhodopsin is catalysed by rhodopsin itself. Although there is no present experimental evidence of autocatalysis in this connection, several reactions are known to be more or less tightly coupled with the regeneration of rhodopsin.

For instance, there is evidence that retinol is exchanged between the retina and the pigment layers. WALD (1935) showed that in frogs most of the retinol released upon bleaching leaves the retina. The disappearance of retinol from the retina is a slow process. It has usually been observed during light adaptation (see also DOWLING, 1960). However, if the adaptation is intense and short, a greater amount of retinol leaves the retina in the subsequent dark period (PESKIN, 1942). Retinol does not leave the eye altogether. It is transferred from the retina to adjacent tissues, the pigment layers, where it is found in esterified form (HUBBARD and COLMAN, 1959; HUBBARD and DOWLING, 1962). During dark adaptation, when rhodopsin is resynthesized, the pigment layer supplies the retina with retinol. HUBBARD and WALD (1951) found that homogenates of bleached frog retinas that had been treated with petroleum ether to remove the retinol, can still regenerate rhodopsin when mixed with freeze-dried pigment layers. Obviously, the latter must have supplied the retinol. Thus, retinol moves back and forth between the retina and the pigment epithelium, the total amount of ocular retinol, if one includes that bound as retinal in rhodopsin, remaining essentially constant during light and dark adaptation (HUBBARD and COLMAN, 1959).

In frogs, not all the ocular retinol is needed for rhodopsin synthesis, the excess being stored (WALD, 1935). Dark adapted *R. pipiens*, for instance, stores about 2 μgm retinol ester per eye in the pigment epithelium (HUBBARD and

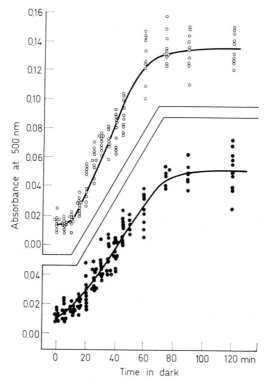

Fig. 3. Regeneration of rhodopsin in the intact eye of the frog at 25° C. The concentration is measured as absorbance at 500 nm. *Plain circles*, rhodopsin concentration following light adaptation to 9500 millilambert; *filled circles*, the same following light adaptation to 1700 milli-lambert. Each point records a measurement with 8 retinas. The curves are drawn through the averages. (From PESKIN, 1942)

DOWLING, 1962). These retinol esters represent 95 % of the stored retinol, a con-siderable fraction of which is in the 11-*cis* form. When, in HUBBARD and DOWLING's experiments, the frogs were dark adapted for a minimum of 24 hours, 42 % of the retinol esters were found to have the 11-*cis* form. Even after bleaching most of the rhodopsin by intense light, the amount of the 11-*cis*-ester remained nearly the same, though since the total amount of esters increased markedly its proportion fell to about 25 %. If the frogs were then returned to darkness, they re-synthesized all their rhodopsin within about 2 hours. At the end of this period, the 11-*cis* and all-*trans*-isomers of the retinol esters were found to be still in the same proportion as they were in the light adapted eye (25 : 75). This means that the 11-*cis*-isomer had not been drawn on preferentially and "suggests that the isomerization from all-*trans* to 11-*cis* is not the rate-limiting step in the utilization of vitamin A ester for rhodopsin synthesis" (HUBBARD and DOWLING, 1962). After completion of dark adaptation, the fraction of 11-*cis*-retinol esters in the pigment layers increases slowly up to about 42 %, the value found after a dark period of at least 24 hours.

Reactions that may be relevant to the process of regeneration are shown in the following scheme —

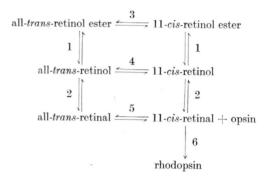

Some of these reactions have been extensively studied; others are merely speculative. The scheme is not confined to the frog retina. Reaction 1, for instance, is known to occur also in the eyes of several animals other than frogs. DOWLING (1960) found retinol esters in the rat eye and FUTTERMAN and ANDREWS (1964) studied the composition of retinol esters isolated from retinal tissue of the calf, sheep, rabbit, cat, frog and trout. A cell-free enzyme system capable of esterifying retinol has been prepared from cattle eye tissues by KRINSKY (1958). Some of this enzyme activity is localized in the retina itself (see also ANDREWS and FUTTERMAN, 1964); but the pigment layers are a much more active source of the esterifying enzyme. However, the pigment layers alone, unlike retinal preparations alone, were found to be ineffective in the hydrolysis of the retinol esters. Clearly the term "reaction 1" in the above scheme is an oversimplification for, in the living eye, esterification appears to occur in a location (pigment layer) that is different from that of hydrolysis (retina). The mechanism of transfer between the two locations is completely unknown. Similarly, it is not known whether the enzyme responsible for the reversible esterification process is stereospecific or not, as is suggested in the above scheme.

Reaction 2 is a reversible reduction of retinal to retinol (BLISS, 1948, 1951a; WALD and HUBBARD, 1949; FUTTERMAN, 1965). The alcohol dehydrogenase involved in this reaction is situated in the outer segments of visual cells (WALD and HUBBARD, 1949; FUTTERMAN and SASLAW, 1961). According to WALD and HUBBARD, NADH is the coenzyme of this reaction. More recently, FUTTERMAN (1963, 1965) has shown that NADPH can also function as a reducing agent. It is known that in the (rat) retina NAD is predominantly in the oxidized form and NADP is largely in the reduced form (SLATER, HEATH, and GRAYMORE, 1962). It seems likely, therefore, that NAD mediates the oxidation of retinol, and NADPH the reduction of retinal. As noted above, the reversible retinol/retinal conversion reaction is only slightly stereospecific (HUBBARD and WALD, 1951).

Reaction 3, the reversible interconversion of all-*trans*- and 11-*cis*-retinol ester can be inferred from the results of Hubbard and Dowling (1962) (see above) and also from the work of Krinsky (1958) who found in the pigment layers of cattle 65 % of retinol esters having the 11-*cis*-configuration.

Reaction 4 is hypothetical. Its existence is inferred from the fact that the other isomerizing reactions appear to be either very slow (reaction 3) or (so far as the formation of the 11-*cis* form is concerned) not very effective (reaction 5).

Reactions 5 and 6 have already been described in detail (see pp. 401 and 399).

The scheme of reactions relevant to the formation of rhodopsin in the living eye is thus a rather complex process accompanied by a not less complex kinetics. If more details of the reactions 1 to 5 were known (e.g. the rate constants *in situ*), it would be possible to calculate the kinetics of rhodopsin regeneration. This should follow the same curve as that found by Peskin (1942) in the living frog's eye (Fig. 3). It is worth mentioning, however, that systems less complicated than those we have discussed could also produce sigmoid curves. If, for instance, three consecutive reactions of the type

$$A \xrightarrow{k_1} B \xrightarrow{k_2} C \xrightarrow{+ D}{k_3} E$$

are considered (the constants k_1, k_2 and k_3 having the same order of magnitude), the accumulation of E will follow a sigmoid curve with a marked initial delay (the above sequence of reactions is tantamount to rhodopsin's being formed exclusively from 11-*cis*-retinol ester via 11-*cis*-retinol and 11-*cis*-retinal).

A characteristic of regeneration *in situ* is the initial delay. This delay could arise, as we have seen, if several reactions contribute to the final synthesis. In addition purely topographical factors, e.g. the time required for transfer of retinol from the pigment layers to the retina, may also contribute. Again, the mode of bleaching can also influence the kinetics of regeneration. This can be seen in Fig. 3 which shows the time course of regeneration following 10 min light adaptation to 9500 milli-lamberts (top) or to 1700 millilamberts (bottom). The onset of regeneration is much more delayed at the higher intensity. Although Zewi (1939) reported that only short periods of light adaptation (e.g. 6 min) were followed by a delay in subsequent rhodopsin formation, this was not confirmed by Peskin (1942) nor by Reuter (1996) who observed delays after longer periods (20 min or more).

b) Rat. The regeneration of rhodopsin in the rat eye is fairly well known from several studies carried out during the last five decades. Fridericia and Holm (1925) used the above-mentioned colour standards to estimate the rhodopsin content of rat eyes; Tansley (1931) and Dowling (1960, 1963) extracted the pigment and measured its concentration spectrophotometrically. Lewis (1957) used the method of fundus reflectometry to follow the time course of rhodopsin accumulation after a substantial bleach. The data of Tansley (1931) and Dowling (1963) agree and may be approximated by an expression of the form $x_t/x_0 = \exp(-kt)$, where x_t/x_0 is the fraction of rhodopsin still in the bleached state at time t. k is a constant; its value is 0.016—0.018 min^{-1}. Thus 50% regeneration is accomplished in about 40 mins. The data of Fridericia and Holm, although less accurate, also agree fairly well with these results. The time course of regeneration, observed by Lewis (1957), however, was remarkably slow, taking more than 5 hours to virtual completion. Lewis worked with anaesthetized animals, however, and it is possible that the anaesthetic had slowed down the rate of regeneration (see also Dowling 1963).

It was mentioned above that several processes are linked to the re-synthesis of rhodopsin from 11-*cis*-retinal and opsin. Among them is an exchange of retinol between the retina and the pigment layers. Details of this migration in the rat eye have been worked out by Dowling (1960). As in the frog eye (Hubbard and Colman, 1959), the total amount of retinal plus retinol remains constant during light and dark adaptation. The distribution of these two substances between the retina and the pigment epithelium undergoes remarkable changes however (Fig. 4).

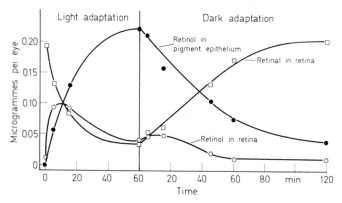

Fig. 4. Topographic distribution of retinal and retinol in the eyes of albino rats during light and dark adaptation. (From Dowling, 1960)

In the fully dark-adapted state of the animal, practically no retinol is found in the pigment epithelium (filled circles, Fig. 4). This means that, unlike the frog, the rat is unable to store retinol in this tissue. A small amount (5 % of the potential content) is stored in the retina (plain circles, Fig. 4). The bulk of the retinol is bound as retinal in rhodopsin (plain squares, Fig. 4). On bleaching the retina (95 %) retinal is liberated and quickly reduced to retinol. Consequently the retinal content of the retina falls, and a corresponding increase of retinol is observed. After about 10 min light adaptation, the retina contains its maximum amount of retinol (about 30 % of the total) which is then gradually diminished since, at this time, the rate of migration of retinol out of the retina exceeds the rate of its formation by reduction of retinal. The retinol that leaves the retina accumulates in the pigment layer until, at the end of light adaptation, it reaches about 80 % of the total ocular retinol. As in other animals, most of the retinol entering the pigment layer is esterified (92 %). Among these esters there is no fraction that contains retinol in the 11-*cis* form (it will be remembered that in frog pigment layers up to 42 %, and in cattle pigment layers up to 65 %, 11-*cis*-retinol esters were found). In darkness, all the processes go in the reverse direction. Retinol is oxidized to retinal which then combines with opsin to form rhodopsin. Thus, all the retinol — the small fraction still present in the retina as well as the bulk that returns to the retina from the pigment epithelium — is consumed. The reason for the exchange of retinol between the two tissues is unknown.

c) **Cat.** By comparison with that in the rat, the regeneration of rhodopsin in the cat is a rather fast process. Thus GRANIT, MUNSTERHJELM, and ZEWI (1939) found that when the rhodopsin in the cat retina was reduced by bleaching to about 40 % of its original value, only 30 min in the dark was necessary for full restoration. This was confirmed by WEALE (1953) who used the method of fundus reflectometry to study the recovery of pigment in bleached retinas (GRANIT and his co-workers extracted the pigment). He found that regeneration was virtually complete after 35—40 mins the half return period being about 15 mins. WEALE (1953, 1957) also observed yet another regeneration process that proceeds very rapidly. This process (observed in both cat and frog) needs about 1 minute to complete and its difference spectrum peaks at between 540 and 550 nm. WEALE (1965) has discussed the possibility that this rapid reaction may relate to a precursor (such as prelumirhodopsin, $\lambda_{max} = 543$ nm) of rhodopsin and that an isomerizing effect of the bleaching light is somehow involved.

d) **Rabbit.** Regeneration of rhodopsin in the eye of the intact rabbit has been studied by HAGINS and RUSHTON (1953) and by RUSHTON, CAMPBELL, HAGINS, and BRINDLEY (1955). The experiments were performed with RUSHTON's retinal densitometer (see Chapter 9, p. 370) and a typical result is given in Fig. 5. The regeneration proceeds at a uniform speed for the first half-hour and is virtually complete in about 80 mins. The initial "linear increase in the dark suggests saturation at some stage of rhodopsin synthesis, e.g. a very high affinity between enzyme and substrate" (HAGINS and RUSHTON, 1953).

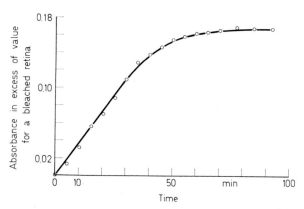

Fig. 5. Time course of rhodopsin regeneration in the retina of the decerebrate rabbit. (Redrawn after RUSHTON, CAMPBELL, HAGINS, and BRINDLEY, 1955)

e) **Fishes.** Two old papers on regeneration in the eye of the living bream (KÜHNE and SEWALL, 1880; ABELSDORFF, 1897) were mentioned earlier. The bream retina probably contains only porphyropsin [this may be inferred from the studies of KÖTTGEN and ABELSDORFF (1896) and GARTEN (1906)]. After bleaching, the porphyropsin is regenerated with remarkable speed (virtually complete in 30 to 40 mins). This figure is at variance with recent results of BAUMANN (1971) who found, in the eyes of crucian carp, a slow regeneration of porphyropsin (virtually complete after no less than 5 hours).

In the retinas of certain fishes, porphyropsin is found paired with rhodopsin, and the relative amounts of these two pigments may vary in response to several factors, principally the light environment. Thus if these animals are kept in light for a prolonged period, they convert most of their porphyropsin into rhodopsin, while in darkness rhodopsin is converted back to porphyropsin. This phenomenon may add an additional complication to future studies on the regeneration of the paired pigments. For details of the rhodopsin-porphyropsin interconversion the reader is referred to Chapter 11, p. 417.

f) Cone Pigments. All the pigments so far mentioned in this section are rod pigments serving the scotopic apparatus of the eye. The regeneration of cone pigments in living animals can hardly be investigated with present methods of extraction since cone pigments, although extractable, are present in very small quantities in most retinas and no method of separation from the preponderant rod pigment has yet been devised. The method of partial bleaching is not applicable unless the cone pigments form a substantial fraction of the extract (e.g. iodopsin). Thus one is left with two possibilities: regeneration studies (if monitored by extraction techniques) must be restricted to pure cone retinas; alternatively, a method other than that of extraction must be used, e.g. retinal densitometry. The application of this method to the rod-free fovea of the living human eye allows the kinetics of regeneration of cone pigments to be followed quantitatively. For the results of these measurements, the reader is referred to Chapter 9, p. 381 which deals with the visual pigments in man.

4. Factors Known to Influence Regeneration *in situ*

a) Intact Blood Circulation. A normal blood supply appears to be necessary for regeneration in the eyes of mammals. Thus AYRES and KÜHNE (1882) detected no regeneration in the excised eyes of rabbits. Similarly, eyes from light-adapted albino rats do not regenerate rhodopsin even when incubated in a tissue culture medium at 37° C in the dark (HUBBARD and DOWLING, 1962). On the other hand, the excised eyes of frogs (KÜHNE, 1878), fishes (KÜHNE and SEWALL, 1880) and crocodiles (ABELSDORFF, 1898) are well able to regenerate bleached photopigment. Recently, REUTER (1966) studied this problem quantitatively and found that excised opened eyes of frogs regenerated their bleached photopigment as completely and as quickly as did eyes in the living animal.

b) Oxygen Pressure. Several authors have found that unless the excised eyes are opened the regeneration of rhodopsin is greatly reduced (ZEWI, 1939; HUBBARD and DOWLING, 1962). There can be little doubt that this observation has to do with the oxygen supply of the retina, which clearly shows signs of oxygen deficiency unless the isolated (un-opened) frog eye is kept in an atmosphere containing at least 80 to 90 % oxygen (BAUEREISEN, LIPPMANN, SCHUBERT, and SICKEL, 1958). The opened frog eye, however, needs hardly more oxygen than is normally present in the air (REUTER, 1966). Application of pure nitrogen (instead of normal air) to such preparations is followed by a substantially diminished capacity to regenerate rhodopsin (ZEWI, 1939).

LEWIS (1957) found that the rate of regeneration in the eyes of anaesthetized rats was lowered if the animals were in respiratory difficulties because of excessive tracheal mucous secretion, which occasionally led to an early death. It may be assumed that the retina was in a state of oxygen deficiency in these experiments.

c) **Temperature.** The temperature dependence of regeneration has been studied by a number of authors who have mainly used frog eyes. The classic work of GATTI (1901) has already been mentioned. Table 1 gives a short list of the Q_{10} values taken from several more recent papers. ZEWI (1939) made the extraordinary observation that temperature did not affect the rate of regeneration in the excised opened eye (from 7.2 to 22.4° C) but DONNER and REUTER (1967) found nearly the same Q_{10} in well prepared excised eyes as that obtained by ZEWI in living frogs (within a comparable temperature range; cf. Table 1).

Table 1. *Temperature dependence of rhodopsin regeneration in frog eyes*

Preparation	Temperature range, °C	Q_{10}	Authors
Intact eye	7.2—17.2	4.1	ZEWI, 1939
Excised opened eye	8.5—18.0	4.6	DONNER and REUTER, 1967
Intact eye	12.2—22.1	2.8	ZEWI, 1939
Intact eye	15.0—25.0	1.8	PESKIN, 1942

d) **Vitamin A supply.** A continuous supply to the body of a certain amount of vitamin A is a necessary condition for normal visual function, including normal regeneration of bleached photopigments. In vitamin A deficient animals regeneration can be seriously disturbed (FRIDERICIA and HOLM, 1925; TANSLEY, 1931). This point, however, will not be further commented on since it belongs to the field of pathological physiology. The reader will find more information about this particular problem in DOWLING and WALD (1958).

IV. Renewal of Visual Pigment Molecules

The essence of regeneration is the repair of previously damaged molecules. In addition to this *re*-synthesis, *new* pigment molecules are formed as outer segment material is continuously renewed in the living eye. This process does not result in the formation of new cells nor is it a growth of developing cells. Instead it is an exchange of material in mature tissues, and it does not influence the morphological feature of the cells involved.

Radioautographic work has provided the main evidence for the existence of this renewal process. Working with a mixture of tritiated amino acids, DROZ (1963) identified the myoid portion of the inner segment of photoreceptors in rats and mice as the site of protein synthesis. A considerable fraction of the newly synthesized protein was reported to migrate into the outer segment. Later YOUNG (1967) and YOUNG and DROZ (1968) followed the fate of the radioactive material over a time range between ten minutes and several weeks after injection of the animals. The method of quantitative electron microscopic autoradiography enabled YOUNG and DROZ to localize the radioactive constituents in the different intracellular organelles of frog photoreceptors (*Rana esculenta*). Ten minutes after injection, most of the radioactivity was found in the ergastoplasm of the myoid. The labelled material migrates as far as the connecting cilium in about 2 hours (cf. Young, 1968) and begins to accumulate at the base of the outer segment within the fourth hour following the injection. At this stage, the newly synthesized proteins already form a part of the basal discs of the rods (it should be remembered that outer segments contain many hundreds of densely packed membranous discs). The next step is a gradual movement of the disc-shaped unit of radioactive material along the axis of the outer segment. First discernible after 8 hr, this sclerical displacement then proceeds for several weeks until the labelled discs finally reach the apical end of the outer segment, when they are detached from it and may later be found within inclusion bodies of the retinal pigment epithelium (Young and Bok, 1969). The whole migratory process, starting at the base and ending at the top of the outer segment, has been reported to last 8.5 weeks in *Rana pipiens* (Hall, Bok, and Bacharach, 1969). If it is assumed that the observed phenomena reflect the formation of new discs, 36 of these organelles are formed per day in the red rods, and 25 in the green rods of *R. esculenta*. These figures refer to room temperature; they may vary according to a Q_{10} of about 2 within the temperature range of 4 to 34° C. There is also an effect due to illumination which, if it is intense and continuous, may slightly hasten the displacement (Young, 1967). This interpretation, i.e. the renewal of whole discs, is applicable to rods but not to cones where in similar experiments the radioactivity was found to be diffusely distributed throughout the outer segment. The mechanism governing the renewal of cone outer segments is not yet understood.

All the morphological studies cited above refer to the outer segment material in general. They leave unanswered the question whether the specific protein of the visual pigment takes part in the renewal process and, if so, to what extent. This aspect of the problem has recently been elucidated by the work of three independent groups (Hall, Bok, and Bacharach, 1968; Matsubara, Miyata, and Mizuno, 1968; Bargoot, Williams, and Beidler, 1969). As in the morphological investigations, tritiated amino acids were used and their incorporation into the proteins of photoreceptors was studied. The labelled substances were injected into the lymph or blood vessel system of frogs (*R. pipiens* or *R. catesbeiana*). After one or two weeks the animals were killed, and their rhodopsin extracted from the isolated and washed rod outer segments. A substantial fraction of the radioactivity in the outer segments was found to be associated with rhodopsin (although Matsubara and co-workers found fractions of less than 20 %, values as high as 70 or 80 % were obtained by the two other groups). Hall, Bok, and Bacharach (1969) found this proportion (80 %) to remain fairly constant for 8.5 weeks; then it dropped suddenly, obviously because of the detachment of groups of (labelled) discs from the apex of the outer segment.

As the visual pigment molecules are continuously renewed, retinal (or 3-dehydroretinal) must be supplied. In fact, Bridges and Yoshikami (1969) found a turnover of visual pigment prosthetic groups in dark-adapted animals. They injected rats with labelled retinal and kept the animals in absolute darkness for 1,7 or 14 days. The rhodopsin that was extracted after these various intervals, when bleached released considerable and progressively greater amounts of labelled retinal. The incorporation of the radioactive prosthetic groups cannot be attributed to a regenerative process, for no light-induced decomposition of the visual pigment had taken place. Instead, the continuous renewal of rhodopsin, even in the dark-adapted animal, is implied by these results. In fishes (BRIDGES and YOSHIKAMI, 1968, 1970), a similar process was discovered. However, the renewal process in fish retinas is complicated by the fact that in certain fishes the prosthetic group of rhodopsin is replaced in darkness by its 3-dehydro derivative (see also Chapter 11 by BRIDGES, p. 417).

References

ABELSDORFF, G.: Die ophthalmoskopische Erkennbarkeit des Sehpurpurs. Z. Psychol. Physiol. Sinnesorg. **14**, 77—90 (1897).
— Physiologische Beobachtungen am Auge der Krokodile. Arch. Anat. u. Physiol. (Physiol.) **1898**, 155—167.
ANDREWS, J. S., FUTTERMAN, S.: Metabolism of the retina. V. The role of microsomes in vitamin A esterification in the visual cycle. J. biol. Chem. **239**, 4073—4076 (1964).
ARDEN, G. B., IKEDA, H.. SIEGEL, I. M.: Effects of light adaptation on the early receptor potential. Vision Res. **6**, 357—371 (1966a).
— — — New components of the mammalian receptor potential and their relation to visual photochemistry. Vision Res. **6**, 373—384 (1966b).
AYRES, W. C., KÜHNE, W.: Über Regeneration des Sehpurpurs beim Säugethiere. Unters. physiol. Inst. Heidelberg **2**, 215—240 (1882).
BARGOOT, F. G., WILLIAMS, T. P., BEIDLER, L. B.: The localization of radioactive amino acid taken up into the outer segments of frog (Rana pipiens) rod. Vision Res. **9**, 385—391 (1969).
BAUEREISEN E., LIPPMANN, H. G., SCHUBERT, E., SICKEL, W.: Bioelektrische Aktivität und Sauerstoff-Verbrauch isolierter Potentialbildner bei Sauerstoffdrucken zwischen 0 und 10 Atm. Pflügers Arch. ges. Physiol. **267**, 636—648 (1958).
BAUMANN CH.: Die Photosensitivität der Sehpurpurs in der isolierten Netzhaut Vision Res. **5**, 425—434 (1965).
— Regeneration of rhodopsin in the isolated retina of the frog (Rana esculenta) Vision Res. **10**, 627—637 (1970).
— Regeneration of porphyropsin in vivo. Nature (Lond.) **233**, 484—485 (1971).
— ERNST, W.: Formation of isorhodopsin in isolated frog retinae by intense nanosecond flashes. J. Physiol. (Lond.) **210**, 156—157 P (1970).
BLISS, A. F.: The chemistry of daylight vision. J. gen. Physiol. **29**, 277—297 (1946).
— The mechanism of retinal vitamin A formation. J. biol. Chem. **172**, 165—178 (1948).
— The equilibrium between vitamin A alcohol and aldehyde in the presence of alcohol dehydrogenase. Arch. Biochem. **31**, 197—204 (1951a).
— Properties of the pigment layer factor in the regeneration of rhodopsin. J. biol. Chem. **193**, 525—531 (1951b).
BOLL, F.: Zur Anatomie und Physiologie der Retina. Monatsber. Akad. Wiss. Berlin **1876**, 783—787.
BRIDGES, C. D. B.: Studies on the flash photolysis of visual pigments. 4. Dark reactions following the flash irradiation of frog rhodopsin in suspensions of isolated photoreceptors. Vision Res. **2**, 215—232 (1962).
— YOSHIKAMI, S.: Mechanism of rhodopsin-porphyropsin interconversions in fish. Abstr. Fifth Int. Congr. Photobiol. (1968), p. 112, Dartmouth College, Hanover, N. H., U.S.A.
— — Uptake of tritiated retinaldehyde by the visual pigment of dark adapted rats. Nature (Lond.) **221**, 275—276 (1969).
— — The rhodopsin-porphyropsin system in freshwater fishes. 2. Turnover and interconversion of visual pigment prosthetic groups in light and darkness — role of the pigment epithelium. Vision Res. **10**, 1333—1345 (1970).

Brown, P. K., Brown, P. S.: Visual pigments of the octopus and cuttlefish. Nature (Lond.) **182**, 1288—1290 (1958).

Chase, A. M.: An accessory photosensitive substance in visual purple regeneration. Science **85**, 484 (1937).

— Smith, E. L.: Regeneration of visual purple in solution. J. gen. Physiol. **23**, 21—39 (1939).

Collins, F. D., Green, J. N., Morton, R. A.: Studies in rhodopsin. 6. Regeneration of rhodopsin. Biochem. J. **53**, 152—157 (1953).

— — — Studies in rhodopsin. 7. Regeneration of rhodopsin by comminuted ox retina. Biochem. J. **56**, 493—498 (1954).

Cone, R. A.: Early receptor potential: photoreversible charge displacement in rhodopsin. Science **155**, 1128—1131 (1967).

— Brown, P. K.: Spontaneous regeneration of rhodopsin in the isolated rat retina. Nature (Lond.) **221**, 818—820 (1969).

Crescitelli, F., Dartnall, H. J. A.: A photosensitive pigment of the carp retina. J. Physiol. (Lond.) **125**, 607—627 (1954).

— Sickel, E.: Delayed off-responses recorded from the isolated frog retina. Vision Res. **8**, 801—816 (1968).

— Wilson, B. W., Lilyblade, A. L.: The visual pigments of birds. 1. The turkey. Vision Res. **4**, 275—280 (1964).

Donner, K. O., Reuter, T.: Dark-adaptation processes in the rhodopsin rods of the frog's retina. Vision Res. **7**, 17—41 (1967).

Dowling, J. E.: Chemistry of visual adaptation in the rat. Nature (Lond.) **188**, 114—118 (1960).

— Neural and photochemical mechanisms of visual adaptation in the rat. J. gen. Physiol. **46**, 1287—1301 (1963).

— Hubbard, R.: Effects of brilliant flashes on light and dark adaptation. Nature (Lond.) **199**, 972—975 (1963).

— Wald, G.: Vitamin A deficiency and night blindness. Proc. nat. Acad. Sci. (Wash.) **44**, 648—661 (1958).

Droz, B.: Dynamic condition of proteins in the visual cells of rats and mice as shown by radioautography with labelled amino acids. Anat. Rec. **145**, 157—167 (1963).

Ewald, E., Kühne, W.: Untersuchungen über den Sehpurpur. II. Entstehung der Retinafarbe. Unters. physiol. Inst. Heidelberg **1**, 248—290 (1878).

Frank, R. N.: Photoproducts of rhodopsin bleaching in the isolated, perfused frog retina. Vision Res. **9**, 1415—1433 (1969).

Fridericia, L. S., Holm, E.: Experimental contribution to the study of the relation between night blindness and malnutrition. Amer. J. Physiol. **73**, 63—78 (1925).

Futterman, S.: Metabolism of the retina. 3. The role of reduced triphosphopyridine nucleotide in the visual cycle. J. biol. Chem. **238**, 1145—1150 (1963).

— Stoichiometry of retinal vitamin A metabolism during light adaptation. In: Biochemistry of the retina; p. 16—21. (C. N. Graymore, Ed.). London-New York: Academic Press 1965.

— Andrews, J. S.: Metabolism of the retina. IV. The composition of vitamin A ester synthesized by the retina. J. biol. Chem. **239**, 81—84 (1964).

— Saslaw, L. D.: The estimation of vitamin A aldehyde with thiobarbituric acid. J. biol. Chem. **236**, 1652—1657 (1961).

Garten, S.: Über die Veränderungen des Sehpurpurs durch Licht. Albrecht v. Graefes Arch. Ophthal. **63**, 112—187 (1906).

Gatti, A.: Intorno all' influenza della temperatura sulla formazione della porpora retinica. Ann. Ottal. Clin. ocul. **30**, 377—419 (1901).

Granit, R., Munsterhjelm, A., Zewi, M.: The relation between concentration of visual purple and retinal sensitivity to light during dark adaptation. J. Physiol. (Lond.) **96**, 31—44 (1939).

Hagins, W. A., Rushton, W. A. H.: The measurement of rhodopsin in the decerebrate albino rabbit. J. Physiol. (Lond.) **120**, 61 P (1953).

Hall, M. O., Bok, D., Bacharach, A. D. E.: Visual pigment renewal in the mature frog retina. Science **161**, 787—789 (1968).

— — — Biosynthesis and assembly of the rod outer segment membrane system. Formation and fate of visual pigment in the frog retina. J. Mol. Biol. **45**, 397—406 (1969).

HAMDORF, K., SCHWEMER, J., TÄUBER, U.: Der Sehfarbstoff, die Absorption der Rezeptoren und die spektrale Empfindlichkeit der Retina von *Eledone moschata*. Z. vgl. Physiol. **60**, 375—415 (1968).

HECHT, S., CHASE, A. M., SHLAER, S., HAIG, C.: The regeneration of visual purple in solution. Science **84**, 331—333 (1936).

HOSOYA, Y., SASAKI, T.: Über die Regeneration des extrahierten Sehpurpurs. Tohoku J. exp. Med. **32**, 447—459 (1938).

HUBBARD, R.: Retinene isomerase. J. gen. Physiol. **39**, 935—962 (1956).

— BOWNDS, D., YOSHIZAWA, T.: The chemistry of visual photoreception. Cold Spring Harbor Symp. Quant. Biol. **30**, 301—315 (1965).

— COLMAN, A. D.: Vitamin-A content of the frog eye during light and dark adaptation. Science **130**, 977—978 (1959).

— DOWLING, J. E.: Formation and utilization of 11-*cis*-vitamin A by the eye tissues during light and dark adaptation. Nature (Lond.) **193**, 341—343 (1962).

— ST. GEORGE, R. C. C.: The rhodopsin system of the squid. J. gen. Physiol. **41**, 501—528 (1958).

— WALD, G.: The mechanism of rhodopsin synthesis. Proc. nat. Acad. Sci. (Wash.) **37**, 69—79 (1951).

— — Cis-trans isomers of vitamin A and retinene in the rhodopsin system. J. gen. Physiol. **36**, 269—315 (1952).

KÖTTGEN, E., ABELSDORFF, G.: Absorption und Zersetzung des Sehpurpurs bei den Wirbeltieren. Z. Psychol. Physiol. Sinnesorg. **12**, 161—184 (1896).

KRINSKY, N. I.: The enzymatic esterification of vitamin A. J. biol. Chem. **232**, 881—894 (1958).

KÜHNE, W.: Vorläufige Mittheilung über optographische Versuche. Zbl. med. Wiss. **15**, 33—35 (1877).

— Zur Photochemie der Netzhaut. Unters. physiol. Inst. Heidelberg **1**, 1—14 (1878).

— Chemische Vorgänge in der Netzhaut. In: Handbuch der Physiologie, S. 235—342 (L. HERMANN, Ed.). Leipzig: Vogel 1879.

— SEWALL H.: Zur Physiologie des Sehepithels, insbesondere der Fische. Unters. physiol. Inst. Heidelberg **3**, 221—277 (1880).

LEWIS, D. M.: Regeneration of rhodopsin in the albino rat. J. Physiol. (Lond.) **136**, 624—631 (1957).

MATSUBARA, T., MIYATA, M., MIZUNO, K.: Radioisotopic studies on renewal of opsin. Vision Res. **8**, 1139—1143 (1968).

OROSHNIK, W.: The synthesis and configuration of neo-b vitamin A and neoretine b. J. Amer. chem. Soc. **78**, 2651—2652 (1956).

PAK, W. L., BOES, R. J.: Rhodopsin: responses from transient intermediates formed during its bleaching. Science **155**, 1131—1133 (1967).

PESKIN, J. C.: The regeneration of visual purple in the living animal. J. gen. Physiol. **26**, 27—47 (1942).

REUTER, T.: Kinetics of rhodopsin regeneration in the eye of the frog. Nature (Lond.) **202**, 1119—1120 (1964a).

— Formation of isorhodopsin in the frog's eye during continuous illumination. Nature (Lond.) **204**, 784—785 (1964b).

— The synthesis of photosensitive pigments in the rods of the frog's retina. Vision Res. **6**, 15—38 (1966).

RIPPS, H., WEALE, R. A.: Rhodopsin regeneration in man. Nature (Lond.) **222**, 775—777 (1969).

RUSHTON, W. A. H.: Apparatus for analysing the light reflected from the eye of the cat. J. Physiol. (Lond.) **117**, 47 P (1952).

— The difference spectrum and the photosensitivity of rhodopsin in the living human eye. J. Physiol. (Lond.) **134**, 11—29 (1956).

— Blue light and the regeneration of human rhodopsin *in situ*. J. gen. Physiol. **41**, 419—428 (1957).

— CAMPBELL, F. W., HAGINS, W. A., BRINDLEY, G. S.: The bleaching and regeneration of rhodopsin in the living eye of the albino rabbit and of man. Optica Acta **1**, 183—190 (1955).

SLATER, T. F., HEATH, H., GRAYMORE, C. N.: Levels of oxidized and reduced pyridine nucleotides in rat retina. Biochem. J. 84, 37 P (1962).

TANSLEY, K.: The regeneration of visual purple; its relation to dark adaptation and night blindness. J. Physiol. (Lond.) 71, 442—458 (1931).

WALD, G.: Carotenoids and the visual cycle. J. gen. Physiol. 19, 351—371 (1935).

— Photo-labile pigments of the chicken retina. Nature (Lond.) 140, 545—546 (1937).

— Vision. Fed. Proc. 12, 606—611 (1953).

— BROWN, P. K., KENNEDY, D.: The visual system of the alligator. J. gen. Physiol. 40, 703—713 (1957).

— — SMITH, P. H.: Iodopsin. J. gen. Physiol. 38, 623—681 (1955).

— HUBBARD, R.: The reduction of retinene$_1$ to vitamin A$_1$ in vitro. J. gen. Physiol. 32, 367—389 (1949).

— — The synthesis of rhodopsin from vitamin A$_1$. Proc. nat. Acad. Sci. (Wash.) 36, 92—102 (1950).

WEALE, R. A.: Photochemical reactions in the living cat's retina. J. Physiol. (Lond.) 122, 322—331 (1953).

— Observations on photochemical reactions in living eyes. Brit. J. Ophthal. 41, 461—474 (1957).

— Vision and fundus reflectometry. Documenta Ophthalmologica 19, 252—286 (1965).

— On an early stage of rhodopsin regeneration in man. Vision Res. 7, 819—827 (1967).

WEINSTEIN, G. W., HOBSON, R. R., DOWLING, J. E.: Light and dark adaptation in the isolated rat retina. Nature (Lond.) 215, 134—138 (1967).

YOUNG, R. W.: The renewal of photoreceptor cell outer segments. J. Cell Biol. 33, 61—72 (1967).

— Passage of newly formed protein through the connecting cilium of retinal rods in the frog. J. Ultrastruct. Res. 23, 462—473 (1968).

— BOK, D.: Participation of the retinal pigment epithelium in the rod outer segment renewal process. J. Cell Biol. 42, 392—403 (1969).

— DROZ, B.: The renewal of protein in retinal rods and cones. J. Cell Biol. 39, 169—184 (1968).

ZEWI, M.: On the regeneration of visual purple. Acta. Soc. Sci. fenn. N.S.B. 2, 1—56 (1939).

Chapter 11

The Rhodopsin-Porphyropsin Visual System*

By

C. D. B. Bridges, New York, New York (USA)

With 37 Figures

Contents

* This work was supported by PHS Research Grant No. 5 RO 1 EY 00461 (Natl. Eye Institute).

I. Introduction

The light-absorbing properties of visual pigments determine the sensitivity
of the eye to various parts of the spectrum. An animal with a red-absorbing
pigment is sensitive to red light. Conversely, an animal with a blue-absorbing
pigment is relatively more sensitive to blue light. These points are illustrated in
Fig. 1, where the visual pigment spectra and corresponding scotopic sensitivities
of tench (a freshwater fish) and frog are compared. The tench pigment absorbs
maximally at 533 nm, whereas that of the frog is displaced some 30 nm towards
shorter wavelengths. KÖTTGEN and ABELSDORFF (1896) were the first workers
who noted this difference between tench and frog. In fact, all the freshwater
fish they examined had visual pigments that were more violet in colour (i. e.

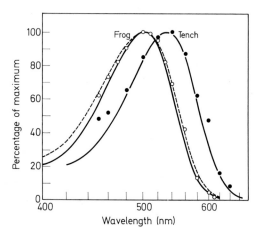

Fig. 1. Visual pigment spectra and spectral sensitivities of frog *(Rana temporaria)* and a
freshwater fish (the tench, *Tinca tinca*). Absorbance spectra are represented by continuous
curves (dashed curve is the percentage light absorption of the frog pigment, calculated from
the *in vivo* absorbance), spectral sensitivities by plain and filled circles (frog and tench respectively). Reproduced with permission from DARTNALL, 1953

absorbed at longer wavelengths) than those from terrestrial vertebrates such as birds, mammals and amphibians.

Forty years later, WALD discovered that whereas fishes from *freshwaters* had visual pigments absorbing near the red end of the spectrum, those of *marine* origin had pigments similar to those of the terrestrial group (WALD, 1936a, b, 1937, 1939a, b). Thus the idea originated of two large classes of visual pigments — the "visual violets" or porphyropsins of freshwater inhabitants and the "visual purples" or rhodopsins of terrestrial and marine forms. This duality was found to have a chemical basis, depending on the particular variety of vitamin A in the pigment molecule. Rhodopsins were derived from "vitamin A_1" or retinol, while in porphyropsins this was replaced by "vitamin A_2" or 3-dehydroretinol.

Subsequently it was found in amphibians that adaptation to a freshwater or terrestrial habitat was manifested by a succession of visual pigments during ontogenesis. Thus tadpoles have red-absorbing porphyropsins, which are transmuted into blue-absorbing rhodopsins in the terrestrial adult frogs. In a related category are the amphibia of the fish world, the migratory lampreys, eels, salmons and trouts, which have mixtures of rhodopsins and porphyropsins, switching from one to the other depending on whether a downstream (seaward) or upstream journey is involved. Thus it was postulated that the retinol-based rhodopsins were confined to terrestrial and marine species, 3-dehydroretinol-based porphyropsins to freshwater species, while mixtures of the two pigments occurred in fishes and amphibians distributing their lives between these environments (a summary of this view is given by WALD, 1960a, b). This generalization still holds true for terrestrial animals and the majority of truly marine fishes. There are some exceptions in migratory fishes and amphibia. However, it is in connexion with the freshwater fishes that our views must be thoroughly revised, for whereas the majority have porphyropsin as expected, in about half of the species examined rhodopsin is also present (for example, see DARTNALL, 1952, 1962; DARTNALL, LANDER, and MUNZ, 1961; BRIDGES, 1965a, b, c; SCHWANZARA, 1967). Although migration is not a feature of the life cycle in these cases, large shifts in the proportions of the two pigments may occur in response to a variety of conditions, often resulting in an overwhelming preponderance of the rhodopsin component. The function of these shifts, the factors controlling them and their underlying mechanisms are discussed in the second half of this chapter.

II. Chemical Basis of the Rhodopsins and Porphyropsins

Since the early studies of EWALD and KÜHNE (1878) it has been recognized that the visual pigments are proteins. Until recently, it was usually accepted that they were better regarded as lipoproteins (for reviews, see ABRAHAMSON and OSTROY, 1967; BRIDGES, 1970a), although now this is less certain. Frog rod outer segments contain a high proportion of lipid, amounting to between 39 and 41 % of the dry weight (SJÖSTRAND, 1959; EICHBERG and HESS, 1967). Two-thirds is phospholipid (COLLINS, LOVE, and MORTON, 1952; EICHBERG and HESS, 1967), which is always present in digitonin extracts of visual pigment (BRODA, 1941; KRINSKY, 1958). However, when bovine rhodopsin is extracted with hexadecyltrimethyl-ammonium bromide and purified by gel-filtration it appears to contain little, if any, phospholipid[1]. Thus, Heller (1968a) concluded that rhodopsin was a conjugated glycoprotein of molecular weight 27,000—30,000 (Shields, Dinovo, Henriksen, Kimbel, and Millar, 1967, found a molecular weight of 28,600: Shichi, Lewis, Irreverre, and Stone, 1969, report 28,000). However, such extracts are abnormal in one respect — after bleaching they are incapable of regeneration when 11-*cis* retinaldehyde is added to them (Snodderly, 1967). A similar situation is found in digitonin extracts of rod outer segments from which most of the phospholipid has been removed (Krinsky, 1958), suggesting that maintenance of structural integrity in the bleached protein (opsin) may be critically dependent on the presence of phospholipid, even though its removal does not alter the absorption properties of the visual pigment.

Pure preparations of visual pigments show several light-absorption bands, one in the visible spectrum (α), another in the ultraviolet (γ) at about 278 nm, as illustrated in Fig. 2. In this example, cattle rhodopsin, the γ-band arises from the summed absorption of 10—11 tyrosine, 19—22 phenylalanine and 5 tryptophan residues (Shields, Dinovo, Henriksen, Kimbel, and Millar, 1967; Shichi, Lewis, Irreverre, and Stone, 1969; Heller, 1968a). In other pigments it is possible that these proportions are different. The α-band arises from the combina-

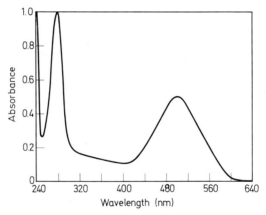

Fig. 2. Absorbance spectrum of purified bovine rhodopsin. Reproduced with permission from Heller (1968a). One important feature of this curve, which distinguishes it from previously published spectra, is the absence of a minor band at 340—350 nm. This band is known as the β-band. Heller claims that the β-band is an artefact attributable to the presence of trace quantities of free retinaldehyde released by part-bleaching of the visual pigment during the preparative procedures of other workers. After this chapter was written, however, Shichi (1970) has cast serious doubt on this argument and suggests that Heller's spectrum is considerably in error in the ultraviolet. One further problem in connexion with Heller's spectroscopic data is his extraordinarily low figure of 23,100 for the molar absorbance coefficient (ε_{max}). This value has not been confirmed by other workers, all of whom report ε_{max} near Wald and Brown's (1953) original figure of about 41,000 (Bridges, 1970c, 1971; Shichi, 1970)

---

[1] There is now further controversy on this point. Since the time of writing Poincelot, Millar, Kimbel, and Abrahamson (1969) have produced evidence that rhodopsin is a true lipoprotein.

tion of retinaldehyde (retinene) with the apoprotein. The primary site of attachment appears to involve condensation of the terminal aldehyde group with an ε-amino group of lysine (AKHTAR, BLOSSE, and DEWHURST, 1967, 1968; BOWNDS, 1967; HELLER, 1968 b)[2]. The retinaldehyde is in the 11-*cis* configuration, and is further linked to the opsin by less well-defined bonds, resulting in some mutual rearrangment of conformations and a bathochromic shift of absorption properties (for reviews, see MORTON and PITT, 1957; DARTNALL, 1962; BRIDGES, 1967a; 1970a). On bleaching, 11-*cis* retinaldehyde changes to all-*trans* retinaldehyde (HUBBARD and WALD, 1952) which is released after hydrolysis of the $-C=N-$ link and is then reduced to all-*trans* retinol ("vitamin A") by the membrane-bound dehydrogenase-NADP system of the photoreceptor outer segments (WALD and HUBBARD, 1949; BLISS, 1948, 1949; FUTTERMAN and SASLAW, 1961; FUTTERMAN, 1963).

As stated in the Introduction, the visual pigments utilising retinaldehyde as prosthetic group are referred to as the *rhodopsins*.

$$\text{Rhodopsin} \xrightarrow{\text{light}} \text{retinaldehyde} + \text{opsin} \xrightarrow{2\,\text{H}} \text{retinol} + \text{opsin}.$$

The rhodopsin cycle in the living vertebrate eye is schematised in Fig. 3.

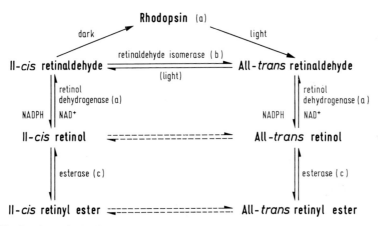

Fig. 3. Rhodopsin cycle in the vertebrate retina (dashed lines indicate speculative reactions). (a) in the outer segments, (b) in cattle retinas and frog pigment epithelium, (c) in cattle retinas. Based on BRIDGES, 1967a, where relevant references are listed

Porphyropsins are based on the 3.4-dehydro derivative of retinaldehyde, and bleach in the retina to products analogous to those found in the rhodopsin system (WALD, 1939a, b).

Porphyropsin $\xrightarrow{\text{light}}$ 3-dehydroretinaldehyde + opsin $\xrightarrow{2\,\text{H}}$ 3-dehydroretinol + opsin.

---

[2] POÏNCELOT, MILLAR, KIMBEL, and ABRAHAMSON (1969) disagree, and suggest that the primary link involves phosphatidyl ethanolamine, retinaldehyde being transferred to the ε-amino group of lysine during bleaching of the visual pigment.

Originally, 3-dehydroretinaldehyde was known as "retinene$_2$" and 3-dehydroretinol as "vitamin A$_2$". The structures of these compounds are illustrated in Fig. 4. Like rhodopsin, porphyropsin is composed of an opsin combined with a *cis*-stereoisomer of the prosthetic group which is transformed to all-*trans* when the pigment is bleached. In 3-dehydroretinaldehyde the *cis*-link probably lies in the 11-position, but this has not been established with certainty (WALD, BROWN, and SMITH, quoted by WALD, 1953). A cycle analogous to that for rhodopsin (Fig. 3) probably occurs in eyes containing porphyropsin.

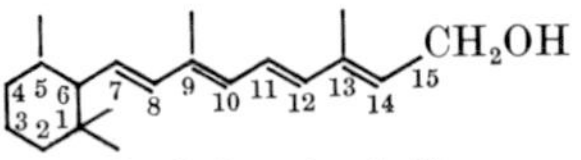

retinol ("vitamin A$_1$")
λ_{max} in ethanol = 325 nm

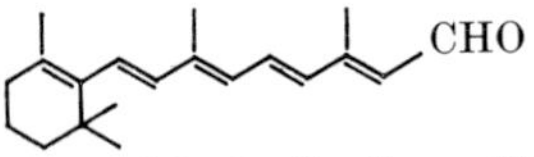

retinaldehyde ("retinene$_1$")
λ_{max} in ethanol = 381 nm

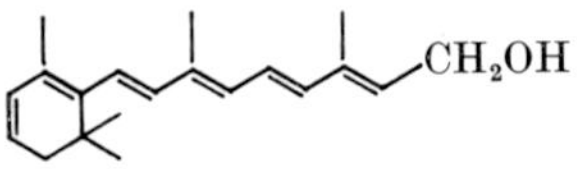

8-dehydroretinol
("vitamin A$_2$")
λ_{max} in ethanol
= 350, 286, 276 nm

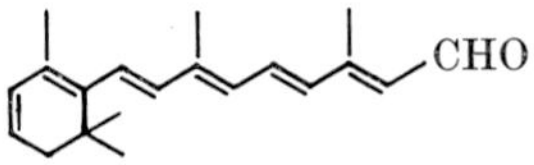

3-dehydroretinaldehyde
("retine$_2$")
λ_{max} in ethanol = 401 nm,
with inflexion at ca 314 nm

Fig. 4

III. Rhodopsins and Porphyropsins — Similar and Contrasting Properties

A. Absorbance Spectra

Incubation of cattle opsin with 11-*cis* retinaldehyde results in the formation of cattle rhodopsin, which has an α-band peaking at 498 nm. The *same* opsin may be incubated with *cis*-3-dehydroretinaldehyde instead, yielding a porphyropsin with maximum at 517 nm (WALD, BROWN, and SMITH, quoted by HUBBARD, 1958b). Opsin from another source (chicken) produces a rhodopsin with maximum at 562 nm and a porphyropsin with maximum at 620 nm (WALD, BROWN, and SMITH, 1953: these pigments are commonly referred to as "iodopsin" and "cyanopsin" respectively). The absorbance spectra of a typical rhodopsin-porphyropsin pair are illustrated in Fig. 5. Spectroscopically, the switch from retinaldehyde to 3-dehydroretinaldehyde, while retaining the same opsin, is accompanied by a bathochromic shift of λ_{max}, augmented absorption on the shortwave side of the main (α) band and a hypochromic reduction of absorbance coefficient to between 70 and 75 % of the rhodopsin value. These effects and their possible structural basis have been discussed in detail elsewhere (BRIDGES, 1965a, 1967b).

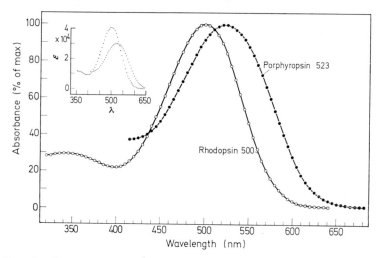

Fig. 5. The absorbance spectrum of a rhodopsin compared with that of its corresponding porphyropsin (maxima at 500 and 523 nm respectively). Inset: the two spectra compared in terms of their molar absorbance coefficients. From BRIDGES, 1967 b

B. Optical Activity

Differences may also be observed in the circular dichroism (CD) spectra[3] (see Chapter 6, p. 180). According to CRESCITELLI, MOMMAERTS, and SHAW (1966), carp porphyropsin and cattle rhodopsin show a CD of identical magnitude in the region of their respective α-bands, but below about 410 nm the CD of porphyropsin drops progressively below that of rhodopsin. Thus although absorption in this region is more intense in porphyropsin, the electronic transitions involved do not seem to be optically active.

C. Thermal Stability

A further consequence of switching prosthetic groups is that porphyropsins are less stable than their homologous rhodopsins, perhaps owing to different steric relationships in their molecules (BRIDGES, 1956; 1967 b).

Thermal stabilities have also been examined by WILLIAMS and MILBY (1968), but with rather equivocal results. These authors did not study rhodopsin-porphyropsin pairs, but selected porphyropsins from four fish species and contrasted them with unrelated rhodopsins from cattle and frog. Even among visual pigments based on the same prosthetic group it was found that the thermal stability was variable, and not all the porphyropsins were found to be less stable than the two rhodopsins. In only one instance was an attempt made to study a possibly homologous pair, i. e. tadpole porphyropsin and adult rhodopsin from *Rana catesbeiana*. Here, the expected result was obtained, for the larval pigment decayed 10 times more rapidly than that of the adult frog (pH 6.5). BRIDGES (1956) had found that

---

[3] Circular dichroism is the difference between absorbances measured with right- and left-circularly polarized light.

rainbow trout porphyropsin decayed 40 times more rapidly than its corresponding rhodopsin in an extract containing a mixture of the two (at pH 8) and Dartnall (1955) reported similar results in extracts from another fish. Regrettably, the *R. catesbeiana* experiment may not have revealed the full extent of the disparity in stabilities, for although Williams and Milby assumed that their extract was homogeneous, they reported the maximum at 516 nm (difference spectrum), whereas according to an earlier report (Crescitelli, 1958a, b) the porphyropsin of this species has λ_{max} close to 523 nm. Moreover, Wilt (1959a) had found that *R. catesbeiana* tadpoles always had rhodopsin as well as porphyropsin in their retinas, the former accounting for as much as 30 % in many instances. Thus it is virtually certain that the "porphyropsin" used by Williams and Milby was really a mixture of rhodopsin and porphyropsin, the separate decay rates remaining undetected and unresolved by the experimental method used.

Schwanzara's (1967) finding that porphyropsins are less common than rhodopsins in warm-water species may be connected with the lower thermal stability of porphyropsin.

D. Intermediates of Photolysis

Rhodopsins and porphyropsins display a parallel sequence of intermediates following absorption of light. At temperatures ranging from $-190°$C down to $3°$K (liquid helium), irradiated cattle rhodopsin yields prelumirhodopsin with λ_{max} at 543 nm ($-190°$C). Above $-140°$ prelumirhodopsin passes over to lumirhodopsin with λ_{max} at 497 nm, which in turn is converted by further warming into meta-rhodopsins I and II with maxima at 478 and 380 nm respectively (for summaries, see Bridges, 1970a; Abrahamson and Ostroy, 1967). Under the same conditions, Yoshizawa and Horiuchi (1969) have shown that carp porphyropsin yields prelumiporphyropsin (λ_{max} 592 nm), lumiporphyropsin (λ_{max} 542 nm) and meta-porphyropsins I and II (λ_{max} at 509 and 410 nm respectively). These reactions are discussed in more detail by T. Yoshizawa in Chapter 5, p. 146. Subsequent steps involve the conversion of meta II to the corresponding N-retinylideneopsin (by way of at least one other intermediate absorbing maximally at 465 nm in the rhodopsin sequence; Matthews, Hubbard, Brown, and Wald, 1963) and final hydrolysis of this compound to the free aldehyde.

IV. Range of λ_{max} in Rhodopsins and Porphyropsins — Analytical Methods

Visual pigments may be characterised by the λ_{max} of their α-bands (the γ-bands vary hardly at all) and by whether they are based on retinaldehyde or its 3-dehydro derivative. In the case of an extract that contains a single pigment and no absorbing impurities, the λ_{max} determination is comparatively simple. If yellow impurities are present, they shift the extract absorbance peak towards shorter wavelengths. Crescitelli and Dartnall (1954) found that a rough correction could be made for this effect, the magnitude of which depended on the ratio

$A_{\min}/A_{\max}$. In this ratio, $A_{\max}$ is the absorbance at the $\lambda_{\max}$ and $A_{\min}$ is the absorbance recorded at the $\lambda_{\min}$ on the blue side of the α-band. Rhodopsins have $A_{\min}/A_{\max}$ of about 0.2 compared with 0.4 for the porphyropsins (see BRIDGES, 1965a; also Fig. 5).

Difference spectra are independent of the presence of photostable impurities, but are sensitive to conditions of bleaching which alter the absorbance spectra of the photoproducts. Examples of various terminal products obtainable by bleaching porphyropsin at room temperature are illustrated in Fig. 6. The lower half of the figure shows the derived difference spectra, with $\lambda_{\max}$ that are identical with the true $\lambda_{\max}$ of the pigment only when the photoproduct bands do not overlap the α-band peak. In Fig. 6 we see that the greatest overlap occurs at pH 6.3, when 3-dehydro-retinaldehyde is released (curve 2, $\lambda_{\max}$ about 408 nm). The least overlap occurs when this material is subsequently reduced to 3-dehydroretinol with sodium boro-hydride (curve 6, $\lambda_{\max}$ about 360 nm), or when bleaching is carried out in the

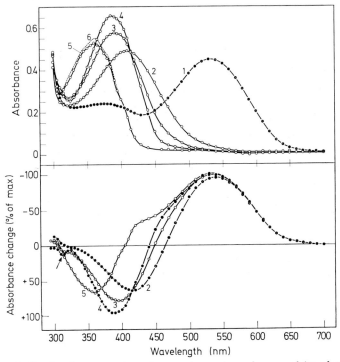

Fig. 6. Upper half: absorbance spectra of a porphyropsin and some of its photoproducts. Curve 1 — porphyropsin extract; curve 2 — result of bleaching at pH 6.3, producing 3-dehydroretinaldehyde; curve 3 — result of bleaching at pH 8.9, producing 3-dehydro-N-retinylidene opsin (better referred to as "alkaline indicator yellow," because the union between aldehyde and opsin is no longer through the original amino group at this pH; cf. MORTON and PITT, 1955); curve 4 — result of bleaching in 0.02M hydroxylamine, producing 3-dehydro-retinaldehyde oxime; curve 5 — result of bleaching in sodium borohydride at pH 9.0, produc-ing 3-dehydro-N-retinyl opsin; curve 6 — the result of sodium borohydride reduction of 3-dehydroretinaldehyde in curve 2, producing 3-dehydroretinol. Lower half: difference spectra constructed from the above absorbance spectra, and numbered correspondingly. From BRIDGES, 1967b

presence of this reagent. In that case, the product is 3-dehydro-N-retinylopsin (curve 5, λ_{max} about 360 nm). Most convenient for routine use, however, are extracts at strongly alkaline pH (curve 5, λ_{max} about 390 nm) or those containing hydroxylamine, which condenses with the aldehyde to form 3-dehydro retinaldehyde oxime. Partly because of the narrowness of the oxime band (curve 4, λ_{max} about 385 nm) and partly because of higher standards of reproducibility attributable to accelerated breakdown of intermediate photoproducts, the use of hydroxylamine is now preferred by most workers. The oxime absorbance may be effectively discounted at wavelengths longer than 480—490 nm, so that porphyropsins with λ_{max} down to within about 10 nm of this point may be safely characterised by the maxima of their difference spectra in this reagent. Rhodopsins with absorption maxima down to about 450 nm may be dealt with in similar fashion.

Difference spectra also tell us whether we are dealing with a rhodopsin or a porphyropsin, as Fig. 7 demonstrates. For rhodopsins bleached in the presence of hydroxylamine, the wavelength of maximum absorbance gain on the positive shortwave branch of the difference spectrum is 367—368 nm, whereas for porphyropsins this wavelength is 386—387 nm. In borohydride this distinction is even more marked, and the respective wavelengths are 328—329 nm and 359—360 nm.

The λ_{max} of a difference or absorbance spectrum may be determined accurately by fitting the curves in whole or in part with some form of polynomial expression, then differentiating (Bridges, 1967b). Most workers, however, have estimated the λ_{max} by eye, which can be done with surprisingly little sacrifice of precision in the majority of cases, as shown in Table 1.

The empirical observation, originally due to Dartnall (1953), that rhodopsin spectra have identical shapes when plotted against frequency instead of wavelength

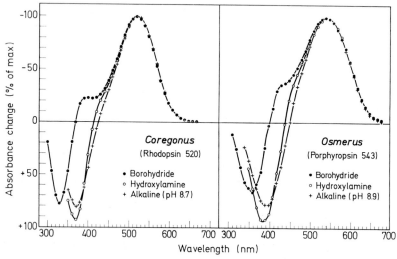

Fig. 7. Contrasted difference spectra of a rhodopsin and a porphyropsin, illustrating the effect of different photoproducts on the shortwave, positive portions of the spectra. From Bridges, 1967b

Table 1. *Determination of λ_{max} of difference spectra by fitting polynomial expressions, or estimating by eye (data of* BRIDGES, *1967 b)*

Species	λ_{max} in nm	
	mean of two fitting procedures	by eye
Mugil cephalus	522.1	522.6
Thymallus thymallus	527.1	527.2
Perca fluviatilis	533.5	533.5
Osmerus eperlanus	543.2	543.0

has simplified procedures. Thus one standard "template" curve of absorbance against frequency describes the spectra of all rhodopsins. Since we know the λ_{max} of this standard, which is based on frog rhodopsin, we can determine the λ_{max} of an unknown (e. g. BRIDGES, 1959; MUNZ, 1964; DARTNALL and LYTHGOE, 1965). Another broader standard curve must be used for porphyropsin absorbance spectra (BRIDGES, 1965a) and has been tabulated recently (BRIDGES, 1967b). A nomogram applicable to difference spectra in hydroxylamine has also been published (MUNZ and SCHWANZARA, 1967).

It frequently happens that extracts do not contain single pigments, but mixtures of two rhodopsins or of a rhodopsin and a porphyropsin. Under these circumstances, one of the pigments absorbs relatively more red light than the other. Irradiation with red light therefore bleaches the red-sensitive component and spares the other. Judicious selection of wavelengths and intensities coupled with analysis of the difference spectra at each phase of the bleaching process enables us to determine the absorbing properties of the two components in the mixture (e. g. DARTNALL, 1952; BRIDGES, 1956; MUNZ, 1958a; CRESCITELLI, 1958a; MUNZ and BEATTY, 1965; SCHWANZARA, 1967). Examples of experiments in which retinal extracts have been analysed by this method are illustrated in Fig. 8.

Rhodopsin absorption maxima range from 433 nm (frog green-rod pigment, DARTNALL 1967) to 562 nm (chicken "iodopsin"; WALD, BROWN, and SMITH, 1955). Human rhodopsin lies roughly midway between these points, at 497 nm according to CRESCITELLI and DARTNALL (1953), 493 nm according to WALD and BROWN (1958) and 493—494 nm according to BRIDGES (1970a). Most mammals have rhodopsins within about 10 nm of this position: thus the rabbit's is at 502 nm (BRIDGES, 1959), the cat's is at 500 nm (BRIDGES, 1970a) and the chimpanzee's at 491 nm (CRESCITELLI, 1958a).

The α-peaks of known porphyropsins are distributed over a more restricted range, from 510 nm (in some labrid fishes, BROWN and BROWN, quoted by WALD, 1960b) to 543 nm (in the fish *Osmerus*, BRIDGES, 1965a), although this is extended if we include "cyanopsin". Cyanopsin was originally discovered as the product of incubating "iodopsin" opsin with *cis*-3-dehydroretinaldehyde (WALD, BROWN, and SMITH, 1953) and has been detected recently in the intact cones of carp, frog tadpole and the freshwater tortoise *Pseudemys* (MARKS, 1965; LIEBMAN and ENTINE, 1967, 1968).

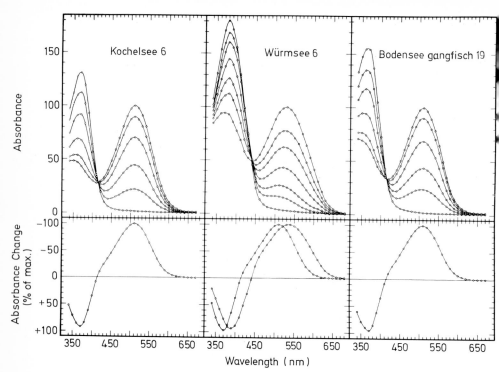

Fig. 8. Analysis by partial bleaching of three extracts from coregonine fishes of southern Germany. Kochelsee 6, Würmsee 6 and Bodensee Gangfisch 19 refer to extracts from single specimens of *Coregonus* from the Kochelsee, Würmsee and Bodensee (Lake Constance) respectively. The Bodensee Gangfisch is *Coregonus macrophthalmus*. All solutions contained hydroxylamine and were bleached in stages by irradiation with red light, followed by a terminal exposure to yellow-orange light. The initial small amounts bleached in the Kochelsee and Bodensee coregonines contained trace quantities of a porphyropsin, but subsequent bleaching operations yielded difference spectra that were all identical and maximal at 509—510 nm, as illustrated in the lower portion of the figure. Since the wavelength of maximum absorbance gain in both cases is at 367—368 nm, these pigments are rhodopsins. The visual pigment of the Würmsee coregonine was obviously heterogeneous, because the initial difference spectra were displaced towards the red when compared with later ones. The lower portion of the figure depicts the difference spectra of the two component pigments, with maxima at 536 nm in one and 509 nm in the other. The respective positive segments are maximal at 387 and 368 nm, showing that we are dealing with a mixture of rhodopsin and porphyropsin. The latter accounts for 84% of the photosensitive material. From Bridges and Yoshikami, 1970a

V. Distribution of Rhodopsins and Porphyropsins According to Photic Environment

The widest variety of visual pigments is found in the fishes, where it is considered to be the result of evolutionary adaptation to correspondingly diverse spectral light distributions in different aquatic habitats (for summaries and reviews, see Dartnall, 1962; Bridges, 1965a; Munz, 1965). The partition of solar radiation between different parts of the spectrum in some of these habitats is illustrated in Figs. 9 and 11. The transmissivities of some freshwaters are plotted in Fig. 10.

Fishes living deep in oceanic waters, where solar radiation is confined to a narrow band of wavelengths centred in the blue-green at about 480 nm (Fig. 9), tend to have visual pigments with maxima in the same spectral region. Fishes in freshwaters and turbid inshore waters, where there is a high proportion of red light (Figs. 10, 11), have pigments displaced towards the red. As might be expected, therefore, fishes in intermediate habitats have pigments absorbing in intermediate positions. The majority of land vertebrates have pigments with peaks near 500 nm, the maximum of solar radiation at the earth's surface. Hence the basis for the distribution of rhodopsins and porphyropsins outlined in the introduc-

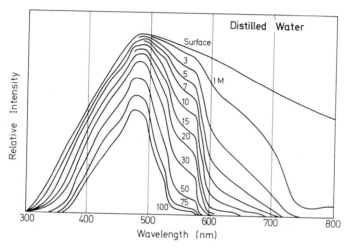

Fig. 9. The spectral distribution of solar energy at the earth's surface and after passage through various depths of distilled water. The latter approximates clearest oceanic waters. After CLARKE (1939), based on data of BIRGE and JAMES

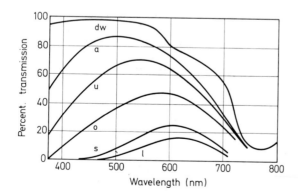

Fig. 10. The spectral transmissivity of a stratum of water 1 metre thick from various bodies of freshwater. dw distilled water; a Achensee (Tyrol); u Lunzer Untersee; o Lunzer Obersee (Lower Austria); s Skärhultsjön (South Sweden); l Lammen: after RUTTNER (1953)

tion to this chapter is obvious. Typically, marine and land vertebrates have rhodopsins, because these pigments as a group tend to absorb nearer the blue end of the spectrum. Typically, the red-absorbing porphyropsins occur only in freshwater forms and in fishes of turbid inshore and brackish habitats. These porphyropsins are sometimes in isolation, as may have been true for the species examined by KÖTTGEN and ABELSDORFF (1896) and WALD (1939b), but are frequently mixed with rhodopsins. Such mixtures occur in about 50% of the freshwater fishes examined, and are nearly always present in diadromous fishes such as the salmons, trouts, eels and lampreys.

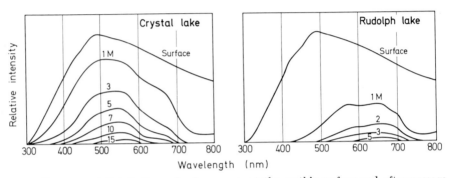

Fig. 11. The spectral distributions of solar energy at the earth's surface and after passage through various depths in two North American lakes. After CLARKE (1939), based on data of BIRGE and JAMES

Because spectral light-habitat is one of the most important factors that determines an animal's visual pigments, and because there is considerable overlap between the λ_{max} of rhodopsins and porphyropsins, it is not surprising that we sometimes find low-λ_{max} porphyropsins in marine environments and high-λ_{max} rhodopsins in freshwater or brackish water species. Examples are the porphyropsins with absorbance maxima at 510 and 512 nm in some marine labrids (BROWN and BROWN, quoted by WALD, 1960b) and the rhodopsins with maxima at 512 and 520 nm in *Gillichthys* and *Coregonus* respectively (MUNZ, 1956; BRIDGES, 1965a).

It is not known whether environmental temperature might be important. A recent report by SCHWANZARA (1967) claims that pure rhodopsins are more common in tropical freshwater fish, but some of these results should be interpreted with circumspection because most specimens originated from dealers, who may have kept them under artificial conditions of light and feeding. Many fishes with mixed rhodopsin-porphyropsin retinas may lose their porphyropsin entirely if kept in unnaturally bright surroundings (p. 457), as could have occurred in this case. Thus *Mollienesia latipinna* Le Sueur (= *Poecilia latipinna* (Le Sueur); BRIDGES, 1964b, 1965b) and *Anableps* (BRIDGES, unpublished) both have appreciable amounts of porphyropsin in their retinas, although SCHWANZARA (1967) subsequently found only rhodopsins. In the investigation by BRIDGES, *Mollienesia* were taken directly from their natural habitat (brackish and freshwaters of Florida) and *Anableps* were examined immediately upon arrival from South America.

VI. Significance of Mixed Rhodopsin-Porphyropsin Systems

The spectra of a rhodopsin and porphyropsin sum to give a unimodal curve with λ_{max} intermediate between those of the two pigments. Does an animal with such a mixture in its retina have the same spectral sensitivity as another possessing one visual pigment with the identical λ_{max}? Probably this is not very far from the truth if we ignore the fact that the mixture has a rather broader spectrum, for in all these cases we believe that the pigments are mingled in the same photoreceptor cell. This cell is most unlikely to be able to distinguish which pigment has trapped the stimulating quantum of light. Admittedly, on a molecule-for-molecule basis, porphyropsins are less efficient light catchers than rhodopsins because their absorbance coefficients are lower (see Fig. 5). In fact, we need about four molecules of porphyropsin to do the work of three molecules of rhodopsin (on the basis of their relative ε_{max}), but this simply has the effect of "weighting" their contributions to the absorbance spectrum of the mixture.

The most important characteristic of such mixtures is that their composition need not be fixed, but may range all the way from a pure porphyropsin condition to one where the retina contains pure rhodopsin, as illustrated in Fig. 12. Fishes

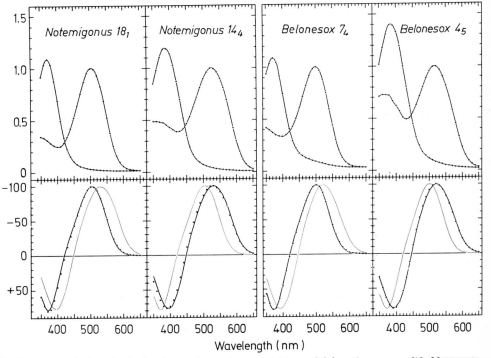

2. Extreme variations in rhodopsin-porphyropsin compositions of fish retinas, exemplified by spectra extracts from specimens of the freshwater cyprinid *Notemigonus crysoleucas* and the poeciliid *Belonesox* *nus*. The difference spectra (white light irradiation, alkaline conditions) are plotted as points in the lower of the figure, the continuous curves representing the pure difference spectrum of the preponderating nt in each case, and the dotted curves that of the pigment in lesser amount (based on BRIDGES, 1965a)

often fluctuate back and forth between these extremes in response to changing environmental influences or endogenous factors, while in amphibia the change is usually unidirectional and irreversible, associated with a permanent change of habitat at metamorphosis[4]. Effectively, from the standpoint of spectral sensitivity, the paired-pigment system is equivalent to a single visual pigment with continuously variable λ_{max}.

The inherent variability of these systems is the outcome of a very special relationship between the pigments of a pair. This becomes apparent if we plot the λ_{max} of rhodopsins against those of the porphyropsins associated with them. As shown in Fig. 13, the points lie close to a straight line which encompasses not only

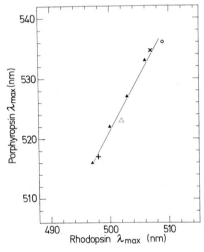

Fig. 13. Relationship between the λ_{max} of rhodopsins and of their corresponding porphyropsins. ▲, four pairs from SCHWANZARA (1967); ○, Coregonus (BRIDGES and YOSHIKAMI, 1970a); ×, Scardinius (BRIDGES and YOSHIKAMI, 1968); △, amphibia (see CRESCITELLI, 1958a, b; DARTNALL, 1962; WALD, 1960a for summaries); +, synthetic pair based on cattle opsin (WALD, BROWN, and SMITH, quoted by HUBBARD, 1958b)

fish visual pigments, but also the amphibian pair (rhodopsin 502 and porphyropsin 523) and, more significantly, the synthetic rhodopsin 497/porphyropsin 517 pair derived by WALD, BROWN, and SMITH from the single opsin of cattle retinas (quoted by HUBBARD, 1958b). In the light of this last observation, it seems that the most likely explanation for these findings is that the pigments of each *natural* pair are based on the same opsin, the only distinguishing feature being that the chromophoric groups differ. Further indirect evidence in support of this conclusion is to be found in results that will be discussed more fully in a later section. Briefly, it is found that whenever there is a change in the percentages of pigments in a pair, then a reciprocal relationship exists between the *quantities* of the two pigments — as one diminishes in amount the other increases (see Fig. 20, p. 454). Thus the total amount of pigment may remain nearly constant, even though the

---

[4] But see footnote no. 5.

proportions alter considerably, indicating that one has been converted directly into the other by a simple process of chromophoric-group replacement.

The various major conditions under which this substitution occurs will now be considered in detail for different groups of animals.

VII. Amphibians

A. Distribution and Metamorphosis of Visual Pigments

Adult terrestrial amphibians have rhodopsins with λ_{max} at 501—505 nm (CRESCITELLI, 1958a, b). In many instances the larval forms possess porphyropsin. Thus CRESCITELLI (1958a, b) showed that in *Hyla regilla* the very young larvae (tails, no limbs) had retinas containing pure porphyropsin (λ_{max} about 522 nm), intermediate larvae (tails, hind limbs) had 83% porphyropsin, advanced larvae (tails, fore and hind limbs) ranged from 75 to 60% porphyropsin while the adults had no porphyropsin at all, their retinas containing only rhodopsin. Similarly, the larvae of *Rana catesbeiana*, *R. esculenta* and *R. temporaria* have porphyropsin, which is absent from the adult retinas (WALD, 1947; CRESCITELLI, 1958a, b; MUNTZ and REUTER, 1966)[5]. However, as indicated in Fig. 14, it is likely that the rhodopsin system is never completely lacking in *R. temporaria*. In this species, unlike *Hyla*, the switch to pure rhodopsin is rather abrupt, and coincides with the emergence of the fore-limbs.[5]

Adult amphibians that have remained in the freshwater habitat where they were hatched have mainly porphyropsin in their retinas. Examples are *Necturus*, which retains many larval features, and *Xenopus*, which undergoes a metamorphic transformation similar to that found in *Rana* spp. (the porphyropsin λ_{max} are at 523 ± 1 nm; CRESCITELLI, 1958a, b; DARTNALL, 1956).

A good example of an amphibian with two habitat changes is the spotted newt *Diemyctylus viridescens*, which begins life as a gilled larva, becomes terrestrial as a red eft then returns to the water after 2—3 years to spawn and live out the remainder of its life. The visual pigments of the larva are unknown, but it appears that the terrestrial eft has a mixture of rhodopsin and porphyropsin (mainly the former) whereas the adult aquatic newt has switched to a (natal?) pure porphyropsin condition (WALD, 1952). On the other hand, *Taricha torosa*, a newt that is terrestrial in its adult form, has only rhodopsin (CRESCITELLI, 1958a).

In contrast to the species discussed above, tadpoles of the toads *Bufo boreas halophilus* and *Bufo bufo* have pure rhodopsin systems, as in the adult forms (CRESCITELLI, 1958a, b; MUNTZ and REUTER, 1966). Both species nevertheless exhibit the succession of metamorphic events and habitat changes characterising the life histories of *Rana* and *Hyla*. CRESCITELLI observes that his

---

[5] Since this was written, several new facts concerning the amphibian system have been discovered. Porphyropsin is not entirely lacking from the retina of the adult *R. catesbeiana*, and appears to be concentrated in the most dorsal one-third of it (T. REUTER, private communication, 1970). In *Rana* tadpoles (three species) exposure to light and darkness causes reversible interconversion of rhodopsin and porphyropsin. Thus in in darkness the amount of rhodopsin increases, while on transfer to the light the effect is reversed (BRIDGES, 1970b). Light-induced changes in the balance of rhodopsin and porphyropsin also occur in fishes (p. 457), although in this instance darkness favours *porphyropsin*.

specimens of *Bufo* and *Hyla* were taken from the same body of water, that their food was presumably the same and that their aquatic period of life was of about the same duration. As adults they are essentially terrestrial and nocturnal animals. According to Crescitelli, "These facts suggest that the possession of a dual system of this kind is an innate characteristic".[6]

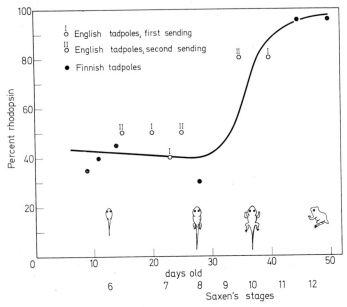

Fig. 14. Variation in the proportion of rhodopsin in retinal extracts of *Rana temporaria* during ontogenesis. Reproduced with permission from Muntz and Reuter (1966)

Recently, the metamorphosis of visual pigments in amphibia has been studied in single photoreceptors by the technique of microspectrophotometry (Liebman and Entine, 1968, see Chapter 12, p. 481). The rods of *R. pipiens* tadpoles contain porphyropsin (difference spectrum λ_{max} 527 nm), whereas those of the adult contain rhodopsin (difference spectrum λ_{max} ca. 502 nm). The absorbances are about the same, 0.016 per μm, in rods of about the same length in both forms. Of particular interest was the finding that at the time when the forelimbs were being completed at the expense of the tail, individual rods had mixtures of rhodopsin and porphyropsin. Cones were not examined at this stage of development, but in young tadpoles the cone pigments had maxima at 527 and 620 nm compared with 502 and 575 nm in the adult. Thus in the cones as well as the rods there appears to be a metamorphic switch from 3-dehydroretinaldehyde to retinaldehyde, while the same opsins are retained throughout life.

B. Mechanism of Visual Pigment Interconversions in Amphibia

The system that has been investigated in detail is that of the bullfrog, *Rana catesbeiana* (Wilt, 1959 a, b; Ohtsu, Naito, and Wilt, 1964). Second-year tadpoles

[6] See footnote no. 5.

have a mixture of 70—85 % porphyropsin and 15—30 % rhodopsin. Thyroxine, either added to the water or administered by intraperitoneal injection, induces not only the anatomical changes of metamorphosis but also a sharp increase in the proportion of rhodopsin, which rises to an average of 51 %.

One of the most interesting findings in WILT's work was the occurrence of parallel alterations in the balance of retinol/3-dehydroretinol stored in the pigmented ocular tissues (presumably mainly pigment epithelium rather than choroid).

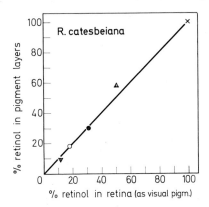

Fig. 15. Relationship between the compositions of retinols stored in the pigmented ocular tissues and the visual pigments in the retina during metamorphosis in *R. catesbeiana* (averaged data of WILT, 1959a). ▼, 1-year tadpoles; o, 2-year tadpoles; ●, tadpoles with ocular thyroid hormone implants; ▲, tadpoles kept in water containing thyroid hormone; ×, adult frogs

Thus the two-year old tadpoles had on average 18 % retinol in the pigmented layers, and this increased to 58 % after induction of metamorphosis. These results have been summarised and plotted in Fig. 15, which suggests that there is a direct proportionality between the rhodopsin/porphyropsin composition in the retina and that of the retinol/3-dehydroretinol supplies elsewhere in the eye.

In comparison, the liver and other tissues of both tadpole and adult contain only retinol, indicating that the ability to synthesise 3-dehydroretinol is a property of the ocular tissues alone. Direct confirmation of this was obtained by OHTSU, NAITO, and WILT (1964), who showed that when isolated eyes were treated with ^{3}H-retinol, there was extensive labelling of the 3-dehydroretinaldehyde prosthetic group of porphyropsin. In one experiment, for example, excised tadpole eyes were injected with ^{3}H-retinol and then incubated in darkness on a special organ culture medium. After 20 hours the visual pigments were extracted. The methods used after this stage involved extraction of 3-dehydroretinaldehyde released by bleaching the porphyropsin (77 %) with red light, followed by extraction of retinaldehyde liberated by bleaching the residual rhodopsin (23 %) with a terminal exposure to white light. Radioassays revealed that the retinaldehyde had a specific activity of 1400 cpm/μgm, while the 3-dehydroretinaldehyde activity was 1070 cpm/μgm.

Because the 3,4-dehydrogenation of retinol can take place in the isolated eye, it might be expected that thyroxine would act specifically at this site in the whole animal. In fact, before the 1964 experiment, this had been demonstrated in 1959 by Wilt, who implanted thyroxine pellets into the eyes of tadpoles. He found that a pellet introduced into one eye could induce a partial "metamorphosis" from porphyropsin to rhodopsin in that eye alone (Wilt, 1959b).

What biochemical changes occur in the eye during metamorphosis that lead to the formation of rhodopsin in preference to porphyropsin? We may discount any alterations in specificity of the water-soluble dehydrogenases and retinaldehyde isomerase, which can use indiscriminately both retinol and 3-dehydroretinol as substrates in the tadpole (Wilt, 1959a). Moreover, tadpole opsin can combine with 11-*cis* retinaldehyde to form a pigment spectroscopically indistinguishable from the adult rhodopsin. The change-over from 3-dehydroretinol to retinol in the ocular stores strongly suggests that thyroxine acts by impairing the ability to manufacture 3-dehydroretinol from retinol. Ohtsu, Naito and Wilt (1964) come to essentially the same conclusion. These authors also present limited evidence in favour of retinaldehyde as an intermediate in the production of 3-dehydroretinaldehyde from retinol (see scheme below), mainly on the basis that when ³H-retinol was injected intraperitoneally, a simultaneous intraocular injection of *unlabelled* retinaldehyde reduced the specific activity of 3-dehydroretinaldehyde extracted 20 hours later. On the other hand, 3-dehydroretinol did not have this effect. This is a rather remarkable finding, because we should expect that the alcohol should be readily converted into its aldehyde, and hence should reduce uptake of label by the porphyropsin.

The metabolic interrelationships of retinol and the visual pigments rhodopsin and porphyropsin are summarised in the scheme below. According to Ohtsu, Naito and Wilt, retinol would be transformed into the 3-dehydroretinaldehyde prosthetic group of porphyropsin by way of steps A, B and C. The other possibility involves steps A', B' and C. Because of its rapid conversion to retinol, free retinaldehyde is not usually detectable in the living eye, although it may have a fleeting existence in the photoreceptors during photolysis of the visual pigment. Thus reactions involving this compound might be restricted to the outer segments of the rods and cones. The alcohols formed from their respective aldehydes are probably speedily transferred to the pigment epithelium (cf. Dowling, 1960: see Fig. 3). A 3,4 *retinaldehyde* dehydrogenase might therefore occur in the retina, but a 3,4 *retinol* dehydrogenase would be found in the pigment epithelium.

Thyroxine would act by inhibiting the dehydrogenase at step A′ or B, which would lead to depletion of the supplies of 3-dehydroretinol and a switch to rhodopsin as the available opsin combines with retinaldehyde.

Failure of some species (e. g. *Bufo:* CRESCITELLI, 1958a; MUNTZ and REUTER, 1966) to manufacture porphyropsin probably reflects a congenital absence of the "terminal-ring" or 3,4-dehydrogenase in the ocular tissues.

VIII. Diadromous Fishes — Lampreys and Eels

The other major vertebrate group whose members make habitat transitions during their lifetimes includes the lampreys, eels and salmonids, which carry out diadromous migrations involving rivers and lakes on the one hand and the ocean on the other. From the standpoint of fish visual pigments, the sea takes the place of the land in the amphibian scheme of things. As in the amphibia, there are important hormonal and physiological changes prior to any major habitat transition.

Because there have been several reviews on the lampreys and eels (WALD, 1960a; CRESCITELLI, 1958a; DARTNALL, 1962), the following is intended to be no more than a brief summary.

A. Lampreys

Sea lampreys *(Petromyzon marinus)* start their lives in freshwater streams as blind ammocoetes which undergo a profound metamorphosis after several years prior to migrating to the ocean. After two or three years they become sexually mature and return upstream to spawn. Upstream migrants have porphyropsin (WALD, 1957). Unfortunately, the sea-running populations of this species have not been examined on their downstream migration, but both CRESCITELLI (1956) and WALD (1957) have reported the occurrence of pure rhodopsin in downstream migrants of *landlocked* populations. The latter swim only as far as the nearest lake, thus spending the whole of their lives in freshwaters. It is probable that sea-run lampreys would also have rhodopsin on their way downstream and that landlocked lampreys would have porphyropsin on their way back upstream from the lakes.

In *Petromyzon*, therefore, the switch from one pigment system to the other may anticipate the habitat change, and appears to be a completely useless or even disadvantageous relic of an earlier existence if the animal simply transfers from a stream to a freshwater lake, where there is no accompanying blue-shift of environmental light. Thus it is difficult to escape the conclusion that these changes are under some form of endocrine control, as in the frog.

In lampreys, as in amphibia, the possession of a dual pigment system is not the rule for all species. CRESCITELLI (1958a) examined downstream migrants of the Pacific Coast lamprey *Entosphenus tridentatus* and found the expected pure rhodopsin system. An unexpected finding, however, was that upstream migrants had rhodopsin also, and no trace of porphyropsin could be detected. CRESCITELLI admits that he has not had the opportunity to examine *Entosphenus* adults at their final destination on the spawning grounds, but at the moment it appears that this species might differ from *Petromyzon* in having lost or failed to acquire the ability to form porphyropsin.

B. Eels

The eel is spawned at depths of about 400 metres below the surface of the Western Atlantic breeding grounds, and as a larval leptocephalus it drifts for two years towards the coast of Europe. Once arrived, the leptocephali undergo metamorphosis to Elvers or Glass Eels and in large numbers commence the ascent of rivers. They then enter upon a prolonged growth phase, during which time they come to be known as Yellow Eels. At the end of this phase they are ready to undergo a second metamorphosis preparatory to the downstream migration and their prodigious 3000—4000 mile journey back to the spawning grounds[7]. The second metamorphosis takes place when the males are 8—10 years old and the females 10—18 years. At this stage they cease to feed, the alimentary tract withers, the reproductive organs develop, the eyes undergo enormous enlargement and the yellowish or greenish body colouration changes to a silvery lustre along the sides. They are now known as Silver Eels.

The sequence of visual pigment changes is no less remarkable (Carlisle and Denton, 1959; Brown and Brown, quoted by Wald, 1960a), although the story is rather patchy and more work needs to be done. Both the American and European species of *Anguilla* have dual pigment systems, with the rhodopsin maximum at 501 and the porphyropsin maximum at 523 nm. The presence of these two pigments in varying amounts characterises the retinas of immature yellow eels. At the stage of metamorphosis to the Silver Eels, but before the downstream expedition has begun, all the porphyropsin has been lost and the retinas contain only rhodopsin. But there is something odd about this rhodopsin. In some silver eels it has λ_{max} near 500 nm, as we would expect, but in others it ranges all the way down to 487 nm, near the position that is typical of the rhodopsins (or "chrysopsins") of deep-sea fish. Thus at least two visual pigment transitions are known to occur in the eel, the first involving replacement of 3-dehydroretinaldehyde by retinaldehyde with an accompanying shift of pigment λ_{max} from 523 to about 500 nm, the second by an *opsin* modification which adjusts the λ_{max} to wavelengths more appropriate to the abyssal blue of the future environment. Again, migratory movements are anticipated, suggesting that visual pigment alterations are governed by the metamorphic process itself, and are not a direct response to environment.

The pigments of the leptocephali and elvers are not known, although there has been some speculation (Wald, 1960a) that the former have the deep-sea rhodopsin of the sexually mature Silver Eels.

C. How do Eels Change their Rhodopsin into "Chrysopsin"?

The mechanism whereby one opsin is switched for another is unknown. Since the visual pigments are important structural components in the photoreceptor outer segments, where they may comprise an appreciable fraction of the dry weight (cf. Hubbard, 1954; see also Bridges, 1970a), the change might be expected

---

[7] The fact that they may not survive to reach these spawning grounds (Tucker, 1959) does not appreciably alter our discussion.

to be associated with massive reorganisation of photoreceptor proteins. Alternatively, there might be outright loss of the rhodopsin 500 cells and growth of new receptors containing rhodopsin 487. At the moment it is difficult to choose between these possibilities because there are no microspectrophotometric data of the kind that demonstrated the direct conversion of rhodopsin into porphyropsin *via* a transition mixture in isolated frog rods (LIEBMAN and ENTINE, 1968). However, if eel photoreceptor outer segments are continually renewed by the combined processes of growth from the inner segment and balanced loss at the opposite end, as occurs in rats, mice, frogs and probably fish (YOUNG, 1967; see p. 473), then the inner segments may simply go over to synthesising a different opsin when the time arrives. Consistent with this notion is the finding that although the eye may more than double its diameter during the yellow-to-silver metamorphosis, the total number of visual cells does not alter (CARLISLE and DENTON, 1959; the rod diameters are different, however, being 3 μm compared with 1.5 μm in the yellow eel condition).

D. Storage of Retinols in the Pigmented Ocular Tissues: Endocrine Factors in Metamorphosis

There is little or no 3-dehydroretinol in the livers of eels or lampreys (WALD, 1939a, 1941, 1942, 1957; CRESCITELLI, 1956). In lampreys, both upstream and downstream migrants were examined, but no difference was detectable. Unfortunately, only scanty information is available on storage of retinols in the ocular tissues. In a batch of eels examined by WALD (1939a) the pigmented layers of the eyes differed from the liver, but paralleled the porphyropsin-dominated retinal visual pigments in having a preponderance of 3-dehydroretinol (see Fig. 34, where this finding has been included). A similar situation was found in lampreys during their upstream journey, but downstream migrants were not investigated.

As noted previously, changes in the pigments of both species probably correspond with metamorphic events rather than with the immediate habitat. During metamorphosis in eels there appears to be increased activity of the pituitary and thyroid glands. In yellow eels the thyroids have large vesicles filled with colloid, whereas in silver eels the vesicles are small, scattered and have very little colloid, suggestive of an extensive discharge of secretion (D'ANCONA, 1960; also BARRINGTON, 1961). If the thyroid hormone acts in the same way as in the frog, then we should expect that the transformation of retinol into 3-dehydroretinol would be suppressed at this stage of development, resulting in the observed switch to a rhodopsin system.

In lampreys, the proper attainment of sexual maturity requires the action of the pituitary (e. g. LARSEN, 1965; HOAR, 1965), and during the spawning migration there are profound changes in endocrine activity. Even in these primitive cyclostomes, therefore, hormonal control of the 3,4-dehydrogenase system may be a means for influencing the rhodopsin-porphyropsin balance in the retinal photoreceptors.

IX. Diadromous Fishes — the Salmonidae

A. Introduction

The salmonidae belong to a suborder of fishes that includes many families with members that have invaded a variety of ecological niches. The families of the suborder Salmonoidei (order Clupeiformes) are the Osmeridae, Salmonidae, Argentinidae, Retropinnatidae, Salangidae, Aplochitonidae and Plecoglossidae. Although not all the families have been examined, it is clear from existing data that the visual pigments in this suborder show the same degree of variety as in the other fishes. The deep-sea Argentinidae *Bathylagus wesethi* Bolin and *B. microphalus* Norman (MUNZ, 1958b; DARTNALL and LYTHGOE, 1965) have deep-sea rhodopsins with maxima at 478 and 468 nm respectively. The grayling, *Thymallus*, is a purely freshwater fluviatile species, and has a porphyropsin with maximum at 527 nm (BRIDGES, 1965a). The smelt, *Osmerus*, is migratory, ascending streams to spawn, although it may never enter purely freshwaters. A group of upstream migrants taken in March/April on the River Conway (N. Wales) had retinas containing pure porphyropsin with the unusually high λ_{max} of 543 nm (BRIDGES, 1965a). It is not known whether this species has rhodopsin at other times (the American smelt has appreciable amounts of rhodopsin; see Table 2, BRIDGES, unpublished).

Until recently, the visual pigments of the Salmonidae received little attention, the only observations being those of WALD (1941), BRIDGES (1956) and DARTNALL (1962) who found rhodopsin-porphyropsin mixtures in some species. In the last few years, however, this group has been studied in considerable detail by several investigators. Fundamentally, fishes of the family are distinguished by the anadromous habit. That is, they live in salt water and spawn in fresh, although

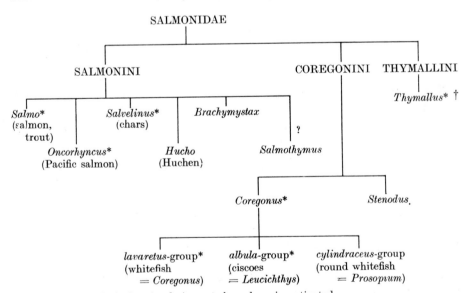

* Genera in which the visual pigments have been investigated.

† Note that *Thymallus* is now included in the Salmonidae (NORDEN, 1961).

some species have become strictly freshwater despite the fact that they derive from anadromous ancestors. The classification of this family is summarised above.

These fishes form a highly plastic group, which appears to be in a state of active evolution and speciation, particularly in the coregonines. The latter form an extremely complex sub-family with members distributed throughout northern Europe, Asia and North America. There is no general agreement on the classification of the coregonines (whitefishes, *sensu lato*). North American workers usually recognise four genera, i. e. *Coregonus*, *Leucichthys*, *Prosopium* and *Stenodus* (cf. SMITH, 1957; KOELZ, 1929, 1931; NORDEN, 1961), while SVÄRDSON (1957, 1965) groups the first three together under the single genus *Coregonus*, as illustrated above.

The major genera of the salmonidae may undergo extensive migrations, always spawning in freshwater. The basic pattern of these migrations is discussed in detail on p. 448. The migratory habit, coupled with a low tolerance for high temperatures, has played an important part in the present-day circumpolar distribution of these fishes, and preference for cooler waters has led to isolation of many species in lakes during the succession of ice ages. Examples are *Coregonus* and *Salvelinus*, originally pushed south in the face of the advancing ice-sheets, which were also creating the conditions for lateral westward migration into Britain from Eurasia by producing ice-dammed lakes in northward-flowing rivers. As warmer conditions prevailed and the ice receded, so many remained as "glacial relicts" trapped in such lakes as Baikal in the U.S.S.R., the Great Lakes in N. America, Bodensee in Germany and Lough Neagh in Northern Ireland. Others are found in Fennoscandia, where they may pass between rivers and the brackish waters of the Baltic Sea.

Some species may be migratory in one area but not in another. Thus *Salmo trutta* includes both the anadromous sea trout and the freshwater brown trout; *S. gairdnerii* includes the freshwater Rainbow and the anadromous Steelhead of Vancouver Island. Land-locking also occurs in populations of *S. salar* (salmon), *Salvelinus* and *Oncorhyncus*. As in lampreys, migratory movements associated with spawning may still take place, but these may involve nothing more than a short trip from lake to tributary as occurs in the kokanee (one of the Pacific salmons) and rainbow trout (see, e.g., CARTWRIGHT, 1961). These isolations play an important role in speciation. Thus after isolation for more than 15,000 years the difference between *Salvelinus* populations in the British Isles and the ancestral *S. alpinus* was sufficient to persuade TATE REGAN (1911) that they represented 15 distinct native species (see also REGAN, 1932). Modern workers, however, tend to place them no higher than subspecies. In *Coregonus* the situation is also complicated. In the British Isles, this genus exists in at least five forms in as many lakes. They are known by the vernacular names of Powan, Pollan, Skelly or Schelly, Gwyniad and Vendace. In the Bodensee there are four co-existing species (degraded by some authors to the status of ecotypes). These are known as Blaufelchen, Gangfisch, Kilch and Sandfelchen (WAGLER, 1950; KARBE, 1964a, b). This situation may arise from the development of sibling species evolved in allopatric isolation during glacial periods followed by sympatric meeting of these species. According to SVÄRDSON (1957, 1958, 1965) introgression may subsequently occur (see also KARBE, 1964a). Human interference has played its part also, by the introduction of new coregonines into lakes where indigenous populations already

Table 2. *Salmonid visual pigments*

Common name	Specific name	Source	λ_{max} (nm)		Autho
			Rhodopsin	Porphyropsin[a]	
Pink salmon	*Oncorhyncus gorbuscha* (Walbaum)	N. America	503	527	[1]
Chum salmon	*Oncorhyncus keta* (Walbaum)	N. America	503	527	[1]
Coho salmon	*Oncorhyncus kisutch* (Walbaum)	N. America	503	527	[1]
Sockeye salmon	*Oncorhyncus nerka* (Walbaum)	N. America	503	527	[1]
King salmon	*Oncorhyncus tshawytscha* (Walbaum)	N. America	503	527	[1]
Cutthroat trout	*Salmo clarkii* Richardson	N. America	503	527	[1]
Rainbow trout	*Salmo gairdneri* Richardson	N. America	503	527	[1]
		England	504	526	[2]
Atlantic salmon	*Salmo salar* L.	N. America	503	527	[1]
Brown trout	*Salmo trutta* L.	N. America	503	527	[1]
		England	503	527	[2]
Brook char, brook trout	*Salvelinus fontinalis* (Mitchill)	N. America	503	527	[2]
		England	503	527	[3]
Dolly Varden	*Salvelinus malma* (Walbaum)	N. America	503	527	[3]
		N. America	512	($\sim$545)	[3]
Lake char	*Salvelinus namaycush* (Walbaum)	N. America	511	540[f]	[2]
Arctic char[b]	*Salvelinus alpinus*, L.	N. America	509	—	[3]
Saibling	*Salvelinus alpinus*, L.	Königsee, (Germany)	508	+	[4]
Torgoch[c]	*Salvelinus perisii* (Günther)[c]	Llyn Padarn (Wales)	508	+	[4]
Willoughby's char[c]	*Salvelinus willughbii* (Günther)[c]	L. Windermere (England)	508	+	[4, 5]
Grayling	*Thymallus thymallus* L.	R. Nadder (England)	—	527	[6]
Powan	*Coregonus clupeoides* Lacépède	L. Lomond (Scotland)	—	536	[5]
Pollan	*Coregonus pollan* Thompson	L. Neagh (N. Ireland)	—	536	[5]
Schelly, skelly	*Coregonus clupeoides stigmaticus* Regan	Ullswater (England)	510	+	[5]
Gwyniad	*Coregonus clupeoides pennantii* C. & V.	Llyn Tegid (Wales)	520	—	[6]
Cumberland vendace	*Coregonus vandesius gracilior* Regan	Bassenthwaite (England)	510	+	[5]
Blaufelchen	*Coregonus wartmannii* (Bloch)	Bodensee (Germany)	510	+	[4]
Gangfisch	*Coregonus macrophthalmus* Nüsslin	Bodensee (Germany)	510	+	[4]
Renke[d]	*Coregonus species*[d]	Würmsee (Germany)	509	536	[4]
Renke[d]	*Coregonus species*[d]	Kochelsee (Germany)	509	+	[4]
Smelt, sparling brwyniad	*Osmerus eperlanus* L.[e]	R. Conway (Wales)	—	543	[5]
American smelt	*Osmerus eperlanus mordax* (Mitchill)	N. America (Canada, P. Q.)	512	543	[2]

Authors: [1] Munz and Beatty (1965); [2] Bridges, unpublished; [3] Munz and McFarland (19
[4] Bridges and Yoshikami, (1970a); [5] Bridges (1967b); [6] Bridges (1965a).

existed (cf. DOTTRENS, 1959). Amid all the phenotypic plasticity displayed by the coregonines, the gill-raker numbers apparently remain fairly constant features, and are used as a basis for classification (SVÄRDSON, 1957).

In summary, the salmonids comprise a family where most genera are of fairly recent origin, evolving in late Pliocene or early Pleistocene times. Unfortunately, we cannot say whether the common ancestor was freshwater or marine. It may have been estuarine. The migratory habit characterises the group, although landlocking plays an important role in speciation.

B. Visual Pigments of the Salmonidae

The visual pigments of the Salmonidae are summarised in Table 2. Examination of this table reveals the existence of certain major groupings. Thus all species of the genera *Salmo* and *Oncorhyncus* possess a rhodopsin with maximum at 503 nm. Always this is mixed in varying amounts with the corresponding porphyropsin 527, which occurs as a pure pigment in the retina of *Thymallus*. We therefore conclude that only one visual protein, that giving rise to the rhodopsin 503/porphyropsin 527 pair, occurs in all species examined in the genera *Salmo*, *Oncorhyncus* and *Thymallus*. There are two species in the genus *Salvelinus* that also possess this protein, but the others have proteins yielding rhodopsins with maxima ranging from 508 to 512 nm. All varieties of *Salvelinus alpinus* (including *S. perisii* and *S. willughbii*) have rhodopsin 508−509, usually mixed with a small amount of an unidentified porphyropsin.

In the genus *Coregonus* the rhodopsin usually absorbs in about the same position as that of *S. alpinus*, the λ_{max} lying at 509−510 nm (Fig. 8). Again, this rhodopsin is always mixed with porphyropsin, frequently in amounts too small to identify. However, in the case of the Renken from the Würmsee, this porphyropsin was present in amounts up to 84 %, thus permitting an accurate analysis which established that its λ_{max} lay at 536 nm (see Fig. 8). The selfsame porphyropsin is found *in isolation* in two British coregonines. Thus one visual protein, that giving rise to rhodopsin 509−510/porphyropsin 536, occurs in eight of the nine coregonines examined. The remaining coregonine, the gwyniad, has evolved a new protein, which is the basis of its rhodopsin 520.

The taxonomic positions of these coregonines are problematical. The vendace is undoubtedly a cisco belonging to the *albula*-group, yet its visual pigment is no different from that possessed by other coregonines which belong to the *lavaretus*-group. Following SVÄRDSON (1957) we classify the coregonines of Table 2 in the following Table 3.

Footnotes to Table 2

[a] The + sign indicates the undoubted presence of a porphyropsin, but in amounts too small to identify its absorption maximum.

[b] A single extract only.

[c] These populations are better regarded as subspecies of *S. alpinus*.

[d] The taxonomic status of these populations is considered in the text.

[e] No longer included in the Salmonidae. Collected in brackish water during their spawning migration upstream in March/April.

[f] Estimated ± 2 nm.

Thus although the gwyniad is the odd member of this series from the standpoint of its visual pigments, its taxonomic position would not lead us to expect this. Even on the basis of the nomenclature used in Table 2, the gwyniad is grouped with schelly and powan under *C. clupeoides*. Although we would hesitate to claim that visual pigments alone should be used as a basis for fish taxonomy, the possession of a distinct visual protein indicates that the gwyniad differs genotypically as well as phenotypically from its British and European neighbours.

Table 3. *Classification of the coregonines of Table 2 according to* Svärdson (1957), *based on gill-raker counts of* Dottrens *and* Wagler

Group	Species	Vernacular name
lavaretus	*C. lavaretus* (L.)	Powan Blaufelchen Renke (Kochelsee)
	C. oxyrhyncus (L.)	Gangfisch Pollan Schelly Gwyniad Renke (Würmsee)
albula	*C. albula* (L.)	Cumberland vendace

C. Inheritance of Visual Pigments in the Genus *Salvelinus*

A fascinating study by McFarland and Munz (1965) has revealed a simple pattern of visual pigment inheritance in two species of *Salvelinus* (Table 4). Thus hybrids ("splake") of Brook char (rhodopsin 503) and Lake char (rhodopsin 512) had mixtures of the two parental rhodopsins. F_2 splake had the pure pigments or mixtures in 1 : 2 : 1 ratios compared with 1 : 1 for the backcross. These results are indicative of single-factor inheritance with codominance. At the moment, we do not know whether this type of inheritance is applicable to all salmonids (and other families).

Table 4. *Frequency distribution of visual pigments in parental and hybrid chars (from* McFarland *and* Munz, 1965). *Only the rhodopsins are considered here: because of the difficulty of analysing two rhodopsins and two porphyropsins in the hybrid it was decided to bleach the mixture and regenerate the rhodopsins alone by the addition of 11-cis retinaldehyde*

	Rhodopsin 503	Rhodopsin 503 + 512	Rhodopsin 512
Brook	7	0	0
Lake	0	0	19
F_1 splake	0	12	0
F_2 splake	4	8	3
Backcross ($F_1 \times$ Brook)	8	7	0

D. Possible Evolutionary Pathways in the Visual Pigments of the Salmonidae

Evolution of visual pigments in the salmonids probably followed several pathways. If the ancestral type was marine, it could have possessed a rhodopsin with maximum in the region of 500 nm, perhaps at 503 nm, in the same position as the present-day *Salmo* and *Oncorhyncus* pigments. Development of the anadromous habit may have involved a sojourn in inshore waters and estuaries. Here, the need for enhanced red-sensitivity could have been met in one of the two ways exemplified by modern non-salmonid inhabitants of these waters, as shown below.

The visual pigments shown for the species in Table 5 are either high-λ_{max} rhodopsins or paired pigments. The latter confer the ability to vary the "effective" λ_{max} from about 500 nm to as high as 523 nm. The maximum of a rhodopsin can be shifted towards the red end of the spectrum by modification of the opsin. The production of porphyropsin in the paired-pigment system, however, required the ability to convert retinol into 3-dehydroretinol, and hence the fish must have evolved a "terminal-ring dehydrogenase" mediating 3,4-dehydrogenation of the β-ionone ring of retinol or retinaldehyde. It is likely that this step has occurred not once but several times in fish evolution.

Table 5. *Visual pigments of fishes frequenting fresh, brackish and turbid marine waters in the coastal zone of N. America (from* BRIDGES, *1965a)*

Species	λ_{max} of		Ref.
	rhodopsin	porphyropsin	
Seriphus politus	504	—	[1]
Embiotoca jacksoni	504	—	[1]
Hyperprosopon argenteum	506	—	[1]
Cyprinodon variegatus	506	—	[2]
Anchoa compressa	508	—	[1]
Atherinops affinis	508	—	[1]
Cottus spp.	511	—	[1]
Leptocottus armatus	511	—	[1]
Clevelandia ios	512	—	[1]
Eucyclogobius newberryi	512	—	[1]
Gillichthys mirabilis	512	—	[3]
Sphoeroides annulatus	500	522	[1]
Belonesox belizanus	498	521	[2]
Mollienesia latipinna	502	525	[2]
Mugil curema	499	522	[2]
Mugil cephalus	499	522	[2]
Dorosoma cepedianum	500	521	[2]

[1] MUNZ, 1958a. [2] BRIDGES, 1964b, 1965b. [3] MUNZ, 1956.

Evidence suggests that opsin modification would not proceed continuously but would occur in steps or jumps (BRIDGES, 1964b, 1965b). As in other proteins, we might expect that each evolutionary jump would represent an amino-acid substitution, perhaps altering the λ_{max} by stabilising a new resonance form of the retinaldehyde chromophore (cf. Hubbard and Kropf, 1965; see also Dartnall and Lythgoe, 1965; Munz and McFarland, 1965; McFarland and Munz, 1965). Discontinuous variation would lead to the evolution of pigments with maxima separated by discrete intervals. For rhodopsins this interval has been estimated at about 6 nm compared with about 10 nm for the porphyropsins (Bridges, 1965b). Although such grouping is not particularly evident in salmonid visual pigments, it is noteworthy that the two porphyropsins have maxima separated by 9 nm, and their two corresponding rhodopsins are separated by 6 nm. Munz and McFarland (1965) suggested that visual pigment proteins were determined by a series of multiple alleles. In the case of *Salvelinus* we know that a change of one of these alleles can result in a shift of rhodopsin λ_{max} amounting to as much as 9 nm. Other changes may produce shifts that are greater or less than this, perhaps averaging 6 nm or some multiple of this figure.

A scheme illustrating the possible relationships of salmonid visual pigments, starting with the rhodopsin 503 of a hypothetically marine ancestor, is given below.

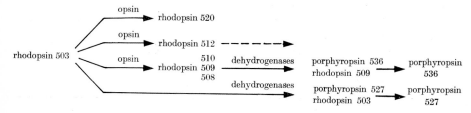

The step from a rhodopsin 509 to a porphyropsin 536 would require development of a terminal-ring dehydrogenase, probably in the pigment epithelium (p. 474). Perhaps several enzymes having different efficacies are involved, determined by a corresponding number of alleles (an example of enzyme polymorphism ?, cf. Harris, 1966). Thus individual variation of the proportions of rhodopsin and porphyropsin in the Würmsee coregonines (11—84 % porphyropsin) might reflect a genetic (rather than phenotypic) variability in the population, where the porphyropsin-rich condition is subject to selection pressure as time goes on, finally culminating in the pollan/powan situation (similar steps may have been involved in development of the *Thymallus* porphyropsin 527, perhaps from an early salmonine with rhodopsin 503). The other coregonines may be at earlier stages of development, as may be the case with some populations of *Salvelinus alpinus*, which differ in their porphyropsin proportions. Thus one specimen of North American *S. alpinus* examined by Munz and McFarland (1965) had pure rhodopsin 509 $\pm$ 2. Bridges and Yoshikami (1970a) found that three landlocked populations had the following compositions: (a) the Königsee group (11 fish) had rhodopsin 508 with no porphyropsin; (b) the Llyn Padarn group (4 fish) had rhodopsin 508 with about 4 % porphyropsin; (c) a group from L. Windermere (5 fish) had rhodopsin 508 and averaged as much as 24 % porphyropsin, with individuals ranging from 0—51 %.

We do not know why one method should be preferred to another in the evolution of a red-sensitive pigment. Sudden appearance of an allele for a high-λ_{max} rhodopsin would obviously reduce selection pressure for a retinol/3-dehydroretinol switch. On the other hand, this allele might confer little or no further advantage in a population that had already evolved an efficient terminal-ring dehydrogenase. At one stage in the investigation of coregonine visual pigments by BRIDGES and YOSHIKAMI (1970a), it was thought that the gwyniad might be unable to synthesise 3-dehydroretinol in any of its tissues. This is not the case, although it is true that the liver of this species contains less 3-dehydroretinol (15 % on average) than found in other coregonines (see curve 1, Fig. 32). However, as pointed out elsewhere (p. 467), there is usually little relationship between eye pigments and liver retinols. Blaufelchen, for example, average over 80 % 3-dehydro-retinol in the liver compared with only 2.5 % porphyropsin in the retina.

An estimate of the time-scale required for evolution of a new pigment raises difficulties[8]. The unit step in evolution is substitution of one allele A^2 for another A^1 by selective death of individuals carrying gene A^1. As discussed above, this can lead to substitution of one amino acid for another in a polypeptide chain. In the cytochromes c, haemoglobins, and triosephosphate dehydrogenases it has been estimated that one evolutionarily effective amino acid substitution has occurred on average once every 28,000,000 years per 100 amino-acid chain (for references, see KIMURA, 1968). Bovine rhodopsin has 235 amino acid residues (HELLER, 1968a), and would therefore substitute one amino acid every 12,000,000 years on the basis of these proteins. However, since fewer amino acids must be implicated in the binding of retinaldehyde to rhodopsin, and since only these amino acids would be expected to influence light-absorption, the time required for evolution of a high-λ_{max} rhodopsin should be even longer. In the haemoglobins, ZUCKERKANDL and PAULING (1965) estimated that the chance for any *given* changeable site to be changed evolutionarily is once in 800,000,000 years, which would take us back to the pre-Cambrian era!

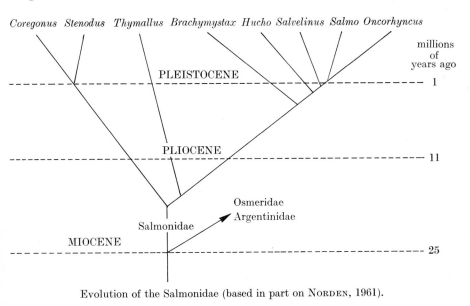

Evolution of the Salmonidae (based in part on NORDEN, 1961).

---

[8] A more recent discussion is presented by BRIDGES and YOSHIKAMI (1970a).

Available fossil evidence indicates that the Osmeridae and Argentinidae (represented now by such genera as *Osmerus* and *Bathylagus*) were separated from the Salmonidae about 25,000,000 years ago, at the beginning of the Miocene era. The salmonini, coregonini and thymallini may have diverged into three phyletic lines later during the Miocene, which ended 11,000,000 years ago, but the modern genera and species probably originated as recently as the late Pliocene or early Pleistocene, perhaps only 1,000,000 years ago. Hence while the coregonines and salmonines have been separated for a possible 18,000,000 years, it appears that a million years or less is sufficient time for development of separate visual proteins in species such as *Salvelinus fontinalis* and *Salvelinus alpinus*. If relicts such as the gwyniad evolved new pigments *subsequent* to isolation at the end of the last glacial epoch, then the period involved is a mere 10,000—20,000 years. While true speciation can occur over such short time periods under similar conditions of isolation (HERRE, 1933; MYERS, 1960), this finding would indicate a remarkably high rate of protein evolution resulting from particularly intensive selection pressure. If visual pigments are always inherited with codominance (McFARLAND and MUNZ, 1965), the presence of only one pigment in the gwyniad suggests that it is now homozygous for this condition. An investigation of other proteins in this species and its close relatives might be particularly rewarding, and would help towards a clearer insight into the problems of protein evolution.

E. The Rhodopsin-Porphyropsin System of the Pacific Salmon

The visual pigments of all five North American species of the Pacific salmon have been subjected to penetrating and exhaustive study by BEATTY (1966) at many stages of their life-history. The sixth known species, *Oncorhyncus masou*, has not been investigated. The visual pigments and vernacular names of these salmons are listed in Table 2.

The life-history of the salmon is basically similar in all species, although the details may differ, particularly with respect to the times spent in different environments, and the distance of the spawning grounds from the sea. After hatching in freshwater, the fry may move down to the sea in some species (pink and chum) or remain in freshwaters for several years. These latter grow to the parr stage and finally undergo a parr-smolt metamorphosis in which a thin layer of guanine is deposited in the scales and physiological changes in preparation for the salt water life occur. This transformation is probably under endocrine control. It is present in Atlantic salmon *(Salmo salar)*, steelhead, coho, king and sockeye but has been suppressed or lost in pink and chum.

A period is now spent in the ocean, feeding and growing until the time comes to pass into the estuaries and upstream to spawn. Once spawned, it is doubtful whether any Pacific salmon survive to re-enter the sea, although spawned kelts of the Atlantic salmon may do so, after which they may return another year to the spawning grounds.

Ocean-caught coho salmon *(O. kisutch)* have retinas dominated by rhodopsin. As the fish moved into tidewater, BEATTY found that there was a gradual switch towards porphyropsin, until at the spawning site after the upstream migration was over, porphyropsin often accounted for over 90 % of the visual pigment. This is clearly illustrated in Fig. 16.

King and pink salmon (*O. tshawytscha* and *O. gorbuscha* respectively) displayed exactly the same transition from a predominantly rhodopsin retina in the ocean to a porphyropsin-dominated condition during their journeys upstream to the freshwater spawning ground.

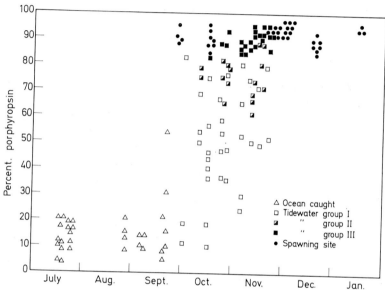

Fig. 16. Variation in the proportion of porphyropsin in individual adult coho salmon during their pre-spawning return to freshwaters. Tidewater group I have external appearances identical with ocean-caught fish. The appearance of tidewater group III is nearly identical with that of adults collected at the spawning site. Tidewater group II is intermediate in appearance. Reproduced with permission from BEATTY (1966)

In the sockeye *(O. nerka)*, however, the retinas always had a predominance of rhodopsin, and only a slight shift to porphyropsin occurred during the upstream migration. The landlocked sibling species, known as the kokanee, likewise possessed a rhodopsin-dominated retina, which shifted only a few percent towards porphyropsin during spawning. BRIDGES (1967c) had found that landlocked Windermere char *(Salvelinus willughbii = S. alpinus)* were similar in having rhodopsin-dominated retinas during spring and autumn spawning, although there is no information on immature or non-spawning specimens of this fish.

Thus, with the exception of the sockeye, BEATTY has obtained clear evidence for a succession of rhodopsin and porphyropsin in the Pacific salmon similar to that found in lampreys and eels, and related to the changes in habitat that this family experiences during its transit to the spawning grounds. As with the lampreys and eels, there is some evidence that the pigment adaptation to freshwater is anticipated, because fish that had only just entered tidewater a few hours before were found to be in possession of a high proportion of porphyropsin.

The switch from a retinaldehyde to a 3-dehydroretinaldehyde prosthetic group is therefore influenced by factors unconnected with the immediate environment.

What is the situation in juvenile salmon, spawned and reared in freshwaters before the migratory urge drives them seaward? Unfortunately we have little information on the situation in the wild. Hatchery-reared king and coho, according to Beatty, start out in winter as fry with relatively high proportions of porphyropsin that diminish to a minimum in summer, but then rise again as winter approaches and the smolt are released for their downstream migration (Fig. 17). Clearly, at some subsequent stage there must be a transformation to rhodopsin, but whether this occurs before the fish enter the sea or afterwards, perhaps this time in response to the immediate habitat, is not known.

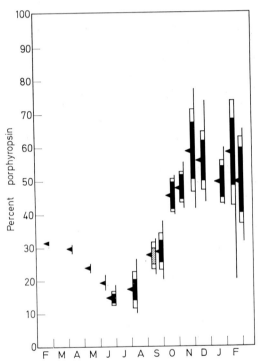

Fig. 17. Changes of retinal porphyropsin in hatchery-reared juvenile coho salmon, starting with sac fry in February and ending with smolt in February of the following year. The shaded bar is a single collection of "wild" juveniles collected near the hatchery. The vertical line represents the range, the white area outlines one standard deviation from the mean, the dark area represents two standard errors of the mean. Reproduced with permission from Beatty (1966)

We noted above that sockeye adults had much less porphyropsin than the other species, even when spawning; the juveniles are similar in that they have comparatively little porphyropsin at all stages of their hatchery lives.

The amount of rhodopsin in the retinas of coho and king salmon increased when Beatty (1966) transferred juvenile fish to outdoor tanks where they were exposed to higher light intensities than was usual in the dimly-lit tanks of the hatchery.

The phenomenon was not dependent on day-length, because both indoor and outdoor groups were exposed to natural daylight, which differed only in intensity. A "light-effect" of this type had been reported for Rainbow and Brown trout by DARTNALL (1962) and has been the subject of very extensive studies in non-migratory paired-pigment cyprinids and a poeciliid, as will be discussed fully in the next section. It is very likely, therefore, that the seasonally varying retinal pigment composition of juvenile king and coho salmon is attributable to the combined action of light intensity and duration, for rhodopsin is present in highest proportion in midsummer, when sunlight is strongest and days are long. In contrast, porphyropsin is the major pigment during the shorter days and weaker light of winter.

The effect of light was not tested in the adults. Inspection of Fig. 16, however, might lead to the supposition that light is the factor that leads to a switch from rhodopsin in July, August and September to porphyropsin during spawning in autumn and winter. BEATTY asserts that this cannot be the case, however, and lists the following supporting evidence. (A) Immature salmon taken from the high seas in winter possess "almost entirely" rhodopsin; (B) adult *spring-run* king salmon taken in freshwaters in June have predominantly porphyropsin. As in the case of eels and lampreys, therefore, it is difficult to escape the conclusion that pigment changes in migrating *Oncorhyncus* are governed by endocrine events associated with the advancement of sexual maturity. This is reinforced by BEATTY's observations in the "tidewater" groups of coho salmon in Fig. 16, where the retinal visual pigment composition seems to be correlated with external appearances of the fish. In the Rainbow trout there is some evidence for hormonal control of visual pigments, where MUNZ and SWANSON (1965) claimed that fish kept in water containing thyroxine increased the proportion of porphyropsin in their retinas (note the opposite effect of thyroxine in frogs, but see also p. 463)[9]. Thiourea apparently had an antagonistic action. In this connexion, it is curious that the visual pigments of juvenile salmon remain completely unaffected during the parr-smolt metamorphosis in the months of November and December (e.g. in Fig. 17). Endocrine changes associated with smolting appear to involve the hypothalamic-pituitary system (if not the thyroid; HOAR, 1965) and result in profound physiological and behavioural reorganisation before the salt water phase of existence commences. Perhaps these changes differ fundamentally from those occurring during the pre-spawning return, or possibly the ocular tissues do not respond for several months, until downstream migration is properly under way.

Further evidence that different systems affect the visual pigments of juveniles is provided by the finding that although there is a clear relationship between rhodopsin-porphyropsin proportions and liver retinols in adult migrants (Fig. 18), none can be detected in the young fish. In this respect they resemble the non-migratory species discussed on p. 461. BEATTY did not analyse the pigment epithelium retinols under these variable circumstances. However, WALD's earlier studies (WALD, 1939a) with the salmonids *Oncorhyncus tshawytscha*, *Salmo gairdnerii*, and *Salvelinus fontinalis* had indicated a close correspondence between

---

[9] Recent work by BEATTY (1969) has convincingly demonstrated that thyroid hormones (tetraiodothyronine and 3:5:3′ triiodothyronine) induce a conversion from rhodopsin to porphyropsin when injected into juvenile kokanee salmon.

their retinal pigment proportions and the composition of the retinol/3-dehydroretinol supplies in the pigment epithelium. This correspondence is also found in other fishes (see Fig. 34, p. 468) and has been noted in the case of the frog on p. 435.

To summarise our discussion up to this point — many adult salmons, eels, lampreys and amphibians switch visual pigments in response to endocrine events associated with metamorphosis or attainment of sexual maturity. These effects serve to adapt the animal to its approaching new environment, which may be terrestrial (rhodopsin) in the case of the frog, freshwater (porphyropsin) in the case of the spawning salmon, the ocean (rhodopsin) in the case of the lamprey or the deep sea ("chrysopsin") in the eel. Light regime can alter the pigments of juvenile salmon, and this is probably effected by the same mechanism as in non-migratory species, which will now be discussed.

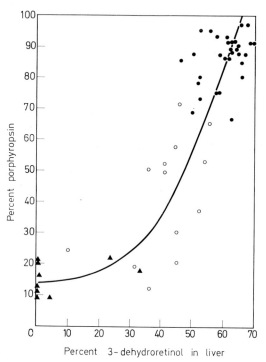

Fig. 18. Comparison of the compositions of retinal visual pigments and liver retinols in individual adult coho salmon during their pre-spawning return to freshwaters. ▲, ocean-caught; ○, tidewater group I; ●, tidewater groups II, III and spawning site fish (see Fig. 16 for explanation of these groups). Reproduced with permission from Beatty (1966)

X. Non-Migratory Fishes

A. Introduction

Some fishes of inshore waters possess the paired-pigment system (see Table 5). Strictly speaking, they are not migratory, although they may pass freely between

fresh and salt waters. Examples of this group are the mullets *(Mugil* spp*)* and
Dorosoma. A dual rhodopsin-porphyropsin system is also characteristic of about
half of the purely freshwater fishes examined to date (for summaries, see BRIDGES,
1965b, c; SCHWANZARA, 1967). The important common feature is that all these
fishes occupy aquatic habitats where there is considerable fluctuation in spectral
light quality from place to place and time to time (see Figs 10, 11, 21). This
fluctuation is attributable to the presence of scattering particles, dissolved products
of vegetable decay (the humic acids) and chlorophyll, all present in varying
amounts. As stated previously, the essential property of the rhodopsin-porphyropsin pair is that its composition is highly variable; hence its presence in
fishes living in habitats with variable spectral light distributions. In the freshwater fishes (the other groups have not been thoroughly investigated) the proportions of these two pigments are influenced by a variety of circumstances. These
are considered below.

B. Variation in the Natural Environment

1. Time of Year

The finding that retinal pigment composition varied in synchrony with the
seasons (DARTNALL, LANDER, and MUNZ, 1961) led to most of the investigations
discussed in this final section. The freshwater cyprinid *Scardinius erythrophthalmus*
has a pair of pigments, where the rhodopsin has λ_{max} at 507 and the porphyropsin

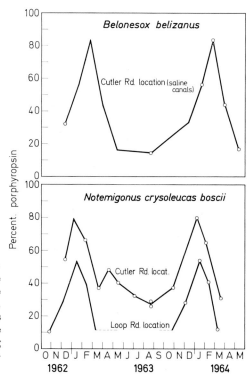

Fig. 19. Seasonal variation of visual pigment composition in the retinas of the
cyprinid *Notemigonus* (from two separate
locations) and the poeciliid *Belonesox*.
Where no points are shown at the angles
in the three graphs, the figures for the
same month of the following or preceding
year have been transposed (from BRID-
GES, 1964a)

at 535 nm (Bridges and Yoshikami, 1968). Dartnall *et al.* showed that batches
of this species taken at various times from the same outdoor pond had maximum
proportions of rhodopsin in the summer and that these dropped to a minimum in
the winter. Similar findings apply to another cyprinid *Notemigonus crysoleucas*
(rhodopsin 503/porphyropsin 529) and a poeciliid *Belonesox belizanus* (rhodopsin
498/porphyropsin 522) as shown in Fig. 19 (Bridges, 1964a, 1965c). Thus the
sequence of visual pigments with time of year is much the same as in juvenile
salmon (Beatty, 1966).

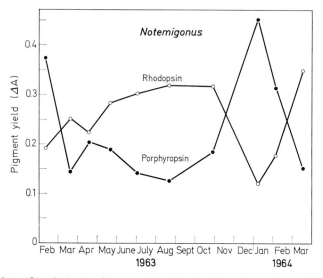

Fig. 20. Reciprocal variation in the amounts of rhodopsin and porphyropsin in *Notemigonus*
retinas throughout the year. ○, rhodopsin; ●, porphyropsin. From Bridges, 1965a

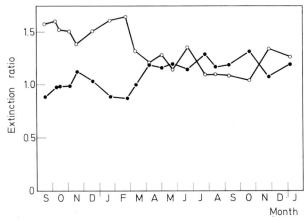

Fig. 21. Variability of extinction ratios $\varepsilon_v^{430}/\bar{\varepsilon}_v$ (●) and $\varepsilon_v^{630}/\bar{\varepsilon}_v$ (○) in Lake Maggiore.
ε_v^{λ} = vertical extinction coefficient for wavelength λ (630 and 430 nm in the present case):
$\bar{\varepsilon}_v = -\ln\left[1/3(T^{630} + T^{530} + T^{430})\right]$, where T^{λ} is the percentage transmission for wavelength
λ of a layer of water 1 metre thick. Based on Vollenweider (1961)

In *Notemigonus* there is clear evidence for a reciprocal relationship between the quantities of the two pigments throughout the year, as shown in Fig. 20 (BRIDGES, 1965a).

The winter porphyropsin increase, or more particularly the red-shifted spectral sensitivity that must accompany it, may be an adaptation to reddening of ambient light due to diminished solar elevation, perhaps coupled with changes in atmospheric and water transmissivities.

Often blue and red vertical extinction coefficients may vary in opposite directions throughout a given year, as exemplified for Lake Maggiore in Fig. 21 (VOL-LENWEIDER, 1961), although in this case the trend is in the "wrong" direction to accord with the seasonal pigment changes of the fish discussed above.

2. Habitat

Fig. 19 also illustrates that fish of a given species from different habitats may differ in the proportions of pigments in their retinas. Thus although both groups of *Notemigonus* in this figure exhibited seasonal variation, there was significantly more rhodopsin in fish from clear waters than in those from a more turbid canal. The difference was probably not due to diet, but may have represented a specific, perhaps short-term adaptation to different light conditions. This finding reinforces the suggestion that the paired-pigment system assists in dealing with an intrinsically variable aquatic light environment.

3. Age

In *Scardinius*, older specimens have more porphyropsin (BRIDGES and YOSHIK-AMI, 1970b). This is illustrated in Fig. 22 for a group of fish taken from the same pond. Even in midsummer, the older fish had up to between 90 and 100 % porphyropsin while the younger ones (3—4 yr old) had no more than 20 % retinal

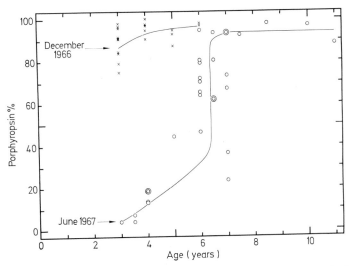

Fig. 22. Variation of retinal visual pigment composition according to age in individuals of *Scardinius*. ×, winter batch; ○, summer batch. Ages were determined by counting rings in the cleared otoliths. From BRIDGES and YOSHIKAMI, 1970b

porphyropsin. In the preceding winter, the retinas of the young fish had contained between 70 and 100 % porphyropsin. Thus it is reasonable to suppose that seasonal fluctuation of visual pigments in this species becomes less and less marked as the fishes age, and their retinas exhibit a progressive increase of porphyropsin over the years. Fortunately, the batches of fish used by Bridges and by Dartnall et al. were all young enough to exhibit a marked seasonal effect.

Age might influence the visual pigments of Belonesox as well. In one case, eyes from the unborn young in this live-bearer were extracted and compared with the mother (Bridges, unpublished). The bulk extract from the eyes of 30—40 fry contained 87 % rhodopsin compared with only 53 % for the mother.

4. Individual Variation

Individuals taken from the same habitat at the same time of year may vary considerably amongst themselves, as exemplified in Fig. 23. These differences are

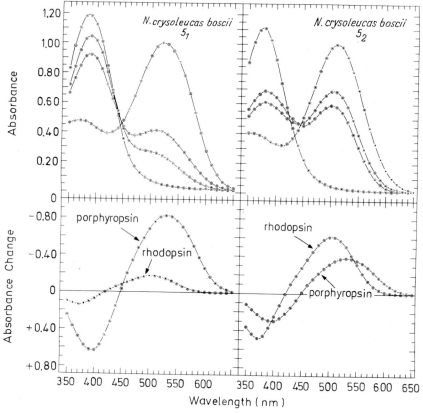

Fig. 23. Two individual minnows *(Notemigonus)* from the same habitat, but with very different visual pigment compositions. — Both extracts were exposed to three identical irradiations, i.e. 1 hour λ660 nm light, 1 hour λ660 nm light, 10 minutes white. In the lower section, difference spectra for the pure pigments are shown scaled according to their proportions in each extract. Fish no. 5_1 had 83% porphyropsin compared with only 39% in fish no. 5_2. Reproduced from Bridges (1964c)

not entirely attributable to age. Thus in Fig. 22, the 7-year old fish in June had retinas containing porphyropsin in percentages ranging from 20 % to 95 %. Similar individual variation had been described earlier for *Notemigonus*, *Belonesox*, *Hybopsis* and *Mugil curema* (BRIDGES, 1964c, 1965c), and also occurs in juvenile salmon (BEATTY, 1966). Variation persists even when fish are kept in the same light environment for as long as 4—5 months (Fig. 25), although it may nearly vanish under conditions where there is an overwhelming tendency to switch to the pure pigment condition (Fig. 24).

Variability seems to be an inherent trait, for both eyes of an individual fish are identical in composition (BRIDGES, 1964c). As suggested in the case of the salmonids (p. 446), individual variation may be due to a polymorphic "terminal-ring" dehydrogenase, and is an expression of genetic variation in a population.

Variation may also be particularly valuable for the schooling species such as the cyprinids and grey mullets, where it might be a means for broadening the spectral sensitivity of the whole school (cf. BRIDGES, 1964c). In the younger fish, of course, the median position would fluctuate according to the time of year.

C. Induced Photopigment Changes in Artificial Environments

1. Light and Darkness

The most important environmental factor controlling the proportions of rhodopsin and porphyropsin, and what is probably the causative agent in seasonal variation, is the intensity and duration of light exposure (DARTNALL, LANDER, and MUNZ, 1961). We have already alluded to this effect in juvenile salmon (p. 450), which increased their rhodopsin when transferred to brighter tanks (BEATTY, 1966). *Belonesox* behaves in much the same way when taken from its natural environment and placed in brightly lit laboratory tanks (BRIDGES, 1965d).

DARTNALL, LANDER, and MUNZ (1961) showed that if *Scardinius* were transferred from daylit tanks to complete darkness, they increased their porphyropsin at the expense of the rhodopsin. Conversely, when returned to the illuminated tanks this porphyropsin decreased and was replaced by rhodopsin. A similar experiment (BRIDGES and YOSHIKAMI, 1970b, c, dealing with extracts from single fish and using tanks exposed to continuous artificial illumination instead of daylight, is illustrated in Fig. 24. Fish could be exposed to our conditions of continuous light or continuous darkness for long periods of time (four months) without any morphological changes becoming apparent in electron microscope pictures of the photoreceptor outer segments (BRIDGES, LOCKET, and YOSHIKAMI, unpublished).

At one time it was suggested (DARTNALL, LANDER, and MUNZ, 1961) that the light effect might be photoperiodic, i.e. depending on the duration of light and dark periods but independent of intensity provided this was above threshold. However, there is no evidence for photoperiodicity in *Belonesox*. Fish from the natural habitat exposed to a $10^1/_2$ hours day were transferred to brightly-lit tanks exposed to an artificial day that was $4^1/_2$ hours shorter. Nevertheless, an *increase* in retinal rhodopsin was found (BRIDGES, 1965d). Similarly, BEATTY's experiments with juvenile salmon kept on the same natural day length but under two brightness conditions do not support a photoperiodic effect. It is more likely that the combination of intensity and duration, or the total light exposure, is the important consideration, as in the photographic process. Further evidence against a photoperiodic effect will be discussed shortly, when we deal with fish that have had one eye occluded.

Intermediate photic conditions were investigated by BRIDGES and YOSHIKAMI (1970b, c). A batch of *Scardinius* was split into four groups. One was kept in

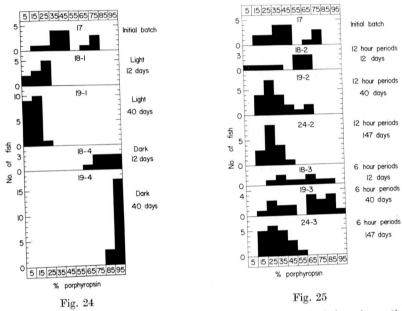

Fig. 24.   Fig. 25.

Fig. 24. Changes of visual pigment composition in *Scardinius* individuals kept in continuous light or continuous darkness. The figures along the abscissa mark the centre of each interval; thus "35" includes all fish with from 30 to 40% porphyropsin. From BRIDGES and YOSHIKAMI, 1970b, c

Fig. 25. Visual pigment composition in *Scardinius* individuals kept under conditions of intermittent illumination (abscissa marked as in Fig. 24). From BRIDGES and YOSHIKAMI, 1970b

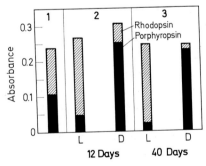

Fig. 26. Yields of visual pigments from *Scardinius* kept in continuous light or continuous darkness. Yields are expressed in terms of average absorbance (1 cm) per fish, with reference to an extract volume of 0.7 ml. From BRIDGES and YOSHIKAMI, 1970b

continuous light, one in darkness. The pigment composition of these two groups sampled at different times has been summarised in Fig. 24. The remaining fish were exposed to alternating equal periods of light and darkness. The period was six hours long for one group and 12 hours for the other. Hence over the 24 hour period each group received exactly the same amount of intermittent light. The pigment compositions of these two groups are summarised in Fig. 25. Assessment of these findings is not easy during the first forty days, because of the high degree of variability in these 3-year old specimens. After about five months, however, the two populations present a more homogeneous picture, when it is clear that on the average there is little difference between the six and twelve hour groups, indicating their ability to integrate light exposure over the 24 hour period. At this time, the retinal pigment composition lies between that of fish kept in darkness and of those kept in continuous light. After these preliminary experiments had revealed the highly variable nature of the material, further work along these lines was discontinued.

On the average, each fish from the 40-day light group yielded 0.0223 absorbance units of porphyropsin and 0.2336 of rhodopsin (i.e. the latter represented 91 % of the mixture) whereas the amount of porphyropsin in the dark group was 0.2308 compared with only 0.0134 for the rhodopsin (i.e. only 5 % of the mixture). These results are summarized in Fig. 26. Thus although these proportions are very different, the total amount of pigment present is much the same, supporting the idea of a direct interconversion.

2. Occlusion of one Eye

If photoperiod were an important factor in pigment interconversions, the eyes of an individual fish should be unable to change their visual pigments independently of one another if exposed to different light conditions, because both would be under the influence of a central control (e.g. pineal and/or pituitary). Recently, BRIDGES and YOSHIKAMI (1968; 1970b, c) induced such independent shifts in specimens of *Scardinius*.

The fish were first kept in light or dark holding-tanks until their retinas became predominantly rhodopsin or porphyropsin. Each specimen was then fitted with an opaque silver or plastic cap which excluded light from one eye (Figs. 27, 28) and was finally placed in a continuously illuminated tank. After 1—2 weeks the fish were killed and the pigment from each eye analysed. Normally both eyes have the same pigment composition. This time, however, a clear difference was found. In the covered eyes of fish that had started out containing mainly rhodopsin there was an increase in the amount of porphyropsin, as shown in Fig. 29. Thus the covered eye had 51.4 % porphyropsin after 28 days compared with only 18.3 % in the "control" eye. In a fish that had been placed in the dark at the same time (neither eye capped) the percentages of porphyropsin were 62.0 and 58.6 for the left and right eyes respectively.

Conversely, in the exposed eyes of fish that had started out with porphyropsin-dominated retinas, the expected increase in rhodopsin was found, as exemplified in Fig. 30. In this case the exposed eye contained 27.8 % porphyropsin after 22 days, while the covered eye had 55.0 %. In another experiment where the cap had been kept on for 18 days the corresponding figures were 40.3 and 71.8 %

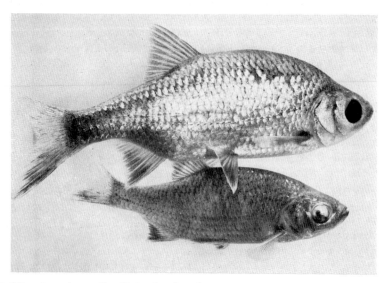

Fig. 27. Side view of two *Scardinius* fitted with monocular caps pressed from black Cobex plastic in one case and metallic silver in the other. From Bridges and Yoshikami, 1970b

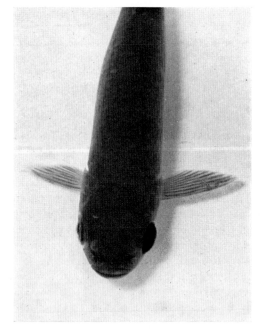

Fig. 28. Top view of a specimen of *Scardinius* fitted with a black Cobex cap. From Bridges and Yoshikami, 1970b

(Fig. 31). However, in such experiments the percentages of porphyropsin found in the capped eyes were sufficiently low to make us believe that even here a shift towards a retina richer in rhodopsin had occurred. We concluded that a small amount of light must have leaked around the cap, or possibly through the translucent skull and then into the eye by way of the sclera and optic nerve insertion.

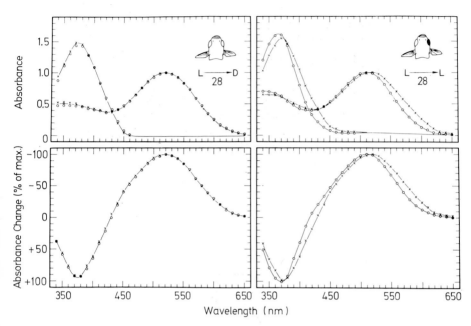

Fig. 29. Visual pigment extracts from left and right eyes of *Scardinius* individuals. ○, left eye; ×, right eye. Absorbance spectra are shown in the top portion, difference spectra below (all solutions were bleached with non-isomerising light in the presence of hydroxylamine). $L \to D$ signifies transfer of a rhodopsin-rich fish from the light tank into darkness. $L \to L$ signifies that the rhodopsin-rich fish has been kept in the light, in this case after a cap had been placed over the right eye, blackened in the inset diagram. The numerals give the duration of the experiment in days. From BRIDGES and YOSHIKAMI, 1970b

In order to test whether the cap itself was influencing the visual pigments, perhaps by pressure, a further experiment was carried out. One eye of a rhodopsin-fish was covered with a black cap, the other with a transparent one. After 21 days in the light, the dark eye had 51.4 % porphyropsin compared with 32.2 % for the eye with the transparent cap.

These results show that the eyes can respond to light independently of each other, and suggest that the whole process of light-induced photopigment conversion in this species occurs within the compass of the ocular tissues without dependence on external hormonal control. This conclusion does not rule out the possibility that endocrine control may be operative under some circumstances, as discussed below.

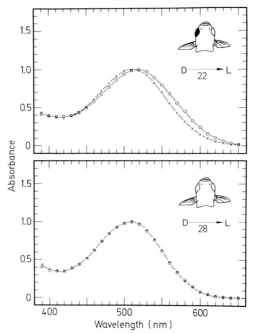

Fig. 30. Visual pigment extracts from left and right eyes of *Scardinius* individuals (absorbance spectra only). Same conventions as in Fig. 29. In these cases, porphyropsin-rich fish were transferred from dark tanks to the light. From BRIDGES and YOSHIKAMI, 1970b

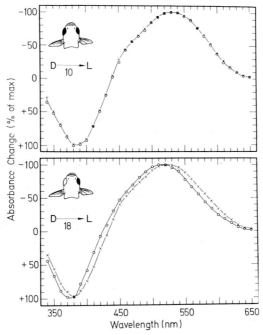

Fig. 31. Visual pigment extracts from left and right eyes of *Scardinius* individuals (difference spectra only). Same conventions as in Figs. 29 and 30 (note that the fish in the upper half has been fitted with caps over *both* eyes). From BRIDGES and YOSHIKAMI, 1970b

D. Possible Effects of Thyroxine?

BRIDGES and YOSHIKAMI (1970b) tested the effect of thyroxine in a group of *Scardinius* by administration of unilateral ocular injections of the hormone. Rhodopsin- and porphyropsin-fish received monocular injections of $1/2$ % agar saturated with L-thyroxine and were placed in darkness for six days. The results, summarised in Table 6, were rather inconclusive. In this experiment, it is clear that the effects of thyroxine were slight. Thus during the six-day period in darkness it appears that the proportion of porphyropsin in the thyroxine-treated eyes of the "rhodopsin group" was slightly higher than in the corresponding untreated eyes. Of course, there is the difficulty that the injection would be expected to leak into the general circulation and minimise any differences between the two eyes (cf. WILT, 1959b). In this connexion it is interesting that the average amount of porphyropsin (left and right eyes) was higher in the two fish that had received thyroxine than in the one that had not.

Table 6. *Possible effect of thyroxine on Scardinius visual pigments* (BRIDGES *and* YOSHIKAMI, 1970b)

| Operation | Fish no. | Predominating pigment at time of injection | Porphyropsin % | | Difference (operated minus non-operated %) |
			Operated eye	Non-operated eye	
Sham	1	Rhodopsin	12.8	15.7	—2.9
Thyrox.	2	Rhodopsin	34.2	27.8	+6.4
Thyrox.	3	Rhodopsin	32.2	23.3	+8.9
Thyrox.	4	Porphyropsin	95.7	94.6	+1.1
Thyrox.	5	Porphyropsin	96.3	97.8	—1.5
Sham	6	Porphyropsin	94.6	94.6	0.0

The "porphyropsin group" showed none of the above effects, perhaps because little further increase of porphyropsin could be induced in retinas that were nearly pure in the pigment.

If these results are significant, the effect of thyroxine is in the same direction as that found by MUNZ and SWANSON (1965) in the Rainbow trout, which increases its porphyropsin when kept in water containing thyroxine[10]. However, experiments by NAITO and WILT (1962) on the eyes of *Lepomis* isolated in organ culture indicated that thyroid hormone suppressed the conversion of retinol to the 3-dehydroretinaldehyde prosthetic group of porphyropsin, as in the tadpole. Thus seven hours after an injection of ^{3}H-retinol (6030 cpm) into isolated eyes, the specific activity of 3-dehydroretinaldehyde, liberated by bleaching the extracted porphyropsin, was 3280—3730 cpm/μgm. On the other hand, the specific activity in a second batch of eyes that had received triiodothyronine in addition to the ^{3}H-retinol was only 1490—1510 cpm/μgm. Since *Lepomis* does not have rhodopsin in its retina at any stage of its life history, however, the situation may not be the same as in paired-pigment species.

[10] See also BEATTY's (1969) study, where he finds a similar effect of thyroid hormone on the visual pigments of juvenile kokanee salmon. The work was published after this chapter was written.

E. Why do Older Fish Have More Porphyropsin?

It is possible that the shift towards a porphyropsin-dominated condition in older specimens of *Scardinius* is under endocrine control. However, sexual maturity may not be the important controlling factor, for this occurs at about 4 years of age, several years before the sharp increase in porphyropsin takes place (Fig. 22). Perhaps there is an association with the full development of deep golden body colour and red fins at about 6 years of age.

One experiment was carried out by Bridges and Yoshikami (1970b, c) to see whether the older fish had become "set" in the high-porphyropsin condition of winter and could no longer revert to rhodopsin in response to more intense illumination. Two 9—10 year old fish were used in this investigation. Initially, one eye from each fish was removed and used as a control. One one-eyed fish was then placed in darkness while the other was kept under continuous illumination. After 3 weeks the fish were killed and the pigments of the remaining eyes were analysed. The results are summarised below in Table 7.

Table 7. *Effect of light on old fish (Scardinius)* (Bridges and Yoshikami, 1970b)

Fish No.	Tank conditions	% porphyropsin in		Difference (test eye minus control)
		control eye	test eye	
28-1	light	44.3	32.2	—12.1
28-2	dark	68.5	80.3	+11.8

Thus there had been a porphyropsin increase in the dark fish and a decrease in the light. It is noteworthy that both these specimens started out with less porphyropsin than was observed in the same age group and batch of Fig. 22. However, the latter had been killed and analysed immediately upon arrival from the pond, whereas the two used in the present experiment had been kept for several months in the relatively bright surroundings of our outdoor holding tanks, thus inducing a shift towards rhodopsin. At present, we cannot say whether these changes proceed more sluggishly than in younger fish (compare the results tabulated above with Fig. 24).

Another possibility is that the older fish tend to seek deeper and darker regions of their pool, thus living under conditions favouring porphyropsin and leaving the younger ones to school in the brighter surroundings favouring rhodopsin near the surface. Observations of these fish in their ponds do not support this idea, however, and in any event it would not account for the findings with *Belonesox* fry (p. 456).

F. Origins and Biogenesis of the 3-Dehydroretinol Prosthetic Group in Fish Porphyropsins

We have seen that the frog liver contains only retinol, irrespective of whether we are dealing with a "porphyropsin tadpole" or a "rhodopsin frog" (p. 435). The livers of *Scardinius* and most other freshwater fishes, however, contain in addition to retinol appreciable quantities of the 3-dehydro derivative (cf. EDISBURY, MORTON, and SIMPKINS, 1937; EDISBURY, MORTON, SIMPKINS, and LOVERN, 1938; LEDERER, ROSANOVA, GILLAM, and HEILBRON, 1937; WALD, 1939a; MORTON and CREED, 1939; CAMA, DALVI, MORTON, SALAH, STEINBERG, and STUBBS, 1952), which may account for nearly 100 % of the liver retinols in some cases (Fig. 32). A little-publicised finding is the widespread occurrence of 3-dehydroretinol in *marine* fish-liver oils also, often amounting to between 4 and 20 % of the total "vitamins A" (COLLINS,

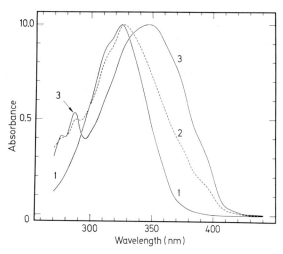

Fig. 32. Absorbance spectra of petroleum ether extracts from saponified coregonine livers. Curve 1 — gwyniad, 8.2% 3-dehydroretinol; curve 2 — Renke from the Kochelsee, 53.6% 3-dehydroretinol; curve 3 — Renke from the Würmsee, 98.4% 3-dehydroretinol. From BRIDGES and YOSHIKAMI, 1970a

LOVE, and MORTON, 1953). There are several ways of obtaining 3-dehydroretinol, e.g. (a) as the preformed compound; (b) from a specific dietary precursor possessing a 3,4- dehydro-β-ionone ring; (c) from other precursors such as β-carotene, by way of retinol as an intermediate.

Preformed 3-dehydroretinol is absent from the eyes and other tissues of all invertebrates that have been examined (cf. MORTON and CREED, 1939; COLLINS, LOVE, and MORTON, 1953; GROSS and BUDOWSKI, 1966), and hence the only dietary source would be other fishes. Carotenoids containing even one 3,4-dehydro-β-ionone ring are unknown in nature, although synthetic substances of this type have been tested in chicks and mice, where there is some evidence for the formation of 3-dehydroretinol (BUDOWSKI, ASCARELLI, GROSS, and NIR, 1963; BUDOWSKI and GROSS, 1965). A suggestion by BUDOWSKI and his colleagues that the dehydration of lutein to anhydrolutein (3,4-dehydro-3'-hydroxy-β-carotene) might be of possible significance in the biogenesis of 3-dehydroretinol has not been substantiated (GROSS and BUDOWSKI, 1966).

There is little doubt that β-carotene itself can act as a precursor of 3-dehydroretinol as well as retinol in fish, as shown by MORTON and CREED (1939), GRAN-

Gaud and Moatti (1958) and Gross and Budowski (1966). This is true of tadpoles also, in which Ohtsu, Naito and Wilt (1964) found that ^{14}C-β-carotene labelled the porphyropsin prosthetic group as effectively as that of rhodopsin (these authors also found similar precursor activity with labelled echinenone, hydroxy-echinenone and myxoxanthophyll). Probably, conversion to retinol is a preliminary step in the process. Thus when ^{3}H-retinol is injected into the single-pigment *Lepomis*, there is extensive labelling of the porphyropsin 3-dehydroretinaldehyde prosthetic group (Naito and Wilt, 1962; see p. 463). There is some evidence that this happens in *Scardinius* as well (p. 472).

In addition to α- and β-carotene (and perhaps ocular retinol), the oxygen-containing carotenoids astaxanthin[11], canthaxanthin[11], cryptoxanthin[11], 3-hydroxy-4-oxo-β-carotene, echinenone[11] and isozeaxanthin[11] abound in lower aquatic life forms such as *Chironomus* larvae and *Daphnia*, which are the major food sources for many freshwater fishes (Gross and Budowski, 1966; Gilchrist, 1968; Herring, 1968). These compounds are readily utilised by *Lebistes* and *Xiphophorus* to form retinol and some 3-dehydroretinol (Gross and Budowski, 1966). Since β-carotene is formed from astaxanthin by *Gambusia*, *Lebistes* and *Xiphophorus*, it is likely that the steps leading from astaxanthin to retinol and 3-dehydroretinol (in the intestine) are as follows: (a) reduction to β-carotene[12]; (b) conversion of β-carotene to retinol; (c) dehydrogenation of retinol to 3-dehydroretinol (cf. Grangaud, Vignais, Massonet, and Moatti, 1957).

Another possible reaction pathway yielding first 3-dehydroretinol and then retinol is summarised below (from Gross and Budowski, 1966).

Barua and Nayar (1966) suggest that dietary hydroxy-carotenoids are converted into 3-dehydroretinaldehyde by way of the intermediate "naturally-occurring anhydrovitamin A$_2$", or 3-hydroxyanhydroretinol, which has been found in

small quantities in some freshwater fish-liver oils. In chloroform this compound has λ_{max} at 357, 375 and 397 nm. It is noteworthy that spectra of digitonin extracts of porphyropsin-rich retinas usually have small irregularities that might indicate the

---

[11] Astaxanthin = 3,3'-dihydroxy-4.4'-dioxo-β-carotene; canthaxanthin = 4,4'-dioxo-β-carotene; cryptoxanthin = 3-hydroxy-β-carotene; iso-zeaxanthin = 4,4'-dihydroxy-β-carotene; echinenone = 4-oxo-β-carotene.

[12] It is of interest to note that this might represent a *reversal* of the metabolic pathways used by food animals such as *Daphnia magna*, which are capable of performing the oxidation sequence: β-carotene (from algae)→echinenone→canthaxanthin→astaxanthin (see e. g. Herring, 1968; Thommen and Wackernagel, 1964).

presence of a substance with peaks at about 360, 380 and ca. 405 nm (BRIDGES, 1965a; unpublished) — whether this is related to 3-hydroxyanhydroretinol is not clear.

As far as the eye is concerned, we may ask whether the 3-dehydroretinaldehyde prosthetic group of porphyropsin originates principally in extraocular sites of synthesis or of storage. The fact that there is often little relationship between composition of visual pigments and that of the liver "vitamins A" (cf. WALD, 1939a) does not rule out the possibility that the liver provides the eye with preformed retinol and 3-dehydroretinol, as we shall see shortly. The lack of correspondence between eye and liver is exemplified by the results tabulated below (Table 8): in *Scardinius* that have been kept in light and darkness until their retinas contain nearly pure rhodopsin or porphyropsin, the liver compositions remain nearly constant (cf. BEATTY's similar findings in juvenile trout, but not in the migrating adults).

Table 8. *Analysis of liver retinols and retinal visual pigments in groups of Scardinius kept under various conditions of light and darkness (from* BRIDGES *and* YOSHIKAMI, *1970b, c)*

No.	% 3-dehydroretinol in liver (av.)	% porphyropsin in eye (av.)	No. of fish	Remarks
17A	81.1	64.1	4	Initial batch[a]
17B	75.7	25.0	4	Initial batch[a]
19-1	79.3	8.4	2	40 days light
19-1A	82.6	10.4	9	40 days light
19-1B	82.1	7.9	9	40 days light
19-4	81.8	94.6	2	40 days dark
19-4A	83.3	95.0	9	40 days dark
19-4B	81.3	94.0	9	40 days dark

[a] Visual pigments were analysed first, while the livers were kept in individual foil wrappers in the deep freeze. Then the livers from high and low porphyropsin fish were bulked together and analysed.

If we transfer our attention from the liver to the pigment epithelium the situation is seen to be very different. We noted earlier that the composition of retinols stored in the pigmented ocular tissues of frogs and tadpoles accurately reflected the retinal pigment compositions (Fig. 15, p. 435). This may be true also for lampreys, eels and salmonids (see pages 439, 451 and Fig. 34 below), and there is now little doubt that *Scardinius* visual pigments and pigment epithelium retinols exhibit a similar relationship. If dissection is carried out carefully, the retina of this species can be removed from the eye cup with the black, single-cell layer of pigment epithelium adhering to it. After freeze-drying, the retinols stored in the pigment epithelium may be extracted with a solvent that does not destroy the visual pigments (e.g. light petroleum). If "clean" retinas are treated similarly, virtually no retinols are extracted. Fig. 33 shows that the pigment epithelium of fish kept in the light contains mainly retinol, while that of fish kept in darkness is dominated by 3-dehydroretinol (BRIDGES and YOSHIKAMI, 1968, 1970 b, c). The maximum amounts were at least three times the total visual pigment[13].

Fig. 34 illustrates the relationship between pigment epithelium stores and retinal visual pigment in three specimens of *Scardinius* kept in light and darkness.

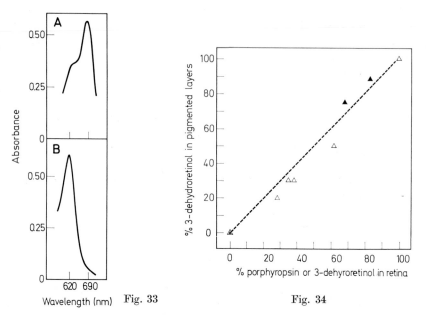

Fig. 33   Fig. 34

Fig. 33. Carr-Price "blues" obtained by reacting antimony trichloride with chloroform extracts from *Scardinius* pigment epithelia. Curve A — fish kept in darkness (porphyropsin-rich condition); curve B — fish kept in the light (rhodopsin-rich condition). The former group yielded a blue colour in which the 693 nm peak of 3-dehydroretinol predominated. The latter group shows only a maximum at about 620 nm characteristic of retinol; there is no trace of a peak that could be attributed to 3-dehydroretinol. The wavelength scale is not linear. From BRIDGES and YOSHIKAMI, 1970 c

Fig. 34. Relationship between the constitution of retinal visual pigment and stored retinols in the pigmented layers of fish eyes. ▲, three specimens of *Scardinius* kept in light or darkness (combined retinas were first freeze-dried and the pigment epithelium retinols extracted in darkness with petroleum ether: then the retinal visual pigments were extracted with digitonin). Unpublished data from BRIDGES and YOSHIKAMI. △, a variety of fish examined by WALD (1939 a), where the retinas were isolated and the pigments bleached to the retinol/3-dehydroretinol stage. Since these substances are absent from the dark-adapted retina, the composition of the mixture reflects the composition of the visual pigment. The remaining ocular tissues (pigment epithelium and/or choroids) were extracted with chloroform or petroleum ether

This figure also summarises some earlier studies of WALD (1939 a) on the retinal visual pigments and the retinols of the pigmented layers in freshwater, marine and diadromous fishes (including salmonids and eel).

The pigment epithelium may act by sequestering one of the retinols preferentially from the circulation, or it may be the primary site of interconversion of the

[13] Compare the lamprey, which has about two equivalents of visual pigment stored as retinol/3-dehydroretinol in the pigmented ocular tissues (WALD, 1942).

two retinols. We have no information on the first possibility (which may not occur at all), but the second is undoubtedly feasible. NAITO and WILT (1962) showed that the isolated eyes of *Lepomis* spp. (family Centrarchidae: a freshwater fish possessing only porphyropsin) can transform injected retinol into 3-dehydro-retinaldehyde after incubation in organ culture. Thus in at least one freshwater fish, as well as in tadpoles, a 3,4-dehydrogenase for retinol or retinaldehyde is present in the ocular tissues, the most likely place being the pigment epithelium. Consequently, by itself the eye can provide some, if not all, of the 3-dehydroretinol required for porphyropsin synthesis and for maintenance of ocular stores: in some species it is even conceivable that a proportion of the *liver* 3-dehydroretinol originates from this source.

There may be occasions, however, when the system is flooded with preformed dietary retinol, which may alter the proportions of rhodopsin and porphyropsin in a paired-pigment species. The changes observed by BRIDGES and YOSHIKAMI were on starved *Scardinius*, but DARTNALL, LANDER, and MUNZ (1961) investigated the effect of feeding and claimed that the dark change towards porphyropsin was retarded in fed fishes. They attributed this effect to the presumed presence of retinol in the food (crushed dog biscuit). Unfortunately, DARTNALL *et al.* were unaware of the existence of individual variation in their fish (as illustrated in Fig. 24), so that the statistical significance of their observations has not been established[14].

BRIDGES and YOSHIKAMI, in the course of another study (p. 470), injected retinyl acetate into rhodopsin-dominated *Scardinius*, producing a rise of liver retinol from about 20 to 60 % of the total "vitamins A". When these fish were placed in darkness, the change to porphyropsin appeared to proceed at much the same rate as observed in other experiments with normal, starved fish. When another batch of these rhodopsin-dominated fish was transferred from strongly to moderately illuminated tanks, a rise in porphyropsin was again observed, although less than in total darkness. Retinyl acetate was also injected into porphyropsin-fish. No changes occurred subsequently if the fish were kept in darkness, and the change towards rhodopsin did not appear to be accelerated in the light. However, the sketchy observations described above provide insufficient evidence on the possible effects of feeding, one way or the other, and a conclusion must await more thorough investigations.

G. Possible Mechanisms of Rhodopsin-Porphyropsin Interconversion in Light and Darkness

How does exposure to light or darkness bring about such radical alterations in the rhodopsin-porphyropsin composition of the eye ? A scheme based on a proposal by DARTNALL (1964) is presented below (see BRIDGES, 1965a).

DARTNALL assumed that the circulation carried at all times a preponderance of retinol, which entered the visual cycle during turnover of the visual pigment prosthetic groups in the light. Any 3-dehydroretinol released by bleaching of por-phyropsin molecules would be lost by way of the same route, thus leading to the

---

[14] In all experiments the eyes of several (usually 10) identically-treated fish were bulked. — Editor.

replacement of porphyropsin by rhodopsin. In darkness, it was supposed that 3,4-dehydrogenation of the retinaldehyde prosthetic group occurred *while it was still bound to opsin*. Thus one might think in terms of a "rhodopsin dehydrogenase" which converted rhodopsin directly into porphyropsin in the lamellae of the outer segments. At the time, this process seemed "very probable, as it is difficult to see how any other type of chromophore replacement could occur in a (presumably)

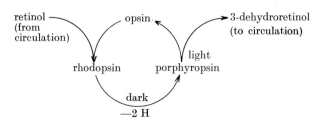

thermally stable pigment in darkness" (Bridges, 1965a).But the scheme outlined above does not take into account the pigment epithelium supplies, and dehydrogenation in the outer segments cannot plausibly explain how these supplies switch from retinol to 3-dehydroretinol in the dark. The maintenance of considerable amounts of 3-dehydroretinol in the pigment epithelium under these conditions shows that it does not "leak" away into the circulation.

Because of recent work by Bridges and Yoshikami (1968; 1969a, b) the assumption that visual pigment molecules are stable entities in the dark-adapted eye must be discarded. The albino rat was selected for preliminary experiments, because it differs from most other animals in that there is no retinol stored in its pigment epithelium. In the dark-adapted eye, virtually all the retinol is bound as aldehyde within the rhodopsin molecules of the outer segments. The retinaldehyde is released during light-adaptation, and is then reduced to retinol which flows into the pigment epithelium. The process reverses in the dark (Dowling, 1960). The two-way interchange between photoreceptor outer segments and pigment epithelium in light and dark-adaptation is probably a generalised phenomenon in all vertebrate retinas (Dowling, 1960).

A group of rats was dark-adapted for 30 hours, then under the weak red illumination of a safelight they were injected intraperitoneally with retinyl acetate labelled with tritium at C(11) and C(12). Half the rats were left in darkness, while the remainder were transferred to illuminated cages. Animals were sampled at intervals of 24 hours, 7 days and 14 days. In darkness, the whole eyes were ground with alum solution, washed, then extracted with light petroleum to remove any small amounts of free retinol. Radioassays of the petrol washings are shown in Fig. 35. The tissue was then wetted, the retinaldehyde prosthetic group first liberated by bleaching in the light, then extracted with light petroleum after redrying. As illustrated in Fig. 35, over the 14-day period there was a progressive increase in the radioactivity of retinaldehyde from the dark-group of rats, indicating an appreciable interchange with the injected labelled material, i.e. a turnover of visual pigment prosthetic groups in darkness.

Next, a similar series of experiments was carried out with *Scardinius* (Bridges and Yoshikami, 1968, 1970b, c). Fig. 36 illustrates an example. This fish had

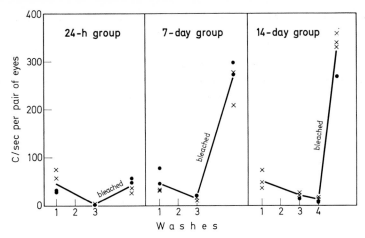

Fig. 35. Labelling of the rhodopsin prosthetic group (retinaldehyde) in rats injected with 11,12-^{3}H$_2$-retinyl acetate and subsequently kept in light or darkness. ×, dark group; •, light group. Reproduced from BRIDGES and YOSHIKAMI (1969a)

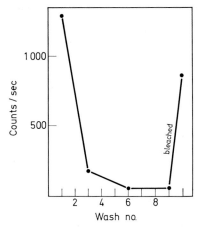

Fig. 36. Labelling of visual pigment prosthetic groups (retinaldehyde, 3-dehydroretinaldehyde) in a dark-adapted, porphyropsin-rich specimen of *Scardinius* injected with 11,12-^{3}H$_2$-retinyl acetate and kept in darkness for seven days. From BRIDGES and YOSHIKAMI, 1970c

been kept in darkness for 3 weeks beforehand, and therefore the retinas contained principally porphyropsin. Seven days in total darkness were allowed to elapse after injection with 11,12-^{3}H$_2$-retinyl acetate, after which the same procedure was used as described above for the rat. In this case, however, it will be noted that there was very high activity in the initial washings, associated with the extraction of an appreciable amount of 3-dehydroretinol (mainly) from the pigment layers. After the dried tissue had been extracted nine times with light petroleum, it was wetted, bleached, dried and re-extracted. The activity released by bleaching amounted to 2/3 of that in the first wash, showing that in darkness the visual pigment of *Scardinius*, like that of the rat, had taken up considerable quantities

of the injected label. Since most of the visual pigment would have been porphyropsin, the label was probably incorporated mainly as 11,12-$^3H_2$-3-dehydro-
retinaldehyde.

In order to obtain a precise analysis of the visual pigment contents, the retinas
were dissected out, dried and exhaustively extracted with light petroleum. This
precaution was necessary for, although the retina itself contained little free retinol,
the pigment epithelium sometimes adhered tenaciously. After final extraction
with digitonin solution, the amounts of rhodopsin and porphyropsin were estimated
from the absorbance spectra. Finally, these solutions were bleached and the
retinaldehyde or its 3-dehydro derivative extracted with methanol/ether. Some of
the results are summarised in Table 9. Although the counts vary a good deal from
fish to fish (possibly owing to the vagaries of intraperitoneal injections in these
animals), the results confirm that there is uptake of the retinol label in darkness,
showing that turnover of visual pigment chromophoric groups is not confined to
the illuminated retina. In the case of those fish that have mainly porphyropsin in
their retinas, the label must be incorporated mainly in the form of the 3-dehydro
derivative. Thus if we were to assume that *all* the activity were attributable to the
rhodopsin alone, then its specific activity (absorbance of 0.1 in 0.6 ml for 1 cm
optical path) would vary from 10,500 cpsec. for the extract with 96 % porphyropsin
down to 800—1,200 for the extracts with 23 % porphyropsin. The first figure would
correspond to a prosthetic group specific activity many times that of the injected
retinol (246 μCi/mg).

Table 9. *Radioassays of visual pigment extracts from Scardinius 2 weeks after injection of tritiated
retinyl acetate* (Bridges *and* Yoshikami, *unpublished*)

	Initially "rhodopsin fish"		Initially "porphyropsin fish"	
	% por-phyropsin	c.p. sec./0.1 absorbance at λ_{max}	% por-phyropsin	c.p. sec./0.1 absorbance at λ_{max}
Illuminated tanks[a]	23.3	882 ⎫	48.0	659 ⎫
	51.4	627 ⎬ = 704	44.3	475 ⎬ = 518
	23.3	602 ⎭	58.6	419 ⎭
Dark tanks	51.4	562 ⎫	95.7	453 ⎫
	65.3	790 ⎬ = 723	85.8	493 ⎬ = 473
	80.3	816 ⎭		
Means		714		496

[a] The fish in these tanks were exposed to moderate conditions of illumination (10—15 ft. c.
at the water surface for 12 hours in 24 hours) compared with the "light" tanks used for
producing rhodopsin fish (continuous exposure to 280 ft. c. at the water surface).

Recently, Hall, Bok, and Bacharach (1968) have carried out similar experiments with frogs, this time injecting with tritiated amino acids and radioassaying
the *opsin* moiety of the visual pigment. In these experiments it was not necessary
to work in darkness, because the opsin should remain as a fixed and integral part
of the outer segment structure, even when the visual pigment is bleached. Nevertheless, uptake of label into the opsin molecule indicated that not only was the

prosthetic group a labile entity under physiological conditions, as had been found by BRIDGES and YOSHIKAMI, but that the whole visual pigment molecule was undergoing breakdown and resynthesis.

The basis for these findings lies in the elegant radioautographic studies of DROZ (1963), YOUNG (1967, 1968), YOUNG and DROZ (1968). After injection of tritiated amino acids into rats, mice and frogs, bands of labelled material moved along the outer segments from their junctions with the inner segments, and finally disappeared into the pigment epithelium. This evidence showed that the outer segments were constantly renewed by growth from the inner segment coupled with balanced attrition at the end nearest the pigment epithelium. In frog at 22.5°C it has been estimated that 36 lamellar discs are synthesised by each rod every day (YOUNG and DROZ, 1968). Synthesis of new lamellae implies synthesis of new visual pigment molecules, and hence there is a requirement for retinaldehyde or 3-dehydroretinaldehyde in the process. These compounds probably emanate from the pigment epithelium, partly from permanent supplies which are kept topped-up from the circulation and perhaps partly from "old" visual pigment, which is probably digested by the pigment epithelium along with the other outer segment components.

Thus in *Scardinius* the rhodopsin-porphyropsin switch in darkness is made possible without the need for a "rhodopsin dehydrogenase", if we assume that in darkness porphyropsin is incorporated into the newly-synthesised lamellae, while the old rhodopsin-lamellae are progressively assimilated at the opposite end of the

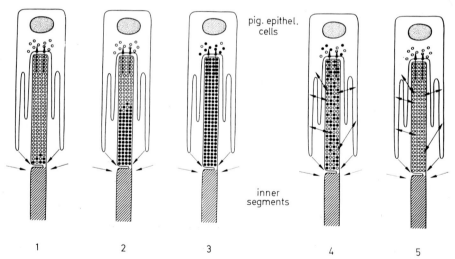

Fig. 37. Diagram illustrating the replacement of rhodopsin molecules (o) by porphyropsin (●) in the dark (1, 2, 3), and the reverse process in the light (4, 5). The cross-hatched area is the inner segment of the rod cell: the outer segment is filled with rhodopsin and/or porphyropsin molecules. As a result of phagocytosis of "old" lamellae, some of these molecules are depicted in the juxtaposed pigment epithelium cell. Arrows indicate direction of prosthetic group flow: in the dark, 3-dehydroretinaldehyde condenses with freshly-synthesised opsin at or near the base of the outer segment and is lost (as visual pigment) at the opposite end; in the light, in addition to this dark process, indiscriminate interchange of retinol/3-dehydroretinol occurs at all points along the outer segment

photoreceptor, as illustrated in Fig. 37-1, 2 and 3. When a porphyropsin-rich retina is exposed to light, 3-dehydroretinaldehyde is liberated from the opsin and is converted to the alcohol in the outer segments. By analogy with rat and frog (Dowling, 1960) we would then expect a transfer to the pigment epithelium. An equilibrium is set up, where bleaching is counterbalanced by regeneration, the latter resulting from a reversed flow from pigment epithelium to photoreceptor. In a paired-pigment fish, we must suppose that the material returning to the outer segment is richer in retinol, so that rhodopsin would gradually replace porphyropsin at all points along the length of the outer segment (Fig. 37-4 and 5).

However, the foregoing considerations do not explain *why* porphyropsin is synthesised in new lamellae in darkness, or why retinol rather than 3-dehydroretinol returns to the outer segment in the light. Several hypotheses might account for our results, but probably the most plausible explanation supposes that the primary site of interconversion of retinol and 3-dehydroretinol is in the pigment epithelium, and that the state of the retinol/3-dehydroretinol supplies in this tissue determines the composition of pigment synthesised by the inner segment or regenerated in the light[15]. How is the composition of the pigment epithelium supplies regulated? The cells may be primitive light detectors in amphibia and fishes, where migration of melanin granules occurs during light and dark adaptation. In such animals, the pigment epithelium cells contain particles composed of accumulations of membranes derived from endoplasmic reticulum. These "myeloid" bodies could be the photoreceptors of melanin migration (Yamada, 1961), and if so they could equally serve as sites where 3,4-dehydrogenation of the β-ionone ring occurred, the process being reversed by light.

An important difference between the light and dark condition is that in darkness the disintegration of the visual pigment molecule must release the prosthetic group in its 11-*cis* conformation [cf. the situation in thermal or chemical destruction of rhodopsin, (Hubbard, 1958a), compared with all-*trans* during photic bleaching (Hubbard and Wald, 1952)]. At any time, we suppose, retinol and 3-dehydroretinol would be in equilibrium with one another by the agency of a 3,4-dehydrogenase. If this enzyme were sterically selective, (Bridges and Yoshikami, 1968) the equilibrium position could be shifted in the direction of retinol for *trans* configurations, or 3-dehydroretinol for 11-*cis*. A verifiable consequence of this idea is that the 3-dehydroretinol which accumulates in the pigment epithelium of "dark" fish should be 11-*cis*, whereas the retinol which replaces it after exposure to light should be all-*trans*. This has not been tested.

In darkness, the minimum time required for replacement of rhodopsin by porphyropsin would be determined by the growth rate of the outer segments, which may be temperature-dependent in cold-blooded vertebrates, requiring about six weeks for complete renewal in frogs at 25°C (Fig. 21 of Young, 1967). In *Scardinius*, it was estimated that the change from rhodopsin to porphyropsin took between 3 and 6 weeks. In the light, on the other hand, turnover of prosthetic

---

[15] This may be demonstrated by bleaching a goldfish retina (pure porphyropsin) placed in contact with a *frog* pigment epithelium. During subsequent dark-adaptation, the pigment regenerated in the goldfish retina contains as much as 71% *rhodopsin*. In a parallel experiment where the goldfish retina was placed in contact with its own pigment epithelium, the pigment regenerated was 100% porphyropsin, as expected (Bridges, unpublished observations).

groups is governed by light-intensity, and this determines the rate at which rhodopsin replaces porphyropsin.

In conclusion, we do not know whether the cone pigments change in the same way as the rod pigments discussed above. LIEBMAN and ENTINE (1968) have shown that this probably happens during metamorphosis in frog (p. 434), but because the phenomenon of outer segment renewal appears to be confined to the rods (of frogs: YOUNG and DROZ, 1968), it is possible that there is no mechanism permitting a dark exchange of prosthetic groups in *Scardinius* cone pigments.

References

ABRAHAMSON, E. W., OSTROY, S. E.: The photochemical and macromolecular aspects of vision. Progr. Biophys. Molec. Biol. 17, 179—215 (1967).

AKHTAR, M., BLOSSE, P. T., DEWHURST, P. B.: The active site of the visual protein, rhodopsin Chem. Commun. 631—632 (1967)

— — — Studies on vision. The nature of the retinal-opsin linkage. Biochem. J. 110, 693—702 (1968).

BARRINGTON, E. J. W.: Metamorphic processes in fishes and lampreys. Amer. Zoologist, 1, 97—106 (1961).

BARUA, R. K., NAYAR, P. G.: Naturally occurring anhydrovitamin A_2. Transformation into retinene$_2$. Biochem. J. 101, 302—307 (1966).

BEATTY, D. D.: A study of the succession of visual pigments in Pacific Salmon *(Oncorhyncus)*. Canad. J. Zool. 44, 429—455 (1966).

— Visual pigment changes in juvenile kokanee salmon in response to thyroid hormones. Vision Res. 9, 855—864 (1969).

BLISS, A. F.: The mechanism of retinal vitamin A formation. J. biol. Chem. 172, 165—178 (1948).

— Reversible enzymic reduction of retinene to vitamin A. Biol. Bull. Woods Hole 97, 221 (1949).

BOWNDS, D.: Site of attachment of retinal in rhodopsin. Nature (Lond.) 216, 1178—1181 (1967).

BRIDGES, C. D. B.: The visual pigments of the rainbow trout *(Salmo irideus)*. J. Physiol. (Lond.) 134, 620—629 (1956).

— Visual pigments of some common laboratory mammals. Nature (Lond.) 184, 1727—1728 (1959).

— Effect of season and environment on the retinal pigments of two fishes. Nature (Lond.) 203, 191—192 (1964a).

— Periodicity of absorption properties in pigments based on vitamin A_2 from fish retinae. Nature (Lond.) 203, 303—304 (1964b).

— Variation of visual pigment amongst individuals of an American minnow, *Notemigonus crysoleucas boscii*. Vision Res. 4, 233—239 (1964c) .

— Absorption properties, interconversions and environmental adaptation of pigments from fish photoreceptors. Cold Spr. Harb. Symp. quant. Biol. 30, 317—334 (1965a).

— The grouping of fish visual pigments about preferred positions in the spectrum. Vision Res. 5, 223—238 (1965b).

— Variability and relationships of fish visual pigments. Vision Res. 5, 239—251 (1965c).

— Visual pigments in a fish exposed to different light-environments. Nature (Lond.) 206, 1161—1162 (1965d).

— Biochemistry of visual processes. In: Comprehensive Biochemistry 27, pp. 31—78. Edited by M. FLORKIN and E. H. STOTZ. Amsterdam: Elsevier 1967a.

— Spectroscopic properties of porphyropsins. Vision Res. 7, 349—369 (1967b).

— Photopigments in the char of Lake Windermere *(Salvelinus willughbii* (Günther), forma *autumnalis* and forma *vernalis)*. Nature (Lond.) 214, 205—206 (1967c).

— Biochemistry of vision. In: Biochemistry of the Eye, pp. 563—644. Edited by C. N. GRAYMORE. London-New York: Academic Press 1970a.

BRIDGES, C. D. B.: Reversible visual pigment changes in tadpoles exposed to light and darkness. Nature (Lond.) **227**, 956—957 (1970b).
— Molar absorbance coefficient of rhodopsin. Nature (Lond.) **227**, 1258—1259 (1970c).
— The molar absorbance coefficient of rhodopsin. Vision Res. **11**, 841—848 (1971).
— YOSHIKAMI, S.: Mechanism of rhodopsin-porphyropsin interconversions in fish. Abstracts Fifth Int. Congr. Photobiol., p. 112. Dartmouth College, Hanover, New Hampshire, U.S.A. (1968).
— — Uptake of tritiated retinaldehyde by the visual pigment of dark-adapted rats. Nature (Lond.) **221**, 275—276 (1969a).
— — Retinaldehyde turnover in rhodopsin of dark-adapted rat eye. Int. Symp.Biochem.of the Eye, Nijmegen, Netherlands (1968). Exp. Eye Res., 8, 251—252 (1969b).
— — Distribution and evolution of visual pigments in salmonid fishes. Vision Res. **10**, 601—606 (1970a).
— — The rhodopsin-porphyropsin system in freshwater fishes. 1. Effects of age and photic environment. Vision Res. **10**, 1315—1332 (1970b).
— — The rhodopsin-porphyropsin system in freshwater fishes. 2. Turnover and interconversion of visual pigment prosthetic groups in light and darkness — role of the pigment epithelium. Vision Res. **10**, 1333—1345 (1970c).
BRODA, E. E.: The role of phospholipin in visual purple solutions. Biochem. J. **35**, 960—965 (1941).
BUDOWSKI, P., ASCARELLI, I., GROSS, J., NIR, I.: Provitamin A₂ from lutein. Science **142**, 969—971 (1963).
— GROSS, J.: Conversion of carotenoids to 3-dehydroretinol (vitamin A₂) in the mouse. Nature (Lond.) **206**, 1254—1255 (1965).
CAMA, H. R., DALVI, P. D., MORTON, R. A., SALAH, M. K., STEINBERG, G. R., STUBBS, A. L.: Studies in vitamin A: 19. Preparation and properties of retinene₂. Biochem. J. **52**, 535—540 (1952).
CARLISLE, D. B., DENTON, E. J.: On the metamorphosis of the visual pigments of *Anguilla anguilla* (L.). J. mar. biol. Ass. U. K. **38**, 97—102 (1959).
CARTWRIGHT, J. W.: Investigation of the rainbow trout of Kootenay Lake, British Columbia with special reference to the Lardeau River. B. C. Fish Wildlife Branch, Management Publ. **7**, 46 pp. (1961).
CLARKE, G. L.: The utilization of solar energy by aquatic organisms. In: Problems in Lake Biology. Amer. Ass. Advanc. Sci. Publ. **10**, 27—38 (1939).
COLLINS, F. D., LOVE, R. M., MORTON, R. A.: Studies in rhodopsin, 5. Chemical analysis of retinal material. Biochem. J. **51**, 669—673 (1952).
— — — Studies in vitamin A: 25. Visual pigments in tadpoles and adult frogs. Biochem. J. **53**, 632—636 (1953).
CRESCITELLI, F.: The nature of the lamprey visual pigment. J. gen. Physiol. **39**, 423—435 (1956).
— The natural history of visual pigments. In: Photobiology, Proc. 19th Ann. Biol. Coll. Oregon State College, Corvallis. pp. 30—51 (1958a).
— The natural history of visual pigments. Ann. N. Y. Acad. Sci. **74**, 230—255 (1958b).
— DARTNALL, H. J. A.: Human visual purple. Nature (Lond.) **172**, 195—196 (1953).
— — A photosensitive pigment from the carp retina. J. Physiol. (Lond.) **125**, 607—627 (1954).
— MOMMAERTS, W. F. H. M., SHAW, T. I.: Circular dichroism of visual pigments in the visible and ultraviolet regions. Proc. nat. Acad. Sci. (Wash.) **56**, 1729—1734 (1966).
D'ANCONA, U.: The life-cycle of the Atlantic eel. Symp. zool. Soc. Lond. **1**, 61—75 (1960).
DARTNALL, H. J. A.: Visual pigment 467, a photosensitive pigment present in tench retinae. J. Physiol. (Lond.) **116**, 257—289 (1952).
— The interpretation of spectral sensitivity curves. Brit. med. Bull. **9**, 24—30 (1953).
— Visual pigments of the bleak *(Alburnus lucidus)*. J. Physiol. (Lond.) **128**, 131—156 (1955).
— Further observations on the visual pigments of the clawed toad, *Xenopus laevis*. J. Physiol. (Lond.) **134**, 327—338 (1956).
— The photobiology of visual processes. In: The eye, **2**, pp. 323—533. Edited by H. DAVSON. New York, London: Academic Press 1962.

DARTNALL, H. J. A.: The visual pigments: a photobiological study. Ann. roy. Coll. Surg. Engl. **35**, 131—150 (1964).
— The visual pigment of the green rods. Vision Res. **7**, 1—16 (1967).
— LANDER, M. R., MUNZ, F. W.: Periodic changes in the visual pigment of a fish. In: Progress in Photobiology, pp. 203—213. Edited by B. CHR. CHRISTENSEN and B. BUCHMANN. Amsterdam: Elsevier 1961.
— LYTHGOE, J. N.: The spectral clustering of visual pigments. Vision Res. **5**, 81—100 (1965).
DOTTRENS, E.: Systématique des Corégones de l'Europe occidentale, basée sur une étude biométrique. Rev. suisse Zool. **66**, 1—66 (1959).
DOWLING, J. E.: Chemistry of visual adaptation in the rat. Nature (Lond.) **188**, 114—118 (1960).
DROZ, B.: Dynamic condition of proteins in the visual cells of rats and mice as shown by radioautography with labelled amino acids. Anat. Rec. **145**, 157 (1963).
EDISBURY, J. R., MORTON, R. A., SIMPKINS, G. W.: A possible vitamin A₂. Nature (Lond.) **140**, 234 (1937).
— — — LOVERN, J. A.: The distribution of vitamin A and factor A₂. Biochem. J. **32**, 118—140 (1938).
EICHBERG, J., HESS, H. H.: The lipid composition of frog retinal rod outer segments. Experientia (Basel) **23**, 994 (1967).
EWALD, A., KÜHNE, W.: Untersuchungen über den Sehpurpur. Untersuch. Physiol. Inst. Heidelberg **1**, 248—290 (1878).
FUTTERMAN, S.: Metabolism of the retina III. The role of reduced triphosphopyridine nucleotide in the visual cycle. J. biol. Chem. **238**, 1145—1150 (1963).
— SASLAW, L. D.: The estimation of vitamin A aldehyde with thiobarbituric acid. J. biol. Chem. **236**, 1652—1657 (1961).
GILCHRIST, B. M.: Distribution and relative abundance of carotenoid pigments in anostraca (crustacea: branchiopoda). Comp. Biochem. Physiol. **24**, 123—147 (1968).
GRANGAUD, R., MOATTI, J. P.: Néoformation de vitamine A₂ chez *Gambusia holbrooki* Grd., après administration de β-carotène ou de vitamine A₁. C. R. Soc. Biol. (Paris) **152**, 1235—1257 (1958).
— VIGNAIS, P., MASSONET, R., MOATTI, J. P.: Recherches sur la biogenèse de la vitamine A des poissons. II Néoformation des vitamines A₁ (rétinol) et A₂ (déhydrorétinol) chez *Gambusia holbrooki* Grd. Bull. Soc. Chim. biol. (Paris) **39**, 1271—1278 (1957).
GROSS, J., BUDOWSKI, P.: Conversion of carotenoids into vitamins A₁ and A₂ in two species of freshwater fish. Biochem. J. **101**, 747—754 (1966).
HALL, M. O., BOK, D., BACHARACH, A. D. E.: Visual pigment renewal in the mature frog retina. Science **161**, 787—789 (1968).
HARRIS, H.: Enzyme polymorphisms in man. Proc. roy. Soc. B**164**, 298—310 (1966).
HELLER, J.: Structure of visual pigments, I. Purification, molecular weight, and composition of bovine visual pigment₅₀₀. Biochemistry **7**, 2906—2913 (1968a).
— Structure of visual pigments, II. Binding of retinal and conformational changes on light exposure in bovine visual pigment₅₀₀. Biochemistry **7**, 2914—2920 (1968).
HERRE, A. W.: The fishes of Lake Lanao: a problem in evolution. Amer. Naturalist **67**, 154—162 (1933).
HERRING, P. J.: The carotenoid pigments of *Daphnia magna* Strauss - I. The pigments of animals fed *Chlorella pyrenoidosa* and pure carotenoids. Comp. Biochem. Physiol. **24**, 187—203 (1968).
HOAR, W. S.: The endocrine system as a chemical link between the organism and its environment. Trans. roy. Soc. Can. III: Ser. IV: Sect. III, **1965**, 175—200 (1965).
HUBBARD, R.: The molecular weight of rhodopsin and the nature of the rhodopsin-digitonin complex. J. gen. Physiol. **37**, 381—399 (1954).
— The bleaching of rhodopsin by light and heat. Nature (Lond.) **181**, 1126 (1958a).
— On the chromophores of the visual pigments. In:Visual problems of colour I. Nat. phys. Lab. Symp. No. 8, 153—169. H.M.S.O., London 1958b.
— KROPF, A.: On the colors of visual pigment chromophores. J. gen. Physiol. **49**, 381—385 (1965).

478   C. D. B. Bridges: The Rhodopsin-Porphyropsin Visual System

Hubbard, R., Wald, G.: Cis-trans isomers of vitamin A and retinene in the rhodopsin System, J. gen. Physiol. **36**, 269—315 (1952).
Karbe, L.: Die Chromosomenverhältnisse bei den Coregonen des Bodensees und einiger weiterer voralpiner Seen, ein Beitrag zum Problem der Speziation in der Gattung *Coregonus*. Z. zool. Systematik u. Evolutionsforsch. **2**, 18—40 (1964a).
— Die Auswirkung der künstlichen Eutrophierung des Bodensees auf das Artgefüge seiner Coregonenpopulation. Mitt. Hamburg Zool. Mus. Inst., Kosswig-Festschrift, Ergänzungsband zu Bd. **61**, 83—90 (1964b).
Kimura, M.: Evolutionary rate at the molecular level. Nature (Lond.), **217**, 624—626 (1968).
Koelz, W.: Coregonid fishes of the Great Lakes. Bull. U.S. Bur. Fish. for 1927, **43**, 297—643 (1929).
— The coregonid fishes of northeastern America. Pap. Michigan Acad. Sci., Arts and Let. **13**, 303—432 (1931).
Köttgen, E., Abelsdorff, G.: Absorption und Zersetzung des Sehpurpurs bei den Wirbeltieren. Z. Psychol. Physiol. Sinnesorg. **12**, 161—184 (1896).
Krinsky, N. I.: The lipoprotein nature of rhodopsin. Arch. Ophthal. **60**, 688—694 (1958).
Larsen, L. O.: Effects of hypophysectomy in the cyclostome, *Lampetra fluviatilis* (L.) Gray. Gen. Comp. Endocrin. **5**, 16—30 (1965).
Lederer, E., Rosanova, V. A., Gillam, A. E., Heilbron, I. M.: Differences in the chromogenic properties of freshwater and marine fish liver oils. Nature (Lond.) **140**, 233 (1937).
Liebman, P. A., Entine, G.: Cyanopsin, a visual pigment of retinal origin. Nature (Lond.) **216**, 501—503 (1967).
— — Visual pigments of frog and tadpole *(Rana pipiens)*. Vision Res. **8**, 761—775 (1968).
Marks, W. B.: Visual pigments of single goldfish cones. J. Physiol. (Lond.) **178**, 14—32 (1965).
Matthews, R. G., Hubbard, R., Brown, P. K., Wald, G.: Tautomeric forms of metarhodopsin. J. gen. Physiol. **47**, 215—240 (1963).
McFarland, W. N., Munz, F. W.: Codominance of visual pigments in hybrid fishes. Science **150**, 1055—1056 (1965).
Morton, R. A., Creed, R. H.: The conversion of carotene to vitamin A_2 by some freshwater fishes. Biochem. J. **33**, 318—324 (1939).
— Pitt, G. A. J.: Studies on rhodopsin 9. pH and the hydrolysis of indicator yellow. Biochem. J. **59**, 128—134 (1955).
— — Visual pigments. Fortschr. Chem. Organ. Naturstoffe XIV, 244—316. Vienna: Springer 1957.
Muntz, W. R. A., Reuter, T.: Visual pigments and spectral sensitivity in *Rana temporaria* and other European tadpoles. Vision Res. **6**, 601—618 (1966).
Munz, F. W.: A new photosensitive pigment of the euryhaline teleost, *Gillichthys mirabilis*. J. gen. Physiol. **40**, 233—249 (1956).
— The photosensitive retinal pigments of fishes from relatively turbid coastal waters. J. gen. Physiol. **42**, 445—459 (1958a).
— Photosensitive pigments from the retinae of certain deep sea fishes. J. Physiol. (Lond.) **140**, system. J. gen. Physiol. **36**, 220—235 (1958b).
— The visual pigments of epipelagic and rocky-shore fishes. Vision Res. **4**, 441—454 (1964).
— Adaptation of visual pigments to the photic environment. In: Colour vision, physiology and experimental psychology. Ciba Foundation Symposium, pp. 27—45. London: J. & A. Churchill 1965.
— Beatty, D. D.: A critical analysis of the visual pigments of salmon and trout. Vision Res. **5**, 1—17 (1965).
— McFarland, W. N.: A suggested hereditary mechanism for visual pigments of chars *(Salvelinus* spp.). Nature (Lond.) **206**, 955—956 (1965).
— Schwanzara, S. A.: A nomogram for retinene₂-based visual pigments. Vision Res. **7**, 111—120 (1967).
— Swanson, R. T.: Thyroxine-induced changes in the proportions of visual pigments. Amer. Zoologist **5**, 683 (1965).
Myers, G. S.: The endemic fish fauna of Lake Lanao, and the evolution of higher taxonomic categories. Evolution **14**, 323—333 (1960).

NAITO, K., WILT, F. H.: The conversion of vitamin A_1 to retinene$_2$ in a freshwater fish. J. biol. Chem. **237**, 3060—3064 (1962).

NORDEN, C. R.: Comparative osteology of representative salmonid fishes, with particular reference to the grayling *(Thymallus arcticus)* and its phylogeny. J. Fish. Res. Bd. Canada **18**, 679—791 (1961).

OHTSU, K., NAITO, K., WILT, F. H.: Metabolic basis of visual pigment conversion in metamorphosing *Rana catesbiana*. Develop. Biol. **10**, 216—232 (1964).

POINCELOT, R. P., MILLAR, P. G., KIMBEL, R. L., ABRAHAMSON, E. W.: Lipid to protein chromophore transfer in the photolysis of visual Pigments. Nature (Lond.), **221**, 256—257 (1969).

REGAN, C. TATE: The freshwater fishes of the British Isles. London: Methuen 1911.

— Guide to the freshwater fishes exhibited in the Department of Zoology, British Museum (Natural History), 2nd. ed. London: British Museum (Natural History) 1932.

RUTTNER, R.: Fundamentals of limnology. Translated by D. G. and F. E. J. FREY. Toronto: University of Toronto Press. 1953.

SCHWANZARA, S. A.: The visual pigments of freshwater fishes. Vision Res. **7**, 121—148 (1967).

SHICHI, H.: Spectrum and purity of bovine rhodopsin. Biochemistry **9**, 1973—1977 (1970).

— LEWIS, M. S., IRREVERRE, F., STONE, A. L.: Biochemistry of visual pigments. 1. Purification and properties of bovine rhodopsin. J. biol. Chem. **244**, 529—536 (1969).

SHIELDS, J. E., DINOVO, E. C., HENRIKSEN, R. A., KIMBEL, R. L., MILLAR, P. G.: The purification and amino acid composition of bovine rhodopsin. Biochim. Biophys. Acta **147**, 238—251 (1967).

SJÖSTRAND, F. S.: The structure of cytoplasm: the organisation of membranous layers. Rev. mod. Phys. **31**, 302—318 (1959).

SMITH, S. H.: Evolution and distribution of the coregonids. J. Fish. Res. Bd. Canada **14**, 599—604 (1957).

SNODDERLY, D. M.: Reversible and irreversible bleaching of rhodopsin in detergent solutions. Proc. natl. Acad. Sci. (Wash.) **57**, 1356—1362 (1967).

SVÄRDSON, G.: The coregonid problem VI. The Palaearctic species and their intergrades. Rept. Inst. Freshwater Res. Drottningholm **38**, 267—356 (1957).

— Interspecific hybrid populations in *Coregonus*. In: Systematics of Today. Uppsala University Årsskrift **6**, 231—239 (1958).

— The coregonid problem VII. The isolating mechanisms in sympatric species. Rept. Inst. Freshwater Res. Drottningholm **46**, 95—123 (1965).

THOMMEN, H., WACKERNAGEL, H.: Zum Vorkommen von Keto-Carotenoiden in Crustaceen. Naturwissenschaften **51**, 87—88 (1964).

TUCKER, D. W.: A new solution to the Atlantic eel problem. Nature (Lond.) **183**, 495—501 (1959).

VOLLENWEIDER, R. A.: Photometric studies in inland waters: I. Relations existing in the spectral extinction of light in water. Mem. Ist. Ital. Idrobiol. **13**, 87—113 (1961).

WAGLER, E.: Die Coregonen in den Seen des Voralpengebietes XI. Herkunft und Einwanderung der Voralpencoregonen. Veröff. Zool. Staatssaml. München **1**, 3—62 (1950).

WALD, G.: Pigments of the retina I. The bull frog. J. gen. Physiol. **19**, 781—795 (1936a).

— Pigments of the retina II. Sea robin, sea bass and scup. J. gen. Physiol. **20**, 45—56 (1936b).

— Visual purple system in fresh-water fishes. Nature (Lond.) **139**, 1017—1018 (1937).

— On the distribution of vitamins A_1 and A_2. J. gen. Physiol. **22**, 391—415 (1939a).

— The porphyropsin visual system. J. gen. Physiol. **22**, 775—794 (1939b).

— The visual systems of euryhaline fishes. J. gen. Physiol. **25**, 235—245 (1941).

— The visual system and vitamins A of the sea lamprey. J. gen. Physiol. **25**, 331—336 (1942).

— The chemical evolution of vision. Harvey Lect. **41**, 117—160 (1947).

— Biochemical evolution. In: Modern Trends in Physiology and Biochemistry pp. 337—376. Ed. by E. S. G. BARRON. New York: Academic Press 1952.

— Vision. Fed.Proc. **12**, 606—611 (1953).

— The metamorphosis of visual systems in the sea lamprey. J. gen. Physiol. **40**, 901—914 (1957).

— The significance of vertebrate metamorphosis. Circulation **21**, 916—938 (1960a).

Wald, G.: The distribution and evolution of visual systems. In: Comparative Biochemistry 1, pp. 311—345. Ed. by M. Florkin and H. S. Mason. New York-London: Academic Press 1960 b.

— Brown, P. K.: Human rhodopsin. Science **127**, 222—226 (1958).

— Brown, P. K.: The molar extinction of rhodopsin. J. gen. Physiol. **37**, 189—200 (1953).

— — Smith, P. H.: Cyanopsin, a new cone pigment of vision. Science **118**, 505—508 (1953).

— — Smith, P. S: Iodopsin. J. gen. Physiol. **38**, 623—681 (1955).

— Hubbard, R.: The reduction of retinene to vitamin A_1 *in vitro*. J. gen. Physiol. **32**, 367—389 (1949).

Williams, T. P., Milby, S. E.: The thermal decomposition of some visual pigments. Vision Res. 8, 359—367 (1968).

Wilt, F. H.: The differentiation of visual pigments in metamorphosing larvae of *Rana catesbiana*. Develop. Biol. 1, 199—233 (1959 a).

— The organ specific action of thyroxin in visual pigment differentiation. J. Embryol. exp. Morph. 7, 556—563 (1959 b).

Yamada, E.: The fine structure of the pigment epithelium in the turtle eye. In: The Structure of the Eye, pp. 73—84. Ed. by G. K. Smelser. New York: Academic Press 1961.

Yoshizawa, T., Horiuchi, S.: Intermediates in the photolytic process of porphyropsin. Int. Symp. Biochem. of the Eye, Nijmegen, Netherlands (1968). Exp. Eye Res. 8, 243—244 (1969).

Young, R. W.: The renewal of photoreceptor cell outer segments. J. Cell Biol. **33**. 61—72 (1967).

— Passage of newly formed protein through the connecting cilium of retinal rods in the frog. J. Ultrastruct. Res. **23**, 462—473 (1968).

— Droz, B.: The renewal of protein in retinal rods and cones. J. Cell Biol. **39**, 169—184 (1968).

Zuckerkandl, E., Pauling, L.: Evolutionary divergence and convergence in proteins. In: Evolving Genes and Proteins, pp. 97—166. Ed. by V. Bryson and H. J. Vogel. New York: Academic Press 1965.

Chapter 12

Microspectrophotometry of Photoreceptors

By

P. A. LIEBMAN, Philadelphia, Pennsylvania. (USA)

With 14 Figures

Contents

I. Methods of Studying Visual Pigments

In truth, the working out of the photochemical system of the cone may long continue to seem the most difficult branch of the physiology of the eye.... With the very sloppiest of technique, we can mount the fresh dark-adapted retina of a frog or a goldfish on the microscope and still see the rich wine of rhodopsin filling its rods. But with the most careful of methods, we can succeed in seeing living cones only as completely colorless structures, whose bland innocence conceals invisible traces of three important somethings — to our utter exasperation. (G. L. WALLS, 1942)

In nearly thirty intervening years we have not overcome the exasperation so poetically expressed by GORDON WALLS, for in achieving the conditions of illumination under which our own cones "see" color, the important somethings of the cones we observe are inevitably destroyed. It would no doubt have been of great satisfaction to WALLS, himself an engineer, to know that the technical revolution, which has steadily progressed since the wedding of the physical sciences with biology, would so soon extend man's senses to make possible the detection of the invisible, and thus, in a fashion perhaps even more satisfactory than detection directly by the experimenter's own eye, enable us to observe the invisible somethings in nearly any of the "completely colorless structures" he spent his life examining. It is an arresting coincidence that it was the very "living cones" of frog and goldfish mentioned in WALLS' rhetoric whose "bland innocence" was first denied through discovery of their contained pigments by microspectrophotometry.

The answer to the question why we cannot directly observe the color of cones is an instructive one, and may well serve to introduce one of the problems in the detection of visual pigments in single cells. It is by now regarded as reasonable to expect that all visual pigments are photosensitive and are bleached by light. At room temperature, each molecule of visual pigment that absorbs a photon will, with near certainty, decompose to colorless products within a few thousandths of a second. For practical purposes, the bleaching is irreversible for all visual pigments — in the absence of the pigment epithelium or of externally supplied 11-cis retinal. (We exclude photoregeneration which does not appreciably occur under conditions of direct observation or spectroscopy.) Even in the presence of rejuvenants, regeneration is a slow process that reaches a significant level only after many seconds or minutes. The efficiency of bleaching is high, and it will later be shown that visual pigments in isolated single cells will not survive an illumination of 5×10^{16} photons/cm²/sec of "white" light for more than about one second.

With this limit in mind we must then ask how much light will be needed to perceive the color of a single cone outer segment visualized in a microscope. Measurements from the several laboratories detecting cone pigments in single cells are in fair agreement that unbleached cone outer segments absorb about 5% of the incident light at λ_{max}, when the measurements are made side-on. To determine whether the color of such a weakly absorbing object can be detected by the human eye at sufficiently dim illuminations, a 1×6 mm piece of a photostable color filter material, Kodak CC 025M, was mounted on a spectrally neutral white surface and illuminated by a tungsten lamp the flux density of which could be varied. The filter material absorbs maximally at 550 nm, 5% of the incident light or about 10% on a reflected double pass at λ_{max}, with a visual-pigment-like band width. The mounted piece of filter was made to subtend the same portion of the observer's retina at 10 inches as does a typical amphibian cone outer segment under adequately magnified microscopic viewing conditions. The minimum illumination that allowed the color of the object to be discerned against a large-field white background in a dark room contained 10^{11} photons/sec/cm^2 of 550 nm light of 12 nm band width and $\sim 10^{12}$ photons/sec/cm^2 integrated over the 400—700 nm range. A cone outer segment 1—2 μm in diameter must be magnified 500—1000 times for adequate visualization. Since a magnified illumination of 10^{12} is required to see color, the required microscope object plane illumination must be about $(1000)^2 \times 10^{12}$ or 10^{18} photons/sec/cm^2. As little as one second of exposure to this intensity would exceed the estimate of illumination sufficient to bleach the cone completely by more than an order of magnitude. For this reason it is clear that one should be surprised indeed at any claim that the color of a visual pigment could be seen in cones. On the other hand, the larger size of amphibian rods allows them to be viewed adequately with 5—10× less magnification. Their larger diameter further yields a more saturated color which allows easier detection. The object-plane illumination for single rods may therefore be reduced to around 10^{16} photons/sec/-cm^2 and an exposure of several seconds will be tolerated. That these calculations are reasonably accurate may be confirmed by watching the rapid fading of a single amphibian rod in the microscope where the illumination is just sufficient to convince one that dark adapted rods are originally pink. Of course it is much easier to see "the rich wine of rhodopsin" in a whole retina, for here, with little or no magnification, the color of many rods together may be seen for some time at light intensities sufficient to bleach only slowly. No retina, however, contains enough cones together in one place, and free of overlying absorbers, e.g. macular pigments or oil drops, to allow the direct visualization of pigment color, so simple in the case of rods. For this and other reasons, microspectrophotometers have come on the scene.

It is perhaps of further empirical interest to note that although one can see the rich wine of goldfish rods in large fields of retina, this color too is absent when individual cells are examined. In view of the previous discussion this comes as no surprise for goldfish rods are only about 1 μm in diameter and, like cones of comparable size, are too quickly bleached in light sufficiently strong for us to see color at the single cell level. Thus it may be confirmed that it is not cone pigments *per se* that are at fault but rather the size of small outer segments in general that sets a limit on what can be observed directly. Microspectrophotometry (MSP) of single goldfish rods on the other hand has directly demonstrated the presence of a pigment absorbing maximally at 522 nm. This confirms earlier evidence based on extraction of a 522 nm pigment but obviates the presumptive logic, which is necessary in extraction experiments, to assign the pigment to a particular cell type.

But before going further into discussion of the technique and results of MSP let us detail and compare the several variations of spectroscopic technique that have been used to define the light-absorbing properties of visual pigments and of their intermediate products of bleaching. Each technique has its own set of assets and liabilities, some of which have been summarized in Table 1. To develop a keener perspective concerning the efficacy of MSP as a tool for the study of visual pigments, a brief discussion of these methodological assets and liabilities is appropriate.

Table 1. *Methods of visual pigment spectroscopy and their associated problems[a]. Method 7 and 8 are included for completeness. 0, does not have the problems specified below, +, does have the problems specified below; ±, may or may not have the problems specified below, depending on the animal, or the problems may be compensated in data reduction*

Method	Problem							
	1	2	3	4	5	6	7	8
1. Extraction	+ +	±	+	±	+ +	0	±	±
2. Fundal Reflectometry	+ +	±	+	0	+ +	+	+	+
3. Macrodensitometry	+ +	±	+	0	+ +	0	±	±
4. Film Densitometry	0	0	±	0	0	0	0	±
5. Microdensitometry (MSP)								
a) end on	0	0	±	0	0	±	0	±
b) side on	0	0	0	0	0	±	0	0
6. ERP	+ +	±	(+ +)	0	+ +	±	±	±
7. Microelectrode								
8. Psychophysical								

Problems
1. Specification of components in mixtures of equally concentrated components.
2. Spectroscopic swamping of minority pigment.
3. Scattering-ultraviolet or visible.
4. Destruction or alteration of pigments by the solubilizer.
5. Identification of pigment with cellular origin.
6. Sensitivity and resolution.
7. Product interference.
8. Interference by extraneous absorbing material.

[a] This list is not intended to be exhaustive but is illustrative of where MSP can fill gaps caused by methodological difficulties.

A. Densitometry of Extracts

Subsequent to visual observations of the ephemeral pink color of excised retinas, the first quantitative spectroscopic studies of visual pigments were done on bile-salt extracts of retina. Extraction by detergents is unique in providing large quantities of visual pigment (of the order of 1 mg/retina and many mgs from pooled retinas) in an accessible *in vitro* form upon which detailed chemical analyses can be pursued. Such massive quantities of single pigments lend themselves to very accurate determinations of spectroscopic parameters such as λ_{max}, ε_{max}, bandwidth, photosensitivity, etc. The absorption traces obtainable from a cuvette of rhodopsin properly prepared under dark-room (red light) conditions are so smooth and reproducible that one can generally be excused for being unmindful of considerations such as signal-to-noise ratio, bleaching by the measuring beam, etc., factors that may properly preoccupy the microspectroscopist. It is clear that the asset of quantity that is peculiar to the solubilisation technique will continue to assure its preference wherever detailed studies on a single pigment must be carried out.

Solubilisation spectroscopy of visual pigment may be complicated by the simultaneous extraction of several visual pigments and of non-visual pigments, which cause distortion of absolute spectra and necessitate special procedures and corrections, such as bleaching difference spectra and differential bleaching. Difference spectra may in turn require correction for the presence of photoproducts formed in the post-bleach state that were not present in the pre-bleach state. The use of hydroxylamine to shift the photoproduct spectrum to shorter wavelengths, where it interferes less with the parent pigment spectrum, has become popular. However, hydroxylamine has been shown to lead to the early spontaneous decay of some pigments present (REUTER, 1966; DARTNALL, 1967). Differential bleaching is progressively less effective in separating two or more visual pigments simultaneously present as the concentration of the pigments become disparate and as their λ_{max} become closer together. One would hope that these restrictions might ultimately be removed by a technique for extracting different pigments separately, or of separating them after extraction, e. g. by electrophoresis, but reports of success in these endeavors have not appeared. Although the resolution of two components in mixtures of rhodopsin and porphyropsin has become a commonplace, only rarely has the resolution of other (minority) pigments proved feasible by differential bleaching. This has certainly been the case in attempts to resolve the contribution of cone pigments to the overall spectrum of extracts, for the cone pigments may contribute only 1% or less of the total and may easily be spectroscopically "swamped out" by the preponderant 99% of rod pigment present. That is, the shape of the overall rod pigment spectrum may be imperceptibly altered by the cone pigment spectrum, and furthermore it may be impossible to find any wavelength for differential bleaching that will bleach a much larger amount of the cone pigment than of the rod pigment present.

Absorption and scattering by the solubilizer or its suspended micelles has little effect on spectra in the visible range but can be a problem in ultraviolet spectroscopy. Since the protein bands (near 280 nm and 233 nm) persist after bleaching, difference spectroscopy is of no value, and indirect estimates of the scattering contribution to the spectrum must be made.

Finally, visual pigment extraction forever removes the identifying link that tells in what type cell the pigment originated. In some cases indirect evidence has been sufficient to establish the cellular origin of a pigment but one can expect much greater difficulty in establishing such connections for extracts containing more than one dominant pigment or several minority pigments.

B. Fundal Reflectometry

In the hands of its principle users, RUSHTON and WEALE, fundal reflectometry has yielded valuable data on intact conscious human subjects. This is the only technique of visual pigment spectroscopy that measures pigments and their behavior under physiologic conditions. Using such results one can correlate visual pigment photochemistry with psychophysical measurements on the same subject and in the animal of most interest to man, man. The major achievements have been measurements of the kinetics of rod and cone pigment regeneration following light adaptation, and the demonstration that more than one cone pigment is present in normal human foveas. These results have been extended to explain several abnormal conditions of retinal performance, and to show to what extent pigment bleaching and neural factors are responsible for light and dark adaption. However, it is seen on perusal of Table 1, that in spite of an unique ability to apprise us of pigment properties under perfectly physiologic conditions, fundal reflectometry has many of the same disadvantages as the extraction method, and, in some regards, its results are even less satisfying. One of its insuperable limitations results from the presence of the pigment epithelium at the back of the eye. This structure allows only one part in 10^4-10^5 of the light striking it to return to the detection apparatus through the pupil. This means that to achieve satisfactory photometric accuracy one must use either brilliant measuring lights, which may bleach too much pigment during measurement, or one must sum the light reflected from large fields of receptors in the retina, which, in turn, results in poor spatial resolution. For example, it has not been possible to record the presence of pigments in regions any smaller than the entire fovea, containing about 100,000 cells. One must therefore employ differential bleaching to detect the presence of more than one pigment. Difference spectra must be used in any event because of the large distortion caused by the presence of the yellow macular pigment and of hemoglobin in the retinal light path. Bleaching products cannot be as satisfactorily dealt with as in solution and the thorny problem of parallel absorbances has led to unfortunate difficulties (Ripps and Weale, 1964; Rushton, 1964). As in solution, uncertainties in assigning pigments to specific cellular morphologies has made it impossible to learn whether the two cone pigments demonstrated in human foveas should be assigned to the same or to different cells. Finally, because of limitations in spatial resolution, it is not possible to determine directly whether cone pigments in the parafoveal retina are the same as those in the fovea.

C. Macrodensitometry

With this technique, the light transmission through small patches of excised retina is measured in a spectrophotometer equipped with a light stop, which allows only a small portion of a retina to be illuminated, or with an interposed low power microscope, which demagnifies the measuring beam of the spectrometer on to a small portion of retina (Brown, 1961). Using excised retina without pigment epithelium, one may regain much of the factor of 10^4-10^5 that is lost in fundal reflectometry without acquiring the liabilities associated with the use of a solubiliser. However, in achieving reasonably high spectral resolution, portions of retina have been examined that contain $100-1000$ cells or more. Thus mixtures of pigments will again appear in the spectrum, simultaneously presenting the problems associated with the resolution of similar mixture-spectra in both the two previously discussed methods. Light scattering is increased in the excised retina and difference spectra may again be a necessity. The chief advantage of this technique is that it obviates the labor, and side effects of solubilisation. It is most useful when only one pigment predominates, and it has the same pitfalls in estimating cellular pigment densities as does fundal reflectometry.

D. Film Densitometry

Though it is generally thought that reliable spectroscopy of visual pigments in single cells was not possible until the advent of S—20 photomultipliers, photographic films of adequate sensitivity have been available for some time. As in microspectrophotometry, film spectrography of photosensitive material must be used with some attention to methodological limitations. Proper experimental design includes the same care to avoid bleaching during preparation of the specimen before measurement that the other methods require. An estimate should be made of the number of photons that can be tolerated in measurement before an unacceptable amount of bleaching is caused by the measuring light. A film is then chosen that is capable of detecting the density difference expected at particular wavelengths upon bleaching, and of rendering density differences in the film image that a densitometer can detect. A microscope magnification is then chosen that will transfer the acceptable photon flux in the object plane to the film at the appropriate value for optimal film performance. This magnification will usually be lower than that for direct visual microscopy since lower magnification means higher photon flux density at the film plane, and consequently less exposure of the object plane, which is bleaching. The magnification must not, however, provide an image whose spread function at the film plane exceeds the resolving power of the film.

Although film spectrography has never been applied to the detection of visual pigments in single cones, DENTON and WYLLIE (1955) used it to obtain end-on, single-cell spectra of the pigments of red and green rods of the frog, using a film plane magnification of 36. A 500× film plane magnification was used by DOBROWOLSKI, JOHNSON and TANSLEY (1955) to measure side-on spectra of single *Xenopus* rods. Though no elaborate theoretical justification was given for the methodological details in either case, the qualitative appreciation of the need for low magnification expressed by DENTON and WYLLIE seems to have been rewarded by a more satisfactory experimental result. It is a pity that this technique has been so little used with other retinas. At least part of the explanation may be in the labor involved, for direct photoelectric recording of single cells by MSP can produce the final spectrum within 0.1—1 min., compared with times of the order of hours for film spectrography. Thus experiments that would require weeks by the latter method could be done in an afternoon using MSP. On the other hand, film recording has the unique feature that data from thousands of cells are registered as quickly as from one cell. Thus a record of topographic distribution, which would be an insuperable task for the microspectrophotometer alone, could be easily provided, the full spectral density data for a large number of cells being obtained in one operation for later densitometric analysis. Since individual pigments stay compartmented in separate cells, problems of discriminating the spectra of minority pigments should not arise except, for example, where tiny frog cones may be hidden deep among the larger outer segments of rods. The practical problems caused by light scattering and photoproduct interference are the same as those associated with end-on MSP of single receptors and are discussed in that section of this chapter.

E. The Early Receptor Potential

The early receptor potential (ERP) has been shown to arise in the visual receptors (BROWN and MURAKAMI, 1964; CONE, 1964). In a dark-adapted retina containing a single visual pigment, the action spectrum of the ERP is found to match exactly the absorption spectrum of the pigment (CONE, 1964), and its amplitude is linearly proportional to the amount of pigment present. Regeneration of bleached pigment is accompanied by directly proportional regeneration of the ERP, and the kinetics of regeneration match those found by earlier techniques (Cone and Cobbs, 1969). It thus seems feasible in principle to use ERP action spectroscopy, in combination with standard differential bleaching techniques, for the discovery and study of visual pigments in excised retinas or in intact eyes, in or removed from the animal. The ERP recorded by wick electrodes from the whole eye in response to a bright flash may be hundreds of microvolts in amplitude. Measurement accuracy is limited by the small amplitude and brief duration of this potential, and tissue approximating the entire retina in size must be utilised. ERP action spectra have thus far been obtained on few retinas but the frog retina illustrates a peculiarity, which may in this case be an asset, though in others a liability. The frog retina has been shown by other techniques to contain a preponderance of rhodopsin, but its ERP action spectrum contains a dominant peak at about 575 nm (Goldstein, 1968), which corresponds to the principal cone absorption spectrum (Liebman and Entine, 1968 a, b). This comes as somewhat of a surprise since more than 90% of the retinal pigment is rhodopsin though little evidence of its existence is seen by ERP spectroscopy. Whatever the reason for this unexpected result, the advantage in thus finding minority pigments that can be spectroscopically separated from more copious amounts of other pigments by such a simple method (recording a voltage across the eye using wick electrodes) is quite obvious. On the other hand, the failure of some cells or pigments to contribute to the ERP cannot always be looked upon as an asset if it is our purpose to discover visual pigments using this technique. Currently, most work with the ERP concerns analysis of its component parts and the mechanism of its generation, and little exploration of visual pigments is being made. Its assets, however, may be expected to be those of a technique that requires no elaborate or expensive spectrophotometer or microdensitometer. Its liabilities will be similar to the other techniques that require large areas of retina rather than single cells to provide adequate signals for spectral analysis.

F. Microspectrophotometry

The potentialities, and many of the limitations, of MSP as applied to single visual receptor outer segments were realised, at least qualitatively, by Hanaoka and Fujimoto (1957) who seem to have been the first to extend the techniques initiated by Caspersson (1940) to the photosensitive visual pigments. Although the precise results they obtained on carp retina are still somewhat difficult to interpret (see later), modern (1962—present) photoreceptor MSP has added only a little refinement and some technological muscle to the laudable foresight of these investigators. Pulse amplitude modulation and feedback control systems used by Yang and Legallais (1954) and by Chance, Perry, Akerman and Thorell (1959) in their microspectrophotometers have added speed, accuracy and automaticity to instruments that have been designed and built in individual laboratories for this work. Automatic wavelength scanning was used by Brown (1961) in his adaption of a commercial instrument, by Liebman (Liebman; 1962; Liebman and Entine, 1964) and by Marks (1963) who made further electronic improvements in their homemade instruments. The list of investigators who have joined in the search for visual pigment spectra from single cells by MSP has grown steadily and includes Strother and WOLKEN (1960), WOLKEN (1962), LANGER and THORELL (1966a), MURRAY (1966), GOLDSMITH, DIZON and FERNANDEZ (1968), and WATERMAN, FERNÁNDEZ and GOLDSMITH (1969).

In MSP, single receptors are visualised in a high-magnification microscope placed in the optical path of a monochomator (Fig. 1). Two submillimeter light beams defined in a field stop are demagnified by an inverted microscope on to the

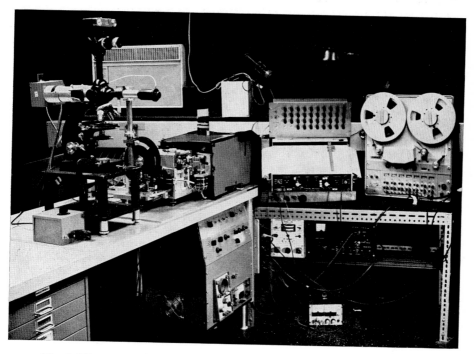

Fig. 1. Microspectrophotometer (Mk. 5) constructed in the author's laboratory

specimen (Fig. 2). One of these beams is made to superimpose on a single outer segment and the other on an area free of cells. The light intensities of the two beams are detected by a photoelectric device (phototube, photomultiplier or phototransistor) and their ratio is formed to give the transmission of the specimen. The wavelength is changed stepwise or continuously and a plot of transmittance (or an equivalent function such as optical density) vs. wavelength is produced on a paper chart. Since MSP is performed directly on optically or mechanically-isolated outer segments, the labors and uncertainties associated with the use of solubilisers are completely obviated. In principle, the spectroscopic swamping of one pigment by another cannot arise and there is no problem of resolving one pigment from another since in nearly all cases it has been found that each different pigment is packaged in a different cell. Cellular morphology is easily correlated with pigment type by direct observation. Interference by non-visual pigments is an infrequent problem, associated in our experience only with the presence of macular pigment in primate retinas and with the oil drops of some receptors in bird and turtle retinas.

Photoproduct distortion of difference spectra, though anticipated, has not been seen in cone spectra, probably because of the very short lifetime of the early intermediates of bleaching and the high surface-to-volume ratio of cones, which leads to the rapid loss of the retinals from the outer segment by diffusion into the large reservoir of surrounding medium. Measurements have been made side-on (receptor long axis perpendicular to direction of light propagation) and end-on. Except for a very small, nearly wavelength-independent reflection from the receptor surfaces, there is virtually no light scattering problem associated with side-on microspectrophotometry of the homogeneous outer segment, even in the ultraviolet to about 200 nm (see Fig. 10). On the other hand, light-scattering may present a severe problem, even in the visible region, to end-on MSP of receptors attached to the retina for, at least in the method so far used, the measuring light beam must pass through the milky neural layers of the excised retina before encountering the outer segments. The scattering of these layers grows intense with time and cannot be eliminated by refractive index matching using e.g. glycerol. In our hands, single receptor spectra obtained from primate retinas are highly suspect for this reason, and inevitably contain contributions from the pigments of the surrounding receptors through which scattered light reaches the detector. Finally, a liability inherent in the technique, which is not likely to find much improvement in the future, is that of the intrinsic limit of sensitivity and resolution set by the small size, limited pigment content and high photosensitivity of the receptor outer segment. These limitations are treated quantitatively in the following section.

II. Theory of Detection of Photosensitive Substances

To detect a substance by its absorption of light one must be able to determine that the difference between the average number of photons transmitted by the sample and the average number of photons incident on the sample (the signal) exceeds by a sufficient amount the random fluctuations (noise) in the combined measuring and measured system. The combined noise may arise from dark noise and photoelectron shot noise in the detector (photomultiplier), from amplifier or other electrical circuit noise, from mechanical vibration, and from biological motion due to Brownian movement or convection currents in the preparation. The last of these is easily eliminated by using 8% gelatin in Ringer's solution as a mounting medium since this solution gels at room temperature to immobilise the preparation without causing apparent changes in absorptive properties of the cells. For the light intensities that must be used in MSP, the relative contribution of photoelectron shot noise (which sets the irreducible intrinsic limit to any photoelectric measurement) should be much larger than any of the remaining possible noise sources, and only a little care in instrument design and in selection and use of components is necessary to ensure that this is the case.

The mean-square photoelectron noise or shot noise current, $\overline{i_n^2}$, at the cathode of a photomultiplier is given by

$$\overline{i_n^2} = 2e^2 k I R \Delta B \tag{1}$$

where e is the charge on the electron, k, the ratio of photoelectrons generated to photons incident at the cathode surface (including contribution of non-total absorption of incident photons and non-total transmission by collecting optics as well as the quantum efficiency for conversion of absorbed photons to electrons), I, the incident photon flux density at the object plane, R, the area of the object illuminated and ΔB, the limiting signal bandwith of the attached electrical circuitry. ΔB may also be regarded as the reciprocal of the detection or observation time, τ, where $\tau = \dfrac{1}{\Delta B} = 2\,rc$ for a single stage filter, where r and c are the resistance and capacitance.

The signal to be detected is $I_i - I_t$ where I_i is the average flux density incident on the sample and I_t the flux density after attenuation by the sample. Since the fraction absorbed by the sample is $A = 1 - T$, where T is the fraction transmitted, it follows that the signal is also $I_i - I_t = A I_i$. This produces an average photoelectric signal current difference, i_s, given by

$$i_s = ek A I_i R .\qquad(2)$$

The total mean-square shot noise involved in a measurement is contributed by both the incident beam I_i, and the transmitted beam I_t. If the absorption is small (20% or less), there is little difference in the two fluxes and the vectorial sum of the noises is

$$\overline{i_{nt}^2} = 2e^2 k \Delta B \, (I_t + I_i) \, R \cong 4 e^2 k \Delta B I_i R .$$

However, the photocurrent from I_i may be used in a separate channel for electronic control of the spectrometer and the relative noise associated with it made smaller through a separate narrower filter bandwidth, ΔB; or by making $R I_i > R I_t$. Thus the total noise may be nearly the same as that associated with I_t alone. We therefore return to expression (1) for $\overline{i_n^2}$. The root-mean-square signal to noise ratio $S/N|_{\mathrm{rms}} = i_s/i_n$ of a photoelectron shot noise limited photometer is then

$$\left.\frac{S}{N}\right|_{\mathrm{rms}} = \frac{ek A I_i R}{\sqrt{2e^2 k I_i R \Delta B}} = \frac{A\sqrt{k I_i \tau R}}{\sqrt{2}} = \frac{A\sqrt{kER}}{\sqrt{2}}\qquad(3a)$$

where $E = I_i \tau$, is the total light exposure density per datum point. Units of E are particles/cm². As most recording systems record noise voltage directly rather than its root-mean-square (rms) value, Eq. (3a) must be modified to give the peak to peak $(P-P)$ signal-to-noise ratio, which has been shown to be about 6.5 times less than the rms S/N. Thus

$$\left.\frac{S}{N}\right|_{P-P} \approx \frac{A}{6\cdot 5}\sqrt{\frac{kER}{2}} \approx \frac{A\sqrt{kER}}{9} .\qquad(3b)$$

Detectivity is quantitatively proportional to the signal-to-noise ratio, and the important features in attaining good detectivity are summarised in Eq. (3b). The chances of detecting a substance that absorbs a fraction, A, of the incident light are improved by selecting a detector with a high quantum efficiency, k, and by using a high flux density, I_i, and a long exposure time, τ. The light flux density may be made larger through the use of a brighter light source. The total flux, ER, may be increased by collecting light from a larger area, R, e.g. by using a larger sample. Finally, if the substance can be concentrated or a longer light path used, the absorption, A, may be increased to improve the accuracy of recording.

When we attempt to apply these principles to the detection of visual pigments in single cells, however, several difficulties arise. Thus both the pathlength and concentration of visual pigments in single cells are small and unalterable. Again, if the exposure is increased by increasing either I_i or τ, there is more bleaching of the visual pigment. Moreover, the rate of pigment bleaching increases in direct proportion to the exposure, whereas detectivity is improved only as the square root of the exposure increase.

When bleaching by the measuring light alters a significant fraction of the molecules originally present, distortion of the recorded absorption spectrum may be expected and this can occur in two ways. If the bleached molecules are quickly replaced by product molecules that absorb little or no visible light, the effect on the recorded curve will be to shift its $\lambda_{\max}$ toward the end of the spectrum from which the scan originated. This is the simple case for which Marks (1963, 1965a) derived his correction procedure which estimates the rate of destruction of unbleached molecules during the scan and adds back to the absorption axis the appropriate quantity estimated to have been lost by bleaching during the entire duration of the scan prior to each point that is corrected. Without such a correction procedure, 50% bleach during a spectral scan will shift the apparent $\lambda_{\max}$ of a 575 nm pigment by about 20 nm.

If the "bleached" molecules are not "colorless" but rather form photoproducts whose spectra differ from that of the unbleached pigment, another kind of distortion occurs, and is much more difficult to correct, for a precise knowledge of the spectrum of the products as well as of the kinetic constants for their decay, one to another, is required.

The need to correct such spectral distortions is obviated if the light exposure used to determine the spectrum is reduced to the point where little visual pigment is bleached. However, this procedure is limited by the finding that one must use so little light to attain this goal that noise fluctuations in the measuring beam limit spectral resolution. Thus, we are faced with an impasse: To obtain good spectral resolution and detectivity for weakly-absorbing cells we need to use high light exposures to reduce the relative noise fluctuations—but the more light we use, the more pigment is bleached with increasing danger of spectral distortion or, in the limit, complete destruction of the pigment being measured!

We have suggested that Eq. (3b), although valid, does not help very much because of the constraint put on the value of E. Since E cannot be a free parameter, it is of some interest to investigate just what value E can have, and whether a condition can be found that leads to an acceptable compromise between detectivity and bleaching. For small densities, the bleaching equation is (see Appendix II for derivation)

$$P_t = P_0 e^{-\Phi E} \tag{4}$$

where P_0 and P_t are respectively the amount of pigment initially present and that present after a time, t, of bleaching exposure, $\Phi E = \varepsilon \gamma$ is the photosensitivity of the pigment, P, where ε is the napierian extinction coefficient and γ the quantum efficiency of bleaching.

At the end of a spectral scan, it is desired to have remaining the major part of the pigment originally present so that

$$\frac{P_t}{P_0} = e^{-\Phi E} \approx 1$$

This is approached as $\Phi E \to 0$.

Expanding $e^{-\Phi E}$ we have

$$e^{-\Phi E} = 1 - \Phi E + \frac{(\Phi E)^2}{2!} + \cdots$$

$$= 1 - \Phi E \text{ to a first approximation.}$$

But

$$\frac{P_t}{P_0} + \frac{P_b}{P_0} = 1$$

where P_b is pigment bleached.

Therefore,

$$\frac{P_b}{P_0} = 1 - \frac{P_t}{P_0} = 1 - (1 - \Phi E)$$

$$= \Phi E \tag{5}$$

For small values of P_b/P_0, which is the experimentally desirable condition, the approximation expressed in Eq. (5) gives the exposure that must not be exceeded for a given majority of pigment molecules to remain unbleached.

We now have two separate equations in E, one that tells the virtues of a large E (Eq. (3b)) and the other that tells the folly of a large E (Eq. (5)). The proper choice is between the two extremes and is easily made as follows: If E is chosen larger than that which bleaches an amount of pigment equivalent to the noise in the measuring beam, the advantage of high S/N will be offset by signal attenuation and spectral distortions caused by bleaching during measurement. However, if E is chosen smaller than that which bleaches the noise-equivalent of pigment, the S/N will suffer needlessly through salvation of a little pigment that the S/N is not good enough to detect. The optimum value of E is therefore that which equates the pigment bleached to the peak-to-peak photoelectron shot noise. Thus combining Eq. (3b) and (5) and assuming $P_0 - P_b \cong P_0$ we have

$$\frac{S}{N} = \frac{P_0}{P_b}$$

$$\text{or } \frac{A\sqrt{kER}}{9} = \frac{1}{\Phi E}$$

and solving for E_0, the optimized value of E,

$$E_0 = \frac{4}{(kR)^{1/3}(\Phi A)^{2/3}} \tag{6}$$

An optimal measurement of any visual pigment of low density is achieved when the measuring light exposure is adjusted to be in inverse proportion to the two-thirds power of the fraction, A, of light absorbed by that pigment. This implies that stronger lights (really exposure density) may be used for measuring small cells (cones) than for large cells (such as frog rods) to gain the optimum achievable compromise between bleaching and noise. Substituting the value of E_0 from Eq. (6) back into Eq. (3b), we can see how the signal-to-noise ratio may be expected to vary in measuring weakly-absorbing, as opposed to strongly-absorbing, cells, when the exposure is optimised as suggested:

$$\left. \frac{S}{N} \right|_{E_0} = \frac{2}{9} \left(\frac{kR}{\Phi} \right)^{1/3} A^{2/3} \tag{7}$$

Using the exposure constraint, therefore, we see that instead of a direct S/N dependence on A, we have a two-thirds power dependence. A pigment absorbing 10% of the incident light can thus be recorded at a signal-to-noise ratio only 4.6 times better than that for a pigment absorbing 1%, when the bleaching is made to equal the noise.

The above equations and discussions have a further interesting consequence. Suppose one has the choice of recording a cylindrical outer segment measuring 2 μm in diameter by 20 μm long either end-on or side-on. Which is to be preferred? Since the end-on path length is 10 times that side-on, the end-on absorption will be about 10 times greater than that measured side-on (the latter in linearly polarised light). This factor will improve the optimised end-on S/N by $10^{2/3}$ or 4.6 over the side-on S/N. However, the cell area that can be made to intercept a measuring light beam without causing any difference in the fraction of pigment bleached is greater for the side-on measurement by a factor of 10. The flux at the photomultiplier can therefore be increased by this factor, and from equation 7 we see that this will improve the resultant side-on S/N by $10^{1/3}$ or 2.2. The relative S/N gain realised in using end-on measurement is therefore at most only a factor of 2, which may be an insignificant improvement when one considers the magnitude of the optical problems (light scattering) that inevitably accompany end-on geometry in some excised retinas. This latter factor is so serious as to preclude end-on measurements for S/N improvement alone unless one has fresh retinas, which can with care be maintained in good optical condition. (See later discussion of primate pigments).

The above mathematical formulation applies to the single wavelength case but if we are still only interested in the S/N near the absorption peak, a computation based on equation 7 should give considerably better than order-of-magnitude estimation of the results to be expected in MSP of outer segments. Using the values 0.1 for k, and 10^{-16} cm²/molecule for Φ, a frog rod absorbing 20% of the incident light side-on in an area measuring 4 μm × 50 μm = 200 μm² should yield a S/N of $\sim 100/1$ using an exposure of 10^6 photons/μm², which will bleach only 1% of the contained pigment (0.2% absorption loss at peak). For a frog cone measured similarly with a beam area 1.5 μm × 4 μm = 6 μm², an absorption of 5% at peak should be detected with a S/N of 14/1 using an exposure of 10^7 photons/μm² which will bleach about 7% of the contained pigment. Using the formulation of Marks (1965a) for computing the amount by which the λ_{max} will be shifted to spurious values by bleaching during recording, we find an expected 3 nm red shift for the frog cone and < 0.5 nm for the frog rod. This degree of accuracy is currently quite adequate.

III. Design and Performance of a Microspectrophotometer

The basic building blocks of our instrument are depicted in Fig. 2 and consist of light source, monochromator with associated optics, aperture plate and chopper to form and pulse the microbeams, a pair of microscopes (inverted and upright), and photomultiplier and electronic circuitry, which deliver their output signal to an X-Y recorder, (Fig. 1).

For visible-spectrum recording, a tungsten ribbon filament lamp is preferred. Operated from a constant current regulated DC power supply, the tungsten ribbon provides the highly stable average quantum flux output so important to the attainment of shot-noise limited performance. The much higher radiance provided by arc lamps, e.g., xenon, is not necessary for our purposes and the fluctuations due to arc wandering, so familiar to those who have worked with these sources, may seriously impair performance to below the shot-noise limit required. For ultra-violet recordings we prefer the deuterium arc lamp to xenon, (LIEBMAN and ENTINE, 1969). The hollow cathode of the small arc deuterium lamp provides excellent arc stability and its low output of visible radiation makes it unnecessary to use double monochromation which is required to eliminate the stray light when a xenon lamp is used in uv recording.

A single diffraction grating monochromator is sufficient with the above sources for recording pigments present at low density in single cells. The wavelength advance is linear with shaft rotation. The shaft can thus be coupled to a linear potentiometer for transmitting the wavelength value in electrical form directly to the X axis of the recorder, thus providing an axis of abscissae that is linear in wavelength. The grating is blazed for the ultraviolet to compensate in part for the diminishing quantum flux of the tungsten lamp with shorter wavelengths. The exit slit of the monochromator is focused on the exit pupil of the ocular of an inverted microscope consisting of the Zeiss $32 \times$ Ultrafluar objective and quartz ocular, together designed to minimise lateral chromatic magnification difference over the spectral region $200-650$ nm. These optics reduce and project on to the object plane of the microscope, an image of the aperture plate which is placed at the field lens of the monochromator. The configuration provides Abbé rather than critical illumination, although either method may in principle be used with the spatially homogeneous tungsten ribbon source. The aperture plate obscures all but two tiny holes, cut in aluminium foil or machined to match the dimensions of specific outer segments when reduced in size by the demagnifying inverted microscope. Each of these holes, the sample and the reference beam, is allowed to transmit light for about 6 msec, sample and reference pulses being separated in time by about 1.5 msec of darkness. This time separation is achieved by a rotating sector disc driven from a synchronous motor (see Fig. 2). Thus the two beams flash in temporal periodic succession on to the specimen plane and are similarly transmitted to the photomultiplier whose output then consists of similar pulses of photocurrent plus dark current separated by pulses of dark current.

The remainder of the microscope consists of a removable pellicle beam combiner placed in the base illuminator of the Zeiss microscope stand to allow simultaneous field illumination and spectrometer beam projection on to the specimen, a rotating-rectilinear stage, upright microscope optics for viewing and beam deflector which allows the light to reach the viewer, the photomultiplier or a 35 mm camera.

The photomultiplier is of course the heart of the detection system and should at this stage of technology be regarded as a necessity for MSP. A single stage phototube is inadequate even if it has the proper type photocathode because without the approximately 10^4-fold (nearly noise free) amplification provided by the electron multiplier section, the signal which contains only photoelectron shot-noise and cathode dark noise cannot be made large compared to the thermal noise generated by the large resistor required at the input to the electronics. Electronic and resistor noise thus become limiting and one could never attain sufficient sensitivity to achieve the goal of retinal receptor MSP. Similarly, photodiodes or phototransistors fail (because of their irreducible dark noise caused by recombination of carriers and edge effects) in spite of their intrinsically high quantum efficiency which exceeds that of photomultipliers. The requirement for low dark noise, high quantum efficiency and noiseless amplification can, at present, only be met by photomultipliers. Among the many types available, those with the S-17 and S-20 cathodes are to be preferred since these give the highest available primary quantum efficiency of up to 30% at peak.

The S-8 cathode, used by Hanaoka and Fujimoto (1957), is still available but its very low quantum efficiency of <1% makes it the least desirable on the present market. On comparative curves, the reflective substrate S-17 has been shown to have the highest efficiency but this is now equalled by the S-20 since its availability on a reflective substrate (RCA-4526 data sheet). The spectral response of the S-17 cuts off steeply at about 550 nm whereas the response of the S-20 makes it preferable to all other types beyond this cutoff to about 800 nm. Even among individual samples of S-20 multipliers there is enormous variation in spectral response. Most manufacturers will supply pre-tested tubes as required to emphasise either the blue or the red end of the spectrum. We have generally used an exceptionally red-sensitive tube when looking for red-sensitive pigments and a blue-sensitive tube for 400—550 nm pigments. The quartz window available on several S-20 tubes makes it unnecessary to change tubes for ultraviolet recording to 200 nm. A Bertrand lens in front of the photomultiplier ensures that the reference and sample beams, which are separated in space in the object plane, are not separated in space when they strike the photocathode. Lack of homogeneity in spectral response with microbeam position on the much larger cathode make this a prudent step. In some cases micrometer translation of the photomultiplier with respect to the light beam allows us to find the most sensitive part of the cathode (Liebman and Entine, 1964).

An infrared image-converter fits over the viewing ocular, and infrared filters are interposed in the illuminating optics to protect the specimen from bleaching light when visible recording is not in progress. Before recording is begun, the specimen is placed on the microscope stage using dim red illumination. The field illuminator and monochromator are turned on and pass through a thin gelatin infrared filter placed above the pellicle beam combiner. The optics are focused and an outer segment located using infrared light. The stage is rotated until the major axis of the outer segment is parallel to the long axis of the sample beam. The cell is then moved with the rectilinear stage until it lies over the sample beam. The condenser focus is changed by about 5 μm to correspond to a previously calibrated position that corrects its focus for longitudinal chromatic aberration in the infrared. The microbeam will then come into focus on the cell at about 700 nm and remain in focus throughout the uv-visible spectrum. The monochromator is set to about 750 nm, the pellicle removed, the field illuminator extinguished, the beams directed to the photomultiplier and the electronics activated. After the electronic feedback circuit comes into regulation, the infrared filter is removed and the automatic wavelength scan mechanism is activated. Thus no bleaching light strikes the cells until the moment of measurement.

The photomultiplier output wave is further amplified, the dark period clamped to ground (Fig. 2) and separated into reference and sample channels through an electromechanical chopper. The signal in each channel is filtered by an RC integrator and the now D.C. value is stored at capacitors F_1 and F_2. The value of the reference voltage at F_2 is compared to a standard voltage in comparator amplifier E, and the amplified difference is used to control the output of a voltage-variable,

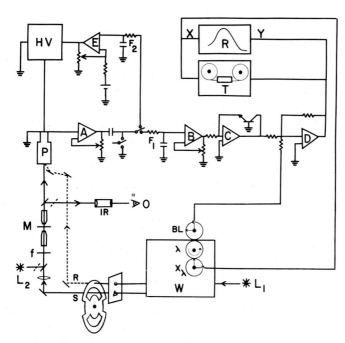

Fig. 2. Schematic diagram of the author's microspectrophotometer. A, B, C, D, E operational amplifiers; F_1 F_2, electrical filters; f, infrared filter; HV, kilovolt power supply; L_1, monochromator light source; L_2, microscope field illuminator with removable beam combiner; M, inverted and upright microscope optics; P, S-20 photomultiplier; R, X-Y recorder; R, S, reference and sample beams formed by aperture plate and time modulated by rotating disc; T, DC tape recorder; W, monochromator; X_λ, wavelength retransmitting potentiometer; λ, wavelength drive motor; BL, baseline compensating function generator; IR, infrared image coverter; O, observer

kilovolt power supply (HV), which in turn supplies the dynode voltage that controls the gain of the photomultiplier. If light becomes weaker at some wavelengths, power fluctuations occur, or the sensitivity of the cathode changes as a function of wavelength, both reference and sample pulses will become smaller, causing a larger difference to be detected at comparator E, and this will cause an increase in dynode voltage until the increase in multiplier gain just exactly offsets the weakening of the pulses. This automatic feedback system is good to 0.1% correction accuracy, responding faster than the speed of the recorder (<5 cps upper band 3 db point). Electronic feedback thus completely compensates for a changing I_i or for fluctuations slower than 10 msec that may affect any other part of the system. Meanwhile, the DC sample voltage passes through a buffer amplifier (B) after which it can drive an operational amplifier log converter (C) from a low impedance source. The output of this device is proportional to log I_t. Since the optical density is by definition $D = \log I_i/I_t = \log I_i - \log I_t$, and the log I_i signal has been made constant by the reference feedback electronics, the output log I_t can be used directly on a calibrated chart to record optical density. Furthermore, since the reference log I_i is a constant, we can make reference I_i anything we want. It is desirable to make I_i larger in the reference beam than in the sample beam for the following reason: If the average reference beam signal is used to control the gain of the sample channel alone, the noise recorded will be the vectorial sum of the photocurrent shot noises of both beams (see p. 491). To achieve the best possible S/N therefore it would be valuable if the reference channel noise could be reduced so that the major contribution came from the sample channel alone. Equation 3a tells how this can be done; by larger $\tau = 2\pi rc$, greater light intensity, I_i, or by larger area R. An increase in the reference circuit rc is a poor choice because this will slow the response speed of the feedback correction of I_i with changing wavelength. Greater I_i is impractical since the reference beam is defined in a field of constant intensity relative to the sample beam. However, R is not fixed for the reference beam, and a larger reference beam can be used to make its relative noise contribution negligible.

When one finally records a baseline with no cell in the sample beam, one finds a line that does not suggest the constant $I_t = I_i (\lambda)$ expected. This is due to the fact that the two beams, sample and reference, do not originate from and pass through identical parts of the entire optical system. In particular, they traverse different paths at the diffraction grating surface and this surface is not homogeneous. However, the differences in $I_i (\lambda)$ between the two beams is constant so long as the apertures are constant in size and continue to correspond to the same part of the grating. Although a constant wiggly baseline can be subtracted from absorbance spectra to obtain the correct spectrum, it is more satisfying to have an immediate display of absolute spectra. The baseline is therefore corrected by generating a function that is the mirror image of the baseline about a horizontal reflection plane passing perpendicular to the chart paper. This correction function $C (\lambda)$ is inserted into a summing amplifier, D, with the log $I_t (\lambda)$ function from log converter, C. The log output of D is therefore log $I (\lambda) + \log J (\lambda)$ or log $I (\lambda) J (\lambda)$ which will now be $K \log I_i (\lambda) = $ constant where $C (\lambda) \equiv \log J (\lambda)$. The function $C (\lambda)$ is generated in 40 linear segments on a 40 tap potentiometer. A different voltage can be inserted into each tap from a master control panel containing an independent control for the voltage of each tap.

The wavelength scan is produced by a variable speed DC motor coupled to the monochromator drive shaft. Scanning speeds of $1-40$ nm/sec can be accomodated. Changing the speed, of course, changes the exposure, E, by altering the time of exposure. Most of our experiments have been done using scans of $10-20$ nm/sec. This keeps the effective exposure time at $10-20$ sec since visual pigments span about 200 nm. Faster scanning speeds must be matched by faster rc's in the electronic circuit filters. Otherwise attenuation and phase shift may result in instrument-induced spectral distortion. One can ensure that this does not occur by recording from a photostable Wratten color filter such as the CC 025 M which has a visual-pigment-like spectrum. Different rc's can be tested with different scan rates to establish the fastest distortion free rates for the rc's.

In recent years we have made increasing use of an external reference beam (dashed line in Fig. 2, bypassing the microscope) in order to obviate the problem of placing simultaneously outer segments in the proper orientation in the sample beam and a space that is free of retinal material in the reference beam. A baseline results that is a measure of the difference in transmission of the microscope and the bypass optics. The loss in violet transmission of the microscope is corrected by the baseline compensator previously discussed.

IV. Results of Microspectrophotometric Investigations on Photoreceptors

A. Early Work on Carp

The 1957 paper of HANAOKA and FUJIMOTO reporting the first known attempt to record signals from single cone outer-segments remains a remarkably prescient document that was not improved upon for at least 5 years. These investigators recognized the impotence of extract spectroscopy to detect cone pigments or to determine whether there were several pigments per cell or different pigments in different cells. They realized that the low pigment density and its high photosensitivity would require precautions against bleaching during preparation and measurement in the microspectrophotometer. They chose a species known to have very large cones in order to minimise these problems. Although they had no infra-red vision equipment, they searched out and aligned outer segments in their instrument using alternately red light or blue light to shield different possible pigments from early destruction. The cells were spared from light exposure, in the intervals between measurements at different wavelengths, by a beam sampling system similar, if less automatic and speedy, to that of current instruments. Our present (side-on) isolation procedure and mounting technique is nearly identical to theirs. Following CASPERSSON (1940), however, they used objectives of very high NA (1.25) and took pains to eliminate high density errors due to optical glare and the small size of very dense objects. These, of course, were quite unnecessary precautions since the authors had by their own recognition to measure low densities of photosensitive substances present in large areas – quite different problems from those that faced CASPERSSON and later investigators of nucleic acids. Today we find little advantage in the use of high NA objectives, for although their resolution (about 0.2 µm at NA 1.25) may be good, all of their other properties (greater spherical, chromatic and higher-order aberrations, lower transmission, and glare leading to poor contrast in an application where contrast for visualisation of outer segments is already a significant problem) make a difficult job in microscopy nearly impossible. Nevertheless examples of spectra were given for frog red rods and green rods as well as for the carp cones. Seventy-three cone spectra were recorded which fell into non-overlapping categories having λ_{max} of 420–430 nm, 490–500 nm, 520–540 nm, 560–580 nm, 620–640 nm, and 670–680 nm – six classes in all. They also reported several instances of two peaks in a single cone outer segment. Most of their cone spectra were narrow and seldom came close to fitting the Dartnall nomogram. Their results were obtained as difference spectra but there is no indication whether or not the pre-bleach spectrum was reproducible. Thus if bleaching occurred during measurement, the spectral maxima would be shifted from their true values and would be variable if the exposure were not quite constant for each cell measured. It will be seen later that there is mounting evidence that not all visual pigments fit the Dartnall nomogram. However, HANAOKA and FUJIMOTO's results are far more extreme. Although their curves for frog and carp rods give about the right λ_{max} in each case, the absolute densities given for side-on measurements (0.1—0.3) challenge credulity and the curve shapes are very peculiar, giving a density at 600 nm of about 0.1 for frog and 0.2 for carp, and near zero at 450 nm for both (see LIEBMAN and ENTINE, 1968b). The unbleachable absolute spectrum of a frog "green" rod showing maximum transmission at 550 nm and densities greater than 0.1 at both 450 nm and at 650 nm must certainly be spurious (see LIEBMAN and ENTINE, 1968b). The recent microelectrode single cone action spectra on *Cyprinus carpio* obtained by TOMITA (1967) show only three separate λ_{max} which agree very well with the MSP data both MARKS and LIEBMAN obtained from the related species *Carassius auratus*. In the admittedly few species that have been examined by MSP since this early work, there has been no evidence of more than three cone pigments in any retina. Furthermore, with the exception of the possible 665—690 nm pigment suggested by RUSHTON (1965), NAKA and RUSHTON (1966) and WITKOVSKY (1967), there is no evidence that makes us believe there may be more than three cone pigments in any one species.

What then is the explanation for HANAOKA and FUJIMOTO's results? It is of course not possible to answer this question with assurance. However, there are two major optical effects in outer segments that the authors may not have considered when they did their measurements. These are linear dichroism and birefringence (SCHMIDT, 1938). Current side-on measurements utilize the predominant orientation of visual chromophores across the long axis of outer segments to increase the absorbance and S/N measured in light that is plane polarized in this same direction. Simultaneously, since the E vector of the measuring light is parallel to one of the major retardation axes (fast axis) of the outer segment, no change in the state of polarisation of the transmitted beam can result from birefringence.

It has been shown that the light emitted from a monochromator (even one without lenses) is elliptically polarised and that the ellipticity may change as a function of wavelength, even to the extent of reversal of its major axis (LIEBMAN and ENTINE, 1964). If such a beam is not made plane polarised as suggested above, it may interact with the cellular dichroism in a manner that increases the fraction of light absorbed in one part of the spectrum (when the major axis of the ellipse crosses the cellular axis) and diminishes it in another (when the axial ratio changes as a function of wavelength). Furthermore, if there is an optical component following the outer segment in the system that can behave as a linear polariser (as e.g., a reflecting surface struck at non-normal incidence or a high NA objective), attenuation of the beam due to anomalous dispersion may superimpose a function that looks like the first derivative of the absorption spectrum onto the already distorted absorbance spectrum. This will yield narrow band spectra.

Thus, while the work of HANAOKA and FUJIMOTO was the forerunner of contemporary work, it must fall short of satisfying the logical demands of present analysis. To bear conviction, data from single receptors must be reproducible, the pigment should be bleachable and full account must be taken of the known properties of both cell and instrument that might lead to distortion.

B. Goldfish

As in the carp, the cone outer segments of the common goldfish, *Carassius auratus* are behemoths of the cone world. It was natural, therefore, and in keeping with the expectation of difficulties caused by bleaching during measurement, that MARKS (1963) and later LIEBMAN and ENTINE (1964) began their attempts to measure cone pigments with this species. Goldfish cone outer segments have a basal diameter that may measure as much as 5μm. They taper to 1 μm within the first 10 μm of length but continue to as much as 40—50 μm in total length (LATIES and LIEBMAN, unpublished data). The 1 μm diameter prolongation of 30 μm length or so is almost always broken off in the preparation of samples for spectroscopy, however, and has been ignored in MSP. In his work, MARKS soon recognized that although the problems of high S/N and bleaching were at odds one with the other, there was additional information to be gained from bleach distorted spectra that might be used to correct the distortion that he exchanged for a higher S/N. MACNICHOL and MARKS (MARKS, 1965a) purport to have shown that the S/N of corrected bleach distorted spectra can exceed by a factor of 3 the S/N expected from minimally bleached cells, if the corrections are based on bleaching data of sufficient accuracy. It is still difficult to decide whether the theoretical advantage of the correct-for-bleach method has been realized in practice, for as MARKS has pointed out, there are a number of sources of inaccuracy. Furthermore, spectra of the quality attained by LIEBMAN and ENTINE on goldfish make the correct-for-bleach method of questionable advantage, at least in this application (Fig. 3). Nonetheless, the data of MARKS and of LIEBMAN and ENTINE were in complete agreement in finding three different cone pigments, each in a separate outer segment. The mean λ_{max} found by MARKS (455 nm, 530 nm and 625 nm) are nearly identical to those found by LIEBMAN and ENTINE (455 nm, 535 nm and 620 nm) and both laboratories have confirmed the goldfish rod pigment at 522 nm. The pigment densities found in the two laboratories are in somewhat poorer agreement, MARKS reporting specific densities of about 0.008/μm and LIEBMAN at least 0.013/μm. As this variation may be ascribed to errors in estimating pathlength through the receptor when only the width of the receptor viewed side-on can be measured directly, or to the tapering outer-segment geometry of goldfish cones, the difference may, perhaps, be overlooked. It should be pointed out, however, that in using a measuring beam that nearly fills the width of an outer segment to gain relative noise reduction, there is concurrent reduction in the absorption measured because the circular cross section of outer segments reduces the average pathlength for wider measuring beams. To achieve the greatest accuracy in estimating pigment concentration in side-on measurements, a beam about $^1/_3$ the width of the outer segment should be used. In our hands, the specific density values so obtained (0.013 ± 0.002 per micron) hold with truly amazing constancy over the large

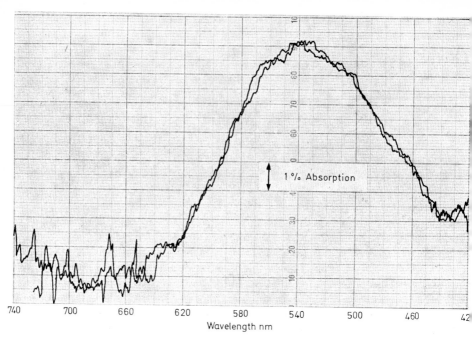

Fig. 3. Two successive absolute spectra recorded from the same goldfish "green" cone, showing the high resolution compatible with minimum bleach that is attainable when using the exposure optimisation technique described in text (from LIEBMAN and ENTINE, 1964)

Table 2. *The wavelengths* (λ_{max}) *of maximum absorbance of visual pigments discovered by MSP in the author's laboratory.* R_1 = *retinal pigments* R_2 = *dehydroretinal pigments. The subscripts R and C indicate whether the pigment was found in an outer segment morphologically identified as a rod or a cone respectively. The* λ_{max} *are placed approximately in their correct positions along a wavelength scale to facilitate grouping into possible classes*

	Wavelength nm.				
	400	450	500	550	600
R_1					
Frog	432_R		$502_{R,C}$	575_C	
Salamander	432_R		$502_{R,C}$	575_C	
Gecko		467_R	518_R		
Turtle	442_C		$502_{R,C}$	562_C	
Pigeon			500_R	562_C	
Chicken			500_R	562_C	
Gull			508_R	562_C	
Monkey	440_C		498_R	535_C	575_C	
Man	440_C		498_R	535_C	575_C	
R_2					
Goldfish		455_C	522_R 535_C		620_C
Mudpuppy			527_R	575_C	
Tadpole	438_R		527_R		620_C
Turtle		450_C	$518_{R,C}$		620_C
	400	450	500	550	600
			Wavelength nm.		

variety of both cones and rods that are listed in Table 2. These densities are measured in light plane polarised across the cellular long axis and must be identical for light propagated linearly down the long axis since the electric vector is in the same plane (that of the disc membranes) for both propagation directions. The extinction coefficient for molecules with only two degrees of orientational freedom is 3/2 larger than that measured in solution. Using this value we find the concentration of visual pigments to be 2—2.5 mM which agrees very well ($\pm 20\%$) with the data of BLASIE, DEWEY, BLAUROCK and WORTHINGTON, (1965) obtained both from X-ray diffraction of rhodopsin and electron microscopic visualisation of antibody-labelled rhodopsin in disc membranes. One of the important assumptions in MARKS' bleaching correction procedure is that no visible-absorbing photoproducts appear during the measurement. Although some small negative absorbances were found in his difference spectra, the close agreement of LIEBMAN and ENTINE'S absolute, minimum-bleach spectra add credibility to the assumption that no serious problem is caused by photoproducts. This is not to say there are no visible-absorbing photoproducts formed in cone pigment bleaching. It does suggest that those formed are quite short-lived on the time scale of these measurements. MARKS' spectra were scanned about 10 times slower ($\sim$ 150 sec/scan), than those of LIEBMAN and ENTINE ($\sim$ 15 sec/scan). The slower scans should allow more time for photoproducts to disappear. Faster scans might be expected to allow detection of photoproducts in the post-bleach (PB) spectra of LIEBMAN and ENTINE if the duration of illumination required to bleach was short and the PB spectrum was recorded immediately. Visible-absorbing photoproducts were never seen under these circumstances and it must therefore be concluded that any formed do not persist for as long as 15 seconds.

Finally, it has been asked whether the not inconsiderable dispersion of λ_{max} reported by MARKS for goldfish cones represents intrinsic biological variation. Our feelings are quite strong on this matter since we have found very little variation ($\sim$ 5 nm) in λ_{max} position in goldfish cones using the minimum bleach technique. This small variation is consistent with the shot-noise fluctuations of the measurements and does not require the hypothesis of biological variability. One of the great advantages of fast-scanning, minimum-bleach recording is that within 10—15 seconds an absolute spectrum is displayed in final form. In the cases where "peculiar" spectra were obtained, we were able to confirm immediately that there was specimen motion in the sample beam, that there was specimen interference with the reference beam or that a refracting cell border was too close to an edge of the measuring beam, causing a chromatic or refraction error. We can only conclude therefore that if MARKS' work was free of these problems, the variation he found must be ascribed to a new technique, not fully grown to maturity.

C. Trout

The interesting studies of DARTNALL, LANDER and MUNZ (1961) and of BRIDGES (1965a) on extracted visual pigments of a number of fish show the presence of mixtures of retinal- and dehydroretinal-based pigments, the proportions of which are sensitive to photic environment. An argument given by DARTNALL and LYTHGOE (1965a, b) suggests that pigment-pairs are indeed based on a common visual protein (or opsin). Retinas of rainbow trout were found by Munz and Beatty (1965) to contain $P527_2$-$P503_1$ mixtures (see also Bridges, 1956). It is of interest to determine whether the mixtures are present in identical proportions in all cells or if there are separate populations of $P527_2$- and of $P503_1$-containing cells. If mixtures occur in individual outer segments, is there more $P527_2$ in one end of the outer segment than in the other? The answer to these questions cannot be found through the extraction technique but is easily amenable to MSP. Measurements were made by Liebman (1969) on the 5×40 μm rod outer-segments of young rainbow trout obtained from a hatchery where they were being reared under very dim light conditions. A 2×6 μm measuring beam was used to allow portions of the outer segments to be sampled from one end to the other. Fish used directly from the hatchery showed spectra of λ_{max} 527 nm in all outer segments and in all parts of the outer segment.

After 4 days of cycled illumination consisting of 16 hours of light per day from three 60 watt bulbs placed adjacent to a small aquarium of trout, a λ_{max} of 515 nm was obtained from all parts of all outer segments examined. The post-bleach spectra were consistent with the presence of a dehydroretinal-based pigment in the first case and of mixtures of retinal and dehydroretinal pigments in the second. The mixture λ_{max} of 515 nm after 4 days' illumination suggests about 50% replacement of $P527_2$ by $P503_1$ homogeneously throughout the outer segment. The total density of pigments present before and after the change of photic environment was constant.

D. Mudpuppy

The cones of the mudpuppy, *Necturus maculosus* are as large as those of the goldfish, and constitute a larger proportion of the total receptor population. The first MSP measurements might have been made on them to advantage but in that case the discovery of the several cone pigments that put the Young-Helmholtz theory of color vision on an experimental basis would have been delayed, for mudpuppies have only one cone pigment. Its spectrum shown in Fig. 4 has $\lambda_{max} = 575$ nm, almost exactly midway between the two long-wave goldfish cone pigments at 535 and 620 nm. This is a very interesting result for it raises several questions. Is this a mixture spectrum of equal amounts of P535 and P620? This possibility can be ruled out by differential bleaching which shows a half bleached spectrum with the same λ_{max} as the original spectrum, and by simple curve construction which shows the bandwidth of *Necturus* P575 too narrow to originate in this way. Although Crescitelli (1958) has shown that the *Necturus* rod pigment is based on dehydroretinal, the possibility that the cone pigment is based on retinal should not be overlooked since a retinal pigment of $\lambda_{max} = 575$ nm has been found in frog cones (Liebman and Entine, 1968 a, b). However, the frog cone pigment (Fig. 5) has a narrower bandwidth than that of Fig. 4 and this is consistent with the rule that retinal pigments have a narrower bandwith than do dehydroretinal pigments (Bridges, 1967; Munz and Schwanzara, 1967). Another possibility is that the *Necturus* cone pigment is based on 9-*cis* instead of 11-*cis* dehydroretinal. A 9-*cis* synthetic pigment reported by Wald, Brown and Smith, (1953) has λ_{max} about 575 nm. This matter might be settled by resynthesis in bleached cells using either 11-*cis* or 9-*cis* dehydroretinal. Though we have not done this experiment, we have

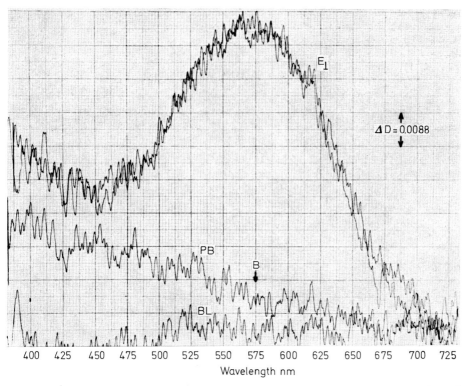

Fig. 4. Side-on absolute spectrum from *Necturus* cone recorded in light plane-polarized across the outer segment's long axis ($E_\perp$). *PB* Post bleach spectrum (after bleaching with 575 nm light). *BL* Baseline, recorded without cone. ΔD Optical density calibration

done regeneration studies on *Necturus* cones using 11-*cis* retinal and find a pigment of λ_{max} about 540 nm. This of course shows that the original pigment was not based on retinal, but there is a further implication. The studies of DARTNALL and LYTH-GOE (1965a, b) and of BRIDGES (1965b) showing a systematic relationship betwene the λ_{max} of retinal- and dehydroretinal-based pigment pairs using the same opsin, have been extended to cone pigments (LIEBMAN and ENTINE, 1968b). When the hypothetical pigment pair $P575_2$–$P540_1$ is placed on the graph of A_2 vs. A_1 pigments (in *R. pipiens*), it falls exactly on the straight line generated by other pigment pairs. This suggests that the *Necturus* P575 cone pigment is based on dehydroretinal and that its opsin is probably different from any of the three goldfish cone opsins.

Examination of Fig. 4 shows that the *Necturus* cone pigment is present at a specific density of about $0.016/\mu m$, somewhat higher than that found in frog rods. We have found *Necturus* rods to give the same specific density, a result that is inconsistent with the contention of BROWN, GIBBONS and WALD (1963) that the porphyropsin of *Necturus* rods is more dilute than the rhodopsin of frog rods. This discrepancy again points out the danger in drawing quantitative conclusions from end-on MSP of patches of retina as well as single receptors (see section on primates).

We also find that the dichroism of *Necturus* receptors is identical to that of frog receptors, at about $4-4.5/1$ for $D_\perp/D_{||}$ (LIEBMAN, 1962; WALD, BROWN and GIBBONS, 1963).

E. Frog and Tadpole

An intensive study of the visual pigments of the adult frog and tadpole (*R. pipiens*) has appeared in the literature (LIEBMAN and ENTINE, 1968a, b) and the results of this work are herein summarised. Both frog and tadpole retinas contain two morphological types of rods (red and green) as well as three types of cones (single, principal and accessory). The red rod pigments for frog and tadpole are, respectively, $P502_1$ and $P527_2$, consistent with values previously obtained by extraction (LYTHGOE, 1937; CRESCITELLI, 1958). The accessory cones in each case contain pigments indistinguishable spectroscopically from the respective red rod pigments. The principal and single cones of the frog contain $P575_1$ (Fig. 5) and the corresponding cones of the tadpole contain $P620_2$. The parallel of these findings to the work of Wald on chicken iodopsin (WALD, BROWN and SMITH, 1955) and on the synthetic pigment cyanopsin (WALD, BROWN and SMITH, 1953) has been pointed out (LIEBMAN and ENTINE, 1968 a, b). The pigments of frog and tadpole green rods are $P432_1$ and $P438_2$. Towards the end of somatic metamorphosis, when

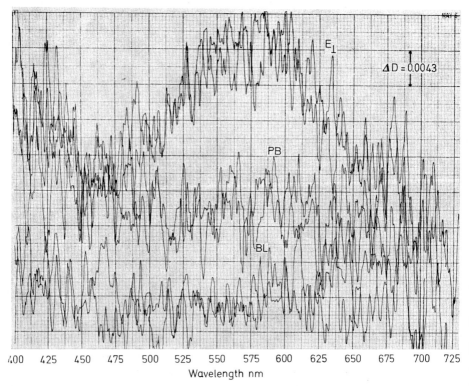

Fig. 5. Frog principal-cone spectrum (from LIEBMAN and ENTINE, 1968b) (note relatively poor S/N due to small size of outer segment)

animals have fully developed all four limbs but still have a tail, "frogpole" red rods containing pigment mixtures (λ_{max} 515 nm) are found (spectra nearly identical to trout). The specific density and photosensitivity of each pigment was found to be similar to that in frog red rods. A bleaching product of frog red rods and accessory cones was found at 387 nm and for corresponding structures in the tadpole at 400 nm. These λ_{max} are consistent with the formation respectively of all-trans retinal and of all-trans dehydroretinal. The peak densities of these products are quite variable, generally because of their rapid diffusion from the outer segment (Fig. 12). The majority of this material before diffusion is oriented in the same way as the original visual pigment, i.e., in the plane of the disc membranes. Whether this implies that these short-wave products are the intermediate, meta-rhodopsin II, rather than "free" retinal is not clear, for vitamin A, which is certainly "free", also shows signs of orientation in rod outer segments (DENTON, 1959). The bandwidths of the frog pigments were compared to the Dartnall nomogram and the tadpole pigments to the Bridges-Munz-Schwanzara (B-M-S) nomogram. $P502_1$ and $P527_2$ fit perfectly but the shortwave pigments were broader and the longwave pigments decidedly narrower than their respective nomograms. This seems to be a systematic deviation for it is shown by "cone-type" pigments in a number of other species. On the assumption that opsins of corresponding cell types for frog and tadpole are identical, pigment-pair points were plotted in the fashion of DARTNALL and LYTHGOE (1965a, b). A linear relationship predicts the λ_{max} of the tadpole pigments from those of the frog and *vice versa*. The significance of the converging difference in λ_{max} of A_1- and A_2- based pigment pairs toward the violet part of the spectrum is discussed later.

F. Salamander

The retina of *Salamandra tigrinum* is indistinguishable from the frog retina. It contains green rods and red rods as well as cones, all of which contain pigments identical to those measured in *R. pipiens* (LIEBMAN, unpublished, 1964).

G. Turtles

The visual pigments of two species of turtle, *Pseudemys scripta scripta* and *Chelonia midas* have been studied by LIEBMAN and GRANDA (1969). These animals have predominantly cone retinas (though by no means pure cone as has been suggested). Numerous rods measuring about 4 μm × 50 μm were seen. The majority of the cone inner segments glitter with a clear or brilliantly colored oil droplet adjacent to the thin outer segment, which measures about 2 μm at the base and quickly tapers to 1 μm for a total length of 40—50 μm. The oil drops are red, orange, yellow and colorless in *Pseudemys*; and orange, yellow (perhaps two types) and colorless in *Chelonia* (Fig. 6). The green oil drops described by early anatomists are colorless drops that appear green when viewed with an objective poorly correc-ted for chromatic aberration. Through a good apochromat, they appear crystal clear and their spectra bear this out. As already demonstrated for several species (STROTHER and WOLKEN, 1960; DONNER, 1960; STROTHER, 1963), the colored oil drops are cutoff filters, whose high density at short wavelengths makes them nearly opaque in these regions. Since light that reaches the outer segment to excite the receptor must first pass through the oil drop, its color must strongly influence spectral sensitivity at the receptor level. The possible consequences of this influence have been the subject of some heated debate in past years (WALLS and JUDD, 1933). The debate has applied to bird retinas as well as to those of reptiles. However, this debate could not be tempered by a certain knowledge of the visual pigment characteristics until just recently.

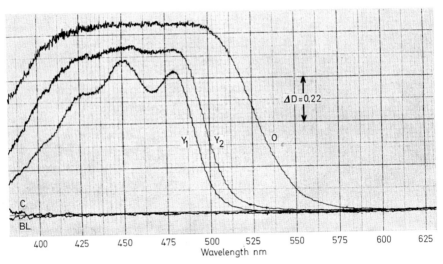

Fig. 6. Spectra of *Chelonia* cone oil drops. *O* orange, Y_1 and Y_2 yellow, *C*, clear

In addition to cones and rods with oil drops, the turtle retina contains accessory cones without drops. As with the accessory cones of frogs and tadpoles, such cones in both species of turtle contained a pigment spectroscopically indistinguishable from that of the rods of the same species. In *Pseudemys*, the rods and accessory cones contain $P518_2$. (A P518 has also been found in cones containing an orange oil drop.) This pigment is designated as of dehydroretinal origin on the basis of its bandwidth, which exceeds that predicted by the Dartnall nomogram and matches that predicted by the B-M-S nomogram. In addition the P518 bandwidth in *Pseudemys* exceeds that in *Gekko*, the latter pigment having been demonstrated to have retinal as its prosthetic group (CRESCITELLI, 1963). A *Pseudemys* cone having a colorless drop may contain P450. This pigment is the least frequently found of the cone pigments in *Pseudemys*. $P620_2$ (so designated because of its correspondence to the P620 pigments of tadpole and goldfish) has been found associated with both orange and red oil drops.

In *Chelonia*, rods and accessory cones contain $P502_1$, which fits the Dartnall nomogram. In addition, P502 is found in cones associated with colourless- and with yellow oil drops, and although $P562_1$ has been found in all types of cone in *Chelonia*, the majority contained an orange or yellow oil drop. Many more cells were studied in *Chelonia* than in *Pseudemys*. The statistics for *Pseudemys* are incomplete largely because of the extreme rarity with which intact cones were found in this species. The attachment of outer segment to inner at the interposed oil drop margin is extremely fragile, and most cones are seen to retain no outer segment under the conditions of the side-on preparation technique.

Several generalisations can be made from existing data, however. The minority population of accessory cones contains rod pigment, as in the case for frogs and tadpoles. The oil drop with the longest cutoff wavelength (red-*Pseudemys*, orange-*Chelonia*) is found only with the "reddest" visual pigment. This is reasonable since these oil drops filter out almost all light below the λ_{max} of the longest wave visual pigment in each species. The species with the cutoff filters of longest wavelength is also the species with the visual pigment of longest λ_{max}. The fresh water species, *Pseudemys*, has pigments based on dehydroretinal whereas the marine *Chelonia* has pigments consistent with a retinal origin, in keeping with Wald's hypothesis (WALD, 1946). The trend demonstrated by DARTNALL and LYTHGOE for the λ_{max} of A_1- and A_2-based pigment pairs to be closer together in the violet than in the red is borne out in a comparison of the pigments of *Chelonia* and *Pseudemys*, even though pigment pairs may not have the same visual protein (A_1 vs A_2 plot is not quite linear either). Finally, calculation of sensitivity curves at receptor level (by multiplying the outer segment axial spectral absorption by the spectral transmission of the associated oil drop) sheds some light on the debated question of oildrop function. The red oil drop of *Pseudemys* moves the effective peak of P620 to about 640 nm, and cuts the receptor sensitivity below 575 nm by a log unit or more. The orange oil drop of *Chelonia* similarly moves the P562 peak to about 575 nm and cuts receptor sensitivity a log unit or more below 500 nm. The oil drops that cut off at shorter wavelengths can only cut out the short wave sensitivity of the long wave pigments and do not affect their peak sensitivities which remain unchanged at 620 nm and 562 nm in the two species. The orange oil drop of *Pseudemys* shifts the effective peak sensitivity of P518 to about 560 nm, reducing the receptor peak absolute sensitivity by a factor of 2 and cutting sensitivity below about 500 nm by a log unit or more. Similarly, yellow oil drops in *Chelonia* shift the effective peak of P502 to 520 nm, reduce peak sensitivity by only 20% but cut the sensitivity below 475 nm by a log unit or more. The violet-absorbing pigment is of course unaffected by colored oil drops in either species.

Thus the constraints imposed by the colored oil drops provide two significantly different receptor sensitivities in each species. These are in addition to the sensitivities provided by the three cone visual pigments whose sensitivities are not much altered in other cells. The majority of receptors studied, with the exception of the violet receptor, have the blue-violet spectrum almost completely cut out by colored oil drops. The above data suggest that turtles may be provided with a five-receptor color vision system, in addition to a mechanism that may reduce the effects of chromatic aberration and scattering. The reduction of short wave sensitivity in many receptors might also be a way of reducing ambiguity in color information analysis by the retina.

The painted turtle, *Chrysemys picta* and the snapping turtle, *Chelydra serpentina*, have also been studied to some extent and their retinas appear to be indistinguishable from that of *Pseudemys* (LIEBMAN, unpublished, 1965).

H. Gecko

Extracted visual pigments of *Gekko gekko* were studied by CRESCITELLI (1963) using hydroxylamine difference spectra. His work showed the presence of two photosensitive pigments; a dominant one at 521 nm, and a minor pigment at 478 nm, demonstrated after bleaching away the dominant pigment. MARKS and DOBELLE (MARKS, 1965b) confirmed a pigment at 520 nm using MSP but could not find the other pigment. As MARKS pointed out, the outer segments of *Gekko*

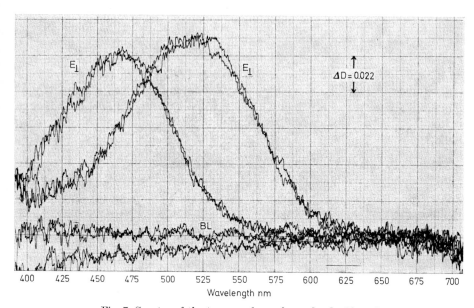

Fig. 7. Spectra of the two members of a gecko double rod

receptors are firmly attached to the pigment epithelium, even in the dark-adapted state, making it difficult to isolate the outer segments. Nevertheless, two visual pigments were found by LIEBMAN (unpublished, 1966) in isolated *Gekko* outer segments. The majority of single and double rods contained P518 while the smaller member of the (presumed) class B double absorbed maximally at 467 nm and the larger member of this double at 518 nm (Fig. 7). The shape of these absorption bands closely match the Dartnall nomogram but are narrower than the B-M-S nomogram. The conclusion therefore that these pigments are derived from retinal is consistent with the product spectra of both the pigments reported by CRESCITELLI for this species and with his surprise at finding such a long-wave rod pigment (P518) that was not a dehydroretinal derivative. The discrepancy between CRESCITELLI's value of 478 nm for the short-wave pigment and the value found by LIEBMAN at 467 nm is attributable to distortion of the bleaching difference spectrum of this pigment, even though determined in the presence of hydroxylamine (CRESCITELLI, personal communication, 1968).

The observation of more than two colors of fluorescence emission originating in different *Gekko* receptors viewed end-on (LIEBMAN and LEIGH, 1969) raises the question whether there are other visual pigments in *Gekko gekko*. The answer to this question must await further MSP.

J. Pigeon, Chicken and Gull

A few measurements have been made on pigeon and chicken retinas by LIEB-MAN (1964, unpublished) and, on the retina of the laughing gull, *Larus atricilla*, by LIEBMAN and HAILMAN (1967, unpublished). Rod outer segments of both chicken and pigeon absorb maximally at 500 nm while those of the gull give a consistently longer λ_{max} of 508 nm. Cone outer segments are very thin and delicate in each of

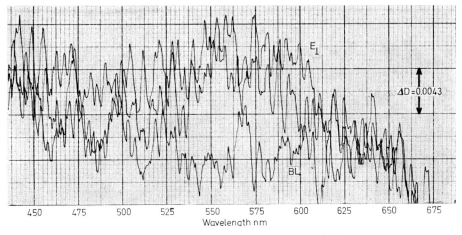

Fig. 8. Cone spectrum of the Laughing Gull

these species and it is difficult to obtain many that are intact and still associated with their inner segments containing the colored oil drop. However, dissociation from the inner segment has so far not impaired correlative results, such as were found for turtles, because only one outer-segment pigment has been found. Cone outer segments of all three species absorb maximally at 560—575 nm (Fig. 8). These results differ from the pigeon pigment ($\lambda_{max} = 544$ nm) of BRIDGES (1962). The spread in λ_{max} can be attributed to optical problems encountered in passing a microbeam through a 1 μm diameter cylindrical or conical outer segment in exactly the same way on each trial using a 0.4 N.A. objective. The MSP spectra of cone outer segments are consistent with WALD's work on chicken retinas (WALD, BROWN and SMITH, 1955) and demonstrate for the first time directly that the iodopsin attributed to cones does actually reside in cone outer segments.

Each of these birds has a system of cone oil drops whose spectra have been measured (DONNER, 1960; STROTHER and WOLKEN, 1960; STROTHER, 1963; LIEB-MAN, unpublished, 1964; LIEBMAN and HAILMAN, unpublished, 1967). The computed peaks of receptor sensitivity for the cones with red oil drops are much displaced to the red in all species, viz. to about 625 nm in the pigeon, 605 nm in the chicken and 590 nm in the gull. Similarly, the pigeon cones with orange oil drops must have a receptor sensitivity peak at about 585 nm. The cutoffs for orange and yellow oil drops in the gull and chicken do not alter peak wavelength sensitivity significantly, though all colored oil drops reduce the blue-violet sensitivity of the outer segments with which they are associated. The receptor sensitivities for all these birds do not have a single sharp peak (as in the case of Turtles) but rather a shoulder of considerable breadth in addition to, and on the short wave side of, the peak. This results from the "mismatch" of the red oil drop and the iodopsin spectra. The "matched" orange oil drop, however, does yield a single sensitivity peak without a shoulder, as is the case for *Chelonia*.

We cannot conclude from present data that there is only one pigment in the cone outer segments of birds, though only one has been found so far. However, colored oil drops provide birds with at least two or three receptor sensitivity curves that are sufficiently different, one from the other, that an engineer might find them attractive as the basis for the design of a color discriminating system.

K. Primates

End-on MSP data from parafoveal cones of monkeys and man have already received a great deal of attention in the literature (MARKS, DOBELLE and MAC NICHOL, 1964; BROWN and WALD, 1964). MARKS, DOBELLE and MACNICHOL reported spectra of eight monkey cones with average λ_{max} of 445 nm, (1 cell), 535 nm (4 cells), and 570 nm (3 cells) and two human cones of λ_{max} 455 nm and 570 nm. A later summary by MACNICHOL (1964) gives "primate" peaks of 447 nm, 540 nm, and 577 nm. Maximum absorption of these pigments was 3–6% (0.013–0.026 optical density). BROWN and WALD report spectra of two human rods with λ_{max} 505 nm and peak density 0.04–0.05. Cone λ_{max} were found at 450 nm (1 cell), 525 nm (2 cells), and 555 nm (1 cell) with peak densities of 0.02, 0.02, and 0.013 respectively. Earlier macrodensitometry on monkey and human foveas and peripheral retinas was reported by BROWN and WALD (1963). The nearly pure rod culture of peripheral retina gave hydroxylamine difference spectra with $\lambda_{max} = 500$ nm for human, and 503 nm for monkey (*Macaca mulatta*). The respective peak densities were 0.15 and 0.1. Foveal difference spectra gave λ_{max} 550 nm and maximum density 0.04. Differential bleaching and some curve matching adjustments yielded two monkey foveal cone pigment spectra with λ_{max} 565 nm and 527 nm and adjusted maximum densities of 0.017 and 0.027, while the similar results λ_{max} 565 nm and 535 nm were obtained for human foveas. These pigments could be partially regenerated after bleaching by adding 11-cis retinal to the preparations. Suggestive but inconclusive evidence was given for the existence of a 440 nm pigment. Both BROWN and WALD and MARKS, DOBELLE, and MACNICHOL have suggested that some cells may contain mixtures of the two longest-wave pigments (single cell data).

In side-on measurements, contemporary with the above, LIEBMAN (unpublished data, 1964) found foveal cones with λ_{max} 535 and 575–580 nm, and some evidence for a pigment of $\lambda_{max} = 440$ nm in end-on measurements of immediately parafoveal cones. Both side-on and end-on densities were about 0.015. MURRAY's (1968) investigation of foveal sonicates yielded pigments of λ_{max} 526 and 573 nm.

If it seems there is more than desirable variability in the primate data from various laboratories, and even within the same laboratory, this must, at least in the main, be attributed to the great experimental difficulties (mostly biological) and our primitive stage of sophistication in dealing with mammalian, and especially human, retinas. Excised dark-adapted monkey retinas can be freshly obtained but deteriorative light-scattering changes set in immediately (ENOCH and GLISS-MANN, 1966). Human' retinas can usually be obtained only under experimentally undesirable conditions of uncertain light exposure and pathology, or many hours after death. Human retinas inevitably must be examined only after severe light scattering changes have ensued. Unfortunately almost none of the original data has even been shown in reports on primate pigments, and no mention has been made of the unacceptable experimental conditions that have been tolerated. Perhaps some of this is due to our having become so dependent on apparatus that we do not take the time to look and see with our own eyes what happens to a microbeam of light as it passes through one of these retinas in end-on geometry. Nevertheless, cursory examination of the one figure of original data that appears in the literature (WALD and BROWN, 1965) will convince one that end-on measurements have been made under extreme scattering conditions. Since this scattering increases as $\sim 1/\lambda^2$ its effect is hardly seen when a cone is aligned with the sample beam in the deep red or infrared, but is enormous in visible light. Thus, using infrared vision equipment to prevent bleaching during alignment, a $1^1/_2$ μm diameter sample beam may appear sharply light-piped up a single parafoveal cone outer segment, only to have almost disappeared on similar examination at 550 nm. At this wavelength, where scattering is already significant, the microbeam has been diffused over an area covering many of the rods that surround parafoveal cones in their rosette-like arrangement, and this diffusion area increases as the wavelength decreases. A great deal of light is also back scattered and never reaches the collecting optics of the microscope. (This is, of course, the cause of the steep $1/\lambda^2$ function seen in the aforementioned original data figure). The effect of the lost light is only to reduce the signal-to-noise ratio according to equation 3 b, and its wavelength dependence can be subtracted away by bleaching difference spectra as has been done in the above investigations. However, that does not correct the more serious problem that the resultant difference spectrum has been obtained not from one cell but from a population of cells, and furthermore that the size and character of this population changes as a function of wavelength. The light scattering exists primarily in the neural layers of the retina and is due to the heterogeneity of refractive index that is common in sick or dead biological tissues. It occurs especially rapidly in tissue with a high metabolic rate or special metabolic requirements, and is quite common in neural tissue. While the scattering of simple systems consisting of a dispersion of particles of one refractive index in another can be cleared by raising the refractive index of the suspending medium, this trick (as by adding glycerin to retinas) does not succeed for retinas, which are apparently not so simply constituted, (LIEBMAN, unpublished, 1964). There are still several other ways of dealing with the scattering problem. One is to do side-on measurements as has been advocated earlier. However, this has the difficulty that cones of primates are difficult to distinguish from rods, and the outer segments alone are absolutely indistinguishable in a light microscope. Side-on measurements of outer segments from the peripheral retina can be expected to yield, on average, hundreds of rhodopsin spectra before a single cone spectrum turns up, in keeping with the known population ratio of these cells. Our side-on measurements were made on cones isolated from excised foveas where it is expected that all the cells are cones. In the peripheral retina the rosette geometry allows the discrimination of cones to be made only for end-on measurements. We must thus deal with this matter more directly, and this can be done in two ways, one biological and one technological.

The biological way is based on the observation that primate retinas kept on ice for several days do not lose their visual pigments but they do aquire a mechanical defect which results in a split through the outer plexiform layer in the plane of the retina. This allows large areas of the photoreceptor layer to separate from the neural retina. About 90% of the light scattering goes with the neural retina and end-on measurements on the residual receptor layer are freed from the scattering impediment.

The technical way to deal with the scattering has been discussed (ENOCH, 1965; LIEBMAN, 1965; and ENOCH, 1966). The idea is that a microscope objective having the same (preferably small) numerical aperature (N.A.) as the illuminating microscope condenser, will collect mainly (but not exclusively) light transmitted by the parafoveal cone illuminated. An objective of larger N.A. will collect predominantly more-scattered light and one of smaller N.A. will exclude preferentially more-transmitted light. Furthermore, an aperture that corresponds in size with the non-scattered illuminating microbeam placed at the focus of the light collecting optics will exclude mainly light that originated away from the cone image, i.e., that scattered in the retinal object space. The N.A. restriction effects angular scattering in the objective plane.

In the language of waveguide optics expressed by ENOCH, these "stops" are placed so as to restrict both the near and far field radiation pattern to that of the cone transmission. ENOCH has constructed a microspectrophotometer based on these principles but has not yet published details.

The above mentioned use of objectives of small numerical aperture deserves further comment. The inclination of many who are engaged in microscopy, especially of single cells, is to use an objective with as high a magnification and N.A. as possible. If this wisdom is incorporated into end-on MSP, two consequences will be certain. First, as a result of the poorer optical corrections of high power lenses, beam definition will suffer and the light that makes the fuzziness of the edges of small apertures will bypass the receptor and reduce the apparent absorption and therefore the S/N. Second, since the existence of the Stiles-Crawford effect tells us that a cone will accept little more than 1/10th of the light striking it at 10° from normal incidence (due to waveguide properties), one must use a correspondingly small angular aperture of illumination to project the sample beam on to a cone to be measured end-on. This angle corresponds to an N.A. of about 0.3. Use of a 100×, 1.25 N.A. objective will assure that 90% or more of the incident light in the sample beam will be excluded from the receptor at which it is aimed, even in an optically clear retina, and that this 90% must either bypass the cone outer segment to dilute the absorption signal of the 10% that is accepted by the cone; or must pass through the surrounding parafoveal rods to distort the cone spectrum with a rhodopsin spectrum, as the scattering does in a milky retina.

The spectroscopic result of end-on measurements with large N.A. objectives or in the presence of scattering is to reduce the optical density of pigments measured, and/or to distort the spectra so that the peaks appear at wavelengths intermediate between the true λ_{max} and that of rhodopsin, and to broaden the absolute spectra so that it appears as though there were more than one pigment present in a single cone. Bleaching difference spectra may yield more complicated combinations that result in spectral narrowing and peak shifts.

Although some of the spectra presented seem to come close to fitting the Dartnall nomogram, others are abnormally narrow or give indication of two pigments that could easily be due to scattering into rods. The very small peak densities reported are entirely out of keeping with results obtained from the rest of the animal world. Furthermore, the specific densities obtained by LIEBMAN in side-on measurements of foveal cones are in agreement $(0.015-1^1/_2$ μm cone diameter) with other data, implying that the small end-on densities are due to 1) bleaching before measurement, 2) scattering past the receptor, 3) leakage out of the receptor from non-normal beam incidence or 4) loss of the major portion of the outer segment length. The last of these possibilities is not to be ignored, for it is impossible to learn the length of a receptor lying in the light propagation axis, and many parafoveal cones look the same whether an outer segment is present or not since the light piping that gives their characteristic appearance begins in the inner segment. The densities reported are consistent with an outer segment fragment $1-3$ μm long for cones, and $10-15$ μm long for rods, if the disc membranes maintain their order, or $1^1/_2$ times these figures if they do not.

In conclusion then, primate data have not been improved upon in the five years since their promulgation. At best, they suggest the existence of three cone pigments in separate cones in confirmation of previous theory. Although arguments for knowledge of greater accuracy can be given and ancillary information has been cited, the MSP data alone cannot be regarded as accurate to better than $20-30$ nm, and published densities cannot be regarded as indicative in the least of what exists in the living eye. The reader is referred to the excellent reviews of ALPERN (1968) and of WEALE (1968) for further critical comment.

L. Oil Drops and Ellipsoids

In addition to the brilliantly colored oil drops already discussed above, the cones and/or rods of a number of species contain clear or pale-yellow oil globules. These, like the easily identified large oil drops of frog pigment epithelium, emit a bright green fluorescence in response to ultraviolet radiation and have been observed, in preliminary investigations, to undergo photochemical alteration as judged by shifts in wavelength and intensity of maximum emission in response to 366 nm Hg arc illumination (LIEBMAN, unpublished experiments). Absorption spectra recorded from oil drops of the frog pigment epithelium (Fig. 9) show the characteristic three fingered blue-violet absorption of β-carotene.

Although there is strong indirect evidence for strict localization of visual pigment to the outer segment, and of respiratory enzymes to the mitochondria-containing ellipsoid, satisfying direct confirmation of this contention comes from MSP. Outer segments that have been bleached and reduced with borohydride to remove visible-absorbing photoproducts contain no spectroscopically detectable cytochrome pigments (LIEBMAN, 1962). In contrast MSP of the ellipsoid region yields

33*

characteristic multipeaked spectra characteristic of the various animal cytochromes and no evidence of the coincident presence of visual pigment (LIEBMAN, 1969).

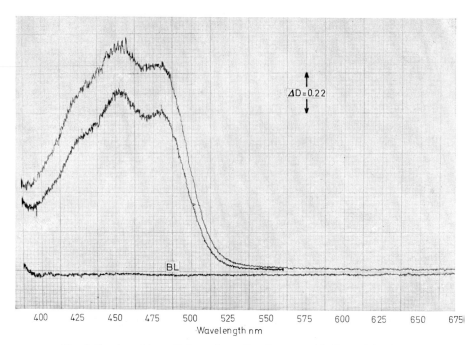

Fig. 9. Spectra of two oil drops from the pigment epithelium of the frog

M. Invertebrate Visual Pigments

MSP has been used by LANGER and THORELL (1966a, b) to detect photosensitive pigments in single rhabdoms of the blowfly, *Calliphora erythrocephala*. Razor-cut tangential slices of the chalky mutant were used in end-on recordings with a 1 μm diameter microbeam. Most rhabdomeres possessed a double peak spectrum (λ_{max} 500—510 nm and 350—380 nm) while No. 7 rhabdomere absorbed maximally at 460—470 nm. There was evidence of weak dichroism (4 : 3) whose major axis varied from rhabdomere to rhabdomere, consistent with electron-microscopic observation of variation in microtubular axis orientation among the rhabdomeres of each rhabdom. The measured dichroism must be regarded as a lower limit because of the very unfavorable optics of the measurements.

Side-on MSP was used by GOLDSMITH, DIZON, and FERNÁNDEZ (1968) to detect two pigments (λ_{max} 555 and 496 nm) present in the same rhabdomere, of the prawn, *Palaemonetes*. The former pigment "bleached" to a stable product, absorbing maximally at 496 nm, the same λ_{max} as the second photosensitive pigment, which bleached away completely on illumination. Similarly, WATERMAN, FERNÁNDEZ, and GOLDSMITH (1969) studied rhabdoms of the crayfish, *Orconectes*, and found two pigments, again simultaneously present in the same cell, at 568 nm and 515 nm. The bandwidth of the long-wave pigment was less than that of a similar retinal nomogram-pigment. Although the 568-nm pigment is evident in electrophysiological recordings, the 515-nm pigment seems to be electrically silent. A 430-nm pigment corresponding to electrophysiological action spectra was not detected by MSP. The peculiar morphology of interdigitating bands of microvilli in adjacent rhabdomeres made possible the proper determinations of dichroic ratio in these side-on preparations. A ratio of 2 : 1, positive with respect to the known microvillar axes, was found. It is a simple matter to compute that this low dichroic ratio could be accounted for by the orientation of the microvilli themselves, while the transition moments (absorption vectors) of the visual pigment molecule had no more than two-dimensional random orientation in the tubular membranes of the microvilli.

Pigment concentrations inferred by the above investigators from their measurements are 0.3—0.4 mM, a factor of 5—10 lower than that found in vertebrate receptors.

MURRAY (1966) has found a photosensitive pigment absorbing maximally at 529±5 nm in large cell bodies scattered along the lateral olfactory nerve of *Limulus polyphemus*. This is similar to the P520, extracted by HUBBARD and WALD (1960) from the lateral eye of *Limulus polyphemus*, and to other studies on the *Limulus polyphemus* median eye. The function of the cells studied by MURRAY is unknown.

N. UV Spectra

It is possible to achieve sufficient signal-to-noise ratio from single cells as large as the rods of frog and *Necturus* to allow spectral recordings to about 330 nm using a tungsten light source. However, as described above in discussion of instrument components, we have used the deuterium arc lamp for recordings primarily directed to the ultraviolet. The results of such recordings are remarkable in their high signal-to-noise ratio and in the absence of significant scattering effects into the 220 nm region (Fig. 10). The later is especially significant for one can obtain absolute spectra throughout the protein region in a single outer segment, which retains the protein geometry present in the native cellular structure.

Although few experiments have thus far been done in the uv, several results may be noted. The strong dichroism of the rhodopsin alpha band has been found as well in the beta or *cis* band in intact outer segments (Fig. 11). In carotenoids, the *cis* band seems to be due to an electronic transition that is polarised perpendicular to the lower-energy alpha transition (ZECHMEISTER and POLGAR, 1943). The alpha-band-transition is polarised along the long axis of the chromophoric chain of conjugated double bonds. Together, the vectors representing the *cis*-band and alpha-band-transitions define a plane in which the entire bent chain of the molecule must lie. These arguments have now been confirmed also for 11-*cis* retinal (SPERLING and RAFFERTY, 1969). The conclusion that can be drawn from Fig. 11 therefore is that the bent chromophores of rhodopsin molecules in rod outer segments lie in the plane of the disc membranes. This fact could not be deduced from determinations of dichroism in visible light alone. (See also DENTON, 1954.)

It comes as no surprise that the protein absorption in the 280-nm region is not dichroic, for the aromatic amino-acid rings responsible for this absorption are expected to be randomly oriented in proteins. It has been shown that none of the

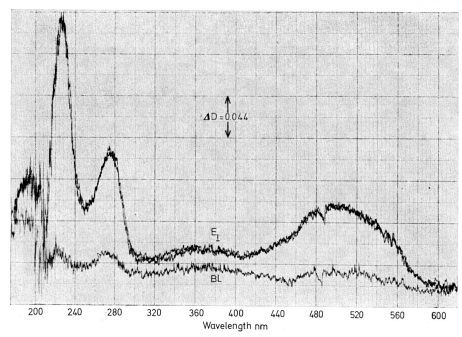

Fig. 10. UV-visible spectrum from single frog rod outer segment using deuterium light source

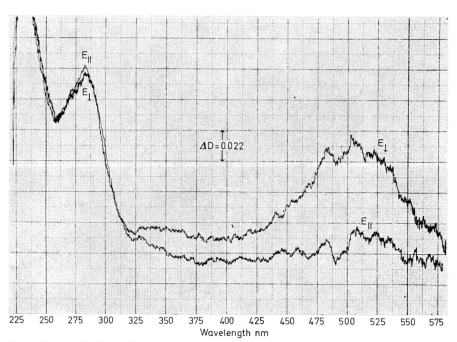

Fig. 11. Frog rod in light polarised across $(E_\perp)$ and along $(E_{||})$ the long axis. Note the dichroism of the *cis* and α-bands and its absence in the protein bands. The jagged structure in the α-band is due to uncompensated spectral lines in the deuterium source (compare baseline, Fig. 10) (from Entine, Liebman, and Storey, 1968)

absorption in the 280 band is due to quinones, which had been hypothesized to be present at high concentration in rod outer-segments (ENTINE, LIEBMAN and STOREY, 1968). When suitable correction is made for the dichroism of the alpha-

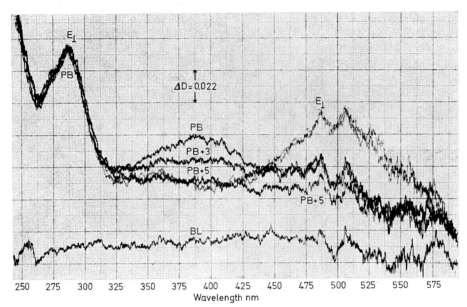

Fig. 12. Frog rod before ($E_\perp$) and 1 min (PB), 3 min ($PB + 3$) and 5 min ($PB + 5$) after bleaching

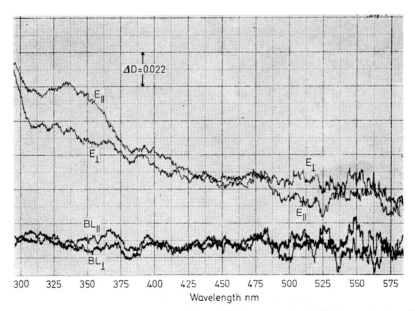

Fig. 13. Frog rod bleached in dissection dish and allowed to stand for 30 min before MSP preparation. $E_{\parallel}$ shows Vitamin A oriented along rod long axis

band transition, it may be seen that the ratio D280/D500 is nearly the same in outer segments as it is for extracted pigment. This implies either that solubilisation removes non-rhodopsin protein in a complex with rhodopsin or that all of the membrane protein in rod outer segments is provided by rhodopsin itself. A third possibility that non-rhodopsin, "structural" protein of rod outer segments contains no aromatic amino acids, is deemed unlikely. Thus, the relevance of possible conformational changes of bleached rhodopsin protein to alterations in the disc membranes associated with visual excitation may be more direct than hitherto imagined.

The 230—235 nm band (Fig. 10) is surprisingly large but its significance in rod outer-segments has not been explored.

In the near ultraviolet, a series of spectra show characteristic changes immediately after rhodopsin is bleached (Fig. 12). Initially, bleached frog rods show a peak at about 387 nm consistent with the formation of retinal or of a mixture of retinal and metarhodopsin II. The magnitude of this product-spectrum is sufficient to account for all of the rhodopsin absorption lost on bleaching. Moreover, it is dichroic like the original rhodopsin. Thus, the molecular entity responsible for this peak has the same transverse molecular orientation as did the original rhodopsin. However, as time passes, the 387 peak diminishes progressively in magnitude. This loss is not due to molecular reorientation along the rod long axis (LIEBMAN and ENTINE, unpublished). It is likewise not due to conversion of retinal to vitamin A, for no vitamin A is formed under these conditions. The loss of retinal must therefore be due to diffusion away from the outer segment, and the rate of this diffusion can be evaluated from records such as that of Fig. 12.

If retinas are bleached and allowed to remain in the dissection dish for 15 minutes before preparations are made for microspectrophotometry, the result shown in Fig. 13 is obtained. A peak is found near 335 nm. This is neither found in unbleached rods nor in previously dark-adapted rods bleached in the microspectrophotometer. It is found almost entirely parallel to the rod long axis. It yields a faint greenish fluorescence on illumination with the spectrophotometer uv source, necessitating the use of visible-light blocking filters if its absorption is to be measured properly. It is undoubtedly vitamin A. Its absorption is less than $1/3$ of that expected if it were stoichiometrically equivalent to the rhodopsin bleached. This implies that some retinene may have diffused away before it could be reduced by NADH, or that some vitamin A had diffused away. In any event, the vitamin A that remains in outer segments under the conditions of these experiments is oriented along the rod long axis, as previously shown by DENTON (1959) and by LIEBMAN (1969) who studied fluorescence polarisation of vitamin A. Why dark adapted rods do not yield vitamin A when bleached in closed preparations has not been studied.

V. Nomenclature and Classification of Visual Pigments

The work of KÖTTGEN and ABELSDORFF (1896) established the existence of two kinds of visual pigment, which were defined in more detail and renamed rhodopsin and porphyropsin by WALD (1937). WALD further showed that the same opsin that was found capable of regenerating rhodopsin in the presence of 11-*cis* retinal also yielded a spectrum close to that of natural porphyropsin when combined with 11-*cis* dehydroretinal (WALD, 1953a). Bleached iodopsin was similarly shown to be capable of generating cyanopsin in the presence of 11-*cis* dehydroretinal (WALD, BROWN, and SMITH, 1953). These relatively clear and simple results led WALD (1956) to formulate his well-known diagram illustrating the formation of four visual pigments from the possible combinatorials of two retinals. WALD viewed interspecies diversity in λ_{max} as a second order effect on the basic classes of pigment. Thus, "rhodopsin like other proteins varies somewhat from one species to another. These differences are reflected in small displacements in its absorption spectrum...498 nm in cattle, rats, dogfish, 500 in sheep and 502 in frogs. Like the hemoglobins, each of these pigments contains the same prosthetic group; it is the protein or the attachment to protein that varies. The term rhodopsin or opsin, therefore, like hemoglobin, designates a family of closely related substances, each of which should be named for the animal of origin" (WALD, 1953b). The discovery of an ever increasing diversity of "rhodopsins" (λ_{max} range 468—528) and "porphyropsins" (λ_{max} range 510—543) has led a number of investigators to question the utility of WALD's nomenclature (DARTNALL, 1952; CRESCITELLI, 1956; MUNZ, 1958; DARTNALL and LYTHGOE, 1965b), and many have adopted the numerical system used in this chapter. WALD, on the other hand, has accommodated to the appearance of λ_{max} diversity by simply expanding his definition of the classes of pigments - - "In vertebrates the two retinals join with the two great *families* of opsins, those of the rods and those of the cones, to form the four *major* pigments of vertebrate vision" (WALD, 1968). There is no contemporary evidence that the hypothesis of two retinals joined with various opsins need be challenged, but although there may be sufficiently strong second order effects to account for the presumptive rod-pigment *inter*species diversity, it is difficult to see what is to be gained by considering the *intra*species diversity of three different cone pigments as a second order effect within a single family of cone opsin. There must rather be at least three "families" of opsin frequently, but not always, found in cones which differ from the opsin usually, but not exclusively, found in rods.

These conclusions are not new, of course, for the "cone-like" green-rod pigment had been studied by DENTON and WYLLIE (1955) and by DARTNALL (1957), and the chlorolabe-erythrolabe pigments had been discovered by RUSHTON (1958) in human foveas. Although erythrolabe might be classified in the iodopsin family, it is clear there is no place for green rods or chlorolabe without significant expansion of WALD's diagram. The results of MSP confirm and extend this view. The data displayed in Table 2 may be interpreted to suggest the existence of several classes of opsin with variation within each class. Thus, violet-absorbing pigments based on retinal occupy the range 432—442 nm, excluding Gecko P467. The next class centers near 500 nm and is found in some cones as well as rods. At longer wavelength is RUSHTON's chlorolabe, confirmed by MSP at about 535 nm. Finally, several pigments in the range 562—575 nm correspond to WALD's iodopsin and RUSHTON's erythrolabe. For visual systems based on dehydroretinal, there are pigments corresponding to the first two and to the last two retinal pigments above. However, there is an additional dehydroretinal pigment, goldfish $P535_2$, that does *not* correspond to any retinal pigment thus far discovered. $P535_2$ is not a porphyropsin in WALD's sense for it is not a rod pigment and it is present in a species that already has a "porphyropsin" at 522 nm in its rods. The latter pigment is the one that corresponds to "rhodopsin" in retinal-based pigments. Neither does $P535_2$ correspond to chlorolabe ($P535_1$) for the latter is the pigment that corresponds to *Necturus* $P575_2$ as shown above by direct resynthesis ($P575_2 \rightarrow P540_1$). The most reasonable hypothesis seems to be that goldfish $P535_2$ belongs to an additional "opsin family", making a total of five opsins for vertebrate retinas. It is not presently clear whether we should regard gecko P467 as a deviant member of the violet pigments, or as representative of yet another class of opsins. It is also possible that a pigment will be found that corresponds to the electrophysiologic sensitivities found near 670 nm by NAKA and RUSHTON (1966) and by WITKOVSKY (1967).

It has been shown that there are a number of invertebrate pigments whose λ_{max} fall readily into the vertebrate classes. It may therefore not be gratuitous to group all animal visual pigments together and to include the presumptive ultraviolet pigment of the bee (GOLDSMITH, 1960; AUTRUM, 1965) and the horseshoe crab (WALD and KRAININ, 1963). Considered in this manner it is likely that there exist seven or more families of opsin in the visual world and that at least 14 visual pigments are possible, utilizing these opsins in combination with the two retinals. It is not altogether clear that the task of finding euphonious names for each of these would be worth the effort. We may in fact do well to take a page from past visual pigment history and expect considerable diversity in each of these hypothesized classes, to the point where it will perhaps not be obvious at all that the hypothesis of classes of opsin is justified. In this twilight zone of our rapidly expanding knowledge, therefore, we should find quite adequate justification in the use of the numerical nomenclature proposed by DARTNALL (1952) as modified by MUNZ (1958).

VI. Visual Pigment Systematics and their Significance

It is well known from organic chemistry that the λ_{max} of conjugated polyenes increases with the number of double bonds or length of the conjugated chain. Thus, since the replacement of the prosthetic group retinal by dehydroretinal increases the number of conjugated double bonds from 6 to 7, one might expect to find a constant energy increment (nearly constant wavelength increment) in whatever pigment this replacement occurs.

However, from WALD's work on the conversion of rhodopsin to porphyropsin and of iodopsin to cyanopsin, it appears that the additional double bond of dehydroretinal influences the λ_{max} of iodopsin much more than that of rhodopsin. This peculiar phenomenon was apparently accorded no attention until DARTNALL and LYTHGOE (1965a, b) studied a number of naturally occuring pairs of presumptive retinal-dehydroretinal pigments, each pair based upon its own single opsin. When the λ_{max} of the pairs were plotted one against the other, it was noticed that the degree of bathochromic shift varied in linear proportion to the λ_{max} of the retinal pigment, at least in the admittedly small range of λ_{max} (493—510 nm) observed. Using data from MSP, it has been possible to extend this interesting result throughout the λ_{max} range of the known vertebrate retinal visual pigments, 432 nm—575 nm (LIEBMAN and ENTINE, 1968b) and to confirm this striking linearity. The importance of this result, namely that the degree of bathochromic shift on adding a double bond to the chromophore of a visual pigment molecule is proportional to the λ_{max} of the starting material, cannot be overemphasized for, in the author's opinion, an understanding of why this happens is the key to understanding why the same prosthetic group—retinal—can yield different visual pigments when combined with different opsins. A challenging explanation of these phenomena is the two-stage theory of BLATZ and LIEBMAN (1967, unpublished). In brief, it is assumed that retinal combines covalently with opsin through a Schiff base linkage, possibly to phosphatidylethanolamine, and forms a protonated or charge-transfer complex. This causes a large bathochromic shift from 380 nm to about 600 nm, the precise amount being subject to the enviroment imposed internally by the part of the lipoprotein that is juxtaposed to the carotenoid at the active site (through Van der Waals forces or internal solvent effect). Secondly, a hyposochromic shift occurs due to truncation of the π cloud of the conjugated polyene, largely localized at the C_6—C_7 bond (Fig. 14). The truncation is presumed

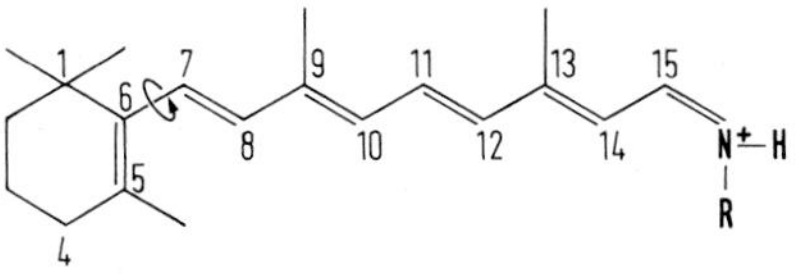

Fig. 14. Proposed model for visual pigments to explain diversity of λ_{max}. π-cloud truncation occurs at C_6–C_7 due to rotation of ring (circular arrow) caused by steric interference of the apoprotein, opsin

to be due either to steric interference by the apoprotein so that the β-ionone ring cannot be coplanar with the side-chain, or to charge localization near C_7 imposed by the lipoprotein (see WIESENFIELD and ABRAHAMSON, 1968). In either event, the effect is to remove the π electrons of the ring from conjugation with the π electrons of the side chain. The effectiveness of the favored steric mechanism of truncation depends on how far the ring is rotated out of coplanarity, being completely effective when the plane of the ring π-cloud is perpendicular to that of the side chain, and completely ineffective when the ring π-cloud is coplanar with that of the side chain. For pigments of low λ_{max} (e.g. frog green-rod pigment) the ring is rotated 70—80° allowing very little conjugation. This produces the short wave pigment ($P432_1$) and also makes it impossible for additional π electrons in the dehydroretinal pigment ring to change the λ_{max} by much ($P438_2$) since these will also be out of coplanarity. On the other hand the opsin of, e.g., frog $P575_1$ does not interfere significantly and the ring is nearly coplanar with the side-chain. This allows the λ_{max} of the retinal pigment to reach nearly to the limit set by the initial bathychromic shift. Furthermore, when more π electrons are added in the dehydroretinal pigment, they can conjugate effectively with the rest and produce nearly the full change in transition energy (ca. 10%) expected for such a system. Pigments such as rhodopsin and porphyropsin are the result of an intermediate degree of ring-twist imposed by their particular opsin. It is a natural corollary of this theory that the displacement in λ_{max} caused by changing from retinal to dehydroretinal should be directly proportional to the λ_{max} of the retinal pigment.

It may further be suggested that if the pigment pair relationship is perfectly linear, as it is within at least one species, *R. pipiens* (Liebman and Entine, 1968b), this implies that the internal solvent or Van der Waals environment for each of the pigments of differing λ_{max} is the same; for if it were different all pigment-pair points would no longer fall exactly on the same line. Similarly, failure of Dartnall and Lythgoe's points to fall exactly on a line may imply that these pigment pairs do not all have the identical internal environment, and it is perhaps this "second order" effect that accounts for the λ_{max} diversity in one "class" of opsin. If the protein primary sequence is the same in all pigments of the same animal except where the steric "knob" that adjusts λ_{max} is placed, the environment should be identical for all pigments, and a linear plot should result. If the primary sequence near the active site differs from pigment to pigment, the pigment-pair points will not all fall *on* the best line. The slope of the pair-plot lines will vary from species to species if the environment varies. Knowledge of one λ_{max} alone does not specify the entire wavelength-shift mechanism for, in the presence of both steric and e.g. solvent effects, one species may achieve a 500 nm pigment through large steric and small solvent effect, and another the reverse for the same λ_{max}. However, a comparison of the intraspecies pigment-pair slopes will indicate the proportions of the mechanisms that have been invoked.

Appendix I

The conservation law for absorption spectroscopy is:

$$I_t + I_a = I_i .$$

Dividing by I_i we have:

$$T + A = 1$$

where

$$T = \frac{I_t}{I_i}, \ A = \frac{I_a}{I_i} .$$

By definition:

$$ln \frac{I_i}{I_t} = \varepsilon P$$

where ε is the napierian extinction coefficient and P is moles per cm².

$$\frac{I_t}{I_i} = T = e^{-\varepsilon P} ,$$

$$A = 1 - e^{-\varepsilon P} . \tag{1}$$

Further, for $\varepsilon P < 0.1$

$$e^{-\varepsilon P} = (1 - \varepsilon P + \ldots \ldots)$$

$$\approx 1 - \varepsilon P$$

and $A = \varepsilon P$ (to about 10% accuracy) . $\tag{2}$

Since $\varepsilon = 2.3 \, \varepsilon'$ and $D = \varepsilon' P$ where ε' is the decadic extinction coefficient

$$A = 2.3 \, D \tag{3}$$

Thus for 1% absorption ($A = 0.01$)

$$D = \frac{0.01}{2.3} = 0.00435$$

Our recorder Y axis and the density axes in the figures of this paper are calibrated in multiples of this basic unit.

Appendix II

The Bleaching Equation

Let there be P moles of photosensitive pigment per cm² absorbing a fraction, A_λ, of incident photons from a monochromatic beam of flux density, F_λ (in mmoles photons/cm²/sec), which bleach with an efficiency of γ mmoles of pigment lost per mmole of photons absorbed. The rate of loss, of pigment is

$$\frac{-dP}{dt} = F_\lambda \gamma A_\lambda \qquad (4)$$

Substituting from equation (1)

$$\frac{-dP}{dt} = F_\lambda \gamma (1 - e^{-\varepsilon P})$$

and using the approximation of Eqn. (2)

$$\frac{-dP}{dt} = F_\lambda \gamma \varepsilon_\lambda P .$$

Integrating

$$P_t = P_o e^{-F t \gamma \varepsilon}$$

$$= P_o e^{-E \phi} \qquad (5)$$

where P_t is pigment concentration at any time, t; P_o is pigment concentration before bleaching; E, the total light exposure and Φ, the photosensitivity.

Acknowledgment

This work was made possible by the support of the USPHS (Grant NB04935) and Fight for Sight Inc., New York City (G-324).

References

ALPERN, M.: Distal mechanisms of color vision. Ann. Rev. Physiol. **30**, 279—318 (1968).

AUTRUM, H.: The physiological basis of colour vision in honeybees in Ciba Symposium on Colour Vision, pp. 286—300. Ed. A.V.S. de Reuck Boston: Little Brown. 1965.

BLASIE, J. K., DEWEY, M. M., BLAUROCK, A. E., WORTHINGTON, C. R.: Electron microscope and low angle x-ray diffraction studies on outer segment membranes from the retina of the frog. J. molec. Biol. **14**, 143—152 (1965).

BRIDGES, C. D. B.: The visual pigments of the rainbow trout (*Salmo irideus*). J. Physiol. (Lond.) **134**, 620—629 (1956).

— Visual pigment 544, a presumptive cone pigment from the pigeon. Nature (Lond.) **195**, 40—42 (1962).

— Visual pigments in a fish exposed to different light-environments. Nature (Lond.) **206**, 1161—1162 (1965a).

— The grouping of fish visual pigments about preferred positions in the spectrum. Vision Res. **5**, 223—238 (1965b).

— Spectroscopic properties of porphyropsins. Vision Res. **7**, 349—369 (1967).

BROWN, K. T., MURAKAMI, M.: A new receptor potential of the monkey retina with no detectible latency. Nature (Lond.) **201**, 626—628 (1964).

BROWN, P. K.: A system for microspectrophotometry employing a commercial recording spectrophotometer. J. Opt. Soc. Amer. **51**, 1000—1008 (1961).

— WALD, G : Visual pigments in human and monkey retinas. Nature (Lond.) **200**, 37—43 (1963).

— — Visual pigments in single rods and cones of human retina. Science **144**, 45—52 (1964).

— GIBBONS, I. R., WALD, G.: Visual cells and visual pigment of the mudpuppy. J. Cell Biol. **19**, 79—106 (1963).

CASPERSSON, T.: Methods for the determination of absorption spectra of cell structures. J. roy. micr. Soc. **60**, 8—25 (1940).

CHANCE, B., PERRY, R., AKERMAN, L , THORELL, B : Highly sensitive recording microspectrophotometer. Rev. sci. Instr **30**, 735—741 (1959).

CONE, R.: Early receptor potential of the vertebrate retina. Nature (Lond.) **204**, 736—739 (1964).

— COBBS, W. H.: Rhodopsin cycle in the living eye of the rat. Nature (Lond.) **221**, 820—822 (1969).

CRESCITELLI, F.: The nature of the gecko visual pigment. J. gen. Physiol. **40**, 217—231 (1956).

— The natural history of visual pigments. Ann. N. Y. Acad. Sci. **74**, 230—255 (1958).

— The photosensitive retinal pigment system of Gecko gecko. J. gen. Physiol. **47**, 33—52 (1963).

DARTNALL, H. J. A.: Visual pigment 467, a photosensitive pigment present in tench retinae. J. Physiol. (Lond.) **116**, 257—289 (1952).

— In: The Visual Pigments, pp. 190—192. London: Methuen 1957.

— The visual pigment of the green rods. Vision Res. **7**, 1—16 (1967).

— LANDER, M. R., MUNZ, F. W.: Periodic changes in the visual pigment of a fish. Progress in Photobiology, pp. 203—213. Amsterdam: Elsevier 1961.

— LYTHGOE, J. N.: The spectral clustering of visual pigments. Vision Res. **5**, 81—100 (1965a).

— — The clustering of fish visual pigments around discrete spectral positions and its bearing on chemical structure, In: Ciba Symposium on Colour Vision, pp. 3—26. Ed. A. V. S. de Reuck. London: Little Brown 1965b.

DENTON, E. J.: On the orientation of molecules in the visual rods of *Salamandra maculosa*. J. Physiol. (Lond.) **124**, 17—18 (1954).

— The contributions of the oriented photosensitive and other molecules to the absorption of whole retina. Proc. roy. Soc. B. **150**, 78—94 (1959).

— WYLLIE, J. H.: Study of the photosensitive pigments in the pink and green rods of the frog. J. Physiol. (Lond.) **127**, 81—89 (1955).

DOBROWOLSKI, J. A., JOHNSON, B. K., TANSLEY, K.: The spectral absorption of the photopigment of *Xenopus laevis* measured in single rods, J. Physiol. (Lond.) **130**, 533—542 (1955).

DONNER, K. O.: The effect of the colored oil droplets on the spectral sensitivity of the avian retina. 12th International Ornith. Congr. 167—172 (1960).

ENOCH, J. M.: Discussion of paper by Wald and Brown in Cold Spr. Harb. Symp. quant. Biol. **30**, 345—361 (1965).

— Retinal microspectrophotometry. J. Opt. Soc. Amer. **56**, 833—835 (1966).

— GLISMANN, L. E.: Physical and optical changes in excised retinal tissue. Invest. Ophthal. **5**, 208—221 (1966).

ENTINE, G., LIEBMAN, P. A., STOREY, B. T.: Ubiquinone in the retina. Vision Res. **8**, 215—219 (1968).

GOLDSMITH, T. H.: The nature of the retinal action potential and the spectral sensitivities of ultraviolet and green receptor systems of the compound eye of the worker honey bee. J. gen. Physiol. **43**, 657—799 (1960).

— DIZON, A. E., FERNANDEZ, H. R.: Microspectrophotometry of photoreceptor organelles from eyes of the prawn, *Palaemonetes*. Science **161**, 468—470 (1968).

GOLDSTEIN, E. B.: Visual pigments and the early receptor potential of the isolated frog retina. Vision Res. **8**, 953—963 (1968).

HANAOKA, T., FUJIMOTO, K.: Absorption spectrum of a single cone in carp retina. Jap. J. Physiol. **7**, 276—285 (1957).

HUBBARD, R., WALD, G.: Visual pigment of the horseshoe crab, *Limulus polyphemus*. Nature (Lond.) **186**, 212—215 (1960).

KÖTTGEN, E., ABELSDORFF, G.: Absorption und Zersetzung des Sehpurpurs bei den Wirbeltieren. Z. Psychol. Physiol. Sinnesorg. **12**, 161—184 (1896). Cited in DARTNALL, H. J. A.: The Visual Pigments. London: Methuen 1957.

LANGER, H., THORELL, B.: Microspectrophotometry of single rhabdomeres in the insect eye. Exp. Cell Res. **41**, 673—677 (1966a).

— — Microspectrophotometric assay of visual pigments in single rhabdomeres of the insect eye. Functional Organization of the Compound Eye; pp. 145—149.Oxford-New York: Pergamon Press 1966b.

LIEBMAN, P. A.: In situ microspectrophotometric studies on the pigments of single retinal rods. Biophys. J. **2**, 161—178 (1962).
— Discussion of paper by Wald and Brown. Cold Spr. Harb. Symp. quant. Biol. **30**, 345—361 (1965).
— Microspectrophotometry of retinal cells. Ann. N. Y. Acad. Sci. **157**, 250—264 (1969).
— ENTINE, G.: Sensitive low-light-level microspectrophotometer detection of photosensitive pigments of retinal cones. J. opt. Soc. Amer. **54**, 1451—1459 (1964).
— — Cyanopsin, a visual pigment of retinal origin. Nature (Lond.) **216**, 501—503 (1968a).
— — Visual pigments of frog and tadpole. Vision Res. **8**, 761—775 (1968b).
— — Radiance of deuterium arc lamps. Applied Optics. **8**, 1502 (1969).
— GRANDA, A. M.: Microspectrophotometric measurements of visual pigments in two species of turtle. In preparation (1969).
— LEIGH, R. A.: Autofluorescence of visual receptors. Nature (Lond.) **221**, 1249—1251 (1969).
LYTHGOE, R. J.: The absorption spectra of visual purple and of indicator yellow. J. Physiol. (Lond.) **89**, 331—358 (1937).
MAC NICHOL, E. F. JR.: Three pigment color vision. Sci. Amer. **211**, 48—56 (1964).
MARKS, W. B.: Difference spectra of the visual pigments in single goldfish cones. Ph. D. Thesis. Johns Hopkins University 1963.
— Visual pigments of single goldfish cones. J. Physiol. (Lond.) **178**, 14—32 (1965a).
— Discussion of the paper by F. Crescitelli on visual system of Gecko gecko, Ciba Symposium on Colour Vision, pp. 323. Ed. A. V. S. de Reuck. Boston: Little Brown and Co. 1965b.
— DOBELLE, W. H., MACNICHOL, E. F. JR.: Visual pigments of single primate cones. Science **143**, 1181—1183 (1964).
MUNZ, F. W.: The photosensitive pigments from the retinae of certain deep sea fishes. J. Physiol. (Lond.) **140**, 220—235 (1958).
— BEATTY, D. D.: A critical analysis of the visual pigments of salmon and trout. Vision Res. **5**, 1—17 (1965).
— SCHWANZARA, S. A.: A nomogram for retinene$_2$-based visual pigments. Vision Res. **7**, 111—120 (1967).
MURRAY, G. C.: Intracellular absorption difference spectrum of *Limulus* extra-ocular photolabile pigment. Science **154**, 1182—1183 (1966).
— Visual pigment multiplicity in cones of the primate fovea. Ph. D. Thesis. Johns Hopkins University 1968.
NAKA, K. I., RUSHTON, W. A. H.: S potentials from colour units in the retina of fish (Cyprinidae). J. Physiol. (Lond.) **185**, 536—555 (1966).
REUTER, T.: The synthesis of photosensitive pigments in the rods of the frog's retina. Vision Res. **6**, 15—28 (1966).
RIPPS, H., WEALE, R. A.: On seeing red. J. opt. Soc. Amer. **54**, 272—273 (1964).
RUSHTON, W. A. H.: The cone pigments of the human fovea in colour blind and normal in Visual Problems of Colour. National Physical Laboratory Symposium No. 8. Her Majesty's Stationery Office, pp. 71—101 (1958).
— Interpretation of retinal densitometry. J. opt. Soc. Amer. **54**, 273 (1964).
— Discussion in Colour Vision, Ciba Symposium. Ed. A. V. S. de Reuck and J. Knight, pp. 271—285. London: Churchill 1965.
SCHMIDT, W. J.: Polarisationsoptische Analyse eines Eiweiß-Lipoid-Systems, erläutert am Außenglied der Sehzellen. Kolloid-Z. **85**, 137—148 (1938).
SPERLING, W., RAFFERTY, C. N.: The relationship between absorption spectrum and different molecular conformations of 11-cis-retinal. Nature (Lond.) **224**, 591—594 (1969).
STROTHER, G. K.: Absorption spectra of retinal oil globules in turkey, turtle and pigeon. Exp. Cell Res. **29**, 349—355 (1963).
— WOLKEN, J. J.: Microspectrophotometry. I. Absorption spectra of colored oil globules in the chicken retina. Exp. Cell Res. **21**, 504—512 (1960).
TOMITA, T., KANEKO, A., MURAKAMI, M., PAUTLER, E. L.: Spectral response curves of single cones in the carp. Vision Res. **7**, 519—531 (1967).

Wald, G.: Visual purple system in freshwater fishes. Nature (Lond.) **139**, 1017—1018 (1937).
— The chemical evolution of vision. Harvey Lect. **41**, 117—160 (1946).
— Vision. Fed. Proc. **12**, 606—611 (1953a).
— The biochemistry of vision. Ann. Rev. Biochem. **22**, 497—526 (1953b).
— The biochemistry of visual excitation. In Enzymes: Units of Biol. Structure and Function, pp. 355—367. Ed. H. Gaebler. London-New York: Academic Press (1956).
— The molecular basis of visual excitation. Nobel Lecture, Dec. 12, 1967. The Nobel Foundation 1968.
— Brown, P. K.: Human color vision and color blindness. Cold Spr. Harb. Symp. quant. Biol. **30**, 345—361 (1965).
— — Gibbons, I. R.: The problem of visual excitation. J. opt. Soc. Amer. **53**, 20—35 (1963).
— — Smith, P. H.: Cyanopsin, a new pigment of cone vision. Science **118**, 505—508 (1953).
— — — Iodopsin. J. gen. Physiol. **38**, 623—681 (1955).
— Krainin, J. M.: The median eye of *Limulus:* an ultraviolet receptor. Proc. nat. Acad. Sci. (Wash.) **50**, 1011 (1963).
Walls, G. L.: The Vertebrate Eye and its Adaptive Radiation p. 103. Michigan: Cranbrook Institute of Science, 1942.
— Judd, H. D.: The intraocular colour-filters of vertebrates. Brit. J. Ophthal. **17**, 641—675 and 705—725 (1933).
Waterman, T. H., Fernández, H. R., Goldsmith, T. H.: Dichroism of photosensitive pigment in rhabdomes of the crayfish, *Orconectes.* J. gen. Physiol. **54**, 415—432 (1969).
Weale, R. A.: Photochemistry and vision. Photophysiology, Vol. II, Chap. 9. London-New York: Academic Press 1968.
Wiesenfield, J. R., Abrahamson, E. W.: Visual pigments: their spectra and isomerizations. Photochem. Photobiol. **8**, 487—493 (1968).
Witkovsky, P.: A comparison of ganglion cell and S-potential response properties in carp retina. J. Neurophysiol. **30**, 546—561 (1967).
Wolken, J. J.: The visual pigments, absorption spectra of isolated single frog retinal rods and cones. Invest. Ophthal. **1**, 327—332 (1962).
Yang, C. C., Legallais, V.: A rapid and sensitive recording spectrophotometer for the visible and ultraviolet region. Rev. sci. Instr. **25**, 801—813 (1954).
Zechmeister, L., Polgar, A.: Cis-trans isomerization and spectral characteristics of carotenoids and some related copounds. J. amer. chem. Soc. **65**, 1522—1528 (1943).

Chapter 13

Inert Absorbing and Reflecting Pigments

By

W. R. A. Muntz, Falmer, Brighton (Great Britain)

With 16 Figures

Contents

I. Introduction

One of the most striking early correlations between physiology and behaviour was König's (1894) demonstration that human scotopic spectral sensitivity resembled the spectral absorptive characteristics (difference spectrum) of a pigment — visual purple, or rhodopsin — that he extracted from the human retina. Later comparisons between such functions (e.g. Hecht and Williams, 1922; Dartnall and Goodeve, 1937; Wald, 1938; Crescitelli and Dartnall, 1953; Dartnall, 1953; Wald and Brown, 1958; Weale, 1961; Dartnall, 1961) have amply confirmed König's hypothesis. No one today doubts that the photosensitive pigments in retinal receptors mediate vision, and the sophisticated comparisons that are now possible serve rather to give some insight into the nature of the visual process.

Spectral sensitivity can be defined as the spectral variation of the reciprocal of the relative numbers of quanta in stimuli that evoke equal responses. These numbers must, of course, refer to the stimuli that reach the visual pigment. The quantal intensities measured are those incident on the cornea, and hence allowance must be made for the substantial losses by absorption in pre-retinal media (e.g. cornea, lens, and humours) and for the (usually small) gains by reflectance and fluorescence of surfaces lying behind the retina. The correlation between human scotopic sensitivity and human visual pigment has improved as each of these effects has been measured and allowed for, until, today, the two sets of measurements agree within the limits of experimental accuracy.

The success of the comparison in the human case has led to numerous other attempts to correlate visual pigment absorbance spectra and measures of spectral sensitivity. These have included, for example, attempts by Wald (1949) and Granit (1955) to identify the pigments underlying scotopic and photopic vision in a variety of animals, as well as attempts to unravel the workings of the retina by hypothesising interactions between receptors that are assumed to contain various visual pigments (e. g. Rushton, 1959).

Work of this type requires a knowledge of the absorption characteristics of all the structures in the eye lying between the photosensitive pigments and the light. It also requires a knowledge of any fluorescence and scattering that may occur, and of any reflecting structures in the eye, such as a tapetum. The purpose of the present chapter is to review the data that are at present available on these questions. This subject was reviewed by Walls and Judd in 1933 (summarised in Walls 1942), and, in general, work previous to that date will not be covered in this chapter.

II. Pre-Retinal Absorption

A. Spectral Characteristics of Lens, Cornea, and Vitreous in Vertebrates

1. Early Work

It has long been known that the lens and cornea of some vertebrates are yellow in colour. Walls and Judd (1933) presented a comprehensive review of the distribution of yellow corneas and lenses in vertebrates. Unfortunately, this early work was qualitative, and does not give spectrophotometric data on the absorbances at different wavelengths, so it cannot be used in assessing the effect of the lens and cornea on an animal's spectral sensitivity. Nevertheless, the work is still useful, since any theory about the function of yellow lenses and corneas must account for their distribution within the animal kingdom, and the data also indicate where, in comparative work, a correction for absorption at this level might be particularly important.

According to WALLS and JUDD, yellow lenses occur in lampreys, squirrels, and diurnal snakes. Among the squirrels, there is a wide variation in the depth of pigmentation, varying from the prairie dog (*Cynomys ludovicianus*) and ground squirrel (*Citellus t. tridecemlineatus*), with deeply pigmented lenses, to the flying squirrel (*Glaucomys v. volans*) and the grey squirrel (*Sciurus carolinensis leucotis*), with pale yellow lenses. There is also a rough correlation with the light levels normally encountered in the animals' environments, the squirrels with pigmented lenses living in the open, and those with pale lenses among trees.

Corneas are usually remarkably transparent, indeed yellow corneas occur only in teleost fish, where they are common. The colour is usually not uniform, being generally much deeper above the pupil than below (cf. Fig. 2a). In many species, only the top of the cornea is coloured, while in others, such as the pike (*Esox*), the colour extends well down over the pupil, shading from an orange colour above to colourless below. WALLS and JUDD state that "eye shades" of this type occur in *Esox lucius*, *E. vermiculatis*, *Amia calva*, *Cottus bairdii*, *Cyprinus carpio*, *Carassius auratus*, *Perva flavescens*, *Poecilichthys coeruleus*, and *Notemigonus crysoleucus*: a recent paper by MORELAND and LYTHGOE (1968) shows that they also occur in *Coris julis*, *Labrus bergylta*, *Julis parvo*, *Labrus viridis*, *Halichoeres centriquadrus*, *Balistapus undulatus*, *Perca fluviatilis*, and four species of *Tilapia*. It is clear in these fishes (and presumably many others are similar) that the correlation of behavioural or physiological data with pigment absorption is going to present special difficulties. These may be aggravated by behavioural idiosyncrasies. Thus goldfish (*Carassius auratus*) are said to rise up to the stimulus in behavioural situations, so that the "eye shade" will be brought actively into play (SUTHERLAND, 1968).

2. Spectrophotometric Data

The data reviewed by WALLS and JUDD are qualitative. Recently, however, detailed spectrophotometric data have become available for a variety of animals. In some cases these data refer to the lens alone; in others they refer to the lens and cornea together, or to all the structures lying between the retina and the incoming light. It seems probable that the lens is the limiting factor in most cases (except in those teleosts where the cornea is coloured) and consequently that the absorption of all the optic media together will not differ greatly from that for the lens alone. In man, the cornea transmits nearly 100% of the incident light down to 310 nm (KINSEY, 1948), while in the infra red the transmission characteristics are very similar to those of water (KENSHALO, 1960). The vitreous body also transmits light well in the near ultraviolet (BALAZ, 1954).

The most detailed determinations are those on man. The original measurements were made by LUDVIGH and MCCARTHY (1938) on excised material, and their data are shown in Fig. 1. In more recent work the transmissions of the lens and optic media have been measured *in vivo* by Said and Weale (1959) and by Alpern, Thompson, and Lee (1965). Said and Weale (1959) estimated the spectral absorbance of the lens by comparing the intensities of light reflected from the aqueous-lens and the lens-vitreous surfaces. Alpern, Thompson, and Lee (1965) used human patients who had portions of the sclera devoid of retina and choroid (scar tissue). The reflectance of monochromatic light from these areas of scar tissue was measured, thus allowing the transmission at different wavelengths to be calculated. The results obtained *in vivo* agree well with Ludvigh and McCarthy's data.

Various complications have also been demonstrated. The most important of these is the effect of age (Wald, 1949; Said and Weale, 1959; Cooper and Robson, 1969b) which is to increase the degree of pigmentation, thus reducing the light transmission at short wave-lengths. This effect is quite large, and is easily detectable in psychophysical experiments on colour vision and spectral sensitivity as a decrease in sensitivity to the blue (Stiles and Burch, 1958; Ruddock, 1965).

Weale (1961) has suggested that a correction should also be applied for the size of the pupil, and has demonstrated that certain psychophysical findings, such as the change in size of the perimetric field and absolute threshold with age, can be explained if this is allowed for. The correction is necessary because the lens is thinner at the edges than it is at the centre, so that the effective thickness of the lens depends on its aperture. The effect of pupil size is also complicated by the Stiles-Crawford effect (Stiles and Crawford, 1933).

Pirenne (1962) has further pointed out that Ludvigh and McCarthy's data include any light loss due to scattering by the optic media, and that such light losses will be less for extended images than for small images. Finally, fluorescence will on occasion be a complicating factor (see below).

Although the spectral characteristics of the lenses of animals other than man have not been studied in the same detail, a considerable body of data has now accumulated. A few examples are shown in Fig. 1. In some cases the measurements

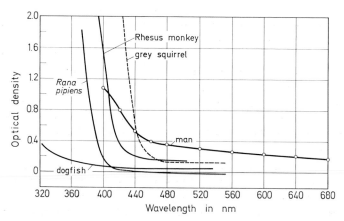

Fig. 1. Spectral absorbances of various vertebrate lenses. Data for dogfish, *Rana pipiens*, and Rhesus monkey from Kennedy and Milkman (1956), for the grey squirrel from Cooper and Robson (1969a), and for man from Ludvigh and McCarthy (1938).

include all the transparent structures of the eye, while in other cases they are restricted to the lens alone. Also, in most cases the measurements include light losses due to scattering, though in a few the scattering component has been allowed for, by using the opal glass technique developed by DARTNALL (1961) for measuring light absorption in suspensions of receptor outer segments.

It is clear from Fig. 1 that lenses absorb short wavelengths, and transmit long wavelengths, and that the point at which they start to transmit varies greatly between animals. This is true of all animals that have been studied so far. In most cases the cut-off is quite sharp, which means that a lens can be characterised with reasonable accuracy by measuring the cut-off point. Table 1 summarises the data available in this way, by showing the wavelengths at which the lenses transmit 0.3 log units less than they transmit at 550 nm (beyond which there is normally little increase in transmissivity). Two points about these data require comment. First, the most pigmented lens measured is that of the grey squirrel. However, as we have seen, the lens of the grey squirrel is one of the palest of the squirrel lenses, so that no strongly pigmented lens has yet been studied. Second, it is interesting to note that the effect of age in cats and cows is the same as in man. In the other species no effort was made to study the individual differences, which may well be considerable. Age has been shown to affect the chemical composition of the lens in rabbits and cattle, causing, among other things, an increase in the protein content and a decrease in the amount of water present (VAN HEYNINGEN, 1962).

Less detailed data have been presented for many other animals. KENNEDY and MILKMAN (1956) state that the calico bass (*Pomoxis sparoides*), sunfish (*Lepomis pallidus*), flounder (*Paralichthys dentatus*), rudderfish (*Seriola zonata*), and sea robin (*Prionotus volans*) all have lenses cutting off at about 400 nm, while the toadfish (*Opsanus tan*) and catfish (*Ameiurus nebulosus*) have lenses that transmit down to about 340 nm. They suggest a rough correlation with habitat: active surface-feeding fishes have lenses cutting out the near ultraviolet, while bottom feeders have lenses transparent down to much shorter wavelengths. The brook trout (*Salvelinus fontinalis*) is interesting because although the lens transmits down to about 320 nm, the cornea cuts off at 400 nm. Tables 1 and 2 show that the cornea is also the limiting structure in two other salmonids, the rainbow trout and the lake trout (McCANDLESS, HOFFERT, and FROMM, 1969).

The lenses of a variety of sea fishes have been studied by DENTON (1956) and MOTAIS (1957). In these experiments a mercury spectrum was photographed through the lenses, thus allowing a rough estimate of the cut-off point to be made. DENTON used the lenses of 28 species in all, and found a wide variation of cut-off points. Among the six deep-sea species investigated (all living at 100 metres or more), the cut-off varied from about 440 nm (*Chlorophthalmus agassizi*) to about 310 nm (*Lepidorhombus bosci*). DENTON suggests that since, in any case, there is no ultraviolet light at these depths, the exact cut-off point is not important. For surface fishes he concludes that nocturnal forms have lenses transparent in the ultraviolet, while the lenses of diurnal predatory fishes absorb in this region. He points out, however, that the correlation is not perfect, and that fishes with very different cut-off points may live in very similar visual environments.

DENTON and WARREN (1968), using the same technique, have reported that deep sea cephalopods have lenses that are transparent to ultraviolet light, while species that live at the surface, such as the squid (*Onychoteuthis banksi*), have yellow lenses cutting off at about 430 nm. The Histioteuthidae are particularly interesting. In these squid one eye is much larger than the other, and the lens of the large eye is yellow in colour, while that of the small eye is colourless. Denton and Warren

Table 1. *Cut-off points for the lens (wavelengths at which the lenses of various animals transmit 0.3 log units less than they transmit at 550 nm)*

Species	cut-off wave-lengths (nm)	Reference		Notes
Fishes				
Dogfish (*Mustelus canis*)	320			
Yellow perch (*Perca flavescens*)	405			
Tautog (*Tautoga onitis*)	350	Kennedy and Milkman	(1956)	
Butterfish (*Poronotus triacanthus*)	350			
Scup (*Stenotomus versicolor*)	410			
Carp (*Cyprinus carpio*)	405	Witkovsky	(1968)	
Goldfish (*Carassius auratus*)	405	Burkardt	(1966)	(2)
Rainbow trout (*Salmo gairdneri*)	322	McCandless, Hoffert and		(3)
Lake trout (*Salvelinus namaycush*)	324	Fromm	(1969)	(4)
Amphibians				
Frog (*Rana pipiens*)	395	Kennedy and Milkman	(1956)	
Mammals				
Grey squirrel	445	Arden and Silver	(1962)	(1)
		Cooper and Robson	(1969a)	(5)
Guinea-pig	360	Cooper and Robson	(1969a)	(5)
Rabbit	390	Weisinger, Schmidt, Williams, Tiller, Ruffin, Guerry, and Ham	(1956)	(2)
Cow	440	Ludvigh and McCarthy	(1938)	(2)
	410	Merker	(1934)	
Calf	395	Merker	(1934)	
Old cat	420	Dodt and Walther	(1958)	
Young cat	320			
Bush baby	410	Dartnall, Arden, Ikeda, Luck, Rosenberg, Pedler, and Tansley	(1965)	(1)
	415	Cooper and Robson	(1969b)	(5)
Macaque	428			
Squirrel monkey	420	Cooper and Robson	(1969b)	(5)
Baboon	420			
Rhesus monkey	420	Kennedy and Milkman	(1956)	
Young man	425	Ludvigh and McCarthy	(1938)	(2)
68 yrs old man	480	Wald	(1949)	

Notes
(1) Scattering allowed for.
(2) Includes all optic media.
(3) Lens transmits 0.3 log units less at 322 nm than at 668 nm.
(4) Lens transmits 0.3 log units less at 324 nm than at 800 nm.
(5) Whole lens characteristics reconstructed from measurements made on thin layers of lens material.

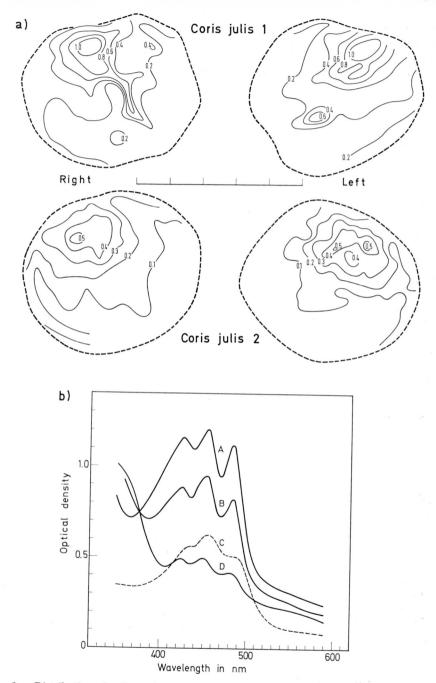

Fig. 2. *a* Distribution of yellow pigmentation in the conea of *Coris julis*. Equal absorbance contours are shown for two specimens in "blue" light. The anterior aspects of each pair of corneas are opposed, the dorsal aspect being uppermost. From MORELAND and LYTHGOE (1968). *b* Spectral absorbance (in region of highest density) of the corneas of four individual fishes
A Labrus viridis; *B Coris julis*; *C Perca fluviatilis*; *D Julis parvo*

suggest that the large eye may be adapted for vision at the surface, and the small eye for vision in deep water.

Comparatively little spectrophotometric work has been done on the cornea. Data are given for the cow and the calf by Merker (1934), and for two species of trout by McCandless, Hoffert, and Fromm (1969). In these animals the spectral absorbance is similar to that for the lens, and the cut off points are summarised in Table 2. Spectrophotometric curves for four species of fishes with yellow corneas are also shown in Fig. 2b (Moreland and Lythgoe, 1968).

Table 2. *Cut-off points for the cornea (wavelengths at which corneas of various animals transmit 0.3 log units less than they transmit at 550 nm)*

Species	cut-off wavelength (nm)	Reference
Rainbow trout (*Salmo gairdneri*)	350	McCandless, Hoffert, and Fromm (1969)
Lake trout (*Salvelinus namaycush*)	360	
Cow	350	Merker (1934)
Calf	330	

3. Fluorescence

Ultraviolet light (< 400 nm) causes the human lens to fluoresce, producing a general veil of bluish light over the retina. The composition of the fluorescent light has been determined by LeGrand in sheep, rabbit and ox (summarised in Wyszecki and Stiles, 1967), and later experiments by Brolin and Cederlund (1958) have extended the work to a variety of other animals (haddock, frog, hen, rat, rabbit, guinea pig, cat, cow, pig, and man). The spectral distribution of the fluorescent light varies little between species, and is centred at about 430 nm. Brolin and Cederland's (1958) data show, however, that the quantum yield varies greatly across species, being low for the haddock, rat, hen, cat, pig and cow, and comparatively high for the rabbit, frog and guinea pig. The quantum yield in the guinea pig is at least thirty times greater than that in the haddock. The amount of fluorescence also increases with age. Merker (1934) likewise reports species variation. He gives the frog, salamander, wild duck, lizard, cow, sheep, and pig as examples of animals with strongly fluorescing lenses, and the toad, alpine salamander, barn owl, wood owl, cat, fieldmouse and woodmouse as examples with weakly-fluorescing lenses.

Dodt and Walther (1958c) have presented data suggesting that fluorescence can affect spectral sensitivity under certain circumstances. They measured the spectral sensitivity of humans, using the electroretinogram (ERG), and found that the sensitivity in the near ultra-violet was greater than would be expected on the basis of Wald's (1945) psychophysical results on aphakic subjects. Furthermore, the extra sensitivity at short wavelengths was greater in old subjects than in young, even though old lenses transmit less light. However, old lenses fluoresce more than do young lenses, and, at the light intensities necessary to obtain an ERG, the lenses both fluoresce visibly in the ultra-violet. Dodt and Walther (1958b) showed a similar effect in cats, in finding that the sensitivity in the near ultraviolet was greater when the lens was present that when it was removed. This effect only occurred with small stimuli, and it seems possible that here also the lens fluoresces, and forms a secondary source that is larger than the original stimulus. This will cause an apparent increase in sensitivity, since the ERG depends strongly on the size of the stimulus.

DODT and WALTHER's results were obtained via the ERG, which necessitates fairly intense stimuli. The effects of fluorescence would, presumably, be less marked at behavioural threshold. Some animals show fluorescence much more strongly than others which will increase the effect. The guinea pig lens, for example, fluoresces exceptionally strongly. This may account, at least in part, for the high blue sensitivity found in the ERG of this animal (GRANIT, 1942a).

4. Function of Yellow Lenses and Corneas

WALLS and JUDD (1933) and WALLS (1942), have put forward various suggestions for the possible function of yellow lenses and corneas. The first suggestion was that they act as a filter, improving visual acuity by reducing chromatic aberration. This could occur because the short wavelengths, which are most strongly dispersed and thus contribute most to chromatic aberration, are preferentially absorbed by the filter. The effect could benefit terrestial animals, but not those teleosts that have yellow corneas, for the lenses of these animals are apparently free of chromatic aberration (PUMPHREY, 1961). The second suggestion was that a yellow lens would improve distance vision by absorbing "blue haze". By this they meant the scattered light of the atmosphere, which limits the range at which distant objects can be seen. If most of the scattered light is of short wavelength a yellow filter will improve vision for such objects.

The maximum distance at which an object can be seen depends on the extinction coefficient of the medium between the object and the observer (MIDDLETON, 1952). The extinction coefficient is the sum of the absorbance and scattering coefficients. The former of these is negligible in air, so that in this case the range at which an object can be seen depends on scattering alone. MIDDLETON (1952) has presented data on the extinction coefficients for red (657—636 nm), green (565—528 nm), and blue (483—462 nm) lights during different atmospheric conditions. Fig. 3 has been constructed from these data, and shows that the visual range is greater for long wavelength light under conditions of good visibility, but that this no longer holds once the visual range drops below about one kilometre.

The spectral characteristics of fogs vary considerably, but MIDDLETON believes that Fig. 3, which was constructed on the basis of data from two different experiments, represents the typical situation when the fog or haze is not of industrial origin. If this is the case, a yellow filter will improve only the visibility of very distant objects on clear days. Such an improvement might be of value to birds (which, although they do not have yellow lenses or corneas, have yellow oil droplets: see below), but it is difficult to believe that very distant visual stimuli are important to prairie dogs, lampreys, or diurnal snakes.

WALLS and JUDD have further suggested that a yellow filter may improve vision by reducing "glare", and also that it may improve contrast for vision against a blue sky. These suggestions are also relevant to the possible functions of the oil droplets, and will be considered at that point.

The simplest hypothesis on the function of the yellow corneas of teleosts is that they reduce the intensity of retinal illumination from above. Fishes that live near the surface are subjected to very large differences in light intensity between the top and the bottom of the visual field. Tyler and Preisendorfer (1962) have studied in detail the distribution of light underwater: they have shown, as one example, that, with an overcast sky and the sun at an altitude of 40°, the difference in illumination from above and below amounts to over 3 log units at a depth of six metres

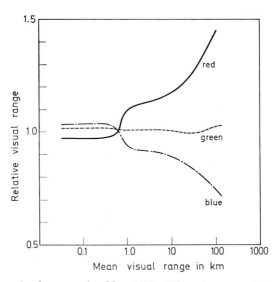

Fig. 3. Relative visual ranges for blue (462—483 nm), green (528—565 nm), and red (636—657 nm) lights as a function of the mean visual range for the three spectral regions (the visual range (V) is the distance over which the contrast of an object drops to 2% of its original value)

in fresh water. The presence of a yellow corneal "eye shade", absorbing preferentially at the top, will help to even out this difference. The data of Moreland and Lythgoe (1968) show that the difference in optical density between the top and bottom of the cornea in *Coris julis* is 0.8 log units or less, so that even with a pigmented cornea a considerable difference in retinal illumination may remain. In some teleosts other mechanisms exist to help even out the retinal illumination. The melanin, for example, is much denser in the ventral half of the eye in many teleosts, such as the rudd and goldfish, and the tapetum may also be more developed in the upper half of the eye.

B. Invertebrate Corneas

The spectral characteristics of the corneas of some arthropod eyes have also been studied (Carricaburu and Chardenot, 1967, Bernhard, Miller, and Møller, 1965; Miller, Bernard, and Allen, 1968). In general, these results are similar to those obtained with vertebrate corneas and lenses, with increasing absorption at short wavelengths (Fig. 4). Many arthropods are sensitive to near ultraviolet light, and the cornea in such cases must be transparent down to very short wavelengths, (e.g. the bee *Apis mellifica* in Fig. 4).

Many of the structural components of the arthropod eye have dimensions near the wavelength of light, and in some cases these cause observable optical effects (MILLER, BERNARD, and ALLEN, 1968). In the compound eyes of many insects the surface is covered with a hexagonal array of conical protuberances, known as corneal nipples. These are approximately 200 nm high, with a similar distance

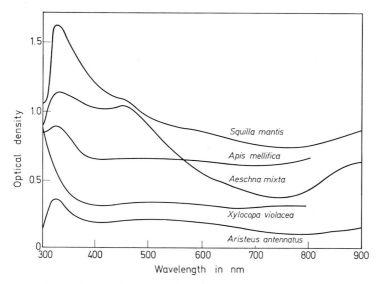

Fig. 4. Spectral absorbance of various invertebrate corneas. Data from CARRICABURU and CHARDENOT (1967). (These data are reproduced as given, but it is clear that the absolute positions of the curves relative to the ordinate axis were not determined)

between them. They act as an antireflection coating, and increase the transmission of light through the cornea by about 5%. Apart from the resulting increase in sensitivity, another possible benefit is the improvement in camouflage that might result from a decrease in corneal reflection.

In some dipterans there is also a specialised system of alternating dense and rare layers located just beneath the corneal surface, the number of layers varying between six and twenty in different species. These act as an interference filter, and the eyes appear coloured from the reflected light when viewed from the same direction as the incident light. The colouring may be uniform over the whole eye, or may be subdivided into different areas of different colours. In the female horse fly (*Hybomitra lasiophthalma*), for example, the eye shows a pattern of five dark bluish stripes alternating with five bright and predominantly orange stripes. The colours that are seen, and the effects of the angle of incident illumination, can be accounted for by the spacing of the corneal layers.

Fluorescence of the cornea also occurs in compound eyes (MERKER, 1934). It has been suggested in the case of *Limulus* (ADOLPH, 1968) that this may increase sensitivity to short wavelengths.

III. Absorption at the Retinal Level

A. Oil Droplets

1. Introduction

The oil droplets are highly refractile bodies, occurring in the cones of many species (Fig. 5). Most such receptors contain a single droplet, but multiple small (red) droplets have also been described in the receptors of the pigeon (WALLS and JUDD, 1933; PEDLER and BOYLE, 1969). The droplets may appear colourless, green, yellow, orange, or red. When they are coloured, they must affect the spectral sensitivity of the receptor in which they are located, since the light has to pass through the droplet to reach the visual pigment in the outer segment.

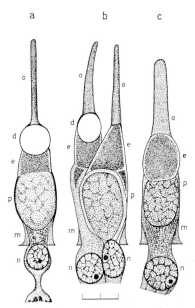

Fig. 5. Single cone (*a*), double cone (*b*), and rod (*c*) of the snapping turtle (*Chelydra serpentina*) Each scale division represents 5 μm. *o*, outer segment; *d*, oil droplet; *e*, ellipsoid; *p*, paraboloid; *m*, myoid; *n*, nucleus. From WALLS (1942)

In general, oil droplets are found only in cones, although they do occur in the rods of a few reptiles (e.g. *Sphenodon*, and certain geckoes; WALLS 1942). The droplets have been shown to contain carotenoids, which have been extracted, isolated, and analysed spectroscopically by various workers (e.g. WALD and ZUSSMAN, 1937; VON STUDNITZ, LOEVINICH and NEWMANN, 1943). In the present chapter, however, we are not concerned with their chemistry, but with their effects on vision. In this respect the most important data are their spectral transmission characteristics.

2. Spectrophotometric Data

The first objective measurements were made by ROAF (1929), who worked on the retina of the domestic hen. Previous to this, knowledge of the spectral characteristics of the droplet had been based on direct visual observation and estimation. ROAF formed the image of a droplet on the slit of a microspectroscope, and then photographed the resulting spectrum. He found that the droplets transmitted long wavelengths and absorbed short wavelengths, and that they fell into three groups: those starting to absorb at 574 nm (red droplets), at 512 nm (yellow droplets), and at 455 nm (pale green droplets).

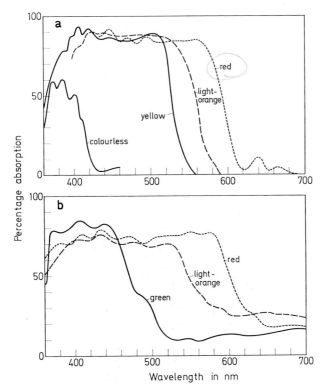

Fig. 6. Absorption spectra of the oil droplets of the swamp turtle (*a*) and the pigeon (*b*). Data from STROTHER (1963)

Some examples of more recent determinations of the absorption of the oil droplets are shown in Fig. 6, which is taken from STROTHER (1963). These spectra were obtained using a microspectrophotometer; details of the procedure and other examples of absorption spectra may be found in Chapter 12. It can be seen that the results substantially confirm ROAF's data, and show that the droplets all act as cut-off filters, transmitting long wavelengths and absorbing short wavelengths. Data were obtained on the pigeon, turkey, swamp turtle (*Pseudemys elegans*), and wood turtle (*Clemmys insculpta*). STROTHER's results may be summarised as follows:

a) The maximum absorption is roughly the same (about 80%) irrespective of the size or colour of the droplet, or the species used.

b) The cut-off wavelength for a given colour of droplet is independent of species. Thus red droplets cut off at about 570 nm, orange at 540 nm, light orange at 530 nm,

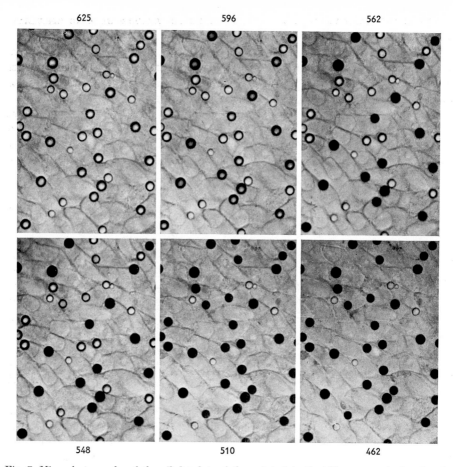

Fig. 7. Microphotographs of the oil droplets of the painted turtle (*Chrysemys picta*), taken in different monochromatic illuminations. The wavelength in nm of the illumination is shown against each photograph

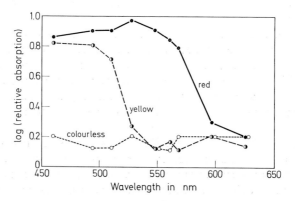

Fig. 8. Spectral absorbances (in logarithmic units) of the oil droplets of the painted turtle, determined from photographs such as those in Fig. 7

yellow at 510 nm, and green at 440 nm. Colourless droplets have an absorption maximum at 380 nm, with lesser peaks on either side.

c) Different species have droplets of different colours. Thus the pigeon has red, light orange, and green droplets; the turkey, red, orange, yellow, and colourless droplets; the swamp turtle, red, light orange, yellow, and colourless droplets, and the wood turtle, red, orange, yellow, and colourless droplets.

Microspectrophotometry clearly provides the most accurate and detailed data on the spectral absorption of the oil droplets. However, as the droplets are cut-off filters, they are relatively easy to classify according to their cut-off point alone. This can also be done by photographing the retina (using near monochromatic light such as can be obtained with interference filters). This procedure has the advantage that a large number of droplets can be characterised rapidly. Fig. 7 shows photographs of the retina of the painted turtle (*Chrysemys picta*), obtained in this way. It can be seen that, unlike the turtles studied by STROTHER, there are only three types of droplet in evidence; red, yellow, and colourless. The film was calibrated by photographing chips of neutral density filter under the same conditions, the absorption at different wavelengths being measured from the density of the image on the negatives. The resulting spectra for three droplets are shown in Fig. 8. The photographic spectra, though presumably less accurate than the microspectrophotometric data, nevertheless characterise the droplets accurately enough for many purposes.

3. Distribution in the Retina

Cones that bear droplets of different colours are found to differ in other characteristics as well. Thus, in many birds, the different colours occur in cones of different lengths, with the colourless and green droplets lying closer to the pigment epithelium than do the yellow, orange, and red droplets (PEIPONEN, 1964). This is not invariable, however: WAELCHI (1883), for example, maintains that the opposite is true for the red area of the pigeon's retina (see below), and PEIPONEN states that all the droplets lie at the same level in the macular region. PEIPONEN also reports that *Anas penelope* has twice as many orange-yellow droplets as red, half of which lie on the same plane as the red droplets, and the other half displaced 4—5 nm toward the pigment epithelium. A similar situation is true for the painted turtle. Here the single cones contain colourless, yellow, and red droplets, but the double cones contain yellow droplets only.

The segregation of different droplets into different cone types can also be shown using the electronmicroscope. MORRIS and SHOREY (1967), working with the chicken retina, described two types of single cone and a double cone, and found that the droplets in the different cone types showed quite distinct staining properties. They suggest, from a comparison with previous data, that the green droplets occur in the principal elements of the double cones, while the yellow and red droplets occur in the two types of single cone.

The distribution of droplets within different cone types suggested by MORRIS and SHOREY disagrees with the findings of MEYER and COOPER (1966), who combined phase contrast microscopy of the chicken retina with direct observation of the colours of the droplets. These authors only describe one type of single cone, containing a red droplet. They also state that the principal element of the double cones contains yellow droplets, and the accessory element green droplets.

In spite of this disagreement, it seems clear that the different colours of droplet are found in different classes of receptor. This finding may well be of considerable importance in the study of retinal function, for it allows the different classes of colour coded receptor to be recognised in histological preparations. In general, this is not possible in species lacking oil droplets. There is thus a real possibility of tracing the connections anatomically between known receptor types, with a view to explaining colour vision.

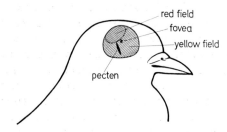

Fig. 9. View of the fundus of the pigeon eye, showing positions of the red and yellow fields

Apart from the distribution of different colours of droplet in different receptors there is, in many species, a difference in the proportions of the different droplet colours in different parts of the retina. According to Peiponen, in many birds the proportion of red droplets is much greater in the dorsal part of the retina than in the ventral part (experimental consequences and possible functional correlations of this distribution are considered in Section 7 below). This distribution is well marked, for example, in the pigeon, where there is a large yellow field with comparatively small and scarce red droplets, and a smaller red field, where the red droplets are much more frequent, as well as being larger (Fig. 9). According to Walls and Judd, red droplets are also missing from the fovea in some hawks. Not all animals, however, have such regional differences; there is no sign of them, for example, in the turtle.

4. Phylogenetic Distribution

Oil droplets occur in the retinas of chondrosteans, dipnoeans, amphibians, reptiles, birds, monotremes, and marsupials. All of these groups have colourless droplets. In amphibians, reptiles, and birds, yellow droplets occur as well. The presence of red droplets is restricted to birds and turtles.

Most of the comparative data on the relative proportions of different droplets relate to birds, and a smaller amount to turtles [summaries in Walls and Judd (1933), and in Peiponen (1964)]. The data are usually qualitative, since in most cases the droplets are characterised by the colour that they appear to have under the microscope. Although Strother (1963) found that, in the species he studied, the appearance of a droplet was a good guide to its spectral characteristics, this need not necessarily be true of all species. A further defect of the data is that there is seldom an accurate distinction between orange and yellow droplets, or between colourless and green droplets, and in some cases even no distinction between yellow and red droplets. Finally, the retinal position of the counts is often not specified. Nevertheless, certain general conclusions seem warranted.

a) In nocturnal birds, the number of coloured droplets is greatly reduced. Thus only about 10% of the droplets are red or yellow in *Caprimulgus europaeus* (PEIPONEN, 1964), while *Strix aluco* and *Tylo alba* lack coloured droplets altogether (ERHARD, 1924).

b) The swallows and swifts also have very few red and orange droplets. KRAUSE (1894) has estimated that only 6% of the droplets are red or orange in *Micropus apus* (the swift) and 10% in *Hirundo rustica* (the swallow). PEIPONEN gives about 2—3% red and yellow droplets for the dorsal nasal retina of the former, and 12% for the latter: he also finds low percentages in *Riparia riparia* [the sand martin (9—10%)], and in *Delichon urbica*, the house martin (14—15%).

c) Birds that fly above water, and need to see through the surface, have a large proportion of red droplets. In the European kingfisher, 60% of the droplets are red, compared with a mean figure of about 20% for passerines in general (ERHARD 1924). PEIPONEN's (1964) data also show this effect: 80% red or yellow droplets in *Larus fuscus* (the lesser black-backed gull), 78% in *L. canus* (the common gull), and 76% in *Sterna hirundo* (the common tern). In another gull, *L. ridibundus* (the black-headed gull), the high proportion of red and yellow droplets is less marked (63%), but this species spends a considerable amount of its time inland.

Birds that live on the water, but do not commonly fly above it and hence do not need to look through the surface, lack this development of the red droplets. In

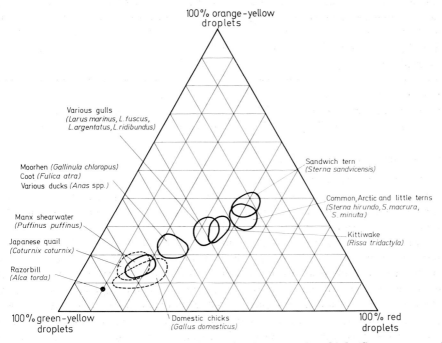

Fig. 10. Percentage of different colours of oil droplets in various birds (CULLEN, personal communication). The diagram shows the relative proportions of red (cut-off above 558 nm), orange-yellow (cut-off at 535—520 nm), and green-yellow (cut-off below 470 nm) droplets for different species. The counts were taken in all cases from an area dorsal and anterior to the optic nerve

Nycora fuligula (a duck) 20% of the droplets are red, and in the European water ousel 24% are red. The heron is a special case, for it has to look through the water surface, but only does this from short range. In one species (*Ardea c. cinerea*), 20% of the droplets are red, which is not high.

This relationship between environment and red oil droplets has recently been confirmed and extended by DR. J. M. CULLEN (personal communication). Fig. 10 shows the proportion of green-yellow (cut-off below 470 nm), yellow-orange (cut-off at 520—535 nm), and red (cut-off above 558 nm) droplets in various groups of birds. The relationship described above can be clearly seen, with aquatic birds that swim underwater in search of food having relatively few red and yellow droplets (lower lefthand corner), compared with plunge divers at the other extreme. The figure also shows that the red and yellow droplets occur in approximately equal numbers in these species, so that the results fall on a line that passes through the centre of the figure, which justifies our considering the red and yellow droplets together. In view of this CULLEN has characterised droplets simply according as they cut off at wavelengths longer or shorter than 521 nm. This can be done by photographing the retinas in illumination of this wavelength, and counting the droplets that appear opaque (red or orange-yellow), and those that appear transparent (green or colourless). In Table 3 some further results of CULLEN's are summarised,

Table 3. *Red and orange-yellow oil droplets (cut-off points above 521 nm) in various aquatic birds (counts from an area dorsal and anterior to the optic nerve in all cases. In some species several counts are given. Data from J. M. CULLEN, personal communication)*

Species	Droplets cutting off above 521 nm (% of total)
Arctic tern (*Sterna macrura*)	73
Kittiwake (*Rissa tridactyla*)	53
Herring gull (*Larus argentatus*)	58, 50, 59, 54, 66
Black-headed gull (*Larus ridibundus*)	56
Gannet (*Sula bassana*)	57, 55, 50
Shag (*Phalacrocorax aristotelis*)	19
Oyster catcher (*Haematopus ostralegus*)	43, 31
Knot (*Calidris calidris*)	46, 44
Manx shearwater (*Puffinus puffinus*)	16, 19
Mallard duck (*Anas platyrhyncus*)	41
Moorhen (*Gallinula chloropus*)	25, 46

in which this technique was used. The relationship remains clear, with a high proportion of red droplets in the tern, gulls and gannet. The gannet and the shag are closely related, belonging to the same sub-order (Pelecani), but the percentage of red and orange-yellow droplets is very different in the two cases. The gannet is a plunge diver, while the shag pursues fish underwater.

d) Turtles are the only other animals, apart from birds, that have red oil droplets. In these animals there is little variation in the proportion of droplets in different parts of the retina, and the percentage of red, orange, and yellow droplets is high. Some of the data on turtles are summarised in Table 4.

Table 4. *Oil droplets in the retinas of various turtles*

Species	Retinal location if known	Percentage of total droplets			Reference
		red	orange/ yellow	colourless	
Emys lutaria	—	43	45	12	Birukow (1939)
Testudo graeca	—	35	51	14	Birukow (1939)
Testudo graeca	Dorsal central	51	22	27 ⎫	
	Dorsal peripheral	44	26	30 ⎬	Peiponen (1964)
	Ventral lateral	44	28	28 ⎭	
Pseudemys scripta elegans	—	36	45	19	Peiponen (1964)
Chrysemys picta belli	Peripheral	42	42	16 ⎫	Muntz (unpublished)
	Central	40	43	17 ⎭	

5. Development

There is general agreement that during development the droplets initially appear colourless under the microscope. There is almost complete disagreement, however, between different workers on the timing and sequence of appearance of the different colours. The literature has been reviewed by COOPER and MYER (1968), who suggest that the disagreement is largely due to the fact that the pigments are initially present in very low concentrations, thus making their identification by microscopic examination uncertain. COOPER and MYER found that three pigments, (presumably associated with three colours of droplet) could be detected in chromatographically separated extracts of chick retina. These pigments could be detected before the droplets themselves were visible under the microscope. The golden yellow pigment appeared first, at a stage when the retina consisted of a thick unstratified neuro-epithelial layer lacking visual cells. The greenish yellow pigment could only be detected at a later stage, by which time the retina was organised into several layers, though still without photoreceptor cells. The red pigment appeared last, at a stage when the retina possessed adult stratification, and oil droplets. All these droplet pigments were detectable before any visual pigments could be extracted from the retinas.

6. Effect on Spectral Sensitivity

Owing to their position in the receptors, the oil droplets must affect spectral sensitivity. Since many animals have several types of droplets, and may well have several visual pigments as well (see Section 7 below), and since the proportions of the various droplets may also differ with retinal location, any interpretation of spectral sensitivity is clearly subject to numerous difficulties. One fact is clear, however; the sensitivity will necessarily be altered by the droplets. This means, for example, that GRANIT's (1941) demonstration that the photopic dominator of the tortoise agrees well with the spectral absorbance of cyanopsin is probably fortuitous.

The effects of the droplets on spectral sensitivity can be detected in various ways. In one type of study the spectral sensitivities of different species are compared, and correlated with the oil droplets found in the retinas. An experiment by BIRUKOW (1939), for example, compared the spectral sensitivity of *Testudo graeca* and *Emys lutaria*, using the optomotor response. According the BIRUKOW the latter species has a greater number of red oil droplets than the former, and, as expected, its spectral sensitivity is displaced towards long wavelengths. In this experiment coloured papers were used as stimuli, and accurate spectral sensitivity curves were not presented, though the difference between the two species is clear. More recent work using the ERG has clearly demonstrated a similar difference between *Testudo* and *Pseudemys* (Fig. 11). Likewise the behavioural photopic spectral sensitivity curve for the starling and the pigeon have been correlated with the proportions of the red droplets in the two species (BLOUGH, 1957; ADLER and DALLAND, 1959).

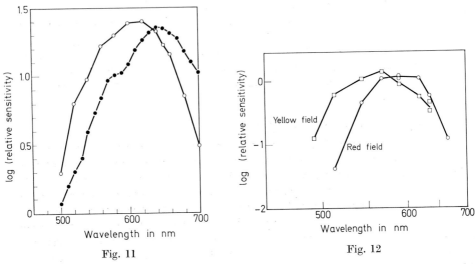

Fig. 11

Fig. 12

Fig. 11. Spectral sensitivity of *Testudo graeca* (*plain circles*, data from GRANIT, 1941) and *Pseudemys scripta* (*filled circles*, data from GRANDA, 1962)

Fig. 12. Spectral sensitivity curves for single tectal neurones in the pigeon having receptive fields in the yellow and red fields respectively of the retina (KING-SMITH, personal communication)

The effect of the droplets can also be demonstrated in some cases by comparing different parts of the retina. Fig. 12 shows two spectral sensitivity curves obtained by Dr. P. E. KING-SMITH (personal communication) from the pigeon. The curves show the average sensitivities of tectal neurones having receptive fields in different parts of the retina: as we should expect, the relative sensitivity at short wavelengths is much less in the red field.

The spectral sensitivity of the pigeon has been measured by several workers, both behaviourally (BLOUGH, 1957), and electro-physiologically (GRANIT, 1942b; DONNER, 1953; IKEDA, 1965). Other aspects of its vision have also been studied, such as the wavelength discrimination function (HAMILTON and COLEMAN, 1933), and stimulus generalisation along the spectrum (GUTTMAN and KALISH, 1956). In most cases, however, the retinal locus stimulated was not controlled though this is clearly important. In behavioural situations that involve pecking it may be a reasonable assumption that the pigeon is using the red field, though this is much less certain for a jumping stand such as the one used by HAMILTON and COLEMAN. IKEDA (1965) compared axial and peripheral stimulation, in a study that used the ERG, but (see Fig. 9) this is not a very appropriate comparison to make in the pigeon. Similar considerations apply to the chicken, for which various determinations of spectral sensitivity have also been carried out (HONIGMANN, 1921; ARMINGTON and CRAMPTON, 1958).

The most direct method of demonstrating the effects of the droplets on spectral sensitivity is to compare the results obtained when the retina is normally illuminated, with those obtained when it is illuminated from behind. This can be done with cold-blooded vertebrates, in which the retina can be removed from the eye cup and still remain capable of responding electrically to light. The experiment has been done on a lizard (*Agama caucasia*) by ORLOV and MAXIMOVA (1964), using the ERG. They found, as expected, that the spectral sensitivity curve was narrower, and its maximum displaced slightly towards long wavelengths, when the retina was normally illuminated. A similar result has been reported by PAUTLER (1967) for a turtle (*Clemmys japonica*).

7. Theories of Oil-Droplet Function

a) **Role in Colour Vision.** The fact that the oil droplets of turtles and birds are brightly coloured inevitably leads to speculation on their function in colour vision. In particular, it has frequently been suggested that the cones of such animals contain one visual pigment only, and that wavelength discrimination is achieved by the presence of different coloured filters (the droplets) lying between this pigment and the stimulating light. This hypothesis appears to have been put forward originally by KRAUSE (1863), and several other writers have subsequently also held this view (ROAF, 1933; WALD, 1938; DONNER, 1960; HAILMAN, 1964).

There is not very much evidence in favour of this hypothesis however. One approach has been made by HAILMAN (1964), who worked on the colour preferences shown in pecking by gull chicks. He found that the chicks preferred short or long wavelength stimuli, and seldom pecked at objects of intermediate green wavelengths. He was also able to show that this was a genuine example of colour vision, and not merely a case of spectral sensitivity. His data were quantitatively described by a simple model that assumed the birds to have two classes of receptor, both containing the same photosensitive pigment, one associated with a red and the other with a yellow droplet.

A more direct test of this hypothesis was made by ORLOV and MAXIMOVA (1964), using the retinas of reptiles, and stimulating from the vitreal or receptor sides as described in Section 6 above. They used the technique of "silent substitution", in which a monochromatic light is suddenly replaced by a mixture. If a mixture can be found that allows this to be done without any electrical response, it is assumed that it is identical to the monochromatic light in stimulus value. They found, for a lizard (*Agama caucasia*), that any monochromatic light could be matched in this way by a suitable mixture of two primaries, thus suggesting that the animal is dichromatic. When the stimuli were given from the receptor side, however, the animals appeared to have monochromatic vision, for any light could be substituted for any other without causing a response if the intensities were suitably adjusted. The situation was more complicated in a turtle (*Emys orbicularis*). In this case four primaries were needed to match monochromatic lights when they were normally presented, but two were sufficient when presented from behind. These results suggest, for the lizard, that dichromatic vision is achieved through the oil droplets, while in the turtle the droplets convert dichromatic vision to tetrachromatic vision.

It is now known from microspectrophotometric work that, at any rate in turtles, there are several visual pigments as well as several oil droplet types

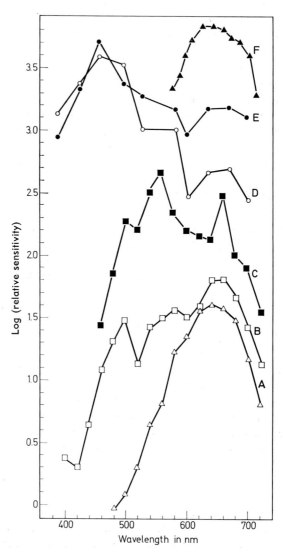

Fig. 13. Various spectral sensitivity curves of freshwater turtles of the family Emydidae. *A* and *B*, results from Granda (1962) and Granda and Stirling (1966) using the ERG; *C*, results from Granda and Stirling (1965) for evoked potentials at the tectum; *D* and *E*, behavioural results from Muntz and Sokol (1967) and Sokol and Muntz (1965); *F*, behavioural results from Graf (1967)

(Chapter 12). Thus in *Pseudemys* cone pigments absorbing maximally at 450 nm, 518 nm, and 620 nm have been described, and several pigments are also found in other species. Fig. 13 shows various spectral sensitivity curves that have been obtained with North American freshwater turtles. There are clear indications of three maxima, at about 460 nm, 550 nm, and 640 nm. These are also clearly shown by an experiment of LISENBY's (1965), in which a spectral response curve (as opposed to a spectral sensitivity curve) was obtained. The 460 nm peak is presumably due to receptors containing 450 nm pigment and colourless droplets. This association between pigment and droplet has been found microspectrophotometrically (Chapter 12), and indeed on theoretical grounds we should not expect to find the 450 nm pigment associated with any other droplet type, since these do not transmit appreciable amounts of short wavelength light.

At the other extreme we can calculate what pigment could, if associated with a red droplet, account for the sensitivity maximum at 640 nm. A good accounting can be made by a 620 nm pigment associated with the red droplet (STROTHER, 1963), but no pigment with λ_{max} shorter than this will do. A pigment absorbing maximally at this wavelength is now known to occur in turtle retinas, in association with either red or orange droplets. Finally, the 550 nm maximum in the turtle's spectral sensitivity curve is presumably due to the 518 nm pigment in association with an orange droplet, since the effective maximum of this combination (which has been found microspectrophotometrically) is at about 560 nm.

In birds also it is unlikely that colour vision can rest on the basis of one pigment and several oil droplets. LE GRAND (1962) has calculated the form of the colour mixing triangle that would be expected on this basis for the chicken, and finds that colour vision would be very poor. LE GRAND's work is open to criticism, however, since he used the spectral absorbances of pigments that had been extracted from the droplets, instead of the effective absorbances of the droplets *in situ*. DR. P. E. KING-SMITH (personal communication) has pointed out that, on the single pigment theory, the pigeon should be unable to discriminate between the spectral extremes, e.g. 470 nm and 640 nm, for in the former case all the droplets are absorbing equally about 80% of the incoming light, and in the latter case they are all transparent (STROTHER, 1963). There would thus be no difference between the relative activity of the three receptor types at the two extremes of the spectrum. A behavioural study, however, demonstrated that pigeons performed the discrimination readily (KING-SMITH and MUNTZ, unpublished). Finally, BRIDGES (1962) has extracted a pigment, presumed to be a cone pigment, with $\lambda_{max} = 544$ nm, from pigeons. If this is the only cone pigment they possess, they could not have a blue receptor, for as we have seen the droplets can only shift the effective absorbance of the receptors towards long wavelengths.

FRIEDMAN (1967) has shown that the Virginia oppossum has colour vision. Marsupials, however, only have colourless oil droplets (WALLS and JUDD, 1933), so here also the discrimination cannot depend on a single visual pigment.

Apart from the possibility, suggested by ORLOV and MAXIMOVA's results, that colour vision can be enriched by the oil droplets, these latter are bound to alter the effective spectral sensitivity of the receptors. In particular, they will make the short wavelength arms of the curves steeper. This should improve wavelength discrimination at those spectral positions where it increases the change in a receptor's output for a given change in wavelength.

b) Other Theories. Walls and Judd (1933) presented a unified view of the function of yellow filters in the eye. The oil droplets were considered as one type of yellow filter, with basically the same function as yellow lenses and corneas. In their view, most of the possible functions of yellow lenses and corneas, some of which have already been discussed, would also apply to the yellow oil droplets. These include the improvement of visual acuity (by reducing chromatic aberration and the effects of scattered light), and of contrast against certain backgrounds. The distribution of oil droplets in the bird retina is particularly striking in the latter respect, for the bottom half of the retina is often dominated by yellow oil droplets and the top half by red. It seems possible, therefore, that the yellow droplets improve vision against the sky in the same way as a yellow filter on a camera lens brings out details in the sky (Walls and Judd, 1933; Peiponen, 1964). This idea is supported by the finding that the retinas of swallows and swifts have predominantly yellow droplets and very few red droplets.

However, most objects when viewed against the sky are much darker than their background, and appear as silhouettes. This will be especially true for the insects, which are preyed on by the swallows and swifts, and it will also be true for bird predators such as hawks seen against the sky from below. A yellow filter, by darkening the sky, will reduce the contrast between such objects and the background, and so will be maladaptive. Such a filter is used with a camera to improve the rendering of the clouds, which are brighter than the background, but it decreases the contrast of other objects. Since, to a bird, the detection of insects and other birds must be more important than the detection of clouds, it seems unlikely that the function of the yellow droplets is to improve contrast. It is more probable that the lack of red droplets in swallows and swifts, and in the ventral retinas of some other birds, is associated with a reduction in colour vision. Colour vision is useful when an object cannot be discriminated from its background on a brightness basis, but this is seldom the case for objects seen against the sky, when very large brightness differences almost invariably exist. Middleton (1952) has shown that when both brightness and colour differences exist the limits of visual detection usually depend on the former.

On this view the lack of red droplets in swallows and swifts has the same underlying cause as the lack of red droplets in nocturnal birds. In this case also colour vision is of relatively small importance compared with the loss of sensitivity associated with it (some of the receptors must be inhibitory if colour vision is to be achieved).

It has also been suggested that the red droplets in the dorsal retinas of some birds are associated with increased contrast sensitivity against the green vegetation. Here again, however, it is not clear whether the presence of such a filter would be adaptive. A red filter will make the grass appear darker, and will improve the detection of light-coloured objects, but at the same time it will make the detection of dark objects more difficult. It seems probable that the presence of red droplets is simply associated with better colour vision, which will be valuable in these circumstances since brightness will often not be a reliable cue.

WALLS and JUDD (1933) have also suggested that red droplets may be associated with the reduction of "glare" and "dazzle". They admit that this factor is intangible, and that the reduction of glare may be achieved as well with a neutral filter as with a red one. The idea receives some support from the great development of red droplets in birds that have to see through the water surface, where glare and dazzle may well be a serious problem.

Finally, attempts have been made to correlate the colours of droplets with the plumage, or other specific markings of the animals concerned (PEIPONEN, 1964), or with their food preferences (DUCKER, 1963). These correlations, however, are not very convincing.

B. Blood Vessels

WALLS and JUDD (1933) consider that the retinal blood vessels which lie between the stimulus and receptors also act as yellow filters, along with the lens, cornea, and oil droplets. In their opinion the effect of the blood vessels may well be uniform, because they are out of focus. A network of capillaries, that might act in this way, occurs in many mammals, and in eels. WALLS and JUDD also point out that the retinal capillaries are missing from the fovea of diurnal primates but are replaced by the macular pigment in this area.

Whether or not the blood vessels can be considered as a uniform filter is open to question. There is no doubt, however, that blood can affect spectral sensitivity in certain cases. This has been shown for albino rabbits by DODT and WALTHER (1958a, 1959), and for albino rats by DODT and ECHTE (1961). In these experiments spectral sensitivity was measured using the ERG as index. It was found that albino rabbits were relatively more sensitive to long wavelengths than were pigmented rabbits. The difference between the curves for albino and pigmented animals agreed very well with the absorbance spectrum of blood. Further work showed that the greater sensitivity in the red shown by the albino animals depended on the stimulus size, being much less marked with large stimuli. DODT and WALTHER interpret this as an effect of light diffusely reflected back from the fundus in the albino animals to form a secondary source of larger size. In another experiment (DODT, 1958) sodium fluorescein was injected into pigmented rabbits, and this was also found to increase the sensitivity to small stimuli and not to large stimuli. This again was interpreted as the affect of a secondary source, which effectively increases the size of the stimulus.

The effect of blood on spectral sensitivity has been demonstrated by experiments of this sort with albino rats, rabbits, and guinea pigs. It does not seem probable, however, that blood in general can have a great effect on spectral sensitivity, for no effect is detectable in pigmented animals, and moreover, with the exception of the eel, mammals are the only vertebrates that have a network of retinal capillaries.

C. The Macular Pigment

In man and other diurnal primates the central area of the retina contains a photostable yellow pigment, the macular pigment. Its presence may be detected in several ways. Thus, since it is restricted to a central area, an estimate of its spectral absorbance may be made by comparing the spectral sensitivities of central and peripheral areas of the retina. This is so provided it can be assumed that the spectral sensitivity of the two areas would have been the same in the absence of the pigment. Such an approach has been made by WALD (1945) and STILES (1953). The absorbance spectrum of the pigment can also be determined objectively, though less accurately, by measuring the reflection of monochromatic lights from foveal and peripheral areas (BRINDLEY and WILLMER, 1952). Finally, the absorbance may be measured by making use of the fact that the macular pigment appears to be dichroic. If an observer looks at a uniform white field that is plane polarised he sees, on the fovea, a faint cross, two arms of which are yellowish, and two bluish in appearance (HAIDINGER's brushes). The macular pigment absorbs maximally when the electric vector of the stimulating light lies along any line radiating from the centre of the fovea. The spectral density of the oriented pigment can then be estimated by comparing the brightnesses of the two narrow elongated stimuli, polarised at right angles to each other (DE VRIES, SPOOR, and JIELOF, 1953; NAYLOR and STANWORTH, 1954).

All these various methods of estimation are in substantial agreement (Fig. 14). They also agree with the data obtained from a chloroform extract of the macular pigment, and, incidentally, with the absorbance spectrum of lutein or leaf xanthophyll (WALD, 1945).

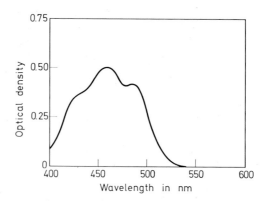

Fig. 14. Spectral absorbance of human macular pigment. The curve is WYZECKI and STILES' (1967) best estimate from various data sources

D. Photopigments and Photoproducts

Since light must be absorbed by the visual pigments to cause visual responses, the spectral absorbances of these pigments are the major determinants of spectral sensitivity. The photosensitive pigments can, in theory, also affect spectral sensitivity in other ways. In the first place, the parent pigment itself acts as a filter, affecting the spectral composition of any light that penetrates to deeper layers of pigment in the same receptor. This is known as "self-screening". In the second place, when the pigment absorbs light, it decomposes into a photoproduct that may be coloured.

This could also act as a filter, and change the effective absorption of the residual parent pigment in the receptor.

The effects of photoproduct on spectral sensitivity were estimated by DARTNALL (1948), for the case of indicator yellow. He was able to show that the effective absorption spectrum of rhodopsin could be greatly changed in this way, and even approach the form of the human *photopic* spectral sensitivity curve. However, as DARTNALL was aware, these sensitivity changes could only be obtained by assuming very high concentrations of photoproduct, which are now known to be unreasonable (GOLDSTEIN and WILLIAMS, 1966).

GOLDSTEIN and WILLIAMS (1966) have considered in some detail the effects of self-screening and screening by photoproducts on the effective absorption of rhodopsin. They calculated the effects of (1) the distribution of the photoproduct within the receptor, (2) the λ_{max} of the photoproduct, (3) the ratio of the photoproduct to the parent pigment, and (4) the overall pigment density. They concluded that, for effects to be appreciable, three conditions have to be satisfied:

a) the photoproduct must be long-lived, so that appreciable amounts can accumulate.

b) the spectrum of the photoproduct must have a considerable overlap with that of the parent pigment.

c) the total optical density must be greater than about 0.15.

They conclude that such effects are not likely to occur in man, since condition c) is not fulfilled. However, in other animals, such as the frog, salamander, gecko, conger eel, and some deep-sea fishes, pigment densities are high (DENTON, 1958), and effective screening by photoproducts could occur. Screening by photoproducts could also affect spectral sensitivity in the rat (MUNTZ, 1967). In this animal it has been shown that the photopic spectral sensitivity curve is shifted slightly towards long wavelengths by comparison with that for the scotopic sensitivity (DODT and ECHTE, 1961; SILVER, 1967; MUNTZ, 1967). The total pigment density in the rat is high (optical density at least 0.32; LEWIS, 1957), and GOLDSTEIN and WILLIAMS's calculations show that, with this density, the small change in spectral sensitivity between photopic and scotopic conditions could easily be caused by a photoproduct having $\lambda_{max} = 470$ nm.

Self-screening has been put forward as a hypothesis to explain the breakdown of colour matches with high intensity adapting lights (BRINDLEY, 1953). Irrespective of the wavelength of the adapting light, the effect is to increase the amount of the red primary and to decrease the amount of the green primary required to make a given match. The increase in red is about five times the decrease in green. According to BRINDLEY, this is only compatible with a three-pigment hypothesis of colour vision if the adapting lights produce or destroy some screening pigment in front of one of the receptors. He showed that the results could be explained if self-screening occurred for the red receptor alone, and if the receptor contained pigment with an optical density of about 0.98, a very high value. BRINDLEY also had to suppose that the optical density of the red pigment is much greater than that of the green pigment. Neither of these assumptions has been confirmed by later objective measurements of these pigments *in situ* (RUSHTON, 1958; WEALE, 1959).

IV. Absorption and Reflection Behind the Retina

A. Introduction

After light has passed through the retina, it reaches the pigment epithelium and the choroid. Some of this light is reflected back, and passes through the retina a second time. Even in eyes where the pigment epithelium contains melanin a small proportion is reflected back in this way, and this, indeed, forms the basis of the reflex densitometry measurements on human visual pigments carried out by Rushton (1958), Weale (1959), and others. In many animals the choroid is modified to form a reflecting tapetum, and the proportion of reflected light is large. The spectral characteristics of the pigment epithelium and choroid may thus also affect the spectral sensitivity appreciably.

B. Melanin

The pigment epithelium usually contains a black or dark brown pigment, melanin, that absorbs most of the light not absorbed by the retina. Browness and Morton (1952) have measured the absorbance spectrum of melanin suspensions and found, for the perch and the frog, that the absorbance is spectrally non-selective. A pigment of similar function is present in most invertebrate eyes, but whereas that from the compound eye of *Limulus* is spectrally neutral (Wasserman, 1967), the corresponding pigment of the fly (*Musca domestica*) transmits long wavelengths (Strother, 1966). It has been shown that this is responsible for the secondary sensitivity maximum in this spectral region (Goldsmith,1965), previously thought to be due to a red receptor. The secondary maximum is located at 615—620 nm and arises from the recruitment of additional ommatidia through leakage of long wave light between them. The second maximum is absent in a white-eyed mutant, which lacks the screening pigment, and the difference between the sensitivity curves of white-eyed and normal flies agrees very well with a direct microspectrophotometric determination of the spectral absorption of the screening pigment (Strother, 1966). A similar situation occurs in *Calliphora*. In vertebrates, however, there is no evidence for any effect of melanin on spectral sensitivity.

C. The Tapetum

Reflecting tapeta may be of various types, being formed in some cases by modification of the choroid, and in others by modification of the pigment epithelium. The anatomy of the different forms is described in detail by Walls (1942) and only a brief summary will be given here, together with more recent data on their effectiveness in increasing absolute sensitivity, and modifying spectral sensitivity. Tapeta are usually located in the upper half of the eye, thus tending to counteract the difference in light intensity reaching the animals from above and below.

1. The Tapetum Fibrosum

The tapetum fibrosum is characteristic of ungulates and, according to Walls, also accurs in *Aotes* (a nocturnal monkey), elephants, whales, and possibly a few fishes. The reflective power arises from the conversion of a portion of the choroid from an alveolar type of connective tissue to a tendinous type, composed of dense, regular, fibrous tissue.

No experimental data are available on the spectral characteristics of the tapetum fibrosum. Electrophysiological data on spectral sensitivity have been obtained on *Aotes* by JONES (1966): the results are complicated, however, by the presence of more than one visual pigment, and do not give any information on this question.

2. The Tapetum Cellulosum

The tapetum cellulosum also is formed by modification of the choroid, and is found in prosimians and carnivores (especially seals). It is formed by layers of thin tile-like epithelial cells that are packed with crystalline rods or plates. The number of layers varies greatly in different animals.

The tapetum of the cat has been studied in detail (GUNTER, HARDING, and STILES, 1951; WEALE, 1953). WEALE (1953) measured the reflectance of the cat tapetum *in situ*, after removing the front of the eye. He found that reflection was not specular, but diffuse, and did not show interference colours. The spectral characteristics were greatly affected by dehydration, and WEALE believes that because of this the earlier data of GUNTER, HARDING, and STILES (1951), which were obtained *in vitro*, are not relevant to the normal functioning of the tapetum.

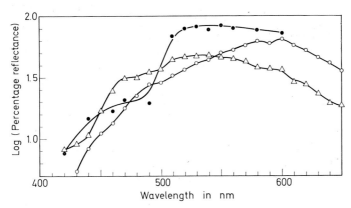

Fig. 15. Spectral reflectance of the tapetum of the cat (*plain symbols*, data from WEALE, 1953) and bush baby (*filled circles*, data from DARTNALL, ARDEN, IKEDA, LUCK, ROSENBERG, PEDLER, and TANSLEY, 1965)

WEALE found considerable variation, especially of colour, in different cats, and also between different parts of the tapetum in any individual cat. He presented average tables for the reflection at different wavelengths for tapeta that appeared yellow in colour, and for those that appeared green. These data are summarised in Fig. 15.

Several behavioural experiments have shown that the absolute threshold of the cat is between 5 and 10 times lower than that of man (BRIDGEMAN and SMITH, 1942; GUNTER, 1951), and WEALE believes that this difference can be accounted for by the tapetum. The optical power of the cat's eye is also greater than man's, and according to Vakkur and Bishop (1963) the retinal image of a given object, when the pupil is maximally dilated, will be 5.2 times brighter in cat than man. These two factors between them are certainly sufficient to account for the difference in sensitivity in cat and man, without any need to suppose that the retina itself is more sensitive in the former animal. Dodt and Walther (1958a) found, using the ERG, that the sensitivity of the cat eye was between 0.45 and 0.75 log units better for tapetal than non-tapetal regions. These results did not show any difference in spectral sensitivity between the two areas, however, which is surprising in view of Weale's results.

The structure and spectral characteristics of the tapetum, and its effect on vision, have also been studied in detail in the bush-baby (*Galago crassicaudatus agisymbanus*) (Dartnall, Arden, Ikeda, Luck, Rosenberg, Pedler, and Tansley, 1965). The tapetum in this animal is very similar to that of the cat, except that the interior of the tapetal cells contains regularly spaced lamellae, as opposed to the arrays of rodlets that occur in the cat. These lamellae are apparently composed of crystals of riboflavin (Pirie, 1959; Dartnall et al., 1965). The spectral reflectance, measured in excised portions of the tapetum, is shown in Fig. 15. These measurements were made with the incident light reaching the tapetum at an angle of 45°: there was no apparent colour change with change in this angle.

The absorption of radiation by riboflavin causes fluorescence centred at 520 nm, at a quantum yield of 0.26. Since the tapetum absorbs short-wave light one would expect the fluorescence to increase sensitivity to this part of the spectrum. Dartnall et al. (1965) found that, in order to get the best fit between an electrophysiologically-determined spectral sensitivity curve and the absorption spectrum of the visual pigment of this animal, contribution from both tapetal reflectance and fluorescence had to be included. Behavioural data (Silver, 1966) suggest that the bush baby may have an absolute threshold somewhat better than that of man, although this difference is not as clear as it is in the case of the cat.

3. Choroidal Tapeta

Choroidal tapeta containing guanin occur in sturgeons and elasmobranchs. In elasmobranchs, the guanin occurs in plates, and the choroid contains pigment cells with processes that lie between these plates. In some elasmobranchs, but not all, these processes are mobile, and can move out between the guanin plates, thus cutting off their reflective power and reducing sensitivity in the light (Franz, 1905; Nicol, 1961).

Two characteristic spectral reflectance curves for an elasmobranch tapetum are shown in Fig. 16. The elasmobranch tapetum, unlike those considered so far, is highly specular, and the spectral composition of the reflected light varies with the angle of the incident light. This suggests that the spectral characteristics depend on interference phenomena. Denton and Land (1967) have shown that the dimensions of the tapetal plates in the elasmobranch eye are exactly right to account for the spectral reflectance curves. The variation in spectral reflectance with angle of incidence will not affect the animal's spectral sensitivity, however, since the tapetal plates are so arranged behind the retina that they are always perpendicular to incident light rays entering the eye (Denton and Nicol, 1964).

DENTON and NICOL (1964) also discuss the effect of the elasmobranch tapetum on absolute sensitivity. They have shown that the optical densities of the visual pigments in elasmobranchs that have tapeta are much lower than they are in species lacking tapeta, and it appears that the sensitivity will be no greater in the former case than in the latter. It seems that the presence of a tapetum does not make the animal more sensitive, but allows it to reach the same sensitivity with

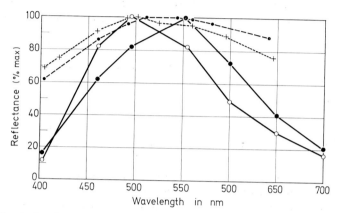

Fig. 16. Spectral reflectance curves of interference tapeta. Dots and crosses, tapetum of *Scyliorhinus canicula* measured with the incident light at 10° and 20° respectively from the normal (data from DENTON and NICOL, 1964); *plain* and *filled circles*, two individual tapeta of *Pecten* (data from LAND, 1966)

a smaller concentration of visual pigment. One possible advantage of this arrangement is that the amount of "retinal noise", which is assumed to have an effect on performance near absolute threshold, may be reduced (assuming that "retinal noise" is due to thermal breakdown of the visual pigment molecules).

4. Retinal Tapeta

Retinal tapeta containing guanin occur in both freshwater and marine teleosts (WALLS, 1942; O'CONNELL, 1953). In these tapeta processes of the pigment epithelial cells, containing crystals of guanin, extend between the receptors. Such tapeta are usually occusible; in the light the melanin migrates out into the processes of the pigment epithelial cells and masks the guanin crystals. No detailed work has been done on the effectiveness of such tapeta.

5. Invertebrate Tapeta

Reflecting tapeta also occur in some invertebrates. In the scallop (*Pecten*) the back of every eye forms a concave mirror, the argentea, which is responsible for image formation. The argentea consists of 30—40 layers of high refactive index (guanin crystals), separated by layers of low refractive index (cytoplasm). The spectral characteristics are similar to those of the elasmobranch tapetum, and depend on the angle of the incident light (LAND, 1966). Two examples of spectral reflectance curves are shown in Fig. 16. LAND points out that, due to the structure of the scallop eye, the incident light normally reaches the argentea at an angle, so that the maximum of the effective reflectance curve will be slightly displaced towards shorter wavelengths.

Reflecting tapeta also occur in many Lepidoptera (Miller, Bernhard, and Allen, 1968). The reflecting structures in these cases are situated in the tracheole layer just beneath the rhabdomes, and consist of layers of cytoplasmic platelets separated by spaces containing air. Generally the eyeshine of different moths and butterflies is predominantly of short-wave light in the upper half of the eye, and of longer-wave light in the lower. The dimensions of the platelets and the spaces between the platelets agree with this distribution of colours, on the assumption that the reflection depends on interference phenomena. It is interesting that the red and orange colours occur in the ventral part of the eye. Since there is no inversion of the image in the compound eye, this may be analogous to the predominance of red oil droplets in the dorsal retina of some birds (see above).

V. Summary

By far the most striking general conclusion about the optical properties of the various structures that have been described is that they almost all reduce the relative effectiveness of short wavelength stimuli compared with long. This occurs in many cases because the optical density of these structures (lens, cornea of various teleosts, blood, oil droplets, photopigments, melanin in *Musca*) is greater at short wavelengths. It also occurs in the tapetum cellulosum, where the reflection of long wavelengths is better than that of short. The only exceptions to this general rule are structures where the spectral characteristics depend on interference phenomena (the corneas of some insects, and various tapeta), and those that fluoresce to give a modest increase in sensitivity in the blue.

The general characteristics of the inert absorbing and reflecting pigments of the eye led Walls and Judd (1933) to suggest that a single hypothesis might be sufficient to explain the function of them all. They suggested that reduction in chromatic aberration, increase in visibility by reduction in scatter, reduction of "glare" and "dazzle", and increased contrast against certain backgrounds, might all be beneficial consequences of such yellow filters. These possibilities have already been considered above. It is also possible, however, that in some cases the spectral characteristics do not have any beneficial consequences, but arise as a limitation in the transparency that can be achieved by biological materials. Proteins, for example, all absorb heavily in the ultraviolet, and thus limit the possibilities of short wavelength vision. Moreover the pigmentation of the lens increases with age, probably through the accummulation of degradation products of proteins (McEwen, 1959), and it is difficult to imagine that this has any function. Similarly, the yellow colour of teleost corneas and the lenses of certain animals may have no correlation with the spectral characteristics of the animals' environment, but may simply be the most convenient way of achieving an increase in effective density in a transparent structure.

The great prevalence of substances absorbing short wavelengths means that, in general, discrepancies between spectral sensitivity curves and the spectral absorbances of the underlying photosensitive pigments are greatest at short wavelengths. Furthermore, since such effects are often not evenly distributed over the retina (yellow cornea of teleosts, oil droplets in birds, tapeta in many species), and may vary considerably between different individuals (effects of ageing on the lens, yellow cornea of teleosts), the variability of the spectral sensitivity curve will likewise tend to be greatest in the blue.

References

ADLER, H. E., DALLAND, J. I.: Spectral thresholds in the starling *(Sturnus vulgaris)*. J. comp. physiol. Psychol. **52**, 438—445 (1959).

ADOLPH, A. R.: Thermal and spectral sensitivities of discrete slow potentials in *Limulus* eye. J. gen. Physiol. **52**, 584—599 (1968).

ALPERN, M., THOMPSON, S., LEE, M. S.: Spectral transmission of visible light by the living human eye. J. opt. Soc. Amer. **55**, 723—727 (1965).

ARDEN, G. B., SILVER, P. H.: Visual thresholds and spectral sensitivities of the grey squirrel *(Sciurus carolinensis leucotis)*. J. Physiol. (Lond.) **163**, 540—557 (1962).

ARMINGTON, J. C., CRAMPTON, G. H.: Comparison of spectral sensitivity at the eye and the optic tectum of the chicken. Amer. J. Ophthal. **46**, 72—87 (1958).

BALAZ, E. A.: Studies on the structure of the vitreous body. 1. The absorption of ultraviolet light. Amer. J. Ophthal. **38**, No. 1, pt. II, 21—28 (1954).

BERNHARD, C. G., MILLER, W. H., MØLLER, A. R.: The insect corneal nipple array. Acta physiol. scand. **63**, suppl. 243 (1965).

BIRUKOW, G.: Beobachtungen über Reizwertverteilung in reinen Zapfennetzhäuten. Z. vergl. Physiol. **27**, 322—334 (1939).

BLOUGH, D. S.: Spectral sensitivity in the pigeon. J. opt. Soc. Amer. **47**, 827—833 (1957).

BRIDGEMAN, C. S., SMITH, K. U.: The absolute threshold of vision in cat and man with observations on its relation to the optic cortex. Amer. J. Physiol. **136**, 463—466 (1942).

BRIDGES, C. D. B.: Visual pigments of the pigeon *(Columba livia)*. Vision Res. **2**, 125—137 (1962).

BRINDLEY, G. S.: The effects on colour vision of adaptation to very bright lights. J. Physiol. (Lond.) **122**, 332—350 (1953).

— WILLMER, E. N.: The reflection of light from the macular and peripheral fundus oculi in man. J. Physiol. (Lond.) **116**, 350—356 (1952).

BROLIN, S. E., CEDERLUND, C.: The fluorescence of the lens of the eyes of different species. Acta Ophthal. (Kbh.) **36**, 324—328 (1958).

BROWNESS, J. M., MORTON, R. A.: Distribution of copper and zinc in the eyes of fresh-water fishes and frogs. Occurrence of metals in melanin fractions from eye tissues. Biochem. J. **51**, 530—535 (1952).

BURKHARDT, D. A.: The goldfish electroretinogram: relation between photopic spectral sensitivity functions and cone absorption spectra. Vision Res. **6**, 517—532 (1966).

CARRICABURU, P., CHARDENOT, P.: Spectres d'absorption de la cornée de quelques arthropodes. Vision Res. **7**, 43—50 (1967).

COOPER, G. F., ROBSON, J. G.: The yellow colour of the lens of the grey squirrel *(Sciurus carolinensis leucotis)*. J. Physiol. (Lond.) **203**, 403—410 (1969a).

— — The yellow colour of the lens of man and other primates. J. Physiol. (Lond.) **203**, 411 to 418 (1969b).

COOPER, T. G., MYER, D. B.: Ontogeny of retinal oil droplets in the chick embryo. Exp. Eye Res. **7**, 434—442 (1968).

CRESCITELLI, F., DARTNALL, H. J. A.: Human visual purple. Nature (Lond.) **172**, 195—196 (1953).

DARTNALL, H. J. A.: Visual purple and the photopic luminosity curve. Brit. J. Ophthal. **32**, 793—811 (1948).

— The interpretation of spectral sensitivity curves. Brit. med. Bull. **9**, 24—30 (1953).

Dartnall, H. J. A.: Visual pigments before and after extraction from visual cells. Proc. roy. Soc. B **154**, 250—266 (1961).

— Arden, G. B., Ikeda, H., Luck, C. P., Rosenberg, M. E., Pedler, C. M. H., Tansley, K.: Anatomical, electro-physiological and pigmentary aspects of vision in the bush baby: an interpretative study. Vision Res. **5**, 399—424 (1965).

— Goodeve, C. F.: Scotopic luminosity curve and the absorption spectrum of visual purple. Nature (Lond.) **139**, 409—411 (1937).

Denton, E. J.: Recherches sur l'absorption de la lumière par le cristallin des poissons. Bull. Inst. Océanog. Monaco **1071**, 1—10 (1956).

— Light absorption by the intact retina. In: Visual problems of colour. Nat. Phys. Lab., G. Brit., Proc. Symp. No. 8, H.M.S.O., London 1958.

— Land, M. F.: Optical properties of the lamellae causing interference colours in animal reflectors. J. Physiol. (Lond.) **191**, 23P (1967).

— Nicol, J. A. C.: The choroidal tapeta of some cartilaginous fishes *(Chondrichthyes)*. J. marine biol. Assoc. U.K. **44**, 219—258 (1964).

— Warren, F. J.: Eyes of Histioteuthidae. Nature (Lond.) **219**, 400—401 (1968).

De Vries, H., Spoor, A., Jielof, R.: Properties of the eye with respect to polarised light. Physica **19**, 419—432 (1953).

Dodt, E.: Physical factors in the correlation of electroretinogram spectral sensitivity curves with visual pigments. Amer. J. Ophthal. **46**, 87—90 (1958).

— Echte, K.: Dark and light adaptation in pigmented and white rat as measured by electro-retinogram threshold. J. Neurophysiol. **24**, 427—445 (1961).

— Walther, J. B.: Spektrale Sensitivität und Blutreflexion. Pflügers Arch. ges. Physiol. **266**, 187—192 (1958a).

— — Netzhautsensitivität, Linsenabsorption und physikalische Lichtstreuung. Pflügers Arch. ges. Physiol. **266**, 167—174 (1958b).

— — Fluorescence of the crystalline lens and electroretinographic sensitivity determinations. Nature (Lond.) **181**, 286—287 (1958c).

Donner, K. O.: The spectral sensitivity of pigeon's retinal elements. J. Physiol. (Lond.) **122**, 524—537 (1953).

— On the effect of the coloured oil droplets in the spectral sensitivity of the avian retina. Proc. XIIth Int. Ornithol. Congress, Helsinki 1958, 167—172 (1960).

Ducker, G.: Spontane Bevorzugung arteigener Farben bei Vögeln. Z. Tierpsychol. **20**, 43—65 (1963).

Erhard, H.: Messende Untersuchungen über den Farbensinn der Vögel. Zool. Jahrb., Allg. Zool. Physiol. **41**, 489—552 (1924).

Franz, V.: Zur Anatomie, Histologie und funktionellen Gestaltung des Selachierauges. Z. Naturwiss. **40**, 697—840 (1905).

Friedman, H.: Colour vision in the Virginia opossum. Nature (Lond.) **213**, 835 (1967).

Goldsmith, T. H.: Do flies have a red receptor? J. gen. Physiol. **49**, 265—287 (1965).

Goldstein, E. B., Williams, T. P.: Calculated effects of "screening pigments". Vision Res. **6**, 39—50 (1966).

Graf, V.: A spectral sensitivity curve and wavelength discrimination for the turtle *(Chrysemys picta picta)*. Vision Res. **7**, 915—928 (1967).

Granda, A. M.: Electrical responses of the light- and dark-adapted turtle eye. Vision Res. **2**, 343—356 (1962).

— Stirling, C. E.: Differential spectral sensitivity in the optic tectum and eye of the turtle. J. gen. Physiol. **48**, 901—917 (1965).

— — The spectral sensitivity of the turtle's eye to very dim lights. Vision Res. **6**, 143—152 (1966).

Granit, R.: The "red" receptor of *Testudo*. Acta physiol. scand. **1**, 386—390 (1941).

— Spectral properties of the visual receptor elements of the Guinea pig. Acta physiol. scand. **3**, 318—328 (1942a).

— The photopic spectrum of the pigeon. Acta physiol. scand. **4**, 118—124 (1942b).

— Receptors and sensory perception. New Haven: Yale Univ. Press 1955.

Gunter, R.: The absolute threshold for vision in the cat. J. Physiol. (Lond.) **114**, 8—15 (1951).

GUNTER, R., HARDING, H. G. W., STILES, W. S.: Spectral reflexion factor of the cat's tapetum. Nature (Lond.) 168, 293—294 (1951).

GUTTMAN, M., KALISH, M. I.: Discriminability and stimulus generalisation. J. exp. Psychol. 51, 79—88 (1956).

HAILMAN, J. F.: Coding of the colour preference of the gull chick. Nature (Lond.) 204, 710. (1964).

HAMILTON, W. F., COLEMAN, T. B.: Trichomatic vision in the pigeon as illustrated by the spectral discrimination curve. J. comp. Psychol. 15, 183—191 (1933).

HECHT, S., WILLIAMS, R. E.: The visibility of monochromatic radiation and the absorption spectrum of visual purple. J. gen. Physiol. 5, 1—34 (1922).

HEYNINGEN, R. VAN: The lens. In: The eye, Vol. 1, ed. H. DAVSON, New York, London: Academic Press 1962.

HONIGMANN, H.: Untersuchungen über Lichtempfindlichkeit und Adaptierung des Vogelauges. Pflügers Arch. ges. Physiol. 189, 1—72 (1921).

IKEDA, H.: The spectral sensitivity of the pigeon (Columba livia). Vision Res. 5, 19—36 (1965).

JONES, A. E.: Wavelength and intensity effects on the response of single lateral geniculate nucleus units in the owl monkey. J. Neurophysiol. 24, 125—138 (1966).

KENNEDY, D., MILKMAN, R. D.: Selective light absorption by the lenses of lower vertebrates, and its influence on spectral sensitivity. Biol. Bull. 111, 375—386 (1956).

KENSHALO, D. R.: Comparison of thermal sensitivity of the forehead, lip, conjunctiva, and cornea. J. appl. Physiol. 15, 987—991 (1960).

KINSEY, V. E.: Spectral transmission of the eye to ultraviolet radiations. Arch. Ophthal.(N.Y.) 39, 508—513 (1948).

KÖNIG, A.: Über den menschlichen Sehpurpur und seine Bedeutung für das Sehen. S. B. Akad. Wiss. Berlin 577—598 (1894).

KRAUSE, W.: Über die Endigung der Muskelnerven. Z. rationelle Med. 20, 1—18 (1863).

— Die Retina. V. Die Retina der Vögel. Int. Mschr. Anat. Physiol. 11, 69—122 (1894).

LAND, M. F.: A multilayer interference reflector in the eye of the scallop (Pecten maximus). J. exp. Biol. 45, 433—447 (1966).

LE GRAND, Y.: Colorimétrie du poulet théorique. Vision Res. 2, 81—83 (1962).

LEWIS, D. M.: Retinal photopigments in the albino rat. J. Physiol. 136, 615—623 (1957).

LISENBY, D.: Spectral sensitivity in the turtle. J. Psychol. 59, 95—100 (1965).

LUDVIGH, E., McCARTHY, E. F.: Absorption of visible light by the refractive media of the human eye. Arch. Ophthal. 20, 37—51 (1938).

McCANDLESS, R. L., HOFFERT, J. R., FROMM, P. O.: Light transmission by corneas, aqueous humor and crystalline lenses of fishes. Vision Res. 9, 223—232 (1969).

McEWEN, W. K.: The yellow pigment of human lenses. Amer. J. Ophthal. 47, No. 5 pt. II, 144—146 (1959).

MERKER, E.: Die Sichtbarkeit ultravioletten Lichtes. Biol. Rev. 9, 49—78 (1934).

MEYER, D. B., COOPER, T. G.: The visual cells of the chicken as revealed by phase contrast microscopy. Amer. J. Anat. 118, 723—734 (1966).

MIDDLETON, W. E. K.: Vision through the atmosphere. Toronto: Toronto Univ. Press 1952.

MILLER, W. H., BERNARD, G. D., ALLEN, J. L.: The optics of insect compound eyes. Science 162, 760—767 (1968).

MORELAND, J. D., LYTHGOE, J. N.: Yellow corneas in fishes. Vision Res. 8, 1377—1380 (1968).

MORRIS, V. B., SHOREY, C. D.: An electron microscope study of types of receptor in the chick retina. J. comp. Neurol. 129, 313—339 (1967).

MOTAIS, R.: Sur l'absorption de la lumière par le cristallin de quelques poissons de grande profondeur. Bull. Inst. Océanog. Monaco, No. 1094, 1—4 (1957).

MUNTZ, W. R. A.: A behavioural study on photopic and scotopic vision in the hooded rat. Vision Res. 7, 371—376 (1967).

— SOKOL, S.: Psychophysical thresholds to different wavelengths in light adapted turtles. Vision Res. 7, 729—741 (1967).

NAYLOR, E. J., STANWORTH, A.: Retinal pigment and the Haidinger effect. J. Physiol. (Lond.) 124, 543—552 (1954).

NICOL, J. A. C.: The tapetum in Scyliorhinus canicula. J. Marine Biol. Assoc. U.K. 41, 271 to 277 (1961).

O'Connell, C. P.: The structure of the eye of *Sardinops caerulea, Engraulis mordax*, and four other pelagic marine teleosts. J. Morph. **113**, 287—329 (1963).

Orlov, O. I. U., Maximova, E. M.: On the role of the intra-bulbar light filters. Dokl. Akad. Nauk SSSR u Otd. Biol. Ch. **154**, 463—466 (1964) (in Russian).

Pautler, E. L.: Directional sensitivity of isolated turtle retinas. J. opt. Soc. Amer. **57**, 1267 to 1269 (1967).

Pedler, C. M. H., Boyle, M.: Multiple oil droplets in the photoreceptors of the pigeon. Vision Res. **9**, 525—528 (1969).

Peiponen, V. A.: Zur Bedeutung der Ölkugeln im Farbensehen der Sauropsiden. Ann. Zool. Fenn. **1**, 281—302 (1964).

Pirenne, M. H.: Spectral luminous efficiency of radiation. In: The Eye, Vol. 2, ed. H. Davson, New York, London: Academic Press 1962.

Pirie, A.: Crystals of riboflavin making up the tapetum lucidum in the eye of a lemur. Nature (Lond.) **183**, 985—986 (1959).

Pumphrey, R. J.: Concerning vision. In: The cell and the organism, ed. J. A. Ramsey and V. B. Wigglesworth, Cambridge Univ. Press 1961.

Roaf, H. E.: The absorption of light by the coloured globules in the retina of the domestic hen. Proc. roy. Soc. B **105**, 371—374 (1929).

— Colour vision. Physiol. Rev. **13**, 43—79 (1933).

Ruddock, K. H.: The effect of age upon colour vision — II. Changes with age in light transmission of the ocular media. Vision Res. **5**, 47—58 (1965).

Rushton, W. A. H.: The cone pigments of the human fovea in colour blind and normal. In: Visual Problems of colour, Nat. Phys. Lab. G. Brit., Proc. Symp. No. 8, London: H.M.S.O. 1958.

— Excitation pools in the frog's retina. J. Physiol. (Lond.) **149**, 327—345 (1959).

Said, F. S., Weale, R. A.: The variation with age of the spectral transmissivity of the living human crystalline lens. Gerontologica **3**, 213—223 (1959).

Silver, P. H.: Spectral sensitivity of a trained bush baby. Vision Res. **6**, 153—162 (1966).

— Spectral sensitivity of the white rat by a training method. Vision Res. **7**, 377—384 (1967).

Sokol, S., Muntz, W. R. A.: The spectral sensitivity of the turtle *(Chrysemys picta picta)*. Vision Res. **6**, 285—292 (1966).

Stiles, W. S.: Further studies of visual mechanisms by the two-colour threshold technique. Colloquio sobre problemas opticas de la vision. Union internationale de physique pure et appliquée, Madrid 1953.

— Burch, J. M.: N.P.L. colour-matching investigation: final report 1958. Opt. Acta **6**, 1—26 (1959).

— Crawford, B. H.: The luminous efficiency of rays entering the eye pupil at different points. Proc. roy. Soc. B **112**, 428—450 (1933).

Strother, G. K.: Absorption spectra of retinal oil globules in turkey, turtle and pigeon. Exp. Cell Res. **29**, 349—355 (1963).

— Absorption of *Musca domestica* screening pigment. J. gen. Physiol. **49**, 1087—1088 (1966).

Sutherland, N. S.: Shape discrimination in the goldfish. In: The central nervous system and fish behaviour, ed. D. Ingle, Chicago: Univ. Chicago Press 1968.

Studnitz, G. von, Loevinich, H. K., Newmann, H. J. Über die Löslichkeit und Trennbarkeit der Farbsubstanzen. Z. vergl. Physiol. **30**, 74—83 (1943).

Tyler, J. E., Preisendorfer, R. W.: Transmission of energy within the sea. 8. Light. In: The Sea, Vol. 1, ed. M. N. Hill. New York: Interscience Publishers 1962.

Vakkur, G. J., Bishop, P. O.: The schematic eye in the cat. Vision Res. **3**, 357—381 (1963).

Waelchi, G.: Zur Topographie der gefärbten Kugeln der Vogelnetzhaut. Arch. Ophthal. **29**, 205—223 (1883).

Wald, G.: On rhodopsin in solution. J. gen. Physiol. **21**, 795—832 (1938).

— Human vision and the spectrum. Science **101**, 653—658 (1945).

— The photochemistry of vision. Doc. Ophthal. **3**, 94—137 (1949).

— Brown, P. K.: Human rhodopsin. Science **127**, 222—226 (1958).

— Zussman, H.: Carotenoids of the chicken retina. Nature (Lond.) **140**, 197 (1937).

Walls, G. L.: The vertebrate eye and its adaptive radiation. Michigan. Cranbrook Inst. of Science, 1942.

WALLS, G. L., JUDD, H. D.: The intra-ocular colour-filters of vertebrates. Brit. J. Ophthal. 17, 641—675; 705—725 (1933).

WASSERMAN, G. S.: Density spectrum of *Limulus* screening pigment. J. gen. Physiol. 50, 1075—1077 (1967).

WEALE, R. A.: The spectral reflectivity of the cat's tapetum measured *in situ*. J. Physiol. 119, 30—42 (1953).

— Photosensitive reactions in foveae of normal and cone-monochromatic observers. Optica Acta 6, 158—174 (1959).

— Notes on the photometric significance of the human crystalline lens. Vision Res. 1, 183—191 (1961).

WEISINGER, H., SCHMIDT, F. H., WILLIAMS, R. C., TILLER, C. O., RUFFIN, R. S., GUERRY, D., HAM, W. T.: The transmission of light through the ocular media of the rabbit eye. Amer. J. Ophthal. 42, 907—910 (1956).

WITKOVSKY, P.: The effect of chromatic adaptation on colour sensitivity of the carp electroretinogram. Vision Res. 8, 823—837 (1968).

WYSZECKI, G., STILES, W. S.: Color science. New York: Wiley & Sons Inc. 1967.

Chapter 14

The Adaptation of Visual Pigments
to the Photic Environment

By

John N. Lythgoe, Falmer, Brighton (Great Britain)

With 18 Figures

Contents

I. Introduction

In 1936 CLARKE wrote: "These results [clear ocean water selectively transmits blue light] raise the question of the possibility of a shift in sensitivity of the eyes of a deep water fish towards the blue end of the spectrum." This prediction must be one of the most accurate in biology, for twenty-one years later DENTON and WARREN (1957) and MUNZ (1957) published papers showing that bathypelagic fishes did indeed possess large quantities of visual pigments with λ_{max} located in the blue region of the spectrum.

This prediction and its confirmation laid the guidelines for the bulk of the subsequent work on the adaptation of the visual pigments to the photic environment, and the resulting hypothesis that an animal tends to possess visual pigment that will render it most sensitive to the ambient light has been a most useful one.

On the other hand the observed variability of visual pigment in the animal kingdom cannot be explained in terms of sensitivity alone, and it now seems likely that the spectral location of the visual pigment may be important in the perception of brightness contrast, and certainly important in the perception of colour.

Much of this chapter is concerned with the ways in which a particular visual pigment may affect the visual performance of an animal that possesses it. In attempting this I have presumed it is more important for an animal to detect its prey or predator at a sufficient range for some action to be taken, than for the visual scene to appear very bright or very contrasty. It is true that poor sensitivity or contrast perception can limit the capacity of an animal to survive in nature, but a study of the ecology of visual pigments must be integrated with the study of vision as a whole.

Lack of data imposes a considerable limitation on the ecological approach, which is attempted here. Rather unexpectedly the greatest paucity of information is to be found in such subjects as the optics of the leafy forest or of the shallow lake rather than in the photochemistry of visual pigments or the physiology of vision. Moreover we scarcely ever know what visual tasks a species must perform with great efficiency if it is to survive; without that knowledge the study of visual ecology must rely on generalisations.

Finally, almost all of what follows is devoted to scotopic vision, for the simple reason that our present techniques of pigment extraction do not usually yield measurable amounts of cone pigments. The technique of microspectrophotometry (see Liebman in this volume) is now doing much to fill this great gap in our knowledge, and it is a safe prediction that a decade hence a similar chapter to this will have its emphasis set firmly upon colour vision.

II. The Spectral Distributions of Natural Light

1. Daylight

The sun, overwhelmingly the brightest source of light that illuminates our planet, burns with an almost constant brightness and colour, but in reaching the surface of the earth the sunlight must penetrate the atmosphere, in which it is both scattered and absorbed. The spectral distribution of total daylight differs significantly from that of the sun and shows a large variation with meteorological conditions and time of day.

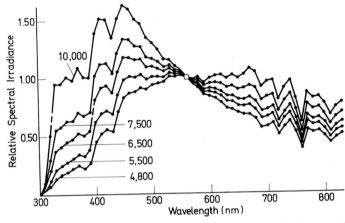

Fig. 1. Relative spectral distributions of average daylight irradiances for the five colour temperatures 4,800 °K, 5,500°, 6,500°, 7,500° and 10,000 °K (Judd, MacAdam, and Wyszecki, 1964)

The spectral irradiances ($Wm^{-2}\mu m^{-1}$) of sunlight both above the atmosphere and also at the surface of the earth were compiled by Moon in (1940) from a variety of sources then available, and are given in Table 1. It should be noted, however, as Dartnall and Goodeve (1937) pointed out, that in vision (as in other photochemical processes) it is the number of quanta (not the intensity in energy units) absorbed by the light-sensitive area that determines the effectiveness of the light. Since the energy of a quantum is inversely proportional to the wavelength, it follows that an energy unit of long-wave light contains more quanta than one of short wave light.

The average relative spectral irradiances of typical daylights for a series of colour temperatures have been calculated by Judd, MacAdam and Wyszecki (1964) (Table 2 and Fig. 1). These spectral distributions (in energy units, the values at 560 nm being adjusted arbitrarily to 1000) were derived from an analysis of 622 experimental curves of daylight measured by Condit and Grum (1964), and

Table 1. *Spectral irradiance (Wm^{-2} μm^{-1}) of direct sunlight; normal incidence, mean solar distance. (From* MOON, *1940)*

λ(nm)	Above atmosphere (solar constant = 1322 Wm^{-2})	At sea level (solar constant = 739.8 Wm^{-2}; air mass = 2)	λ(nm)	Above atmosphere (solar constant = 1322 Wm^{-2})	At sea level (solar constant = 739.8 Wm^{-2}; air mass = 2)
300	450	0.081	500	2061	1215
05	540	1.91	10	2000	1206
10	616	11.0	20	1954	1199
15	676	30.0	30	1912	1188
20	726	54.0	40	1894	1198
325	762	75.0[a]	550	1878	1190
30	796	101	60	1861	1182
35	826	130[a]	70	1841	1178
40	856	151	80	1819	1168
45	886	170[a]	90	1795	1161
350	916	188	600	1762	1167
60	976	233	10	1727	1168
70	1046	279	20	1690	1165
80	1121	336	30	1653	1176
90	1202	397	40	1616	1175
400	1304	470	650	1579	1173
10	1728	672	60	1543	1166
20	1766	733	70	1508	1160
30	1788	787	80	1473	1149
40	1939	911	90	1439	978
450	2036	1006	700	1405	1108
60	2096	1080	10	1371	1070
70	2119	1138	20	1337	832
80	2127	1183	30	1304	965
90	2103	1210	40	1270	1041
			750	1236	867
			60	1205[a]	566
			70	1175[a]	968

[a] Interpolated by WYSZECKI and STILES (1967) from MOON's (1940) table. To convert these quantities into relative quantal intensities multiply by λ.

Table 2. *Spectral distribution of typical day-light for colour temperatures 4800 °K, 5500 °K, 6500 °K, 7500 °K and 10,000 °K (*JUDD, MACADAM, *and* WYSZECKI, *1964)*

Wavelength (nm)	Correlated colour temperature (°K)				
	4800	5500	6500	7500	10000
300	0.2	0.2	0.3	0.4	0.6
310	23	21	33	52	97
320	68	112	202	298	506
330	132	207	371	550	943
340	163	240	400	573	952
350	190	279	450	627	1011

Table 2 (Continued)

Wavelength (nm)	Correlated colour temperature (°K)				
	4800	5500	6500	7500	10000
360	218	307	467	630	977
370	246	344	522	703	1091
380	215	326	500	668	1010
390	267	382	547	700	1006
400	446	610	828	1019	1388
410	516	686	916	1119	1515
420	554	716	935	1128	1503
430	537	679	868	1033	1346
440	704	856	1049	1211	1518
450	827	981	1171	1330	1628
460	864	1004	1178	1323	1594
470	878	999	1149	1272	1503
480	916	1026	1159	1269	1469
490	894	980	1088	1177	1344
500	936	1007	1094	1165	1300
510	949	1008	1078	1137	1246
520	959	1000	1049	1086	1156
530	1011	1042	1077	1105	1153
540	1002	1021	1044	1063	1097
550	1020	1030	1040	1049	1064
560	1000	1000	1000	1000	1000
570	979	973	964	956	943
580	995	977	957	942	914
590	945	914	886	870	848
600	993	944	900	873	835
610	1012	951	896	862	816
620	1014	942	876	836	780
630	983	904	833	787	726
640	1020	923	837	785	716
650	990	889	800	748	683
660	1021	903	802	745	673
670	1075	940	822	755	671
680	1037	900	783	717	638
690	912	797	697	640	567
700	960	829	716	652	573
710	969	849	743	681	602
720	801	702	616	565	500
730	901	793	699	643	572
740	963	850	751	692	617
750	814	719	636	587	524
760	601	528	464	427	379
770	864	759	668	614	545
780	815	718	634	584	520
790	828	729	643	592	527
800	764	674	594	548	488
810	665	587	519	480	429
820	736	650	574	530	472
830	775	683	603	556	496

by HENDERSON and HODGKISS (1963). The C.I.E. Standard Source C for overcast skylight is approximately 6740 °K (DAVIS and GIBSON, 1931). Although there does not seem to be any very significant differences in the spectral distribution of daylight at different geographical locations, the colour temperature of daylight can vary from 4,000 to 40,000 °K for various phases throughout the day, and under different meteorological conditions (SASTRI and DAS, 1968). In general clouds tend to reduce the colour temperature. The marked effect of solar altitude on the colour temperature of daylight is shown in the figure published by CONDIT and GRUM (1964) and reproduced here as Fig. 2.

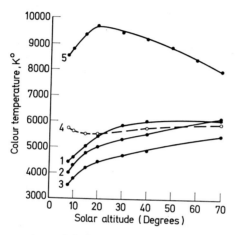

Fig. 2. The colour temperatures of skylight and daylight for different atmospheric conditions as a function of solar altitude. 1. Clear skylight, 15. VI. 1962 (morning) and 27. VI. 1962 (morning). 2. Daylight, heavy overcast sky. 20. VI. 1962. 3. Daylight, clear sky, 26. VI. 1962. 4. Daylight, clear sky, 3. VII. 1962. 5. Daylight, hazy sky, 15. VI. 1962 (afternoon). (CONDIT and GRUM, 1964)

2 Nightlight

The visual pigments, discussed later, must chiefly be contained in the rods, for present extraction procedures rarely yield cone pigments in detectable amounts (DARTNALL, 1960). Thus we are most interested in the quantum intensity distribution of natural radiance once the sun has sunk beneath the horizon, or at depths in the sea where the penetrating daylight is too dim for photopic vision. Unfortunately the low radiances at night make sufficiently detailed measurements difficult and there are few, if any, data sufficient for a quantitative approach.

Nevertheless, it is true to say that the light from the twilight and night sky is "redder"[1] than from a clear sky during the day. ROZENBERG (1966) has reviewed the very complex changes that occur in the radiance of the twilight sky as the sun sinks further beneath the horizon. Initially the sky at the zenith becomes richer in long wavelength light. There follows a phase, as the sun sinks from about 5° to about 10° beneath the horizon, when the sky becomes somewhat more "blue"

---

[1] These terms are used to indicate that the maximum irradiance may be displaced to longer ("redder") or shorter ("bluer") spectral regions. The actual intensity of irradiance, however, may be below the photopic level so that these terms are sensually meaningless.

(although still redder than the clear daytime sky), until finally with the onset of night the sky becomes redder yet again.

There seem to be few systematic data on the total radiation of the night sky, although there is a considerable literature on the radiance of small elements of it. The moon itself has a colour temperature of about 4,100 °K (Le Grand, 1957) and an almost flat reflectance curve; the spectral radiance of the total night sky is very much redder than the daytime sky, Fig. 3 (Richardson, 1969).

At night the airglow from the earth's own atmosphere becomes relatively more important (see Chamberlain, 1961, for a review). Barbier (1955) finds that the airglow in the direction of the celestial pole is about 40% of the total night sky emission, with extreme values ranging between 20 and 54%. In particular, one component of this earthlight — the green auroral line at 557.5 nm — is very prominent. This line which is the result of the "forbidden" transition $^1D_2-^1S_0$ of oxygen contains about one third of the energy of the airglow spectrum between 496 and 600 nm (Dufay, 1929), and between 6 and 9% of the total brightness of the night sky. Rayleigh (1930) in another estimate thought that 7% of the light seen by the dark adapted eye comes from the green line.

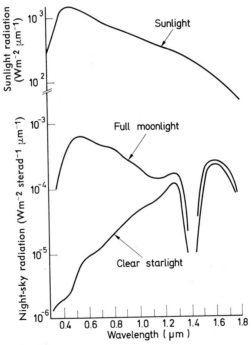

Fig. 3. The spectral energy distributions of sunlight, moonlight and starlight. Note interruption of scale (Richardson, 1969)

3. Bioluminescence

There is a large amount of information about the apparent colour of bioluminescent organisms (see Harvey, 1952, 1955) and some data on the relative spectral emission curves of the light (Fig. 4 and Table 3). Much of the available data on the optical and physiological aspects of bioluminescence has been reviewed by NICOL (1958e, 1962). There are few direct observations of luminescent marine animals in their natural habitat, however, and very few serious attempts to relate the observed properties of the luminescence to other biological parameters. Thus there seem to be only two instances where the emission spectra for bioluminescence are known

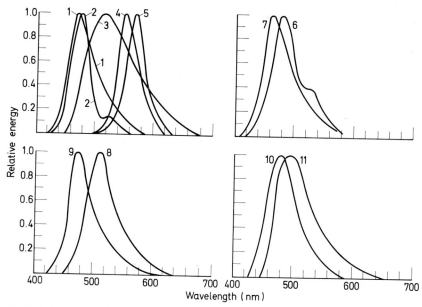

Fig. 4. Relative spectral emission curves of the bioluminescent light from: 1. *Noctiluca miliaris* (NICOL, 1958c). 2. *Euphausia pacifica* (KAMPA and BODEN, 1957). 3. *Polynoid* worms (NICOL, 1957a). 4. *Photuris pennsylvanica* (from COBLENTZ, 1912). 5. *Photinus pyralis* (COBLENTZ, 1912). 6. *Pyrosoma atlanticum* (from KAMPA and BODEN, 1957). 7. *Chaetopterus variopedatus* (NICOL, 1957b). 8. *Pennatula phosphorea* (NICOL, 1958d). 9. *Myctophum punctatum* (NICOL, 1960). 10. *Gonyaulax polyedra* (from HASTINGS and SWEENEY, 1957). 11. *Pholas dactylus* (NICOL, 1958b). (From NICOL, 1962)

for species from which visual pigment has been extracted (NICOL, 1962). The first example is *Euphausia pacifica* for which KAMPA and BODEN (1957) measured an emission maximum of 476 nm and a rhodopsin of λ_{max} 462 nm (KAMPA, 1955). The second is for the bathypelagic fish *Myctophum punctatum* where NICOL (1960) records an emission maximum at 470 nm and DENTON and WARREN (1957) found a visual pigment of about 485 nm. In the latter case the visual pigment was not tested for homogeneity and may contain more than one pigment.

Very recently DENTON, GILPIN-BROWN, and WRIGHT have reported that the mesopelagic fish *Pachystomias* both emits, and is apparently exceptionally sensitive to, red light. *Pachystomias* has photophores emitting blue-green light along the belly, but close to the eyes there are large photophores that are covered with red tissue and thus emit only red light. The maximum retinal absorbance is at a wavelength around 575 nm with a maximum density of about 1.0. It is, therefore,

Table 3. *The wavelengths of maximum light emission for various marine animals*

		Emission maximum (nm)	
Protozoa	*Noctiluca miliaris*	470	Nicol (1958 c)
	Gonyaulax polyedra	478	Hastings and Sweeney (1957)
Coelenterata	*Pennatula phosphorea*	510	Nicol (1958 d)
	Vogtia glabra	470, 570[a]	Nicol (1958 e)
	Atolla wyvellei	470, 545[a]	Nicol (1958 e)
	Beroe ovata	510	Nicol (1958 e)
Annelida	*Chaetopterus variopedatus*	465	Nicol (1957 b)
	Acholoe astericola	515	Nicol (1958 a)
	Lagisca extenuata	515	Nicol (1957 a)
	Polynoe scolopendrina	515	Nicol (1957 a)
	Gattyana cirrosa	515	Nicol (1957 a)
	Harmothoe longisetis	515	Nicol (1957 a)
Crustacea	*Euphausia pacifica*	476, c. 530[a]	Kampa and Boden (1957)
	Thysanoessa raschii	476, 500—530[a]	Boden and Kampa (1959)
	Cypridina sp.	469	Harvey (1952)
	Cypridina sp.	470	Harvey, Chase and McElroy (1957)
	Metridia lucens	480	David and Conover (1961)
Mollusca	*Pholas dactylus*	490	Nicol (1958 b)
Tunicata	*Pyrosoma atlanticum*	480, 525[a]	Kampa and Boden (1957)
Pisces	*Myctophum punctatum*	470	Nicol (1960)
	Malacocephalus laevis	510	Haneda (1938)

[a] Secondary emission maximum.

reasonable to conclude that the fish is exceptionally sensitive to the bioluminescence from others of the same species.

The paucity of such comparable environmental and optical data is unfortunate, for few are likely to dispute Beebe's (1935) observation that in deep oceanic water the light from bioluminescent organisms is the major if not the only visual stimulus present. This is also true during full daylight in shallow and coastal water for, where the water is turbid with suspended matter, full daylight is attenuated so rapidly that at a depth of 30 m a dark-adapted human eye may be able to detect bioluminescent organism, which can appear much brighter than the down-welling daylight (Hemmings and Lythgoe, 1964).

There is little doubt that an understanding of the visual functions of marine fishes must involve a thorough study of bioluminescence. This must include both the spectral distribution of the emission, and also the kind of information that can be imparted by it to other animals. Royal Navy divers, for instance, have told me that they can distinguish seals from divers by their respective wakes. Near the bottom, when there is a current running, stationary objects can be detected by the luminous organisms that kindle their lights when they collide with the obstacle. These flashes of light may last from a few milliseconds to more than 10 seconds (see Nicol, 1962), and the observer sees long streaks of light that accurately trace the direction of the water flow around the object.

The visibility of a bioluminescent object in the dark sea is simpler to calculate than is the visibility of objects in daylight, for at night there is no "veiling brightness" and the diffuse attenuation coefficient K (see p. 577) can be ignored. Thus in Eq. (5) (p. 585) the second term on the right is zero and only the beam attenuation coefficient α, the inherent radiance of the photophore, $_tN_0$, and, of course, the sensitivity of the eye for the solid angle subtended by the photophore need to be considered. However, it must not be forgotten that for very small distant objects the inverse square law becomes significant (NICOL, 1962).

A. Selective Absorption by Natural Filters

1. The Vegetable Canopy

All the higher green plants contain chlorophyll — chiefly chlorophyll a — and this substance absorbs red and blue light for photosynthesis leaving a "window" in the green. The result is that light in penetrating through a canopy of vegetation becomes relatively rich in green (Fig. 5). It is worth noting that the wavelength of maximum transmission of chlorophyll is about 540 nm and that the bright aurora line (p. 572) is at 557 nm. There is thus every reason to expect that at night the light on the forest floor will be particularly rich in light of wavelengths around 550 nm. Yet many animals living under these conditions have rhodopsins of λ_{max} around 500 nm. The adaptive significance (if any) of this apparent paradox will be discussed later (p. 599).

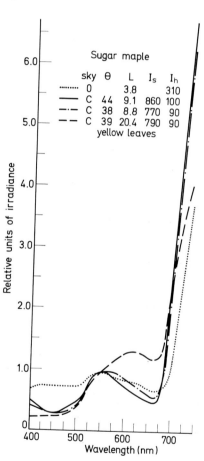

Fig. 5. The spectral distribution of shade light within a Sugar Maple plantation for overcast (O) and clear (C) sky conditions with various solar elevations (θ in degrees). L, the light within the plantation, I_s the direct sunlight above the stand and I_h, the diffuse sky light above the stand, are given for 550 nm in mwatts m^{-2} nm^{-1}. (FEDERER and TANNER, 1966)

2. Natural Waters

On a dull and rainy day the Mediterranean or Caribbean can look just as grey as the Baltic Sea or the English Channel. Yet even in the dirtiest weather the Mediterranean will be a clear blue to a diver whilst the Baltic is always yellow-green. The colour of the surface depends in large part on the light reflected from the sky, but beneath the waves it is the colour of the water itself that is dominant, the quality of the daylight incident at the surface being relatively unimportant to vision (Lythgoe, 1966).

Measurement of the spectral absorbance of pure water in the laboratory (Hulburt, 1945) shows that it is most transparent to light at about 460 nm and strongly absorbs light at shorter and longer wavelengths. In particular there is a sharp increase in absorbance at wavelengths greater than 580 nm (Smith and Tyler, 1967).

Chlorophyll contained in the phytoplankton and the yellow products of vegetable decay are very important colouring agents in natural water. The so-called "yellow substance" or "Gelbstoff" is a complex mixture of substances formed from carbohydrates by a "Muillard" reaction as part of the decay processes of natural vegetation (Kalle, 1966). The end products are yellow or brown, soluble melanoidines that are very stable. The "yellow substance" may either be formed by the phytoplankton itself or have its origin in rotting humus on land. When "Gelbstoff" is dissolved the long wave light is filtered out by the water and the yellow substance filters out the shorter wavelengths. Intermediate wavelengths are not absorbed and the green colour of much inshore water is the result. "Yellow substance" is particularly important in north-temperate coastal waters where the many rivers bring down humus derivatives to the sea, which thereby is stained green for many miles offshore.

Chlorophyll is another important colouring medium in natural water (Tyler, 1965; Tyler and Smith, 1967), especially where there are sufficient nutrients for the phytoplankton to grow. Measurements of the radiance of the underwater spacelight by these authors has sufficiently fine detail to determine the type of chlorophyll most abundantly present in the water (Fig. 11).

The colour of pure water is a fixed physical property of the water molecule itself, but the contributions of "Gelbstoff", chlorophyll and suspended matter are extremely variable, and depend on factors such as the time of year, tidal state, and the weather. It is hardly surprising, therefore, that the colours of inland and inshore waters defy rigid classification, although this has been attempted (Sauberer, 1942; Jerlov, 1964). Furthermore, data obtained in the field are few and generally unsystematic. Any attempt to relate the visual properties of fishes to their photic environment must, therefore, be tentative. There must also be a certain allowance made for the tendency of authors (this one included) to treat a particular set of measurements from a locality as applying equally to neighbouring areas, and all the time.

3. Intra-ocular Filters

Many animals have coloured lenses, corneas, or a tapetum that selectively reflects light back through the visual cells. These intra-ocular filters must be taken into account when calculating the importance of lights of different spectral radiance, and are discussed fully by Muntz in this volume (Chap. 13).

B. Measurement of the Spectral Absorbances of Natural Waters

A satisfactory analysis of the adaptation of visual pigments to the photic environment has to take into account the optics of radiance transfer through the water, both by the downwelling daylight and the image-forming and scattered light travelling through the water in other directions. The aim of the analysis should be, after all, to estimate the ability of the animal in question to use its vision for the various tasks of its life under some particular range of conditions. It is perhaps less important to know whether the animal, on looking upwards, can detect some dim smudge of daylight penetrating down from the surface.

The measurement of the spectral absorbance of natural water has been reviewed by TYLER and PREISENDORFER (1962) and by JERLOV (1968). From the biological point of view the two most useful quantities are the total beam attenuation coefficient α and the diffuse attenuation coefficient K. Both quantities are strongly wavelength-dependent but K is always smaller than α.

1. The Beam Attenuation Coefficient, α

When a parallel beam of light is shone (in any direction) through a volume of water its intensity is progressively weakened, both by the true absorption and by scattering out of the direction of the beam. This weakening is quantitatively expressed by the beam attenuation coefficient α which is defined in Eq. (1) by the relations,

$$N_0 = N_r \, e^{-\alpha r}, \tag{1}$$

where N_0 is the spectral radiance of the source, r is the thickness of water traversed by the beam and N_r is the radiance of the beam at distance r.

As already mentioned the loss of radiance is due partly to loss by absorption and partly to loss by scattering out of the direction of the beam, i.e.

$$\alpha = a + b, \tag{2}$$

where a is the attenuation coefficient by scattering and b is the attenuation coefficient by absorption. The wavelength-dependence of absorption and scattering has been summarised by JERLOV (1968).

2. The Diffuse Attenuation Coefficient, K

Natural daylight under water is substantially diffuse and it requires a different mathematical treatment from that given to a parallel beam through the water for light can be scattered into a given volume of water as well as out of it. The spectral attenuation of diffuse light is quantified by the diffuse absorption coefficient K, which enables calculations to be made affecting the light available for vision or photosynthesis.

Thus if two photocells are placed one beneath the other separated by a depth z, the spectral irradiance falling on the deeper one, I_z, will be related to the spectral irradiance falling on the shallower by the relation

$$I_z = I_0 \, e^{-Kz}. \tag{3}$$

The light-collecting surface in all such irradiance measurements must be such as to collect flux according to the cosine law:

$$J_\theta = J_0 \cos \theta \tag{4}$$

where J_θ is the radiant intensity of a beam of light at an angle θ from the normal.

C. Types of Natural Water

a) The Clearest Known Natural Water. Crater Lake, Oregon, is one of the clearest known natural waters and is a natural analogue of distilled water. Smith and Tyler (1967) have studied the *in situ* optical properties of this water in great detail and their data for the diffuse attenuation coefficient and the downwelling irradiance in this lake (Fig. 6) come close to describing the optical properties of pure water.

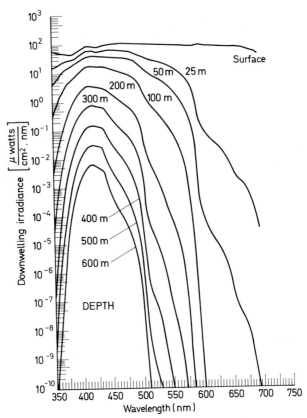

Fig. 6. Downwelling irradiance in the very pure water of Crater Lake, Oregon. These values have been calculated from field measurements made at 0, 5, 15 and 25 metres and assume that the lake water is homogeneous. Note that the units are μwatts cm^{-2} nm^{-1}.
(Smith and Tyler, 1967)

b) Oceanic Water. The dissolved salts in ocean water make virtually no difference to the absorption of visible light (Clarke and James, 1939; Sullivan, 1963). The differences in spectral absorbance of water from various bodies of natural water can be attributed to differences in dissolved and suspended matter.

Jerlov (1951, 1964) has drawn up a very useful classification of water types (Fig. 7, Table 4) but it should be noted that this classification strictly applies only to shallow water. The absorption characteristics of offshore open waters is relatively

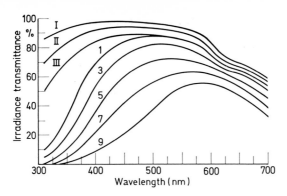

Fig. 7. JERLOV's classification of marine waters. I, II, III are oceanic waters; 1, 3, 5, 7, 9 are coastal waters (the numerical values are given in Table 4). (JERLOV, 1968)

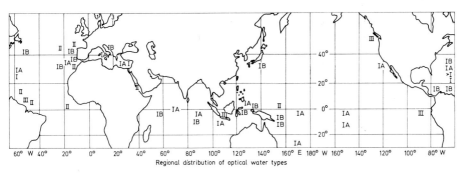

Fig. 8. Distribution of water of different optical types (JERLOV, 1968). See Fig. 7 and Table 4

Table 4. *Jerlov's classification of different surface water types according to their spectral transmittance (I−III, oceanic water; 1−9 coastal water). The table shows the percentage of downwelling daylight irradiance transmitted by 1 m of water* (JERLOV, 1968)

310	350	375	400	425	450	475	Wavelength (nm) 500	525	550	575	600	625	650	675	700
86	94	96.3	97.2	97.8	98.1	98.2	97.2	96.1	94.2	92	85	74	70	66	59
83	92.5	95.1	96.3	97.1	97.4	97.5	96.6	95.5	93.6	91	84	73.5	69.5	65.5	58.5
80	90.5	94	95.5	96.4	96.7	96.8	96.0	95.0	93.0	90.5	83	73	69	65	58.0
69	84	89	92	93.5	94	94	93.5	92.5	90.5	87.5	80	71	67.5	63.5	56
50	71	79	84	87	88.5	89	89	88.5	86.5	82.5	75	68	65	61	54
16	32	54	69	79	84	87.5	88.8	88.5	86.5	82.5	75	68	65	61	54
9	19	34	53	66	75	80	82	82	81	78	71	65	62	57	51
3	10	21	36	50	60	67	71	73	72	70	67	62	58	52	45
	5.0	12	22	32	42	50	56	61	63	63	62	58	53	46	40
	1.5	4.7	9	15	21	29	37	46	53	56	55	52	47	40	33

well known in comparison to coastal waters and a map of the distribution of the different oceanic waters is shown in Fig. 8.

Other measurements of the downwelling diffuse light in deep and clear water suitable for calculations of visual capability have been made by Boden, Kampa, and Snodgrass (1960) for the Bay of Biscay (Fig. 9), by Kampa (1961) for the Californian coast, Bermuda, and the Gulf of Lion and by Kampa (1970) for the eastern Atlantic.

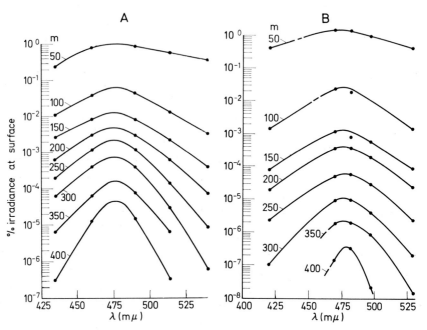

Fig. 9. Spectra of transmitted sunlight at 50 m intervals of depth in the Bay of Biscay (lat. 46° 29′ N, long. 7° 59′ W) on 25th September, 1958. A, 10.30—11.30 h G.M.T; B, 13.25—14.10 h G.M.T. (Boden, Kampa, and Snodgrass, 1960)

c) Coastal Water. Ocean water is relatively pure and thus has fairly stable optical properties. Coastal water, on the other hand, contains large quantities of suspended sand and silt as well as chlorophyll-containing phytoplankton and dissolved "Gelbstoff". Silt and sand in particular vary greatly with the state of the sea and the set of the tides, while rainstorms on land will swell the rivers bringing yellow substance down into the sea. The plankton also varies in density with the time of year, water temperature and the presence of nutrients in the water. It is hardly surprising, therefore, that divers in coastal waters report dramatic changes in water colour and transparency from day to day and from hour to hour.

There has been little systematic measurement of the spectral absorbance of coastal water sufficiently detailed for our purposes. Measurements made *in situ* of natural water are summarised in Table 5, and there is the expected variation in water colour. These data, with the obvious exception of the later measurements by Tyler and Smith (1967, 1970) and Smith and Tyler (1967) were used by Jerlov

Table 5. *The wavelengths of maximum light transmittance for various bodies of natural water*

Station	Depth (m)	Wavelength for minimum value of K	Authority
N. Pacific	0— 5	515 nm	UTTERBACK (1936)
N. Pacific	0— 5	520 nm	UTTERBACK (1936)
N. Pacific	0— 5	490 nm	UTTERBACK (1936)
Norwegian Fjord	0— 4	520 nm	ÅLVIK (1937)
English Channel	10—15	530 nm	POOLE and ATKINS (1937)
Gullmar Fjord	0— 1	590 nm	JERLOV and KULLENBERG (1946)
Gullmar Fjord	0— 2	570 nm	JERLOV and KULLENBERG (1946)
Gullmar Fjord	0— 1	560 nm	JERLOV and KULLENBERG (1946)
Gullmar Fjord	2— 3	530 nm	JERLOV and KULLENBERG (1946)
Gullmar Fjord	0— 2	540 nm	JERLOV and KULLENBERG (1946)
Bornholm Deep	1— 3	520 nm	JERLOV and KULLENBERG (1946)
Mexico San Vincente Reservoir	6	580 nm	TYLER and SMITH (1967, 1970)
Mexico San Vincente Reservoir	8	585 nm	TYLER and SMITH (1967, 1970)
Mexico San Vincente Reservoir	10	575 nm	TYLER and SMITH (1967, 1970)
Mexico Isla Coronado (West)	11.5	580 nm	TYLER and SMITH (1967, 1970)
Mexico Isla Coronado (North East)	16.5	520 nm	TYLER and SMITH (1967, 1970)
Puerto Don Juan	11.5	570 nm	TYLER and SMITH (1967, 1970)
N. Portugal (41° 50.4′ N; 09° 24′ W)	50—130	480 nm	KAMPA (1970)
	210	486 nm	KAMPA (1970)
Madeira (32° 34′ N; 16° 15.7′ W)	50	460 nm	KAMPA (1970)
	50— 90	464 nm	KAMPA (1970)
	137	470 nm	KAMPA (1970)
	240	472 nm	KAMPA (1970)
	332	476 nm	KAMPA (1970)
Teneriffe (28° 07.5′ N; 16° 22′ W)	80—190	470 nm	KAMPA (1970)
	190—615	474 nm	KAMPA (1970)
Fuertaventura (28° 04.5′ N; 14° 11.1′ W)	68—100	470 nm	KAMPA (1970)
	120	472 nm	KAMPA (1970)
	154	474 nm	KAMPA (1970)
	173—511	476 nm	KAMPA (1970)

and KULLENBERG (1946) as the basis for their classification of coastal water types that foreshadowed JERLOV's 1951 classification given here in Table 4. Natural water tends to become stratified into layers according to its density and this is particularly obvious near the surface. A particularly sharp discontinuity can often be seen where low density fresh or brackish water, which contains a high concentration of yellow substance, overlies the more saline sea water. The tidal water of tropical reef flats and lagoons can become very warm in the sun and at the same time becomes stained with a brown or yellow tint. When the tide ebbs the warm water overlies the cooler (and bluer) ocean water outside the reef but in this case the horizontal discontinuity does not seem to be so sharp as in the fresh water case. It is thus reasonable to suppose that fishes such as the Grey Mullets *(Mullidae)* living near the surface in shallow inshore water experience a somewhat redder light-climate than do fishes that live a few metres deeper.

d) Fresh Water. Lake and river waters are exceedingly variable in spectral absorption characteristics and range from the clearest known natural water of Crater Lake, Oregon (Smith and Tyler, 1967) to the almost red waters of some northern lakes (Reuter, 1969). As in the sea the dominant colouring materials are the "yellow substance" produced by vegetable decay and the chlorophyll contained in the phytoplankton, but fresh water differs from the sea in having no bioluminescent organisms. In addition the fresh water can become extremely turbid with suspended particles of mud and sand washed into the rivers and lakes by natural drainage. The presence of phytoplankton is highly seasonal and the plankton-bloom during the warmer months can radically alter the colour and transparency of the water (Talling, 1957). It is not surprising therefore that lakes located in the same geographical area can show great variation in colour even when sampled during the same season (Lundquist, 1936). Measurements of natural lake waters have been made by Clark (1939), Sauberer (1942), Aberg (1943), Tyler (1965), Smith and Tyler (1967), and Spence, Campbell and Chrystal (1971).

At present there are not enough data to show how the light climate in natural fresh water varies with the season. However, the transmission maximum of fresh water probably moves nearer to 550 nm during the plankton blooms in the warmer months, while during the winter, especially when the lakes become frozen, the water becomes purer (and thus bluer) as suspended matter gradually sinks to the bottom.

III. The Scattering of Natural Light under Water

a) Visually Important Characteristics of Natural Light under Water. Pure water scatters light according to the Rayleigh λ^{-4} law (Dawson and Hulburt, 1937; Morel, 1966). However, natural water usually contains large quantities of particulate matter sufficiently large in size to scatter light independently of wavelength (see Jerlov, 1968, for a review).

The scattering of light is important to vision when it is the visual pigments that are under scrutiny. First, the scattering properties of water (together with its absorption) determines the polar distribution of light in the sea and hence the conditions of illumination under which an object is seen. Secondly, scattered light reduces the visible range of objects both by interposing a bright veil of light between the eye and the object, and by blurring its otherwise sharp outline when it is seen at a distance. This is important for it is in part the visible range of an object that determines the visual pigment most suited for its detection (p. 587). Thirdly, Rayleigh scattering results in a marked polarization of the underwater spacelight and this may have important visual consequences for those invertebrate animals that have visual pigments so ordered that they distinguish light polarized in different planes.

b) **The Directional Distribution of Light under Water.** Light does not come equally from all directions under water but chiefly from above. Typical values for the angular distribution of light in the sea are shown in Fig. 10, and TYLER and PREISENDORFER (1962) have published detailed measurements for lake water at different depths for clear and overcast skies. In optically deep water the radiance assumes a fixed angular distribution (the asymptotic radiance distribution). At these depths, the ambient light is essentially monochromatic and light

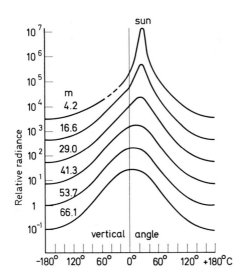

Fig. 10. The directional distribution of radiance of daylight at different depths in Lake Pend, Oreille. (JERLOV, 1968, after TYLER, 1960)

from all directions will have almost the same spectral distribution. At lesser depths the downwelling light will have travelled a shorter path through the water than light arriving from other directions. Measurements of the spectral distribution of the underwater spacelight have been made by several authors (see JERLOV, 1968, for a review) but the most relevant measurements of this phenomenon have been made by TYLER (1965), Fig. 11. A non-luminous object suspended in the water will derive most of its radiance by reflection of the downwelling light but it will usually be viewed against the somewhat more monochromatic radiance of the water spacelight (LYTHGOE, 1968). The consequences of this for vision are discussed below, p. 585—589.

c) **The Polarization of Light through Scattering Media.** Both the daytime sky and the underwater spacelight have a significant component of plane polarized light resulting from Rayleigh scattering. The plane of maximum polarization is at right angles to the apparent direction of the sun (Fig. 12) although in optically deep water the plane of maximum polarization is nearly horizontal. Large particles, such as water droplets in the atmosphere, and sand and plankton in the sea, reduce the amount of polarization; thus any effects of polarization on vision are most likely to be found in clear conditions. Such effects are to be expected when a

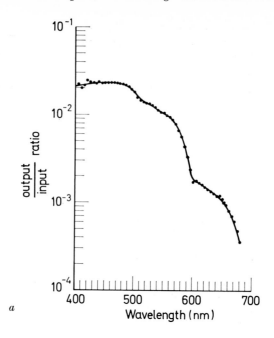

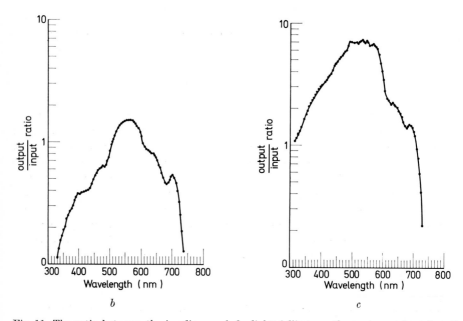

Fig. 11. The ratio between the irradiance of daylight falling on the water surface (input) and the radiance of the water background spacelight in the hemisphere away from the sun's direction (output). The spectrophotometer was mounted at a depth of 33 inches. *a* Crater Lake, Oregon (very pure fresh water). *b* A large volume culture of mixed phytoplankton. The band at 675 nm is characteristic of chlorophyll a. Concentration of chlorophyll a was 1.73 µg per litre. *c* Pacific Coast Water. Concentration of chlorophyll a was 1.24 µg per litre (Tyler, 1965)

diffusely reflecting object is suspended in a scattering medium for it will tend to depolarize the light it reflects, but should an animal viewing it be differentially sensitive to the plane of polarized light there will then be important effects on visibility range.

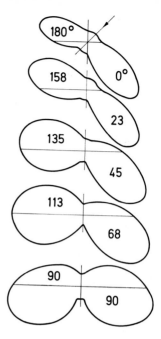

Fig. 12. Cross sections, in various vertical planes, of the distribution of polarized light in light-scattering water space near the surface. In the top sketch the distribution is shown in the vertical plane that includes the solar bearing (arrowed line). The other sketches show distributions in other vertical planes at various angles of rotation to that plane in steps of $22\frac{1}{2}°$. (In the sketches the angles have been rounded up to the nearest degree.) Note the non-symmetrical distributions for all angles except 90°.
(TIMOFEEVA, 1962)

IV. Visual Pigments and Vision through Turbid Media

1. The Reduction of Visual Contrast with Distance

The pioneer work on the theory of contrast reduction through the atmosphere was by KOSCHMIEDER (1924) and this has been amplified by MIDDLETON (1941). DUNTLEY (1950, 1951, 1962, 1963) has extended the atmospheric studies to describe contrast reduction underwater, and has also included paths of sight that are at right angles to the sun's azimuth. The basic situation for horizontal paths of sight is shown in Fig. 13. Image-forming light is reduced in its passage between the object and the eye both by absorption and by scatter out of its original path. This loss of image-forming light is described in Eq. (1). Simultaneously there is a gain in the veiling brightness from the light that is scattered into the eye by the intervening air or water. For horizontal paths of sight the relationship between the apparent spectral radiance, $_tN_r$, of an object and its inherent spectral radiance, $_tN_0$, when seen at a distance r, through the water can be written thus:

$$_tN_r = {}_tN_0(e^{-\alpha r}) + {}_bN(1 - e^{-\alpha r}),\tag{5}$$

where $_bN$ is the spectral radiance of the water background. In this equation the first term on the right represents the loss of image-forming light by absorption and scatter and the second on the right the gain in radiance from light scattered into the eye from other directions.

It must be stressed that Eq. (5) represents the simplest form of the radiance transfer equation and applies only to horizontal paths of sight. A more rigorous theory including paths of sight in all directions is given by DUNTLEY (1962, 1963).

The apparent radiance contrast C_r at distance r between an object and its water background may be defined as:

$$C_r = \frac{{}_tN_r - {}_bN}{{}_bN} \tag{6}$$

${}_tN_r$ and ${}_bN$ are actual radiances at a particular wavelength, which can be measured with a photocell. But calculations on the visual capability of an animal require a knowledge of the number of quanta actually absorbed by the eye from the direction of the target and the background spacelight. This visual contrast $({}_{vis}C_r)$ can be calculated using Eq. (7),

$$_{vis}C_r = \frac{\int {}_tN_r \cdot V_p \cdot P \cdot d\lambda - \int {}_bN \cdot V_p \cdot P \cdot d\lambda}{\int {}_bN \cdot V_p \cdot P \, d\lambda} \tag{7}$$

where V_p is the absorptance of the visual pigment at λ, and P is the corresponding transmittance of the pre-retinal media.

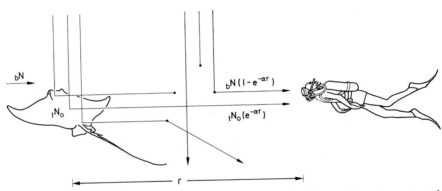

Fig. 13. Diagram to show the visually important features of horizontal radiance transfer through water. In the absence of bioluminescence all light reaching the eye comes ultimately from the daylight that penetrates into the sea. The radiance, ${}_tN_0$, that is reflected by the object into the direction of the eye is partly absorbed, partly scattered out of the direction of the eye and partly reaches the eye. The expression for the radiance reaching the eye is ${}_tN_0(e^{-\alpha r})$, where α is the beam attenuation coefficient and r is the length of the path of sight. Simultaneously there is a gain in brightness due to the light scattered from other directions into the eye. The amount of this so-called "veiling brightness" reaching the eye is described by the expression ${}_bN(1-e^{-\alpha r})$, where ${}_bN$ is the radiance of the water background. The radiance ${}_tN_r$ reaching the eye from the object is thus: ${}_tN_r = {}_tN_0(e^{-\alpha r}) + {}_bN(1 - e^{-\alpha r})$. See Duntley (1962, 1963) when the path of sight is not horizontal

2. Visual Pigments and the Perception of Contrast

In the familiar polychromatic environment of the land the visual scene contains elements of very various spectral distribution; but under water the variety of spectral radiances to be expected is much reduced, for the selective absorption of natural water effectively reduces the band width of light passing through it. This of course remains true irrespective of the direction that the light is travelling. Thus light from above, having travelled a relatively short path from the surface, will have a broader spectral radiance distribution than will light travelling horizontally or from below (see p. 583). At great depths the downwelling light is effectively monochromatic (TYLER, 1959) and there will be little difference in the spectral distribution of light arriving from any direction. Under these conditions the spectral absorptive properties of the visual pigment can have little effect on the perceived brightness contrast of objects suspended in the water. At less extreme depths, however, the spectral qualities of the visual pigment will have a marked effect on the perception of brightness contrast and hence the range that objects can be detected through the water (LYTHGOE, 1966, 1968).

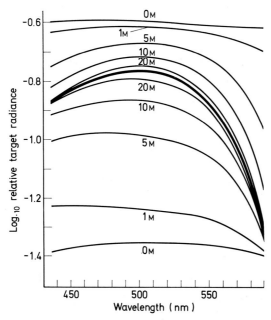

Fig. 14. The relative spectral radiance of the water background in rather turbid inshore Medit-terranean water just below the water surface (heavy line) and the apparent spectral radiance of two matt grey targets, one slightly brighter than the water background (curves above heavy line) and one slightly darker than the water background (curves below heavy line) at various target ranges (M = metres). Both families of curves approach the water background as the range increases. (LYTHGOE, 1968)

The situation where the visual pigment λ_{max} has a marked effect on the visual range of underwater objects is illustrated in Fig. 14. A visual pigment having a λ_{max} offset from the wavelength of maximum water spacelight radiance (c. 510 nm in this case) will absorb less light from both the object and the background space-light, but more light will be absorbed from the object than from its background. The relative brightness of the object will thus be enhanced, and if the object be brighter than the water background it will, accordingly, be more easily seen, but if it be darker it will be less visible.

The apparent contrast of an object seen horizontally against an optically infinite water background decreases exponentially as the visual range increases, for when the right hand side of Eq. (5) is substituted for $_tN_r$ in Eq. (6), it follows that:

$$C_r = C_0 e^{-\alpha r}. \tag{8}$$

It is evident that C_r is small when α is large and it follows that brightness contrasts are reduced most rapidly at those wavelengths where the object appears relatively bright compared to the water background. This has been illustrated diagrammatically in Fig. 15 for two visual pigments, and for white, light-grey, dark grey and black targets. Actual values for two rhodopsins are given in Fig. 16.

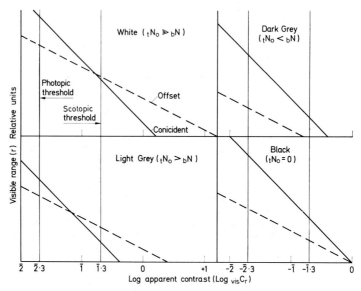

Fig. 15. Diagram to show the visibility range of grey targets of different albedo, both for a visual pigment whose λ_{max} is coincident with wavelength of maximum water transparency (continuous line) and for a visual pigment of λ_{max} offset from the wavelength of maximum water transparency (interrupted line). The optical properties of the water are identical in each case. (The threshold for contrast perception is larger if the object is small or the illumination is dim). For large objects the smallest contrast that can be perceived is approximately 0.02 ($\log_{10} = \bar{2} \cdot 3$) for photopic vision and 0.2 ($\log_{10} = \bar{1} \cdot 3$) for scotopic vision. (See also Table 6)

3. Visual Pigments and Visibility Range under Water

The precise range at which an object becomes invisible can be found by calculating the visual contrast it presents when viewed against its water background [Eq. (7)], taking into account the eye's ability to detect contrast for the prevailing background illumination and the angle subtended by the object at the eye. It will be found that an offset visual pigment would be best for detecting small bright objects, and a coincident visual pigment would be best for detecting any large object naturally visible at a longer range. These conclusions are summarised in Table 6.

The expected magnitudes of these effects under a particular set of conditions are shown in Fig. 16. Here the visual range of large grey targets varying in albedo from white, through greys, to black have been calculated for two different rhodopsins. It is clear that in this shallow water the spectral location of visual pigments can have a significant effect on the visual range of underwater objects and that an object invisible to an eye with one visual pigment would be visible with another.

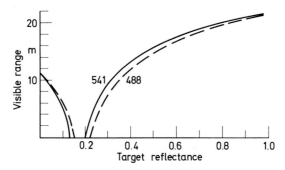

Fig. 16. The horizontal range at which large grey targets of various reflectances can be seen by a diver in rather turbid shallow inshore Mediterranean water when vision is mediated by hypothetical rhodopsins of λ_{max} 541 (offset) and 488 nm (nearly coincident) respectively. The contrast perception threshold is taken as 0.2 — a reasonable value for scotopic vision (LYTHGOE, 1968)

Table 6. *The most suitable visual pigment for detecting different types of object when viewed horizontally against a water background. An "offset" visual pigment is one where the wavelength of maximum absorbance of the pigment does not coincide with the wavelength of maximum transmission of the sea. A "coincident" visual pigment is one where the wavelength of maximum absorbance is approximately equal to the wavelength of maximum transmission of the water.* $_bN$ *is the radiance of the water background*

	Visual range at which the apparent contrast becomes subliminal in shallow water	
	Short (Inherent contrast is small, Object is small, $_bN$ is small)	*Long* (Inherent contrast is large, Object is large, $_bN$ is large)
Objects appear darker than the water background	Coincident	Coincident
Objects appear brighter than the water background	Offset	Coincident

In deep water a coincident visual pigment is always the most effective

4. Polarized Light and the Perception of Distant Objects

The spacelight both in the atmosphere and under water is plane-polarized as a result of Rayleigh scattering (p. 583). Many animals utilise this phenomenon as a navigational aid (see WATERMAN, 1966, for a review) but there is also a strong possibility that it could be useful in improving the visibility of distant objects, especially under water (LYTHGOE and HEMMINGS, 1967).

The underwater spacelight is plane-polarized at all depths although the effect appears to be more pronounced near the surface in clear water. Underwater objects that are of visible size and are not specular reflectors will tend to depolarize any light that they reflect. Thus the radiance reaching the eye from such objects will not be polarized whilst the background spacelight will be, especially if the path of sight is at right angles to the sun's direction. If a diver holds a plane-polarizing filter up to his eye and rotates it, the brightness of the background will appear to fluctuate but that of the object will remain relatively constant. The result is that the contrast between background and object will be enhanced in some orientations of the filter and the object will become visible at a greater range through the water.

Vertebrates are not able to distinguish the plane of polarized light except presumably, where there is the birefringent adipose eyelid found in some pelagic fishes (Stewart, 1962). But many invertebrates are able to distinguish it by reason of the structure of their eyes (p. 703), and the arrangement of the visual pigment therein. It is therefore possible, although not experimentally demonstrated, that the ability of aquatic invertebrates to detect the plane polarized light may be important to their vision.

V. Visual Pigments and Visual Sensitivity

Should the number of quanta absorbed by the eye fall below a certain level, contrast perception and visual acuity are impaired, and when the number of absorbed quanta becomes too small the eye can perceive nothing at all. The relationship between the spectral absorbance of the visual pigment and the spectral characteristics of the photic environment has been the subject of most of the work on the ecology of visual pigments because low sensitivity implies poor contrast perception and visual acuity. This in turn means that morsels of food may be missed, mates may not be found, and finally predators may not be seen until it is too late.

A. The Sensitivity Hypothesis

1. The Purkinje Shift

Most terrestrial animals possess extractable rhodopsins of λ_{max} clustered around 500 nm (Dartnall and Lythgoe, 1965). These rhodopsins are probably scotopic pigments (Dartnall, 1960), and the scotopic sensitivity curve, where it has been measured, shows the animal to be most sensitive in that region. On the other hand photopic sensitivity curves often show a maximum at rather longer wavelengths (557 nm in man). The reason for the shift in sensitivity to longer wavelengths remains obscure, for nightlight is redder than daylight (p. 571) and even if it had the same spectral distribution Dartnall (1962) has shown that when the spectral energy curve of daylight is calculated in the visually correct quantum-intensity terms the photopic pigments are more efficient at trapping the incident quanta than are the scotopic pigments.

2. Sensitivity of Aquatic Animals

a) **Marine Fishes.** It was a coincidence that in the same year BAYLISS, LYTHGOE, and TANSLEY (1936) and CLARKE (1936) published the prediction that there might be a shift in the spectral sensitivity of deep-living fishes to render them more sensitive to the homochromatic blue light available for vision. It was a second coincidence that DENTON and WARREN (1957) and MUNZ (1957, 1958) independently, and almost simultaneously, decided to find out if deep-sea fishes really did possess visual pigments with λ_{max} shifted towards the shorter wavelengths.

DENTON and WARREN (1957) caught their bathypelagic fishes from depths between 200 and 2,000 m. They opened the eyes of 15 species and observed that the retinas were not the usual reddish purple or purple colour found in fishes from shallower water but instead were a golden colour (hence the name "Chrysopsin" for the visual pigment) which bleached when exposed to light. These authors also measured the spectral absorbances of the excised retinas before and after bleaching in white light. The difference spectra resembled that of visual purple (rhodopsin) but the λ_{max} was displaced by some 20 nm to shorter wavelengths. The λ_{max} of the visual pigment in the retinas of these deep-sea fishes is thus around 480 nm – a figure that is significant in view of JERLOV's (1951) report that the maximum penetration by light into ocean water is achieved at 475 nm.

MUNZ (1957, 1958) collected his fishes from between 513 and 696 m in the Pacific near Guadalupe Island, Baja, California. He extracted the visual pigment from the retinas with digitonin, and examined them by the technique of partial bleaching. MUNZ's results are amongst those set out in Table 7. Five of his species had homogeneous visual pigments falling in the range 478–490 nm, but one (*Bathylagus wesethi*) is not included in the table since it has two visual pigments, the main one at 478 nm and a subsidiary one at 501 nm.

At the time that DENTON and WARREN, and MUNZ began working on the visual pigments taken from different habitats it was still very much an open question whether the distribution of visual pigments in fishes might correlate with the taxonomic relationships of the fishes, the salinity of the water, the thermal stability of visual pigments, or the adaption of the visual pigments to the spectral quality of the ambient light.

Table 7. *The visual pigments of fishes caught in various types of natural water. Data have only been included from fishes that were analysed immediately after capture, and where partial bleaching revealed significant amounts of a single pigment only.*
(See Chap. 15 for taxonomic and experimental data)

Bathypelagic fishes

Argyropelecus affinis Garman	478_1	MUNZ (1958)
Sternoptyx obscura Garman	485_1	MUNZ (1958)
Searsia koefoedi Parr	477_1	DARTNALL and LYTHGOE (1965)
Lampanyctus mexicanus Gilbert	490_1	MUNZ (1958)
Lampanyctus sp.	485_1	DARTNALL and LYTHGOE (1965)
Antimora rostrata Gunther	485_1	DARTNALL and LYTHGOE (1965)
Melamphaes bispinosa Gilbert	488_1	MUNZ (1958)

Table 7 (continued)

Epipelagic fishes

Caranx hippos	499₁	Munz (1964)
Trachurus symmetricus	497₁	Munz (1964)
Scomber japonicus	491₁	Munz (1964)
Sarda chiliensis	488₁	Munz (1964)

Rocky Shore, Mediterranean

Zeus faber	492₁	Dartnall and Lythgoe (1965)
Serranus cabrilla (L)	493₁	Dartnall and Lythgoe (1965)
Corvina nigra (Bloch)	500₁	Dartnall and Lythgoe (1965)
Oblada melanura (L)	500₁	Dartnall and Lythgoe (1965)
Oblada sp.	505₁	Dartnall and Lythgoe (1965)
Spondyliosoma cantharus (L)	498₁	Dartnall and Lythgoe (1965)

Rocky Shore, California

Chromis punctipinnis	498₁	Munz (1957)
Axoclinus carminalis	500₁	Munz (1964)

English Channel

Clupea sprattus (L)	500₁	Dartnall and Lythgoe (1965)
Gadus merlangus (L)	500₁	Dartnall and Lythgoe (1965)
Gadus minutus (L)	493₁	Dartnall and Lythgoe (1965)
Gadus morrhua Day	499₁	Dartnall and Lythgoe (1965)
Capros aper (L)	493₁	Dartnall and Lythgoe (1965)
Caranx trachurus Day	498₁	Dartnall and Lythgoe (1965)

Bay and Estuarine

Anchoa compressa	508₁	Munz (1958)
Seriphus politus Ayres	504₁	Munz (1958)
Embiotoca jacksoni Agassiz	506₁	Munz (1958)
Hyperprosopon argenteum Gibbons	506₁	Munz (1958)
Clevelandia ios (Jordon and Gilbert)	512₁	Munz (1958)
Eucyclogobius newberryi Girard	512₁	Munz (1958)
Gillichthys mirabilis Cooper	512₁	Munz (1958)
Atherinops affinis Ayres	508₁	Munz (1958)
Cottus sp.	511₁	Munz (1958)
Leptocottus armatus Girard	511₁	Munz (1958)
Osmerus eperlanus (L)	543₂	Bridges (1965a, b)

Fresh Water

Ameiurus nebulosus marmoratus (Holbrook)	534₂	Bridges (1965a, b)
Chaenobryttus coronarius Bartram	524₂	Bridges (1965a, b)
Lepomis microlophus Gunther	525₂	Bridges (1965a, b)
L. macrochirus purpurescens Cope	525₂	Bridges (1965a, b)
Micropterus salmoides floridianus (La Sueur)	525₂	Bridges (1965a, b)
Lepisosteus platyrhincus De Kay	523₂	Bridges (1965a, b)
Amia calva (L)	525₂	Bridges (1965a, b)
Coregonus clupeoides pennantii (C et V)	520₁	Bridges (1965a, b)

N.B. For the reasons explained in p. 621, footnote a the λ_{max} of all visual pigments reported by Lythgoe and Dartnall (1965) have been reduced here by 1 nm.

Munz (1957, 1958, 1964) clearly recognised that, if the visual pigments of fishes are adapted to capture the greatest possible number of quanta in any particular light climate under water, the correlation must be sought between visual pigment λ_{max} and the spectral irradiance at the point of capture rather than with the depth of water *per se* that the fish is caught at. In his wide-ranging investigation he analysed the visual pigments of fishes from water varying in colour from the blue of the deep oceans to the yellow green of turbid inshore bays and estuaries. Munz found that the visual pigments extracted from fishes living in the various habitats had λ_{max} within the following limits:

Deep sea	478–490 nm,
Surface waters	486–499 nm,
Rocky shore	497–500 nm,
Bays and Estuaries	504–512 nm.

The clustering of the deep-sea rhodopsins around 480 nm has been amply confirmed by Denton and Shaw (1963) and by Dartnall and Lythgoe (1965).

Dartnall and Lythgoe also made collections from rocky-shore Maltese waters and from the coastal waters of the English channel. In both these groups the visual pigment λ_{max} tended to centre around 500 nm. At first glance this might seem a tidy result fully consistent with the "Sensitivity Hypothesis". However, the water around Malta is of oceanic clarity and probably has a transmittance maximum in the blue between 470 and 490 nm, although on one day when the water was particularly turbid Lythgoe (1968) located the maximum transmittance at about 520 nm. In contrast the English Channel is always green or yellow-green in colour although only one set of data is available on its spectral transmittance (Poole and Atkins, 1937). On the sensitivity hypothesis a difference in the λ_{max} of rhodopsins from the Mediterranean and the English Channel was to be expected, but was not found.

b) Fresh-Water Fishes. The range in colour of different bodies of fresh water is at least as wide as that found in the sea and probably much wider. Nevertheless the optically clear water of the deep ocean is only rarely found in fresh water, and most fresh water, which contains high concentrations of phytoplankton and yellow substance, is green or yellow-green in colour. A most important difference between fresh and sea water is that the former contains no bioluminescent organisms. The importance of this is difficult to overstate for at depths in the sea where little daylight penetrates, or at all depths during the night, bioluminescent organisms provide the only visual clues.

In 1896 Köttgen and Abelsdorff noticed that the extracted photopigments of fresh water fishes were more violet in colour (and hence absorbed longer waves) than did those of terrestrial vertebrates. This finding was confirmed by Wald (1936) who also showed that these violet pigments which he named Porphyropsins were related to vitamin A_2, not to vitamin A_1. It is now apparent that porphyropsins are only found in fresh-water fishes and amphibia (exceptions are some of the marine Wrasses) but that rhodopsins and porphyropsins frequently occupy the same retina and perhaps the same outer segments of the rod (see Chapter 11 by Bridges).

The ease with which porphyropsins and rhodopsins are interconverted presents something of a problem, for not only may the interconversion take place from season to season, but also in response to local lighting conditions. Fishes containing both types of pigment present the further difficulty that it is not yet known whether the pigments occur mixed in each outer segment or are segregated in different receptors. These difficulties can be side-stepped by considering only those cases where a single visual pigment has been extracted from a recently caught fish. This selection excludes much excellent data, but enough remain for some conclusions to be formed.

A glance at Fig. 17 will show that fresh water fishes do possess visual pigments with rather longer λ_{max} than those of sea-caught fishes. However, the improvement in sensitivity to be gained by having a porphyropsin instead of the homologous rhodopsin is small or indeed absent. First, the shift towards longer wavelengths is less than would be expected if sensitivity were the only criterion. Secondly, the photosensitivity of porphyropsin is only about 70 % that of rhodopsin (see p. 143) and must be set against any gain in sensitivity resulting from the shift of λ_{max}.

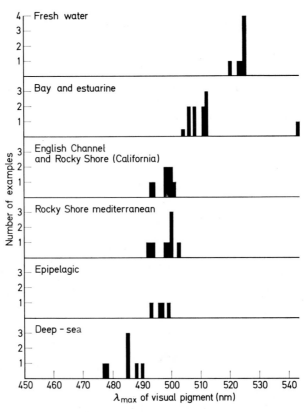

Fig. 17. The λ_{max} of visual pigments extracted from eyes of fishes caught in various types of natural water (see Table 7). Only data where partial bleaching analysis indicated that a single visual pigment was present in significant amounts have been included. Data from fishes kept for prolonged periods in the aquarium have not been included

3. The Optical Densities of Visual Pigments

The number of quanta absorbed by a visual pigment increases with the optical density of that pigment. As the optical density of the pigment increases, so its spectral absorptance curve becomes broader and if it were possible for the pigment to have a near infinite optical density, light of all wavelengths would be equally and totally absorbed.

The optical density of visual pigment in man lies between 0.09 and 0.15 (RUSHTON, 1956) compared to values of 1.0 and more in deep-sea fishes and 0.5 in fishes of the Continental slope (DENTON, 1959; DENTON and NICOL, 1964). It is not really understood why the density of pigment in the retina is not increased further; for example, if the *in situ* density of human rhodopsin were increased from 0.1 to 0.5 there would be an increase in sensitivity by a factor of 3.3. However, increase in optical density brings diminishing returns: a density of 1.0 at a particular wavelength corresponds to 90% absorption leaving little scope for further improvement at that wavelength no matter how great the density.

Some fishes, chiefly elasmobranchs, possess a silvery chorioidal tapetum, which reflects back into the outer segments light that has escaped absorption on the first traverse and would otherwise have been lost to vision. DENTON and NICOL (1964) have shown that, all else being equal, fishes possessing a chorioidal tapetum would have nearly double the sensitivity to be expected in its absence, but instead the retinal rods are reduced to about half the length found in fishes that do not have tapeta but live in the same habitat. Thus a fish possessing a tapetum will have about the same sensitivity as one without.

VI. Visual Pigments and Colour Vision

Until recently visual pigments had to be taken into solution before they could be characterised, and in general the cells of origin of a particular pigment were unknown. Indeed, evidence for the presence of cone pigments was rarely found. More recently the technique of microspectrophotometry (see Chapter 12, p. 481 by LIEBMAN) has allowed the *in situ* measurement of cone pigments.

The presence of visual pigments of different absorptive properties has been deduced from psychophysical evidence since HELMHOLTZ's (1896) classical work on the trichromatic theory of colour vision. A considerable amount of work has since been devoted to building a mathematical theory that would accurately explain the observed characteristics of human colour vision (see WYSZECKI and STILES, 1967, for a review). From our present point of view the most useful of these formulations is the Line Element Equation (Eq. (11)) proposed by STILES (1946), which is only slightly modified from HELMHOLTZ's original equation.

HELMHOLTZ postulated that the visual process is governed by three independent mechanisms each with a characteristic response function — r_λ, g_λ, and b_λ for the red, green, and blue mechanisms respectively. These mechanisms can here be approximated to the absorptance of the pigments contained in the three primate cones discussed by LIEBMAN in Chapter 12. The responses of the respective mechanisms are then:

$$R = \int P_\lambda \cdot \bar{r}_\lambda \cdot d\lambda \,,$$
$$G = \int P_\lambda \cdot \bar{g}_\lambda \cdot d\lambda \,, \tag{9}$$
$$B = \int P_\lambda \cdot \bar{b}_\lambda \cdot d\lambda \,.$$

Where P_λ is the energy of the radiant flux, between wavelengths λ and $\lambda + d\lambda$, reaching the visual pigment.

Hᴇʟᴍʜᴏʟᴛᴢ assumed that for lights of moderate brightness the Weber fractions

$$\frac{R-R'}{R}\,,\quad\frac{G-G'}{G}\,,\quad\frac{B-B'}{B}$$

(where $R - R'$, $G - G'$, $B - B'$ are the just noticeable increments or decrements) were all equal. Sᴛɪʟᴇs, 1946, has since shown that the experimental data are not fitted unless a different Weber fraction is assumed for each mechanism. Hᴇʟᴍ-ʜᴏʟᴛᴢ went on to suppose that the smallest perceptible difference between two radiances is obtained by combining the three fractions in a sum-of-squares relationship thus:

$$\left(\frac{R-R'}{R}\right)^2 + \left(\frac{G-G'}{G}\right)^2 + \left(\frac{B-B'}{B}\right)^2 = (ds)^2 . \tag{10}$$

When ds rises above a certain liminal value the two radiances can be distinguished because they differ either in hue or in brightness. In this form the Helmholtz line element does not fit the experimental data, but if different Weber fractions proportional to ϱ, γ, β are inserted for each mechanism:

$$\left(\frac{R-R'}{\varrho R}\right)^2 + \left(\frac{G-G'}{\gamma G}\right)^2 + \left(\frac{B-B'}{\beta B}\right)^2 = (ds)^2 , \tag{11}$$

there is a remarkably good fit with the observed human photopic response data (Sᴛɪʟᴇs, 1946).

In its basic form the Stiles-Helmholtz line element requires only that the fundamental response mechanisms act independently and that the three mechanisms are additive on a sum-of-the-squares basis. It is reasonable to assume that other vertebrate eyes function in the same basic way as man's and the Stiles-Helmholtz line element can be used in conjunction with the radiance-transfer equations given on pp. 585–586 to predict the advantages of particular sets of visual pigments for different visual tasks.

The major part of this chapter has been concerned with scotopic vision, for our ignorance about the precise disposition and nature of the cone pigments and the huge volume of calculation involved has prevented any comparable study of colour vision. But the way has now been opened by the computer and microspectro-photometric techniques and the ecology of colour vision will surely attract great interest in the future.

VII. The Ecology of Visual Pigments

A. Migratory Fishes

The eel *Anguilla anguilla* spends most of its immature life feeding in fresh and brackish water, but when it is about to embark on its breeding migration to the deep clear water of the Sargasso Sea its visual pigment changes from a mixture of 502_1 and 523_2 to a homogeneous rhodopsin of λ_{max} 487 nm (see Chapter 8, p. 299).

All the other known examples of pigment changes in migratory fishes involve a shift in the relative amounts of porphyropsin and the analogous rhodopsin.

Many fishes, especially lampreys and some salmonids, unquestionably possess a greater proportion of rhodopsin immediately prior to a migration to the sea, and produce some porphyropsin on their return to fresh water. On the other hand, a shift in the balance between rhodopsin and porphyropsin can be observed in land-locked and non-migratory fishes, and changes in the day length or overall light intensity can also induce such changes. It is very difficult to decide whether the observed changes in visual pigments arise from changes in day length, from the depth at which the fishes live, from increased sediment in the water, or indeed from an adaptation to some difference in the spectral distribution of light penetrating into the water (see Chapter 11, p. 417 for a discussion).

B. Deep-Sea Animals

There is an excellent correspondence between the λ_{max} of the rhodopsins from deep-sea fishes and crustacea and the spectral transmission of the water where they live (see Fig. 17 and Table 7). Recently the elephant seal *Mirounga leonina* has also yielded a homogeneous rhodopsin of λ_{max} 485 nm and this mammal is supposed to live a pelagic life in the deep ocean where it dives to considerable depths in search of food (LYTHGOE and DARTNALL, 1970).

It has also been pointed out that the absorptive properties of visual pigments might make the eye very sensitive to the bioluminescence of many marine animals (DENTON and WARREN, 1957; MUNZ, 1957; WALD, BROWN, and BROWN, 1957). A glance at the Table 3 shows that the emission maximum of bioluminescent light can vary widely from source to source but, because its radiance is often below the photopic threshold for the human eye, may appear a uniform blue-grey colour under the conditions that the phenomenon is usually seen on ship-board. In fact there is only one species where the spectral emission of bioluminescence is known and a partial bleaching analysis has also been carried out on the visual pigment. This is in *Euphausia pacifica* where the rhodopsin has a λ_{max} of 462 nm and the bioluminescence an emission maximum of 476 nm (KAMPA, 1955).

C. Inshore, Estuarine, and Fresh-Water Fishes

A glance at Fig. 17 leaves little doubt that fishes living in the predominantly blue or blue-green waters of the Mediterranean do possess visual pigments that are more blue-sensitive than those fishes living in green, yellow-green or brown fresh and land-locked waters. But on closer study (Fig. 18) it is apparent that with the possible exception of very clear Mediterranean water, the fishes have visual pigments that absorb light of shorter wavelengths than might be expected for maximum sensitivity.

D. Terrestrial Vertebrates

Most terrestrial vertebrates have rhodopsins of λ_{max} near 500 nm. PIRENNE (1951) noted that the wavelength of maximum energy of sunlight has a maximum at 480 nm. Yet DARTNALL (1962) has pointed out that when the spectral distribution of sunlight is re-calculated to the more relevant quantum-intensity basis a visual pigment of λ_{max} near 555 nm would confer the greatest sensitivity. Further-

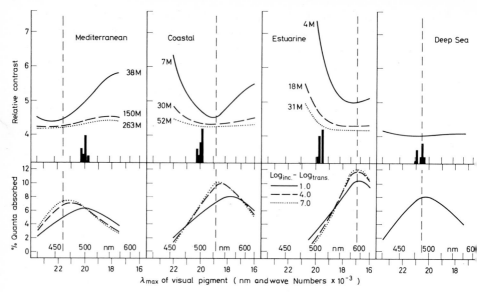

Fig. 18. The advantage in sensitivity and the estimated advantage in the perception of visual contrast (presented by a white target very close to the eye and viewed horizontally against an infinite water background) that are conferred by rhodopsins of varying λ_{max} in four types of water at equivalent optical depths. The actual depths corresponding to an optical density of overlying water are given for Mediterranean, coastal and estuarine water (Jerlov, type II, 5 and 9 respectively). The deep-sea case (Type III) is calculated for an optical density of 7 and is equivalent to a depth of 138 m. The vertical interrupted lines represent the wavelengths at which the water is most transparent. The curves are calculated for rhodopsins of optical density of 0.1 and the daylight above the sea has a colour temperature of 4800 °K. The histogram plots represent the λ_{max} of visual pigments extracted from fishes caught in each water type. (From Lythgoe, 1966)

more the spectral energy of total daylight, as distinct from sunlight alone, is very variable (Figs. 1, 2) and the light from the night sky contains more red light than does daylight (p. 571). There is thus no purely visual explanation for the Purkinje shift presently available although rhodopsins of λ_{max} around 500 nm may be particularly suitable in detecting contrast differences in green vegetation.

E. Larval and Adult Amphibia

Bridges (Chapter 11, p. 483), Crescitelli (Chapter 8, p. 303), and Liebman (Chapter 12, p. 504) have discussed the distribution and location of rhodopsin and porphyropsins in the amphibia. It only remains to note here that in general amphibia whilst in the aquatic phase possess porphyropsins and the terrestrial adults have rhodopsins.

It is obvious from the data outlined above that no simple explanation of contrast perception or sensitivity alone will explain the visual pigments observed in animals. Instead it is clear that there may be many factors, some environmental, some perhaps purely chemical, that influence the visual pigments possessed by an animal.

The only instance where there is a close correlation on a sensitivity basis between visual pigment λ_{max} and the spectral distribution of the ambient light is in the deep-sea fishes. Their example may be instructive, for in the absence of bioluminescence the spectral distribution of the ambient light is essentially the same irrespective of direction. Under these circumstances the possession of an offset visual pigment will not enhance contrast perception. Furthermore at night or at depths too great for daylight to penetrate in visually significant amounts, bioluminescent organisms will appear as bright spots against a dark background and in this case an offset visual pigment will not improve vision. Deep-sea creatures require visual pigments that confer upon them the greatest possible sensitivity, and these they possess.

Since an offset visual pigment, which is required for good contrast perception, will result in loss of sensitivity LYTHGOE (1966) suggested that the visual pigments actually found in fishes might represent a compromise between the rival demands of contrast perception and sensitivity. It is also possible that the almost universal possession of rhodopsin of λ_{max} near 500 nm in land vertebrates provides a means under scotopic conditions for distinguishing a brightness contrast between different species of green plants, which have spectral radiances dominated by the optical properties of chlorophyll.

VIII. Non-Visual Explanations for the Distribution of Visual Pigments

Visual pigments can be bleached by thermal processes as well as by light. Since, on energetic grounds (STILES, 1948), one might expect a low λ_{max} visual pigment to be more thermally stable than a high λ_{max} one, BARLOW (1957) suggested that low λ_{max} visual pigments would produce less visual noise (it being tacitly assumed that the visual process could be as well triggered by a thermal bleaching as by a photochemical one). However, this view was not supported by HUBBARD'S (1958) finding that whereas the absorption of a quantum of light results in the isomerisation of retinal (an essential step in the visual process), heat bleaching occurs by the denaturation of the opsin, the retinal remaining unisomerised and hence not contributing to the visual response.

There is an almost total absence of porphyropsins in purely marine animals (some Wrasses are exceptions) whereas both porphyropsins and rhodopsins occur in fresh water species. At present there is little evidence that either type of pigment would significantly alter the visual performance of the animal providing it is present in adequate amounts and is of suitable λ_{max}.

There is also the possibility that the evolutionary history of a species might be important in determining its visual pigments. This may be true for closely related species (BRIDGES, Chapter 11, p. 445) but taking a broader view of the animal kingdom in general, the evolutionary explanation is not helpful (CRESCITELLI, Chapter 8, p. 347). On balance, therefore, it seems even more difficult to explain the distribution of visual pigments on purely chemical grounds than on purely visual ones.

References

Aberg, B.: Physiologische und ökologische Studien über die pflanzliche Photomorphose. Symb. Botan. Upsaliensis 8, 1—189 (1943).

Ålvik, G.: Über Lichtabsorption von Wasser und Algen in nat. Gewässern. Bergens Museums Årsbok. Naturv. rekke 2. (1937).

Barbier, D.: Analyse du spectre du ciel nocturne. Ann. géophys. 11, 181—208 (1955).

Barlow, H. B.: Purkinje shift and retinal noise. Nature (Lond.) 179 255—256 (1957).

Bayliss, L. E., Lythgoe, R. J., Tansley, K.: Some new forms of visual purple found in sea fishes, with a note on the visual cells of origin. Proc. roy. Soc. B. 816, 95—113 (1936).

Beebe, W.: Half Mile Down. London: John Lane 1935.

Boden, B. P., Kampa, E. M.: Spectral composition of the luminescence of the euphausiid. *Thysanoessa raschii.* Nature (Lond.) 184, 1321—1322 (1959).

— — Planktonic bioluminescence. Oceanogr. Mar. Biol. Ann. Rev. 2, 341 (1964).

— — Snodgrass, J. M.: Underwater daylight measurements in the Bay of Biscay. J. Mar. biol. Ass. U.K. 39, 227—238 (1960).

Bridges, C. D. B.: Absorption properties, interconversions, and environmental adaptation of pigments from fish photoreceptors. Cold Spr. Harb. Symp. quant. Biol. 30, 317—334 (1965a).

— The grouping of fish visual pigments about preferred positions in the spectrum. Vision Res. 5, 223—238 (1965b).

Chamberlain, J. W.: Physics of the Aurora and Airglow. New York-London: Academic Press 1961.

Clarke, G. L.: On the depth at which fishes can see. Ecology 17, 452—456 (1936).

— The utilization of solar energy by aquatic organisms. In: Problems of lake biology. Amer. Ass. Advanc. Sci. 10, 27—38 (1939).

— James, H. R.: Laboratory analysis of the absorption of light by sea water. J. opt. Soc. Amer. 29, 43—55 (1939).

Condit, H. R., Grum, F.: Spectral energy distribution of daylight. J. opt. Soc. Amer. 54, 937—943 (1964).

Dartnall, H. J. A.: Visual pigments of colour vision. In: Mechanisms of Colour Discrimination, pp. 147—161. Ed. by Y. Galifret. Oxford: Pergamon Press 1960.

— Extraction, measurement and analysis of visual photopigment. In: The Eye, pp. 323—365. Ed. by H. Davson. New York-London: Academic Press 1962.

— Goodeve, C. F.: Scotopic luminosity curve and the absorption spectrum of visual purple. Nature (Lond.) 139, 409—411 (1937).

— Lythgoe, J. N.: The spectral clustering of visual pigments. Vision Res. 5, 81—100 (1966).

David, C. N., Conover, R. J.: Preliminary investigation of the physiology and ecology of luminescence in the copepod, *Metridia lucens.* Biol. Bull. 121, 92 (1961).

Davis, R., Gibson, K. S.: Filters for the reproduction of sunlight and daylight and the determination of colour temperature. Bur. Standards misc. Pub. 114, (1931).

Dawson, L. H., Hulburt, E. O.: The scattering of light by water. J. opt. Soc. Amer. 27, 199—201 (1937).

Denton, E. J.: The contributions of the orientated photosensitive and other molecules to the absorption of the whole retina. Proc. roy. Soc. B 150, 78—94 (1959).

— Gilpin-Brown, J. B., Wright, P. G.: On the "filters" in the photophores of mesopelagic fish and on a fish emitting red light and especially sensitive to red light. Proc. Physiol. Soc. (in press).

— Nicol, J. A. C.: The chorioidal tapeta of some cartilagenous fishes (Chondrichthyes). J. mar. biol. Ass. U.K. 44, 219—258 (1964).

— Warren, F. J.: Photosensitive pigments in the retinae of deep-sea fish. J. mar. biol. Ass. U.K. 36, 651—662 (1957).

— Shaw, T. I.: The visual pigments of some deep-sea elasmobranchs. J. mar. biol. Ass. U.K. 43, 65—70 (1963).

Dufay, J.: Spectre, couleur et polarisation de la lumière du ciel nocturne. J. phys. Radium (Paris) 10, 219—240 (1929).

Duntley, S. Q.: The visibility of submerged objects I. Proc. armed Forces nat. res. Council Vision Comm. 27, 57 (1950).

Duntley, S. Q.: The visibility of submerged objects II. Proc. armed Forces nat. Res. Council Vision Comm. **28**, 60 (1951).
— Underwater visibility. In: The Sea, pp. 452—455. Ed. by M. N. Hill. New York-London: Interscience Publ. 1962.
— Light in the sea. J. opt. Soc. Amer. **53**, 214—233 (1963).
Federer, C. A., Tanner, C. B.: Spectral distribution of light in the forest. Ecology **47**, 555—560 (1966).
Haneda, Y.: Über den Leuchtfisch, *Malacocephalus laevis* (Lowe). Jap. J. med. Sci. III, **5**, 355 (1938).
Harvey, E. N.: Bioluminescence. New York: Academic Press 1952.
— Survey of luminous organisms. In: Luminescence of biological systems, pp. 1—24. Ed. by F. H. Johnson. Washington, D. C.: Amer. Assoc. Adv. Sci. 1955.
— Chase, A. M., McElroy, W. D.: The spectral energy curve of luminescence of the ostracod crustacean, *Cypridina* and other luminous organisms. J. cell. comp. Physiol. **50**, 499 (1957).
Hastings, J. W., Sweeney, B. M.: The luminescent reaction in extracts of the marine dino-flagellate *Gonyaulax polyedra*. J. cell. Comp. Physiol. **49**, 209—226 (1957).
Helmholtz, H. von: Handbuch der Physiologischen Optik, 2nd Ed. Hamburg: Voss 1896.
Hemmings, C. C., Lythgoe, J. N.: Better visibility for divers in dark water. Triton **9**, 28—31 (1964).
Henderson, S. T., Hodgkiss, D.: The spectral energy distribution of daylight. Brit. J. appl. Phys. **14**, 125 (1963).
Hubbard, R.: Bleaching of rhodopsins by light and heat. Nature (Lond.) **181**, 1126 (1958).
Hulburt, E. O.: Optics of distilled and natural waters. J. opt. Soc. Amer. **54**, 937—944 (1945).
Jerlov, N. G.: Optical studies of ocean water. Rept. swedish deep-sea Exped. **3**, 1—59 (1951).
— Optical classification of ocean water. In: Physical Aspects of Light in the Sea, pp. 45—49. Honolulu: Univ. of Hawaii Press 1964.
— Optical Oceanography. Amsterdam-London-New York: Elsevier 1968.
— Kullenberg, B.: On radiant energy measurements in the sea. Svenska hydr. biol. Kommissionens skrifter 3e ser. Hydrogrophie Bd. 1, H. 1 (1946).
Judd, D. B., MacAdam, D. L., Wyszecki, G.: Spectral distribution of typical daylight as a function of correlated color temperature. J. opt. Soc. Amer. **54**, 1031—1040 (1964).
Kalle, K.: The problem of Gelbstoff in the Sea. Oceanog. marine Biol. ann. Rev. **4**, 91—104 (1966).
Kampa, E. M.: Euphausiopsin, a new photosensitive pigment from the eye of euphausiid crustaceans. Nature (Lond.) **175**, 996—997 (1955).
— Daylight penetration measurements in three oceans. Union Géod. Geophys. intern. Monogr. **10**, 91—96 (1961).
— Underwater daylight and moonlight measurements in the eastern North Atlantic. J. mar. biol. Ass. U. K. **50**, 391—420 (1970)
— Boden, B. P.: Light generation in a sonic scattering layer. Deep-sea Res. **4**, 73—92 (1957).
Koschmieder, H.: Theorie der horizontalen Sichtweite. Beitr. Phys. freien Atm. **12**, 33—53 and 171—181 (1924).
Köttgen, E., Abelsdorff, G.: Absorption und Zersetzung des Sehpurpurs bei den Wirbel-tieren. Z. Psychol. Physiol. Sinnesorg. **12**, 161—184 (1896).
Le Grand, Y.: Light Colour and Vision. New York: John Wiley & Sons p. 123, 1957.
Lundquist, G.: Sjöarnas transparens, farg och areal. Sveriges Geol. Unders. Afh. ser. C. No. **397**, 1—28 (1936).
Lythgoe, J. N.: Visual pigments and underwater vision. In: Light as an Ecological Factor, pp. 375—391. Ed. by R. Bainbridge, G. C. Evans and O. Rackham. Oxford: Blackwell 1966.
— Visual pigments and visual range underwater. Vision Res. **8**, 997—1012 (1968).
— Dartnall, H. J. A.: A deep-sea rhodopsin in a mammal. Nature (Lond.) **227**, 955—956 (1970).
— Hemmings, C. C.: Polarized light and underwater vision. Nature (Lond.) **213**, 893—894 (1967).
Middleton, W. E. K.: Visibility in Metereology, pp. 28—42. Toronto: Univ. of Toronto Press 1941.

Moon, P.: Proposed standard solar radiation curves for engineering use. J. Franklin Inst. **230**, 583 (1940).

Morel, A.: Etude expérimental de la diffusion de la lumière par l'eau, les solutions de chlorure de sodium et l'eau de mer optiquement pures. J. Chim. Phys. **10**, 1359—1366 (1966).

Munz, F. W.: The photosensitive retinal pigments of marine and euryhaline teleost fishes. Ph. D. Thesis, Univ. of California. Los Angeles (1957).

— Photosensitive pigments from the retinae of certain deep sea fishes. J. Physiol. **140**, 220—225 (1958).

— The visual pigments of epipelagic and rocky shore fishes. Vision Res. **4**, 441—454 (1964).

Nicol, J. A. C.: The spectral composition of the light of Polynoid worms. J. mar. biol. Ass. U.K. **36**, 529—538 (1957a).

— Spectral compositions of the light of *Chaetopterus*. J. mar. biol. Ass. U.K. **36**, 629—642 (1957b).

— Luminescence in Polynoids IV. Measurements of light intensity. J. mar. biol. Ass. **37**, 33—41 (1958a).

— Spectral composition of the light of *Pholas dactylus* L. J. mar. biol. Ass. U.K. **37**, 43—47 (1958b).

— Observations on luminescence in *Noctiluca*. J. mar. biol. Ass. U.K. **37**, 535—549 (1958c).

— Observations on the luminescence of *Pennatula phosphorea*, with a note on the luminescence of *Virgularia mirabilis*. J. mar. biol. Assoc. **37**, 551—563 (1958d).

— Observations of luminescence in pelagic animals. J. mar. biol. Ass. U.K. **37**, 705—752 (1958e).

— Spectral composition of the light of the lantern-fish, *Myctophum punctatum*. J. mar. biol. Ass. U.K. **39**, 27—32 (1960).

— Animal luminescence. Advan. comp. physiol. Biochem. 217—273 (1962).

Pirenne, M. H.: Limits of the visible spectrum. Research **4**, pp. 508—515 (1951).

Poole, H. H., Atkins, W. R. G.: The penetration into the sea of various wavelengths as measured by emission or rectifier photo-electric cells. Proc. roy. Soc. London B **123**, 151—165 (1937).

Rayleigh, Lord (Strutt, R. J.): Absolute intensity of the aurora line in the night sky and the number of atomic transitions. Proc. roy. Soc. Lond. A **129**, 458—467 (1930).

Reuter, T.: Visual pigments and visual cell activity in the retinae of tadpoles and adult frogs (*Rana temporaria* L.). Acta zool. Fenn. **122**, 1—64 (1969).

Richardson, E. A.: Contrast enhancement imaging devices by selection of input photosurface spectral response. Advan. Electronics and Electron Phys. **28** B, 661—675 (1969).

Rozenberg, G. V.: Twilight — a Study in Atmospheric Optics. Plenum Press, N. Y. (1966).

Rushton, W. A. H.: The rhodopsin density in the human rods. J. Physiol. **134**, 30—46 (1956).

Sastri, V. D. P., Das, S. R.: Typical spectral distributions and colour for tropical daylight. J. opt. Soc. Amer. **58**, 391—398 (1968).

Sauberer, F.: Bemerkungen über optische Untersuchungen an Gewässern. Bioklim., Beiblat. Band **9**, (1942).

Smith, R. C., Tyler, J. E.: Optical properties of clear natural water. J. opt. Soc. Amer. **57**, 589—595 (1967).

Spence, D. H. N., Campbell, R. M., Chrystal J.: Spectral intensity in some Scottish freshwater lochs. Freshwater Biol. **1**, in *press* (1971).

Stewart, K. W.: Observations on the morphology and optical properties of the adipose eyelid of fishes. J. fish. Res. Bd. Canada **19**, 1161—1162 (1962).

Stiles, W. S.: A modified Helmholtz line element in brightness-colour space. Proc. phys. Soc. (Lond.) **58**, 41 (1946).

— The physical interpretation of the spectral sensitivity curve of the eye. Trans. Optical Convention of the Worshipful Company of Spectacle Makers **1948**, 97—109.

Sullivan, S. A.: Experimental study of the absorption in distilled water, artificial sea water, and heavy water in the visible region of the spectrum. J. opt. Soc. Amer. **53**, 962—967 (1963).

Talling, J. F.: Photosynthesis and underwater radiation. New Phytol. **56**, 1—132 (1957).

Timofeeva, V. A.: Spatial distribution of the degree of polarization of natural light in the sea. Izv. Akad. Nauk. S.S.S.R. Geofiz. **6**, 1843—1851 (1962).

Smith, R. C., Tyler, J. E.: Optical properties of natural water. J. opt. Soc. Amer. **57**, 589—601 (1967).

Tyler, J. E.: Natural water as a monochromator. Limnol. Oceanog. **4**, 102—105 (1959).

— Radiance distribution as a function of depth in an underwater environment. Bull. Scripps. Inst. Oceanog. Univ. Calif. **7**, 363—412 (1960).

— *In situ* spectroscopy in ocean and lake waters. J. opt. Soc. Amer. **55**, 800—805 (1965).

— Preisendorfer, R. W.: Transmission of energy within the sea. In: The Sea, Vol. 2. pp. 397—451. Ed. by M. N. Hill. New York-London: Interscience Publ. 1962.

— Smith, R. C.: Spectroradiometric characteristics of natural light under water. J. opt. Soc. Amer. **57**, 595—601 (1967).

— — Measurements of Spectral Irradiance Underwater. New York, London, Paris: Gordon and Breach, pp. 1—103 (1970).

Utterback, C. L.: Spectral bands of submarine solar radiation in the North Pacific. Int. p. l'Explor. Mer., Rapp et Procés-Verbaux C. **1**, 2 (1936).

Wald, G.: Pigments of the retina II. Sea robin, sea bass and scup. J. gen. Physiol. **20**, 45—56 (1936).

— Brown, P. K., Brown, P. S.: Visual pigments and depth of habitat of marine fishes. Nature (Lond.) **180**, 969—971 (1957).

Waterman, T. H.: Systems analysis and the visual orientation of animals. Amer. Sci. **54**, 15—45 (1966).

Wyszecki, G., Stiles, W. S.: Colour Science. New York-London-Sydney: John Wiley & Sons 1967.

Chapter 15

List of Vertebrate Visual Pigments[*]

By

John N. Lythgoe, Falmer, Brighton (Great Britain)

Contents

Introduction

Visual pigments have been included in the list that follows if they have either been tested for homogeneity by the technique of partial bleaching (Dartnall, 1952) or if they have been characterized by microspectrophotometry (M.S.P.); (see Liebman, Chapter 12).

Most of the pigments reported here were measured in solution. Digitonin (Lythgoe, 1937) is the most commonly used extractant but other substances (Bridges, 1957) can be used instead. There is no evidence that the extractant used affects the light-absorbing properties of visual pigments. Very pure extracts can be obtained if the outer segments are first separated by flotation in sucrose solution (Saito, 1938). Williams (1968) has described a technique for obtaining extremely concentrated solutions of visual pigment. For a review of extracting procedures see Dartnall (1962).

Hydroxylamine is often added to the solutions, both because it prevents regeneration after bleaching and because the products of bleaching formed in its presence (the oximes) have spectral absorbance curves that are narrower than those of the retinals and are, moreover, slightly displaced to shorter wavelengths — thus exerting less influence on the λ_{max} of the difference spectra.

It is certain that most of the non-M.S.P. measurements have failed to reveal, let alone characterize, all the visual pigments present in retinas. This is partly because it is difficult, with present photometric techniques, to detect a "minor" pigment that is present as only a small percentage of the total, and partly because the conditions of extraction may differentially destroy some pigments. For example, hydroxylamine is known to destroy the 433_1 pigment (green rod pigment) of the frog, leaving the 502_1 pigment (rhodopsin) intact (Dartnall, 1967).

The animals are listed in systematic order and the Authority who first described each species is given after the specific name in the usual way. The temptation to add the Authority where none was given in the reference has been resisted since it can happen that different Authorities give the same name to different species.

---

[*] For the visual pigments of Invertebrates, see Goldsmith, Chapter 17, this volume.

Taxon	Species	Common name	Pigment type and λ_{max} in nm			Reference
			A_1	A_2	not known	
Class Cyclostomata						
Order Petromyzontia	*Petromyzon marinus*	Lamprey	497		518	Crescitelli, 1956a; Wald, 1957
Class Chondrichthyes						
Order Pleurotremata						
Family Carcharinidae	*Mustelus californicus*		497			Crescitelli, Chapter 8
Family Squalidae	*Squalus suckleyi*	Pacific dogfish	497.5			Beatty, 1969a
Order Hypotremata						
Family Rhinobatidae	*Rhinobatos productus*	Shovel-nosed guitar fish	497			Crescitelli, Chapter 8.
Family Raiidae	*Raja binoculata*	Big skate	497			Beatty, 1969a
Order Chimaeroidei						
Family Chimaeridae	*Hydrolagus colliei*	Ratfish	484			Beatty, 1969a; Crescitelli,1969
	Callorhinchus callorynchus Lacépède	Elephant fish	499			McFarland, 1970
Class Osteichthyes						
Super-Order Holostei						
Order Protospondyli						
Family Amiidae	*Amia calva* L.	Bowfin			525	Bridges, 1964
Order Ginglymodi						
Family Lepisosteidae	*Lepisosteus platyrhinchus* De Kay	Florida spotted gar			523	Bridges, 1964
Order Isospondyli						
Family Alepocephalidae	*Xenodermichthys copei* Gill		479 [a, b]			Dartnall and Lythgoe, 1965
Family Clupeidae	*Dorosoma cepedianum* (Le Sueur)		500	521		Bridges, 1964
	Anchoa compressa		508			Munz, 1958b

Taxon	Species	Common name	Pigment type and λ_{max} in nm			Reference
			A_1	A_2	not known	
Family Clupeidae	*Alosa pseudoharengus* (Wilson)	Alewife	504	528		MUNZ ex SCHWANZARA, 1967
	Clupea sprattus L.	Sprat	500[a]			DARTNALL and LYTHGOE, 1965
Family Salmonidae[d]	*Oncorhynchus gorbuscha* (Walbaum)	Pink salmon	503	527		MUNZ and BEATTY, 1965
	O. keta (Walbaum)	Chum salmon	503	527		MUNZ and BEATTY, 1965
	O. kisutch (Walbaum)	Coho salmon	503	527		MUNZ and BEATTY, 1965
	O. nerka (Walbaum)	Sockeye salmon	503	527		MUNZ and BEATTY, 1965
	O. tshawytscha (Walbaum)	King salmon	503	527		MUNZ and BEATTY, 1965
	Salmo clarkii Richardson	Cutthroat trout	503	527		MUNZ and BEATTY, 1965
	S. gairdneri Richardson	Rainbow trout	503	527		MUNZ and BEATTY, 1965
			504	526		BRIDGES, Chapter 11, this volume
	S. salar L.	Atlantic salmon	503	527		MUNZ and BEATTY, 1965
	S. trutta L.	Brown trout	503	527		MUNZ and BEATTY, 1965
			503	527		BRIDGES, Chapter 11, this volume
	Salvelinus fontinalis (Mitchill)	Brook char, Brook trout	503	527		MUNZ and McFARLAND, 1965
			503	527		BRIDGES, Chapter 11, this volume
	S. malma (Walbaum)	Dolly Varden	503	527		MUNZ and McFARLAND, 1965
	S. namaycush (Walbaum)	Lake char	512	(545)		MUNZ and McFARLAND, 1965
	S. alpinus L.	Arctic char	509			MUNZ and McFARLAND, 1965
	S. alpinus L.	Saibling	508		e	BRIDGES and YOSHIKAMI (1970a)
	S. perisii (Günther)	Torgoch	508		e	BRIDGES and YOSHIKAMI (1970a)
	S. willughbii (Günther)	Willoughby's char	508[c]		e	BRIDGES and YOSHIKAMI (1970a)
	Thymallus thymallus L.	Grayling	—	527		BRIDGES, 1967
	Coregonus clupeoides Lacépède	Powan	—	536		BRIDGES, 1965
	C. pollan Thompson	Pollan	—	536		BRIDGES, 1967
	C. clupeoides stigmaticus Regan	Schelly, skelly	510		e	BRIDGES, 1967

Taxon	Species	Common name	Pigment type and λ_{max} in nm — A_1	A_2	not known	Reference
Family Salmonidae [d] [continued]	*C. clupeoides pennantii* C. et V.	Gwyniad	520			BRIDGES, 1965
	C. vandesius gracilior Regan	Cumberland vendace	510		[e]	BRIDGES, 1967
	C. wartmannii (Bloch)	Blaufelchen	510		[e]	BRIDGES and YOSHIKAMI (1970a)
	C. macrophthalmus Nüsslin	Gangfisch	510		[e]	BRIDGES and YOSHIKAMI (1970a)
	Coregonus sp.	Renke	509	536		BRIDGES and YOSHIKAMI (1970a)
	Coregonus sp.	Renke	509		[e]	BRIDGES and YOSHIKAMI (1970a)
	Osmerus eperlanus L.	Smelt, Sparling, Brwyniad		543		BRIDGES, 1967
Family Argentidae	*Searsia koefoedi* Parr		477[a]			DARTNALL and LYTHGOE, 1965
	Nansenia groenlandica (Reinhardt)		491[a]			DARTNALL and LYTHGOE, 1965
	Bathylagus microphthalmus Norman		467[a] 497[a]			DARTNALL and LYTHGOE, 1965
	B. wesethi Bolin		478 501			MUNZ, 1958a
Family Sternoptychiidae	*Sternoptyx obscura* Garman	Hatchet fish	485			MUNZ, 1958a
	Argyropelecus affinis Garman	Hatchet fish	478			MUNZ, 1958a
Family Osteoglossidae	*Osteoglossum bicirrhosum* Vandelli		503	527		SCHWANZARA, 1967
Family Notopteridae	*Xenomystus nigri* (Günther)		503	527		SCHWANZARA, 1967
Order Haplomi Family Esocidae	*Esox lucius* L.	Pike		533		DARTNALL, 1952
Family Umbridae	*Umbra limi* (Kirtland)	Central mud-minnow		526		BRIDGES, 1964

Taxon	Species	Common name	Pigment type and λ_{max} in nm			Reference
			A_1	A_2	not known	
Order Iniomi						
Family Myctophidae	*Lampanyctus mexicanus* Gilbert		490			MUNZ, 1958a
	Lampanyctus sp.		485[a]			DARTNALL and LYTHGOE, 1965
Order Ostariophysi						
Family Gasteropelecidae	*Gasteropelecus levis* (Eigenmann)	Silver hatchetfish	503	527		SCHWANZARA, 1967
Family Characidae	*Arnoldichthys spilopterus* (Boulenger)	Red-eyed characin	503	527		SCHWANZARA, 1967
	Colossoma nigripinnis (Cope)	Pacu	503	527		SCHWANZARA, 1967
	Copeina arnoldi Regan	Spraying characin	503	527		SCHWANZARA, 1967
	Ctenobrycon spilurus (C. et V.)	Silver tetra	503	527		SCHWANZARA, 1967
	Exodon paradoxus Müller and Troschell		503	527		SCHWANZARA, 1967
	Gymnocorymbus ternetzi (Boulenger)	Black tetra	503	527		SCHWANZARA, 1967
	Hemigrammus rhodostomus Ahl	Rummy-nosed tetra	503	527		SCHWANZARA, 1967
	Hyphessobrycon sp.	Bleeding-heart tetra	503	527		SCHWANZARA, 1967
	Metynnis schreitmuelleri Ahl		503	530		SCHWANZARA, 1967
	Micralestes interruptus Boulenger	Congo tetra	503	527		SCHWANZARA, 1967
	Moenkhausia oligolepis (Günther)	Glass tetra	503	527		SCHWANZARA, 1967
	Rooseveltiella nattereri (Kner)	Red piranha		527		SCHWANZARA, 1967
Family Anostomidae	*Abramites microcephalus* Norman	Headstander	503	527		SCHWANZARA, 1967
	Anostomus anostomus (L)	Striped anostomus	503	527		SCHWANZARA, 1967
	Prochilodus insignis Schomburgk		503	527		SCHWANZARA, 1967
Family Hemiodontidae	*Hemiodus semitaeniatus* Kner		503	527		SCHWANZARA, 1967

Taxon	Species	Common name	Pigment type and λ_{max} in nm			Reference
			A_1	A_2	not known	
Family Cyprinidae	*Ptychocheilus oregonensis* (Richardson)		506			MUNZ ex SCHWANZARA, 1967
	Rutilus rutilus (L.)	Roach		535		DARTNALL, 1962
	Scardinius erythrophthalmus (L.)	Rudd	507	535		BRIDGES and YOSHIKAMI (1970b)
	Gobio gobio (L.)	Gudgeon		535		DARTNALL, 1962
	Tinca tinca auratus (L.)	Golden tench		533		DARTNALL, 1962
	T. tinca (L.)	Green tench	467	533		DARTNALL, 1952
	Pimephales notatus (Rafinesque)	Bluntnose minnow	505	535		BRIDGES, 1964
	Notropis cornutus frontalis (Agassiz)		505	536		BRIDGES, 1964
	Notemigonus crysoleucas boscii (Valenciennes)	Southeastern golden shiner	502	529		BRIDGES, 1964
	N. crysoleucas auratus (Rafinesque)		504	532		BRIDGES, 1964
	Hybopsis biguttata (Kirtland)	Honeyhead chub	505	535		BRIDGES, 1964
	Alburnus lucidus Day	Bleak	510	533		DARTNALL, 1955
	Cyprinus carpio L.	Carp		c.-550		CRESCITELLI and DARTNALL, 1954
	Carassius carassius (L.)	Crucian carp		523		DARTNALL, 1962
	C. auratus (L.)	Goldfish		523		SCHWANZARA, 1967
	C. auratus	Goldfish		522	530[g,j] 544[g,j] c. 625[g,j]	MARKS, 1965
	Balantiocheilus melanopterus (Bleeker)	Bala shark		522		SCHWANZARA, 1967
	Barbus conchonius (Hamilton-Buchanan)	Rosy barb	502			SCHWANZARA, 1967
	B. everetti Boulenger	Clown barb	500			SCHWANZARA, 1967
	B. fasciolatus Günther	African banded barb	500	522		SCHWANZARA, 1967

Taxon	Species	Common name	Pigment type and λ_{max} in nm			Reference
			A_1	A_2	not known	
Family Cyprinidae [continued]	B. schwanenfeldi Bleeker	Schwanenfeld's barb	500	522		Schwanzara, 1967
	Brachydanio rerio (Hamilton-Buchanan)	Zebra danio	500			Schwanzara, 1967
	Chela mouhoti Smith		501			Schwanzara, 1967
	Danio malabaricus (Jerdon)	Giant danio	502			Schwanzara, 1967
	Morulius chrysophekadion (Bleeker)	Black shark		522		Schwanzara, 1967
	Rasbora lateristrata elegans (Volz)	Yellow rasbora	501			Schwanzara, 1967
Family Catostomidae	Catostomus commersonii (Lacépède)	Whitesucker		524		Bridges, 1964
Family Pimelodidae	Pimelodella gracilis (C. et V.)			527		Schwanzara, 1967
Family Bagridae	Mystus tengera (Hamilton-Buchanan)			535		
Family Ictaluridae	Ictalurus nebulosus marmoratus (Holbrook)	Southern brown bullhead		534		Bridges, 1964
Family Mochokidae	Synodontis nigriventis David	Upside-down catfish		533		Schwanzara, 1967
Order Apodes Family Anguillidae	Anguilla anguilla (L)	Eel	487 502	523		Brown and Brown ex Wald, 1958, 1960
Family Congridae	Conger conger (L)	Conger eel	487			Walker, 1956
Order Microcyprini Family Cyprinodontidae	Aplocheilus lineatus (C. et V.)		501			Schwanzara, 1967
	Jordanella floridae Goode et Bean	American flagfish	500	522		Schwanzara, 1967
	Cyprinodon variegatus variegatus (Lacépède)	Sheepshead minnow	506			Bridges, 1964
Family Poeciliidae	Belonesox belizanus Kner		498			Bridges, 1964
	Poecilia latipinna Le Sueur	Sailfin molly	502	521		Schwanzara, 1967

Taxon	Species	Common name	Pigment type and λ_{max} in nm			Reference
			A_1	A_2	not known	
Family Poeciliidae [continued]	P. reticulata Peters	Guppy	500			SCHWANZARA, 1967
	P. sphenops Valenciennes	Molly	502			SCHWANZARA, 1967
	Xiphophorus helleri Heckel	Green swordtail	500			SCHWANZARA, 1967
	X. maculatus (Günther)	Southern platyfish	500			SCHWANZARA, 1967
	X. variatus (Meek)	Variable platyfish	501			SCHWANZARA, 1967
Family Anablepidae	Anableps sp.	Four-eyed fish	506			SCHWANZARA, 1967
Order Anacanthini Family Gadidae	Gadus macrocephalus	Pacific cod	498			BEATTY, 1969b
	G. morrhua Day	Cod	499[a]			DARTNALL and LYTHGOE, 1965
	G. minutus L.	Poor cod	493[a]			DARTNALL and LYTHGOE, 1965
	G. merlangus L.	Whiting	500[a]			DARTNALL and LYTHGOE, 1965
	G. aeglifinus L.	Haddock	494[a]			DARTNALL and LYTHGOE, 1965
	Microgadus proximus	Tomcod	499			BEATTY, 1969b
	Theragra chalcogrammus	Walleye pollack	498			BEATTY, 1969b
	Antimora rostrata Günther		485[a]			DARTNALL and LYTHGOE, 1965
	Lota lota	Burbot	523			BEATTY, 1969b
Family Melamphaidae	Melamphaës bispinosus Gilbert		488		527	MUNZ, 1958a
Order Zeomorphi Family Zeidae	Zeus faber L.	John Dory	492[a]			DARTNALL and LYTHGOE, 1965
Family Caproidae	Capros aper (L.)	Boar fish	493[a]			DARTNALL and LYTHGOE, 1965
Order Percomorphi Family Serranidae	Serranus cabrilla (L.)	Comber	493[a]			DARTNALL and LYTHGOE, 1965
	Paracentropristis scriba (L.)	Painted comber	492[a], 498[a]			DARTNALL and LYTHGOE, 1965
	Morone labrax (L.)	Sea bass	502	534		DARTNALL and LYTHGOE, 1965
	Epinephelus guaza (L.)	Grouper	494[a], 501[a]			DARTNALL and LYTHGOE, 1965
	E. alexandrinus (C. et V.)	Grouper	494[a], 499[a]			DARTNALL and LYTHGOE, 1965

Taxon	Species	Common name	A_1	A_2	not known	Reference
Family Centrarchidae	Pomoxis nigromaculatus (Le Sueur)			525		MUNZ, 1965
	P. annularis Rafinesque	White crappie		527		SCHWANZARA, 1967
	Micropterus salmoides floridanus (Le Sueur)	Florida largemouth bass		525		MUNZ, 1965
				525		BRIDGES, 1964
	Lepomis microlophus (Günther)	Shellcracker		525		BRIDGES, 1964
	L. macrochirus purpurescens Cope	Bluegill		525		BRIDGES, 1964
	Chaenobryttus coronarius (Bartram)	Warmouth		524		BRIDGES, 1964
Family Carangidae	Trachurus symmetricus Ayres	Jack mackerel	495			MUNZ, 1957
	Caranx trachurus Day	Scad, horse mackerel	498a			DARTNALL and LYTHGOE, 1965
Family Centropomidae	Chanda ranga (Hamilton-Buchanan)	Indian glassfish	500			SCHWANZARA, 1967
	Lates niloticus	Nile perch	499			LYTHGOE, unpublished
Family Sciaenidae	Seriphus politus Ayres	Queenfish	504	520		MUNZ, 1958b
	Johnius umbra (= Corvina (Sciaena) nigra)	Drumfish	500a			DARTNALL and LYTHGOE, 1965
Family Sparidae	Spondyliosoma cantharus (L)	Black bream	498a			DARTNALL and LYTHGOE, 1965
			518a			DARTNALL and LYTHGOE, 1965
	Sarpa salpa (L)	Salp	500a			DARTNALL and LYTHGOE, 1965
	Pagellus erythrinus (L)	Pandora	493a			DARTNALL and LYTHGOE, 1965
			499a			DARTNALL and LYTHGOE, 1965
	Oblada melanura (L)	Saddle bream	500a			DARTNALL and LYTHGOE, 1965
	Oblada sp.		505a			DARTNALL and LYTHGOE, 1965
Family Centracanthidae	Merolepis maena (L)		501a	522		DARTNALL and LYTHGOE, 1965
	M. chryselis (C. et V.)		512a			DARTNALL and LYTHGOE, 1965
			501a			DARTNALL and LYTHGOE, 1965
Family Monodactylidae	Monodactylus argenteus (L)	Fingerfish	502			SCHWANZARA, 1967
Family Scatophagidae	Scatophagus argus (Gmelin)	Scat	500			SCHWANZARA, 1967

Taxon	Species	Common name	Pigment type and λ$_{max}$ in nm			Reference
			A_1	A_2	not known	
Family Cichlidae	Aequidens portalegrensis (Hensel)	Black acara	500	522		SCHWANZARA, 1967
	Apistogramma sp.		500			SCHWANZARA, 1967
	Astronotus ocellatus (Cuvier)	Oscar's cichlid	500	522		SCHWANZARA, 1967
	Cichlasoma meeki (Brind)	Fire-mouth cichlid	500	522		SCHWANZARA, 1967
	Pelmatochromis guentheri (Sauvage)		500	522		SCHWANZARA, 1967
	P. pulcher Boulenger		500	522		SCHWANZARA, 1967
	Pterophyllum eimekei Ahl	Lesser angelfish	500	522		SCHWANZARA, 1967
	Symphysodon aequifasciata Schultz	Brown discus	497	516		SCHWANZARA, 1967
	Tilapia nilotica (L)	Nile mouthbrooder	503	527		SCHWANZARA, 1967
	T. zilli (Gervais)		[k]	519		LYTHGOE, unpublished
	T. leucosticta Trewavas			519		LYTHGOE, unpublished
	T. variabilis Boulenger			520		LYTHGOE, unpublished
	T. melanopleura		499	520		LYTHGOE, unpublished
	Haplochromis melanopleura		499	520		LYTHGOE, unpublished
Family Embiotocidae	Hyperprosopon argenteum	Wall-eye surf perch	506			MUNZ, 1958b
	Embiotoca jacksoni Agassiz	Bay black perch	506			MUNZ, 1958b
Family Pomacentridae	Chromis punctipinnis (Cooper)	Blacksmith	495[l]			MUNZ, 1957
Family Labridae	Pimelometopon pulchrum (Ayres)	Californian sheep head	497, 520			MUNZ, 1958c
	Labrus mixtus L.	Cuckoo wrasse	486[a], 527[a]			DARTNALL and LYTHGOE, 1965
	L. merula	Brown wrasse	492	510		WALD, 1960
	Crenilabrus festivus	Green wrasse		513		WALD, 1960
	C. massa	Grey wrasse		513		WALD, 1960
	Paralabrax clathratus		500, 520			MUNZ, 1964
Family Scaridae	Sparisoma cretense (L)	Parrot fish	485[a]	520		DARTNALL and LYTHGOE, 1965

Taxon	Species	Common name	Pigment type and λ_{max} in nm			Reference
			A_1	A_2	not known	
Family Scombridae	Pneumatophorus japonicus diego (Ayres)		491			Mᴜɴᴢ, 1957
	Scomber scombrus L.	Mackerel	521[a]			Dᴀʀᴛɴᴀʟʟ and Lᴙᴛʜɢᴏᴇ, 1965
			487[a]			
	S. japonicus		491			Mᴜɴᴢ, 1964
	Scomberomorus concolor		485			Mᴜɴᴢ, 1957
	S. sierra		486			Mᴜɴᴢ, 1964
			(530)			
	Sarda chiliensis		488			Mᴜɴᴢ, 1964
Family Gobiidae	Gillichthys mirabilis Cooper	Mudsucker	512			Mᴜɴᴢ, 1956
	Eucyclogobius newberryi	Tidewater goby	512			Mᴜɴᴢ, 1958b
	Clevelandia ios	Arrow goby	512			Mᴜɴᴢ, 1958b
	Coryphopterus nicholsii (Bean)	Crested goby	500			Mᴜɴᴢ, 1958b
Family Callionymidae	Callionymus lyra L.	Dragonet	485[a]			Dᴀʀᴛɴᴀʟʟ and Lᴙᴛʜɢᴏᴇ, 1965
			511[a]			
Family Tripterygiidae	Axoclinus carminalis		500			Mᴜɴᴢ, 1957
Family Anabantidae	Helostoma temmincki (C. et V.)	Kissing gourami	500		522	Sᴄʜᴡᴀɴᴢᴀʀᴀ, 1967
	Macropodus opercularis concolor Ahl	White paradise fish	500		522	Sᴄʜᴡᴀɴᴢᴀʀᴀ, 1967
Family Atherinidae	Atherinops affinis (Ayres)	Topsmelt	508			Mᴜɴᴢ, 1958b
	Melanotaenia nigrans	New Guinea rainbow	501			Sᴄʜᴡᴀɴᴢᴀʀᴀ, 1967
Family Mugilidae	Mugil curema C. et V.	White mullet	499		522	Bʀɪᴅɢᴇs, 1964
	M. cephalus L.	Striped mullet	499		522	Bʀɪᴅɢᴇs, 1964
Order Scleroparei						
Family Scorpaenidae	Scorpaena guttata Girard		500			Mᴜɴᴢ, 1957
Family Triglidae	Trigla gurnardus L.	Grey gurnard	491[a]			Dᴀʀᴛɴᴀʟʟ and Lᴙᴛʜɢᴏᴇ, 1965
			511[a]			
	T. cuculus L.	Red gurnard	492[a, m]			Dᴀʀᴛɴᴀʟʟ and Lᴙᴛʜɢᴏᴇ, 1965
Family Cottidae	Leptocottus armatus Girard	Staghorn sculpin	511			Mᴜɴᴢ, 1958b
	Cottus sp.	Sculpin	511			Mᴜɴᴢ, 1958b

Taxon	Species	Common name	Pigment type and λ_{max} in nm			Reference
			A_1	A_2	not known	
Family Gasterosteidae	*Gasterosteus aculeatus* L.	Three-spined stickleback	501	522		Munz, 1957
Order Heterosomata						
Family Bothidae	*Rhombus maximus* Day	Turbot	499[a] 517[a]			Dartnall and Lythgoe, 1965
	R. laevis Day	Brill	497[a]			Dartnall and Lythgoe, 1965
	Arnoglossus megastoma Day	Megrim	486[a]			Dartnall and Lythgoe, 1965
Family Pleuronectidae	*Pleuronectes microcephalus* Day	Lemon sole	493[a] 492[a] 501[a]			Dartnall and Lythgoe, 1965
	P. limanda Day	Dab	499[a] 506[a,n]			Dartnall and Lythgoe, 1965
	P. flesus Day	Flounder	507[a] 510[a]			Dartnall and Lythgoe, 1965
Family Soleidae	*Solea vulgaris* Day	Sole	501[a]			Dartnall and Lythgoe, 1965
Order Plectognathi						
Family Tetraodontidae	*Sphaeroides annulatus* (Jenyns)	Network puffer	500	522		Munz, 1958b
	Tetraodon schoutedeni Pellegrin		503	527		Schwanzara, 1967
Class Amphibia						
Order Caudata						
Family Salamandridae	*Taricha torosa*	Pacific Coast newt	502			Crescitelli, 1958
Family Proteidae	*Necturus maculosus*	Mud puppy		522		Crescitelli, 1958
	N. maculosus	Mud puppy			527[f,j] 575[g,j]	Liebman, Chapter 12
Order Salientia[s]						
Family Pipidae	*Xenopus laevis*	Clawed toad	502	523		Dartnall, 1956
Family Ranidae	*Rana temporaria*	Common frog	502			Lythgoe, 1937
	R. temporaria		502			Dartnall and Lythgoe, 1965
	R. temporaria		433°			Dartnall, 1967
	R. temporaria		440°			Reuter, 1966

Taxon	Species	Common name	Pigment type and λ_{max} in nm			Reference
			A_1	A_2	not known	
Family Ranidae[s] [continued]	R. temporaria	(tadpole)	502			Muntz and Reuter, 1966
	R. cancrivora Gravenhorst	Crab-eating frog	433		523	Dartnall, 1967
	R. esculenta	Edible frog	c. 430 502			Dartnall, 1957
	R. aurora		501			Crescitelli, 1958
	R. clamitans		502			Dartnall, 1962
	R. muscosa		501			Crescitelli, 1958
	R. pipiens	Leopard frog	502			Crescitelli, 1958
					432[f,i] 502[g,i] 575[g,i]	Liebman and Entine, 1968
	R. pipiens	(tadpole)			438[f,i] 527[f,g,j] 620[g,j]	Liebman and Entine, 1968
Family Bufonidae	Bufo boreas halophilus	Western toad	502			Crescitelli, 1958
	B. bufo	(tadpole)	502			Muntz and Reuter, 1966
	B. marinus		501			Crescitelli, 1958
	B. terrestris		503			Crescitelli, 1958
	Hyla regilla	Pacific tree frog	501			Crescitelli, 1958
	Microhyla olivacea		504			Crescitelli, 1958
Class Reptilia						
Order Chelonia Family Chelonidae	Chelonia midas				440[g,i] 502[f,g,i] 562[g,i]	Liebman and Granda, 1971
Family Emydidae	Pseudemys scripta scripta				450[g,j] 518[f,g,j] 620[g,j]	Liebman and Granda, 1971

Taxon	Species	Common name	Pigment type and λ_{max} in nm			Reference
			A_1	A_2	not known	
Order Crocodilia						
Family Crocodylidae	*Crocodylus niloticus*	Nile crocodile	526			DARTNALL and LYTHGOE, 1965
Family Alligatoridae	*Alligator mississippiensis*	Mississippi alligator	c. 506 499			CRESCITELLI, 1956b, 1958 WALD, BROWN and KENNEDY, 1957
Order Sauria						
Family Eublepharidae	*Coleonyx variegatus* Gray		c. 516			CRESCITELLI, 1958, 1963a
Family Sphaerodactylidae	*Sphaerodactylus parkeri* Grant		c. 528			CRESCITELLI, 1958, 1963a
Family Gekkonidae	*Aristelliger praesignis* (Hallowell)		c. 500[p] 530[p]			CRESCITELLI, 1958, 1963a
	Oedura lesueuri (Dum. et Bib.)		518			CRESCITELLI, 1958
	O. monilis		457 518			CRESCITELLI, 1958, 1963a
	O. robusta		c. 490			CRESCITELLI, 1956b, 1958, 1963a
	Phyllurus milii (White)		524			CRESCITELLI, 1958, 1963a
	Gehyra mutilata (Wiegmann)		518[p]			CRESCITELLI, 1958, 1963a
	G. variegatus Dum. et Bib.		528[p]			CRESCITELLI, 1958, 1963a
	Gekko gekko (L.)		478 521			CRESCITELLI, 1963b
	G. gekko				467[f,i] 518[f,i]	LIEBMAN, Chapter 12.
	Hemidactylus frenatus Dum. et Bib.		c. 490 520			CRESCITELLI, 1958, 1963a
	H. turcicus (L.)		520—523[p]			CRESCITELLI, 1958, 1963a
	Tarentola mauritanica (L.)		528[p]			CRESCITELLI, 1958, 1963a
Order Serpentes						
Family Crotalidae	*Crotalus viridis helleri*	Rattlesnake	500			CRESCITELLI, 1958

Taxon	Species	Common name	Pigment type and λ_{max} in nm			Reference
			A_1	A_2	not known	
Class Aves						
Order Pelecaniformes						
Family **Pelecanidae**	*Pelicanus occidentalis*	Pelican	502			CRESCITELLI, 1958
Order Anseriformes						
Family **Anatidae**	*Anas boschas*	Duck	502			BRIDGES, 1962
Order Galliformes						
Family **Phasianidae**	*Gallus gallus*	Chicken	500 563			BLISS, 1946 (see DARTNALL, 1952)
	G. gallus	Chicken	500 560			WALD, BROWN and SMITH, 1955
	G. gallus	Chicken			500[4,i] 562[a,i]	LIEBMAN, Chapter 12.
	Colinus virginianus	Bobwhite quail	500			SILLMAN, 1969
	Lophortyx californicus	California quail	500			SILLMAN, 1969
Family **Meleagrididae**	*Meleagris* sp.	Broad breasted bronze turkey	c. 505 562			CRESCITELLI, WILSON and LILYBLADE, 1964
Order Charadriiformes						
Family **Laridae**	*Larus occidentalis*	Gull	501			CRESCITELLI, 1958
	L. atricilla	Laughing gull			508[4,i] 562[a,i]	LIEBMAN and HAILMAN *ex* LIEBMAN, Chapter 12.
Order Columbiformes						
Family **Columbidae**	*Columba livia*	Pigeon	502 544			BRIDGES, 1962
	C. livia	Pigeon			500[4,i] 562[a,i]	LIEBMAN, Chapter 12.
	C. livia	Pigeon	502			SILLMAN, 1969
	Zenaidura macroura	Mourning dove	502			SILLMAN, 1969
	Streptopelia risoria	Ringneck dove	502			SILLMAN, 1969

Taxon	Species	Common name	Pigment type and λ_{max} in nm			Reference
			A_1	A_2	not known	
Order Psittaciformes						
Family Psittacidae	Melopsittacus undulatus	Parakeet	504-505			SILLMAN, 1969
Order Strigiformes						
Family Strigidae	Bubo virginianus	Great horned owl	502			CRESCITELLI, 1958
	Otus asio	Screech owl	503			CRESCITELLI, 1958
	Speotyto cunicularia	Burrowing owl	503			SILLMAN, 1969
Order Caprimulgiformes						
Family Caprimulgidae	Phalaenoptilus nuttallii	Poor-will	506			SILLMAN, 1969
Order Passeriformes						
Family Icteridae	Molothrus ater	Cowbird	501			SILLMAN, 1969
Family Fringillidae	Carpodacus mexicanus	House finch	502			SILLMAN, 1969
	Zonotrichia leucophrys	White crowned sparrow	502			SILLMAN, 1969
Family Estrildidae[r]	Poephila castanotis	Zebra finch	502			SILLMAN, 1969
	Lonchura domestica[r]	Bengalese finch	c. 490			SILLMAN, 1969
			502			SILLMAN, 1969
Class Mammalia						
Order Marsupiala						
Family Didelphidae	Didelphis marsupialis virginiana	Opossum	494			CRESCITELLI, 1958
Order Edentata						
Family Bradypodidae	Bradypus tridactylus	Three-toed sloth	493			CRESCITELLI, 1958
Order Primates						
Family Lorisidae	Galago crassicaudatus agisymbanus Coquerel	Bush tailed bush baby	502			DARTNALL, ARDEN, IKEDA, LUCK, ROSENBERG, PEDLER and TANSLEY, 1966
Family Cercopithecidae	Macaca mulatta	Rhesus monkey	497			BRIDGES, 1959
	M. mulatta	Rhesus monkey			503[t.i] 527[g.i] 565[g.i]	BROWN and WALD, 1963
Family Simiidae	Pan sp.	Chimpanzee	491			CRESCITELLI, 1958

Taxon	Species	Common name	Pigment tape and λ_{max} in nm			Reference
			A_1	A_2	not known	
Family Hominidae	*Homo sapiens*	Man	497			Crescitelli and Dartnall, 1953
	H. sapiens	Man	493			Wald and Brown, 1958
	H. sapiens	Man			450[g,i] 505[g,i] 525[g,i] 555[g,i]	Brown and Wald, 1963
	H. sapiens	Man			440[g,i] 498[f,i] 535[g,i] 575[g,i]	Liebman, Chapter 12.
Order Lagomorpha						
Family Leporidae	*Oryctolagus cuniculus*	Rabbit	502			Bridges, 1959
Order Rodentia						
Family Heteromyidae	*Perognathus lengimembris*	Little pocket mouse	501[p]			Crescitelli, 1958
	Dipodomys deserti	Desert kangaroo rat	501			Crescitelli, 1958
	D. merriami	Merriam kangaroo rat	501			Crescitelli, 1958
	D. mohavensis	Mohave kangaroo rat	501			Crescitelli, 1958
Family Sciuridae	*Sciurus carolinensis leucotis*	Grey squirrel	502			Dartnall, 1960
Family Caviidae	*Cavia porcellus*	Guinea pig	497			Bridges, 1959
Family Muridae	*Cricetus auratus*	Golden hamster	502			Bridges, 1959
	Onychomys torridus	Grashopper mouse	500			Crescitelli, 1958
	Neotoma lepida	Wood rat	498			Crescitelli, 1958
	Rattus rattus	Rat	498			Bridges, 1959
	Mus musculus domesticus	Mouse	498			Bridges, 1959
Order Cetacea						
Family Balaenopteridae	*Megaptera nodosa*	Hump-backed whale	492			Dartnall, 1962
Family Eschrichtiidae	*Eschrichtius gibbosus*	Gray whale	496.9			McFarland, 1971
Family Ziphiidae	*Berardius bairdii*	Beaked whale	481.1			McFarland, 1971

Taxon	Species	Common name	Pigment type and λ_{max} in nm			Reference
			A_1	A_2	not known	
Family Delphinidae [continued]	*Pseudorca crassidens*	False killer whale	486.5			McFarland, 1971
	Cephalorhynchus commersoni	Piebald dolphin	485.4			McFarland, 1971
	Delphinus delphis	Saddle backed dolphin	488.9			McFarland, 1971
	Lagenorhynchus australis	Dusky dolphin	485.9			McFarland, 1971
	Lagenorhynchus obliquidens	Pacific whitesided dolphin	485.5			McFarland, 1971
	Stenella attenuata	Narrow-snouted dolphin	485.7			McFarland, 1971
	Stenella sp	Hawaiian spinning porpoise	485.4			McFarland, 1971
	Tursiops truncatus gilli	Pacific bottlenose dolphin	486.0			McFarland, 1971
Order Pinnepedia Family Phocidae	*Mirounga leonina* L.	Southern elephant seal	485.5			Lythgoe and Dartnall, 1971
	Leptonychotes weddelli (Lesson)	Weddell seal	495.5			Lythgoe and Dartnall, 1971
Order Carnivora Family Procyonidae	*Procyon lotor psora*	Raccoon	500[a]			Crescitelli, 1958
Order Artiodactyla Family Hippopotamidae	*Hippopotamus amphibius*	Hippopotamus	499			Dartnall and Lythgoe, 1965
Family Bovidae	*Bos taurus*	Ox	499			Collins and Morton, 1950
			499			Dartnall, 1962

Notes

  [a] The λ_{max} of this visual pigment is now considered to be one nm shorter in wavelength than originally described by Dartnall and Lythgoe, 1965. The difference spectra published in this paper was referenced to an extract of frog rhodopsin then considered to have a λ_{max} of 502 nm but now considered to have a λ_{max} of 501 nm.

  [b] This extract also contained small amounts of an A_1-based visual pigment, λ_{max} about 471 nm.

  [c] This extract contained a minor amount of a pigment of undetermined category and of λ_{max} about 505 nm.

  [d] The list of Salmonid visual pigments has been copied from the list given by Bridges in this volume (Chapter 11).

Notes (continued)

  e A$_2$-based pigment also present, but in too small amount for λ_{max} determination.

  f Microspectrophotometric measurements from cells identified as rods.

  g Microspectrophotometric measurements from cells identified as cones.

  h Microspectrophotometric measurements from cells not certainly identified.

  i Visual pigment believed, from evidence other than microspectrophotometry, to be A$_1$-based.

  j Visual pigment believed, from evidence other than microspectrophotometry, to be A$_2$-based.

  k Trace of A$_1$-based pigment present in extract, but in too small amount for λ_{max} determination.

  l λ_{max} (with 13 nm correction) reported as 496 nm; mean λ_{max} of difference spectrum reported as 497 nm.

  m WALKER (1956) gives $\lambda_{max} = 497$ nm.

  n An A$_1$-based pigment was also present but its λ_{max} could only be approximately located in the region 499 nm.

  o REUTER (1966) considered that the λ_{max} for the green-rod pigment of *Rana temporaria* was 440 nm since this was the λ_{max} of the difference spectrum after bleaching with 462 nm light. However, DARTNALL (1967) has shown that spectral overlap between pigment and photoproduct absorption bands would have displaced the difference spectrum to longer wavelengths; and by direct comparison with *Rana cancrivora* the green-rod pigment should have λ_{max} at c. 433 nm.

  p Where the relevant data exists for Geckoes there seems to be no difference in λ_{max} between difference spectra obtained with and without hydroxylamine. In these cases, therefore, the 2-nm correction normally subtracted from the observed difference spectrum obtained in the absence of hydroxylamine (DARTNALL, 1962) has not been applied.

  q In contrast to footnote p, where birds and mammals are concerned, the presence of hydroxylamine does indeed lower the λ_{max} of the difference spectra. Thus a 2 nm correction has been applied to the results obtained in the absence of hydroxylamine.

  r SILLMAN also reports experimental data from other members of the Passeriformes, namely the Red eared waxbill *Estrilda troglodytes*, the African silverbill *Lonchura cantans*, the Chestnut mannikin *L. ferruginosa* and the White browed weaver *Plocepasser mahali*, which suggest that these birds also possess visual pigments in the region of 502 nm and a secondary pigment at 480—490 nm.

  s Unless otherwise stated, the visual pigments reported from the order Salientia are from the adult animal.

References

BEATTY, D. D.: A study of the succession of visual pigments in Pacific salmon (*Oncorhynchus*). Canad. J. Zool. **44**, 429—455 (1966).
— Visual pigments of three species of cartilaginous fish. Nature (Lond.) **222**, 285 (1969a).
— Visual pigments of the burbot *Lota lota* and seasonal changes in their relative proportions. Vision Res. **9**, 1173—1183 (1969b).
BLISS, A. F.: The chemistry of daylight vision. J. gen. Physiol. **29**, 277—297 (1946).
BRIDGES, C. D. B.: The visual pigments of the rainbow trout (*Salmo irideus*). J. Physiol. (Lond.) **134**, 620—629 (1956).
— Cationic extracting agents for rhodopsin and their mode of action. Biochem. J. **66**, 375—383 (1957).
— The visual pigments of some common laboratory mammals. Nature (Lond.) **184**, 1727—1728 (1959).

BRIDGES, C. D. B.: Visual pigments of the pigeon (*Columba livia*). Vision Res. **2**, 125—137 (1962).
— Periodicity of absorption properties in pigments based on vitamin A_2 from fish retinae. Nature (Lond.) **203**, 303—304 (1964).
— Absorption properties, interconversions and environmental adaptation of pigments from fish photoreceptors. Cold Spr. Harb. Symp. quant. Biol. **30**, 317—334 (1965).
— Spectroscopic properties of porphyropsins. Vision Res. **7**, 349—369 (1967).
— YOSHIKAMI, S.: Distribution and evolution of visual pigments in Salmonid fishes. Vision Res. **10**, 609—626 (1970a).
— — The rhodopsin-porphyropsin system in freshwater fishes — I. Effects of age and photic environment. Vision Res. **10**, 1315—1332 (1970b).
BROWN, P. K., WALD, G.: Visual pigments in human and monkey retinas. Nature (Lond.) **200**, 37—43 (1963).
COLLINS, F. D. and MORTON, R. A.: Studies on rhodopsin. I. Methods of extraction and the absorption spectrum. Biochem. J. **47**, 3—10 (1950).
CRESCITELLI, F.: The nature of the lamprey visual pigment. J. gen. Physiol. **39**, 423—435 (1956a).
— The nature of the gecko visual pigment. J. gen. Physiol. **40**, 217—231 (1956b).
— The natural history of visual pigments. In: Photobiology, pp. 30—51. Corvallis: Oregon State College 1958.
— The duplicity theory; a phylogenetic view. In: The general physiology of cell specialization. (Ed. by D. MAZIA and A. TYLER), pp. 367—392. New York: McGraw Hill 1963a.
— The photosensitive retinal pigment system of *Gekko gekko*. J. gen. Physiol. **47**, 33—52 (1963b).
— The visual pigment of chimaeroid fish. Vision Res. **9**, 1407—1414 (1969).
— DARTNALL, H. J. A.: Human visual purple. Nature (Lond.) **172**, 195—196 (1953).
— — A photosensitive pigment of the carp retina. J. Physiol. (Lond.) **125**, 607—627 (1954).
— WILSON, B. W., LILYBLADE, A. L.: The visual pigments of birds. 1. The turkey. Vision Res. **4**, 275—280 (1964).
DARTNALL, H. J. A.: Visual pigment 467, a photosensitive pigment present in tench retinae. J. Physiol. (Lond.) **116**, 257—289 (1952).
— Visual pigments of the bleak (*Alburnus lucidus*). J. Physiol. (Lond.) **128**, 131—156 (1955).
— Further observations on the visual pigments of the clawed toad Xenopus laevis. J. Physiol. **134**, 327—338 (1956).
— The Visual Pigments. London: Methuen & Co. Ltd. 1957.
— Visual pigment from a pure-cone retina. Nature (Lond.) **188**, 475—479 (1960).
— The photobiology of visual processes. In: The Eye, Vol. 2, (Ed. H. Davson) pp. 523—533. New York-London: Academic Press 1962.
— The visual pigment of the green rods. Vision Res. **7**, 1—16 (1967).
— ARDEN, G. B., IKEDA, H., LUCK, C. P., ROSENBERG, M. E., PEDLER, C. M. H., TANSLEY, K.: Anatomical electrophysiological and pigmentary aspects of vision in the bush baby: an interpretative study. Vision Res. **5**, 399—424 (1966).
— LYTHGOE, J. N.: The spectral clustering of visual pigments. Vision Res. **5**, 81—100 (1965).
DONNER, K. O., REUTER, T.: The spectral sensitivity and photo-pigment of the green rods in the frog's retina. Vision Res. **2**, 357—372 (1962).
LIEBMAN, P. A., ENTINE, G.: Cyanopsin: a visual pigment of retinal origin. Nature (Lond.) **216**, 501—503 (1968).
— GRANDA, A. M.: Microspectrophotometric measurements of visual pigments in two species of turtle, *Pseudemys scripta* and *Chelonia mydas*. Vision Res. **11**, 105—114 (1971).
LYTHGOE, J. N., DARTNALL, H. J. A.: A "deep-sea rhodopsin" in a mammal. Nature (Lond.) **227**, 955—956 (1971).
LYTHGOE, R. J.: The absorption spectrum of visual purple and of indicator yellow. J. Physiol. (Lond.) **89**, 331—358 (1937).
MCFARLAND, W. N.: Visual pigment of *Callorhinchus callorynchus*, a southern hemisphere chimaeroid fish. Vision Res. **10**, 939—942 (1970).
— Cetacean visual pigments. Vision Res. **11**, 1065—1076 (1971).
MARKS, W. B.: Visual pigments of single goldfish cones. J. Physiol. (Lond.) **178**, 14—32 (1965).

Muntz, W. R. A., Reuter, T.: Visual pigments and spectral sensitivity in *Rana temporaria* and other European tadpoles. Vision Res. **6**, 601—618 (1966).

Munz, F. W.: A new photosensitive pigment of the euryhaline teleost, *Gillichthys mirabilis*. J. gen. Physiol. **40**, 233—249 (1956).

— The photosensitive retinal pigments of marine and euryhaline teleost fishes. Ph. D. thesis. University of California, L.A., 1957.

— Photosensitive pigments from the retinae of certain deep-sea fishes. J. Physiol. (Lond.) **140**, 220—235 (1958a).

— The photosensitive retinal pigments of fishes from relatively turbid coastal waters. J. gen. Physiol. **42**, 445—459 (1958b).

— Retinal pigments of a labrid fish. Nature (Lond.) **181**, 1012—1013 (1958c).

— The visual pigments of epipelagic and rocky-shore fishes. Vision Res. **4**, 441—454 (1964).

— Adaptation of visual pigments to the photic environment. Ciba foundation symposium. Colour Vision, Physiology and Experimental Psychology, pp. 27—45. London: J. & A. Churchill 1965.

— Beatty, D. D.: A critical analysis of the visual pigments of salmon and trout. Vision Res. **5**, 1—17 (1965).

— McFarland, W. N.: A suggested hereditary mechanism for visual pigments of chars (*Salvelinus* spp.). Nature (Lond.) **206**, 955—956 (1965).

Reuter, T.: The synthesis of photosensitive pigments in the rods of the frog's retina. Vision Res. **6**, 15—28 (1966).

Saito, Z.: Isolierung der Stäbchenaußenglieder und spektrale Untersuchung des daraus hergestellten Sehpurpurextraktes. Tohoku J. exp. Med. **32**, 432—446 (1938).

Sillman, A. J.: The visual pigments of several species of birds. Vision Res. **9**, 1063—1077 (1969).

Schwanzara, S. A.: The visual pigments of freshwater fishes. Vision Res. **7**, 121—148 (1967).

Wald, G.: The metamorphosis of visual systems in the sea lamprey. J. gen. Physiol. **40**, 901—914 (1957).

— The significance of vertebrate metamorphosis. Science **128**, 1481—1490 (1958).

— The distribution and evolution of visual systems. In: Comparative Biochemistry, Vol. I. New York-London: Academic Press 1960.

— Brown, P. K.: Human rhodopsin. Science **127**, 222—226 (1958).

— — Kennedy, D.: The visual system of the alligator. J. gen. Physiol. **40**, 703—713 (1957).

— — Smith, P. H.: Iodopsin. J. gen. Physiol. **38**, 623—681 (1955).

Walker, M. A.: Homogeneity tests on visual pigment solutions from two sea fish. J. Physiol. (Lond.) **133**, 56 p. (1956).

Williams, T. P.: On the preparation of very concentrated solutions of visual pigments. Vision Res. **8**, 315—316 (1968).

Chapter 16

Structure of Invertebrate Photoreceptors

By

RICHARD M. EAKIN, Berkeley, California (USA)

With 59 Figures

Contents

Every explorer is thrilled by the unique and the beautiful. How great must have been the wonder of the first men to view the Grand Canyon of the Colorado, Victoria Falls, Fujiyama on a brilliant winter day, or the planet Earth from outer space. So has it been for me in my explorations of photoreceptors. The last time I conducted a tour of them it was down uncertain and treacherous evolutionary streams (EAKIN, 1968). On the present expedition I shall follow a different route and invite the traveler's attention only to the unique and the beautiful. I hope that he will be impressed with the astounding diversity in nature. Our journey excludes vertebrate photoreceptors. This is fortunate because, from the standpoint of variation in architecture, they are dull and uninteresting. True, there are minor differences between most rods and cones, but all are constructed on the same plan, a stack of disks — even the receptors of the ancient third eye. The pattern is still magnificent, but invertebrate photoreceptors offer a much greater variety.

Our itinerary calls for the subdivision of a photoreceptoral cell into three parts: the receptoral organelle, the cell body including any extensions of the cell from which the light-sensitive apparatus arises, and the neurite. In addition, we shall examine briefly three important structures associated with receptors, namely, lenses, pigmented or supportive cells, and tapeta (reflecting layers).

I. Receptoral Organelles

Nature has produced light-sensitive organelles in most animals in one of two fashions. Either a cilium is modified in various ways, or the plasma membrane of the sensory cell is evaginated to form villi or lamellae. The first pattern I have termed ciliary; the second, rhabdomeric (EAKIN, 1963, 1966, 1968). In the final analysis both types are derivatives of the cell membrane, for the membrane of a cilium is actually the everted plasma membrane of the receptoral cell. It is probable that the membranous character of animal photoreceptors has physiological significance, namely, to provide an extensive surface on which a photopigment may be spread in a monomolecular layer and in a fixed orientation for maximal effectiveness in capturing photons (WALD, BROWN, and GIBBONS, 1963). Indeed, other photoreceptors that lie beyond the scope of this chapter, such as the thylakoids of chloroplasts and the chromophores of bacteria, are also systems of membranes. This does not imply that cells without membranous receptors are unresponsive to light. Amphibian melanophores, for example, are photosensitive, and electrical responses can be recorded from simple skin upon illumination with intense flashes of light (BECKER and CONE, 1966). These early receptor potentials are thought to be caused by heat-activation of a sodium pump (BECKER and GOLDSMITH, 1968). And so-called dermal light sensitivity is widespread among invertebrates (see MILLOT, 1968).

A. Ciliary Photoreceptors

It is not surprising that nature has adapted the cilium as a photoreceptor because cilia are ubiquitous, ranging from algae and protozoa to the ginkgo tree and man. Moreover, this adaptation is probably a very early one for, as we shall see, light-sensitive cilia are thought to exist in certain protists. In this essay no distinction is made between a cilium and a flagellum. The external surfaces of

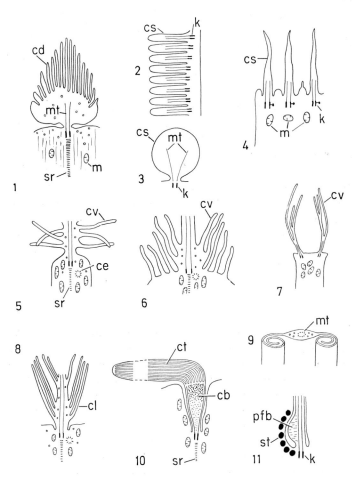

Figs. 1—11. Ciliary photoreceptors. Fig. 1. Ascidian, EAKIN and KUDA, unpublished; Figs. 2 and 3. Sabellid annelid, based on KRASNE and LAWRENCE, 1966; Fig. 4. Scallop, modified from BARBER, EVANS, and LAND, 1967; Fig. 5. Hydromedusan, modified from EAKIN and WESTFALL, 1962b; Fig. 6. Sea star, based upon EAKIN and WESTFALL, unpublished; Fig. 7. Nereid annelid, modified from DHAINAUT-COURTOIS, 1965; Fig. 8. Amphioxus, based on EAKIN and WESTFALL, 1962a; Fig. 9. Comb-jelly (ctenophore), based on HORRIDGE, 1964; Fig. 10. Arrowworm (chaetognath), based on EAKIN and WESTFALL, 1964b; Fig. 11. *Euglena*, based on LEEDALE, MEEUSE, and PRINGSHEIM, 1965. *cb*, conical body; *cd*, ciliary disk; *ce*, centriole; *cl*, ciliary lamella; *cs*, ciliary sac; *ct*, ciliary tubules; *cv*, ciliary villi; *k*, kinetosome (ciliary basal body or axial centriole); *m*, mitochondria; *mt*, microtubules; *pfb*, paraflagellar body; *sr*, striated rootlet; *st*, stigma (eyespot)

lower organisms are clothed with these motile organelles; they constitute the frontier of the organism; photic, chemical and mechanical stimuli reach them first; and nature has modified them into photoreceptors, chemoreceptors, and mechano-receptors. The alterations consist of remodelling the ciliary membrane in various ways, to be detailed below, and usually in a reduction of the complex of microtubules within the cilium. Instead of nine peripheral doublets of microtubules and two central singlets — the typical pattern in motile cilia — sensory cilia, with few exceptions, have an arrangement of nine peripheral doublets but no central tubules (9 + 0 pattern). Moreover, modified cilia typically lack the ATPase-containing arms (GIBBONS, 1965) commonly found on the inner microtubules (microtubule a) of the peripheral doublets. Consequently, they are presumed to be non-motile.

1. Disks

One way in which the ciliary membrane has been transformed into a photo-receptive organelle is by multiple infolding to form a stack of disks. The classic examples are the rods and cones of vertebrate eyes. The only invertebrates so far known to have ciliary disks are larval ascidians. DILLY (1961, 1964) observed stacks of 15 to 20 nm-thick plates in the ocelli of three species of ascidians, *Ciona intestinalis*, *Phallusia mammillata* and *Ascidia nigra*. A series of disks constitutes an outer segment of a receptoral process that extends from the distal end of a sensory cell. No evidence was presented that the disks are derived from a cilium. The so-called tubular part of the cell, which he homologizes with the connecting piece of a cilium, is not typically ciliary; it contains 50 to 100 filaments instead of the usual ring of 9 doublets of microtubules. DILLY (personal communication) has found centrioles in the sensory cells, but whether they are kinetosomes (ciliary basal bodies) is not clear.

To clarify the nature of the ascidian photoreceptor for the purpose of this chapter we (EAKIN and KUDA) have examined the ocellus in the tadpole of an ascidian, *Distaplia occidentalis*. The sensory cells are arranged in relation to the pigmented cup and the lens cells as in the tunicates studied by DILLY. Bulb-like photoreceptoral processes, clearly ciliary in nature (Figs. 1, 12), project from the distal ends of the sensory cells into the ocellar cavity, a narrow space between pigmented cup and lens cells. Each lobate process is attached to the cell proper by a narrow connecting piece through which runs the 9 + 0 assembly of microtubules from a kinetosome. The process is deeply dissected by infoldings (or disks) of the ciliary membrane which do not lie at right angles to the cilium as do vertebrate rod and cone disks. The infoldings (perhaps they should be called lamellae, see below) are open to the ocellar cavity. Note in Fig. 12 the long striated rootlet from the base of the kinetosome, a part of an accessory centriole, and numerous microtubules oriented lengthwise in the sensory cell body. The microtubules are probably the filaments described by DILLY.

Since I first wrote this chapter the above-mentioned study of the ocellus in tadpoles of two ascidians, *D. occidentalis* and *Ciona intestinalis*, has been published (EAKIN and KUDA, 1971). And I have been privileged to read a paper in proof by BARNES (1971) on the fine structure of photoreceptors in the tadpole of *Amaroucium constellatum*. We are in agreement on all major aspects of the ultrastructure of the ascidian photoreceptors studied, as illustrated by Figs. 1 and 12 of this chapter.

Another example of an invertebrate photoreceptor constructed of disks has been described recently in a publication by DILLY (1969) on the eye of a prosobranch mollusk, *Pterotrachea mutica*. This remarkable photoreceptor resembles the outer segment of a vertebrate rod or cone, being a stack of several hundred "folded membranes" (I prefer to call them disks) oriented at right angles to the longitudinal axis of the sensory cell and to the direction of

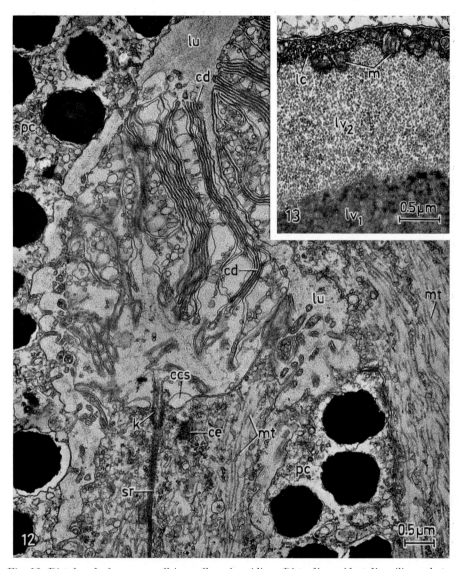

Fig. 12. Distal end of sensory cell in ocellus of ascidian, *Distaplia occidentalis*; ciliary photo-receptor cut lengthwise. *ccs*, circumciliary space; *cd*, ciliary disks; *ce*, accessory centriole; *k*, kinetosome (basal body or axial centriole); *lu*, lumen; *mt*, microtubules; *pc*, pigmented cell; *sr*, striated rootlet. EAKIN and KUDA, hitherto unpublished

Fig. 13. Part of lens cell of *D. occidentalis*. *lc*, thin layer of lens cell cytoplasm; lv_1, dense core of lens vesicle; lv_2, less dense cortex of lens vesicle; *m*, mitochondria. EAKIN and KUDA, hitherto unpublished

incident light. Whereas the disks of a vertebrate rod or cone are derived from a single cilium, the disks in each stack in *Pterotrachea* are said by DILLY to develop from an estimated 75 to 100 cilia.

There are several aspects of DILLY's study that are unclear to me. He speaks of "ciliary bases with a 9 + 0 arrangement of filaments" and of the usual association of this pattern with "cilia that subserve a sensory function." His so-called ciliary bases appear to be kinetosomes, which like all centrioles have a pattern of nine triplets of microtubules but no central ones. I do not observe an axoneme in his figures, that is, ciliary tubules distal to the kinetosome. The ciliary processes which are said to give rise to one disk each, or possibly more by branching, arise from the cell membrane beside or above the centriole. They do not bear microtubules. Accordingly, without more information, I would hesitate to call the receptor truly ciliary in type. I admit, however, that this interpretation may be hair-splitting (cilia-splitting!) because with undeniable centrioles present one has the makings of cilia or perhaps remnants of cilia. A study of the development of this photoreceptor would be instructive in resolving the question.

I puzzle also over the relationship of the distalmost disks to the kinetosomes. They lie 15 μm away from the base of the stack without any apparent connection to the parent cell. I suggest the possibility that the processes develop as outfoldings of the cell membrane, flatten to become disks, bend over to form an array, and then separate from the cell surface. However, centrioles may serve as organizers, inducing the formation of the processes. The procedure is repeated and new disks are added to the base of the stack. If true, the growth of the pile of disks would be somewhat analagous to the growth of vertebrate rods, so elegantly demonstrated by YOUNG (for references see YOUNG, 1971).

2. Sacs

These organelles have been found in the unique eyes on the branchial filaments of certain polychaete worms, *Branchiomma vesiculosum* by KRASNE and LAWRENCE (1966) and *Dasychone bombyx* by KERNÉIS (1968)[1]. The ciliary sacs (Figs. 2, 3) in these annelids differ from the ciliary disks of tunicates just considered. The latter are like rod and cone disks in being derived from the ciliary membrane; each disk is *part* of a cilium, namely, one invagination of its membrane. An individual sac (Fig. 3) in these sabellids, on the other hand, is a *whole* cilium expanded and flattened into a membranous saccule, the cavity of which is usually 3 to 6 nm in depth. About 450 sacs in *B. vesiculosum* (70—100 in *D. bombyx*) are piled upon one another (Fig. 2) to constitute the proximal segment of the photoreceptoral cell. Every sac attaches to a kinetosome from which the microtubules (9 + 0 pattern) splay out within the intra-saccular space. At present we can only presume that the ciliary sacs are photosensitive, although there is no reason to doubt the assumption (see KRASNE and LAWRENCE, 1966).

A lamellibranch mollusk, *Pecten maximus*, also possesses ciliary sacs in its remarkable eyes — a row of 60 blue "lights" on both upper and lower borders of the mantle. The retina of each ocellus has two layers of sensory cells: distal (closer to lens) and proximal. It is the former that exhibits ciliary photoreceptors; the latter has the rhabdomeric type (see below). The sacs (Fig. 4) arise from the inner ends of the distal cells, that is, facing the lens (BARBER, EVANS, and LAND, 1967). Whereas in the sabellid worms just mentioned the ciliary sacs are stacked vertically in a column, in *Pecten* (also in a cockle, *Cardium edule*, see BARBER and LAND, 1967) the sacs stand on edge in a row. Frequently groups of them form whorls as first

---

[1] According to HARTMAN (1959) *Branchiomma vesiculosum* should be *Megalomma vesiculosum* (MONTAGU) 1915 and *Dasychone bombyx* should be *Branchiomma bombyx* (DALYELL) 1853.

noted by MILLER (1958) in *Pecten irradians*. The sacs are attached by short stalks to the surface of the cell immediately above their kinetosomes. The microtubules (9 + 0 pattern) emerge from the kinetosomes and spread out into the sacs as in the branchial ocelli of sabellids. The function of the distal sensory cells will be mentioned later in connection with the proximal cells.

3. Microvilli

The sensory cells in the ocelli of hydromedusae and sea stars possess prominent cilia to which microvilli connect. In a hydromedusan, *Polyorchis penicillatus*, the microvilli (Figs. 5, 14, 15) project from the sides of the ciliary shaft (EAKIN and WESTFALL, 1962b; EAKIN and BRANDENBURGER, unpublished). The microvilli are neither straight nor regularly arranged, and they intermingle with villous processes from adjacent pigmented cells. Consequently, the eyecup contains a mass of tangled tubules, which earlier workers incorrectly regarded as a lens (LITTLE, 1914) or as a vitreous body (LINKO, 1900). The pattern of microtubules (Fig. 15) in the ocellar cilia is 9 + 2!

The fine structure of several species of sea stars has been studied (see EAKIN, 1968, for references). The small, usually red, eyecups are situated on a so-called optic cushion on the oral side and near the tip of every arm. Extending from the distal ends of the sensory cells are long cilia that project into the lumen of the ocellus. Irregular microvilli arise from the base of the cilium and from the surface of the cell proper (Fig. 6). The pattern of microtubules appears to vary (see EAKIN, 1968).

Evidence that coelenterate and echinoderm ocelli are actually light-sensitive rests largely upon observations of behavior and on the changes in phototactic responses following extirpation of the eyecups (see HYMAN, 1940, 1955). For example: a hydromedusan coelenterate, *Sarsia*, exhibits positive phototaxis, aggregating in a beam of light; ablation of the ocelli abolishes the response (HYMAN, 1940). Removal of the optic cushion from an arm of a sea star, *Asterias amurensis*, raises the threshold of sensitivity of the tip of the arm by a factor of ten (YOSHIDA and OHTSUKI, 1966). Finally, photolabile pigments can be extracted from ocelli of medusae and sea stars (see GOLDSMITH, this volume, p. 685).

A third example of villous branches of cilia that probably serve a photoreceptoral function is to be found in the brain of nereid annelids (DHAINAUT-COURTOIS, 1965, 1968). A certain type of cell (type IV of DHAINAUT-COURTOIS) possesses multiple cilia at the distal end of a slender extension (sensory fiber) of the cell. Shortly above their kinetosomes the cilia are said to branch and rebranch into filaments that are circular or oval in cross sections (Fig. 7). At the bases of the sensory cilia the microtubules are ordered in the typical 9 + 0 pattern, but the nine doublets become distributed to the branches, each receiving a doublet that assumes a central position in the filament. Theoretically, each cilium should have nine branches.

An even more remarkable instance of a villous cilium that might be photosensitive is provided by the recent studies of CHAIGNEAU (1969, 1971) on the organ of Bellonci in an isopod crustacean, *Sphaeroma serratum*. This organ lies beneath the integument of the animal's head and is connected to the brain by a nerve. Each principal cell has a so-called outer segment connected to the cell by a ciliary structure. The ciliary features are a basal body that looks like a kinetosome (cross sectional views not given) from which extends proximally a distinct striated rootlet. Beyond the basal body distally there is a large number of microtubules, which do not form a typical ciliary axoneme. The microtubules terminate at the distal surface of the outer segment from which arises a multitude of long, narrow microvilli projecting in parallel array into the lumen of the organ. I say remarkable because of the large number of microtubules in

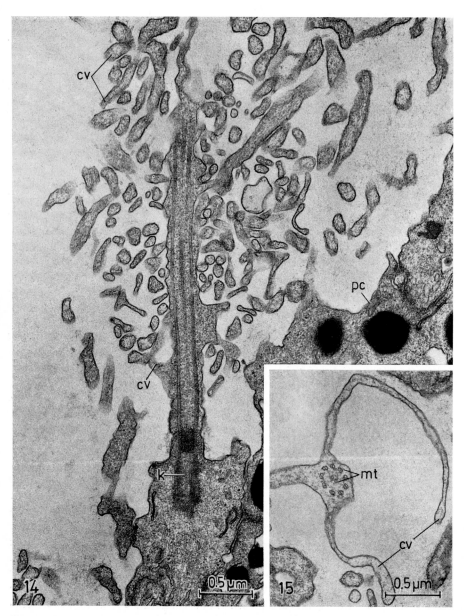

Fig. 14. Distal end of sensory cell in ocellus of hydromedusan, *Polyorchis penicillatus*, with ciliary photoreceptor cut longitudinally. *cv*, ciliary villi; *k*, kinetosome; *pc*, pigmented cell.
EAKIN and BRANDENBURGER, hitherto unpublished

Fig. 15. Cross section of ciliary photoreceptor of *P. penicillatus*. *cv*, ciliary villi; *mt*, 9 + 2 microtubules. EAKIN and BRANDENBURGER, hitherto unpublished

the outer segment and because this will be the first discovery of a ciliary photoreceptor in an arthropod if further research proves CHAIGNEAU's hypothesis that the organ of Bellonci is a photoreceptor.

4. Lamellae

Whereas the ciliary appendages just discussed appear to be cylindrical, and hence villous, in some forms they seem to be flattened extensions of the ciliary membrane and these I propose to call lamellae. Whether the distinction is real or the result of a fixation artifact needs to be determined. The branches of cilia from certain, presumably light-sensitive, cells in the brain of amphioxus (Fig. 8) are thought to be lamellae (addendum of EAKIN and WESTFALL, 1962a; EAKIN, 1963; NAKAO, 1964). The microtubules in the ciliary shaft have a 9 + 0 arrangement.

Another instance of lamellar elaborations of the ciliary membrane is to be found in the apical organ of a ctenophore or comb-jelly, *Pleurobrachia pileus*, studied by HORRIDGE (1964). He observed laminated bodies in the floor of the organ that are composed of whorls of double membranes extending laterally from one or both sides of the cilia (Fig. 9). Cross sections of the ciliary shafts reveal a 9 + 0 arrangement of microtubules. There is no biochemical or physiological evidence that these uniquely modified cilia are light-sensitive. Indeed, according to HYMAN (1940) the reaction of ctenophores to light is not very definite.

The laminated bodies observed by YANASE and SAKAMOTO (1965) in the dorsal ocelli of a gastropod, *Onchidium verruculatum*, are composed of cilia with coiled membranous lateral extensions similar to those in the ctenophore just cited. The ciliary microtubules exhibit a 9 + 0 pattern. The dorsal eyes give a distinct "off" response upon illumination and are believed to be related to the shadow reaction of the animal (FUJIMOTO, YANASE, OKUNO, and IWATA, 1966). Incidentally, the stalked eye of *Onchidium* has rhabdomeric photoreceptors (see below) and may serve as brightness discriminators (FUJIMOTO, YANASE, OKUNO, and IWATA, op. cit.). And BOYLE (1969) has recently reported whorls of membranes derived from 9 + 2 cilia at the periphery of the eye of a polyplacophoran mollusk, *Onithochiton neglectus*.

5. Tubules

In the above modifications of cilia the area of membrane, which may contain a photopigment, has been increased by various forms of outfolding. In the eye of a chaetognath or arrowworm, *Sagitta scrippsae*, the same end is served by an array of long but very narrow (50 nm) cylindrical tubules *within* the cilium (EAKIN and WESTFALL, 1964b). The manner of differentiation of the tubules has not been determined. They form the distal segments of the cilia (Figs. 10, 16, 17) which emerge from the inner ends of sensory cells, one cilium per cell, and project toward the single pigmented cell lying at the center of the eye, making it inverted in type (see p. 649). The tubules are tightly packed and longitudinally arranged and may number as many as 800 per cilium. There is little evidence, beyond analogy to other photoreceptors, that the ciliary tubules are photoreceptoral organelles (see p. 657).

The basal segments of the photosensory cilia of this chaetognath are also intriguing to morphologist and physiologist alike. Each cilium contains a cone-shaped body, the base of which abuts the tubular segment of the cilium whereas its apex adjoins the terminal plate of the kinetosome (Fig. 10, 16, 17). The nine doublets of microtubules spread out from the kinetosome and run along the surface of the conical body. The cone is composed of granules, which grade from fine in

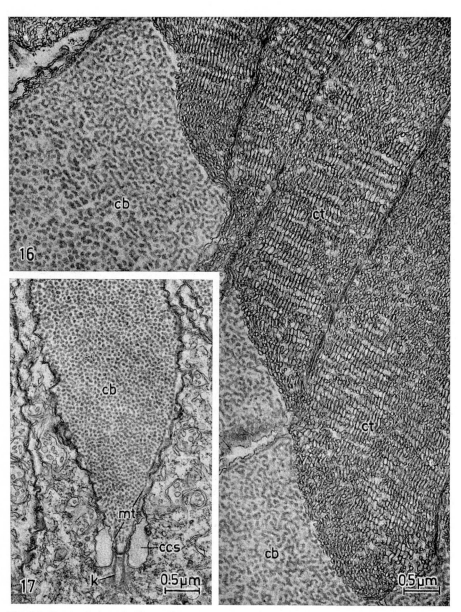

Fig. 16. Parts of several ciliary photoreceptors from eye of arrowworm, *Sagitta scrippsae*. *cb*, conical body or proximal part of cilium; *ct*, distal part of cilium composed of tubules (cut obliquely). EAKIN and WESTFALL, hitherto unpublished

Fig. 17. Basal part of conical body (*cb*) in ciliary photoreceptor of *S. scrippsae*. *ccs*, circumciliary space; k, kinetosome; *mt*, microtubules. EAKIN and WESTFALL, hitherto unpublished

the proximal half (next to the kinetosome) to coarse in the distal half. The function of this structure is an enigma. We (EAKIN and WESTFALL, 1964 b) have suggested the possibility that it has wave guide effects.

6. Paraflagellar Body

The principal or locomotory flagellum of several protists bears a basal swelling, termed paraflagellar body (Fig. 11), that appears to be a photoreceptor (see EAKIN, 1968, for references). Electron microscopy by LEEDALE, MEEUSE, and PRINGSHEIM (1965) has shown that the paraflagellar swelling in *Euglena spirogyra* lies inside the flagellar membrane and that it exhibits uniform electron density except for some striations. Further fine structural studies are urgently needed to clarify and enlarge our understanding of the nature of this organelle. It is the simplest photoreceptoral apparatus among the eukaryotes and perhaps the first evolutionary modification of a cilium (flagellum) into a light-sensitive structure, retaining meanwhile its locomotory function. Later the motile character of the organelle is absent coincidently with the disappearance of central microtubules and, probably more importantly, of the arms containing ATP-ase on the *a* tubules of the peripheral doublets.

WAGER (1900) suggested many years ago that the paraflagellar swelling was a photoreceptor rather than the eyespot (stigma), which is usually a curved plate of droplets. DIEHN (1969) concludes from studies on *Euglena gracilis* that there are two kinds of perpendicularly oriented pigment molecules shading the photoreceptor: a long-wavelength system of carotenoids and a short-wavelength system of flavonols. The stigma merely casts a shadow upon the paraflagellar body which rests in the concavity of the stigma — a conclusion borne out by the behavior of mutants. Those mutants that lack a stigma react to light; those without a paraflagellar body but with a stigma show no phototaxis (see GRELL, 1968). As a consequence of the rotational swimming movements of *Euglena* the eyespot intermittently shades the flagellar swelling from a unilaterally directed light. If the organism redirects the path of advancement toward the light (positive phototaxis) the receptor is continuously illuminated.

7. Unmodified Cilia

It has been suggested by several investigators (see EAKIN (1968), discussion, p. 215) that unmodified cilia may be light-sensitive. By unmodified, I mean without elaborations of the ciliary membrane into villi, lamellae, disks, or tubules and without a loss of the features of axonemes characteristic of motile cilia (kinocilia). They would be modified, of course, to the extent that they contain a photopigment, probably on or within the ciliary membrane or in small ciliary vesicles.

I have been privileged to read a manuscript by WOOLLACOTT and ZIMMER (1972) on the fine structure of a potential photoreceptor in the larva of a bryozoan, *Bugula neritina*. This larva, which is positively phototactic after release from the brooding parent, possesses two laterally positioned pigmented spots. Within each spot is a pit, at the base of which lies one sensory cell bearing a remarkable globular mass of recurved cilia. The cilia are said to be structurally identical with kinocilia found elsewhere on the larva, with 9 + 2 axonemes and with arms from microtubule *a* of each peripheral doublet. The ciliary membrane is fluted along the basal third of each cilium, but smooth distally. WOOLLACOTT and ZIMMER could find no other likely photoreceptoral organelle in this bryozoan larva.

I am informed by correspondence that Thomas and Boyle of Aberdeen, Scotland, have just completed a paper, which I have not seen, on the siphon spots of a tunicate, delicately colored bodies which have been thought to be light-sensitive. Not knowing of the work in progress in Aberdeen, Miss Aileen Kuda and I recently examined these structures in *Ciona intestinalis* by means of electron microscopy. Again, the only candidate for a photoreceptor seemed to be cilia in the groove at the center of the spot. I am increasingly impressed with the possibility that relatively little structural modification may be necessary to endow a kinocilium with light-sensitivity.

Professor Vinnikov and his students have stressed the catholicity of cilia in connection with not only vision and general light sensitivity but also with the other senses (see Vinnikov, 1966, 1969). There is, however, a constellation of non-ciliary photoreceptors to which we now turn.

B. Rhabdomeric Photoreceptors

The eyes of many invertebrates contain one or more arrays of microvilli or lamellae termed rhabdomeres (from the Greek ραβδος, rod, and μερος, part). The microvilli are endowed with light sensitivity by the possession of a photopigment. Although most of the evidence supporting the last statement is presumptive, it is generally accepted. More easily demonstrated, however, is the remarkable variety in pattern of form and arrangement of rhabdomeres, a stunning example of nature's versatility, as we shall see from the following selected samples.

1. Lateral Straight Microvilli

The photoreceptors of arthropods and cephalopod mollusks are classic illustrations of this pattern. Indeed, the Greek root, ραβδος, was first used by Grenacher (1879) for the prismatic rod, which he called a rhabdom, formed by clusters of retinal cells in the eyes of spiders, insects, crustaceans, octopuses, and squids. Electron microscopy has resolved this refractile rod into sectors or rhabdomeres, each composed of closely packed microvilli (Fig. 32—36). For an historical account of the analysis of the ultrastructure of a rhabdomere the reader is referred to Moody's review (1964).

Microvilli of lateral rhabdomeres (Figs. 18—26) vary in length from 500 to 5,000 nm and in diameter from 20 to 100 nm. The microvilli, sometimes called tubules, arise as outfoldings of the sensory cell membranes. When first formed they are short and irregularly disposed, but when fully differentiated they are long, finger-like, and ordered in straight arrays (Fig. 32). In some instances, as in a lobster, *Homarus vulgaris*, studied by Rutherford and Horridge (1965), a rhabdomere consists of groups of about nine microvilli joined together at their bases (Fig. 20). Each packet of villi is connected to the retinular cell by a common stem.

The extent to which the villi clothe the lateral surfaces of a retinal cell varies. In some instances (crustaceans, insects) they are restricted to one side of a sensory cell (Figs. 18, 21, 33, 34); in other animals (arachnids, cephalopods) they form on two sides, opposite to each other (Figs. 19, 32, 35, 36), and in still other forms in the groups just named they occur on three or four sides of a cell. In the epistellar body of octopods the microvilli arise from the entire perimeter of neurite-like processes of photoreceptoral cells (Nishioka, Hagadorn, and Bern, 1962). In regions where epistellar processes are in contact with one another the arrangement of their rhabdomeres resembles that (Fig. 35) in the octopus eye (Zonana, 1961). That the

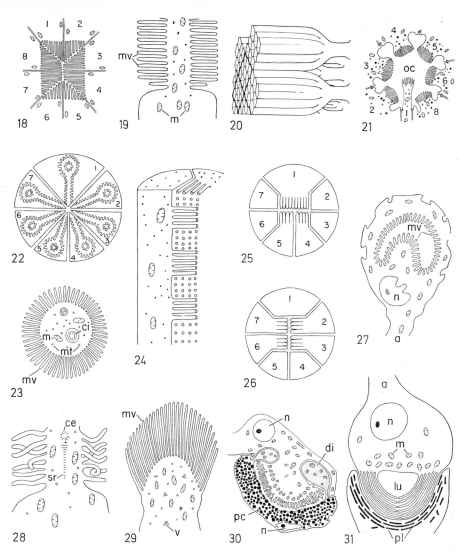

Figs. 18—31. Rhabdomeric photoreceptors. Fig. 18. Honeybee, based on GOLDSMITH, 1962; Fig. 19. Squid, based on ZONANA, 1961; Fig. 20. Groups of nine microvilli with common stalk in eye of lobster, from RUTHERFORD and HORRIDGE, 1965; Fig. 21. Fruit fly, based on Fig. 34, EAKIN and BRANDENBURGER, unpublished; Fig. 22. Spiny lobster, from EGUCHI and WATERMAN, 1966; Fig. 23. Peripatus, based on EAKIN and WESTFALL, 1965b; Fig. 24. Longitudinal sector of an ommatidium of a crayfish showing interdigitating microvilli, from EGUCHI, 1965; Figs. 25 and 26. Cross sections of ommatidia of a crayfish at different levels, from EGUCHI, 1965; Fig. 27. Photosensory cell of a leech with intracellular vesicle lined with microvilli, from RÖHLICH and TÖRÖK, 1964; Fig. 28. Nereid annelid, based on EAKIN and WESTFALL, 1964a; Fig. 29. Snail, based on EAKIN and BRANDENBURGER, 1967a; Fig. 30. Lateral ocellus of polychaete worm, from HERMANS and CLONEY, 1966; Fig. 31. Rotifer, based on EAKIN and WESTFALL, 1965a. Numbers refer to retinular cells. *a*, axon; *ce*, centriole; *ci*, cilium in peripatus unconnected to microvilli; *di*, diaphragm; *lu*, lumen of ocellus; *m*, mitochondria; *mt*, microtubules; *mv*, microvilli; *n*, nuclei; *oc*, ommatidial cavity; *pc*, pigmented cell; *pl*, plates (reflecting ?); *sr*, striated rootlet; *v*, vesicles

epistellar body is indeed photoreceptoral is borne out by the demonstration that it contains rhodopsin (NISHIOKA, YASUMASU, PACKARD, BERN and YOUNG, 1966) and that it exhibits electrophysiological activity when it is illuminated (MAURO and BAUMANN, 1968). In this connection mention should be made of the paraolfactory vesicles of decapod mollusks, which are also presumptively photo-receptive because they have rhabdomeres similar to those in the epistellar bodies and because they too possess rhodopsin (NISHIOKA, YASUMASU, PACKARD, BERN, and YOUNG, 1966). Another example in which microvilli cover all surfaces of a

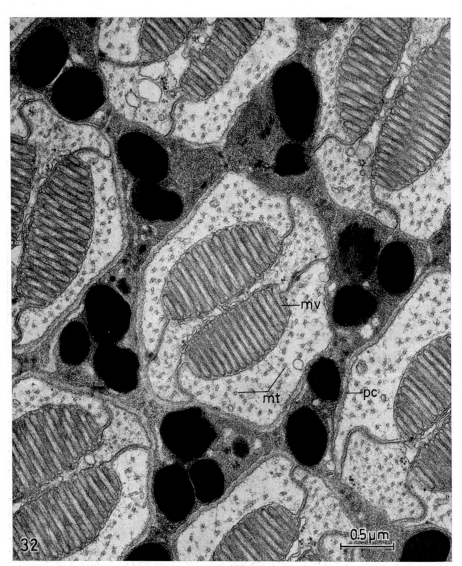

Fig. 32. Cross section of several retinal units in antero-lateral eye of jumping spider, *Phidippus johnsoni*. *mt*, microtubules; *mv*, microvilli; *pc*, pigmented cell. EAKIN and BRANDENBURGER, hitherto unpublished

cell process is the photosensitive neuron in a ganglion of a barnacle, studied by
FAHRENBACH (1965). There are seven of these neurons, the dendrites of which
branch and rebranch several times before ending in digitiform processes bearing
rhabdomeres.

In the eyes of many arthropods the rhabdom is an axial structure encircled by
retinular cells, each of which contributes a rhabdomere to the rhabdom. The cluster
of associated retinular cells and ancillary structures constitute an ommatidium. Eyes
composed of ommatidia are termed compound eyes, in contradistinction to simple
eyes and ocelli in which the retina is not subdivided into ommatidial units. In the
compound eyes of some arthropods (lobster) there are several thousand ommatidia
(EGUCHI and WATERMAN, 1966); at the other extreme, in a copepod, *Copilia
quadrata*, the eye or ocellus has but one ommatidium (WOLKEN and FLORIDA, 1969).
The number of retinular cells in an ommatidium varies greatly among arthropods,
from four in a cladoceran, *Leptodora kindtii*, studied by WOLKEN and GALLIK
(1965) to seventeen in an isopod, *Oniscus asellus*, according to DEBAISIEUX (1944),
and even twenty in some specimens of *Limulus*, as reported by FAHRENBACH
(1969).

Eyes with apposed rhabdomeres are termed *closed* (e.g., honeybee, Figs. 18, 33).
In other instances (e.g., *Drosophila*, Figs. 21, 34) the rhabdomeres are not in contact
with one another (*open* type), and the center of the ommatidium is a cavity into
which project the microvilli of the several rhabdomeres. Although GRENACHER

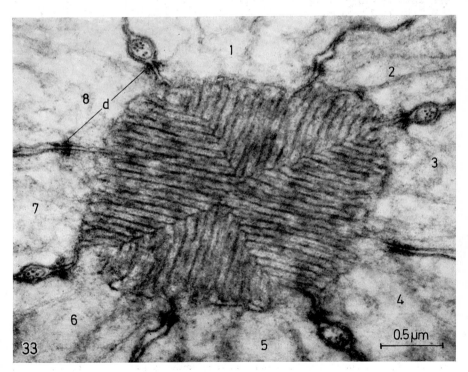

Fig. 33. Cross section of closed rhabdom of honeybee, *Apis mellifera*. Numbers 1—8, retinular
cells, each bearing a rhabdomere; *d*, desmosomes. From GOLDSMITH, 1962

(1879) used the term rhabdom for the refractile rod in closed types, its usage has been extended to include the assembly of disjunct rhabdomeres in open-type ommatidia. The significant difference between these two types may lie in their light-gathering powers, the effective cross-sectional area of closed rhabdoms being larger than that of open ones. In support of this hypothesis are the observations that, in general, ommatidia of arthropods which are active at low intensities of light (e.g., moths) are closed whereas those of diurnal forms (e.g., most dipterans) are open. An instructive exception is the open-type rhabdom of *Copilia quadrata*, which lives at a depth of 200 m in the sea where the incident light is weak. An analysis of its optical system by WOLKEN and FLORIDA (1969) showed that the one ommatidial ocellus has remarkable light-gathering power by virtue of the size, form and position of its two lenses, which may compensate for any inefficiency in the arrangement of its rhabdomeres. On the other hand, the occurrence of closed-type rhabdoms in

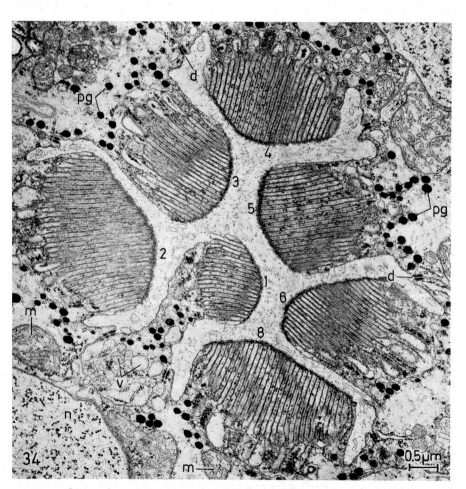

Fig. 34. Cross section of open rhabdom of fruit fly, *Drosophila melanogaster*. Numbers 1—6, 8, rhabdomeres; *d*, desmosomes; *m*, mitochondria; *n*, nucleus; *pg*, pigment granules in retinular cells; *v*, pinocytotic vesicles. EAKIN and BRANDENBURGER, hitherto unpublished

some diurnal insects (e.g., honeybee) may have arisen from evolutionary selection of a rhabdomeric pattern highly adapted for the detection of polarized light (see p. 644). Finally, there is evidence that the open-type rhabdom permits the resolution of an image by the several rhabdomeres since each one is looking at a slightly different point in space (see KUIPER, 1962).

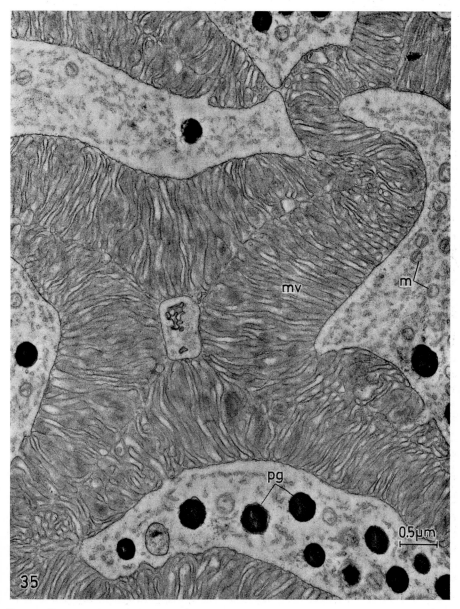

Fig. 35. Cross section of rhabdom in the eye of octopus, *Octopus bimaculatus* (?). *m*, mitochondria; *mv*, microvilli; *pg*, pigment granules in sensory cells. COURTESY of R. NISHIOKA

Since the above was written SHAW (1969) has studied the optics of open and closed rhabdoms in arthropods. He concludes that although the closed-type rhabdom is much more effective in detecting polarized light than is the open type, increase in PL sensitivity is probably of

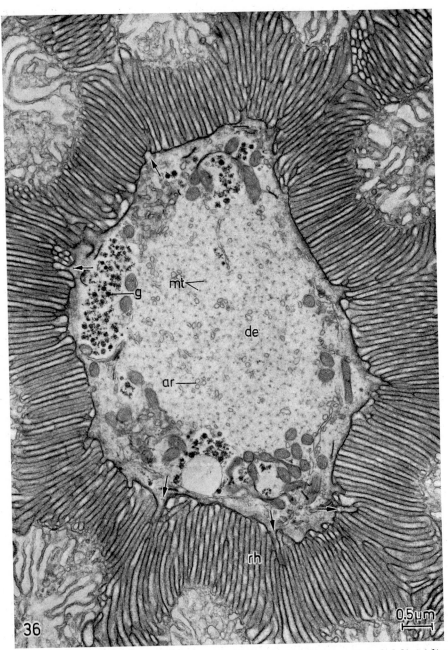

Fig. 36. Cross section of eccentric cell dendrite (*de*) and part of surrounding rhabdom (*rh*) of *Limulus* sp. *ar*, agranular reticulum; *g*, glycogen; *mt*, microtubules; arrows, short stubby microvilli of dendrite. From FAHRENBACH, 1969

secondary importance to an increase in light-gathering power. The rhabdomeres of the open type are optically distinct, light being kept inside by internal reflection. The whole rhabdom in the closed type, on the other hand, acts as a single light guide.

An eye of considerable interest to physiologists, because of a unique morphological feature, is that of a xiphosuran arthropod, *Limulus*. Each ommatidium of its compound eye is composed of 4 to 20 retinular cells (FAHRENBACH, 1969) bearing straight lateral microvilli, as first shown by MILLER (1957), *and* an eccentric cell that sends a dendritic process up the axial canal of the ommatidium. At first it was thought that the dendrite of this cell lacked microvilli, but LASANSKY (1967) found them in *Limulus polyphemus* interdigitating with those from the retinular cells, and he made the suggestion that the eccentric cell may have a photoreceptoral function. Meanwhile, EGUCHI (1962) had discovered that the eccentric cells in ommatidia of a moth, *Bombyx mori*, possess rhabdomeres. In a recent study of the compound eye of *Limulus polyphemus*, however, FAHRENBACH (1969) draws the conclusion that the microvilli of the eccentric cell provide mechanical support to the rhabdom because they are short and stubby (Fig. 36). They constitute less than 1% of the total rhabdomeric surface; therefore, they are not likely to have a significant role in photoreception, if any.

PAULA NEMANIC, currently preparing a doctoral thesis in my laboratory on the fine structure of the eye of an isopod, *Porcellio scaber*, finds an eccentric cell that is the topographic counterpart of that in *Limulus*. It lies not at the base of the ommatidium but distally beneath a *two-cell* cone (see below). The eccentric cell sends a neurite down the center of the rhabdom and into the bundle of nerve fibres from the retinula cells. This fiber bears short stubby processes which Mrs. NEMANIC believes are merely supportive in function.

The ultimate in complexity of organization of lateral arrays of straight microvilli appears to be that described by EGUCHI and WATERMAN (1966) in a spiny lobster, *Panulirus argus*, in which the disposition of microvilli along the medial sides of the seven retinular cells is like that just presented, but in the distal part only of the rhabdom. Basally the medial, villus-bearing surface of each retinular cell is invaginated; moreover, there projects distad between the infolded arrays of microvilli a villus-clothed core from the base of every retinular cell (Fig. 22). The significance of this complicated pattern is not known.

Outside the Arthropoda and Cephalopoda lateral rhabdomeres of straight microvilli have been reported from only a few organisms: from three species of peripatus (Onychophora) (EAKIN and WESTFALL, 1965b); from a turbellarian, *Dendrocoelum lacteum* (see RÖHLICH and TÖRÖK, 1961); from various larval trematodes (ISSEROFF and CABLE, 1968); and from several leeches (see CLARK 1967, for references). The microvilli in peripatus (Fig. 23) and in some flatworms arise from all sides of a sensory process. A rhabdomere in a leech ocellus is unique; the villi project into an intracellular cavity (Fig. 27), an arrangement that raises questions on development and function. Do the microvilli arise by outgrowths of a cytomembrane into some internal cisterna and then by enlargement of the cavity and elongation of the projections reach the adult pattern? And how does a light-induced excitation on or in the microvilli pass to the neurite of the sensory cell? Membranous interconnections between the intracellular vesicle and the external cell membrane have been observed recently in *Hirudo* by A. W. CLARK (personal communication). This discovery is a clue to the probable developmental story, which

Clark is now analyzing, that the villi arise from the surface of a vesicle formed by invagination of the cell membrane. The line of infolding persists as a septate junction.

As a postscript I add that there is now good evidence that the above interpretation is correct. White and Walther (1969) have demonstrated the connection between the vesicle (or phaosome) to extracellular space by lanthanum impregnation. The phaosome membrane and microvilli are indeed continuous with the external membrane of the receptor cell. The cleft formed by the infolding of the cell membrane contains zig-zag bridges.

Röhlich, Aros, and Virágh (1970) have recently studied the fine structure of photo-receptoral cells in the epidermis, branches of the prostomial nerve, and cerebral ganglion of an earthworm, *Lumbricus terrestris*. The picture is similar to that just described in leeches, except that the intracellular cavity (called phaosome) is labyrinthine and there are 9 + 0 cilia in addition to microvilli. The authors regard the microvilli as the primary photoreceptoral organelles, but they believe that the cilia may also be sensory. They did not observe a connection of the intracellular chambers to the exterior.

2. Two-Plane Rhabdomeres

In many arthropods and cephalopod mollusks the rhabdomeres are so ordered that the longitudinal axes of the microvilli of some rhabdomeres are perpendicular to those of other rhabdomeres. This pattern may be regarded as a subtype of straight lateral microvilli. The arrangement endows an organism with an intraretinal analyzer of plane polarized light. It has been demonstrated experimentally that many arthropods and cephalopods can detect the polarization of light (see Autrum, 1961; Waterman, 1966). In the honeybee, upon which von Frisch (e.g., 1964) conducted his brilliant studies, the rhabdom of each ommatidium is a mosaic of microvilli oriented in two planes perpendicular to each other. The rhabdomeres of retinular cells numbered 1, 2, 5, and 6 (see Figs. 18, 33) are normal to those of retinular cells 3, 4, 7, and 8 (Goldsmith, 1962). The closed-type rhabdom perhaps ensures a precise alignment of the microvilli. Incidentally, Perrelet (1970) has recently shown that there are 9 retinular cells in each ommatidium of drone bees.

The molecular basis for the sensitivity to the *e*-vector of plane polarized light is presumably the dichroism of the photopigment on or within the microvilli. The molecules of photopigment (rhodopsin or some related retinal-containing compound) are thought to have their major dichroic axes in agreement with the longitudinal axes of the microvilli (see Waterman, 1966). The alignment of the molecules of photopigment could be achieved if their opsin moieties were structural proteins of the microvillar membranes.

There is yet another variation in pattern of two-plane rhabdomeres, namely, an organization of the microvilli of a given rhabdomere into layers (25 to 450) that are interleaved at right angles with layers of villi of adjacent rhabdomeres. This pattern is found in crustaceans such as a lobster (Rutherford and Horridge, 1965), a crab (Eguchi and Waterman, 1966), and a crayfish (Eguchi, 1965). A diagram of this pattern is shown in Figs. 24—26. Note that seven retinular cells contribute to the rhabdom. Cell number 1 is double the size of the others, and it takes the position of two cells in ommatidia of eight retinular cells (honeybee). An explanation for this difference in size is not apparent. Conceivably the large cell might be an organizer in the development of the ommatidium or perhaps it has a special functional role. It is probable that the interleaving of layers of microvilli from neighboring retinular cells gives a more rigid rhabdom and maintains a more precise perpendicular alignment of microvilli than in less tightly interknit arrays.

In ommatidia of the open type the orientation of the rhabdomeres is not precisely in two planes (Figs. 21, 34). Indeed there are several planes. The same holds true for retinular cells that are three-sided or polygonal. In cephalopods (octopus, for example, Fig. 35) the microvilli are predominantly oriented in two planes, perpendicular to each other, but there are arrays of these organelles that lie in other planes; moreover, the microvilli are not invariably straight. Perhaps these animals with less precisely ordered rhabdomeres have a lower sensitivity to polarized light than those with almost perfect alignment of their retinal analyzers.

In the instance of the dipteran compound eye, more needs to be added. TRUJILLO-CENÓZ and MELAMED (1966) and MELAMED and TRUJILLO-CENÓZ (1968) have studied the rhabdomeres of *Sarcophaga bullata*, *Lucilia* sp. and *Chrysomia* sp. The Uruguayan authors clearly demonstrated that there are six large, long, peripheral rhabdomeres (renumbered 2—6, 8, see Fig. 21, 34) and two small, short, central ones (numbered 1, 7). The latter lie one (no. 1, Fig. 21,34) above the other (no. 7), but at right angles to each other, and are termed respectively superior central and inferior central rhabdomere. The axons from the central cells have unique pathways (see p. 667). The authors conclude that they constitute intra-ommatidial analyzers of plane polarized light.

A recent beautiful paper by SCHNEIDER and LANGER (1969) analyzes the orientation of rhabdomeres in the eye of a water strider, *Gerris lacustris*. Dorso-lateral and ventral ommatidia (open type; rectangular in cross section) differ from one another in the size, number, and orientation of the rhabdomeres. Space does not permit details. Suffice it to say, however, that the former are structured so that they could analyze plane polarized light from the sky. The latter, which view the surface of the water, are "constructed for preferable perception of polarized light with a fixed position" permitting these ommatidia to screen against reflected light and to obtain a better view into the water. And still more recently BOHN and TÄUBER (1971) have analyzed ERG responses of dorsal, lateral, and ventral regions of the eye of the same strider to polarized light, and have related them to the ultrastructural differences in the ommatidia described by SCHNEIDER and LANGER.

3. Lateral Irregular Microvilli

It may seem unnecessary to segregate ordered and unordered lateral rhabdomeres, but it is probable that the difference in arrangement of the microvilli is of functional significance. The eyes of polychaete annelids, examples of irregular rhabdomeres, are inferior in visual performance to those of arthropods and cephalopod mollusks. There is no evidence that an annelid eye can do more than detect the presence and direction of light. In nereid worms the bent and twisted microvilli (Fig. 28) form a tangle of intermingled villi from adjacent sensory cells (for references see FISCHER and BRÖKELMANN, 1966; and EAKIN, 1968). Micrographs of thin sections of adult eyes show the spaces between the receptoral cells to be filled with circular and oval profiles — the outlines of microvilli cut in different planes. Only by tracing through serial sections can one reconstruct a picture of the intertwined and tortuous villi and their attachments to the sensory cells.

The microvilli in the eyes of a lamellibranch mollusk, *Pecten maximus*, appear to belong to this category, judging from the figures and description of BARBER, EVANS, and LAND (1967). The villi are borne by the proximal retinal cells that project backward toward the tapetum, a layer of flat reflecting crystals (see p. 676). The free ends of the proximal cells are clothed on all sides and at their tips by short, somewhat irregular microvilli. The distal cells, on the other hand, have ciliary receptors (see above). The two types appear to differ not only in structure but in physiological role: the distal cells give an "off" response whereas the proximal cells yield an "on" response. The former function in shadow response, the latter in monitoring light intensity (see LAND, 1968, for references).

Recent intracellular recordings obtained from single visual cells of *Pecten irradians* have shown that the rhabdomeric ("on") receptors give depolarizing responses to light, whereas ciliary ("off") receptors give a hyperpolarizing response (GORMAN and McREYNOLDS, 1969; McREYNOLDS and GORMAN, 1970a, b). The former are more sensitive to light, by 2—3 log units, and have a longer latency than the latter. In view of the fact that vertebrate photoreceptors respond to light by hyperpolarization of the cell membrane (see TOMITA, 1970), it appeared that one might generalize: ciliary photoreceptors are hyperpolarizing, rhabdomeric types depolarizing. But nature is not always so simple and neatly categorized as biologists would like it to be to fit their schemes. GORMAN, McREYNOLDS, and BARNES (1971) have just shown that in a group of primitive chordates, the tunicates, both ciliary and rhabdomeric photoreceptors occur and that both give hyperpolarizing responses to light. The former are to be found in the Class Ascidacea; the latter — the exception — have been discovered in *Salpa democratica*, a member of Class Thalicea. The eye of this pelagic tunicate is lensless and not homologous with the eyes of other urochordates and vertebrates. It possesses several hundred elongate sensory cells, each with an irregular arrangement of microvilli. Intracellular recording revealed hyperpolarization graded in amplitude (up to 70 mv) with light intensity.

4. Terminal Arrays of Microvilli

Another pattern of microvilli is a corona of these narrow organelles at the distal end of a sensory cell. Rhabdomeres of pulmonate snails illustrate this arrangement (Figs. 29, 37). (The term rhabdomere has been extended to include any array of microvilli or lamellae presumed to be light-sensitive (EAKIN, 1963, 1966, 1968). The terminal villi arise, as do the lateral ones discussed above, as evaginations of the cell membranes facing the lumen of the embryonic optic vesicle (EAKIN and BRANDENBURGER, 1967a). In the course of development the distal end of the sensory cell becomes cone-shape, so that the villi actually project from the sides of a low cone or hillock. A similar receptoral apparatus is found in a slug, *Agriolimax reticulatus* (NEWELL and NEWELL, 1968).

The eyes in the brain of a sipunculid, *Phascolosoma agassizii*, studied recently by HERMANS and EAKIN (1969) have a retinal arrangement similar to that in the eye of a pulmonate snail. The two sipunculid ocelli, at the proximal ends of the ocular tubes, are symmetrical cups (Figs. 38, 39) composed of sensory and pigmented cells. A crown of microvilli arises from the distal end of each sensory cell. There are several noteworthy structural differences, however, between the eye of *Phascolosoma* and that of *Helix*. The sensory villi of the former are highly irregular, those of the latter straight. Villi of the pigmented cells in the sipunculid are long and supported by bundles of tonofilaments, and form a mesh within the ocellar cavity, whereas in the pulmonate snail they are short, blunt, and without tonofilaments. Thirdly, among the villi, both sensory and supportive, of *Phascolosoma*, there are numerous cilia that arise from sensory and pigmented cells and bundle together as a tuft in the center of the ocellar cavity. In the eye of *Helix*, on the other hand, cilia are few and rudimentary. The presence of cilia in the eye of *Phascolosoma* does not invalidate the assignment of this sipunculid to the rhabdomeric type, because the presumed photoreceptoral organelles, the microvilli, are not morphologically connected to the cilia.

In the ocelli of certain flatworms (e.g., *Dugesia*) the disposition of the microvilli is like that in pulmonate snails, namely, an array from the distal end of the receptor

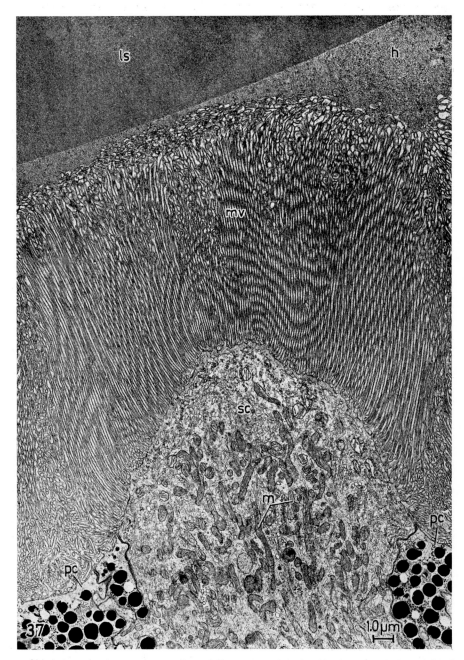

Fig. 37. Longitudinal section through tip of photosensory cell (*sc*) of snail, *Helix aspersa*. *h*, humor; *ls*, lens; *m*, mitochondria; *mv*, microvilli; *pc*, pigmented cells. EAKIN and BRANDEN-BURGER, from EAKIN, 1968

cell. The microvilli are straight basally, as shown by WETZEL (1961), but distally they are bent and tortuous, as described and figured in *Notoplana articola* by MACRAE (1966). The ocelli of ribbon worms (Phylum Rhynchocoela or Nemertina) are similar to those of *Dugesia*: simple eyecups bearing arrays of straight microvilli

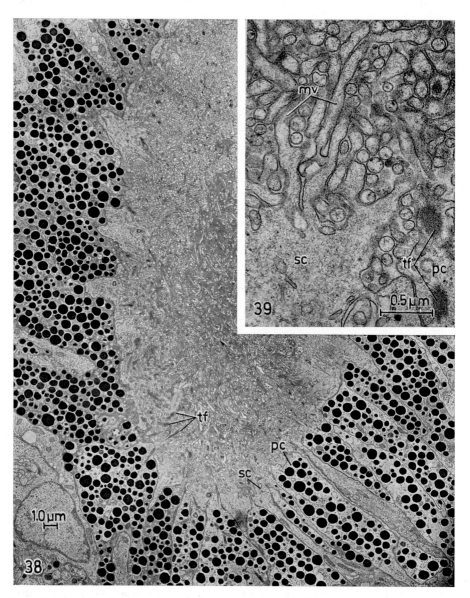

Fig. 38. Longitudinal section through eyecup of sipunculid, *Phascolosoma agassizii. pc*, pigmented cell; *sc*, sensory cell; *tf*, tonofilaments. HERMANS and EAKIN, 1969

Fig. 39. Distal end of sensory cell (*sc*) with microvilli (*mv*) of *P. agassizii. pc*, supportive cell; *tf*, tonofilaments. HERMANS and EAKIN, 1969

at the tips of sensory cells, judging from our recent study (EAKIN and WESTFALL, 1968) of three species of nemerteans (e.g., *Emplectonema gracile*). Finally, in amphioxus the photoreceptoral villi of Hesse cells in the neural tube and of Joseph cells in the cerebral vesicle are fairly straight arrays of microvilli projecting from the distal end of the sensory cell (EAKIN and WESTFALL, 1962 a; EAKIN, 1963; NAKAO 1964; WELSCH, 1968).

The distinction between lateral and terminal rhabdomeres is highly artificial. Whereas the arrangement of microvilli as a corona in a pulmonate snail is strikingly different from the phalanxes of villi along the sides of retinular cells in arthropods, there are many instances in which one or both sides and tips of receptor cells bear these minute processes. Mention has already been made of this pattern in a turbellarian flatworm, *Dendrocoelum*, and the same is to be found in miracidian and cercarian larvae of several species of parasitic flatworms (ISSEROFF and CABLE, 1968); in a nudibranch, *Hermissenda crassicornis*, according to EAKIN, WESTFALL, and DENNIS (1967); and in the prostomial eye of an annelid, *Armandia brevis*, investigated by HERMANS and CLONEY (1966). In some of these forms the villi are relatively straight (e.g., miracidia of *Allocreadium* or cercaria of *Spirorchis*).

The lateral eye of an opheliid polychaete, *Armandia brevis*, also presents an arrangement of lateral and terminal microvilli. In this animal a pair of eyecups are found in each segment from metamere 7 to 17. An ocellus (Figs. 30, 40) consists of a cup of many pigmented cells into which one sensory cell projects via the pupil. Within the ocellus the receptoral cell branches into several cylindrical retinal clubs or processes, each clothed on all sides by relatively straight microvilli. A cross section of a club resembles that of a sensory process in peripatus (Fig. 23). The villi from neighboring clubs appear to interdigitate to some extent as do those from adjacent cell processes in peripatus.

This is an appropriate place to comment on the significance of *converse* and *inverse* eyes. Most of the examples presented so far have been of the converse type, i.e., with the distal ends of the receptor cell oriented toward the source of light. The prostomial and lateral ocelli of the polychaete *Armandia*, the eyes of trematode larvae, fresh-water triclads and nemerteans, and the Hesse cups in amphioxus are inverted, i.e., the receptoral processes project away from the light and toward the pigmented layer. Incidentally, vertebrate rods and cones also belong to this latter type. The explanation for this difference in orientation is to be found in the embryology of eyes. There appears to be no functional advantage to either converse or inverse pattern, because eyes of acute vision (those of insects, octopus and vertebrates) belong to both types.

Limitation on space permits a citation only of very recent studies on microvillar receptors: HUGHES (1970) on a variety of opisthobranch mollusks (in *Aplysia punctata* there are both rhabdomeric and ciliary receptors); KAWAGUTI and MABUCHI (1969) on a giant clam, *Tridacna crocea;* BARBER and WRIGHT (1969) on a cephalopod, *Nautilus macromphalus;* DUDLEY (1969), ELOFSSON (1969), ONG (1970), and VAISSIÈRE and BOULAY (1971) on copepods; FISCHER and HORSTMANN (1971) on a meal moth, *Ephestia kuehniella;* PERRELET and BAUMAN (1969), VARELA and PORTER (1969), and PERRELET (1970) on the honeybee; BRAMMER (1970) on a mosquito, *Aedes aegypti;* TRUJILLO-CENÓZ and MELAMED (1971) on a cockroach, *Periplaneta americana;* CLARK, MILLECCHIA, and MAURO (1969) and FAHRENBACH (1970) on *Limulus polyphemus;* JOLY (1969) and BÄHR (1971) on a chilopod, *Lithobius forficatus;* CURTIS (1969) on a harvestman, *Mitopus morio.*

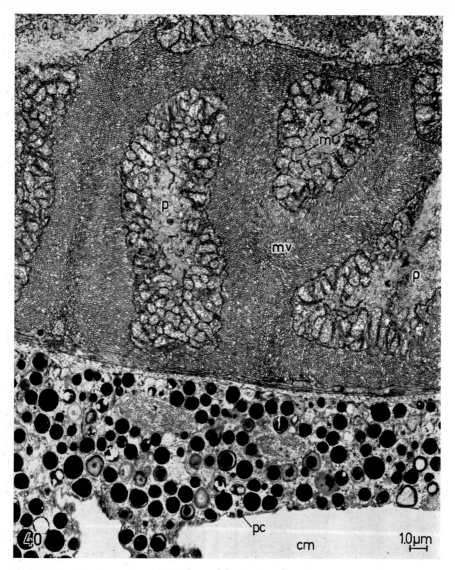

Fig. 40. Part of lateral ocellus of polychaete worm, *Armandia brevis*. *cm*, coelom; *m*, mito-chondria; *mv*, microvilli; *p*, processes of sensory cell; *pc*, pigmented cell. From Hermans, 1969

5. Lamellae

There is at least one eye, that of a rotifer, *Asplanchna brightwelli*, in which the presumed light-sensitive organelles are broad, flat processes about 12 in number and 50 nm in thickness (Eakin and Westfall, 1965a). The lamellae are curved and overlap one another like the petals of an unopened flower. Together they form a laminated hillock on the distal end of the sensory cell which fits into the concavity of an accessory cell. The two cells constitute the cerebral ocellus, (Figs. 31, 41)

situated on the postero-ventral surface of the brain. The lamellae are connected to
the body of the receptoral cell by broad stalks, two of which may be seen in Fig. 41
(arrows). A space, presumably filled with a fluid, separates the innermost lamellae

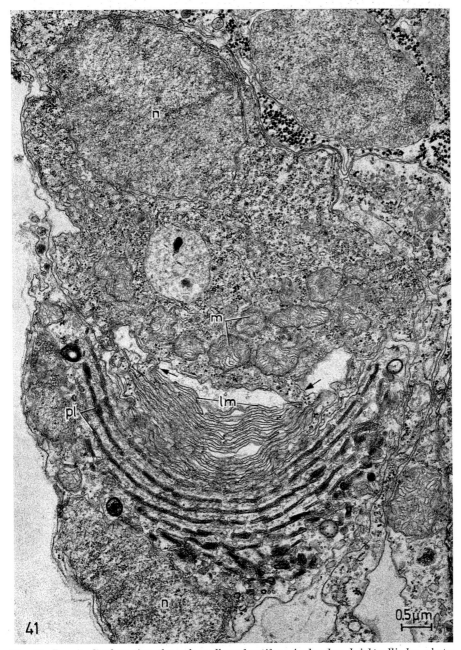

Fig. 41. Longitudinal section through ocellus of rotifer, *Asplanchna brightwelli*. *lm*, photoreceptoral lamellae; *m*, mitochondria; *n*, nuclei; *pl*, plates (reflecting ?); arrows, stalks of
lamellae. From EAKIN and WESTFALL, 1965a

from the body of the sensory cell, and extensions of this space as clefts separate the slightly undulating lamellae from one another. The eyes of other species of rotifers should be examined with the electron microscope to determine if the pattern in *Asplanchna brightwelli* is characteristic of the Rotifera.

6. Tiered Receptors

In most retinas the photoreceptors are arranged in a single layer, but there are instances of stratification. In dragonflies each ommatidium has eight retinula cells ordered in distal and proximal rows of four cells each. The rhabdomeres are fused to give an exceptionally long rhabdom. HORRIDGE (1969b) who studied three species of dragonflies, concluded that this anatomical arrangement permits a high percentage absorption of light and allows color vision. In the dragonfly *Aeschna cyanea*, studied recently by EGUCHI (1971) distal retinula cells (numbered 1, 3, 4, and 6) are thought to be green receptors, and proximal cells (2 and 5) may be UV receptors. No hypothesis was advanced for the function of distal cell number 7. Cell 8 has no rhabdomere. In damsel flies (e.g., *Ishunura senegalensis*) there are three tiers of receptoral elements in each ommatidium which permit, according to the authors (NINOMIYA, TOMINAGA, and KUWABARA, 1969) a "discrimination of succession of images." But retinular cells do not need to be tiered for the perception of different colors by a single ommatidium. MOTE and GOLDSMITH (1971) impaled individual retinular cells in the eye of a cockroach, *Periplaneta americana*, recorded the spectral responses, marked the cells with dye-filled microelectrodes, and showed that at least two kinds of receptors (green and UV) occur in the same ommatidium.

GRIBAKIN (1969) has advanced a cellular basis for color vision in honeybees. He studied the ultrastructural changes in retinular cells resulting from illumination of the compound eye with certain wavelengths. Depending upon the wavelength used, these changes (e.g., swelling or shortening or even disintegration of microvilli, formation of vacuoles in the retinular cells, etc.) are produced in particular cells (classified into three types, see GRIBAKIN, 1967). In an ommatidium the distribution of receptor cells is as follows: 2 UV, 2 blue and 4 green-yellow or 0 blue and 6 green-yellow.

A tiered retina is possessed by another insect, an aquatic beetle, *Dytiscus marginalis*, studied ultrastructurally and electrophysiologically by HORRIDGE, WALCOTT, and IOANNIDES (1970). One retinula cell bears a distal rhabdomere connected to the cone by a crystalline thread, and six large retinula cells contribute to a closed-type rhabdom at the proximal end of each ommatidium. Distal and proximal receptors are separated by $200\,\mu m$ of non-pigmented tissue, and no light pipes lead to the deep rhabdomeres. The authors conclude that the distal receptors have directional acuity, essential for detection of movement, whereas the proximal receptors are without visual acuity, but they have high light-sensitivity by virtue of their ability to capture as much light as possible, no matter by which facet it enters the eye.

A more elegant example of stratification of photoreceptors is to be found in the antero-median eyes of several species of jumping spiders studied by LAND (1969a, b; 1971) and recently by EAKIN and BRANDENBURGER (1972), using electron microscopy. The receptors are arranged in four layers. Focused images with red wavelengths fall on the deepest layer (number 1); the next layer receives focused images with green and blue light; layer 3 is conjugate with violet and near ultraviolet; and layer 4, just below the dioptric apparatus, could receive a focused image with ultraviolet only. Jumping spiders are known to have color vision. We have shown additionally that central and peripheral rhabdomeres are oriented perpendicularly to the direction of incident light but at right angles to one another. Layer 4 could, therefore, function as an analyzer of plane polarized light.

C. An Exceptional Photoreceptor

The erection of a system of pigeon holes usually presents a problem of what to do with the pigeon that does not fit any of the holes. An instance is a protistan photoreceptor that is neither ciliary nor rhabdomeric, although it resembles the latter in some respects. The fantastic eyelets (Fig. 42) of certain dinoflagellates (e.g., *Erythropsis pavillardi* and *Warnowia pulchra*) possess a presumably light-sensitive organelle that is an amazing array of lamellae (Fig. 43) at the back of the eye (GREUET, 1968). The membrane-bounded plates measure 38 nm in thickness and are separated from one another by 10 nm-wide spaces. They constitute the "palisade" layer of a retinette ("corps retinien"). The lamellae are probably light-sensitive structures considering their organization and their position. The eyelet as a whole is composed of two parts: the "hyalosome" which protrudes from the surface of the dinoflagellate and functions as a refractive body, (see p. 673), and the shallow cup-shaped "melanosome" which includes the retinette just mentioned. As the lamellae do not appear to be elaborations of the cell membrane they are not assigned to the category of rhabdomeres, which are, by definition, outfoldings of cell membranes. These remarkable photoreceptors presumably enable the marine dinoflagellate possessing them to detect the direction of light; the organism then swims to levels rich in autotrophs (GRELL, 1968).

Since the above was written, a study of another dinoflagellate, *Glenodinium foliaceum*, by DODGE and CRAWFORD (1969) has appeared. This organism possesses an eyespot similar to that in *Euglena* (see section on paraflagellar body), consisting of a cup-shaped double layer of lipoidal droplets. Adjacent to this orange colored stigma is a unique lamellar body composed of a stack of about 50 flattened vesicles, which are connected to the endoplasmic reticulum in certain places. The lamellar body roughly resembles the outer segment of a vertebrate rod. The authors suggest that the sigma and lamellar body may act together as organelles for determining the direction of light as it strikes the organism, passes through a gap in the eyespot, and stimulates the lamellar body. It is postulated further that a stimulus is passed in some unknown manner to the nearby pair of flagella to elicit a rapid phototactic response.

II. Localization of Photopigments

At this point it may be useful to review present information on the correlation between the morphology and the chemistry and physiology of photoreceptors. Evidence for the presence of photopigments in or on the membranes of rhabdomeric and ciliary receptors of invertebrates is neither so extensive nor so convincing as that for the localization of rod and cone pigments in the disks of the outer segments of vertebrate receptors. As pointed out by MOODY (1964) the biochemistry and physiology of vision is a difficult study in most invertebrates because of the small size of their eyes and because the photoreceptors are often enclosed by pigmented

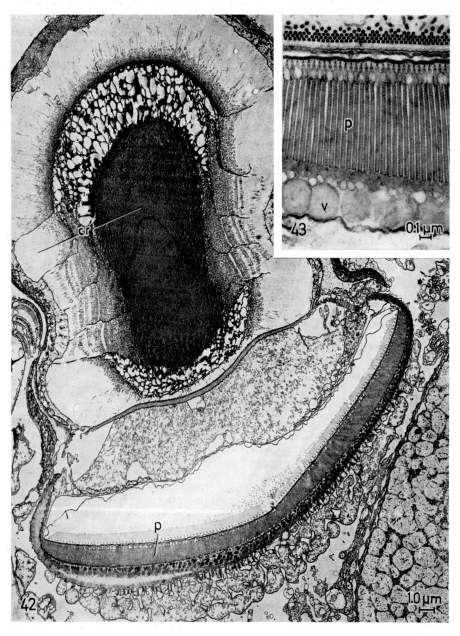

Fig. 42. Longitudinal section through the eyelet of a dinoflagellate, *Erythropsis pavillardi*. *cr*, crystalline (lens) body; *p*, palisade layer of retinette. COURTESY of C. GREUET

Fig. 43. Enlargement of palisade layer in eyelet of *Warnowia pulchra*. *p*, lamellae in palisade layer; *v*, vesicles behind the lamellae. From GREUET, 1968

cells and in addition, in the arthropods, by chitinous coverings. The identification of rhodopsin in the rhabdomeres of certain arthropods (see WOLKEN, 1968) and cephalopods is the best documented instance of anatomical and chemical correlation among invertebrate photoreceptors.

GOLDSMITH (1958) was among the first to demonstrate the presence of retinal, and later retinol (GOLDSMITH and WARNER, 1964), in an invertebrate, but the localization was limited to the head of the organism studied (honeybee).

Investigations on larger arthropods (lobsters and *Limulus*) and on cephalopods, the latter lacking the disadvantages noted above, have narrowed the localization of the photopigment to the rhabdomeres. By centrifuging homogenates of large numbers of eyes of these animals in a sucrose gradient a membranous fraction was isolated (WALD and HUBBARD, 1957, to cite one early paper). It contained rhodopsin.

Second, microspectrophotometry of single rhabdomeres in a blow fly, *Calliphora erythrocephala*, provides about as good evidence (LANGER and THORELL, 1966) as a court of law would need to adjudge this structure as light sensitive. Incidentally, the fly used was not red-headed but a mutant, "chalky" that lacks all screening pigments. The open type rhabdom of diptera facilitates microspectrophotometry of individual rhabdomeres. Extinction curves of six of the rhabdomeres show two maxima: one at about 500 nm and another between 350 and 380 nm. They are very similar to the curves for rhodopsin. The curve for a central rhabdomere (see p. 645) differs from that for the peripheral rhabdomeres in having a maximum absorbence at about 460 nm. The difference is attributable to the protein component of the photopigment.

Third, an embryological study can offer testimony in this trial of the rhabdomere. EGUCHI, NAKA, and KUWABARA (1962) correlated the development of rhabdoms in a moth, *Bombyx mori*, and electrical responses to photic stimulation. No response was obtained from compound eyes of pupae in which rhabdomeres had not yet differentiated, but as soon as microvilli appeared electrical recordings could be made. The amplitude of the response increased progressively with further development of the rhabdomeres.

A fourth line of evidence comes from the first results currently being obtained from studies on vitamin-A deficiency in insects. CARLSON, STEEVES, VANDEBERG, and ROBBINS (1967) have found pathological changes in the eye of *Manduca sexta*, as a result of rearing the moths for several generations on vitamin-A deficient medium. Severe visual impairment in the experimental animals was reported. Light microscopy of their eyes showed rhabdoms that were said to be diffuse, swollen and more lightly stained than those of animals reared on tobacco, their normal food, or on the medium supplemented with β-carotene. The authors state that the histological picture is like that in vitamin A-deficient rats where disks break into vesicles and tubules. CARLSON, GEMNE, and ROBBINS (1969) have recently conducted an electron microscopic study of the changes in the photoreceptors of this nocturnal moth maintained for 20 generations on a vitamin-A deficient diet. The microvilli become misaligned and shortened, sometimes vesiculated and whorled, and vacuoles and multivesicular bodies form in the retinular cells.

BRAMMER and WHITE (1969) have studied the effects of vitamin A deficiency on the ultrastructure of the eyes of mosquitoes. *Aedes aegypti* was reared aseptically for one generation on a diet lacking vitamin A and β-carotene. The fine structure of the rhabdomeres in these mosquitoes was reported to be normal although perhaps smaller in size, especially after prolonged exposure to light. There were two prominent abnormalities, however, in other parts of the sensory cells: masses of smooth cytomembranes appeared in the vicinity of the nuclei, and multivesicular bodies, normally present, were absent. Function (electrical response to light) in the deficient mosquitoes was severely impaired. The authors point out that the mosquitoes were probably not totally lacking in vitamin A, having been reared on the deficient diet for only one generation. Perhaps, breakdown of the rhabdomeres would occur if the experiment were extended over many generations with precautions against trace contamination with retinol through the synthetic activities of microorganisms (see GOLDSMITH and FERNANDEZ, 1966).

Fifth, our study (EAKIN and BRANDENBURGER, 1968b) on the uptake of radioactive retinol by the eye of a pulmonate snail, *Helix aspersa*, further points to the rhabdomere as the functional site of a photopigment. We injected tritiated retinol acetate into the hearts of the animals and after one or two days prepared their eyes for light- and electron microscopy. The microvilli projecting into the lumen of the eyecup showed high tritium activity. The microvilli, as in the rhabdomeres of arthropods and cephalopods, are so tightly compacted that there is little humor bathing them, except at their tips. We concluded, therefore, that the radioactivity was in the rhabdomeres, suggesting that they possess a retinal-based photopigment. This pigment is probably rhodopsin, for GILLARY and WOLBARSHT (1967) showed in another pulmonate gastropod, *Otala lactea*, that the sensitivity curve of its retina, determined by electrical recording, is similar to the spectral absorbance of rhodopsin, having a λ_{max} of 490 nm. Moreover, EAKIN and KING (unpublished) obtained evidence of retinol in the eye of *Helix aspersa* by thin layer chromatography of an extract of approximately 1200 eyes (what a chore to dissect and stockpile so many!). The major component of the extract had the same R_f value, UV fluorescence, and deep-blue staining with antimony trichloride as known retinol.

Sixth, the structural modifications in the rhabdomeres resulting from illumination, or, on the other hand, from absence of light indicate further that the microvilli are light-sensitive organelles. These morphological changes will be considered in detail later.

Seventh, support for the assertion that rhabdomeres bear photopigment comes from the studies of WATERMAN and EGUCHI (see WATERMAN, 1968 for references) correlating the organization of the rhabdomeres in an arthropod's ommatidium with the animal's ability to analyze polarized light. They showed that the two directions of the microvilli (see Figs. 24—26) were parallel to the vertical and horizontal axes of an animal (crab, for example) and they demonstrated by electrophysiological experiments that these directions coincided with those of maximal effectiveness of the *e*-vector of the adapting light. Then they studied the effects of several hours exposure to linearly polarized light upon the fine structure of the rhabdomeric microvilli of a spider crab (*Libinia emarginata*). When the *e*-vector is parallel to the vertical microvilli, namely the villi of cells 2, 3, 6 and 7, only those cells showed light-induced ultrastructural changes (increase in pinocytotic vesicles and complex bodies). On the other hand, with a horizontal adapting *e*-vector cells 1, 4, and 5 showed the syndrome of changes, and 45° oblique *e*-vector affected both groups of cells equally. As there is no structure in the ommatidium, other than the microvilli, arranged in a two-dimensional pattern, the rhabdomere must be the analyzer of polarized light. Furthermore, as WATERMAN concludes, this function of the microvilli is probably dependent upon the dichroism of rhodopsin.

The line of argument above has been entirely restricted to rhabdomeric photo-receptors. There is little to say about localization of visual pigments in the ciliary photoreceptors of invertebrates. In the eyes of chaetognaths, as we have seen, the distal segments of the ciliary processes consist of arrays of longitudinally arranged tubules, believed to be the light-sensitive organelles. BURFIELD (1927) noted in living *Sagitta bipunctata* that the region of the eye corresponding to the arrays of tubules revealed by electron microscopy (EAKIN and WESTFALL, 1964 b) exhibited a faint pink color. This observation suggests the presence of a photopigment in the distal segments of the ciliary processes. Studies on photopigments in the ocelli of sea stars and anthomedusans have been made, notably by YOSHIDA and associates at the Tamano Marine Laboratory (see, for example, YOSHIDA, 1963 and YOSHIDA and OHTSUKI, 1966). As yet no report has been made on a specific localization of these pigments within the ocelli of asteroids and medusae.

Now, can one say anything about structure of invertebrate photoreceptors and color vision ? A little. It has been established from several lines of evidence that many insects can distinguish colors, and there are indications that color-sensitive cells are neither randomly nor uniformly distributed in a compound eye (see AUTRUM, 1961 and GOLDSMITH, 1961). For example, AUTRUM and BURKHARDT (1961) found by electrical recording from individual retinular cells in a blowfly, *Calliphora erythrocephala*, that the dorsal part of the eye is color blind, as in other insects. The sensitivity curves show a maximum at 490 nm. The ventral areas, on the other hand, possess color receptors of three types with the following relative numbers: green 18, blue 4, and yellow-green 3. These authors postulate that each ommatidium may have 5 green, 1 blue and 1 yellow-green sensitive retinular cells, assuming that there are seven units in an ommatidium. From the studies of MELA-MED and TRUJILLO-CENÓZ (1966, 1968) we know now that flies have 8 retinular cells per ommatidium. The ratio 6:1:1 fits the frequencies found by AUTRUM and BURKHARDT just as closely. Are the two central cells of an ommatidium sensitive to blue and yellow-green in addition to functioning as analyzers of polarized light ?

One further example. Superb studies by MICHAEL LAND (1969 a, 1969 b) correlate color perception in jumping spiders with the structure of the retina. He has analyzed the principal (antero-medial) eyes of *Metaphidippus aeneolus* by light microscopy. LAND finds that there are four layers of retinal cells which he designates 1 to 4 from posterior to anterior. He postulates that this layering of receptors permits the spider to examine objects at different distances with sharp images and/or to monitor light of different wave lengths. He has made critical optical measurements and concludes that either theory is possible, but the second one is the more probable. Jumping spiders are known to have color vision (see LAND, 1969 a, for references). LAND suggests that the retinal strata have the following photosensitivities: layer 1 (the deepest), red; layer 2, blue-green; and layer 3, violet-ultraviolet. And what does layer 4 do — the one nearest to the dioptric apparatus ? It may be an analyzer of polarized light according to LAND. This superficial layer of receptors is not con-jugate with any plane for any visible wave length, suggesting that it is not resolving an image. The microvilli lie at right angles to the long axes of the terminals of the sensory cells and also perpendicular to the path of light entering the eye (EAKIN and BRANDENBURGER, unpublished). Since dorsal and ventral terminals of the cells in layer 4 are oriented at different angles in relation to the frontal plane, the spider could analyze sky-light polarized in various planes by the rhabdomeres of this stratum (LAND, 1969a).

III. Soma of Receptoral Cell

This rubric includes not only the perikaryon but all of the regions of the sensory cell except the photoreceptoral apparatus, just discussed, and the neurite to follow. In some instances (e. g., insects, cephalopods, onychophorans, polychaetes, flat-worms, etc.) extensions of the cell — called processes, clubs, hillocks and even dendrites, depending on their size and shape — bear the ciliary or rhabdomeric light-sensitive organelles. For the purpose of this discussion these extensions are considered as parts of the body of the cell.

A. Mitochondria

It is almost an invariable rule that mitochondria occur in greater abundance in the immediate vicinity of the photoreceptoral apparatus, whether it be ciliary or rhabdomeric, than elsewhere in the body of a sensory cell. Sometimes the concentration of mitochondria is almost as great as that in the inner segment of rods and cones, which is about the most dense population of these organelles known in the animal kingdom. The precise role of these transformers of energy is not understood, but one may speculate that the metabolic pathways, which the mito-chondrial enzymes implement, facilitate the generation and amplification of light-induced impulses and, more certainly, the maintenance of the structural integrity and functional state of the business-end of the receptor.

The shape and arrangement of mitochondria in the receptoral cell in the branchial eyes of a polychaete worm, Branchiomma vesiculosum (see above), deserve special comment. The exceedingly long, cylindrical mitochondria are ordered at right angles to the optic axis of the eye (KRASNE and LAWRENCE, 1966). They are so closely packed together that they present a hexagonal pattern of circular profiles in cross-sectional view. They number about 3,000 per cell. The cristae are few and consist of villus-like projections of the inner mitochondrial membrane. Their re-markably ordered arrangement and their position between the lens of the ocellus and the presumed light-sensitive organelles (ciliary sacs) indicate that they have a special function. KRASNE and LAWRENCE (1966) suggest that they endow the photoreceptoral cell with dichroic properties, which would permit it to function as an analyzer of polarized light. I add the possibility that they might have some wave-guidance function. Strangely, this array of mitochondria is absent in the eye of a related sabellid, Dasychone bombyx (KERNÉIS, 1966, 1968).

B. Endoplasmic Reticulum

In many if not most instances both rough and smooth ER are well developed in the nuclear region of the receptoral cell, suggesting a high degree of synthetic activity. Additionally, there are many free ribosomes in the cytoplasm, which in mosquito larvae (*Aedes aegypti*) are long, possibly helical polysomes (see p. 664). Golgi centers are frequently multiple, and occur in both supra and infranuclear parts of the receptoral cell body. Secretory vesicles of Golgi origin are abundant in some instances. An example of the extreme is the remarkable masses of uniform vesicles in the eye of a pulmonate snail, *Helix aspersa*.

The vesicles in *H. aspersa* were first noted by DR. WESTFALL and me in 1962, but at that time we were preoccupied with the photoreceptoral apparatus of the snail and deferred a study of the vesicles until later. Subsequently, similar spherules were discovered in the eye of a European snail, *Helix pomatia*, by SCHWALBACH, LICKFELD, and HAHN (1963) and RÖHLICH and TÖRÖK (1963). JEAN BRANDEN-BURGER and I more fully characterized the vesicles in *H. aspersa* (EAKIN and BRANDENBURGER, 1967a, b) and demonstrated their origin from Golgi saccules (Fig. 44) in an embryological study. The mature vesicles are spherical (about 80 nm in diameter) unless compacted, in which instance they are ovoid. The large aggregations occur above and below the nuclei and exhibit a paracrystalline arrangement (Fig. 45). After preservation with common fixatives the vesicles appear electron-lucent with only faint central densities, but after long osmification (two or three days at 40° C) the lumen of each vesicle appears filled with material (EAKIN and BRANDENBURGER, 1969). Scattered among the vesicles are dense 35 nm-granules. Considering the size, morphology (they occur in rosettes in the pigmented cells), stainability with lead, and digestibility with alpha amylase we concluded that the grains are glycogen (EAKIN and BRANDENBURGER, 1967b). Like vesicles have been noted in the retinal cells of other mollusks, such as a nudibranch, *Hermissenda crassicornis* (see EAKIN, WESTFALL, and DENNIS, 1967) and a sea hare, *Aplysia californica* (JACKLET, 1969).

What is the function of these vesicles? We entertained two hypotheses (EAKIN and BRANDENBURGER, 1967c): 1. they are bearers of photopigment, or precursors thereof, to the rhabdomeres, and 2. they are agents of neurotransmission. At the time of writing I favor the first alternative for several reasons. We have some evidence that these vesicles increase in number at the distal ends of sensory cells of *H. aspersa* after brief illumination of the eyes of a dark-adapted animal (EAKIN and BRANDENBURGER, 1968a). A definitive publication has not been made because of subsequent inconsistencies in the results of our experiments. I surmise that the discrepancies are due to unequal illumination of the various sectors of the retina. Further study is needed to confirm our first observations that the vesicles move from the synthetic centers deep within the cell to the sensory hillock from which the villi arise. Within the hillock we believe that the vesicles break down and that their products move into the villi. Second, the vesicles became radioactive after a snail was injected via the heart with tritiated retinol (EAKIN and BRANDENBURGER, 1968b). After one or two days the counts of silver grains per unit area over the vesicles in a section of a radioactive eye were greater than counts over any other part of the eye. The rhabdomere was second in order of radioactivity. As there is evidence that the eyes of pulmonate snails have a rhodopsin-like photopigment, the accumulation of retinol or retinaldehyde by the vesicles implicates them in the transportation of materials needed by the photoreceptoral apparatus. A recent further study by us (BRANDENBURGER and EAKIN, 1970) shows that radioactive vitamin A is first incorporated by the rough ER and Golgi apparatus of the receptor cell and

42*

that subsequently the photic vesicles and rhabdomere become radioactive. Jacklet (1969) suggests that similar vesicles in *Aplysia californica* "may participate in a kind of intracellular coupling between rhabdomere and the receptor membrane."

A third point of evidence, admittedly weak, that links vesicles to the transportation of photopigment is the stainability of their contents by long osmification

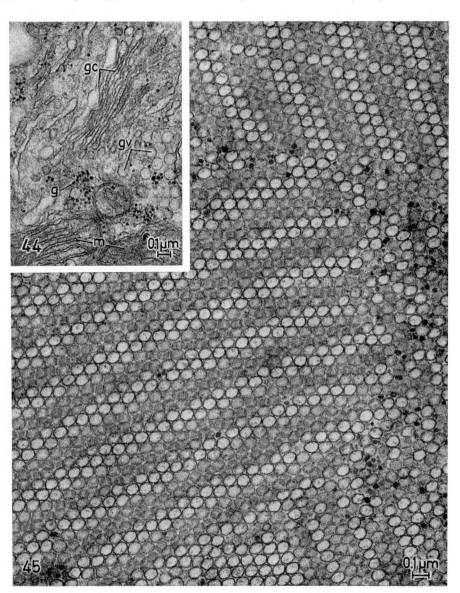

Fig. 44. Golgi apparatus in photosensory cell of snail, *Helix aspersa. g*, glycogen; *gc*, Golgi cisternae; *gv*, Golgi vesicles; *m*, mitochondria. Eakin and Brandenburger, hitherto unpublished

Fig. 45. Paracrystalline array of vesicles in photosensory cell of *H. aspersa*. From Eakin and Brandenburger, 1967a

at 40° C (EAKIN and BRANDENBURGER, 1970). FRIEND and MURRAY (1965) have shown that the formation of osmium black occurs in Golgi lamellae and vesicles of mouse epididymis and in Brunner's gland after prolonged exposure to osmium tetroxide. The nature of the reducing substances is not known, but HANKER, SEAMAN, WEISS, UENO, BERGMAN, and SELIGMAN (1964) state that aldehydes reduce osmium rapidly. Retinal, the prosthetic group of rhodopsin, is an un-saturated aldehyde. It should be mentioned that the rhabdomeric microvilli also show deposits of osmium black in eyes of *H. aspersa* incubated in osmium tetroxide at 40° C for several days.

C. Phaosomes

There are instances of abundant condensations of rough endoplasmic reticulum, called phaosomes. An example is the three ocellar nauplius eye of a copepod, *Macrocyclops albidus*, in which the phaosomes are fusiform or lenticular bodies of closely packed, ribosome-encrusted membranes that are continuous with dispersed ER (FAHRENBACH, 1964). The number and nature of the phaosomes may vary with alterations in illumination. VAISSIÈRE (1961) noted that these bodies are refractive, and suggested that they may serve as light-concentrating structures within the retinular cells of the ocelli.

D. Pinocytotic Vesicles

An increasing number of studies of photoreceptoral cells, especially in rhab-domeric eyes, are revealing pinocytosis (e.g., MELAMED and TRUJILLO-CENÓZ, 1966; EGUCHI and WATERMAN, 1967; WHITE, 1967). Pinocytosis is especially active at the bases of the sensory villi (see Fig. 34). The pinocytotic vesicles are coated, although vesicles of similar size situated deeper within the receptoral cell are devoid of coating. If the latter are pinocytotic in origin they must lose their coats as they move into the cell. An attractive hypothesis for their function is that of removing microvillar membrane and intravillar material as well, perhaps, as incorporating extracellular substances (see p. 665).

E. Microtubules

Cytoplasmic tubules in the order of 20—30 nm in diameter are frequently observed running lengthwise through the distal part of a photoreceptoral cell (Fig. 12). In some instances they continue into the extension of the cell that bears the receptoral organelles (Fig. 23). Note their abundance in the photoreceptoral cells in the antero-lateral eyes of a jumping spider, *Phidippus johnsoni* (Fig. 32). The microtubules might be serving as a cytoskeleton, although in most eyes this function seems adequately provided by the supporting cells, to be considered shortly. Another possibility, which seems more tenable, is transport of materials — perhaps of low molecular weight — to or from the light-sensitive apparatus.

F. Pigment Granules

As a rule sensory cells lack pigment, but there are several exceptions. For example, the retinular cells of *Drosophila* (Fig. 34) and other arthropods have numerous granules of black pigment, presumably melanin, as do the photoreceptoral cells of cephalopods (Fig. 35). Photosensory cells of a polychaete worm, *Platynereis dumerilii*, have orange pigment granules in the central parts of the cells, whereas the pigment in the supporting cells is dark blue (Fischer, 1963). Eakin and West-fall (unpublished) made similar observations on *Nereis vexillosa*. In some instances, as in peripatus, pigment granules are only occasionally seen in the sensory cells (Eakin and Westfall, 1965b).

G. Miscellaneous Structures

Photoreceptoral cells contain a variety of multivesicular bodies, laminated vesicles, vacuoles, secretory granules, lysosomes, dense bodies, *et cetera*. Some of these vary quantitatively with amount of illumination (see below). In some instances as in sensory cells in the eyes of peripatus (*Perpatonder novaezealandiae*) one sees large granules or droplets, a micrometre or more in diameter, of varying density (Eakin and Westfall, 1965b), and beta granules of glycogen are commonly observed, often in abundance as in *Helix aspersa* (Eakin and Brandenburger, 1967b).

IV. Effects of Light and Darkness on Photoreceptors

1. Receptoral Organelles

I stated earlier (p. 656) that one of the points of evidence supporting the conclusion that ciliary and rhabdomeric organelles are indeed light-sensitive is the effect of light (or darkness) upon their fine structure. I shall be quick to add, however, that there is disagreement among investigators, including some studying the same organisms and using similar techniques.

On the one hand there are investigations that demonstrate an impairment of the receptoral apparatus either from absence of light or from very strong light. Thus Eguchi (1965) found that crayfish (*Procambarus clarkii*) maintained in the dark for three months exhibited derangement of microvilli in the rhabdomeres and an increase in the thickness of the microvillar membranes. The receptor potentials of the retinular cells in such animals were abnormal, consisting only of the slow phase. Eguchi and Waterman (1966) confirmed the above observations on crayfish and showed further that if a branchiopod, *Artemia salina*, was kept in darkness for three months the regular arrangement of the microvilli became "virtually destroyed." White (1967) stated that in a mosquito (*Aedes aegypti*) "the surface area of the rhabdom membrane is two to three times greater in mosquito larvae grown in darkness than it is in larvae grown in light." Röhlich and Törö (1965) reported that in a cladoceran, *Daphnia pulex*, strong light causes disintegration of rhabdomeres after 20 to 60 minutes exposure.

On the other hand, Kuwabara and his associates (Kabuta, Tominaga, and Kuwabara, 1968) have conducted a study of the effects of total darkness upon the rhabdomeres of seven species of arthropods, including *Procambarus clarkii* and *Artemia salina* mentioned above. In all instances, if the eyes of the animals were fixed with glutaraldehyde, the arrangement and morphology of the rhabdomeres were found to be normal, even in *Drosophila melanogaster* raised under "completely dark conditions" for 312 generations or crayfish "kept in a completely darkened room for 247 days" or in a shrimp, cricket, and crab living in caves. If the eyes of crayfish and fruit flies (dark-reared and controls alike) were preserved with osmium fixative, however, some of the rhabdomeres showed atypical microvilli, with spi-

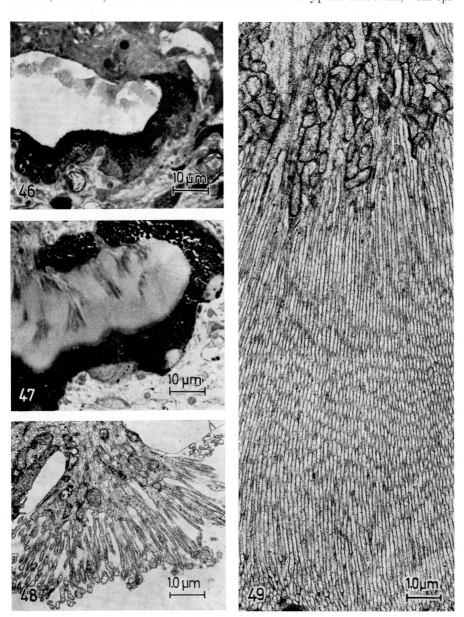

Figs. 46—49. Comparison of dark-adapted (Figs. 46, 48) and light-adapted (Figs. 47, 49) ocelli of planarian, *Dugesia tigrina*. Figs. 46, 47, light micrographs; Figs. 48, 49, electron micrographs. From Röhlich and Tar, 1968

ralling membranes and vesicles. In the instance of *Drosophila* it was found that the degree of membrane abnormality increased with higher concentrations of OsO_4 and also with longer periods of fixation. Further research is obviously needed to clarify the picture of the effects of total darkness on photoreceptors in arthropods.

But now let us look at another animal, a flatworm. Röhlich and Tar (1968) have shown in a very convincing paper that absence of light for three weeks induces a profound atrophy of the eyes of a planarian, *Dugesia tigrina*. In specimens fixed with glutaraldehyde the retinal clubs become reduced in number and to one-fifth normal size, and their microvilli also decrease in both number and length (Figs. 46—49). Moreover, exposure to light after long dark-adaptation leads to rapid regeneration of retinal clubs. The number and length of microvilli are considerably increased after only six hours of illumination. It is instructive, moreover, that fixation with osmium tetroxide does indeed give artifactual vesicle formation in dark-maintained but not in light-maintained planarians. The longer the period of darkness, the greater the susceptibility to artifacts of fixation. Röhlich and Tar consider the artifact "meaningful," indicating a change in the stability of the microvillar membranes in animals deprived of light. In discussing a cellular mechanism for the atrophy of the retinal clubs the authors suggest the possibility that absence of light slows down some synthetic process — production of membrane proteins perhaps — so that the microvilli first lose their stability and then atrophy. This hypothesis is strengthened by the demonstration of Young (1967) that renewal of outer segments of vertebrate rods is accelerated by an increase in retinal illumination.

Investigations by Finnish workers (see Tuurala and Lehtinen, 1967) have shown that in an isopod, *Oniscus asellus*, the angles formed by microvilli in relation to the long axis of a rhabdomere change upon light or dark adaptation. In the light the angle is reduced (30—45°, if specimen is fixed with OsO_4; 40—55°, if fixed with glutaraldehyde); in the dark the angle becomes large (up to 90°, with both fixatives). The authors suggest that the changes in angle, which are relatively rapid, may have something to do with the detection of polarized light. Paula Nemanic of my laboratory has confirmed, in general, the above observations in her study of the eye of another isopod, *Porcellio scabra* (unpublished).

2. Soma of Sensory Cell

In addition to structural changes in the receptoral apparatus reported above, light affects other parts of the sensory cell. In the first place the synthetic organelles (ribosomes and endoplasmic reticulum) appear to be stimulated by light. Eguchi and Waterman (1967) found that in retinular cells of a spider crab, *Libinia emarginata*, both free ribosomes and rough endoplasmic reticulum increase upon light-adaptation. White and Sundeen (1967) report that linearly aggregated ribosomes having, possibly, a helical configuration fill the retinular cells of mosquito larvae (*Aedes aegypti*) after thirty minutes of illumination. The polysomes largely disappear, however, after two hours of light-adaptation, but the amount of endoplasmic reticulum continues to rise, reaching a maximal density after twelve hours. The above authors postulate that these changes signify a high rate of protein synthesis in excited photoreceptors and that the proteins formed may be incorporated into the membranous receptoral organelles. In a later study WHITE (1968) found that the formation of multivesicular bodies is dependent upon light. They form adjacent to the rhabdomeres, move proximally in the cell, and become lamellar and dense bodies. If ferritin is injected into the heads of the larval mosquitoes it is taken up by pinocytotic vesicles and subsequently sequestered in the multivesicular bodies. The role of uniform vesicles in a snail, *Helix aspersa*, has already been discussed.

Light may stimulate a system of cytoplasmic structures which could function to remove rhabdomeric metabolites, according to EGUCHI and WATERMAN (1967). They observed increased pinocytosis at the bases of rhabdoms in *L. emarginata*. The microvesicles formed were about 100 nm in diameter and coated externally with an electron-dense material. Light also increased the number of three kinds of cytoplasmic bodies. Incidentally, cytoplasmic vacuoles are reversely affected; increased by dark-adaptation, decreased by illumination. BURTON and STOCK-HAMMER (1969) have recently studied the eye of a toadbug, *Gelastocoris oculatus*, and report that light stimulates the production of multivesicular bodies in the retinular cells. The vesicles are believed to form by invagination of the vacuolar membrane.

Light may increase the uptake of extracellular material by photoreceptoral cells. RÖHLICH and TÖRÖ (1965) observed bristle-coated vesicles produced at the bases of rhabdomeric microvilli in *Daphnia pulex* after only 5 minute exposure to bright light. WHITE (1967) noted the formation of coated vesicles at the bases of rhabdoms in larvae of a mosquito (*Aedes aegypti*) upon illumination, similar to those described by EGUCHI and WATERMAN (1967) and mentioned above. He believes that these and like vesicles formed in the proximal parts of the retinular cells are engaged in the incorporation of extracellular fluid and macromolecules from the intercellular spaces, which in turn communicate with the hemocoel. MELAMED and TRUJILLO-CENÓZ (1966) attributed the same function to pinocytotic vesicles of photosensory cells in the eyes of certain spiders (*Lycosa erythrognatha* and *L. thorelli*), and they suggested, further, that the material incorporated may be precursors of the photolabile substance that have been synthesized by the pigmented supportive cells.

A dramatic difference between light and dark-adapted retinular cells in a locust, *Locusta migratoria*, has been described by HORRIDGE and BARNARD (1965). In the dark-adapted state the rhabdom (closed type) is surrounded by a so-called palisade layer, 2000—4000 nm thick, of expanded cisternae of endoplasmic reticulum, beyond which is a zone of mitochondria. In light-adapted animals, however, mitochondria are aggregated about the rhabdom, and the palisade layer has become dispersed as vacuoles in the peripheral cytoplasm of the retinular cells. The authors suggest that the palisade layer may increase the acceptance angle of light and keep the light within the rhabdom by internal reflection. PERRELET (1970) has also found swelling of the agranular endoplasmic reticulum adjacent to the rhabdom of dark-adapted drone bees and rapid contraction of the same organelle in the light-adapted state.

In many eyes there are shifts in the position of pigment granules within photosensory cells with presence or absence of light. Only one example will be cited: the photomechanical changes in pigment in the retinal cells of a spider crab, *Libinia emarginata* (Eguchi and Waterman, 1967). In the light-adapted state the granules of melanin (?) are scattered along the entire length of the retinular cells (thus screening the rhabdoms) whereas in the dark the granules separate into two aggregations: one at the distal (nucleated) ends of the cells and the other at the proximal or basal ends, thus exposing the greater part of the rhabdoms.

Last, in some animals (e.g., cephalopods) there are changes in length of sensory cells — increased by as much as 30% upon dark adaptation and decreased by almost the same amount upon exposure of an excised eye to bright light (see Wells, 1966).

V. Neurites

In most photosensitive cells a nerve fiber emerges from the basal end of the cell, that is, the end opposite the receptoral apparatus. In converse eyes, in which the ciliary or rhabdomeric organelles project toward the incident light, the neurites depart from the back of the retina and converge to form a bundle, the optic nerve. The eyes of insects, snails, nereid worms, and peripatus and the ocelli of hydromedusae and sea stars provide examples. In animals with an inverted retina, as in certain flatworms, nemerteans, chaetognaths, and a polychaete annelid, *Armandia* (see Fig. 40), the cell bodies pass forward through the "pupil" of the eyecup and lie to a large extent outside the ocellus. The neurites, although arising from the basal ends of the cells, are consequently never inside the eye proper.

There are numerous exceptions to the usual basal attachment of neurites. In the ocelli of scallops, *Pecten maximus* for example, the retina has two layers of sensory cells: proximal rhabdomeric receptors that follow the rule stated above, and distal ciliary receptors from which axons leave distally, i.e., just below the receptoral organelle (Barber, Evans, and Land, 1967). The neurites then arch above the ciliary sacs, join like fibers to form an optic nerve that passes over the rim of the retina and behind the pigmented epithelium to combine at the back of the eye with the nerve fibers from the proximal sense cells (see Dakin, 1910). As noted elsewhere the fibers from the distal retina carry "off" responses, those from the proximal retina transmit "on" responses. Another arrangement is seen in a copepod, *Macrocyclops albidus*, in which the axons emerge from the sides of the retinular cells (Fahrenbach, 1964). And among the spiders there are many variations in the connections of axons to receptoral cells (see Bullock and Horridge, 1965).

The most common organelles in photoreceptoral neurites are microtubules (neurotubules) and mitochondria. The former are oriented lengthwise and are most abundant centrally. Sometimes they appear to be absent for reasons not clearly understood. For example, few tubules were reported in the optic neurites of lycosid spiders by Melamed and Trujillo-Cenóz (1966), but we (Eakin and Brandenburger, unpublished) find the optic axons of jumping spiders (*Metaphidippus harfordi* and *Phidippus johnsoni*) loaded with microtubules. Perhaps, they were lost in fixation of the lycosid spiders. The mitochondria are often very long, as in a spider crab, *Libinia emarginata* (Eguchi and Waterman, 1967), and they are usually peripheral in position, i.e., just under the plasma membrane of the fiber.

Vesicles are sometimes observed in the axons of photoreceptoral cells. For example, we found several kinds of vesicles in nerve fibers from the eye of a snail, *Helix aspersa* (EAKIN and BRANDENBURGER, 1967 a). Some, between 80 and 100 nm in diameter, have dense centers; others, varying in size from 50 to 130 nm, are relatively clear. Nerve fibers in pulmonate gastropods have been classified according to the kind of vesicle carried (see GERSCHENFELD, 1963). We believe, however, that the fibers in the optic nerve of *H. aspersa* are of one type, and that the variation seen may be attributed to developmental and physiological fluctuations, because we found all kinds of vesicles along the course of a single fiber. A similar or even greater diversification of vesicles was noted in a peripatus, *Perpatonder novaezealandiae*, by EAKIN and WESTFALL (1965 b), and vesicles with dark centers and also clear ones were observed in the single neurite from the ocellus in a rotifer, *Asplanchna brightwelli* (see EAKIN and WESTFALL, 1965 a). Axonal vesicles are believed to be formed by Golgi centers in the sensory cell body and to function as neurotransmitters.

Finally, there is a miscellany of other organelles and inclusions in the axons of photoreceptoral cells: massive aggregations of alpha and beta granules of glycogen (e.g., in barnacles, *Balanus cariosus* and *B. amphitrite*, according to FAHRENBACH, 1965); lines of tubular and vesicular endoplasmic reticulum reported in *Libinia emarginata*, a spider crab, by EGUCHI and WATERMAN (1967); pleomorphic dense bodies (e.g., an onychophoran, *Epiperipatus braziliensis*, see EAKIN and WESTFALL, 1965 b); and unusual pigment granules (e.g., in several species of flies, MELAMED and TRUJILLO-CENÓZ, 1968). The last named are dense osmiophilic particles about 200 nm in diameter, seemingly without membranes, which congregate with mitochondria in the centers of the fibers.

Very few workers have traced optic axons in invertebrates to their terminals. TRUJILLO-CENÓZ and MELAMED (1966, 1968) have recently conducted splendid studies of optic fibers in three dipterans (*Lucilia*, *Chrysomia* and *Sarcophaga*). The axons have been followed to their synapses with the second order neurones in the optic cartridges (first neuropile) below the peripheral retina. The terminals are characterized by an increase in the density of the axoplasm, a greater number of mitochondria, the unusual pigment granules just mentioned, and by invaginations of the cell membrane into which fit capitate projections of glial cells. The synaptic loci are identified by T-shaped structures.

Although I intended to leave neural pathways outside this discussion, I have succumbed to the temptation to refer briefly to two studies. First, MELAMED and TRUJILLO-CENÓZ (1968) observed the configuration of the axons emerging from the eight retinular cells of an ommatidium in three species of flies. The axons are arranged in a bundle of six peripheral fibers and two central ones, the latter from the superior and inferior central cells (see p. 645 and Fig. 34). The peripheral fibers are distributed to six different optic cartridges (each of which receives fibers from six different ommatidia) where they synapse with the second order of neurones; the long central fibers, on the other hand, bypass the first synaptic relays and continue to higher centers. As noted earlier the axons from the central cells probably carry information on polarized light.

The second work is that of LAND (1969a) on jumping spiders, referred to earlier in connection with perception of color. He correlated the four layers of the retina in the antero-medial eyes of *Phidippus johnsoni* with parts of the first optic glomerulus, a horse-shoe shaped body of neuropile lying on the dorsal aspect of the brain immediately behind the eyes. In this body the axons of the receptoral cells synapse with the second order neurones, the cell bodies of which lie to one side of the glomerulus. Without going into details it will suffice to state that LAND found the axons from each retinal layer to be apparently distributed to a specific part of the glomerulus.

VI. Accessory Structures

A. Lenses

The term lens is here used for any structure that gathers and concentrates light. There is almost as great a diversity in types of invertebrate lenses as there is in kinds of photoreceptoral organelles. Lenses can be made in various ways.

1. Aggregations of Cells

First, they can be formed from an aggregation of whole cells, the vertebrate method of lens development. One example: the lenses in the ocelli of a scallop, *Pecten maximus*, are cellular biconvex bodies (Fig. 50) attached to the undersurface of the cornea (see BARBER, EVANS, and LAND, 1967, for references). The lens cells vary from irregular flattened elements peripherally to rectangular or semi-globular ones centrally; they fit closely together without intercellular spaces. Electron microscopy (BARBER, EVANS, and LAND, 1967) reveals a sparse population of mitochondria and cisternae of endoplasmic reticulum in a lightly granular cytoplasm. The lens does not form an image on the retina (see p. 676).

And there are examples of lenses consisting of single cells. The lens in each branchial eye of a sabellid annelid (*Branchiomma vesiculosum*), discussed earlier, is a large cell with a dish-shaped nucleus basally, an ovoid mass of vesicles centrally, and many cytoplasmic protrusions which pass from the distal surface of the cell through the cuticle (KRASNE and LAWRENCE, 1966).

A component of the dioptric apparatus of many arthropods lying beneath a lens or cornea is called a cone. Space does not permit a discussion of the different kinds of cones (see GOLDSMITH, 1964). In some instances, as in spiders and some insects, the cone is an aggregation of cells; in other instances it is a secreted body (see below). In a jumping spider, *Phidippus johnsoni*, the cone cells are wedge-shaped elements, somewhat radially arranged, consisting almost entirely of fine granules (150 Å in diameter) and filaments (EAKIN and BRANDENBURGER, 1972). The nucleus and cytoplasmic organelles are restricted to a narrow layer beneath the outer cell membrane. In a toadbug, *Gelastocoris oculatus*, the cone cells are almost entirely lacking in mitochondria (BURTON and STOCKHAMMER, 1969).

2. Cellular Processes

A second kind of lens is formed by a ball of tangled membrane-bounded cellular processes, illustrated here by lenses of nereid annelids (EAKIN and WESTFALL, 1964a). In two species, *Neanthes succinea* and *Nereis limnicola*, we observed the early formation of the lens from lobate extensions of the distal ends of pigmented

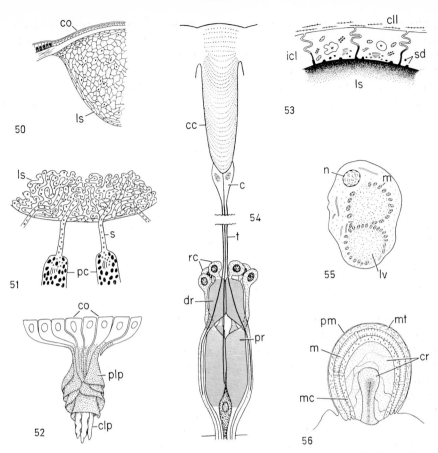

Figs. 50—56. Types of lenses. Fig. 50. Multicellular lens of a scallop, modified from DAKIN, 1910; Fig. 51. Lens formed by processes of pigmented cells in a nereid worm, based on EAKIN and WESTFALL, 1964a; Fig. 52. Developing lens from processes of corneal cells in a squid, from ARNOLD, 1967; Fig. 53. Secreted lens in a peripatus, modified from EAKIN and WESTFALL, 1965b; Fig. 54. Secreted lens or crystalline cone in a firefly, modified from HORRIDGE, 1968; Fig. 55. Intracellular lens vesicles in an ascidian, modified from DILLY, 1961; Fig. 56. Intracellular lens made of scales in a dinoflagellate, modified from GREUET, 1968. *c*, cone cells; *cc*, crystalline cone; *cll*, collagenous layer; *clp*, central lentigenic processes; *co*, cornea; *cr*, crystalline (lens) body; *dr*, distal rhabdomere; *icl*, inner layer of cornea; *ls*, lens; *lv*, lens vesicle; *m*, mitochondria or mitochondrial layer; *mc*, microcrystalline layer; *mt*, microtubular layer; *n*, nucleus; *pc*, pigmented cells; *plp*, peripheral lentigenic processes; *pm*, plasmalemma; *pr*, proximal rhabdomere; *rc*, retinular cell; *s*, stalk; *sd*, secretory droplet; *t*, crystalline threads

(supportive) retinal cells. These processes are filled with multiform osmiophilic bodies or secretory droplets of Golgi origin. As the processes grow they arch above the developing rhabdomeres from sensory cells, and later intertwine with one another to form a lenticular mass that is roughly spherical, except for an irregular distal surface. Figure 51 shows in a small segment of an adult lens in *Nereis vexillosa* that the organ is composed of highly folded and interdigitating processes filled with droplets or vesicles. The processes retain their connections with the parent cells, the supportive elements of the retina, by slender stalks which were seen by light microscopists (see EAKIN and WESTFALL, 1964a, for references). The stalks probably serve as a means of continual renewal of the lenticular processes through the flow of vesicles from the supportive cells. Whether this organ should be called a lens or a vitreous body (or Füllmasse) is open to debate (PFLUGFELDER, 1932; EAKIN and WESTFALL, 1964a; FISCHER and BRÖKELMANN, 1965; HERMANS and CLONEY, 1966). Although it does not appear to form an image, it probably gathers light. FISCHER (1963, 1964) has shown that in the dark-adapted eye of *Platynereis dumerilii* more of the distal surface of the lens is exposed than in the

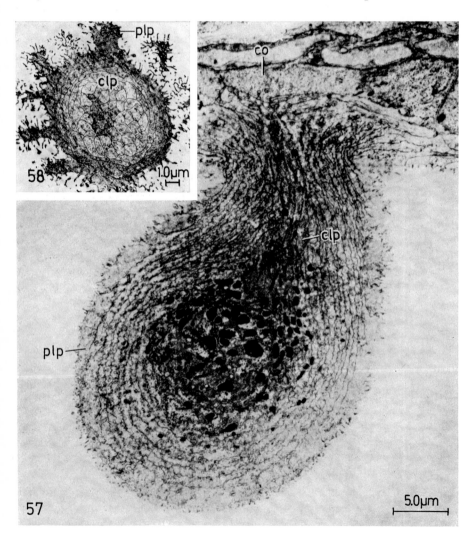

Fig. 57. Section through developing lens of squid, *Loligo pealii*. *clp*, central lentigenic processes; *co*, corneal cell; *plp*, peripheral lentigenic processes. From ARNOLD, 1967

Fig. 58. Cross section through developing lens of *L. pealii*. *clp*, central lentigenic processes; *plp*, peripheral lentigenic processes bearing many microvilli. From ARNOLD, 1967

light-adapted eye by a manifold enlargement of the pupil. The lens in this form is proteinaceous (FISCHER, 1963).

The squid and octopus are other examples of animals with lenses formed by processes of cells. In these instances, however, the processes come not from retinal but from corneal cells. The details of development of the lens in a squid, *Loligo pealii*, and an octopus, *Octopus vulgaris*, have been published by ARNOLD (1967). Cytoplasmic extensions from corneal cells aggregate to form a bulb-like lens primordium that projects into the optic vesicle (Figs. 52, 57, 58). The lentigenic processes enlarge and new ones from other corneal cells are added to the primordium to form additional concentric layers. The outermost one is characterized by prominent microvilli. The lens material is packaged by Golgi centers into granules that fuse, eventually filling the processes. The deposition of the lens material (chemical nature unknown) proceeds from the center to the periphery. The adult lens is a solid, crystalline, spheroidal body that accommodates by movement backward by ciliary muscles and forward by muscles of the eyeball.

3. Extracellular Secretions

The lenses of many gastropods, onychophorans, and arthropods are formed by extracellular aggregations of secretory products. An example is the large spherical lens of a pulmonate snail, *Helix aspersa* (EAKIN and BRANDENBURGER, 1967a). Electron microscopy of the developing eye in embryos of varying age showed that the lens in this mollusk arises from condensations of granular material within the lumen of the early eyecup. Growth is achieved by deposition of more particles at the surface. Meanwhile, the granules fuse internally. A section through the lens at this stage (Fig. 59) shows a gradient in size of units from small densities at the periphery, like those in the lumen of the optic vesicle, through concentric zones of droplets of increasing size to the center of the young lens where the droplets are amalgamated. The adult lens appears completely homogeneous (Fig. 37), although medulla and cortex have different staining properties.

What is the source of the lentigenic material in *H. aspersa*? We noted large numbers of membrane-bounded secretory granules within presumptive corneal cells and prospective supportive cells of the retina. The granules are produced in Golgi centers deep within the cells near their nuclei and large concentrations of rough endoplasmic reticulum. The granules then move, we believe, to the luminal surface, fuse with the plasma membrane of the cells, and discharge the secretion into the cavity of the optic vesicle. Arrows in Fig. 59 direct the reader's attention to the secretory granules in developing cornea (right) and retina (left) and to released granules in the lumen of the eyecup and on the surface of the lens. Less dense humor, similarly produced, fills the rest of the opticoel.

The above account appears to apply also to the structure and development of lenses in a nudibranch, *Hermissenda crassicornis*, and in several species of onychophorans (Fig. 53) (EAKIN, WESTFALL, and DENNIS, 1967; EAKIN and WESTFALL, 1965b).

The secreted lenses and cones of arthropods are highly variable. As merely one example, we may consider the light-refracting and -conducting apparatus of a firefly, *Photuris versicolor*, recently studied by HORRIDGE (1968). Each ommatidium of the compound eye has a long tapering corneal cone (a secreted lens) that is strongly laminated with about 200 concentric paraboloids that bend the light toward the apex of the cone (Fig. 54). Below the tip of the cone is a group of four hyaline cone cells from the proximal ends of which extend very long filaments along the outer surface of the rhabdom[2] to the basement membrane of the

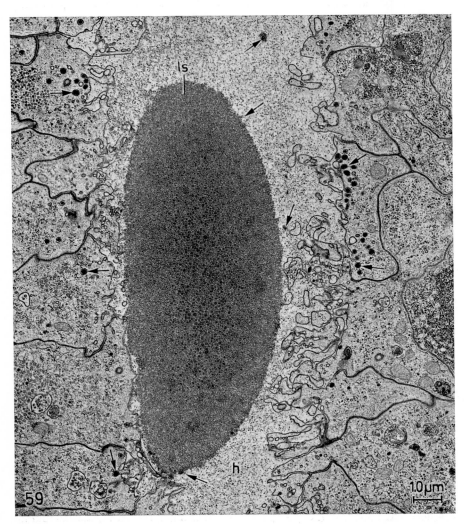

Fig. 59. Section through young optic vesicle of snail, *Helix aspersa*. *h*, humor; *ls*, lens in early stage of development (note gradient in droplets); arrows, secretory droplets in presumptive corneal (right) and retinal (left) cells, in lumen and on lens. From EAKIN and BRANDENBURGER, hitherto unpublished

---

[2] Dr. HORRIDGE informs me that his figure 1 (HORRIDGE, 1968), reproduced here as Fig. 54, should show only one instead of two distal rhabdomeres. He reports, moreover, that the basal cell has a rhabdomere. The eight neurites from each ommatidium arise from one distal retinular cell, six proximal retinular cells, and one basal cell with a small rhabdomere. Postscript in proof: see HORRIDGE (1969a) for a revised figure of the ommatidium of the firefly and for additional information and interpretation.

ommatidium. According to Horridge: "It is directly observable that light entering the corneal facets is channeled along the crystalline threads." Similar threads have been observed in other arthropods (see Röhlich and Törö, 1965). This dioptric and channeling system in *Photuris*, together with the hypertrophied receptor layer and the photomechanical movement of pigment in the supporting cells probably permits the creature to capture the faint flashes of light from other fireflies. The chemical nature of this lens is not known; in other arthropods it is chitinous whereas the crystalline cone or posterior lens of a copepod, *Copilia quadrata*, resembles glycogen (Wolken and Florida, 1969). The optics of the dioptric apparatus of the firefly *Phausis spendidula* has been recently analyzed by Seitz (1969).

Burton and Stockhammer (1969) studied the crystalline threads of a toadbug, *Gelastocoris oculatus*, and their junctional relationships with the retinular cells. It is suggested that these cell junctions have both desmosomal and synaptic properties. In other insects (e.g., skipper butterflies and night-flying moths) the crystalline threads or tracts are distal extensions of retinular cells. The function of crystalline tracts as light guides is discussed by Miller, Bernard, and Allen (1968).

4. Intracellular Organelles

Yet another kind of dioptric device is exemplified by certain vesicles and crystalline bodies within a cell. For example, Dilly (1961, 1964) described and figured lens vesicles in the ocellus of an ascidian tadpole (*Ciona intestinalis*). Above the eyecup lies a single cell containing a vertical row of three vesicles, the diameters of which vary from 6,000 to 12,000 nm. The vesicles are not bounded by a membrane and are filled with finely granular, electron-lucent material. Many mitochondria border the vesicle (Fig. 55), a picture similar to that in the cellular lens of *Daphnia pulex*, a cladoceran (Röhlich and Törö, 1965; Güldner and Wolff, 1970). Eakin and Kuda (1971) described granular bodies in *three* lens cells in the larval ocellus of two ascidians, *Ciona intestinalis* and *Distaplia occidentalis*. Barnes (1971) reports the same in his study of the tadpole of *Amaroucium constellatum*. The granules in the lens cells have the ultrastructure of beta particles of glycogen. We have recently obtained further evidence of their glycogen nature: they give a positive PAS reaction and they are digestible with alpha amylase (Eakin and Kuda, unpublished). Glycogen has also been demonstrated in the cone cells of the honeybee drone (Perrelet, 1970).

A second illustration of an intracellular structure serving in all probability as a condenser takes us from the Chordata to the Protozoa and to the eyelets of certain dinoflagellates (*Erythropsis pavillardi* and *Warnowia pulchra*). Greuet (1968) describes the "corps cristallinien" as a multilaminal bulb, resembling an onion, lying distal to the sensory part of the ocellus. The lens and its covering, the cornea, project forward and above the surface of the organism. The lens consists of a central element, which looks like a pestle, and 6 to 8 flattened scales tightly applied in layers to the core (Figs. 42, 56). A so-called mitochondrial layer situated between lens and cornea is thought to elaborate the lens substance.

No organized lens is present in the eyes of many invertebrates, such as the chambered nautilus, certain annelids, sea stars, certain sipunculids, flatworms, nemerteans, chaetognaths, rotifers, and medusae. Light microscopists thought that a lens was present in some of these (e.g., hydromedusan and echinoderm ocelli), but in those eyes studied by electron microscopy it appears that the lumen of the eyecup is filled only with the processes of sensory and supportive cells, and humor.

5. Corneal Properties

Transmission and scanning electron microscopy have revealed structural features on the surface of many cuticular lenses which have observable optical effects. Miller and his associates (see Miller, Møller, and Bernhard, 1966, for references) have shown that some insects (e.g., the moth *Sphynx*), but not others (e.g., the grasshopper *Melanoplus*), possess arrays of nipples projecting into the air above the corneal surface, which reduce the intensity of reflected radiant energy. The nipples, invisible with light microscopy, are conical rods about 200 nm high and hexagonally spaced, about 200 nm center-to-center. They develop in the pupa of a moth, *Deilephila elpenor*, from an extracellular membrane above the microvilli of young cornea-secreting cells (Gemne, 1966). In still other insects (e.g., the fly *Calliphora*) the nipples are subsurface, being embedded in a cortical layer of the cornea. The finding of subsurface nipples in an Eocene dipteran from Baltic amber demonstrates that corneal nipples are not a modern invention of nature.

Spectrophotometric measurements of the intensity of light reflected from corneal surfaces of various insects and experiments with models showed that nipples reduce the intensity of reflected light and increase the transmission of radiant energy through the cornea (Miller, Møller, and Bernhard, 1966). The advantages of corneal nipples to the insect are: camouflage under conditions of bright light, enhanced visibility in dim light, and reduction of back reflectance in eyes with tapeta.

Another structural feature, lamination of the cornea, has been shown by the same group of workers (see Bernard and Miller, 1968, and Miller, Bernard, and Allen, 1968) to endow the corneas of some dipteran insects with the properties of a transmission interference filter. Certain wavelengths are reflected, thus accounting for the colored bands of the compound eye of a horsefly *(Hybomitra)* or the variously colored corneas of other insects. The wavelengths reflected depend upon the thickness of the alternating laminae and their refractive indices. The greenish cast of the antero-median eyes of jumping spiders (e.g., *Phidippus johnsoni*) appears to be due to lamination in their corneas (Eakin and Brandenburger, 1972). Corneas in this animal are distinct subparts of cuticular lenses. The spacing of the layers is in the correct order of magnitude (1/4 wave length) to reflect green, assuming the refractive index of the cornea to be that of chitin. The lateral eyes, on the other hand, reflect no color, and their corneal laminae are narrower and would give interference transmission in the ultraviolet range only. The value of corneal reflections to an organism would be increased color contrast. In the instance of the AM eyes of a jumping spider, which are color-sensitive (see above), objects against a green background (leaves and grass) would have enhanced contrast if some of the green wavelengths were reflected from the surface of the cornea.

B. Pigmented Cells

The eyes of most invertebrates have pigment-bearing cells closely associated with photoreceptoral cells. In small, simple ocelli there is usually only one pigmented cell, which forms a cup about the light-sensitive organelles of the receptor cells. The prostomial ocelli of an annelid, *Armandia brevis* (Fig. 30) is an example. In the eye of an arrowworm, *Sagitta scrippsae*, there is one pigmented cell at the center of the organ, but it has five concavities, each accommodating a battery of photoreceptors (references in EAKIN and WESTFALL, 1964b). Pigmented cups, such as the stigma of *Euglena* permit illumination of the photoreceptors from certain directions only. The pattern of excitation of the individual receptors may be used by the organism to orient itself in relation to the source of light. Moreover, light having entered the eye and passed through the sensory cell or cells will be absorbed by the pigmented cup. In contrast to these simple eyecups, numerous pigmented cells are found in larger and more complex eyes, such as those of mollusks, arthropods, onychophorans, many annelids, and echinoderms, where they are arrayed with sensory cells to constitute the retina. In many instances the pigment can be moved to permit more or less light to reach the photoreceptors (see p. 666).

Although a chemical identification is usually lacking, the pigment in many ocelli is probably melanin. The pigment in the ocelli of sea stars, however, is not melanin. The pigment is red and the granules differ in appearance in the electron microscope from those in other eyes. The granules in the species of sea stars studied by JANE WESTFALL, JEAN BRANDENBURGER and me are without membranes and are very pale when fixed with glutaraldehyde. VAUPEL von HARNACK (1963) found granules of two kinds in the ocelli of *Asterias rubens*: small ones that are similar in size to those observed by us, and large ones bounded by a membrane and containing vacuoles. The latter may not be pigment granules but cytoplasmic bodies like ones seen by us in Pacific Coast sea stars (e.g., *Pycnopodia helianthoides*) which vary greatly in size and in appearance. YOSHIDA and OHTSUKI (1966) found a water-soluble red substance in the ocelli of a sea star, *Asterias amurensis*, that yielded carotenoids upon denaturation.

Pigment cells function not only as light absorbers but also as supportive elements. They are usually bound tightly to sensory cells and to one another by gap junctions and desmosomes along the luminal border of the retina, and often by septate desmosomes laterally. They characteristically contain bundles of tonofilaments extending lengthwise of the cells. Additionally, their microvillar processes give support in many instances to the receptoral organelles. Examples: in the ocellus of an ascidian, *Distaplia occidentalis*, villi of the pigmented cells project between the disks or lamellae of the receptor cells (EAKIN and KUDA, unpublished); in the eyecup of a sipunculid, *Phascolosoma agassizii*, long processes with tonofilaments (Figs. 38, 39) make a feltwork about the microvilli of the sensory cells (HERMANS and EAKIN, 1969); and slender extensions containing pigment granules (Fig. 32) enclose the rhabdomeric segments of receptor cells in the antero-lateral eyes of a jumping spider, *Phidippus johnsoni*, and in the antero-median eyes of the same animal non-pigmented processes form a dense mesh about the rhabdomeres, especially those (LAND's number 4 layer) just behind the vitreous body (EAKIN and BRANDENBURGER, 1972).

Third, pigmented cells serve as nutritive and metabolic centers for the eye. Mention has already been made of their role in some animals in the secretion of material from which lens and humor form (e.g., nereid worms and pulmonate snails). They usually have well-developed rough endoplasmic reticulum, Golgi apparatus, glycogen granules, secretory vesicles — morphological evidence of synthetic activity. As noted earlier, whether these cells are concerned with the cycling of photopigment, as in the vertebrate retina, has yet to be determined.

In most eyes pigmented cells and sensory cells arise together from embryonic ectoderm. The external germ layer invaginates to form a cup or a vesicle. Some cells differentiate into receptors, others into supportive elements; yet others into corneal cells. To say that the fate of a cell is the function of its position offers little insight into the enigma of differentiation. There is an exception to the rule that pigmented and sensory cells develop from a common source. In the lateral eye of *Armandia brevis* (Fig. 40) studied by HERMANS (1969) the pigmented cell is mesodermal in origin. The evidence for this statement is not embryological but histological. Between the pigmented and receptoral cells lies a basal lamella and some flattened glial cells, and the undersurface of the pigmented cup is bathed with coelomic fluid.

C. Tapeta

Our tour of invertebrate photoreceptors comes to an end with a bright and shining subject: the reflecting layer, at the back of the eye, known as the tapetum or argenteum. Eyes, here and there among invertebrates, have this novel structure, as do, of course, some vertebrates. A few examples will be described.

In the nauplius eye of a copepod, *Macrocyclops albidus*, two tapetal cells in each ocellus form a reflecting cup behind the sensory cells. The reflecting cells are filled with tightly packed, flat square crystals stacked 20 to 60 deep and oriented with their sides toward the inside surface of the cup (FAHRENBACH, 1964). The crystalline platelets fall out on sectioning. They fluoresce strongly in ultraviolet light. FAHRENBACH suggested that they are composed of guanine, although the reflecting pigment in the eye of a lobster was found by other workers to be xanthopterin, xanthine, etc., but not guanine (see FAHRENBACH, 1964).

Second, lycosid spiders possess bands of reflecting cells containing crystals similar to those just described. The strips lie beneath the rhabdomeric parts of the sensory cells, parallel to one another, and at right angles to the long axis of the retinal cells (BACCETTI and BEDINI, 1964; MELAMED and TRUJILLO-CENÓZ, 1966). The chemical nature of the crystals is not known.

Tapeta clearly function as mirrors but the only analysis known to me is that of Land on the eyes of a scallop, *Pecten maximus*. Each ocellus of this animal, described earlier, has a prominent reflecting layer that is composed of a single row of cells containing up to 30 layers of square, flat crystals. LAND (1966) concluded that they were guanine on the basis of a few tests (solubility, refractive index, chromatography). In a series of optical studies LAND (1965, 1966) made the brilliant induction that the tapetum of *Pecten* focuses an image on the distal sensory cells of the retina (see p. 630). The lens alone would form an image outside the eye. The distal retina is nearly a sector of a sphere and parallel with the tapetum so that it can receive a reflected image over its whole area. No image is formed on the proximal retina.

Finally, there is a possibility that the red pigmented cup of a rotifer, *Asplanchna brightwelli*, may be a reflector. DR. MICHAEL LAND suggested to me that the thickness of the plates of the cup and the distance between rows of them might be approximately one quarter of the wave length of maximal reflectivity making this a multilayered interference reflecting system. The plates (Fig. 41) are about 50 nm thick and the six or more rows are separated by spaces approximately 100 nm wide (EAKIN and WESTFALL, 1965a), measurements corresponding closely to those obtained by LAND (1966) on the tapetum of *Pecten*. It appears then that on morphological grounds the eyecup of this rotifer is a reflector. If true, light passes through the receptoral lamellae of the sensory cell on entering the ocellus and again after reflection.

If I were a Hamlet I would say to the reader, my companion on this sight-seeing trip: "What think you now, Horatio, of the versatility of nature ?"

Acknowledgments

I am grateful for a generous grant-in-aid (GM 10292) from the United States Public Health Service, for an appointment this year in the Miller Institute for Basic Research in Science of the University of California, and for general support and encouragement by my department. Of the many persons to whom I am indebted I can cite only a few: Mrs. JEAN L. BRANDEN-BURGER, highly valued research associate, who has assisted on all phases of the preparation of this chapter including new research for this review; Dr. JANE A. WESTFALL who collaborated with me on earlier projects and again last summer on a restudy of coelenterate and echinoderm eyes and on a new investigation of nemertean ocelli; Miss BARBARA WESTREE and Miss AILEEN KUDA, research assistants; Miss DOTTIE EAKIN and the UCLA Brain Information Service, supported by contract DHEW PH-43-66-59, for bibliographic assistance; Mrs. EMILY REID who transformed my sketches into finished drawings; JOHN ARNOLD, HENNER FAHRENBACH, TIMOTHY GOLDSMITH, C. GREUET, COLIN HERMANS, RICHARD NISHIOKA, and P. RÖHLICH for micrographs used as figures in this chapter; and two postdoctoral fellows: COLIN O. HERMANS and MICHAEL F. LAND who participated in the study of the fine structure of other new eyes (sipunculid and jumping spider, respectively) and who gave a critical reading of the manuscript.

References

ARNOLD, J.: Fine structure of the development of the cephalopod lens. J. Ultrastruct. Res. **17**, 527—543 (1967).

AUTRUM, H.: Physiologie des Sehens. In: Fortschr. Zool. **13** (BAUER, H., Ed.). Stuttgart: Fischer Verlag 1961.

— BURKHARDT, D.: Spectral sensitivity of single visual cells. Nature (Lond.) **190**, 639 (1961).

BACCETTI, B., BEDINI, C.: Research on the structure and physiology of the eyes of a lycosid spider. I. Microscopic and ultramicroscopic structure. Arch. ital. Biol. **102**, 97—122 (1964).

BÄHR, R.: Die Ultrastructur der Photorezeptoren von *Lithobius forficatus* L. (Chilopoda: Lithobiidae). Z. Zellforsch. **116**, 70—93 (1971).

BARBER, V. C., EVANS, E. M., LAND, M. F.: The fine structure of the eye of the mollusc *Pecten maximus*. Z. Zellforsch. **76**, 295—312 (1967).

— LAND, M. F.: Eye of the cockle, *Cardium edule*: anatomical and physiological investigations. Experientia **23**, 677—678 (1967).

— WRIGHT, D. E.: The fine structure of the sense organs of the cephalopod mollusc *Nautilus*. Z. Zellforsch. **102**, 293—312 (1969).

BARNES, S. N.: Fine structure of the photoreceptor and cerebral ganglion of the tadpole larva of *Amaroucium constellatum* (Verrill) (subphylum: Urochordata; class: Ascidiacea). Z. Zellforsch. **117**, 1—16 (1971).

Becker, H. E., Cone, R. A.: Light-stimulated electrical responses from skin. Science 154, 1051—1053 (1966).
— Goldsmith, T. H.: Light stimulation on the sodium pump in epithelia. Nature (Lond.) 220, 1236—1239 (1968).
Bernard, G. D., Miller, W. H.: Interference filters in the corneas of Diptera. Invest. Ophthal. 7, 416—434 (1968).
Bohn, H., Täuber, U.: Beziehungen zwischen der Wirkung polarisierten Lichtes auf das Elektroretinogramm und der Ultrastruktur des Auges von Gerris lacustris L. Z. vergl. Physiol. 72, 32—53 (1971).
Boyle, P. R.: Fine structure of the eyes of Onithochiton neglectus (Mollusca: Polyplacophora). Z. Zellforsch. 102, 313—332 (1969).
Brammer, J. D.: The ultrastructure of the compound eye of a mosquito Aedes aegypti L. J. exp. Zool. 175, 181—196 (1970).
— White, R. H.: Vitamin A deficiency: effect on mosquito eye ultrastructure. Science 163, 821—823 (1969).
Brandenburger, J. L., Eakin, R. M.: Pathway of incorporation of vitamin A ^{3}H$_2$ into photoreceptors of a snail, Helix aspersa. Vision Res. 10, 639—653 (1970).
Bullock, T. H., Horridge, G. A.: Structure and function in the nervous systems of invertebrates, Vol. I—II. San Francisco & London: Freeman 1965.
Burfield, S. T.: Sagitta. Proc. Trans. Liverpool Biol. Soc. Memoir. 28, 41, App. ii, 1—104 (1927).
Burton, P. R., Stockhammer, K. A.: Electron microscopic studies of the compound eye of the toadbug, Gelastocoris oculatus. J. Morph. 127, 233—258 (1969).
Carlson, S. D., Gemne, G., Robbins, W. E.: Ultrastructure of photoreceptor cells in a vitamin A-deficient moth (Manduca sexta). Experientia (Basel) 25, 175—177 (1969).
— Steeves, III., H. R., Vandeberg, J. S., Robbins, W. E.: Vitamin A deficiency: effect on retinal structure of the moth Manduca sexta. Science 158, 268—270 (1967).
Chaigneau, J.: Etude ultrastructurale de l'organe de Bellonci de Sphaeroma serratum, (Fabricius), Crustacé Isopode Flabellifere. C. R. Acad. Sci. (Paris) 268, 3177—3179 (1969).
— L'organe de Bellonci du Crustacé Isopode Sphaeroma serratum (Fabricius) ultrastructure et signification. Z. Zellforsch. 112, 166—187 (1971).
Clark, A. W.: The fine structure of the eye of the leech, Helobdella stagnalis. J. Cell Sci. 2, 341—348 (1967).
— Millecchia, R., Mauro, A.: The ventral photoreceptor cells of Limulus. I. The microanatomy. J. gen. Physiol. 54, 289—309 (1969).
Curtis, D. J.: The fine structure of photoreceptors in Mitopus morio (phalangida). J. Cell Sci. 4, 327—351 (1969).
Dakin, W. J.: The eye of Pecten. Quart. J. micr. Sci. 55, 49—112 (1910).
Debaisieux, P.: Les yeux de crustacés — Structure, développement, réactions à l'éclairement. Cellule 50, 9—122 (1944).
Dhainaut-Courtois, N.: Sur la présence d'un organe photorécepteur dans le cerveau de Nereis pelagica L. (Annélide polychète). C. R. Acad. Sci. (Paris) 261, 1085—1088 (1965).
— Étude histologique et ultrastructurale des cellules nerveuses du ganglion cérébral de Nereis pelagica L. (Annélide polychète). Comparison entre les types cellulaires I—VI et ceux décrits antérieurement chez les Nereidae. Gen. comp. Endocr. 11, 414—443 (1968).
Diehn, B.: Two perpendicularly oriented pigment systems involved in phototaxis of Euglena. Nature (Lond.) 221, 366—367 (1969).
Dilly, P. N. (or N.): Electron microscope observations of the receptors in the sensory vesicle of the ascidian tadpole. Nature (Lond.) 191, 786—787 (1961).
— Studies on the receptors in the cerebral vesicle of the ascidian tadpole. 2. The ocellus. Quart. J. micr. Sci. 105, 13—20 (1964).
— The structure of a photoreceptor organelle in the eye of Pterotrachea mutica. Z. Zellforsch. 99, 420—429 (1969).
Dodge, J. D., Crawford, R. M.: Observations on the fine structure of the eyespot and associated organelles in the dinoflagellate Glenodinium foliaceum. J. Cell Sci. 5, 479—493 (1969).

DUDLEY, P. L.: The fine structure and development of the nauplius eye of the copepod *Doropygus seclusus* Illg. Cellule **68**, 7—42 (1969).

EAKIN, R. M.: Lines of evolution of photoreceptors. In: General physiology of cell specialization (MAZIA, D., TYLER, A., Eds.). New York: McGraw-Hill 1963.

— Evolution of photoreceptors. Cold Spr. Harb. Symp. quant. Biol. **30**, 363—370 (1966).

— Evolution of photoreceptors. In: Evolutionary Biology, Vol. II, (DOBZHANSKY, T., HECHT, M. K., STEERE, W. C., Eds.). New York: Appleton-Century-Crofts 1968.

— BRANDENBURGER, J. L.: Differentiation in the eye of a pulmonate snail *Helix aspersa*. J. Ultrastruct. Res. **18**, 391—421 (1967a).

— — Vesicles and granules in the retina of a snail, *Helix aspersa*. Proc. Electron Microscopy Soc. America, 25th meeting, Baton Rouge, La.: Claitors Book Store 1967b.

— — Functional significance of small vesicles in photoreceptoral cells of a snail, *Helix aspersa*. J. Cell Biol. **35**, 36A (1967c).

— — Light-induced ultrastructural changes in eyes of pulmonate snail, *Helix aspersa*. J. Ultrastruct. Res. **21**, 164 (1968a).

— — Localization of vitamin A in the eye of a pulmonate snail. Proc. nat. Acad. Sci. (Wash.) **60**, 140—145 (1968b).

— — Osmic staining of amphibian and gastropod photoreceptors. J. Ultrastruct. Res. **30**, 619—641 (1970).

— — Fine structure of the eyes of jumping spiders. J. Ultrastruct. Res. (1972) (in press).

— KUDA, A.: Ultrastructure of sensory receptors in ascidian tadpoles. Z. Zellforsch. **112**, 287—312 (1971).

— WESTFALL, J. A.: Fine structure of photoreceptors in amphioxus. J. Ultrastruct. Res. **6**, 531—539 (1962a).

— — Fine structure of photoreceptors in the hydromedusan, *Polyorchis penicillatus*. Proc. nat. Acad. Sci. (Wash.) **48**, 826—833 (1962b).

— — Further observations on the fine structure of some invertebrate eyes. Z. Zellforsch. **62**, 310—332 (1964a).

— — Fine structure of the eye of a chaetognath. J. Cell Biol. **21**, 115—132 (1964b).

— — Ultrastructure of the eye of the rotifer *Asplanchna brightwelli*. J. Ultrastruct. Res. **12**, 46—62 (1965a).

— — Fine structure of the eye of peripatus (Onychophora). Z. Zellforsch. **68**, 278—300 (1965b).

— — Fine structure of nemertean ocelli. Amer. Zool. **8**, 803 (1968).

— — DENNIS, M. J.: Fine structure of the eye of a nudibranch mollusc, *Hermissenda crassicornis*. J. Cell Sci. **2**, 349—358 (1967).

EGUCHI, E.: The fine structure of the eccentric retinula cell in the insect compound eye (*Bombyx mori*). J. Ultrastruct. Res. **7**, 328—338 (1962).

— Rhabdom structure and receptor potentials in single crayfish retinular cells. J. cell. comp. Physiol. **66**, 411—430 (1965).

— Fine structure and spectral sensitivities of retinular cells in the dorsal sector of compound eyes in the dragonfly *Aeschna*. Z. vergl. Physiol. **71**, 201—218 (1971).

— NAKA, K. I., KUWABARA, M.: The development of the rhabdom and the appearance of the electrical response in the insect eye. J. gen. Physiol. **46**, 143—157 (1962).

— WATERMAN, T. H.: Fine structure patterns in crustacean rhabdoms. In: Proc. internat. symp. on the functional organization of the compound eye. Oxford-New York: Pergamon Press 1966.

— — Changes in retinal fine structure induced in the crab *Libinia* by light and dark adaptation Z. Zellforsch. **79**, 209—229 (1967).

ELOFSSON, R.: The ultrastructure of the nauplius eye of *Sapphirina* (Crustacea: Copepoda). Z. Zellforsch. **100**, 376—401 (1969).

FAHRENBACH, W. H.: The fine structure of a nauplius eye. Z. Zellforsch. **62**, 182—197 (1964).

— The micromorphology of some simple photoreceptors. Z. Zellforsch. **66**, 233—254 (1965).

— The morphology of the eyes of *Limulus*. II. Ommatidia of the compound eye. Z. Zellforsch. **93**, 451—483 (1969).

— The morphology of the *Limulus* visual system. III. The lateral rudimentary eye. Z. Zellforsch. **105**, 303—316 (1970).

Fischer, A.: Über den Bau und die hell-dunkel-Adaptation der Augen des Polychäten *Platynereis dumerilii*. Z. Zellforsch. **61**, 338—353 (1963).
— Über Adaptation in den Augen von *Platynereis dumerilii*. Zool. Anz. Supp. **27**, 204—208 (1964).
— Brökelmann, J.: Morphology and structural changes of the eye of Platynereis dumerilii (Polychaeta). In: The structure of the eye. II. Symposium (Rohen, J. W., Ed.) Stuttgart: F. K. Schattauer-Verlag 1965.
— — Das Auge von *Platynereis dumerilii* (Polychaeta): sein Feinbau im ontogenetischen und adaptiven Wandel. Z. Zellforsch. **71**, 217—244 (1966).
— Horstmann, G.: Der Feinbau des Auges der Mehlmotte *Ephestia kuehniella* Zeller. (Lepidoptera, Pyralididae). Z. Zellforsch. **116**, 275—304 (1971).
Friend, D. S., Murray, M. J.: Osmium impregnation of the Golgi apparatus. Amer. J. Anat. **117**, 135—150 (1965).
Frisch, K. von: Aus dem Leben der Bienen. Berlin-Göttingen-Heidelberg-New York: Springer 1964.
Fujimoto, K., Yanase, T., Okuno, Y., Iwata, K.: Electrical response in the Onchidium eyes. Memoirs Osaka Gakugei Univ. **15**, 98—108 (1966).
Gemne, G.: Fine structure of the insect cornea and corneal nipples during ontogenesis. In: Sixth international congress for electron microscopy, 511—512. Tokyo: Maruzen Co. 1966.
Gerschenfeld, H. M.: Observations on the ultrastructure of synapses in some pulmonate molluscs. Z. Zellforsch. **60**, 258—275 (1963).
Gibbons, I. R.: Chemical dissection of cilia. Arch. Biol. (Liège) **76**, 317—352 (1965).
Gillary, H. L., Wolbarsht, M. L.: Electrical responses from the eye of a land snail. Rev. canad. Biol. **26**, 125—134 (1967).
Goldsmith, T. H.: The visual system of the honeybee. Proc. nat. Acad. Sci. (Wash.) **44**, 123—126 (1958).
— The color vision of insects. In: Light and life (McElroy, W. D., Glass, B., Eds.). Baltimore: Johns Hopkins Press (1961).
— Fine structure of the retinulae in the compound eye of the honey-bee. J. Cell Biol. **14**, 489—494 (1962).
— The visual system of insects. In: The physiology of insecta, Vol. I (Rockstein, M., Ed.). New York: Academic Press 1964.
— Fernandez, H. R.: Some photochemical and physiological aspects of visual excitation in compound eyes. In: Proc. internat. symp. on the functional organization of the compound eye. Oxford-New York: Pergamon Press 1966.
— Warner, L. T.: Vitamin A in the vision of insects. J. gen. Physiol. **47**, 433—441 (1964).
Gorman, A. L. F., McReynolds, J. S.: Hyperpolarizing and depolarizing receptor potentials in the scallop eye. Science **165**, 309—310 (1969).
— — Barnes, S. N.: Photoreceptors in primitive chordates: fine structure, hyperpolarizing receptor potentials, and evolution. Science **172**, 1052—1054 (1971).
Grell, K. G.: Protozoologie, 2nd ed. Berlin-Heidelberg-New York: Springer 1968.
Grenacher, H.: Untersuchungen über das Sehorgan der Arthropoden, insbes. der Spinnen, Insecten und Crustaceen. Göttingen: Vandenhoeck und Ruprecht 1879.
Greuet, C.: Organisation ultrastructurale de l'ocelle de deux peridiniens *Warnowiidae*, *Erythropsis pavillardi* Kofoid et Swezy et *Warnowia pulchra* Schiller. Protistologica **4**, 209—230 (1968).
Gribakin, F. G.: Types of photoreceptor cells in the compound eye of the worker honey-bee *Apis mellifera* as revealed by the electron microscope. (In Russian). Tsitologiia **9**, 1276—1280 (1967).
— Cellular basis of color vision in the honey bee. Nature (Lond.) **233**, 639—641 (1969).
Güldner, F. H., Wolff, J. R.: Über die Ultrastruktur des Komplexauges von *Daphnia pulex*. Z. Zellforsch. **104**, 259—274 (1970).
Hanker, J. S., Seaman, A. R., Weiss, L. P., Ueno, H., Bergman, R. A., Seligman, A. M.: Osmiophilic reagents: new cytochemical principle for light and electron microscopy. Science **146**, 1039—1043 (1964).
Hartman, O.: Catalogue of the polychaetous annelids of the world. Vol. II, Allan Hancock Foundat. Publ. (occasional paper) no. 23, 537 (1959).

HERMANS, C. O.: Fine structure of the segmental ocelli of *Armandia brevis* (Polychaeta: Opheliidae). Z. Zellforsch. **96**, 361—371 (1969).
— CLONEY, R. A.: Fine structure of the prostomial eyes of *Armandia brevis* (Polychaeta: Opheliidae). Z. Zellforsch. **72**, 583—596 (1966).
— EAKIN, R. M.: Fine structure of the cerebral ocelli of a sipunculid, *Phascolosoma agassizii*. Z. Zellforsch. **100**, 325—339 (1969).
HORRIDGE, G. A.: Presumed photoreceptive cilia in a ctenophore. Quart. J. micr. Sci. **105**, 311—317 (1964).
— Pigment movement and the crystalline threads of the firefly eye. Nature **218**, 778—779 (1968).
— The eye of the firefly *Photuris*. Proc. roy. Soc. B **171**, 445—463 (1969a).
— Unit studies on the retina of dragonflies. Z. vergl. Physiol. **62**, 1—37 (1969b).
— BARNARD, P. B. T.: Movement of palisade in locust retinula cells when illuminated. Quart. J. micr. Sci. **106**, 131—135 (1965).
— WALCOTT, B., IOANNIDES, A. C.: The tiered retina of *Dytiscus*: a new type of compound eye. Proc. roy. Soc. B **175**, 83—94 (1970).
HUGHES, H. P. I.: A light and electron microscope study of some opisthobranch eyes. Z. Zellforsch. **106**, 79—98 (1970).
HYMAN, L. H.: The invertebrates: Protozoa through Ctenophora, Vol. I. New York: McGraw-Hill 1940.
— The invertebrates: Echinodermata, Vol. IV. New York: McGraw-Hill 1955.
ISSEROFF, H., CABLE, R. M.: Fine structure of photoreceptors in larval trematodes. Z. Zellforsch. **86**, 511—534 (1968).
JACKLET, J. W.: Electrophysiological organization of the eye of *Aplysia*. J. gen. Physiol. **53**, 21—42 (1969).
JOLY, R.: Sur l'ultrastructure de l'oeil de *Lithobius forficatus* L. (Myriapode Chilopode). C. R. Acad. Sci. (Paris) **268**, 3180—3182 (1969).
KABUTA, H., TOMINAGA, Y., KUWABARA, M.: The rhabdomeric microvilli of several arthropod compound eyes kept in darkness. Z. Zellforsch. **85**, 78—88 (1968).
KAWAGUTI, S., MABUCHI, K.: Electron microscopy on the eyes of a giant clam. Biol. J. Okayama Univ. **15**, 87—100 (1969).
KERNÉIS, A.: Photorécepteurs du panache de *Dasychone bombyx* (Dalyell) annélides polychètes. Morphologie et ultrastructure. C. R. Acad. Sci. (Paris) **263**, 653—656 (1966).
— Nouvelles données histochimiques et ultrastructurales sur les photorécepteurs "branchiaux" de *Dasychone bombyx* (Dalyell) (Annélide Polychète). Z. Zellforsch. **86**, 280—292 (1968).
KRASNE, F. B., LAWRENCE, P. A.: Structure of the photoreceptors in the compound eyespots of *Branchiomma vesiculosum*. J. Cell Sci. **1**, 239—248 (1966).
KUIPER, J. W.: The optics of the compound eye. Symp. Soc. exp. Biol. **16**, 58—71 (1962).
LAND, M. F.: Image formation by a concave reflector in the eye of the scallop, *Pecten maximus*. J. Physiol. (Lond.) **179**, 138—153 (1965).
— A multilayer interference reflector in the eye of the scallop, *Pecten maximus*. J. exp. Biol. **45**, 433—447 (1966).
— Functional aspects of the optical and retinal organization of the mollusc eye. Symp. Zool. Soc. Lond. **23**, 75—96 (1968).
— Structure of the retinae of the principal eyes of jumping spiders (Salticidae: Dendryphantinae) in relation to visual optics. J. exp. Biol. **51**, 443—470 (1969a).
— Movements of the retinae of jumping spiders (Salticidae: Dendryphantinae) in response to visual stimuli. J. exp. Biol. **51**, 471—493 (1969b).
— Orientation of jumping spiders in the absence of visual feedback. J. exp. Biol. **54**, 119—139 (1971).
LANGER, H., THORELL, B.: Microspectrophotometry of single rhabdomeres in the insect eye. Exp. Cell Res. **41**, 673—677 (1966).
LASANSKY, A.: Cell junctions in ommatidia of *Limulus*. J. Cell Biol. **33**, 365—384 (1967).
LEEDALE, G. F., MEEUSE, B. J. D., PRINGSHEIM, E. G.: Structure and physiology of *Euglena spirogyra*. I and II. Arch. Mikrobiol. **50**, 68—102 (1965).
LINKO, A.: Über den Bau der Augen bei den Hydromedusen. Mem. Acad. Imp. Sci. St. Petersbourg, Ser. VIII, **10**, No. 3, 1—23 (1900).

Little, E. V.: The structure of the ocelli of *Polyorchis penicillata*. Univ. Calif. Publ. Zool. **11**, 307—328 (1914).

MacRae, E. K.: The fine structure of photoreceptors in a marine flatworm. Z. Zellforsch. **75**, 469—484 (1966).

Mauro, A., Baumann, F.: Electrophysiological evidence of photoreceptors in the epistellar body of *Eledone moschata*. Nature (Lond.) **220**, 1332—1334 (1968).

McReynolds, J. S., Gorman, A. L. F.: Photoreceptor potentials of opposite polarity in the eye of the scallop, *Pecten irradians*. J. gen. Physiol. **56**, 376—391 (1970a).

— — Membrane conductances and spectral sensitivities of *Pecten* photoreceptors. J. gen. Physiol. **56**, 392—406 (1970b).

Melamed, J., Trujillo-Cenóz, O.: The fine structure of the visual system of *Lycosa* (Araneae: Lycosidae). I. Retina and optic nerve. Z. Zellforsch. **74**, 12—31 (1966).

— — The fine structure of the central cells in the ommatidia of dipterans. J. Ultrastruct. Res. **21**, 313—334 (1968).

Miller, W. H.: Morphology of the ommatidia of the compound eye of Limulus. J. biophys. biochem. Cytol. **3**, 421—428 (1957).

— Derivatives of cilia in the distal sense cells of the retina of *Pecten*. J. biophys. biochem. Cytol. **4**, 227—228 (1958).

— Bernard, G. D., Allen, J. L.: The optics of insect compound eyes; microcomponents with dimensions near a wavelength of light cause observable optical effects. Science **162**, 760—767 (1968).

— Møller, A. R., Bernhard, C. G.: The corneal nipple array. In: Proc. internat. symp. on the functional organization of the compound eye. 21—33. Oxford-New York: Pergamon Press 1966.

Millott, N.: The dermal light sense. Symp. Zool. Soc. Lond. **23**, 1—36 (1968).

Moody, M. F.: Photoreceptor organelles in animals. Biol. Rev. **39**, 43—86 (1964).

Mote, M. I., Goldsmith, T. H.: Compound eyes: localization of two color receptors in the same ommatidium. Science **171**, 1254—1255 (1971).

Nakao, T.: On the fine structure of the amphioxus photoreceptor. Tohoku J. exp. Med. **82**, 349—369 (1964).

Newell, P. F., Newell, G. E.: The eye of the slug, *Agriolimax reticulatus* (Müll). Symp. Zool. Soc. Lond. **23**, 97—111 (1968).

Ninomiya, N., Tominaga, Y., Kuwabara, M.: The fine structure of the compound eye of a damsel-fly. Z. Zellforsch. **98**, 17—32 (1969).

Nishioka, R. S., Hagadorn, I. R., Bern, H. A.: Ultrastructure of the epistellar body of the octopus. Z. Zellforsch. **57**, 406—421 (1962).

— Yasumasu, I., Packard, A., Bern, H. A., Young, J. Z.: Nature of vesicles associated with the nervous system of cephalopods. Z. Zellforsch. **75**, 301—316 (1966).

Ong, J. E.: The micromorphology of the nauplius eye of the estaurine calanoid copepod *Sulcanus conflictus* Nicholls (Crustacea). Tissue and Cell **2**, 589—610 (1970).

Perrelet, A.: The fine structure of the retina of the honey-bee drone. Z. Zellforsch. **108**, 530—562 (1970).

— Baumann, F.: Presence of three small retinula cells in the ommatidium of the honey-bee drone eye. J. Mikroscopie 8, 497—502 (1969).

Pflugfelder, O.: Über den feineren Bau der Augen freilebender Polychäten. Z. wiss. Zool. **142**, 540—586 (1932).

Röhlich, P., Aros, B., Virágh, S.: Fine structure of photoreceptor cells in the earthworm, *Lumbricus terrestris*. Z. Zellforsch. **104**, 345—357 (1970).

— Tar, E.: The effect of prolonged light-deprivation on the fine structure of planarian photoreceptors. Z. Zellforsch. **90**, 507—518 (1968).

— Törö, I.: Fine structure of the compound eye of daphnia in normal, dark- and strongly light-adapted state. In: The structure of the eye. II. Symposium (Rohen, J. W., Ed.). Stuttgart: F. K. Schattauer-Verlag 1965.

— Török, L. J.: Elektronenmikroskopische Untersuchungen des Auges von Planarien. Z. Zellforsch. **54**, 362—381 (1961).

— — Die Feinstruktur des Auges der Weinbergschnecke (*Helix pomatia* L.). Z. Zellforsch. **60**, 348—368 (1963).

Röhlich, P., Török, L. J.: Elektronenmikroskopische Beobachtungen an den Sehzellen des Blutegels, *Hirudo medicinalis* L. Z. Zellforsch. **63**, 618—635 (1964).

Rutherford, D. J., Horridge, G. A.: The rhabdom of the lobster eye. Quart. J. micr. Sci. **106**, 119—130 (1965).

Schneider, L., Langer, H.: Die Struktur des Rhabdoms im „Doppelauge" des Wasserläufers *Gerris lacustris*. Z. Zellforsch. **99**, 538—559 (1969).

Schwalbach, G., Lickfeld, K. G., Hahn, M.: Der mikromorphologische Aufbau des Linsenauges der Weinbergschnecke (*Helix pomatia* L.). Protoplasma **56**, 242—273 (1963).

Seitz, G.: Untersuchungen am dioptrischen Apparat des Leuchtkäferauges. Z. vergl. Physiol. **62**, 61—74 (1969).

Shaw, S. R.: Sense-cell structure and interspecies comparisons of polarized-light absorption in arthropod compound eyes. Vision Res. **9**, 1031—1040 (1969).

Tomita, T.: Electrical activity of vertebrate photoreceptors. Quart. Rev. Biophys. **3**, 179—222 (1970).

Trujillo-Cenóz, O., Melamed, J.: Electron microscope observations on the peripheral and intermediate retinas of dipterans. In: Proc. internat. symp. on the functional organization of the compound eye. Oxford-New York: Pergamon Press 1966.

— — Spatial distribution of photoreceptor cells in the ommatidia of *Periplaneta americana*. J. Ultrastruct. Res. **34**, 397—400 (1971).

Tuurala, O., Lehtinen, A.: Über die Wandlungen in der Feinstruktur der Lichtsinneszellen bei der Hell- und Dunkeladaptation im Auge einer Asselart, *Oniscus asellus* L. Ann. Acad. Sci. fenn. A, IV. (Biol.) **123**, 1—8 (1967).

Vaissière, R.: Morphologie et histologie comparées des yeux des crustacés copépodes. Arch. Zool. exp. gen. **100**, 1—125 (1961).

— Boulay, M. F.: Ultrastructures et formation de la région lamellaire des yeux médians de Copépodes Pontellides (*Pontella mediterranea* Claus et *Anamalocera patersoni* Templeton). C. R. Acad. Sci. (Paris) **272**, 610—613 (1971).

Varela, F. G., Porter, K. R.: Fine structure of the visual system of the honeybee (*Apis mellifera*) 1. the retina. J. Ultrastruct. Res. **29**, 236—259 (1969).

Vaupel-v. Harnack, M.: Über den Feinbau des Nervensystems des Seesterns (*Asterias rubens* L.) III. Mitt. Die Struktur der Augenpolster. Z. Zellforsch. **60**, 432—451 (1963).

Vinnikov, Ya. A.: Principles of structural, chemical, and functional organization of sensory receptors. Cold Spr. Harb. Symp. quant. Biol. **30**, 293—299 (1966).

— Special senses. In: The structure and function of nervous tissue. Vol. II, 265—392 (Bourne, G. H., Ed.). New York: Academic Press 1969.

Wager, H.: On the eye-spot and flagellum in *Euglena viridis*. J. Linnean Soc. Zool. **27**, 463—481 (1900).

Wald, G., Brown, P. K., Gibbons, I. R.: The problem of visual excitation. J. Opt. Soc. Amer. **53**, 20—35 (1963).

— Hubbard, R.: Visual pigment of a decapod crustacean: "the lobster". Nature (Lond.) **180**, 278—280 (1957).

Waterman, T. H.: Systems analysis and the visual orientation of animals. Amer. Scientist **54**, 15—45 (1966).

— Systems theory and biology — view of a biologist. In: Systems theory and biology (Mesarović, M. D., Ed.). New York: Springer 1968.

Wells, M. J.: Cephalopod sense organs. In: Physiology of mollusca, Vol. II, (Wilbur, K. M., Yonge, C. M., Eds.). New York: Academic Press 1966.

Welsch, U.: Die Feinstruktur der Josephschen Zellen im Gehirn von *Amphioxus*. Z. Zellforsch. **86**, 252—261 (1968).

Wetzel, B. K.: Sodium permanganate fixation for electron microscopy. J. biophys. biochem. Cytol. **9**, 711—716 (1961).

White, R. H.: The effect of light and light deprivation upon the ultrastructure of the larval mosquito eye: II. The rhabdom. J. exp. Zool. **166**, 405—425 (1967).

— The effect of light and light deprivation upon the ultrastructure of the larval mosquito eye. 3. multivesicular bodies and protein uptake. J. exp. Zool. **169**, 261—267 (1968).

White, R. H., Sundeen, C. D.: The effect of light and light deprivation upon the ultra-structure of the larval mosquito eye. I. Polyribosomes and endoplasmic reticulum. J. exp. Zool. **164**, 461—478 (1967).
— Walther, J. B.: The leech photoreceptor cell: ultrastructure of clefts connecting the phaosome with extracellular space demonstrated by lanthanum deposition. Z. Zellforsch. **95**, 102—108 (1969).
Wolken, J. J.: The photoreceptors of arthropod eyes. Symp. Zool. Soc. Lond. **23**, 113—133 (1968).
— Florida, R. G.: The eye structure and optical system of the crustacean copepod, *Copilia*. J. Cell Biol. **40**, 279—285 (1969).
— Gallik, G. J.: The compound eye of a crustacean, *Leptodora kindtii*. J. Cell Biol. **26**, 968—973 (1965).
Woollacott, R. M., Zimmer, R. L.: Fine structure of a potential photoreceptor organ in the larva of *Bugula neritina* (Bryozoa). Z. Zellforsch. (1972) (in press).
Yanase, T., Sakamoto, S.: Fine structure of the visual cells of the dorsal eye in molluscan, *Onchidium verruculatum*. Zool. mag. **74**, 238—242 (1965).
Yoshida, M.: A photolabile pigment from the ocelli of *Spirocodon* an anthomedusa. Photochemistry and Photobiology, **2**, 39—47 (1963).
— Ohtsuki, H.: Compound ocellus of a starfish: its function. Science **153**, 197—198 (1966).
Young, R. W.: The renewal of photoreceptor cell outer segments. J. Cell Biol. **33**, 61—72 (1967).
— An hypothesis to account for a basic distinction between rods and cones. Vision Res. **11**, 1—5 (1971).
Zonana, H. V.: Fine structure of the squid retina. Bull. Johns Hopk. Hosp. **109**, 185—205 (1961).

Chapter 17

The Natural History
of Invertebrate Visual Pigments[*]

By

Timothy H. Goldsmith, New Haven, Connecticut (USA)

With 9 Figures

Contents

I. Introduction

The invertebrates comprise a large and diverse array of animals. In lower forms
responses to light are frequently marked but are mediated by relatively simple

---

[*] In memory of my friend and colleague Philip Ruck.

eyes (ocelli) or anatomically unspecialized receptors in the dermis or nervous system. In two phyla, however, conspicuous image-forming eyes have evolved. For obvious reasons, most of our knowledge of photoreception in the invertebrates has been derived from those species with a well developed visual apparatus.

The relatively large eyes of cephalopod molluscs and arthropods are anatomically very different and have independent evolutionary origins. They nevertheless have two features in common. As is generally true among invertebrates, the photo-receptor organelle of the light-sensitive cells of both cephalopods and arthropods is composed of a compact array of microvilli. This structure, usually called a rhabdom, is different from the typical receptor organelle of vertebrates (see Eakin, this volume, p. 636).

The second common characteristic of cephalopod and arthropod photoreceptors may be even more fundamental, for it is shared with all classes of vertebrates: the prosthetic group of the visual pigment is based on retinal, the aldehyde of vitamin A (retinol). (Dehydroretinal has never been obtained from an invertebrate). More-over, where further identification has been achieved, the retinal is in the 11-*cis* configuration. These considerations suggest that certain basic molecular and cellular characteristics were perfected early in the evolution of photoreceptors, and have been modified but little since.

A comparative approach to the study of photoreception has two complementary aims. A similar photochemistry in different animals suggests a common mechanism for transducing the energy of absorbed photons into messages that are meaningful to neurons. What this mechanism may be remains a mystery, but the fact that organisms have differences permits us to examine the problem from several angles, always looking for what is essential, and seeking vantage points from which impor-tant features can be best observed.

On the other hand, differences between organisms are frequently interesting in their own right. One example will suffice to make the point. Under most conditions the vertebrate eye is an ineffective analyzer of plane polarized light; yet many invertebrates discriminate different orientations of the plane of polarization. It now seems quite clear that this ability is based on the dichroism of the visual pigments.

In vertebrates the chromophores lie randomly in the planes of flat, disk-shaped membranes which are in turn perpendicular to the direction of propagation of naturally incident light (*e.g.* Liebman, 1962; Wald, Brown, and Gibbons. 1962). Rods and cones *in situ* therefore exhibit no dichroism. In arthropods (or, at least in spider crabs and crayfish), the chromophores also seem to be randomly distributed in the surfaces of the membranes of the receptor organelle. But because the mem-branes are rolled into microvilli and the microvilli are oriented in two mutually perpendicular masses (which are also orthogonal to the path of naturally incident light), the rhabdom functions as a polarization analyzer (Waterman, Fernán-dez, and Goldsmith, 1969; Hays and Goldsmith, 1969). In squid rhabdoms, the chromophores show some preferential alignment with the microvillar axes, which amplifies the dichroism and makes the rhabdom an even more effective analyzer (Hagins and Liebman, 1963).

II. Motile Algae and the Lower Invertebrates

There is scarcely a single group of organisms that fails to respond to light in some fashion. Mobile and motile forms frequently exhibit phototaxes, whereas sessile species react by bending toward or away from a source of light or by moving some part of their body in response to illumination.

The anatomical sites of photoreception are not so obvious as in higher animals. For example, the photoreceptor involved in the phototaxis of unicellular flagellates is almost certainly not the "eye spot", which seems instead to be an inert shading device (HALLDAL, 1958; 1964). Among coelenterates, flatworms, annelids, and echinoderms the general body surface is sensitive to light. In addition, some members of all these groups also possess small eyes of varying anatomical complexity. Even arthropods with large compound eyes may have additional small photoreceptors that are not composed of numerous ommatidial subunits. These are known as ocelli or "simple" eyes (although the inappropriateness of this latter term is indicated by HARTLINE's aphorism: "if it's simple, it's not an eye"). Finally, in the central nervous systems of both molluscs and arthropods, cells have been observed that are themselves apparently sensitive to light.

Among the lower phyla, the only clues we have to the nature of the photoreceptor pigment come from action spectra. Table 1 summarizes the wavelengths of maximum sensitivity for a variety of responses from the major groups of lower organisms. Not included are the photokinesis and phobophototaxis of bacteria and other responses related to photosynthesis, as well as the photo-tropism of fungi and higher plants. Nor are all the figures recorded in Table 1 based on action spectra of equivalent quality. What is clear, however, from this assembled information is that most of these responses are based on receptors maximally sensitive in the blue or blue-green region of the spectrum. Where action spectra have been determined, they appear to be broad, single-peaked curves with little if any fine structure, for the most part suggestive of rhodopsins.

The molecular basis of photoreception in lower organisms is unknown. From time to time attention has been drawn to various substances because they occur near the site of reception, have absorption spectra similar to the action spectrum for the response, or in some cases are affected by light. Examples are naphtaquinone, which has been isolated from sea urchins (cf. MILLOTT, 1960); ommochrome in the ocelli of anthomedusae (YOSHIDA, OHTSUKI, and SUGURI, 1967); carotenoids, thought to be present in the eye spot of Euglena (cf. WOLKEN, 1967); and accessory pigments of fly ommatidia (BOWNESS and WOLKEN, 1959). Before it is possible to conclude that one is dealing with the photoreceptor molecule, however, there must be direct evidence that the pigment is located in the photoreceptor organelle (if there be one) and is causally responsible for the physiological response to light. In none of the examples of Table 1 is such evidence now available.

If a rhodopsin-like pigment is present in an invertebrate and its spectral properties can account for the photoresponse of the receptor, there is reasonable precedent for presuming that it is the receptor pigment. There is ample reason to regard other substances with caution. Simple photoreceptors are frequently shielded on one or more sides with dense screening pigment. This decreases stray light and imparts an element of directional sensitivity to the receptor. These

Table 1. *Wavelengths of maximum sensitivity of some relatively unspecialized photoreceptive system*

Group	Organism	Response	λ_{max} (nm)	Author
Euglenophyta	*Euglena*	positive phototaxis	470—490	Engelmann. 1882
		positive and negative phototaxis	483	Mast, 1917
		positive phototaxis	490—500	Bünning and Schneidi höhn, 1956
Chlorophyta	*Chlamydomonas*	positive phototaxis	504	Mast, 1917
	Dunaliella	positive and negative phototaxis	493	Halldal, 1958
	Platymonas	positive and negative phototaxis	493	Halldal, 1958
	Stephanoptera	negative phototaxis	493	Halldal, 1958
	Ulva gametes	positive phototaxis	493	Halldal, 1958
Pyrrophyta (dinoflagellates)	*Prorocentrum*	positive phototaxis	570	Halldal, 1958
	Peridinium	positive phototaxis	475	Halldal, 1958
	Gonyaulax	positive phototaxis	475	Halldal, 1958
Protozoa	*Amoeba*	suppression of movement	515($\pm$)	Hitchcock, 1961
Coelenterata	*Eudendrium*	bending of polyps	474	Loeb and Wasteneys,
Platyhelminthes	*Dendrocoelom*	negative phototaxis	475	Marriott, 1958
	planaria (sp ?)	sensitivity of ocellar potential	508	Brown and Ogden, 196
Annelida	*Arenicola* (larvae)	positive phototaxis	483	Mast, 1917
	Lumbricus	negative phototaxis	483	Mast, 1917
Echinodermata	*Diadema*	movement of the urchin's spines	465—475	Millot and Yoshida, 1
	Asterias	arm movement; eye-spot present	485	Yoshida and Ohtsuki,
		arm movement; eye-spot removed	504	
Arthropoda	*Procambarus*	firing of photoreceptor neurons in the 6th abdominal ganglion	500	Bruno and Kennedy, 1
	Apis	retinal action potential of dorsal ocellus	490, 340	Goldsmith and Ruck, 1
	blowfly (larvae)	negative phototaxis	503	Mast, 1917
	Calliphora (larvae)	negative phototaxis	504	Strange, 1961
Mollusca	*Spisula*	inhibition of firing of unit in the pallial nerve	540	Kennedy, 1960

accessory screening pigments are usually either black, with neutral absorption, or reddish orange to match the absorption of the receptor pigment. Either way they are efficient curtains. In extracts, however, it may be difficult to distinguish an orange screening pigment from the receptor pigment on the basis of spectral absorption alone. The pigment of the eye spot of *Euglena* (probably carotenoid, but the spectral evidence from different laboratories is not in good agreement: *cf.* KRINSKY and GOLDSMITH, 1960; STROTHER and WOLKEN, 1961; COBB, 1963; BATRA and TOLLIN, 1964) and the ommochromes and pteridines of insect eyes (which clearly have nothing to do with visual excitation, *cf.* GOLDSMITH, 1965) provide fair warning.

On the other hand, the unifying hypothesis that all primitive light reactions of animals involve a carotenoid derivative in their photochemistry may lock future investigations into too restrictive a framework. In fact, there is one instance known in which the photoreceptor appears not to employ a carotenoid-based pigment. The circadian rhythm of eclosion of *Drosophila* can be phase-shifted by light. The eyes are not involved, and the sensitivity of this reaction remains unchanged in animals reared on a carotenoid-free diet, a regimen that raises the thresholds of the visual photoreceptors by three log units (ZIMMERMAN and GOLDSMITH, 1971).

The diffuse nature and small size of the photoreceptors of lower organisms has made a direct attack on their photochemistry seem discouragingly difficult. The technique of microspectrophotometry, however, may provide a realistic method for studying this problem.

III. Cephalopod Molluscs

The eyes of cephalopod molluscs, like those of vertebrates, are constructed on the same optical plan as a camera. Phylogenetically, of course, the groups are unrelated, and the cytological organization of their retinas is consequently very different. The cephalopod retina is arranged so that the receptors face the light. The distal segments ("rods") of the receptor cells are several hundred μm in length by several μm in width. They consist of a central strip of cytoplasm which is filled with granules of screening pigment, and two wedge-shaped rhabdomeric borders running the full length of the distal segment. Groups of four rhabdomeres are surrounded by columns of pigment from the four parent receptor cells, and each cell contributes a rhabdomere to two such clusters. Supporting cells are also interspersed between the distal segments of the receptors (see p. 85, Fig. 9).

The distal segments of the receptors project through a basal lamina, below which are located the cell bodies of the receptors. The vertebrate retina contains second and third order neurons in addition to the receptors. The cephalopod retina, by contrast, contains no higher order neurons. The fine axons of the receptors run directly for several millimeters to the optic lobe of the brain. The retina is not so simple as this comparison might suggest, however, for there is a plexus of centrifugal fibers and collaterals of the receptor axons immediately adjacent to the cell bodies of the receptors.

A. Cephalopod Rhodopsins

The visual pigment of squid (*Loligo*) does not bleach in the retina. Moreover, the retinas of squid contain little retinol even in the light-adapted state, and most of the retinaldehyde that is present is bound as rhodopsin (WALD, 1941). These differences from vertebrates notwithstanding, traditional techniques for isolating vertebrate rod outer segments and extracting rhodopsin also work when applied to squid and other cephalopod molluscs.

Under the action of light, and at temperatures below 15° C, squid rhodopsin is converted into a long-lived metarhodopsin which can in turn exist in either of two forms, depending on the concentration of hydrogen ions (Hubbard and St. George, 1958). These relationships are summarized as follows:

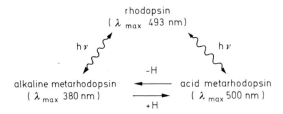

Irradiation of rhodopsin at neutral or acid pH (or in the retina) yields acid metarhodopsin which is spectrally similar to the visual pigment; thus there is no bleaching. If the solution is then made basic, the acid metarhodopsin is converted to the alkaline form, with peak of absorbance at 380 nm in the near ultraviolet. On the other hand, if the initial irradiation is performed in basic solution, alkaline metarhodopsin is the product, and this in turn can be titrated to the acid form. The light reaction in either case is photoreversible. As a consequence, in alkaline solution an orange light (which is absorbed by rhodopsin but not by alkaline metarhodopsin) will convert all of the rhodopsin to alkaline metarhodopsin. By contrast, in neutral or mildly acidic solution the same orange light will form a steady state mixture of rhodopsin and acid metarhodopsin. The pK for the conversion of acid and alkaline metarhodopsin is 7.7.

These relationships are shown in the experiment of Figure 1, which is from Hubbard and St. George (1958). Initially, a solution of rhodopsin at pH 9.7 was irradiated with orange light until it had been converted into alkaline metarhodopsin (pH 9.7). The solution was then acidified stepwise and spectra recorded at pH 8.3, 7.3, 6.4, and 5.5. The fall in extinction at 380 nm is accompanied by a rise at 500 nm with an isosbestic point at 420 nm. This represents the conversion of alkaline to acid metarhodopsin. The final curve (pH 5.5) has a greater height than the initial spectrum of rhodopsin. This is because the molar absorbance coefficient for metarhodopsin is about 1.5 times greater than for rhodopsin.

Squid rhodopsin contains retinal in the 11-*cis* configuration. This has been established by releasing the retinaldehyde of squid rhodopsin by thermal denaturation and reacting it with opsin from cattle retinas to yield cattle rhodopsin. Metarhodopsin, on the other hand, contains all *trans* retinaldehyde. If squid metarhodopsin is denatured with 0.1 molar HCl, a product involving Schiff-base linkage of retinaldehyde and amino groups is formed with peak absorbance at 440 nm. If this is then irradiated with blue light, the absorbance falls and shifts somewhat to shorter wavelengths, indicating the formation of *cis* isomers from all *trans* retinal (Hubbard and St. George, 1958).

It is worth emphasizing the distinction between alkaline metarhodopsin and free retinal that has been hydrolyzed from the protein. 1) In basic solution,

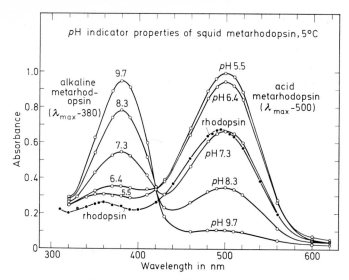

Fig. 1. Absorbance spectra of squid rhodopsin; alkaline metarhodopsin, produced by bleaching with orange light at pH 9.7; mixtures of alkaline and acid metarhodopsin, produced by subsequent gradual acidification in the dark (pH 8.3, 7.3, and 6.4); and, finally, pure acid metarhodopsin (pH 5.5). From HUBBARD and ST. GEORGE, 1958

alkaline metarhodopsin absorbs maximally at 380 nm and has a molar extinction coefficient of 60,900; an alkaline solution of retinaldehyde and protein absorbs maximally at 365 nm, and the molar extinction is about 47,000. 2) Neutralization of a solution of alkaline metarhodopsin yields acid metarhodopsin with peak absorbance at 500 nm; neutralization of other Schiff base linkages of retinal (alkaline indicator yellow) is accompanied by hydrolysis of retinal and a modest spectral shift to 385 nm. 3) Finally, alkaline metarhodopsin reacts with neither hydroxylamine nor alcohol dehydrogenase, whereas retinaldehyde forms the oxime with the former and vitamin A (retinol) in the presence of the latter.

At temperatures above about 15° C, squid metarhodopsin slowly breaks down to yield free retinal. The opsin, however, becomes inactivated so that it fails to yield rhodopsin when an excess of 11-*cis* retinal is added. The dark mechanisms that lead to the regeneration of rhodopsin in the living retina are unknown.

If squid rhodopsin is irradiated at the temperature of liquid nitrogen, prelumirhodopsin (λ_{max} 543 nm) is observed. On warming to $-170°$ C this goes over to lumirhodopsin (λ_{max} 530 nm), and finally, above $-20°$ C, to metarhodopsin (YOSHIZAWA and WALD, 1964). Moreover, under conditions of very low temperature the formation of isorhodopsin (retinal in the 9-*cis* configuration) is also observed (YOSHIZAWA and WALD, 1964).

The rhodopsins of other cephalopods behave in similar fashion to that of squid, although there are differences in the wavelengths of maximal absorbance (Table 2). As is the case with species variation in the spectral locations of vertebrate rhodopsins, the differences in absorption are based on differences in the protein constituent of the visual pigment.

44*

Table 2. *Rhodopsins and metarhodopsins of some cephalopod molluscs*

	Rhodopsin		Acid metarhodopsin		Alkaline metarhodopsin	
	λ_{max} (nm)	molar absorbance	λ_{max} (nm)	molar absorbance	λ_{max} (nm)	molar absorbance
Decapoda						
Loligo pealii[a]	493	40,600	500	59,700	380	60,900
Todarodes pacificus[b]	480	—	—	—	—	—
Sepia officinalis[a]	492	37,000	497	47,700	380	54,500
Sepia esculenta[b]	486	—	—	—	—	—
Sepiella japonica[b]	500	—	—	—	—	—
Octopoda						
Octopus vulgaris[a]	475	37,000	503	44,400	380	56,200
Octopus ocellatus[b]	477	—	—	—	—	—
Eledone moschata[c]	470	—	516	—	380	—

[a] From Brown and Brown, 1958.
[b] From Hara and Hara, 1967.
[c] From Hamdorf, Schwemer, and Täuber, 1968.

B. Squid and Vertebrate Metarhodopsins

Squid and cattle metarhodopsins differ in several ways. The titration of squid metarhodopsin from the acidic to the basic form involves a single acid-binding site with pK 7.7. This may be the Schiff-base linkage of retinaldehyde with the protein (Hubbard, 1959), but if so, in both tautomers there persists sufficient interaction between the protein and the chromophore to shift the spectrum to longer wavelengths from an unenhanced Schiff base. Thus acid indicator yellow has λ_{max} at 443 nm and acid metarhodopsin at 500 nm; alkaline indicator yellow at 367 nm and alkaline metarhodopsin at 380 nm (Brown and Brown, 1958). Furthermore, although the Schiff base of metarhodopsin can apparently be titrated, it is less susceptible to hydrolysis. And last, conversion of acid to alkaline metarhodopsin is accompanied by a small decrease in entropy (-8 e.u.).

This behavior stands in contrast to several characteristics of cattle metarhodopsin (Matthews, Hubbard, Brown, and Wald, 1963). Here the path of bleaching is from metarhodopsin I (λ_{max} 478 nm) to metarhodopsin II (λ_{max} 380 nm), but it is the *latter* form that predominates in acidic solution. The pK for the conversion is 6.4. Moreover, the conversion involves an increase in entropy ($+$ 46.5 e.u.), as though significant unfolding of the protein were occurring. The relationship of the cattle metarhodopsins to other intermediates and to N-retinylidene opsin is discussed elsewhere (Matthews, Hubbard, Brown, and Wald, 1963; Abrahamson and Ostroy, 1967; Bridges, 1967).

C. Retinochrome

A second light-sensitive pigment has recently been extracted from the retinas of cephalopods (Hara and Hara, 1965, 1967, 1968, Hara, Hara, and Takeuchi, 1967). This substance differs from rhodopsin on a number of counts (see Chapter 18 in this volume for a more detailed description), and it has been named retino-chrome.

If the distal segments of the receptor cells and their associated shielding pigments are detached from the retina by mechanical means, the remainder of the retina yields a red pigment with λ_{max} at 13—22 nm longer than the rhodopsin of the same species. This retinochrome contains about 25 per cent of the retinaldehyde of the retina. It bleaches in the light to a photoproduct with λ_{max} at 365 nm, even at neutral pH and 5°C, conditions where acid metarhodopsin forms from rhodopsin.

Retinochrome contains retinal in the all *trans* configuration, and the retinaldehyde is isomerized to *cis* in the light. Thermal denaturation of retinochrome liberates an isomer of retinal that will not react with cattle opsin. Moreover, retinochrome can be regenerated by mixing all *trans* retinal with a bleached sample of retinochrome. And finally, when retinochrome is attacked by NH_2OH the resulting retinaldehyde oxime has a higher absorbance than when the retinochrome is first destroyed by light.

Retinochrome apparently catalyzes the photo-isomerization of retinal from *trans* to *cis*. If a mixture of retinochrome and all *trans* retinaldehyde is exposed to hydroxylamine, the all *trans* oxime results. On the other hand, if the same mixture is irradiated with an orange light, which is absorbed by retinochrome but not by free retinal, and then subjected to hydroxylamine, the resulting oxime is *cis*. By incubating the irradiated solution with cattle opsin rather than hydroxylamine, much of the retinal is shown (by the formation of cattle rhodopsin) to be 11-*cis*.

It has also been reported that bleached retinochrome will regenerate if the source of *trans* retinaldehyde is acid metarhodopsin. The implication of these experiments is that retinochrome is involved in the system for regenerating rhodopsin from metarhodopsin. It is curious, however, that the rhodopsin and metarhodopsin are located in the distal segments of the receptors and the retinochrome scores to hundreds of μm deeper in the retina.

IV. Crustacea

The crustacea, like most other arthropods, possess compound eyes containing several hundred to several thousand sensory units known as ommatidia. Each ommatidium is an elongate structure consisting of a cluster of usually eight photoreceptor (retinular) cells, surrounded by a sleeve of pigment cells containing dense screening pigment, and capped by transparent dioptric structures that give the cornea its minutely faceted appearance. Each cluster of retinular cells (collectively known as a retinula) surrounds the photoreceptive structure or rhabdom. A rhabdom is composed of tightly packed microvillar projections of the retinular cell membranes (see EAKIN, this volume) and contains the visual pigment. It is therefore analogous in function to the outer segments of vertebrate rod and cone cells.

Compound eyes occur in two morphological types: photopic ("apposition") eyes have long rhabdoms that traverse the length of the ommatidium and abut against the internal surface of the dioptric elements, and their accessory screening pigment is relatively stable in position with changes in the environmental illumination: scotopic ("superposition") eyes have short, stout rhabdoms located at the basal ends of the ommatidia and separated from the dioptric structures by inert light-conducting tracts, and the accessory pigment migrates dramatically. Pigment migrations control the sensitivity of the eye over at least 2 log units (e.g. Höglund, 1966), and scotopic eyes are found in species that spend part of their time under conditions of very weak illumination.

A. Vitamin A in Crustacea

Vitamin A has been found in a number of crustacea (see Fisher and Kon, 1959, for review and references). Those species that store vitamin A have more in the eyes than elsewhere in their bodies. The eyes of euphausiids are particularly rich in vitamin A, and subdissection of the eye, fluorescence microscopy, and antimony chloride reactions on lyophilized sections all indicate that the vitamin is preferentially concentrated in the basal ends of the ommatidia, where the rhabdoms are located. In *Meganyctiphanes norvegica* the concentration in the inner ends of the retinulae is estimated to be very high: 4.6 mg gm^{-1} fresh weight (Fisher and Kon, 1959), or more than is found in the livers of most fish (Moore, 1957).

The vitamin A of euphausiids was early recognized as having a lower biopotency than was anticipated from the intensity of the Carr-Price reaction. The explanation is that most of the vitamin A exists as the 11-*cis* isomer, as shown by Wald and Burg (1955) for the lobster *Homarus* and by Wald and Brown (1957) for the euphausiid *Meganyctiphanes*. Both the anatomical location and the isomeric composition of retinol bespeak a role in vision.

B. Extracts of Pigment

The same techniques that have been applied successfully to the extraction of vertebrate visual pigments yield results with crustacea. Rhabdoms, as do outer segments, consist largely of lipo-protein membranes. Consequently, when eyes are macerated in dense sucrose solutions and centrifuged under a layer of buffer, visual pigment can be extracted from the material that rises to the interface. As with vertebrates, surface-active agents are required to effect the extraction. For some as yet unknown reason macrurans (lobsters, crayfish) yield spectrally cleaner and more concentrated solutions of visual pigment than do brachyurans (crabs).

Table 3 is a summary of results obtained in this manner. The spectral data condensed in Table 3 vary in quality and in the detail with which they are reported in the original literature. One can nevertheless draw several conclusions from this information. The prosthetic group of crustacean visual pigments has invariably been retinal; 3-dehydroretinal has not been observed, even though the limited survey now spans fresh water and marine forms as well as terrestrial species. The isomeric form of the retinal has not been directly identified in any instance; however, the observations on the vitamin A of crustacean eyes that were cited in the preceding section provide strong reason to believe that the form is 11-*cis*.

As can be seen from Table 3, a characteristic feature of some, but not all, crustacean visual pigments is that on exposure to light they yield an intermediate of bleaching that absorbs at relatively long wavelengths (near the parent pigment) and that is relatively stable at room temperature. These metarhodopsins decay slowly in the dark over a time course of many minutes, comparable to the decay time of metarhodopsin II (λ_{max} 380 nm) from cattle (*cf.* ABRAHAMSON and OSTROY, 1967). They have not been studied as thoroughly as the metarhodopsins of squid and cattle.

The spiny lobster *Panulirus argus* is an example of an animal whose visual pigment exhibits this behavior (FERNÁNDEZ, 1965; GOLDSMITH and FERNÁNDEZ, 1966), as is illustrated by the experiment shown in Figure 2. The initial absorbance of the extract of dark-adapted eyes is shown by the plain circles. On exposure for

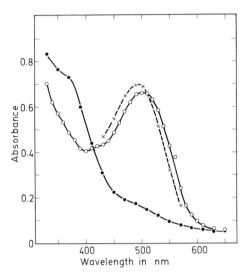

Fig. 2. Spectral changes in a digitonin extract of visual pigment from the eyes of the spiny lobster *Panulirus argus*. The spectral absorbance of the extract, prepared in darkness, is shown by the plain circles. After three minutes exposure to a 30 watt incandescent lamp at 25°C, absorbance increased and shifted about 8 nm to shorter wavelengths (x's, broken curve) indicating the formation of a metarhodopsin. This intermediate decayed slowly in the dark, and after 3 hours the spectral absorbance followed the filled circles. The rise in absorbance at wavelengths below 410 nm reflects the liberation of retinaldehyde. From FERNÁNDEZ, 1965, and GOLDSMITH and FERNÁNDEZ, 1966

3 minutes to a white light at 25°C, the maximal absorbance increased slightly and shifted in position about 8 nm to shorter wavelengths, as shown by the crosses and the broken curve. This represents the conversion of visual pigment to a metarhodopsin. The absorbance then fell slowly in the dark, and after 3 hours had reached the position shown by the filled circles. The rise in absorbance at wavelengths shorter than 410 nm is caused by the liberation of retinal. The positions of the wavelengths of maximum absorbance recorded in Table 3 were determined from difference spectra based on similar experiments.

The conclusion that such light-sensitive pigments as are listed in Table 3 are visual pigments rests on comparisons of their absorbance spectra with the spectral sensitivity functions of the corresponding animals. Table 4 shows those comparisons that are presently possible. In four cases (*Limulus* [not a crustacean], lobster, and

Table 3. *Crustacean visual pigments*

Species	Morphology[a]	Habits
Order Isopoda		
Porcellio scaber (woodlouse)	(P)	terrestrial
Order Euphausiacea		
Euphausia pacifica	S	deep sea
Meganyctiphanes norvegica	S	deep sea
Nematoscelis megalops	(S)	deep sea
Stylocheiron maximum	(S)	deep sea
Thysanoessa raschii	(S)	deep sea
Thysanopoda acutifrons	(S)	deep sea
Order Decapoda		
Suborder Natantia		
Acanthephyra haeckeli (bathypelagic shrimp)	(S)	deep sea
Sergestes arcticus (penaeid shrimp)	(S)	deep sea
Sergestes robustus (penaeid shrimp)	(S)	deep sea
Palaemonetes palludosus (fresh water prawn)	S	fresh water, arhythmic
Penaeus duorarum (pink shrimp)	S	marine, nocturnal
Suborder Reptantia		
Section Macrura		
Homarus americanus (American lobster)	S	marine
Procambarus clarkii (swamp crayfish)	S	fresh water, apparently arhythmic
Orconectes virilis (northern crayfish)	(S)	fresh water
Panulirus argus (spiny lobster)	S	marine, nocturnal
Section Brachyra		
Callinectes ornatus (blue crab)	P	marine or brackish water
Callinectes sapidus (blue crab)	P	marine or brackish water
Hemigrapsus edwardsii (mud crab)	(P)	marine
Leptograpsus variegatus (rock crab)	(P)	marine
Ocypode quadrata (ghost crab)	P	adults terrestrial, active at low tide
Uca pugnax and *U. pugilator* (fiddler crab)	P	marine beaches, active at low tide

[a] P = photopic or "apposition" morphology; S = scotopic or "superposition" morphology. Where the letter is placed in parentheses I was unable to examine histological sections of the eye or to locate an adequate description, and the designation of the morphological type is based on knowledge of near relatives of the species. I am grateful to Professor T. H. WATERMAN and Mrs. MABELITA CAMPBELL for making available their slides of crustacean eyes.

the two genera of crayfish) the agreement between chemistry and physiology is reasonably good. For *Homarus* and *Procambarus* it has been suggested that the spectral sensitivity function is displaced somewhat to longer wavelengths by a filtering effect of astaxanthin (WALD, 1968). In the case of the isopod *Porcellio* and the blue crab *Callinectes* there is a larger discrepancy between absorbance and sensitivity.

Recent unpublished microspectrophotometric measurements of *Callinectes* rhabdoms made in our laboratory, however, show much better agreement between

as they appear in extracts

λ_{max} (nm) of pigment(s)	Metarhodopsin (λ_{max}, nm) appears as intermediate of bleaching at room temperature	Chromophoric group	Author
480	?	ret.[1][c]	Briggs, 1961a
462	?	probably ret[1]	Kampa, 1955
460—465	no	ret.[1][d]	Fisher and Goldie, 1960[b]
465	no	ret.[1][d]	Fisher and Goldie, 1960[b]
470	no	ret.[1][d]	Fisher and Goldie, 1960[b]
460—465	no	ret.[1][d]	Fisher and Goldie, 1960[b]
480	no	ret.[1][d]	Fisher and Goldie, 1960[b]
480	yes	ret.[1][d]	Fisher and Goldie, 1960[b]
475	yes	ret.[1][d]	Fisher and Goldie, 1960[b]
470	yes	ret.[1][d]	Fisher and Goldie, 1960[b]
539 and 512	497 and possibly not	ret.[1][d]	Fernández, 1965
516	475	ret.[1][c, d]	Fernández, 1965
515	490	ret.[1][c, d]	Wald and Hubbard, 1957
556 and 525	yes and no	ret.[1][c, d]	Wald, 1967
562 and 510	515 and no	ret.[1][c, d]	Wald, 1967
504	495	ret.[1][c, d]	Fernández, 1965
484	possibly not	ret.[1][c, d]	Fernández, 1965
476; 480	possibly not	ret.[1][c, d]	Fernández, 1965; Goldsmith and Waterman, unp.
495	495	ret.[1][c, d]	Briggs, 1961b[b]
513	495	ret.[1][c, d]	Briggs, 1961b[b]
478	?	ret.[1][c, d]	Fernández, 1965
480	possibly not	ret.[1][c, d]	Goldsmith and Purple, unpublished

[b] Only maxima are cited; absorbance or difference spectra are not published.
[c] Determined by the Carr-Price reaction.
[d] Determined by the spectral location of the product of bleaching.
(This table is modified from Goldsmith and Fernández, 1966).

pigment absorption and spectral sensitivity. This suggests that the absorbance spectrum of crab rhodopsin is altered when the molecules of pigment are removed with detergents from the rhabdomeric membranes.

Several more general conclusions can be drawn from the data of Table 3. There is no correlation between the spectral location of the visual pigment and the presence of scotopic or photopic morphology. The type of eye is fairly constant within any major subgroup of crustacea, but there is some correlation between the λ_{max} of the pigment and the spectral distribution of energy in the natural environment. For example, the crustaceans studied by Fisher and Goldie yield pigments

Table 4. *Comparison of pigment extracts with physiological measurements of spectral sensitivity*

	λ_{max} of pigment (nm)[a]	λ of maximum sensitivity (nm)[b]
Merostomata: Xiphosurida		
Limulus polyphemus	520[c]	520[d, e]
Crustacea: Isopoda		
Porcellio scaber	480	515[f]
(wood louse)		
Crustacea: Decapoda		
Homarus americanus	515	525[e]
(American lobster)		
Procambarus clarkii	556 and 525	570[e, g]
(swamp crayfish)		
Orconectes virilis	562 and 510	565[e, f]
(northern crayfish)		
Callinectes sapidus	480	505[f]
(blue crab)		

   [a] Reference, unless otherwise noted, is given in Table 3.
   [b] For the most part based on the retinal action potential.
   [c] Hubbard and Wald, 1960.
   [d] Graham and Hartline, 1935.
   [e] Wald, 1968.
   [f] Goldsmith and Fernández, 1968b.
   [g] Kennedy and Bruno, 1961.

with maximum absorbance in the region 462—480 nm. These species all inhabit the open ocean at depths where the transmission of natural light is greatest at 470—480 nm. In contrast, species inhabiting shallower, more turbid waters (with transmission spectra shifted to longer wavelengths) show maximum sensitivity at 500—535 nm. The crabs are an apparent exception to this rule but, as pointed out in the preceding paragraph, with crabs there is a problem in relating spectral sensitivity to the absorbance of the extracted pigment, and more work needs to be done.

Among the crustaceans whose photopigments and spectral sensitivity have been most thoroughly studied are the crayfishes (*Orconectes*, *Procambarus*). Digitonin extracts contain two light sensitive substances: a 562 nm pigment that bleaches to retinal through a long-lived metarhodopsin with λ_{max} at about 515 nm, and a 510 nm pigment that bleaches in the light directly to retinal without detectable intermediates at room temperature (Wald, 1967). The 562 nm pigment is selectively destroyed at pH 9, and the 510 nm pigment is selectively bleached by 0.06 M hydroxylamine.

The spectral sensitivity of the dark-adapted eye is dominated by a peak around 565 nm; however, under the influence of a steady red background adapting light and for retinal action potentials close to threshold, the eye is maximally sensitive at about 430 nm (Wald, 1968; Goldsmith and Fernández, 1968b). There thus seems to be a relatively large number of receptors maximally sensitive at about 565 nm and a smaller number of violet receptors, thereby providing the substrate for a dichromatic color vision. This inference is supported by single unit recordings from the receptors (NOSAKI, 1969; WATERMAN and FERNÁNDEZ, 1970). Color vision may reasonably be assumed to be present in at least some other crustaceans as well (HORRIDGE, 1967).

The 562 nm pigment accounts well for the long wavelength receptor and for the sensitivity of the dark-adapted eye through most of the spectrum. The pigment of the violet receptor has not yet been observed, but what is even more perplexing, no physiological function has been identified for the 510 nm pigment.

C. Microspectrophotometry

The method of microspectrophotometry is described in detail elsewhere in this volume (see the chapter by LIEBMAN). It has the great advantage of providing information on the distribution of pigments in individual receptors. Such information is crucial to an understanding of the peripheral basis of color vision and cannot be obtained by analyzing extracts of whole eyes. Moreover, microspectrophotometry allows the comparison of reactions *in situ* with those observed in solution.

The rhabdoms of decapod crustacea consist of microvilli oriented at right angles to the ommatidial axis. The rhabdom is divided into layers much like the slices in a loaf of bread. Each layer consists of tightly packed, parallel microvilli whose long axes are at right angles to the microvilli in the immediately adjacent layers. A rhabdom that has been detached from its surrounding retinular cells can be studied with small beams of light passing through it transversely. Moreover, in crayfish the layers of microvilli are unusually thick (about 5 μm), and one can position a measuring beam within a single layer.

When the rhabdom is also oriented properly with respect to rotation about its long axis, the measuring beam will be incident at right angles to the microvillar axes in half the layers and will be parallel to the microvilli when placed in any one of the alternate bands (*cf.* the inset diagram in Fig. 6). This condition permits the measurement of dichroism.

When light passes down the axis of the rhabdom, as it does in the living eye, it is always propagating at right angles to the microvillar axes. Therefore, absorption measured with a transverse beam at right angles to the microvilli is the same, for a given path length within a given layer, as absorption of naturally incident light in a functioning eye.

When fresh rhabdoms of the spider crab *Libinia emarginata* are irradiated, the visual pigment (λ_{max} 493 nm) forms a metarhodopsin with absorptance[1] displaced several nm to longer wavelengths (Fig. 3). This metarhodopsin is very stable and does not bleach if the rhabdom is left for many minutes in the dark or is irradiated further.

---

[1] The spectra drawn by the microspectrophotometer give the fractions of light absorbed (absorptance) by pigment. Absorptance — here defined as $(I_i - I_t)/I_i$ where I_i is the incident, and I_t the transmitted, light — is to be distinguished from absorbance, or optical density, defined as $\log I_i/I_t$. Absorbance (or density) spectra (when "normalized", i.e. plotted as fractions or percentages of the maximum absorbance) have shapes that are independent of concentration. Absorptance spectra, on the other hand, become broader with increasing concentration.

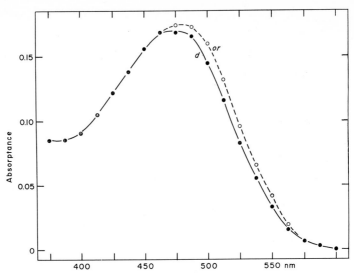

Fig. 3. Absorptance of a freshly isolated rhabdom of the spider crab *Libinia emarginata*: *d*, dark-adapted; *or*, after 1 min. exposure to bright orange light (wavelengths longer than 550 nm). The small spectral shift reflects the formation of a stable metarhodopsin with λ_{max} at a slightly longer wavelength than the visual pigment. This graph was obtained from an original record similar to that of Fig. 5 by subtracting the instrumental base line from the absorptance spectrum of the rhabdom. As rhabdoms are non-homogeneous objects, "absorptance" here includes light scattering. The rhabdom was suspended in artificial sea water at neutral pH and 23°C. From Hays and Goldsmith, 1969

The pattern of bleaching of fresh rhabdoms of the prawn *Palaemonetes vulgaris* and the crayfish *Orconectes virilis* is different and is shown in Figure 4. The two species behave in similar fashion. Absorptance of the dark-adapted rhabdom (*d*, Figure 4) is maximal in the green. Irradiation of the rhabdom for one or two minutes with a bright red light (wavelengths longer than 620 nm) causes a fall in absorptance at wavelengths longer than about 540 nm and a rise at shorter wavelengths (spectrum *r*, Figure 4). These spectral changes indicate the conversion of a visual pigment into metarhodopsin, as observed in solution (Wald, 1967).

If the rhabdom is now irradiated for 2 minutes with a bright yellow light (wavelengths longer than 470 nm), the absorptance falls to the position shown in Figure 4 by y_1. The remaining absorptance decays slowly in the dark, but may require further exposure to light before it disappears completely. In Figure 4A, spectrum y_2 was recorded one hour later. During that hour, two additional 1.5 minute exposures to the yellow bleaching light were given. In the experiment of Figure 4B, spectrum y_2 was recorded after the rhabdom had been exposed for one hour to a dim yellow light, and spectrum y_3 was recorded after an additional 36 minutes of the same treatment.

When the rhabdoms are suspended in glutaraldehyde, the pattern of bleaching is altered in an interesting manner. Figure 5 shows an experiment similar to that of Figure 3, performed on a rhabdom of *Libinia* suspended in 5% glutaraldehyde. The first four spectra were recorded over a two hour period while the rhabdom was

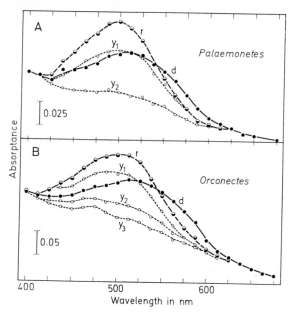

Fig. 4. Changes in spectral absorptance in single rhabdoms of crustacea as studied by microspectrophotometry: d, absorptance of rhabdoms of dark-adapted animals; r, immediately following 1 min exposure to bright red light; y_1, after 2 min exposure to bright yellow light; y_2, y_3, after additional yellow light and time in darkness. See the text for further details and description. *Palaemonetes vulgaris* is a prawn and *Orconectes virilis* is a crayfish. The rhabdoms of both species seem to contain two pigments. The long-wavelength species is converted by red light into a metarhodopsin absorbing maximally at shorter wavelengths. This is the reaction that is indicated by the change in spectrum between d and r. In each case the short-wavelength pigment originally present in the rhabdom has similar absorptance to the metarhodopsin

kept at 26°C in the dark. The slow fall in absorptance during this time represents an attack on the visual pigment by glutaraldehyde. This thermal decay does not occur to a significant extent at 4°C.

Fifteen seconds of bright yellow (or orange) light — which would have bleached a frog rod completely — caused the spectrum to fall to *5* (first dashed line in the inset), from which point absorptance declined further in the dark (spectra *6* and *7*). Clearly the photoproducts that were present after the 15 second exposure to the yellow light were attacked more rapidly by glutaraldehyde than the visual pigment. The experiment ended with additional irradiations with the yellow light (spectra *8-10*), until bleaching was complete. It thus appears that in the presence of glutaraldehyde the metarhodopsin can be bleached by light (HAYS and GOLDSMITH, 1969).

Partial bleaching of the rhabdom with different colored lights yields identical difference spectra with λ_{max} at 493 nm. The rhabdoms therefore contain a single pigment, and comparisons with spectral sensitivity indicate that it is the visual pigment (HAYS and GOLDSMITH, 1969).

Bleaching of prawn and crayfish rhabdoms is also hastened in the presence of glutaraldehyde, but because the rhabdoms seem to contain a mixture of two pigments in the dark-adapted state (in crayfish these probably correspond to the

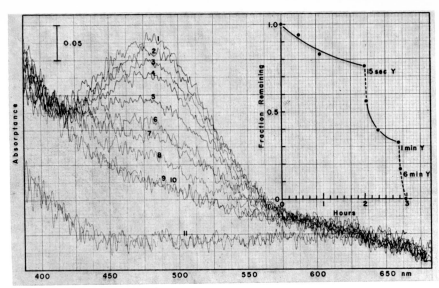

Fig. 5. Original record of the bleaching of a single *Libinia* rhabdom in 5% glutaraldehyde at 26°C. Spectra *1-4* were recorded at 0, 25, 56, and 120 minutes after mounting the rhabdom and locating it under the microscope. Spectrum *5* followed a 15 second exposure to bright yellow light (wavelengths longer than 470 nm), and *6* and *7* were recorded after additional intervals in the dark of 15 and 30 min. Complete bleaching was then effected with irradiation by the yellow source for 1 min (spectrum *8*) and two 6 min exposures (*9* and *10*). The measuring beam was $4 \times 8 \, \mu m$ and passed through the rhabdom transversely, the scanning speed was 20 nm sec^{-1}, and the spectral band width was 3.8 nm. The inset figure shows the remaining absorption *vs* time. Solid portions of the curve indicate when the rhabdom was in the dark (except for the *ca.* 15 sec periods required to measure the spectrum); the broken segments show immediate changes in absorptance produced by the bleaching light. Thermal decays of the original pigment and of the photoproducts were clearly occurring at different rates. From HAYS and GOLDSMITH, 1969

510 and 562 nm pigments reported by WALD, 1967), analysis is more complicated and has not been accomplished in a completely satisfactory manner.

When crayfish rhabdoms have been stabilized by treatment with 2.5% glutaraldehyde and the excess fixative removed by several washes with Ringer, the pattern of bleaching is similar to that of fresh material in that a metarhodopsin which forms in the presence of a red light persists in the dark. Rhabdoms treated in this manner are structurally more stable than fresh material, and the dark reactions of the metarhodopsin seem to be suppressed. Under these conditions, a blue light that follows a red irradiation will photoregenerate some of the longer wavelength pigment (GOLDSMITH, unpublished).

Figure 6 shows the absorptance spectra of 4 consecutive bands of a favorably oriented crayfish rhabdom. As indicated by the diagram on the figure, bands B and D contained microvilli that were illuminated from the side, whereas bands A and C consisted of microvilli that were irradiated end on. The two orientations of the plane of polarization are indicated by the double-headed arrows. Those layers where the microvilli were illuminated from the side show positive dichroism, for the absorptance

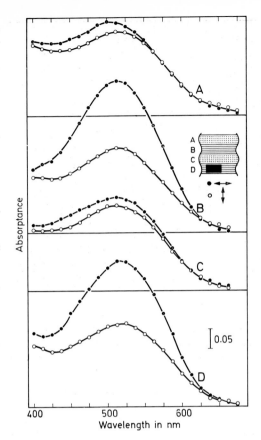

Fig. 6. Spectral absorptance of four adjacent bands of microvilli in a fresh rhabdom of *Orconectes* mounted in Ringer. The rhabdom was so oriented with respect to rotation about its long axis that the measuring beam (black rectangle in the inset) entered the organelle either parallel to the microvilliar axes (bands A and C) or perpendicular to the microvilli (bands E and D). Bands B and D were dichroic, showing maximum absorption with the measuring beam polarized parallel to the microvillar axes (bands B and D, filled circles). The dichroic ratio is 2, with absorptance of isotropic bands equal to absorptance in the minor axis of anisotropic bands. These latter points are shown quantitatively in other experiments in which the pigments are bleached. (WATERMAN, FERNÁNDEZ, and GOLDSMITH, 1969)

is maximal when the light is polarized parallel to the axes of the microvilli (Figure 6 B and D). For those layers illuminated axially, absorptance is essentially independent of the plane of polarization and is about the same in magnitude as that recorded in bands B and D with the plane of polarization oriented perpendicular to the axes of the microvilli. These measurements were made on a fresh rhabdom; however, identical results have been obtained from glutaraldehyde-fixed material (WATERMAN, FERNÁNDEZ, and GOLDSMITH, 1969).

The dichroic ratio in bands B and D is clearly about 2. Moreover, quantitative measurements of the changes in absorptance produced by bleaching confirm this figure for both pigments. Analogous measurements have been made on *Libinia*

(Hays and Goldsmith, 1969). The simplest explanation is that the intrinsic dichroism of the chromophores is reasonably high and that the chromophores lie with their major absorption axes randomly oriented in the surface of the microvillar membranes. The dichroic ratio of 2 thus results from the geometry of the microvilli (Waterman, Fernández, and Goldsmith, 1969).

V. Insects

Insects, in addition to their compound eyes (similar to those of crustacea described on p. 693), generally also possess two or three ocelli. Larvae of the higher insects lack compound eyes, but many have ocelli (stemmata) that are different from the ocelli of the imago. Compound eyes have received more attention, and this discussion will be limited to them; some references to work on ocelli can be found in Goldsmith (1964).

A. Carotenoids and Receptor Sensitivity

The identification of the prosthetic group of insect visual pigments rests on relatively indirect evidence. Efforts have been made to identify retinal and retinol by chemical means in extracts of insect tissue, and more recently the physiological and cytological effects of carotenoid-free diets have been examined.

1. Extracts

After lipid extracts of dark-adapted honeybees, *Apis mellifera*, are chromatographed, the Carr-Price reaction shows the presence of retinaldehyde (Goldsmith, 1958). The thoraces and abdomens have no detectable retinaldehyde, but the heads contain as much as 0.22 μgm gm^{-1} fresh weight. Retinal has been reported in houseflies, *Musca* (Wolken, Bowness, and Scheer, 1960) but the spectral evidence is equivocal. Briggs (1961 c) reports confirmation of the results on bees and flies as well as the presence of retinaldehyde in the heads of other species from the orders Odonata, Orthoptera, Coleoptera, Lepidoptera, and Hymenoptera, but no spectral evidence is given. Wolken and Scheer (1963) present evidence for retinaldehyde in cockroaches (*Blatta orientalis*) in the amount of 0.08 μgm gm^{-1} fresh weight of heads.

When the carotenoids of light- and dark-adapted bees are compared, retinol (vitamin A) is also found (Goldsmith and Warner, 1964). Only traces of retinol are obtained from dark-adapted animals, but when the bees are light-adapted before killing, the amount of retinal that can be extracted falls and is replaced by retinol. Moreover, the heads of honeybees contain an NADH-dependent enzyme capable of reducing retinal to retinol. This is the only instance among the invertebrates where there is evidence for the participation of vitamin A in the visual cycle.

2. Effects of Carotenoid-free Diets

If flies (*Musca domestica*) are reared on a carotenoid-free diet, the sensitivity of the photoreceptor cells decreases (Goldsmith, Barker, and Cohen, 1964). In order to maximize the rise in threshold, it is necessary to rear the flies on the defined diet for several generations and to prevent microbial contamination of the food (GOLDSMITH and FERNÁNDEZ, 1966). When this is done, the threshold can be elevated by at least 10^4, both in the visible and near ultraviolet regions of the spectrum (Figure 7). Furthermore, the rise in threshold can be reversed by the addition of β-carotene (a provitamin A) to the larval diet. Clearly the receptor responsible for sensitivity in the region of 350 nm is just as dependent on carotenoids as the receptor functioning at longer wavelengths.

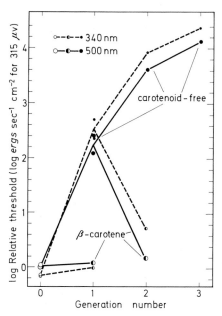

Fig. 7. The effect of carotenoid-free diet on the sensitivity of the retinal action potential of the housefly *Musca domestica*. Filled circles: log relative threshold of flies reared for three successive generations on a carotenoid-free diet under conditions designed to minimize microbial contamination. Half-filled circles: the effect of supplementing the larval diets of F_1 and F_2 flies with β-carotene. Plain circles: control flies. Small circles and broken curve show sensitivities to 340 nm; large circles and solid curve, to 500 nm; note that the threshold rises in both spectral regions. Each point represents an average of 6—12 animals (GOLDSMITH and FERNÁNDEZ, 1966)

Cytological correlates of carotenoid deficiency have been noted for both larval and adult mosquito eyes (BRAMMER and WHITE, 1969; JOLIE and WHITE, 1968). The principal effects of one generation of a deficient diet are an absence of otherwise characteristic multivesicular bodies (regardless of preillumination) and the presence of abnormal masses of cisternal membranes around the nucleus, particularly after exposure to light. The rhabdom, at least in adult eyes, is normal. The structural integrity of dipteran rhabdomeres may therefore be less dependent on a dietary source of retinaldehyde or its precursors than are the outer segments of rat rods (DOWLING and WALD, 1958).

The preceding observations are compatible with the hypothesis that carotenoid deficiency leads to a decreased amount of visual pigment, just as in the vertebrate eye. The results on the tobacco hornworm moth, *Manduca sexta*, however, are more difficult to accommodate under this umbrella. Carotenoid-deficient animals do not exhibit positive phototaxis (Carlson, 1968), yet intracellular and extracellular recording from the retinulae indicate that the receptors have nearly normal sensitivity (Boëthius, Carlson, Höglund, and Struwe, 1968). Cytological effects of deficiency are present, however, including derangement and proliferation of the rhabdomeric microvilli (Carlson, Gemne, and Robbins, 1969).

B. Action Spectra

Measurements of spectral sensitivity have run well ahead of direct measurements of absorption by insect visual pigments, and in most cases provide the only information available on the nature of the visual pigments. The determination of action spectra of insect receptors is complicated by a number of factors, not the least being the presence of color vision in many species. Therefore, techniques capable of resolving the contributions of individual pigments and receptors are required.

In the species so far studied, different color receptors seem to vary in spectral sensitivity because they contain different visual pigments rather than because of the presence of intraocular filtering devices. Certain Diptera, however, have colored corneas that function as broad-band interference filters (Bernard and Miller, 1968). The transmission properties of the corneal facets vary in different regions of the eye and, although the effect has not been studied, these filters must influence the spectral sensitivities of the underlying receptor cells. Under certain conditions the accessory screening pigments also can influence spectral sensitivity (e.g. Goldsmith, 1965), and the tracheal tapetum, which produces the colored "glow" in the eyes of Lepidoptera (Miller, Bernard, and Allen, 1968), may do likewise.

Two methods of measuring action spectra have been successfully employed. The first is to adapt selectively the mass response, or retinal action potential, by using colored lights. This approach has the advantage of relative simplicity. Stable extracellular recordings of responses, which can be ascribed with considerable certainty to the receptors, can be obtained; and fair precision of measurement can be achieved. By this technique it is possible to adapt selectively one or more pigments and measure, indirectly, the absorption of what pigment remains. The disadvantage of this method is that only crude localization of the pigment within the eye is possible.

The alternative approach is to measure the spectral sensitivities of single photoreceptor cells with intracellular microelectrodes. This kind of experiment, although technically more difficult, yields the physiologically important information on what the receptors are reporting to the central nervous system about wavelength. Spectral sensitivity measured in this manner may or may not describe the absorption of individual pigments. One must also know the extent to which the cell impaled is, under the conditions of the experiment, electrotonically coupled to other retinular cells, which perhaps contain different visual pigments. Second, it has not always proved possible to argue convincingly, even in instances where electrotonic coupling is absent, that the cell in question contains a single visual pigment. This point will be illustrated below.

Table 5 is a summary of those insects with multiple sensitivity maxima in which the spectral sensitivity curves have been best described. The selection is not intended to be an exhaustive survey of the literature. The honeybee, *Apis mellifera*, is the species to which both selective adaptation of the mass response and single unit analyses have been most successfully applied. There are three classes of receptors present in the compound eyes of drones, and perhaps four in the compound eyes of workers. There is good agreement between the results obtained by selective adaptation and recording from single units (Table 5; Figure 8). Moreover, the spectral band width of the sensitivity curves is approximately correct for rhodopsin-like pigments, as described by DARTNALL's (1953) nomogram. The back swimmer *Notonecta glauca* has a similar visual system (BRUCKMOSER, 1968).

Table 5. *Presence of multiple sensitivity maxima in the compound eyes of insects[a]*

mal	λmax	(nm)			Method[b]	Author
ellula	<380	420		520	selective adaptation	RUCK, 1965
(dragonfly)		410		450—550[c]	single unit analysis	HORRIDGE, 1969
iplaneta	365			510	single unit analysis	MOTE and GOLD-SMITH, 1970
(cockroach)						
usta		430(515)			single unit analysis	BENNETT, TUNSTALL, and HORRIDGE, 1967
(locust)						
onecta	350	420	464 ?	567	single unit analysis	BRUCKMOSER, 1968
(backswimmer)						
liphora	345(470)		490(345)	520(345)	single unit analysis	BURKHARDT, 1962
(fly)						
is ♀	345			535	selective adaptation	GOLDSMITH, 1960
(honeybee)	340	430	460	530	single unit analysis	AUTRUM, 1965
is ♂	345	440		535	selective adaptation	GOLDSMITH, 1961b
	340	450		530	single unit analysis	AUTRUM, 1965

[a] Figures in parentheses refer to second absorption bands in the same cell.

[b] Selective adaptation of the retinal action potential, recorded extracellularly, or single unit analysis of retinular cells with intracellular micropipette electrodes.

[c] Results variable. See also AUTRUM and KOLB, 1968.

In the locust, all cells have their peak sensitivity at 430 nm, but they differ from one another in seeming to contain varying amounts of a second pigment absorbing maximally at 515 nm (BENNETT, TUNSTALL, and HORRIDGE, 1967). As locust cells in the same retinula do not appear to be electrotonically coupled (SHAW, 1967), the authors suggest that two pigments are present in each rhabdomere.

The fly *Calliphora* has also been studied with intracellular microelectrodes with still different results (BURKHARDT, 1962). Three classes of cells were identified, with sensitivity maxima at 470, 490, and 520 nm. Each cell invariably had a second sensitivity maximum at 345 nm, and in the case of the 470 nm units the ultraviolet maximum was actually the larger. The two peaks could not be made to vary in relative height by selective adaptation with long wavelengths, and the question

45*

remains open as to whether these results indicate the presence of two pigments in a single cell (*cf.* Bennett, Tunstall, and Horridge, 1967), or, as Burkhardt suggests, whether they reflect the existence of visual pigments with two peaks of absorption.

C. Special Problems Raised by the Ultraviolet Receptor

One of the most intriguing features of insect eyes is the frequent presence of sensitivity to near ultraviolet wavelengths. In the honeybee *Apis*, the back swimmer *Notonecta*, and the cockroach *Periplaneta* this sensitivity is clearly based on a specific ultraviolet receptor. As discussed above, the situation is a little less clear in flies. Ultraviolet sensitivity is also present in the median ocellus of *Limulus* (Wald and Krainin, 1963; Chapman and Lall, 1967; Nolte, Brown, and Smith, 1968) and in several groups of arachnids (mites, Naegele, McEnroe, and Soans, 1966; lateral eyes of scorpions, Machan, 1968; and certain spiders, De Voe, Small, and Zvargulis, 1969).

Ultraviolet sensitivity is not widely distributed among the crustacea, being absent in crayfish (*Orconectes*) and the blue crab (*Callinectes*). An uv receptor is present in the prawn *Palaemonetes*, but it is maximally sensitive at longer wavelengths than the receptors of insects, at about 380—390 nm (Goldsmith and Fernández, 1968b; Wald and Seldin, 1968). Unlike most crustacea, insects keep their corneas free of near-ultraviolet-absorbing materials and exploit the shortest wavelengths available in the natural environment (Goldsmith and Fernández, 1968a, b).

In insects, ultraviolet light has an especially high efficiency in directing phototaxis (Goldsmith, 1961a), and it is perceived as a distinct color by honeybees (Daumer, 1956). Sensitivity to ultraviolet light therefore can not be based on fluorescence of the accessory pigments of the eye. The experiments with carotenoid-free flies (see p. 704) implicate retinal as the chromophoric group, and in all likelihood reception of ultraviolet light involves a photochemical mechanism similar to that employed by the longer wavelength receptors.

Free retinal (all *trans*) absorbs at about 389 nm (in aqueous environments), and the alkaline form of Schiff bases at 365—370 nm. The ultraviolet receptors of insects are maximally sensitive at distinctly shorter wavelengths, as low as 345 nm. In vertebrate systems, condensation of retinal to opsin to form a visual pigment shifts the spectrum of the chromophoric system to longer, not shorter, wavelengths. It therefore seems likely that in producing a 345-nm visual pigment, the resonant structure of the chromophore must be shortened. This in turn suggests that in the ultraviolet receptors of insects retinaldehyde is not joined to the rest of the molecule through an amino group to form a Schiff base.

The linkage of retinal with the sulfhydryl group of cysteine is an interesting alternative possibility. Wald and Brown (unpublished experiments cited in Wald and Brown, 1952) report that retinal will condense spontaneously with cysteine and glutathione, with a shift in spectrum to shorter wavelengths. The reaction was studied further by Peskin and Love (1963), who present evidence that the product formed from retinaldehyde and cysteine is the thiazolidine carboxylic acid of the following structure:

$$\begin{array}{c} \qquad\qquad S\!-\!CH_2 \\ \nearrow \qquad\quad \\ C_{19}H_{27}\!-\!CH \qquad\quad \diagdown \\ \diagdown \qquad\qquad \\ NH\!-\!CH\!-\!COOH \end{array}$$

The shift in spectrum to shorter wavelengths reflects the loss of the carbonyl group from the conjugated chain. Because the imino nitrogen is not in conjugation with the polyene chain, the spectrum does not change when the solution is acidified.

The spectral absorbances of this compound and retinaldehyde are compared in Figure 8 with the spectral sensitivity of the 345 nm receptors of the compound eye of the honeybee. The spectral shift from retinal to the thiazolidine carboxylic acid is somewhat more than adequate and the band width of the latter substance precisely right to account for the ultraviolet receptor of this species.

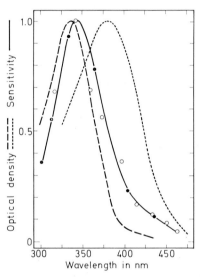

Fig. 8. The ultraviolet receptor of honeybees compared with the spectral absorbances of two relevant compounds. Filled circles and solid curve: the spectral sensitivity of the retinal action potential of the compound eyes of worker honeybees (*Apis mellifera*) measured in the presence of a bright yellow adapting light. Under these conditions, the sensitivity of the eye is determined primarily by the uv receptors. (GOLDSMITH, 1960.) Plain circles: average spectral sensitivity of the ultraviolet receptor as measured with intracellular microelectrodes in single retinular cells (AUTRUM and VON ZWEHL, 1964). The two methods agree very well in defining the sensitivity of this class of units. Dotted curve: spectral absorbance of retinaldehyde. Dashed curve: spectral absorbance of the thiazolidene carboxylic acid formed by condensing retinaldehyde with the sulfhydryl amino acid cysteine. See the text for discussion

The involvement of the nitrogen atom in the ring suggests that this specific compound is a relevant model for the visual pigment of insect uv receptors only if the cysteine occurs as the N-terminal residue in its polypeptide chain. However, there are other possibilities with similar spectral consequences in which the cysteinyl residue would not have to be placed at the end of the polypeptide:

i) a probably less stable hemithioacetal (Shubert, 1936)

$$C_{19}H_{27}—CHOH—S—CH_2—\overset{\displaystyle NH}{\underset{\displaystyle C=O}{CH}}$$

or ii) a linkage requiring both an SH group and an NH_2 group, but from different regions of the lipoprotein, which are brought together by appropriate folding of the molecule.

$$C_{19}\,H_{27}\,-CH\overset{\displaystyle S}{\underset{\displaystyle NH}{}}$$

The merit of these suggestions awaits the results of further work.

Recently measurements of ultraviolet sensitivity have been extended to 250 nm in an attempt to discover whether energy absorbed by the protein component of the visual pigment can contribute to visual excitation (Goldsmith and Fernández, 1968a). A white-eye mutant of the fly *Musca* was employed in order to minimize absorption and fluorescence by the accessory screening pigments. The results are shown in Fig. 9. The log of the reciprocal of the relative number of photons required to produce a constant electrical response from the receptors is

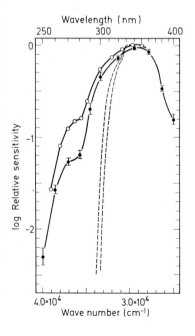

Fig. 9. The spectral sensitivity of housefly (*Musca*) photoreceptors in the near and mid ultraviolet, showing physiological evidence for intramolecular energy transfer. Filled circles ($\pm$ S.E.): spectral sensitivity uncorrected for energy loss in the dioptric elements. Plain circles: after correction for absorption in the cornea. Dashed curves: relative attenuation by the earth's atmosphere of the spectral energy of sunlight. Ordinate (for the sensitivity curves) is the log of the reciprocal of the relative number of photons required to produce a constant contribution of the receptors to the retinal action potential. As discussed in the text, the correction for corneal absorption accounts for only part of the energy lost to inert screening substances lying between the photoreceptive pigment and the external surface of the cornea. (Goldsmith and Fernández, 1968a)

shown by the filled circles. The main peak is at 350 nm, but a distinct shoulder is evident at about 270—280 nm. When the curve is corrected for energy loss in the cornea, the short wavelength shoulder becomes even more prominent, as shown by the plain circles in Fig. 9. The correction was based on microspectrophotometric measurements of absorption of individual corneal facets. As a measure of energy loss in the dioptric apparatus it is conservative, for it does not include absorption by the crystalline cone nor by inert proteins in the structure of the rhabdom itself. The 280 nm shoulder in the spectral sensitivity function is believed to represent intramolecular energy transfer from protein to chromophore, such as has been observed in the bleaching of vertebrate rhodopsin (KROPF, 1967, see pp. 55 and 141).

D. Direct Measurements of Visual Pigments

At present there exist only a few reports of absorbance spectra of what might, with any justice, be called insect visual pigments.

1. Extracts

When the heads of freshly killed bees are ground in a large volume of neutral phosphate buffer, the retinaldehyde that they contain comes into solution. It can be recovered from this aqueous environment by the addition of sufficient acetone to denature protein, followed by extraction with a nonpolar organic solvent such as hexane or petroleum ether.

The retinal is bound to protein in the original buffer solution, for it can be reversibly precipitated with ammonium sulphate. By applying this and other techniques for protein fractionation, the retinal-protein complex can be separated from most of the contaminating ommochrome pigments, and spectrophotometric evidence for light sensitivity obtained. When the partially purified solution is exposed for several minutes to a yellow light, there is bleaching around 450 nm and the formation of a photoproduct at 370 nm. The photoproduct is believed to be retinal, for when the pigment is bleached by potassium borohydride, a reducing agent known to convert retinal to retinol, the product shows maximal absorbance at about 330 nm. The maximum decrease in the difference spectrum is then at about 440 nm. At least one-half of the retinal originally present in the tissue can be ascribed to the 440 nm pigment (GOLDSMITH, 1958). In unpublished experiments, a partial regeneration of the photobleached pigment was achieved by adding 11-*cis* retinal.

The difference spectrum for the 440-nm pigment fits well the spectral sensitivity of the 440 nm receptor of the compound eye of the drone bee. The difficulty is that the pigment was extracted from a mass of worker bees containing only a fraction of a per cent drones. The dominant receptor of the compound eye of the worker is at 535 nm, with smaller contributions from the 340 nm unit. The behavioral work on trained honeybees (DAUMER, 1956) indicates that worker bees have a trichromatic system of color vision, but physiological experiments indicate that the violet receptor is present in relatively small numbers. It was not detected in the experiments on selective adaptation of the retinal action potential (GOLDSMITH, 1960), and in single unit recordings only a few cells were found with peak sensitivity at 430 or 460 nm (AUTRUM and VON ZWEHL, 1964).

Thus there is some doubt whether the 440-nm photopigment is a native visual pigment. It may be that removal of the pigment from the structure of the rhabdom so alters the tertiary structure of the pigment molecule that the enhancement of resonance, which is required to move the absorption to 535 nm, is partially destroyed. Although there is no precedent for this in work on vertebrates, there is also no other known instance of a rhodopsin-like pigment's being brought into solution without the use of some solubilizing agent such as digitonin.

WOLKEN and SCHEER (1963) have described a light-sensitive rhodopsin in extracts of cockroach heads *(Blatta orientalis)*. Heads were ground in 45 % sucrose, centrifuged under phosphate buffer, and the interfacial material extracted with 1.8 % digitonin. On exposure to light the absorbance fell at long wavelengths, maximally at about 500 nm, and a photoproduct formed with λ_{max} at 375 nm. It is not clear from the original description whether more than about 20 % of the pigment bleached. Nevertheless, this pigment behaves more like a conventional rhodopsin than the 440-nm pigment of honeybees, and the shape and λ_{max} of the difference spectrum have the correct properties to account for a 500-nm receptor. Such a receptor is known from electrophysiological evidence (GOLDSMITH and RUCK, 1958; WALTHER, 1958; MOTE and GOLDSMITH, 1970) to be present in *Periplaneta americana*, another species of cockroach.

MARAK, GALLIK, and CORNESKY (1970) obtained a small amount of rhodopsin from 100 grams of housefly heads *(Musca)* that had been previously extracted with buffer and petroleum ether. (Aliquots of the starting material had also been digested with trypsin, lipase, and chitinase.) A digitonin extract of the residue contained a pigment absorbing maximally at 510 nm which bleached in the light, yielding a photoproduct with λ_{max} at 380 nm. Like the pigment from cockroach heads, this presumptive rhodopsin fits well a known spectral sensitivity function of flies (cf. Table 5).

GOGALA, HAMDORF, and SCHWEMER (1970) have extracted with digitonin what appears to be the visual pigment of the ultraviolet receptor of the neuropteran *Ascalaphus*. It absorbs maximally at 345 nm. If the pigment is heat denatured in the presence of hydroxylamine, a product forms with peak absorption at 360 nm. Consequently, retinaldehyde is implicated as the chromophore. When the pigment is irradiated with uv light at pH 5.2, a photoproduct forms with λ_{max} at 483 nm. This reaction is photoreversible. If the solution containing the photoproduct is made basic (pH 9.3), the metarhodopsin with λ_{max} at 483 nm is converted into a form absorbing at 375 nm. The metarhodopsin therefore can exist in stable acid or alkaline forms, similar to the metarhodopsins of cephalopod molluscs.

The observation that the metarhodopsin of this uv pigment absorbs at 483 nm suggests that the linkage of chromophore to protein may involve a Schiff base as in other rhodopsins. The final version of the model proposed in the preceding section could nevertheless apply if participation of the sulfur atom and ring closure were, for steric reasons involving conformation of the protein, possible only when the chromophore is in the *cis* configuration.

2. Microspectrophotometry

LANGER and THORELL (1965) made the first microspectrophotometric measurements of the visual pigment of an invertebrate. Slices of eyes from the white eye mutant "chalky" of the fly *Calliphora* were studied by passing 1.5 μm beams of light down single rhabdomeres. The rhabdomeres of fly ommatidia are unusual in that they are not fused into a single rhabdom. In each retinula there are six peripheral rhabdomeres and a seventh central one. The latter is in fact two rhabdomeres lying end to end so that only one appears in any cross section of the ommatidium. The six peripheral rhabdomeres absorb maximally at about 510 nm and have a smaller peak near 360 nm. The central rhabdomeres contain a pigment with $\lambda_{\max}$ at 470 nm and also show smaller absorption in the near uv. Bleaching is accompanied by fading of the long wavelength peak but with only smaller changes in the near ultraviolet. It may be that bleaching of an ultraviolet absorption band is nearly compensated by the formation of retinaldehyde, so that only small changes in absorption occur in the region around 370 nm. It remains to be demonstrated, however, whether individual dark-adapted rhabdomeres contain one or two pigments. Individual rhabdomeres are also weakly dichroic.

These pigments correspond to two of the three types of receptor that were observed by BURKHARDT (1962, see also Table 5). On the other hand, they do not offer an explanation for why the dark-adapted eyes of flies are maximally sensitive at about 350 nm, as judged from the retinal action potential (WALTHER and DODT, 1957; GOLDSMITH and FERNÁNDEZ, 1968a; but see also HOFFMANN and LANGER, 1961).

The observations of GOGALA, HAMDORF, and SCHWEMER (1970) on extracts of the ultraviolet pigment of *Ascalaphus* have been confirmed by the same authors using microspectrophotometry of rhabdoms, but few details of the experimental procedure or the results have been reported.

VI. Visual Excitation in Rhabdomeric Photoreceptors

As the mechanism of transduction is the central unsolved biophysical problem in vision, it seems desirable to close this chapter with a brief account of where the matter stands.

In general, the pigment is located scores of μm from the site at which nerve impulses arise in the photoreceptor cell axons (squid) or presynaptic endings of the retinular cells (most arthropods), and the cell membrane is the structure that provides the functional connection. Slow, depolarizing potentials have been recorded with intracellular microelectrodes from the photoreceptor cells of a number of species, principally arthropods (*e.g.*, FUORTES, 1959; WASHIZU, 1964) and their electrotonic spread into the axons has been observed (EICHENBAUM and GOLD-SMITH, 1968; JÄRVILEHTO and ZETTLER, 1970; IOANNIDES and WALCOTT, 1971). Other sorts of depolarizing potentials have been observed close to threshold (*e.g.*, DOWLING, 1968). In squid it has been possible to show that the site of inward current is restricted to the illuminated region of the outer segments of the receptor (HAGINS, ZONANA, and ADAMS, 1962). In most cases the changes in membrane potential are believed to reflect increases in membrane conductance, but modulation of the sodium pump has also been suggested for the retinular cells of the ventral eye of *Limulus* (SMITH, STELL, BROWN, FREEMAN, and MURRAY, 1968).

The means by which absorption of light by rhodopsin leads to increases in ionic conductance of the adjacent cell membrane is unknown, but HAGINS (1965) has calculated that for each effective photon, 10^5-10^6 electronic charges pass through the membrane within several μm of the site of absorption. Because of the time relations, attention has been directed to changes in the opsin occurring between lumirhodopsin and metarhodopsin (in vertebrates, metarhodopsin II), although what the relevant changes may be is a matter for conjecture (*cf.* Abrahamson and Ostroy, 1967).

As all rhodopsin molecules are thought to be equally capable of triggering a response (Hecht, Shlaer, and Pirenne, 1942) there is also the problem of how absorption of a photon in the center of a rhabdom produces conductance changes in a region of membrane apparently several μm distant. Various processes for energy transfer have been considered, all of which seem to have difficulties. The distance between chromophores is said to be too great for inductive resonance energy transfer (Hagins and Jennings, 1959), and the probability of formation of triplet states too small for their involvement in significant fashion (Abrahamson and Ostroy, 1967).

A recent study by Perrelet and Baumann (1969) suggests, however, that all the visual pigment of even the most compact rhabdoms may be located in membranes adjacent to extracellular space. According to these authors, lanthanum (but not ferritin) penetrates into the rhabdom and surrounds each microvillus. Moreover, Lasansky and Fuortes (1969) present evidence that in the leech light causes an inward, depolarizing current across the membranes of the microvilli.

VII. Summary

1. Action spectra for behavioral responses of lower invertebrates, and spectra sensitivity measurements of relatively unspecialized photoreceptors indicate receptor pigments with broad absorption maxima centered in the blue or green regions of the spectrum, much like the rhodopsins of vertebrate rod cells. Aside from cephalopod molluscs and arthropods, however, there are no direct measurements of invertebrate visual pigments.

2. The chromophore of the visual pigments of the higher invertebrates (cephalopod molluscs and arthropods) is retinaldehyde. In the rhodopsin of cephalopod molluscs, the chromophore is in the 11-*cis* configuration. The isomeric configuration of the visual pigments of crustacea has not been determined, but the large amounts of 11-*cis* vitamin A in the eyes of a number of species is suggestive.

3. In honeybees, light adaptation is accompanied by a conversion of retinaldehyde to vitamin A. This is the only invertebrate in which this is known to happen as a normal part of the visual cycle.

4. The photoreceptor cells of flies that have been reared on carotenoid-free diets show a loss in sensitivity to light. This is the only "vitamin A deficiency" known among the invertebrates.

5. The visual pigments of cephalopod molluscs are converted by light into long-lived metarhodopsins that, in neutral or acid solution, absorb maximally near the parent pigment (around 500 nm) and, in basic solution, at 380 nm. In the retinas of squid, there are no further thermal reactions that would lead to liberation of the retinaldehyde and bleaching. The light reaction is the isomerization

of retinal from 11-*cis* to all *trans*. The means by which the visual pigment is reconstituted (the chromophoric group is reisomerized) is not known, but attention has recently been drawn to a second pigment (retinochrome) that seems to have the capacity for catalyzing the photoisomerization of all-*trans* retinal to 11-*cis*.

6. The study of the visual pigments of arthropod eyes in extracts has been complicated by the presence of relatively great amounts of accessory screening pigments and the need to start with large quantities of material. More success has been obtained with crustacea (Table 3) than with insects.

7. The technique of microspectrophotometry shows that the visual pigments of arthropods are located in the rhabdoms, but the pattern of distribution of pigments in eyes of animals with color vision is only beginning to be understood. In the ommatidia of Diptera there are seven separate and distinct rhabdomeres evident in any cross section. One of these (the central one) contains a visual pigment with λ_{max} at 470 nm, and the other six contain a pigment with λ_{max} at 510 nm. The rhabdoms of certain decapod crustaceans may contain a mixture of two light-sensitive pigments, only one of which seems to be coupled to visual excitation.

8. Many insects have ultraviolet receptors maximally sensitive at 340—350 nm. Although the chromophore in this receptor is apparently retinaldehyde, its mode of linkage to the protein part of the visual pigment may be different from the Schiff-base attachment presumably found in most other visual pigments.

9. The means by which isomerization of the chromophore leads to visual excitation is not any clearer in invertebrate eyes than it is in vertebrate receptors. The first physiological manifestation is an increase in conductance and consequent lowering of membrane potential in the photoreceptor cells, but the causal molecular events intervening between absorption of light and changes in permeability of the cell membrane have not been identified.

References

ABRAHAMSON, E. W., OSTROY, S. E.: The photochemical and macromolecular aspects of vision. Progr. Biophys. Mol. Biol. **17**, 181—215 (1967).

AUTRUM, H.: The physiological basis of colour vision in honeybees. In: Ciba Foundation Symposium on Physiology and Experimental Psychology of Colour Vision. Boston: Little, Brown and Co. 1965.

— KOLB, G.: Spektrale Empfindlichkeit einzelner Sehzellen der Aeschniden. Z. vergl. Physiol. **60**, 450—477 (1968).

— ZWEHL, V. VON: Die spektrale Empfindlichkeit einzelner Sehzellen des Bienenauges. Z. vergl. Physiol. **48**, 357—384 (1964).

BATRA, P., TOLLIN, G.: Phototaxis in *Euglena*. I. Isolation of the eye-spot granules and identification of the eye-spot pigments. Biochim. biophys. Acta (Amst.) **79**, 371—378 (1964).

BENNETT, R. R., TUNSTALL, J., HORRIDGE, G. A.: Spectral sensitivity of single retinula cells of the locust. Z. vergl. Physiol. **55**, 195—206 (1967).

BERNARD, G. D., MILLER, W. H.: Interference filters in the corneas of diptera. Invest. Ophthal. **7**, 416—434 (1968).

BOETHIUS, J., CARLSON, S. D., HÖGLUND, G., STRUWE, G.: Electrophysiological response to light in a moth species *(Manduca sexta)* reared from a vitamin A deficient diet. Acta physiol. scand. **73**, 27 A (1968).

BOWNESS, J. M., WOLKEN, J. J.: A light-sensitive yellow pigment from the housefly. J. gen. Physiol. **42**, 779—792 (1959).

BRAMMER, J. D., WHITE, R. H.: Vitamin A deficiency: effect on mosquito eye ultrastructure. Science **163**, 821—823 (1969).

Bridges, C. D. B.: Biochemistry of visual processes. In: Comprehensive Biochemistry, Vol. 27, pp. 31—78 (Florkin, M., and Stotz, E. H., eds.). Amsterdam: Elsevier Publishing Co. 1967.

Briggs, M. H.: The visual pigment of an isopod crustacean. Aust. J. biol. Sci. **41**, 487—488 (1961a).

— Visual pigment of grapsoid crabs. Nature (Lond.) **190**, 784—786 (1961b).

— Retinene-1 in insect tissues. Nature (Lond.) **192**, 874—875 (1961c).

Brown, H. M., Ogden, T. E.: The electrical response of the planarian ocellus. J. gen. Physiol. **51**, 237—253 (1968).

Brown, P. K., Brown, P. S.: Visual pigments of the octopus and cuttlefish. Nature (Lond.) **182**, 1288—1290 (1958).

Bruckmoser, P.: Die spektrale Empfindlichkeit einzelner Sehzellen des Rückenschwimmers *Notonecta glauca* L. (Heteroptera). Z. vergl. Physiol. **59**, 187—204 (1968).

Bruno, M. S., Kennedy, D.: The spectral sensitivity of photoreceptor neurons in the sixth ganglion of the crayfish. Comp. Biochem. Physiol. **6**, 41—46 (1962).

Bünning, E., Schneiderhöhn, G.: Über das Aktionsspektrum der phototaktischen Reaktionen von *Euglena*. Arch. Mikrobiol. **24**, 80—90 (1956).

Burkhardt, D.: Spectral sensitivity and other response characteristics of single visual cells in the arthropod eye. Symp. Soc. exp. Biol. **16**, 86—109 (1962).

Carlson, S. D.: Personal communication (1968).

— Gemne, G., Robbins, W. E.: Ultrastructure of photoreceptor cells in a vitamin A-deficient moth *(Manduca sexta)*. Experientia (Basel) **25**, 175—177 (1969).

Chapman, R. M., Lall, A. B.: Electroretinogram characteristics and the spectral mechanisms of the median ocellus and the lateral eye in *Limulus polyphemus*. J. gen. Physiol. **50**, 2267—2287 (1967).

Cobb, H. D.: An *in vivo* absorption spectrum of the eyespot of *Euglena mesnili*. Tex. J. Sci. **60**, 231—235 (1963).

Dartnall, H. J. A.: The interpretation of spectral sensitivity curves. Brit. med. Bull. **9**, 24—30 (1953).

Daumer, K.: Reizmetrische Untersuchung des Farbensehens der Bienen. Z. vergl. Physiol. **38**, 413—478 (1956).

De Voe, R. D., Small, R. J. W., Zvargulis, J. E.: Spectral sensitivities of wolf spider eyes. J. gen. Physiol. **54**, 1—32 (1969).

Dowling, J. E.: Discrete potentials in the dark-adapted eye of *Limulus*. Nature (Lond.) **217**, 28—31 (1968).

— Wald, G.: The biological function of vitamin A acid. Proc. nat. Acad. Sci. (Wash.) **46**, 587—608 (1960).

Eichenbaum, D. M., Goldsmith, T. H.: Properties of intact photoreceptor cells lacking synapses. J. Exp. Zool. **169**, 15—32 (1968).

Engelmann, T. W.: Über Licht- und Farbenperception niederster Organismen. Arch. ges. Physiol. **29**, 387—400 (1882).

Fernández, H. R.: A survey of the visual pigments of decapod crustacea of South Florida. Ph. D. Thesis, University of Miami, Coral Gables, Florida 1965.

Fisher, L. R., Goldie, E. H.: Pigments of compound eyes. Progress in Photobiology, Proc. 3rd Internat. Congr. Photobiol., 153—154 (1960).

— Kon, S. K.: Vitamin A in the invertebrates. Camb. Phil. Soc. Biol. Rev. **34**, 1—36 (1959).

Fuortes, M. G. F.: Initiation of impulses in visual cells of *Limulus*. J. Physiol. **148**, 14—28 (1959).

Gogala, M., Hamdorf, K., Schwemer, J.: UV-Sehfarbstoff bei Insekten. Z. vergl. Physiol. **70**, 410—413 (1970).

Goldsmith, T. H.: The visual system of the honeybee. Proc. nat. Acad. Sci. (Wash.) **44**, 123—126 (1958).

— The nature of the retinal action potential, and the spectral sensitivities of ultraviolet and green receptor systems in the compound eye of the worker honeybee. J. gen. Physiol. **43**, 775—799 (1960).

— The color vision of insects. In: Light and Life, pp. 771—794 (McElroy, W. D., and Glass, B., eds.). Baltimore: The Johns Hopkins Press 1961a.

GOLDSMITH, T. H.: The physiological basis of wave-length discrimination in the eye of the honeybee. In: Sensory Communication, pp. 357—375 (ROSENBLITH, W. A., ed.). New York: The MIT Press and John Wiley and Sons, Inc. 1961 b.
— The visual system of insects. In: The Physiology of Insecta, Vol. 1, 397—462 (ROCKSTEIN, M., ed.). New York: Academic Press 1964.
— Do flies have a red receptor? J. gen. Physiol. 49, 265—287 (1965).
— BARKER, R. J., COHEN, C. F.: Sensitivity of visual receptors of carotenoid-depleted flies: a vitamin A deficiency in an invertebrate. Science 146, 65—67 (1964).
— FERNÁNDEZ, H. R.: Some photochemical and physiological aspects of visual excitation in compound eyes. In: The Functional Organization of the Compound Eye, pp. 125—143 (BERNHARD, C. G., ed.). New York: Pergamon Press 1966.
— — The sensitivity of housefly photoreceptors in the mid-ultraviolet and the limits of the visible spectrum. J. exp. Biol. 49, 669—677 (1968a).
— — Comparative studies of crustacean spectral sensitivity. Z. vergl. Physiol. 60, 156—175 (1968b).
— RUCK, P. R.: The spectral sensitivities of the dorsal ocelli of cockroaches and honeybees. J. gen. Physiol. 41, 1171—1185 (1958).
— WARNER, L. T.: Vitamin A in the vision of insects. J. gen. Physiol. 47, 433—441 (1964).
GRAHAM, C. H., HARTLINE, H. K.: The response of single visual sense cells to lights of different wave lengths. J. gen. Physiol. 18, 917—931 (1935).
HAGINS, W. A.: Electrical signs of information flow in photoreceptors. Cold Spr. Harb. Symp. quant. Biol. 30, 403—418 (1965).
— JENNINGS, W. H.: Radiationless migration of electronic excitation in retinal rods. Disc. Faraday Soc. 27, 180—190 (1959).
— LIEBMAN, P. A.: The relationship between photochemical and electrical processes in living squid photoreceptors. Biophys. Soc. Abstr. ann. Meeting, ME 6 (1963).
— ZONANA, H. V., ADAMS, R. G.: Local membrane current in the outer segments of squid photoreceptors. Nature (Lond.) 194, 844—847 (1962).
HALLDAL, P.: Action spectra of phototaxis and related problems in Volvocales, Ulva-gametes and Dinophyceae. Physiol. Plant. 11, 118—153 (1958).
— Phototaxis in protozoa. In: Biochemistry and Physiology of Protozoa, Vol. 3, 277—296 (HUTNER, S., ed.). New York: Academic Press 1964.
HAMDORF, K., SCHWEMER, J., TÄUBER, U.: Der Sehfarbstoff, die Absorption der Receptoren und die spektrale Empfindlichkeit der Retina von Eledone moschata. Z. vergl. Physiol. 60, 375—415 (1968).
HARA, T., HARA, R.: New photosensitive pigment found in the retina of the squid Ommastrephes. Nature 206, 1331—1334 (1965).
— — Rhodopsin and retinochrome in the octopus retina. Nature (Lond.) 214, 572—573 (1967).
— — Regeneration of squid retinochrome. Nature (Lond.) 219, 450—454 (1968).
— — TAKEUCHI, J.: Rhodopsin and retinochrome in the squid retina. Nature (Lond.) 214, 573—575 (1967).
HAYS, D., GOLDSMITH, T. H.: Microspectrophotometry of the visual pigment of the spider crab Libinia emarginata. Z. vergl. Physiol. 65, 218—232 (1969).
HECHT, S., SHLAER, S., PIRENNE, M. H.: Energy, quanta, and vision. J. gen. Physiol. 25, 819—840 (1942).
HITCHCOCK, L., JR.: Color sensitivity of the amoeba revisited. J. Protozool. 8, 322—324 (1961).
HÖGLUND, G.: Pigment migration, light screening and receptor sensitivity in the compound eye of nocturnal lepidoptera. Acta physiol. scand. 69, 1—56 (1966).
HOFFMAN, C., LANGER, H.: Die spektrale Augenempfindlichkeit der Mutante „chalky" von Calliphora erythrocephala. Naturwissenschaften 48, 605 (1961).
HORRIDGE, G. A.: Perception of polarization plane, colour and movement in two dimensions by the crab, Carcinus. Z. vergl. Physiol. 55, 207—224 (1967).
— Unit studies on the retina of dragonflies. Z. vergl. Physiol. 62, 1—37 (1969).

Hubbard, R.: On the chromophores of the visual pigments. In: Visual problems of colour. Nat. Physical Lab. Symp. no. 8. London: H.M.S.O. 1958.

— St. George, R. C. C.: The rhodopsin system of the squid. J. gen. Physiol. **41**, 501—528 (1958).

— Wald, G.: Visual pigment of the horseshoe crab, *Limulus polyphemus*. Nature (Lond.) **186**, 212—215 (1960).

Ioannides, A. C., Walcott, B.: Graded illumination potentials from retinula cell axons in the bug *Lethocerus*. Z. vergl. Physiol. **71**, 315—325 (1971).

Järvilehto, M., Zettler, F.: Micro-localisation of lamina-located visual cell activities in the compound eye of the blowfly *Calliphora*. Z. vergl. Physiol. **69**, 134—138 (1970).

Jolie, M. A., White, R. H.: Personal communication 1968.

Kampa, E. M.: Euphausiopsin, a new photosensitive pigment from the eyes of euphausiid crustaceans. Nature (Lond.) **175**, 996—998 (1955).

Kennedy, D.: Neural photoreception in a lamellibranch mollusc. J. gen. Physiol. **44**, 277—299 (1960).

— Bruno, M. S.: The spectral sensitivity of crayfish and lobster vision. J. gen. Physiol. **44**, 1089—1102 (1961).

Krinsky, N. I., Goldsmith, T. H.: The carotenoids of the flagellated alga, *Euglena gracilis*. Arch. biochem. Biophys. **91**, 271—279 (1960).

Kropf, A.: Intramolecular energy transfer in rhodopsin. Vision Res. **7**, 811—818 (1967).

Langer, H., Thorell, B.: Microspectrophotometry of single rhabdomeres in the insect eye. Exp. Cell Res. **41**, 673—677 (1966).

Lasansky, A., Fuortes, M. G. F.: The site of origin of electrical responses in visual cells of the leech, *Hirudo medicinalis*. J. Cell Biol. **42**, 241—252 (1969).

Liebman, P. A.: *In situ* microspectrophotometric studies on the pigments of single retinal rods. Biophys. J. **2**, 161—178 (1962).

Loeb, J., Wasteneys, H.: The relative efficiency of various parts of the spectrum for the heliotropic reactions of animals and plants. J. exp. Zool. **19**, 23—35 (1915).

Machan, L.: Spectral sensitivities of scorpion eyes and the possible role of shielding pigment effect. J. exp. Biol. **49**, 95—105 (1968).

Marak, G. E., Gallik, G. J., Cornesky, R. A.: Light-sensitive pigment in insect heads. Ophthal. Res. **1**, 65—71 (1970).

Marriott, F. H. C.: The absolute light-sensitivity and spectral threshold curve of the aquatic flatworm *Dendrocoelum lacteum*. J. Physiol. **143**, 369—379 (1958).

Mast, S. O.: The relation betwen spectral color and stimulation in the lower organisms. J. exp. Zool. **22**, 471—528 (1917).

Matthews, R. G., Hubbard, R., Brown, P. K., Wald, G.: Tautomeric forms of metarhodopsin. J. gen. Physiol. **47**, 215—240 (1963).

Miller, W. H., Bernard, G. D., Allen, J. L.: The optics of insect compound eyes. Science **162**, 760—767 (1968).

Millott, N.: The photosensitivity of sea urchins. In: Comparative biochemistry of photoreactive systems, Vol. I (Allen, M. B., ed.). New York: Academic Press 1960.

— Yoshida, M.: The spectral sensitivity of the echinoid *Diadema antillarum* Philippi. J. Exp. Biol. **34**, 394—401 (1957).

Moore, T.: Vitamin A. Amsterdam: Elsevier Publishing Co. 1957.

Mote, M. I., Goldsmith, T. H.: Spectral sensitivities of color receptors in the compound eye of the cockroach *Periplaneta*. J. exp. Zool. **173**, 137—145 (1970).

Naegele, J. A., McEnroe, W. D., Soans, A. B.: Spectral sensitivity and orientation response of the two-spotted spider mite, *Tetranychus urticae* Koch, from 350 mμ to 700 mμ. J. Insect Physiol. **12**, 1187—1195 (1966).

Nolte, J., Brown, J. E., Smith, T. G., Jr.: A hyperpolarizing component of the receptor potential in the median ocellus of *Limulus*. Science **162**, 677—679 (1968).

Nosaki, H.: Electrophysiological study of color encoding in the compound eye of crayfish, *Procambarus clarkii*. Z. vergl. Physiol. **64**, 318—323 (1969).

Perrelet, A., Baumann, F.: Evidence for extracellular space in the rhabdome of the honeybee drone eye. J. Cell Biol. **40**, 825—830 (1969).

PESKIN, J. C., LOVE, B. B.: The reaction of L-cysteine with all-*trans*-retinene. Biochim. biophys. Acta (Amst.) **78**, 751—753 (1963).

RUCK, P. R.: The components of the visual system of a dragonfly. J. gen. Physiol. **49**, 289—307 (1965).

SHAW, S. R.: Simultaneous recording from two cells in the locust retina. Z. vergl. Physiol. **55**, 183—194 (1967).

SHUBERT, M. P.: Compounds of thiol acids with aldehydes. J. biol. Chem. **114**, 341—350 (1936).

SMITH, T. G., STELL, W. K., BROWN, J. E., FREEMAN, J. A., MURRAY, G. C.: A role for the sodium pump in photoreception in *Limulus*. Science **162**, 456—458 (1968).

STRANGE, P. H.: The spectral sensitivity of *Calliphora* maggots. J. exp. Zool. **38**, 237—248 (1961).

STROTHER, G. K., WOLKEN, J. J.: *In vivo* absorption spectra of *Euglena*: chloroplast and eyespot. J. Protozool. **8**, 261—265 (1961).

WALD, G.: Vitamin A in invertebrate eyes. Amer. J. Physiol. **133**, P 479—P 480 (1941).

— Visual pigments of crayfish. Nature (Lond.) **215**, 1131—1133 (1967).

— Single and multiple visual systems in arthropods. J. gen. Physiol. **51**, 125—156 (1968).

— BROWN, P. K.: The role of sulfhydryl groups in the bleaching and synthesis of rhodopsin. J. gen. Physiol. **35**, 797—821 (1952).

— — The vitamin A of a euphausiid crustacean. J. gen. Physiol. **40**, 627—634 (1957).

— — GIBBONS, I. R.: Visual excitation: achemo-anatomical study. Symp. Soc. Exp. Biol. **16**, 32—57 (1962).

— BURG, S. P.: The vitamin A of the lobster. J. gen. Physiol. **40**, 609—625 (1957).

— HUBBARD, R.: Visual pigment of a decapod crustacean: the lobster. Nature (Lond.) **180**, 278—280 (1957).

— KRAININ, J. M.: The median eye of *Limulus*: an ultraviolet receptor. Proc. nat. Acad. Sci. (Wash.) **50**, 1011—1017 (1963).

— SELDIN, E. B.: Spectral sensitivity of the common prawn, *Palaemonetes vulgaris*. J. gen. Physiol. **51**, 694—700 (1968).

WALTHER, J. B.: Changes induced in spectral sensitivity and form of retinal action potential of the cockroach eye by selective adaptation. J. Insect Physiol. **2**, 142—151 (1958).

— DODT, E.: Elektrophysiologische Untersuchungen über die Ultraviolettempfindlichkeit von Insektenaugen. Experientia (Basel) **13**, 333—334 (1957).

WASHIZU, Y.: Electrical activity of single retinula cells in the compound eye of the blowfly *Calliphora erythrocephala* Meig. Comp. Biochem. Physiol. **12**, 369—387 (1964).

WATERMAN, T. H., FERNÁNDEZ, H. R.: E-vector and wavelength discrimination by retinular cells of the crayfish *Procambarus*. Z. vergl. Physiol. **68**, 154—174 (1970).

— — GOLDSMITH, T. H.: Dichroism of photosensitive pigments in rhabdoms of the crayfish *Orconectes*. J. gen. Physiol. **54**, 415—432 (1969).

WOLKEN, J. J.: *Euglena*, an experimental organism for biochemical and biophysical studies. New York: Meredith Publishing Co. 1967.

— BOWNESS, J. M., SCHEER, I. J.: The visual complex of the insect: retinene in the housefly. Biochim. Biophys. Acta (Amst.) **43**, 531—537 (1960).

— SCHEER, I. J.: An eye pigment of the cockroach. Exp. Eye Res. **2**, 182—188 (1963).

YOSHIDA, M., OHTSUKI, H.: Compound ocellus of a starfish: its function. Science **153**, 197—198 (1966).

— — SUGURI, S.: Ommochrome from anthomedusan ocelli and its photoreduction. Photochem. Photobiol. **6**, 875—884 (1967).

YOSHIZA, T., WALD, G.: Transformations of squid rhodopsin at low temperatures. Nature (Lond.) **201**, 340—345 (1964).

ZIMMERMAN, W. F., GOLDSMITH, T. H.: Photosensitivity of the circadian rhythm and of visual receptors in carotenoid-depleted *Drosophila*. Science **171**, 1167—1169 (1971).

Chapter 18

Cephalopod Retinochrome

By

Tomiyuki Hara and Reiko Hara, Kashihara, Nara (Japan)

With 15 Figures

Contents

Among the marine invertebrates, the dibranchiate cephalopods, which include such familiar forms as squids, cuttlefish, and octopuses, possess the most highly developed type of visual sense organ. This is a large camera-like eye as prominent as that found in vertebrates. Since the Phyla Mollusca and Vertebrata have proceeded separately along their own long routes of evolution, such a close resemblance in the external morphology of the eyes is, perhaps, the prime example of convergent evolution. Closer inspection, however, reveals interesting differences, particularly in retinal structure and in the visual pigment system. Such differences, moreover, are bound to have a direct bearing on the mechanisms of generation and conduction of the visual response. In cephalopods the photoreceptors — unlike those of vertebrates — form the first layer of the retina. The visual pigment is in the rhabdoms (which thus correspond to the outer segments of vertebrate rods) and though behaving differently from vertebrate rhodopsin when exposed to light is sufficiently like it to justify the name "cephalopod rhodopsin". In the course of work on cephalopod rhodopsin, another distinct photosensitive pigment was discovered in a region adjacent to the rhabdoms (HARA and HARA, 1965). We have called this second photopigment "retinochrome". This chapter reviews the evidence that retinochrome, though not a visual pigment, may contribute to the visual mechanism by its co-operative relationship to cephalopod rhodopsin.

I. Retinal Structure and Location of the Two Photopigments

The structure of the retina in dibranchiate cephalopods is much simpler than that in vertebrates. In the light microscope, the cephalopod retina is seen to consist of four layers (Fig. 1A) — the rhabdoms, the black pigment, the visual cell nuclei and a plexus of nerve fibres — and is enclosed by a cartilaginous sclera. Such a construction arises through a markedly different course of development from that of the vertebrate retina (DUKE-ELDER, 1958). The cephalopod eye is derived from the invaginated epithelium which is transformed into an enclosed vesicle sunk beneath the surface ectoderm. The retina is differentiated from the cells lining the proximal portion of this vesicle and, at the final stage, is composed of two kinds of cells, visual and supporting (or basal) cells. Each visual cell is divided by a narrow neck into outer and inner portions, the boundary between the segments forming a distinct basement membrane parallel to the retinal surface. The outer portions of the visual cells then elongate towards the centre of the eye to form a thick layer of rhabdoms. From each of the inner portions, which contain the nuclei of the visual cells, several processes of axonal fibres grow and spread into the nerve plexus (TONOSAKI, 1965). The fibres leave the eyeball through the sclera as short optic nerves, and end within the optic lobes, which contain numerous neuronal elements similar to the amacrine, bipolar and horizontal cells of the vertebrate retina, and finally contact is made with the cerebral ganglion (YOUNG, 1960). In vertebrates the retina itself contains several layers of cells (e.g. amacrine, bipolar, horizontal, ganglion). In cephalopods, on the other hand, the retina is composed in the main of primary sensory cells, and the other neurones are found in the optic lobes. This structural simplicity affords many facilities for investigation of the photoreceptive mechanism of the visual cell.

A tangential or oblique section of the rhabdom layer shows a close packed pattern of cells (Fig. 1C). Such a pattern can be observed in sections right up to the pigmented layer. Electron microscope studies (ZONANA, 1961; YAMAMOTO, TASAKI, SUGAWARA, and TONOSAKI, 1965) have shown that the outer segment of each visual cell carries two rhabdomeres, one on each side. Normally four rhabdomeres of four different visual cells combine face to face to form a rhabdom, which is thus surrounded by four outer segments. This arrangement explains the fact that there are twice as many visual cell nuclei as there are rhabdoms in the retina (YOUNG, 1960). Each rhabdomere is made up of compact piles of microvillous

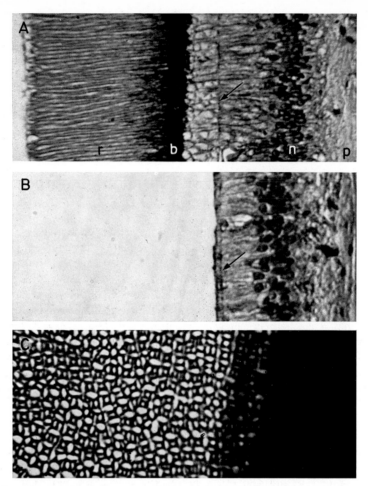

Fig. 1. Microphotographs of the retina of the squid, *Todarodes pacificus* Steenstrup ($\times$ 150).
A. The intact retina: *r*, rhabdoms; *b*, black pigment; *n*, nucleated visual cell bodies; *p*, nerve
plexus; arrows, basement membrane. B. The rhabdom-free retina (used for extraction of
retinochrome) prepared by stirring the eye-cup in buffer solution. C. Oblique section of the
layer of rhabdoms near their proximal ends. (Hara and Hara, 1965)

projections. These are long tubules derived from outgrowths of the rhabdomere
surface. They are perpendicular to the longitudinal axis of the outer segment
(Wolken, 1958; Moody and Robertson, 1960) and are disposed so that in opposite
rhabdomere pairs they are parallel, and in adjacent pairs at right angles, to each
other. This arrangement of microvilli forms a basis for explaining the ability of
some cephalopods to discriminate between different planes of polarization (Tasaki
and Karita, 1966) and suggests also that the molecules of visual pigment are
situated in the microvilli in an ordered way.

On the distal side of the basement membrane, the supporting cells are pigmented
heavily and arranged in a single layer. Black pigment granules are also distributed

within the outer portions of the visual cells, and, in the dark, add to the dense layer of black pigment provided by the supporting cells. In the light, the pigment granules tend to migrate forward in the outer segments, depending on the adaptation of the eye, so as to envelop the rhabdomes in sheaths and thus regulate their exposure to light, or, perhaps, serve to provide substances required by visual pigment. Across the basement membrane, small blood vessels lie adjacent to the supporting cells, which are connected with the neighbouring visual cells by junctions, while at the proximal extremities of the outer segments, the lateral surfaces of the plasma membranes of adjacent outer portions make contact to form a "tight junction" of compound membrane (YAMAMOTO, TASAKI, SUGAWARA, and TONOSAKI, 1965). The close association of the vascular net with these structures in the region of the basement membrane suggests that this could be a centre for adjusting the supply and demand of metabolic materials in the retina.

When the posterior half of an eye is vigorously shaken in a liquid, the outer portions of the visual cells break off at the level of the basement membrane and, together with supporting cells and black pigment, are scattered into the liquid. After this treatment the eye-cup still retains intact the nucleated visual cell bodies and the rest of the retinal structures behind them (Fig. 1B). The surface of such a rhabdome-free retina is light red in colour and fades to pale yellow on exposure to light, thus indicating the presence of a photosensitive pigment. This is retinochrome. When the surface of such a denuded retina is gently wiped with a piece of filter paper, the red pigment adheres to the paper or, if the retina is carefully shaven with a razor blade, it becomes paler and paler as the retinochrome is removed. Histological examination of retinas completely deprived of their retinochrome in this way shows that the nuclei of the visual cells are still present. This means that the retinochrome is contained in the retinal tissues just behind the rhabdoms, viz between the basement membrane and the layer of the nuclei. Since the supporting cells were removed, together with the rhodopsin-bearing rhabdoms and black pigment, during the stirring of the eye-cup, this suggests that retinochrome is concentrated in the inner portion of the visual cell. According to recent investigations (ZONANA, 1961; YAMAMOTO, TASAKI, SUGAWARA, and TONOSAKI, 1965), systems (myeloid bodies) of up to fifty membranes are present in these inner portions of the visual cells. We think it likely that the actual location of retinochrome is in these myeloid bodies, which have a laminated structure similar to those of other pigment-bearing arrangements such as vertebrate outer segments and the chloroplasts of leaves.

II. The Distribution of Rhodopsins and Retinochromes in Cephalopods

A. Extraction of the Photopigments

Since the rhodopsins and retinochromes are photosensitive, extractive procedures must be carried out in a dark-room under a deep-red safe-light. The dark-adapted eye is enucleated from the freshly collected animal, and hemisected to remove its anterior part and lens. The eye-cup so obtained is then violently stirred upside-down in a solution of neutral phosphate buffer, so as to detach the rhabdomes which, with black pigment, enter the liquid. (In some cases (e.g. octopus eyes) where this procedure would not result in complete removal of these structures, prior refrigeration of the fresh eyeball for about a day often results in a satisfactory separation). The suspension so obtained is filtered once through cotton gauze and then centrifuged. The black sediment containing the rhabdomes is collected and stored at $-15°$ C in darkness until needed for extraction of the rhodopsin. In the eye-cup there still remains the rhabdome-free retina containing retinochrome, which is more or less red, probably according to the adaptation of the animal. The eye-cup is spread out on a sheet of filter paper, and the periphery cut away by scissors so as to remove the attached black pigment. The retina is then lifted out and also kept frozen in darkness until required for extraction of the retinochrome.

For the preparation of rhodopsin, it is important to obtain the rhabdomes as clean as possible. This can be done as follows. The frozen mass of tissue containing rhabdomes and black pigment derived (say) from 20 retinas is thawed slowly, ground in a mortar to make a thick paste, and then washed with a large volume of M/15 phosphate buffer (pH 6.2) to dissolve soluble red impurities, and centrifuged. About 50 ml of a 40 per cent sucrose solution (in M/15 phosphate buffer) is then added to the residues, and the whole is shaken to form a suspension. When this suspension is centrifuged for 15 min at 12,000 r.p.m., the rhabdomes float and the unwanted debris sediments. The supernatant, including the rhabdomes, is then withdrawn, diluted with an equal volume of phosphate buffer, and re-centrifuged to yield a residue of rhabdomes at the bottom of the tube. This residue is then resuspended in sucrose solution (say 36 per cent.) and the procedure repeated to get a cleaner product. After the two flotations, the isolated rhabdomes are washed at least three times with M/10 sodium secondary phosphate solution and then several times with ion-free water until, after centrifuging, the supernatant is clear. Finally the rhodopsin is obtained by extracting the rhabdomes for about 1 hour at $4°$ C with a 2 per cent aqueous solution of digitonin. Usually the rhabdomes are re-extracted until they release no further rhodopsin. The combined extract of rhodopsin is weakly acid.

For the preparation of retinochrome, some slight variations of the standard procedure are often required to suit different species. The standard method may be exemplified for the case of the squid *Todarodes*. About fifteen rhabdome-free retinas are cut in pieces, washed with M/15 phosphate buffer solution (pH 6.5) and centrifuged. The tissue fragments are then transferred to 20 ml of 0.5 per cent sodium carbonate solution for mild digestion, and centrifuged for 5 min at 8,000 r.p.m. The slightly turbid supernatant is discarded, and the residue washed with three successive portions of ion-free water, the washings being removed each time by centrifuging at 8,000 r.p.m. for 10 min. This treatment causes the tissues to swell and to release into the washings a pale brown pigment that bears no relation to retinochrome. The tissues are then hardened in 20 ml of M/5 potassium primary phosphate solution, and after a few minutes are collected by centrifuging. The compacted mass of tissue is then ground in a mortar, washed once with neutral phosphate buffer, and kept in 20 ml of Weber-Edsall's solution (0.6 M in KCl, 0.04 M in $NaHCO_3$, and 0.01 M in Na_2CO_3) at $27°$ C for 1 hour. The residue after centrifuging is washed with water, treated again with M/5 potassium primary phosphate solution for a short time, and then washed twice with ion-free water. The retinochrome is then extracted by immersing the pink residue for 1 hour at 18° C in a 2 per cent aqueous solution of digitonin. The retinochrome extract is obtained as the clear supernatant solution by centrifuging for 15 min at 15,000 r.p.m. The pH of the extract is usually between 5 and 6.

Although retinochrome can be easily extracted by digitonin from the tissues after mere digestion with sodium carbonate solution, the solution obtained is usually turbid and inferior in optical purity. To obtain good extracts it is essential to harden the tissues with acid phosphate solution. Some adjustments of the temperature and times of digestion and hardening may be found necessary with different species.

B. Discovery of Retinochrome

Retinochrome was first extracted separately from rhodopsin about six years ago, originally from the retina of the squid *Todarodes pacificus* Steenstrup, which is so plentiful in Japanese waters as to yield about 60 per cent of total landings of cephalopods in all the world (HARA and HARA, 1965). Extracts of rhodopsin and of retinochrome are too alike in colour to distinguish from each other visually. In fact, they have very similar absorbance spectra, though they differ greatly in

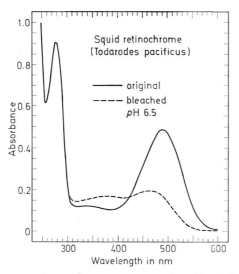

Fig. 2. The absorbance spectrum of a pure extract of squid (*Todarodes*) retinochrome in digitonin solution (pH 6.5) before and after bleaching by orange light

their photolytic behaviour. The absorbance spectrum at pH 6.5 of a pure extract of *Todarodes* retinochrome is shown in Fig. 2. The spectrum is characterized by three absorption bands. The most important of these is in the visible, with λ_{max} at about 490 nm (A-band). On the long-wave side of this maximum the absorbance falls asymptotically to zero, but on the short-wave side, after descending to a minimum around 390 nm, it rises again to form a low peak near 350 nm (B-band) in the near ultraviolet. Absorption of light in either the A- or B-bands causes bleaching. In the ultraviolet, the spectrum rises again to a sharp high maximum at about 280 nm (C-band), due mainly to the protein component of the retinochrome molecule. Although it has been observed that a marked change in absorbance occurs around 231 nm when the *rhodopsin* of the cuttlefish *Sepiella* is irradiated (SEKOGUTI, TAKAGI, and KITÔ, 1964), no such change is observed in the case of retinochrome.

C. Relations Between the Rhodopsins and Retinochromes in Different Species

Following the discovery of retinochrome in the squid *Todarodes*, further investigations with cuttlefish and octopuses showed that retinochrome is widely distributed in the Cephalopoda (HARA and HARA, 1966a; TAKEUCHI, 1966; HARA, HARA, and TAKEUCHI, 1967). The difference spectra of the rhodopsins and retinochromes of various Cephalopoda are shown in Fig. 3. The difference spectra were obtained by bleaching alkaline extracts of the pigments. Although the curves above the axis of abscissae approximate to the true absorbance spectra of the pigments, there is distortion — particularly at short wavelengths — from interference by the product band. In work on vertebrate visual pigments, hydroxylamine is frequently added to the unbleached sample, so that after irradiation all retinal

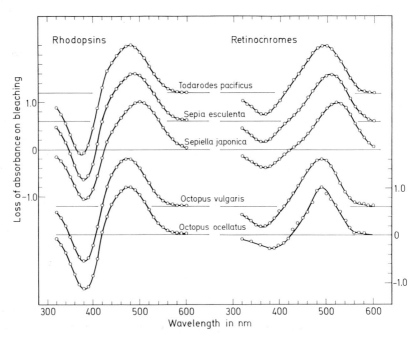

Fig. 3. The difference spectra of rhodopsins and retinochromes from five species of cephalopods; the squid *Todarodes pacificus*, the cuttlefish *Sepia esculenta* and *Sepiella japonica*, and the octopuses *Octopus vulgaris* and *Octopus ocellatus*. All spectra were measured at about pH 10, except for the retinochrome of *Octopus ocellatus* (pH 7.5). All difference spectra have been normalized to a maximum of unity. (Data from HARA and HARA, 1966a; TAKEUCHI, 1966; HARA, HARA, and TAKEUCHI, 1967)

present is converted to the oxime. This, mainly because it has a narrower absorption band than retinal, overlaps less with the A-band of the parent pigment and consequently yields a less distorted difference spectrum, with λ_{max} virtually identical with that of the visual pigment. This technique was not used, however, because retinochrome, unlike rhodopsin, is readily destroyed by hydroxylamine.

Although the retinochromes and rhodopsins have similarly-shaped absorbance spectra their difference spectra, as Fig. 3 shows, are dissimilar in certain respects. This is particularly so for those parts of the difference spectra lying below the axis of abscissae, which are determined by the spectra of the products of bleaching.

The λ_{max} of the cephalopod retinochromes obtained so far are summarized in Table 1, together with those of the corresponding cephalopod rhodopsins. The λ_{max} of the rhodopsins do not depend on pH, but the λ_{max} of the retinochromes tend to shift towards longer wavelengths with increase of pH. The λ_{max} values for the retinochromes listed in Table 1 were obtained from the difference spectra determined at about pH 10.

Table 1. *Wavelengths of maximum absorbance (λ_{max} in nm) of cephalopod rhodopsins and retinochromes*

	Squid	Cuttlefish		Octopus	
	Todarodes pacificus	*Sepia esculenta*	*Sepiella japonica*	*Octopus vulgaris*	*Octopus ocellatus*
Rhodopsin	480	486	500	475	477
Retinochrome	495	508	522	490	490

The retinochromes, like the rhodopsins, are chromoproteins that contain retinal (vitamin A_1 aldehyde) as prosthetic group, and, like the rhodopsins, have λ_{max} that varies from species to species. The λ_{max} of the retinochromes range from 490 to 522 nm and those of the cephalopod rhodopsins from 475 to 500 nm. Thus, the retinochrome λ_{max} is typically $15-20$ nm longer than that of the corresponding rhodopsin.

The retinas of all Decapoda and Octopoda that we have examined have contained this dual system of photosensitive pigments. For this reason we should expect that the squid *Loligo pealii* and the cuttlefish *Sepia officinalis* (which we have not examined) would likewise possess retinochromes of λ_{max} around 510 nm in addition to their rhodopsins of 493 and 492 nm respectively (HUBBARD and ST. GEORGE, 1958; BROWN and BROWN, 1958).

The co-existence in the retina of photopigments with different λ_{max} is sometimes indicative of colour vision, but the rhodopsin-retinochrome system of cephalopods must be associated with a quite different physiological function of the retina. Thus the retinal locations of the photopigments are such as to suggest a visual pigment function for the rhodopsin, but not for the retinochrome. Again the photochemical behaviour and molecular architecture of the two pigments are strikingly different, as will be shown below with particular reference to the squid *Todarodes pacificus*.

III. Properties of the Cephalopod Rhodopsins

A. Effects of Light on Rhodopsin and its Photoproduct (Metarhodopsin)

Cephalopod (squid) rhodopsin differs in certain respects from vertebrate rhodopsin (Hara, 1965; Hara and Hara, 1966b). Thus when exposed to light at ordinary temperature a neutral or acid extract of *Todarodes* rhodopsin ($\lambda_{max} =$ 480 nm) does not bleach; on the contrary it slightly deepens in colour. Only in alkaline solution does it lose its colour when exposed to light (Fig. 4), the λ_{max} moving from 480 nm to 378 nm because of the formation of a product — alkaline metarhodopsin, which has about one and a half times the maximum absorbance of the parent rhodopsin. If now the pH of the bleached solution is brought into the acid range in darkness, the alkaline metarhodopsin is converted to acid metarhodopsin, which has λ_{max} at 488 nm, i.e. close to that of the original rhodopsin. Thus metarhodopsin is an acid-base indicator — being red in acid or neutral, and yellow in alkaline solution. This procedure provides the only way of preparing pure acid metarhodopsin, for direct irradiation of rhodopsin in acid solution results in an equilibrium mixture of the two pigments (see broken-line curve in Fig. 4).

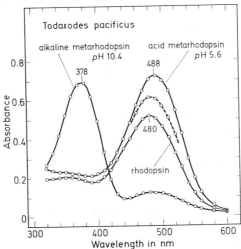

Fig. 4. The spectra of squid rhodopsin and of its alkaline and acid metarhodopsins. Irradiation of either rhodopsin or acid metarhodopsin by yellow light yields an equilibrium mixture of both (broken-line curve). (Hara, 1965)

When acid metarhodopsin ($\lambda_{max} = 488$ nm) is irradiated with yellow light, there is a fall in absorbance and a slight shift of λ_{max} to 484 nm (see broken-line curve in Fig. 4). Continued irradiation has no further effect. Almost the same position of photochemical equilibrium is reached on irradiating an acid extract of rhodopsin with the same light. The spectra of rhodopsin and acid metarhodopsin overlap extensively, and consequently the light, which is absorbed by either, results in mutual conversion. If the pH of the solution is now brought in darkness into the alkaline range, the acid metarhodopsin in the equilibrium mixture is converted to alkaline metarhodopsin to reveal the rhodopsin component. Similarly, if alkaline metarhodopsin is irradiated with near ultraviolet light photoreversal to rhodopsin occurs, the equilibrium being reached when about one half of the original rhodopsin has formed. In addition, however, an approximately equal amount of a photostable pigment with the same λ_{max} (480 nm) as rhodopsin is formed. This gradually fades in darkness — even at $0°$ C — into a photosensitive pigment that resembles alkaline metarhodopsin. Metarhodopsins that can be photoreversed to rhodopsin have their prosthetic group still attached to opsin at the original site. At temperatures near $20°$ C, however, they are slowly hydrolysed to retinal and opsin.

B. The Metarhodopsins in Different Species

Table 1 showed the properties of the rhodopsins from various cephalopods. The acid and alkaline metarhodopsins derived from these are listed in Table 2 (HARA, 1968). The λ_{max} of the acid metarhodopsins vary from species to species, each being somewhat longer than that of its rhodopsin. By irradiation with yellow light, all the acid metarhodopsins can be photoreversed to their original rhodopsins to yield an equilibrium mixture of rhodopsin and acid metarhodopsin free from any contamination by "isorhodopsin". The λ_{max} of the alkaline metarhodopsins hardly vary at all with species (TAKEUCHI, 1966). Nevertheless the irradiation of the alkaline metarhodopsins with near ultraviolet light, yields variable results: sometimes a large amount of a mixture of rhodopsin and isorhodopsin is formed (*Loligo* and *Sepia*), or of rhodopsin and a photostable pigment (*Todarodes*), and sometimes only a small amount of rhodopsin and other pigments (*Sepiella* and *Octopus*).

The dissociation of acid metarhodopsin to the alkaline form releases a hydrogen ion, probably derived from the Schiff's base linkage. The pK values at $3°$ C are also listed in Table 2. Higher temperatures tend to shift the equilibrium slightly towards alkaline metarhodopsin owing to increase of ionization. The large variation in pK (7.3 to 9.1 in different species) is noteworthy and may be of physiological significance. In particular the metarhodopsin of the squid *Todarodes* has such a high pK that the occurence of alkaline metarhodopsin in the living eye is extremely unlikely.

Table 2. *Wavelengths of maximum absorbance (λ_{max} in nm) of acid and alkaline metarhodopsins, and their pK values at $3°C$*

	Squid	Cuttlefish		Octopus	
	Todarodes pacificus	*Sepia esculenta*	*Sepiella japonica*	*Octopus vulgaris*	*Octopus ocellatus*
Acid metarhodopsin	488	495	500	503	512
Alkaline metarhodopsin	378	378	380	380	380
pK	9.1	8.0	8.2	7.4	7.3

C. Isomeric Configuration of the Prosthetic Group

Rhodopsin and metarhodopsin are capable of photochemical interconversion. This capacity is essentially due to photoisomerisation of the prosthetic group (a derivative of retinal). Retinal can exist in several *cis-trans* configurations, and isomerisation can be induced by exposure to near ultraviolet light, which retinal strongly absorbs. When, by combination of retinal with protein, a coloured chromoprotein is formed, isomerisation of the prosthetic group can be induced by visible light. In the visual pigments of vertebrates, the 11-*cis* isomer of retinal is coupled with opsins (Hubbard and Wald, 1952). The visual pigments of cephalopods are also based on 11-*cis* retinal but combined with "rhabdomal" opsins (Hubbard and St. George, 1958; Kropf and Hubbard, 1958), and are usually considered closely akin to the visual pigments of vertebrates. The 11-*cis* configuration in cephalopod rhodopsin is demonstrated by the experiment shown in Fig. 5. *Todarodes* rhodopsin in digitonin solution was bleached by warming it in a water bath at 75° C for 30 sec followed by immediate cooling in ice water. An extract of cattle opsin was then added and the spectrum of the mixture measured

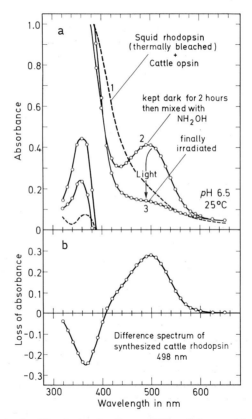

Fig. 5. The synthesis of cattle rhodopsin ($\lambda_{max} = 498$ nm) from cattle opsin (i.e. an extract of bleached retinas) and thermally-bleached squid rhodopsin (i.e. denatured opsin plus retinal in its original configuration). The synthesis shows that squid rhodopsin has an 11-*cis* prosthetic group. (Hara and Hara, 1967)

(curve 1 in Fig. 5a). The mixture was then incubated in darkness for two hours at 25° C, during which time the absorbance at 500 nm gradually rose. After addition of hydroxylamine the product of the incubation was measured (curve 2, Fig. 5a), and again after complete bleaching by light (curve 3). Fig. 5b shows the difference spectrum of the photopigment synthesised during the dark incubation. The wavelength of maximum absorbance is at 498 nm, indicating that cattle rhodopsin had been formed. Thus cattle rhodopsin is produced by the combination of cattle opsin with the retinal liberated by thermal denaturation of cephalopod rhodopsin. Since thermal denaturation does not change the configuration of the prosthetic group it follows that this is the same in *Todarodes* as in cattle rhodopsin (11-*cis*).

On irradiation of cephalopod rhodopsin, its prosthetic group is isomerised from the 11-*cis* to the all-*trans* form, thus initiating a sequence of all-*trans* intermediates in which the prosthetic group is still joined to protein. Although metarhodopsin is one of these intermediates, it is not the first, and prior intermediates are stable only at low temperatures (KROPF, BROWN, and HUBBARD, 1959). Thus the initial photolytic product is pre-lumirhodopsin which is formed immediately on the photoisomerisation of the prosthetic group, and is detectable only near the temperature of liquid air, at which any structural change in the protein is prohibited (YOSHIZAWA and WALD, 1964). At higher temperatures pre-lumirhodopsin changes thermally into lumirhodopsin and then into metarhodopsin, because of conformational changes of the protein opsin.

D. Electrical Conductance Changes on Irradiation

Exposure of the living cephalopod eye to light speedily results in the conversion of its rhodopsin to metarhodopsin. It is probable, therefore, that somewhere within this sequence of changes is the reaction that provides the visual stimulus. The intermediates prelumi-, lumi- and meta-rhodopsin are normally defined by their absorptive characteristics, and these are probably determined in the main by changes in the vicinity of the Schiff's base linkage. At the same time, however, conformational changes to the opsin are occurring that may not have a marked effect on absorptive properties. In this connection it has been found that on irradiation of cattle rhodopsin solutions there are changes in electrical conductance, the time course of which suggests that they are composed of three processes (HARA, 1958; HARA, 1963). Similar studies have since been carried out with squid rhodopsin solutions (HARA, 1965; HARA and HARA, 1966b). As shown by the examples in Fig. 6, on exposure of squid rhodopsin to yellow light there is an initial and immediate fall of conductance (process I) irrespective of the pH of the solution. At pH 6, the initial fall is followed by a rise (process II). At pH's nearer neutrality the initial fall is very slight and is succeeded by a rise to a value that is often above the original conductance level. At alkaline pH, *cattle* rhodopsin shows a slow further decrease (process III) following the initial fall. Process III is never seen in squid rhodopsin, however. Thus, the photolysis of squid rhodopsin to metarhodopsin is accompanied by only two types of conductance change, an initial fall (process I) and a subsequent rise (process II). Conversely when solutions of acid or alkaline metarhodopsin are exposed to lights that they absorb, conductance changes in the reverse sense occur in parallel with the formation of some rhodopsin

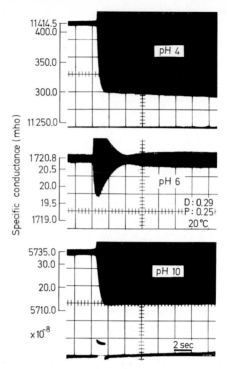

Fig. 6. Conductance changes in extracts of squid rhodopsin following irradiation with yellow light. At all pH's an initial decrease in conductance develops immediately after irradiation. D = optical density at λ_{max}; P = optical purity (Hara and Hara, 1966b)

by photoreversal. At all pH's there is an initial *rise* in conductance while a subsequent *fall* is well shown by acid metarhodopsin solutions at a slightly-acid pH. Thus in the squid rhodopsin system we can observe that the changes in electrical conductance proceed at the same speed (though in opposite directions) whether rhodopsin is converted to metarhodopsin or vice versa. The conductance changes designated 'process I' probably depend on the reversible dissociation of a hydrogen ion from the protein moiety. The initial decrease of conductance, which appears at any pH on photolysis of rhodopsin, can be interpreted as the capture of a hydrogen ion by opsin in the change rhodopsin to acid metarhodopsin, and as the liberation of a hydrogen ion in the change rhodopsin to alkaline metarhodopsin. In the photoreversal of rhodopsin from metarhodopsin these ion movements are reversed. These phenomena suggest that the changes in the protein moiety that accompany photoisomerisation of the prosthetic group have an important bearing on visual excitation. Although we are accustomed to think that visual excitation depends only on the photolysis of photopigment, there is also the possibility (in the present context) that vision may be triggered by the photoreversal of rhodopsin from its intermediate products. It is noteworthy that the conductance changes observed with the visual pigment rhodopsin, are not observed with retinochrome even though it is similarly photosensitive.

IV. Properties of the Cephalopod Retinochromes

A. The Light-sensitive and pH-sensitive Components of Retinochrome

The absorbance maximum of retinochrome prepared from the squid *Todarodes* lies at about 490 nm, i.e. 10 nm longer than the corresponding rhodopsin. This retinochrome is destroyed immediately at pH 12 and very slowly at pH 10. At pH's below 4 it is very rapidly, and irreversibly, denatured. Within the range of pH 4—10, however, retinochrome is stable. If, in the preparation of retinochrome, the tissues are hardened in 4 per cent potassium aluminium sulphate the retinochrome is mildly affected, and its λ_{max} is shifted more than 10 nm towards short wavelengths, though its photosensitivity remains.

The absorbance spectrum of retinochrome is dependent on the hydrogen ion concentration. The spectra of acid and alkaline samples are shown in Fig. 7a. When the pH of the acid extract (pH 5) is adjusted by the addition of sodium carbonate (solid, to avoid dilution of the sample) to pH 10 the absorbance falls near 490 nm, and rises near 370 nm. At the same time, the λ_{max} shifts slightly towards longer wavelengths: on changing the pH from 5 to 10, for example, it moves from 488 to 494 nm in *Todarodes pacificus*, from 490 to 506 nm in *Sepia esculenta*, from 493 to 518 nm in *Sepiella japonica*, but is virtually unaffected in the octopuses. These changes are almost completely reversible.

When exposed to light, retinochrome loses its colour — there being a fall of absorbance at λ_{max}. Fig. 7a also shows the spectra of the photoproducts formed in both acid and alkaline conditions after 5 min of irradiation with orange light (the light of a tungsten lamp (about 10,000 lux) filtered through a glass that transmits longer wavelengths than 530 nm). Although the rhodopsin of cephalopods does not lose its colour on exposure at acid pH's, the retinochrome is readily bleached at any pH, even at temperatures below 20° C, behaving in this respect rather like the rhodopsin of vertebrates. On bleaching, the rise in absorbance near 370 nm is more marked in alkaline than in acid extracts. The bleached extracts have reversible pH indicator properties.

The way in which the spectra of unbleached and bleached retinochrome extracts vary in acid and alkaline conditions (Fig. 7a) suggests that retinochrome may consist of two components, one purely light-sensitive and the other purely pH-sensitive. On this hypothesis, the light-sensitive component would be described by the difference spectrum of bleaching and, as Fig. 7b shows, this is substantially the same — λ_{max} about 495 nm — at pH 5 as at pH 10. The minor differences are attributable to the effect of pH on the photoproduct. Similarly the pH-sensitive component would be described by the difference spectrum of the acid to alkaline change. As Fig. 7c shows this is not very different whether constructed from "unbleached" or "bleached" spectra, the latter being distorted because of the effect of pH on the photoproduct of the *photosensitive* component. The difference spectrum derived from "unbleached" spectra (filled circles in Fig. 7c) indicates that the pH-sensitive component of retinochrome has λ_{max} about 480 nm in acid solution, and about 370 nm in alkaline.

This interpretation is without prejudice to the question whether the light-sensitive and pH-sensitive components are parts of the same molecule or are separate molecules. We incline to the view that the components are both present in the

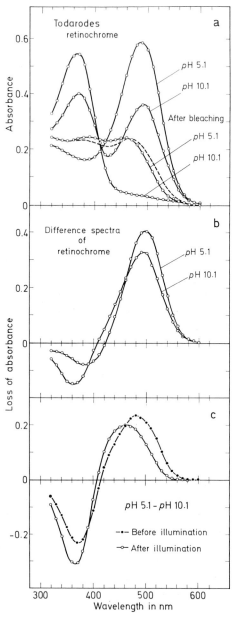

Fig. 7. The light-sensitive and pH-sensitive components of squid retinochrome (*Todarodes pacificus*). a. The spectra of retinochrome at pH 5 and pH 10 before, and after, bleaching by orange light. (Broken-line curve, acid bleached solution after further irradiation by white light). b. Difference spectra of bleaching (related to the light-sensitive component). c. Difference spectra due to pH change (related to the pH-sensitive component). (Hara and Hara, 1968)

single retinochrome molecule, for they are always found in the same ratio (about 2:1, cf. Figs. 7b and c) no matter how the extraction procedure is varied.

Heat irreversibly bleaches retinochrome but whereas cephalopod rhodopsin is thermally bleached at temperatures above 30° C, retinochrome is a little more stable, its threshold for thermal bleaching being 36° C. Retinochrome, unlike rhodopsin, is destroyed by hydroxylamine, the coupling of prosthetic group to protein being readily broken. Formaldehyde attacks the pH-sensitive part of retinochrome more readily than the light-sensitive part. Thus when retinochrome is kept in 4 per cent formalin at pH 6.5 at 15° C, little of the light-sensitive part, but most of the pH-sensitive part, is destroyed.

B. Effects of Light on Retinochrome and its Photoproduct

When an acidified extract of retinochrome that has been bleached to equilibrium by orange light is further exposed to white light (for 3 min), there is a spectral shift in absorption as shown by the broken-line curve in Fig. 7a. This suggests that white light causes a net regeneration of retinochrome. An alkaline extract of retinochrome, when treated in the same way, does not show this effect.

In general, the equilibrium spectrum obtained by exposing retinochrome (or its photoproduct) depends on the wavelength of light used. Fig. 8a shows the resulting spectra (at equilibrium) when an acid extract of retinochrome is exposed successively to near ultraviolet (360 nm) to blue (440 nm) and finally to orange light (> 560 nm). It is clear that, as the wavelength of the bleaching light is increased, the equilibrium shifts towards more net bleaching. Fig. 8b shows the results of a converse experiment: an acid extract of retinochrome that has been completely bleached by orange light (> 560 nm), when exposed exhaustively and successively first to green (500 nm), then to blue (440 nm), then to violet (410 nm) and finally to near ultraviolet (360 nm) lights, shows progressive net regeneration of retinochrome. From a comparison of Figs. 8a and b, it is clear that (in acid solution) it is immaterial whether retinochrome or its photoproduct is irradiated; the same equilibium position (for a given quality of radiation) is eventually reached. The equilibria are, of course, dynamic, i.e. they are reached when the rates of bleaching of retinochrome are just balanced by the respective rates of regeneration from photoproduct. These experiments suggest that in the photoproduct molecule the prosthetic group is still attached to protein at its original site (but has been isomerised into a different configuration). It would be difficult, otherwise, to account for the rapid establishment of equilibria with different specific qualities of radiation.

An alkaline solution of retinochrome (pH 10), on the other hand, is bleached by near ultraviolet light as well as by visible light, and no subsequent exposures can promote the reverse reaction of retinochrome regeneration. However, when an alkaline retinochrome that has been bleached by near ultraviolet light is brought to neutrality the solution immediately turns red through the formation of retinochrome. This can then be bleached normally by orange light (Fig. 8c). The unexpected failure to regenerate in alkaline solution may be due to reversible alterations to the protein surface of the photoproduct molecule under these conditions so that, although the prosthetic group may be isomerised by ultraviolet to a configuration suitable for regeneration, full coupling with protein is not possible.

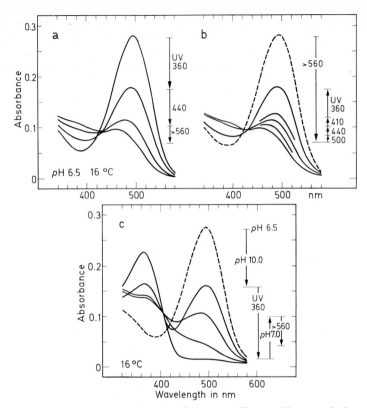

Fig. 8. Photoreversal reactions with retinochrome. a. The equilibria reached at pH 6.5 by exposure first to UV (360 nm), then blue (440 nm), then orange (> 560 nm). b. Similar equilibria reached starting with an extract largely bleached by orange light (> 560 nm) and then exposed successively to 500, 440, 410 and 360 nm. Note that the positions of equilibria are driven towards bleaching by long-wave, and towards regeneration by short-wave light. c. In alkaline solution (pH 10), however, the UV (360 nm) causes complete bleaching (see text)

C. Isomeric Configuration of the Prosthetic Group

The configuration of the prosthetic group of *Todarodes* rhodopsin was shown to be 11-*cis*, because of its capacity to yield cattle rhodopsin when mixed with cattle opsin (i.e. an extract of bleached retinas). Similar experiments have been carried out to examine the configuration of the prosthetic group in the retinochrome molecule (Hara and Hara, 1967). Thus retinochrome was thermally denatured by keeping it at 75° C for 30 sec, chilled immediately in ice, and then incubated in the dark with cattle opsin at 25° C. But, even after some hours, no photopigment was formed. This shows that retinochrome differs from rhodopsin in the configuration of its prosthetic group. However, the mixture of heat-denatured retinochrome and cattle opsin does begin to form cattle rhodopsin in the dark, if first exposed for a few minutes to white light. Since cattle opsin itself yields very little rhodopsin when further irradiated in this way, it seems probable that it is principally the retinal thermally released from retinochrome that is isomerised by further exposure into the 11-*cis* configuration. This is confirmed by the fact if, instead of irradiating the mixture, the heat-denatured retinochrome is irradiated alone before addition to the cattle opsin, then rhodopsin is progressively formed. Even after the heat-denatured retinochrome has been stored for many hours in

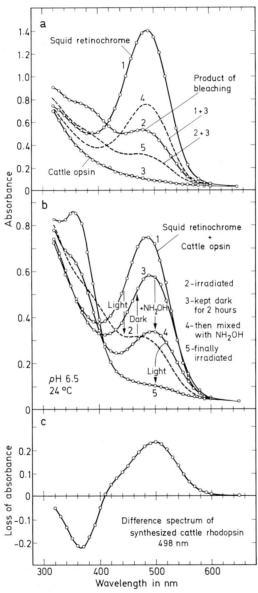

Fig. 9. A mixture of retinochrome and cattle opsin, after irradiation, will form cattle rhodopsin. a. Absorption data for materials used. b. The experiment, for details of which, see text. Curves 1 and 2 ≡ curves 4 and 5 respectively in a. c. Difference spectrum of the synthesised cattle rhodopsin. The experiment shows that 11-*cis* retinal is produced when retinochrome is bleached. (HARA and HARA, 1967)

darkness it retains its capacity (after irradiation) to form rhodopsin with cattle opsin.

These experiments raised the question whether a mixture of squid retinochrome and cattle opsin would form cattle rhodopsin in the dark, after the retinochrome component had been quickly bleached by irradiation. The results of such an experiment are shown in Fig. 9. Fig. 9a gives the absorption data of the materials used. Thus curve 1 is the spectrum of a retinochrome extract at pH 6.5; curve 2, the same after bleaching for 3 min with yellow light; and curve 3, the spectrum of cattle opsin. (Curves 4 and 5 are the sums of curves 1 and 3, and 2 and 3 respectively). In the experiment (Fig. 9b) equal volumes of unbleached retinochrome and cattle opsin were mixed (spectrum 1 ≡ spectrum 4 in Fig. 9a) and then exposed to the yellow light for 3 min (spectrum 2 ≡ spectrum 5 in Fig. 9a). During incubation of this mixture in the dark at 24° C, the absorbance at 500 nm gradually increased exponentially until spectrum 3 was reached after 2 hours. On adding hydroxylamine to block further synthesis and to destroy the remaining fraction of retinochrome, the spectrum changed from 3 to 4 (after correction for the dilution by hydroxylamine). Finally the synthesised pigment was bleached by light (spectrum 5). The difference spectrum for the bleaching is shown in Fig. 9c. It has λ_{max} at 498 nm, and is identical with that for cattle rhodopsin. It is thus clear that on irradiation the prosthetic retinal of retinochrome is changed by light from its original configuration (which is thus not 11-*cis*) into the 11-*cis* form required for rhodopsin synthesis.

Rhodopsin is stable to hydroxylamine, and retinaldehyde oxime is not formed after bleaching until the retinal has been released by hydrolysis of the metarhodopsin. In contrast retinochrome is readily destroyed by low concentrations of hydroxylamine, and retinaldehyde oxime is at once produced. Thus in the retinochrome molecule, the prosthetic retinal seems bound to the protein less

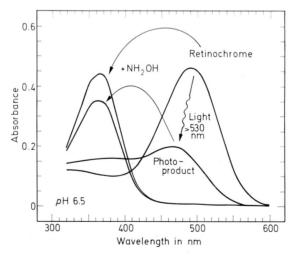

Fig. 10. Comparison between the retinaldehyde oximes formed from retinochrome and from its photoproduct. Note that the "retinochrome oxime" has higher absorbance and λ_{max} than the "photoproduct oxime", suggesting that the former is all-*trans*. (After Hara and Hara, 1967)

tightly than in the rhodopsin molecule. The retinaldehyde oximes formed from non-illuminated and illuminated retinochrome are compared in Fig. 10. The absorbance maximum of retinaldehyde oxime derived from unbleached retinochrome is near 367 nm, while that from bleached retinochrome is shifted towards 360 nm, and is somewhat lower. This suggests that the chromophore in unbleached retinochrome is in the all-*trans* configuration (cf. HUBBARD, 1956a). The spectrum of retinaldehyde oxime derived from heat-denatured retinochrome agrees with that derived from native retinochrome, thus indicating that the original configuration is retained after thermal denaturation.

D. Regeneration of Retinochrome

When a retinochrome extract is divided into two equal portions, one being bleached by orange light for 5 min, and the other by warming at 75° C for 30 sec, and the two portions are then mixed together, progressive regeneration of retinochrome occurs in the mixture when it is kept in the dark at room temperature. In this way, the regeneration of retinochrome can be studied at various acidities, the amount of regeneration being determined by the change in density at 490 nm (ΔD) on exposure to light. Fig. 11 shows that regeneration can occur within the

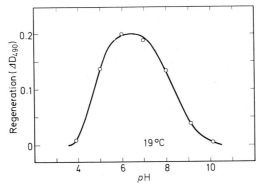

Fig. 11. Influence of pH on the regeneration of squid retinochrome. When aliquots of retinochrome, one bleached by light (i.e. inactive retinal + active protein) and the other by heat (i.e. active retinal + denatured protein) are mixed at different pH's, regeneration occurs in darkness. The ordinates ΔD are the changes in density at 490 nm on bleaching the fully-regenerated mixtures. (HARA and HARA, 1968)

range of pH 4 to 10, the optimum condition being pH 6—7, when there is almost 100 per cent recovery. Below pH 4 little or no regeneration is seen, for the retinochrome is irreversibly broken down. At pH 10 there is likewise little regeneration, but, if the pH of the mixture is brought back towards neutrality considerable regeneration then occurs.

Evidence for believing that the prosthetic group of retinochrome is all-*trans* is provided by direct coupling experiments between all-*trans* retinal and light-bleached retinochrome. The all-*trans* retinal was prepared from all-*trans* retinol (vitamin A₁) by oxidation with active mangenese dioxide, and was crystal-

lised several times. It was then dissolved in an aqueous digitonin solution and
added to an extract of retinochrome (pH 6.5) that had been bleached by exposure
to orange light for 5 min (Fig. 12a). During incubation of this mixture in the dark
(Fig. 12b and c) formation of a photosensitive pigment occurred. After 20 min
the changes were complete, and the mixture was then bleached by the same orange
light to yield a difference spectrum (Fig. 12d) identical in shape with that of the
original retinochrome.

In this experiment it is important to avoid an excess of the all-*trans* retinal for
otherwise, after the final bleaching of the synthesised retinochrome (curve 6,
Fig. 12b), the protein moiety will continue to react with the excess all-*trans* retinal.

The synthesis is extremely fast, being half completed within 30 sec at 19° C
(Fig. 12c). Moreover this is synthesis from all-*trans* retinal and retinochrome
protein that still retains its altered prosthetic group (11-*cis*). If completely free
protein could be used the synthesis would, no doubt, be even faster. In contrast
the synthesis of cattle rhodopsin from cattle opsin and 11-*cis* retinal is only about
one thirtieth as fast (half time of 15 min). Thus retinochrome is very readily
regenerated in the dark near neutrality, when its native protein moiety meets

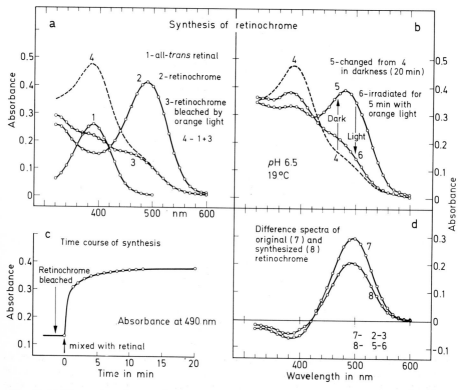

Fig. 12. Evidence that the prosthetic group of retinochrome is in the all-*trans* configuration.
a and b. The synthesis of squid retinochrome from all-*trans* retinal and bleached retinochrome
(i.e., active protein + inactive retinal). c. Note the rapidity of the synthesis. d. Comparison
of synthesised and native retinochrome. (Hara and Hara, 1968)

all-*trans* retinal (HARA and HARA, 1968). This is also the case in the living retina. When a rhabdome-free retina is bleached by light and is then immersed in a solution of all-*trans* retinal in the dark, its surface gradually turns red again.

E. Retinochrome as a Catalyst for Converting all-*trans* Retinal to 11-*cis*

When retinochrome is exposed to light its prosthetic group is changed from the all-*trans* to the 11-*cis* form. If all-*trans* retinal is now added, very rapid regeneration of retinochrome occurs, and this when bleached gives rise to more 11-*cis* retinal and leaves the bleached retinochrome capable of combining with

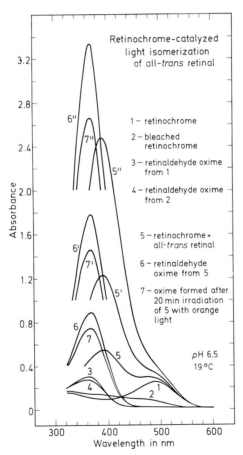

Fig. 13. Irradiated retinochrome as a catalyst for converting all-*trans* retinal to 11-*cis*. Equal portions of a retinochrome extract (curve 1) were mixed with all-*trans* retinal of various concentrations (curves 5, 5' and 5''). When hydroxylamine was added to aliquots of these the all-*trans* oxime was formed (curves 6, 6' and 6''). Other aliquots were then irradiated with orange light (not absorbed by retinal) before adding hydroxylamine (curves 7, 7' and 7''). Note the lower absorbances of the curves 7 compared with those of the curves 6, because of almost complete conversion of all-*trans* retinal to 11-*cis*. (HARA and HARA, 1968)

further all-*trans* retinal, and so on. This suggests that retinochrome, when steadily illuminated, would be able to convert any quantity of all-*trans* retinal into 11-*cis*, i.e. to act as a catalyst.

That this is so is shown by experiments illustrated in Fig. 13. Equal portions of a retinochrome extract (curve 1 in Fig. 13) were mixed with all-*trans* retinal of various concentrations (curves 5, 5′ and 5″). When hydroxylamine was added to aliquots of these the all-*trans* oxime was formed (curves 6, 6′ and 6″). Other aliquots were then irradiated with orange light for 20 min before adding hydroxylamine (curves 7, 7′ and 7″). The lower absorbances in these cases were due to almost complete conversion to the 11-*cis* form (cf. p 739 and Fig. 10). Since retinal does not appreciably absorb orange light the conversion must have proceeded via retinochrome, viz bleaching of retinochrome to yield 11-*cis*, regeneration from excess all-*trans*, followed by bleaching as before, and so on until the excess all-*trans* retinal was expended.

The action of irradiated retinochrome in catalysing the conversion of all-*trans* retinal specifically to 11-*cis* is illustrated in Fig. 14 (Hara and Hara, 1968). A solution of all-*trans* retinal was divided into two equal parts: a trace of retinochrome was added to one (curve 1 in Fig. 14), and an equal volume of water to the other (curve 1′). The former mixture was irradiated with orange light (absorbed by retinochrome alone) until no further changes occurred, and the latter with white light

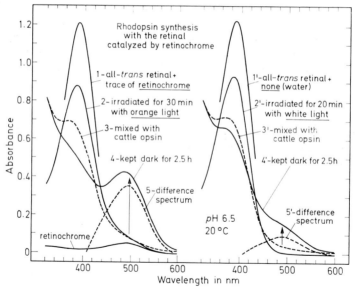

Fig. 14. The synthesis of cattle rhodopsin from cattle opsin and all-trans retinal using a trace of retinochrome to catalyse the conversion of all-*trans* to 11-*cis*. On the left: curve 1, all-*trans* retinal + a trace of retinochrome. Curve 2, after irradiation with orange light (absorbed by retinochrome but not by retinal). Curve 3, after adding cattle opsin. Curve 4, after 2½ hours incubation. Note the large amount of (pure) cattle rhodopsin formed. On the right: curve 1′, all-*trans* retinal alone. Curve 2′, after irradiation with white light (containing short-wave components absorbed by retinal). Curve 3′, after adding cattle opsin. Curve 4′, after 2½ hours incubation. Note the small amount of photosensitive material formed, which is a mixture of cattle rhodopsin and isorhodopsin. (Hara and Hara, 1968)

(containing near ultraviolet light that is directly absorbed by retinal). The absorbance fell almost equally in both solutions due to the isomerisation of retinal (curves 2 and 2'). To each solution was then added an equal volume of cattle opsin (curves 3 and 3'). After incubation in the dark for 2.5 hours at 20° C, curves 4 and 4' were obtained. In both cases the retinal was present in excess so the syntheses were limited by the concentration of opsin. It is clear that curve 4 shows a much higher absorbance around 500 nm than curve 4', indicating that a larger amount of photopigment was synthesised. The difference spectra of the photopigments were obtained by bleaching in the presence of hydroxylamine (curves 5 and 5'). Curve 5, from the solution that contained a trace of retinochrome, has λ_{max} at 497 nm and is indistinguishable from that for cattle rhodopsin, thus showing that only the 11-*cis* isomer of retinal had been produced. Curve 5', however, has λ_{max} near 490 nm and is due to a mixture of rhodopsin and isorhodopsin (9-*cis*). Curve 2 in Fig. 14 must, therefore, be due almost entirely to 11-*cis* retinal, while curve 2' — as one would expect from the ultraviolet irradiation of all-*trans* retinal — represents a mixture of 11-*cis* and 9-*cis*, together with other isomers that do not combine with cattle opsin.

V. The Physiological Function of Retinochrome — an Hypothesis

Although most of the work described here was carried out on the squid *Todarodes*, similar findings have been reported for the cuttlefish, *Sepiella japonica* Sasaki (HARA, 1968; FUJISEKI, 1968), and we believe that the results are applicable to cephalopods in general. These results may be summarised as follows. When cephalopod rhodopsin is converted to metarhodopsin by exposure to light the prosthetic configuration changes from 11-*cis* to all-*trans*. When retinochrome is bleached by light the prosthetic group is changed in the opposite sense, viz. from all-*trans* to 11-*cis*. This suggests that the two pigments could provide a system in which each, when photolysed, assists in the regeneration of the other. Such a system is outlined in the following scheme in which straight lines represent thermal reactions and wavy lines photochemical ones.

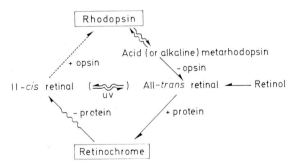

In vertebrate eyes, the isomerisation necessary for the regeneration of visual pigments is in part promoted by the action of "retinal isomerase". This was examined more than ten years ago (HUBBARD, 1956b) and was shown to be an enzyme that, in light, catalysed the conversion of all-*trans* retinal to 11-*cis*. Similarly, in the cephalopod eye we may regard both the rhodopsin and the retinochrome — or more specifically their protein moieties — as enzymatic catalysts or isomerases that are actived by visible light.

It is easy to prepare extracts of cephalopod rhodopsin uncontaminated by metarhodopsin, even when no particular attention is paid to dark adapting the animals prior to killing them. This suggests that the cephalopod retina is provided with a mechanism that quickly converts any metarhodopsin back to rhodopsin. Since this mechanism cannot be photoreversal, which would in any case yield an equilibrium mixture, it seems likely that such regeneration occurs by the coupling of 11-*cis* retinal derived from bleached retinochrome with rhabdomal opsin. However, attempts to carry out this synthesis *in vitro* have had only a limited success, though, as we have seen, there is no difficulty when vertebrate opsin is used (Fig. 14). An attempt to carry out such a synthesis with rhabdomal opsin is illustrated in Fig. 15. Pure acid metarhodopsin was prepared by bleaching an alkaline extract of cephalopod rhodopsin with orange light, and then adjusting the pH to 6.6. An extract of retinochrome was also prepared and bleached by the same orange light. The two

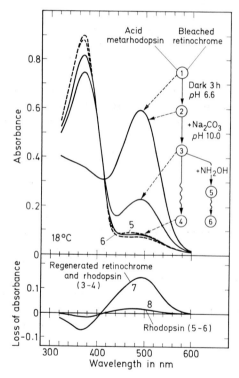

Fig. 15. Attempted synthesis of cephalopod rhodopsin from rhabdomal opsin and bleached retinochrome. Curve 1, a mixture of acid cephalopod metarhodopsin (pH 6.6) and bleached retinochrome. Curve 2, after 3 hours incubation (no apparent change). Curve 3, after bringing the mixture to pH 10. Curve 4, after bleaching one half by orange light. Curve 5, after adding hydroxylamine to the other half to remove retinochrome as oxime. The large fall in absorbance shows that the major part of the regenerated photopigment was retinochrome. Curve 6, after bleaching, showing the small amount of regenerated cephalopod rhodopsin

extracts were mixed and had the spectrum shown as curve 1 in Fig. 15. After a 3-hour incubation in darkness at 18° C the spectrum remained apparently unaltered though, as will appear, changes had taken place. The pH of the mixture was then brought to 10 so that unreacted metarhodopsin and bleached retinochrome were converted to their alkaline forms (curve 3). The mixture was then divided into two parts. One was bleached by orange light (curve 4). The difference spectrum of the change is shown as curve 7, which has λ_{max} near 495 nm. To the other part was added hydroxylamine to remove retinochrome as retinal oxime. The large fall in absorbance (curve 5) shows that the major part of the regenerated photopigment was retinochrome. Nevertheless on exposure to light a small amount of bleaching occurred (curve 6). The difference spectrum for this change (curve 8) had λ_{max} at 480 nm, and was probably due to regenerated cephalopod rhodopsin. This unexpectedly small amount of cephalopod rhodopsin synthesised is not easy to explain. Certainly sufficient 11-*cis* retinal was present from the bleached retinochrome. It is possible that rhabdomal opsin is unstable *in vitro* and becomes denatured more rapidly than does vertebrate opsin.

When cephalopod rhodopsin is irradiated under acid conditions an equilibrium between rhodopsin and acid metarhodopsin is set up (Fig. 4). In this way a preparation containing metarhodopsin that has not passed through the alkaline form can be obtained. If now this is incubated with bleached retinochrome only a trace of retinochrome is regenerated. This suggests that different forms of acid metarhodopsin can exist that can not be distinguished by their absorptive properties but only by their capacities to react with bleached retinochromes. In spite of these difficulties it may be conceded that regeneration of cephalopod rhodopsin via the 11-*cis* retinal derived from bleached retinochrome has been demonstrated *in vitro*, albeit in disappointingly small amount (Fig. 15). Even so there are still problems to be solved before the existence of such a mechanism in the living eye can be proved.

In the first place the location of the retinochrome in tissues that lie behind the rhodopsin-containing rhabdomes and the black pigment layer (Fig. 1) means that little light (necessary for retinochrome to bleach and thus fulfil its hypothetical function) can reach it through the lens of the eye. Nevertheless the amount of retinochrome *in situ* does vary with the level of illumination, and it is possible that light reaches it diffusely through the eyeball. Alternatively, although most of the retinochrome is located in the myeloid bodies some may diffuse forward together with migrating pigment granules. Finally, since the rhodopsin is located in the microvilli of the rhabdomeres, transport of 11-*cis* retinal to this site to regenerate visual pigment and of all-trans retinal from it to regenerate retinochrome is necessary. Nothing, as yet, is known about this.

Acknowledgment

We are greatly indebted to Prof. H. J. A. DARTNALL for his help in the preparation of this chapter.

References

BROWN, P. K., BROWN, P. S.: Visual pigments of the octopus and cuttlefish. Nature (Lond.) **182**, 1288—1290 (1958).

Duke-Elder, S.: System of ophthalmology. Vol. 1, The eye in evolution. London: Henry Kimpton 1958.

Fujiseki, Y.: Studies on rhodopsin and retinochrome in the cuttlefish retina. J. Nara Med. Ass. 19, 161—173 (1968).

Hara, R.: Changes in electrical conductance of rhodopsin on photolysis. J. gen. Physiol. 47, 241—264 (1963).

Hara, T.: The effect of illumination on the electrical conductance of rhodopsin solutions. J. gen. Physiol. 41, 857—877 (1958).

— Vision and rhodopsin. In: Molecular basis of Biological Functions (Biophysics, Vol. 6). Kyoto: Yoshioka 1965.

— Photosensitive pigments in the cephalopod retina. Zool. Mag. (Tokyo) 77, 99—108 (1968).

— Hara, R.: New photosensitive pigment found in the retina of the squid Ommastrephes. Nature (Lond.) 206, 1331—1334 (1965).

— — Photosensitive pigments found in cephalopod retinas. Zool. Mag. (Tokyo) 75, 264—269 (1966a).

— — Electrical conductance of rhodopsin solutions. Jap. J. Ophthal. 10, Suppl. 22—28 (1966b).

— — Rhodopsin and retinochrome in the squid retina. Nature (Lond.) 214, 573—575 (1967).

— — Regeneration of squid retinochrome. Nature (Lond.) 219, 450—454 (1968).

— — Takeuchi, J.: Rhodopsin and retinochrome in the octopus retina. Nature (Lond.) 214, 572—573 (1967).

Hubbard, R.: Geometrical isomerization of vitamin A, retinene and retinene oxime. J. Amer. chem. Soc. 78, 4662—4667 (1956a).

— Retinene isomerase. J. gen. Physiol. 39, 935—962 (1956b).

— St. George, R. C. C.: The rhodopsin system of the squid. J. gen. Physiol. 41, 501—528 (1958).

— Wald, G.: Cis-trans isomers of vitamin A and retinene in the rhodopsin system. J. gen. Physiol. 36, 269—315 (1952).

Kropf, A., Brown, P. K., Hubbard, R.: Lumi- and meta-rhodopsins of squid and octopus. Nature (Lond.) 183, 446—448 (1959).

— Hubbard, R.: The mechanism of bleaching rhodopsin. Ann. N.Y. Acad. Sci. 74, 266—280 (1958).

Moody, M. F., Robertson, J. D.: The fine structure of some retinal photoreceptors. J. biophys. biochem. Cytol. 7, 87—91 (1960).

Sekoguti, Y., Takagi, M., Kitô, Y.: The reversible transconformation of rhodopsin. Ann. Rep. sci. Works, Fac. Sci. Osaka Univ. 12, 67—81 (1964).

Takeuchi, J.: Photosensitive pigments in the cephalopod retinas. J. Nara Med. Ass. 17, 433—448 (1966).

Tasaki, K., Karita, K.: Discrimination of horizontal and vertical planes of polarized light by the cephalopod retina. Jap. J. Physiol. 16, 205—216 (1966).

Tonosaki, A.: The fine structure of the retinal plexus in Octopus vulgaris. Z. Zellforsch. 67, 521—532 (1965).

Wolken, J. J.: Retinal structure. Mollusc cephalopods: Octopus, Sepia. J. biophys. biochem. Cytol. 4, 835—838 (1958).

Yamamoto, T., Tasaki, K., Sugawara, Y., Tonosaki, A.: Fine structure of the octopus retina. J. Cell Biol. 25, 345—360 (1965).

Yoshizawa, T., Wald, G.: Transformations of squid rhodopsin at low temperatures. Nature (Lond.) 201, 340—345 (1964).

Young, J. Z.: Regularities in the retina and optic lobes of octopus in relation to form discrimination. Nature (Lond.) 186, 836—839 (1960).

Zonana, H. V.: Fine structure of the squid retina. Bull. Johns Hopk. Hosp. 109, 185—205 (1961).

Author Index

Page numbers in *italics* refer to the bibliography

Subject Index

Compiled by

PRISCILLA H. SILVER, Falmer, Brighton (Great Britain)

798 Subject Index

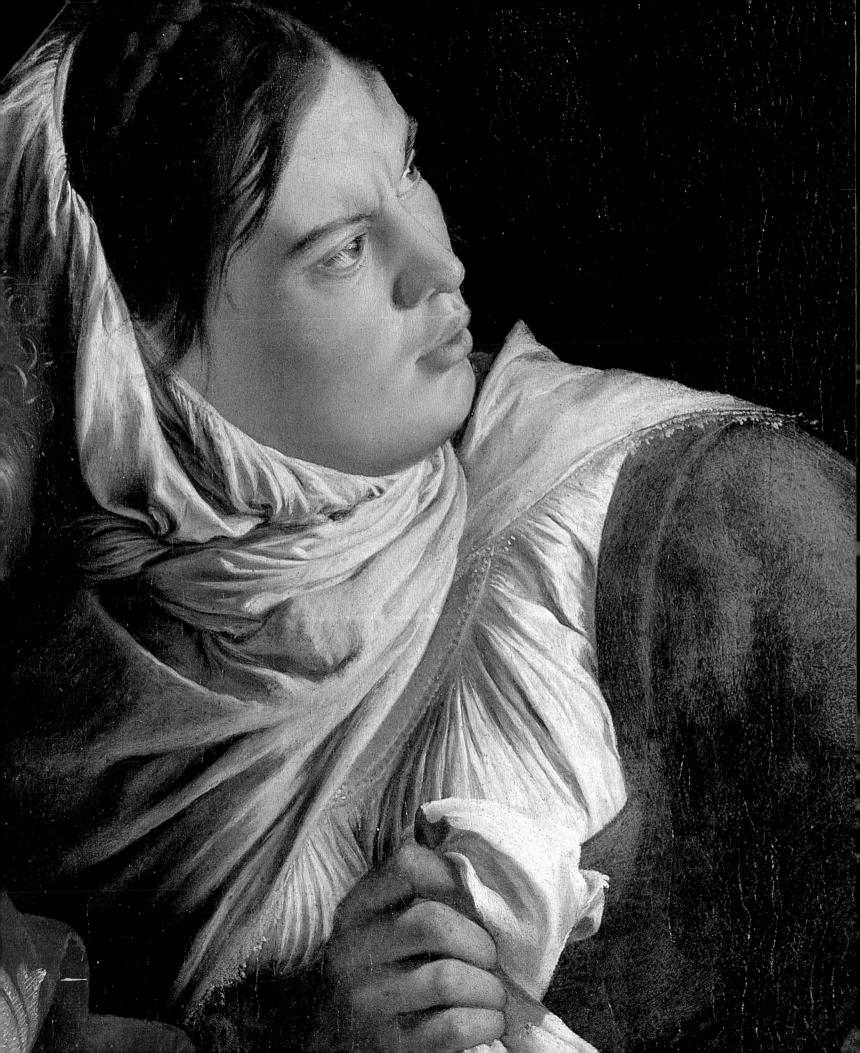

ORAZIO AND ARTEMISIA GENTILESCHI

KEITH CHRISTIANSEN

JUDITH W. MANN

The Metropolitan Museum of Art, New York

Yale University Press, New Haven and London

This catalogue is published in conjunction with the exhibition "Orazio and Artemisia Gentileschi: Father and Daughter Painters in Baroque Italy," held at the Museo del Palazzo di Venezia, Rome, October 15, 2001–January 6, 2002; The Metropolitan Museum of Art, New York, February 14–May 12, 2002; The Saint Louis Art Museum, June 15–September 15, 2002.

This project is supported in part by grants from the National Endowment for the Arts.

In New York, the exhibition is made possible in part by the Gail and Parker Gilbert Fund.

The exhibition has been organized by the Soprintendenza per il Patrimonio Storico Artistico e Demoetnoantropologico di Roma, The Metropolitan Museum of Art, New York, and The Saint Louis Art Museum.

In New York, the exhibition catalogue is made possible by the Doris Duke Fund for Publications.

Published by The Metropolitan Museum of Art, New York

John P. O'Neill, Editor in Chief
Emily Walter, Editor, with the assistance of Jane Bobko
Bruce Campbell, Designer
Gwen Roginsky and Sally VanDevanter, Production
Robert Weisberg, Desktop Publishing
Jean Wagner, Research and Bibliographic Editor

Translations, from the Italian, of the essays by Roberto Contini, Riccardo Lattuada, and Alessandro Zuccari and catalogue entries 11 and 14: A. Lawrence Jenkins; the essay by Livia Carloni, from the Italian, by Erikson Translations; the essay by Jean-Pierre Cuzin, from the French, by Jane Marie Todd.

Set in Dante and Centaur
Printed on 130 gsm R-400
Color separations by Professional Graphics Inc., Rockville, Illinois
Printed and bound by Europrint SNC, Treviso, Italy

Jacket/cover illustration: Orazio Gentileschi (1563–1639). Detail of *Lute Player* (cat. 22)

Back cover illustration: Artemisia Gentileschi (1593–1652/3). Detail of *Susanna and the Elders* (cat. 51)

Frontispiece: Orazio Gentileschi. Detail of *Judith and Her Maidservant with the Head of Holofernes* (cat. 39)

Library of Congress Cataloging-in-Publication Data

Christiansen, Keith.
    Orazio and Artemisia Gentileschi/Keith Christiansen, Judith W. Mann et. al.
        p. cm.
    Catalog of an exhibition held at the Museo del Palazzo di Venezia, Rome, Oct. 15, 2001–Jan. 6, 2002, the Metropolitan Museum of Art, New York, Feb. 14–May 12, 2002, and the Saint Louis Art Museum, June 15–Sept. 15, 2002.
    Includes bibliographical references and index
    ISBN 1-58839-006-3 (hc.:alk. paper)—ISBN 1-58839-007-1 (pbk.:alk. paper)—ISBN 0-300-09077-3 (Yale University Press)
    1. Gentileschi, Orazio, 1563–1639—Exhibitions. 2. Gentileschi, Artemisia, 1593–1652/3—Exhibitions. I. Mann, Judith Walker. II. Gentileschi, Orazio, 1563–1639. III. Gentileschi, Artemisia, 1593–1652/3. IV. Museo di Palazzo Venezia (Rome, Italy). V. Metropolitan Museum of Art (New York, N.Y.). VI. St. Louis Art Museum. VII. Title.

ND623.G36 A4 2001
759.5'09'032074—dc21

                                                                    2001044343

Contents

II. Artemisia Gentileschi (1593–1652/3)

CATALOGUE
Catalogue entries are by Judith W. Mann

DOCUMENTARY APPENDICES

Foreword

Work on this project began in earnest three years ago, when, following the initiative of Judith Mann at The Saint Louis Art Museum, The Metropolitan Museum of Art and the Soprintendenza per il Patrimonio Storico Artistico e Demoetnoantropologico di Roma agreed to collaborate on an ambitious, three-venue exhibition devoted to the work of Orazio and Artemisia Gentileschi, father and daughter. Fascinating figures in their own right, when looked at together these two related but strikingly individual artists define many issues posed by the revolution in painting brought about in early-seventeenth-century Rome by Caravaggio. Orazio was arguably the most singular and inspired of those artists who knew and were directly influenced by the Lombard master (most Caravaggesque artists came to his work indirectly, through the example of Bartolomeo Manfredi), while Artemisia used a Caravaggesque idiom to become the greatest female painter of the century. Surprisingly, Orazio has never been the subject of a monographic exhibition, while the exhibition devoted to Artemisia, held in Florence in 1991, was limited in scope.

Today, much scholarly and popular attention has tended to focus on Artemisia. However, in the seventeenth century Orazio's fame eclipsed that of his daughter, and in the first half of the twentieth century—in the flush of scholarly interest in Caravaggio and his followers—he seemed well on the way to the sort of popularity now enjoyed by Georges de La Tour. In such exhibitions as "The Age of Caravaggio," mounted in New York and Naples in 1985, or the recent "Genius of Rome," in London and Rome, Orazio's pictures stood out for their striking blend of Caravaggesque realism and Raphaelesque classicism—of physical immediacy and abstraction. Of course, Orazio's example was the determining factor in Artemisia's training and has been thought a key element in the art of such non-Italian masters as Hendrick ter Brugghen and even Vermeer. He worked at the courts of Marie de' Medici in Paris and of Charles I in London, and, as Jean-Pierre Cuzin points out in this catalogue, his contribution to French painting was substantial. To those unfamiliar with Orazio's work, the exhibition will be a revelation; his brilliant use of color and his compact, carefully constructed compositions—curiously devoid of the dramatic urgency that lies at the core of Artemisia's paintings—are unforgettable. He is a poet of light—nowhere more so than in the sublime *Annunciation*, in the Galleria Sabauda, Turin (cat. 43)—and on this count alone is a central figure in the history of seventeenth-century painting. Thanks to a number of exceptional loans—among which, mention should be made of the altarpieces from Ancona, Fabriano, Farnese, Rome, Turin, Milan, and Urbino, and the large canvases from Paris and London—it has been possible to present through Orazio's finest paintings a panorama of his career.

Fueled by feminist studies, interest in Artemisia's art has increased enormously over the last quarter of a century: here is a strong female voice in an almost exclusively male chorus. Rejecting the genres of portraiture and still life—the arena deemed suitable to women artists—Artemisia sought to compete (and sometimes collaborate) with her male colleagues, undertaking mythological, allegorical, and biblical themes. Far from shying from violent, erotically charged subjects, she made them the focus of her activity, giving prominence to stories involving a female protagonist-victim. (In this, her work has often been interpreted as an extension of her own biography.) At a time when marriage and the convent were the only respectable alternatives held out to a woman in a Catholic society, Artemisia chose to live by her brush. The audacity of that choice and its implications for the interpretation of her pictures by twenty-first-century viewers are explored by Elizabeth Cropper, in her provocative contribution to this catalogue. Here, it should be stated that despite the groundbreaking monograph by Mary Garrard in 1989 and the recent, indispensable catalogue raisonée by R. Ward Bissell, we are still far from a coherent view of Artemisia's career. There remain basic issues of attribution and dating, and these are best dealt with in the context of a full-scale, monographic exhibition, where pictures can be compared directly. Indeed, it is difficult to imagine a case in which an exhibition could contribute more fruitfully to shaping our views of an artist. The fact that the authorship of a picture of the quality of the *Cleopatra* (cat. nos. 17, 53) is still the subject of debate—it is catalogued here under both Orazio and Artemisia—testifies to the problems that attend the study of her paintings.

Every effort has been made to give the fullest possible representation of Artemisia's work and to deal with some of the thorny problems that beset an understanding of her career. Unfortunately, many of the canvases she painted in Naples are in poor condition, and what are arguably her finest late masterpieces—two splendid canvases in Potsdam—are attached to a wall of the grand gallery of the Neues Palais and thus could not be lent. Despite the presence of the Brno *Susanna and the Elders* (cat. 83), it has proved impossible to do full justice to Artemisia's still undervalued late works. However, as Judith Mann emphasizes in her introductory essay, our understanding of this exceptional artist is still a work in progress and the cumulative effect of this, the most comprehensive display of her work ever assembled, will, we trust, play a vital role in that endeavor.

Doubtless, the experience of seeing the work of father and daughter together will be an enriching one, encouraging a deeper, more subtly shaded appreciation of the very different achievements of each. Our ability to do this is, of course, directly dependent on the generosity of the lenders, to whom we would like to express our profound thanks. We would especially like to note Fernando Cecha, Director of the Museo Nacional del Prado, Madrid; Karl Schütz, Director of the Kunsthistorisches Museum, Vienna; Jan Kelch, Director of the Gemäldegalerie, Berlin; Nicola Spinosa, Soprintendente per i Beni Artistici e Storici in Naples;

Annamaria Petrioli Tofani, Director of the Galleria degli Uffizi, Florence; Serena Padovani, Director of the Galleria Palatina, Florence; Maria Lucrezia Vicini, Director of the Galleria Spada, Rome; Graham W. J. Beal, Director of the Detroit Institute of Arts; Earl A. Powell III, Director of the National Gallery of Art, Washington, D.C.; and Lady Victoria Leatham for agreeing to deprive their collections of two or more works in the interest of furthering our understanding of these artists.

The exhibition was organized by Judith W. Mann, at the Saint Louis Art Museum, Keith Christiansen, at the Metropolitan Museum, and Rossella Vodret, of the Soprintendenza in Rome. They have carried out their tasks with dedication and professionalism and our gratitude to them is great.

This project is supported in part by grants from the National Endowment for the Arts. The Metropolitan Museum gratefully acknowledges the Gail and Parker Gilbert Fund for its generosity toward the exhibition in New York. Our sincere thanks go also to the Doris Duke Fund for Publications for making the exhibition catalogue possible.

Philippe de Montebello
Director
The Metropolitan Museum of Art

Brent Benjamin
Director
The Saint Louis Art Museum

Claudio Strinati
Soprintendente per il Patrimonio Storico Artistico e
Demoetnoantropologico di Roma

Acknowledgments

This catalogue and exhibition would not have been possible without the assistance of numerous friends and colleagues. Special mention should be made of Erich Schleier, to whom we turned again and again for advice and guidance and who acted, in effect, as an unofficial member of the organizing committee. R. Ward Bissell and Mary Garrard—the two leading scholars on Orazio and Artemisia Gentileschi—were no less generous with their counsel and help. Together with Rossella Vodret, Roberta Rinaldi has played an indispensable role in negotiating Italian loans. Richard Spear generously read most of the catalogue and offered invaluable advice.

Keith Christiansen would like, in particular, to thank Andrea Bayer, Patrizia Cavazzini, Gabriele Finaldi, and David Stone, who kindly read his entries and offered their comments. Mary Newcome was his vade mecum in Genoa, while Livia Carloni acted as his mentor in all things Marchigian. He would also like to acknowledge the contribution of the students in a seminar he taught at the Institute of Fine Arts. During the last three years his research was greatly facilitated by the assistance of three young scholars: Laura Zirulnik, Emilie Beck, and Marcello Toffanello.

Judith Mann would like especially to note the contributions of the late Stephen Pepper and to acknowledge the critical support provided by James D. Burke, former director of the Saint Louis Art Museum. She also wishes to express her appreciation for the help of Alexandra Lapierre. She has benefited from fine student assistants: Doug Allebach, Angela Wilcoxson, Heather Maes, Diane Linsin, C. D. Dickerson, Deborah Ruiz, and Susanna Burke. Mary Beth Carosello warrants special thanks for her organizational skills and unflagging ingenuity.

Among the many others to whom we have incurred debts of one kind or another, we would like particularly to acknowledge: Alfred Ackerman, Annette Ahrens, Sivigliano Alloisi, Placido Arango, Luis Arenas, Irina Artemieva, Paola Astrua, Joseph Baillio, Irene Baldriga, Gerd Bartoschek, Alexander Bell, Sergio Benedetti, Carlo Bennati, Carla Bernardini, Rita Bizzotto, Katherine Blaney-Miller, Pietro Boccardo, Babette Bohn, Caterina Bon, Arnauld Brejon de Lavergnée, Claudia Caldari, Piero Cammarota, Francesca Cappelletti, Dawson Carr, Alessandro Cecchi, Costantino Centroni, Matteo Ceriani, Kaliopi Chamonikola, Françoise Chaserant, David Chesterman, William and Marjorie Coleman, Maira Corsinovi, Jon Culverhouse, Jean-Pierre Cuzin, Paolo Dal Poggetto, Mons. Gino Paolo D'Anna, Diane De Grazia, C. Roustan Delatour, Margarita López Diaz, Giampiero Donnini, Jean Edmonson, Yael Even, Everett Fahy, Richard Feigen, Larry Feinberg, Dorothee Feldman, Giancarlo Fiorenza, Sarah Fisher, Michael Foreman, Abramo Galassi, Vittoria Garibaldi, Hans-Joachim Giersberg, Angel Balau Gonxaléx, George Gordon, Burchkhardt Göres, Marco and Matteo Grassi, Mario Guderzo, Ann Guité, Fátima Halcón, Charlotte Hale, Nicholas Hall, Gisela Helmkampf, Sabine Jacob, David Jaffe, Catherine Johnston, J. Richard Judson, George Keyes, Armand Killan, Richard Knight, Teresa Laguna, Jean Laidlaw, Marit Lange, Mario Amedeo Lazzari, Carol Lekarew, Mark Leonard, Knut Ljogodt, Christopher Lloyd, Stéphane Loire, Nannette Maciejeunes, Stefania Macioce, Dorothy Mahon, Eugenio Malgeri, Patrick Matthiesen, Maurizio Marini, Juan Martinez, Don Aldo Mei, Juan Garrido Mesa, Lorenza Mochi Onori, John Morton Morris, Massimo Mossini, José Gabriel Moya, Marina Nelli, Larry Nichols, Bruno Oberhansli, Elke Oberthaler, Father Denis O'Brien, Piero Pagano, Enrica Pagella, Antonio Paolucci, Anna Maria Pedrocchi, Zora Pelousková, George Pepe, Nando Peretti, Silvana Pettenati, Catherine Phillips, Claudio Pizzorusso, Joan Pope, Wolfgang Prohaska, Elizabeth Ravaud, Mons. Cesare Recanatini, Paolo Riani, Eugenio Riccomini, Esperenza Rodriguez, Pierre Rosenberg, Eliot Rowlands, Giorgio Saitta, Timothy Salmons, Ana Sánchez-Lassa, Carla Scoz, Mons. Luigi Scuppa, Michael Shapiro, Michael Simpson, John Somerville, Hubert von Sonnenberg, Carla Enrica Spantigati, Paul van der Spek, Luigi Spezzaferro, Timothy Standring, David Steele, Mahrukh Tarapor, Bonnie Teeter, Marianne Thauré, Katka Tlachová, Letizia Treves, Simona Turriziani, Andrés Ubeda de los Cobos, Jesús Urrea,

Mariella Utili, Maria Rosaria Valazzi, Francesco Virnicchi, Marco Voena, Chrisoph Vogtherr, Robert Wald, Roger Ward, Mark Weil, Clovis Whitfield, Adam Williams, Stephan Wolohojian, Albert Ysequilla, Eric Zafran, Pietro Zampetti, and Don Alfredo Zuccatosta.

For production of the catalogue, we are especially grateful to our editor, Emily Walter, our designer, Bruce Campbell, and to Jean Wagner, Gwen Roginsky, Sally VanDevanter, Robert Weisberg, Ann Lucke, and Jane Bobko, working under the guidance of John P. O'Neill.

For the organization and installation of the exhibition, the following people should be mentioned. At The Metropolitan Museum of Art: Linda M. Sylling, Manager for Special Exhibitions and Gallery Installation; Herbert M. Moskowitz, Chief Registrar; Marceline McKee, Loans Coordinator; Stephanie Oratz Basta, Associate Counsel; Emily Kernan Rafferty, Senior Vice President for External Affairs, and Kerstin Larsen, Deputy Chief Development Officer for Corporate Programs; Michael Langley, Exhibition Designer; Zack Zanolli, Lighting Designer; Barbara Weiss, Graphic Designer; Kent Lydecker, Associate Director for Education; Elizabeth Hammer-Munemura, Associate Museum Educator; Harold Holzer, Vice President for Communications; Andrew Ferren, Senior Press Officer; Barbara Bridgers, Bruce Schwarz, and Paul Lachenauer in the Photograph Studio.

At the Saint Louis Art Museum: Linda Thomas, Assistant Director for Exhibitions; Jeanette Fausz, Registrar; Cornelia Homburg, Assistant Director for Curatorial Affairs; Jim Weidman, Director of Development; Jeff Wamhoff, Installation Designer; Dan Esarey, Head of Building Operations; Ann Thunell, Administrative Assistant, Curatorial; Jon Cournoyer, Graphic Designer; Brett Schott, Corporate Donors; Katie Pope; Kay Porter, Community Relations; Rita Wells, Retail Sales; Louise Cameron, Head of Youth and Family Programs; Victor Simmons, Head of Adult Programs; Stephanie Sigala, Acting Director of Education and Public Programming; Paul Haner, Paintings Conservator; and Mary Ann Steiner, Head of Publications.

Keith Christiansen
Judith W. Mann

Lenders to the Exhibition

Organizing Committee

Claudio Strinati
Rossella Vodret
Livia Carloni
Keith Christiansen
Judith W. Mann

The exhibition has been organized by the Soprintendenza per il Patrimonio Storico Artistico e Demoetnoantropologico di Roma; The Metropolitan Museum of Art, New York; and The Saint Louis Art Museum.

Contributors to the Catalogue

Livia Carloni
Patrizia Cavazzini
Keith Christiansen
Roberto Contini
Elizabeth Cropper
Jean-Pierre Cuzin
Gabriele Finaldi
Riccardo Lattuada
Judith W. Mann
Mary Newcome
Maria Pia d'Orazio
Richard Spear
Jeremy Wood
Alessandro Zuccari

Notes to the Reader

Abbreviated references are used throughout. For full listings, see the bibliography.

Measurements are given in inches and centimeters. Height precedes width.

Unless otherwise noted, entries for Orazio Gentileschi are by Keith Christiansen; those for Artemisia Gentileschi are by Judith W. Mann. The following initials are used:

LC   Livia Carloni
MPdO   Maria Pia d'Orazio

If a picture is not exhibited in all three venues, the venues are designated as follows:

Rome
New York
Saint Louis

The venues reflect loan arrangements as of September 1, 2001.

Chronology

Documented Chronologies of the Life and Work of Orazio and Artemisia Gentileschi

ORAZIO

1563   *July 9*   Orazio Gentileschi is baptized in Pisa, the son of a Florentine goldsmith, Giovanni Battista Lomi. (Carità 81)

ca. 1576–78   Moves to Rome.

1587   Guarantees a loan to his older brother Aurelio Lomi. (Masetti Zannini 1974, 43)

ca. 1588–89   Is part of équipe that decorates the Biblioteca Sistina in the Vatican.

1593   *Presentation of Christ,* Orazio's fresco in Santa Maria Maggiore, Rome, is completed.
Living on via Ripetta near San Giacomo degli Incurabili.

1594   *December 6*   First son, Giovanni Battista, is baptized. (Bissell 1981, 99)

1595   *April 24*   Paid for paintings on the catafalque of Cardinal Marco Sittico Altemps in Santa Maria in Trastevere, Rome. (Toesca 1960)

1596   *June 8*   Working on the *Conversion of Saint Paul,* an altarpiece (destroyed) for San Paolo fuori le Mura, Rome. (Samek Ludovici 1956, 153–54)

1597   *February 27*   Is contracted to decorate two chapels in the Benedictine abbey at Farfa, some twenty-five miles north of Rome, and to carry out other frescoes in the nave of the church. Working with an équipe of artists, he eventually contributes to the decoration of three chapels in the left nave, provides two altarpieces, and decorates the lunettes between the chapels. His personal contribution is limited. Work seems to be completed by February 1599. (Bissell 1981, 135–37)
June 11   Second son, Francesco, is baptized. Living on Piazza di Spagna in the parish of San Lorenzo in Lucina. (Bissell 1981, 100, Lapierre 1998, 430)
August   Angelo Fiorenzuola, a Florentine textile merchant, is pressured to begin the frescoed decoration of the family chapel in San Giovanni dei Fiorentini, Rome. The frescoes are still unfinished in 1604, when funds from revenues are sought; in 1611, Orazio is mentioned as having received four hundred scudi many years ago ("più [anni] fa"). The frescoes are not complete in 1615, and Orazio's actual contribution is limited to frescoes in the vault and the underside of the entrance arch, as noted in an anonymous early-seventeenth-century guidebook. (Suzan Major Germond 1993, 754–59; Christiansen 1994, 621; Dorati da Empoli 2001, 52, 54–55 n. 16)

1598–99   Is paid for work in the Benedictine abbey, Farfa.

1599   *May*   Scaffolding is erected for the frescoed decoration of the transept in San Giovanni in Laterano, Rome, under the direction of the Cavaliere d'Arpino; work is largely completed by August 19, 1600, when the cycle is inspected by Clement VIII; Orazio paints a monumental apostle. (Freiberg 1995, 83, 300–301)

ARTEMISIA

(This chronology is comprised in large part of edited selections from the Register of Documents in R. Ward Bissell, Artemisia Gentileschi and the Authority of Art: Critical Reading and Catalogue Raisonné *[University Park: The Pennsylvania State University Press, 1999], in which full archival and bibliographical references are provided. Reprinted by permission of the author and publisher. Material added by Judith W. Mann appears in brackets.)*

1593   *July 8*   Artemisia Gentileschi is born in Rome.
July 10   Baptized in the Roman church of San Lorenzo in Lucina, the daughter of Orazio Gentileschi and Prudentia Montoni.

July 2 and 29 Is paid for painting four angels in the cupola of the Madonna dei Monti, Rome; four others are painted by Cesare Nebbia. (Tiberia and Barroero)

July 31, 1599–June 5, 1600 Is paid for frescoing the apse of San Nicola in Carcere, Rome, for Cardinal Pietro Aldobrandini. (Abrombson 1981, 355)

September 16 Third son, Giulio, is baptized. Orazio is listed as living on via Paolino (present-day via del Babuino) in the parish of Santa Maria del Popolo. (Hoogewerff 1938, 112)

ca. 1600 Establishes a friendship with Michelangelo Merisi da Caravaggio.

1601 Living in Rome on via del Babuino, at the corner of via dei Greci; he will remain there until 1610. (Bissell 1981, 100; Lapierre 1998, 430)

March 22 Petitions to execute cartoons for the mosaics in the cupola of Saint Peter's (see appendix 2).

September 24 Son Giovanni Battista dies.

October 13 Another son, also named Giovanni Battista, is baptized. (Bissell 1981, 100)

1603 *February 2* Giovanni Battista, the second of Orazio's sons to bear this name, dies.

July Is obliged to pay the Accademia di San Luca, evidently for an evaluation of work he has done in the Ubertini family loggia near his home; he makes the payment on May 30, 1604. (Gallo)

September 12 and 14 Testifies in a libel suit involving the painters Giovanni Baglione and Caravaggio: "I can write, but not very correctly." Caravaggio, in his testimony, denies that Orazio was his friend: "He hasn't spoken to me in over three years." Orazio declares: "I haven't spoken with Caravaggio in about six or seven months, though he sent a request for a Capuchin habit and a pair of wings that I lent him and he returned about ten days ago."

1604 *May 30* Another son, Marco, is born.

1605 Wife, Prudentia Montoni, dies at the age of thirty. (Bissell 1981, 101) Contributes to the Accademia di San Luca (not in 1613, as is often stated). Becomes a member of the Congregazione dei Virtuosi al Pantheon. (Bissell 1981, 101)

1605 *June 12* Confirmation day for the eleven-year-old Artemisia in San Giovanni in Laterano, Rome.

1606 *March 7* Witnesses the will of the sculptor Tommaso della Porta together with Annibale Carracci, Annibale's pupil Giovan Antonio Solari, and the sculptor Domenico Lupo. (Panofsky 1993, 125)

1607 *March 1* Is living on via del Babuino with his four children and his widowed sister, Lucrezia. (Bissell 1981, 101)

March 23 Is contracted by the banker Settimio Olgiati to paint a *Baptism of Christ* for Santa Maria della Pace, Rome (cat. 11). The altarpiece is to be completed within six months. (Maniello 1994)

June 24 Orazio's *Circumcision* (cat. 7) is installed on the high altar of the Gesù, Ancona. It was commissioned at a cost of 303 scudi by Giovanni Nappi sometime after 1605, when construction on the church began. Nappi's son Filippo was rector of the church. (Pirri 1952, 13; Carloni in Fossombrone 1997, 22, 26 n. 31)

November 25 In a record of a pastoral visit by Cardinal Paolo Emilio Sfondrato to Como, Orazio's *Vision of Saint Cecilia* (cat. 9) in the church of Santa Cecilia is described as recently finished. (Rovi 1992)

1608 *May 31* The record of a pastoral visit to the parish church of San Salvatore, Farnese, mentions the altar for which Orazio painted a *Saint Michael* (cat. 14). (Schleier 1970, 177)

1608–9 Artemisia begins her training as a painter.

1609 Date on reverse of *Madonna and Child* (cat. 15).

April 15, July 10, and December 23 Is paid for work on the mosaics in the crossing dome of Saint Peter's.

October 24 Is reported as painting a *Madonna and Child* for the duke of Mantua; it is delivered in February 1610 and returned for retouching. (Luzio 60–61 note; see cat. 15)

1610 *March 20* Living on via del Babuino; moves soon after to via Margutta, where he is certainly listed on February 16, 1611 (*stati di anime:* see appendix 1).
May 28, June 11, July 16, and August 6 Paid for the mosaic of the Madonna in the crossing dome of Saint Peter's. (Orbaan 1919, 84–87)

1610 Artemisia's earliest dated painting, the *Susanna and the Elders* at Pommersfelden (cat. 51).

1611 Works with Agostino Tassi on the decorations of the Sala del Concistoro in the Palazzo del Quirinale. There are payments to Tassi from March 19, 1611; on September 6, 1611, he is paid for having completed the room. Payments to Tassi and Orazio follow in January 1612 for the decorations in Cardinal Lanfranco Margotti's quarters in the Quirinale. A final joint payment to Tassi and Orazio is made in January 1612. (Cavazzini 1998, 219)
April 10 Moves from via Margutta to via della Croce and then, after July 16, to the parish of Santo Spirito in Sassia—not far from Tassi's residence—where he is cited as living in 1612. (Lapierre 1998, 430)
September 13 Payments for the scaffolding for the decoration of Scipione Borghese's Casino delle Muse on the Quirinale, Rome (fig. 6). Payments to both Orazio and Tassi run through April 1612; in October 1612, the frescoes are described as "newly painted." A last payment is made to Orazio on December 6, 1612, and to Tassi on December 15. There are no payments during March or between April and December 1612. (Cavazzini 1998, 218)

1611 *May 6* Raped by Agostino Tassi.
October Designated godmother to the son of the Spaniard Pietro Hernandes (Pedro Hernández), according to testimony presented during perjury proceedings against witnesses at the Tassi trial.

1612 Orazio and Tassi finish the frescoes for the Casino delle Muse (see under 1611).
Date inscribed on the reverse of Orazio's *Judith and Holofernes* (fig. 46), probably the picture confiscated for the trial.
Orazio Griffi founds an oratory at San Girolamo della Carità, Rome, for which Orazio's *Saint Francis with an Angel* (cat. 21) may have been painted. (Vodret 1998, 71–73)
March Files suit against Agostino Tassi for the rape of his daughter, Artemisia. The trial begins on March 2 and ends on October 29, 1612, followed by preliminary sentencing of Tassi on November 27 and definitive sentencing on November 28.
July 3 Writes to the grand duchess of Tuscany to beg her aid in keeping Tassi in prison, offering to send her a sample of Artemisia's work.

1612 *May 14* During her testimony at Tassi's trial, Artemisia speaks of a portrait that she had painted of a cleric named Artigenio.
November 27 "The excellent and very illustrious Hieronimus Felice, judge, condemns [Agostino Tassi] to choose between a punishment of five years of hard labor or banishment from Rome." (Cavazzini 1998, 175–76)
November 28 Tassi chooses banishment; the court sentences him to exile.
November 29 Artemisia marries Pierantonio di Vincenzo Stiattesi, a Florentine, in the church of Santo Spirito in Sassia, Rome.
December 10 Pierantonio Stiattesi assigns power of attorney to his brother, the sometime notary Giovanni Battista, entrusting him with his Roman affairs in a possible preparation for leaving the city.

1613 *October* A roll call of the Accademia di San Luca reports that Orazio is working in the Palazzo (or Monte) Savelli but is at present "outside Rome." (Gallo 1998)

1613 *September 21* In Florence, a son, Giovanni Battista, is born to Artemisia and baptized in the parish of Santa Maria Novella, with Lorenzo di Vincenzo Cavalcanti standing as godfather.

1614 *January* Name appears in the account books of the Savelli family in Rome. (Testa 1998 349)

1614 *November 1* A bill to Pierantonio detailing charges made by Artemisia to a joiner for artist's supplies and household furnishings.

1615 *January 17* Niccolò Tassi, a neighbor and friend of Orazio's, writes to the astronomer Galileo Galilei mentioning Orazio ("pictore insigni"). He encloses an epigram he had written about a *Cleopatra* that Orazio had sent to Cosimo II, grand duke of Tuscany. (Pizzorusso 1987, 70; see cat. 17)
April 6 Name occurs in the account books of the Savelli. (Testa 1998, 349)
March 16 Andrea Cioli, the Florentine secretary of state, writes to Pietro Guicciardini, the Florentine ambassador to Rome, inquiring about Orazio, whose fame has reached Florence, and noting that Artemisia has already established a reputation there. (Crinò 1960, 264)
March 27 Guicciardini responds with a devastating evaluation of Orazio and his art. Stating that the artist is living with Paolo Savelli, he reports that he has located only two pictures on public display in Rome: the Casino delle Muse frescoes (fig. 6) and the Santa Maria della Pace *Baptism of Christ* (cat. 11). (Crinò and Nicolson 1961)

1615 *July 10* In the Florentine parish of San Piero Maggiore, Artemisia stands as godmother at the baptism of a child named after her, born July 9 to Annibale di Nicolò Caroti and Ottavia di Marcantonio Coralli. The painter Cristofano Allori is designated godfather.
August 24 Advance of ten florins from Michelangelo Buonarroti the Younger to Artemisia for the *Allegory of Inclination* (fig. 110).
September 7 Note by Artemisia's husband to Michelangelo Buonarroti the Younger requesting four or five ducats for the "number of misfortunes that had befallen him."
Between September 7 and November 13 Requests of Michelangelo Buonarroti the Younger 21 lire (i.e., three florins), which she claims she will reimburse as she had her previous debts to him.
November 9 A son, Cristofano, born to Artemisia on November 8 and named after his godfather, the painter Cristofano Allori, is baptized in the Florentine parish of Sant'Ambrogio.
November 13 Michelangelo Buonarroti the Younger pays Artemisia three florins; she receives it in bed, "being in childbirth."

	ORAZIO		ARTEMISIA
1616	*July 19* May be in Florence when Artemisia pays her matriculation fee for the Accademia del Disegno. (Bissell 1981, 103)	**1616**	*February 3, April 2, June 18, and August 20* Four payments totaling 16 florins to Artemisia, two stipulated for the *Allegory of Inclination*. *May 9 through January 6, 1617* Itemized account of charges totaling 32 scudi, three baiocchi for goods supplied to Artemisia by a druggist. *July 19* Matriculates at the Accademia del Disegno at Florence. *August 20* *Allegory of Inclination* is delivered. Although Michelangelo Buonarroti the Younger's account with the artist is closed, Artemisia remains indebted to him.
1617	*January* Writes to Don Giovanni de' Medici, the natural son of Duke Cosimo I, and asks his help in securing work in the ducal palace in Venice in place of another artist—probably Carlo Saraceni. (Crinò 1960, 264)	**1617**	*August 2* A daughter, named Prudenza (Prudentia) after her deceased maternal grandmother and born to Artemisia on August 1, is baptized in the Florentine parish of San Salvatore, the Cavaliere Anea di Silvio Piccolomini Aragona standing as godfather. This daughter apparently also answered to the name Palmira. *December 6* Carpenters summoned by the Accademia del Disegno estimate a reduced amount for the bill that Artemisia had run up with another carpenter in 1614 and 1615.
		1618	*January 24* Final judgment against Artemisia for the debt to a carpenter that she had accrued in 1614 and 1615. *March 3* Payment on behalf of the grand duke of Tuscany to Artemisia for paintings executed or to be executed. *June 26–27* Argues successfully before the council of the Accademia del Disegno in Florence that a certain judgment made against her by a Francesco Lomi is invalid, since as an artist she is entitled to the privileges and subject only to the rules of the Accademia. *October 14* A daughter born to Artemisia on October 13 is baptized in the Florentine parish of Santa Lucia sul Prato with the name Lisabella, after her godmother, wife of the dramatist Jacopo Cicognini. The poet Jacopo di Bernardo Soldani stands as godfather.
1619	*February 20 and 27* Is recommended to Duke Francesco Maria della Rovere in Urbino by Cardinal Bonifacio Bevilacqua to fresco the tribune of the church of Sant'Ubaldo, Pesaro. Nothing comes of it. (Gronau 1936, 273–74) *July 24* Applies to decorate the benediction loggia at Saint Peter's, a commission that is instead given to Giovanni Lanfranco (see appendix 2).	**1619**	*February 28* Notice that a *Diana at Her Bath* by Artemisia has entered the collection of the grand duke of Tuscany. *June 5* A letter addressed by Artemisia to Grand Duke Cosimo II of Tuscany requests his intervention in a judgment brought against her by the Accademia for debts incurred by her husband to a Michele *bottegaio*. She claims ignorance of the debts and protests the judgment because "as a woman she could not incur debts while her husband was still with said woman." *June 9* Death of Artemisia's daughter Lisabella. *July 4* In the Florentine parish of Santa Lucia sul Prato, Artemisia stands as godmother at the baptism of a child named after her, a daughter born to Filippo d'Antonio Stinelli and Lisabetta di Alessandro Sapiti. *December (?) 18* The council of the Accademia del Disegno orders Artemisia to pay a creditor 70 lire.
1620	The chapel in San Benedetto, Fabriano, containing Orazio's *San Carlo Borromeo* (fig. 53), is dedicated.	**1620**	Date on *Jael and Sisera* (cat. 61). *January 13* Order to give Artemisia 1½ ounces of ultramarine so that she may finish *Hercules* which the grand duke has ordered. *January 16* Order that Artemisia pay for the aforementioned ultramarine. *February 10* Letter from Artemisia to Cosimo II de' Medici informing him of a proposed trip to Rome and promising to send him within two months a painting for which she has already received 50 scudi. *February 15* Order to return to Artemisia those household goods of hers which had been sequestered because of her failure to pay for the 1½ ounces of ultramarine she had received.
1621	Giovan Antonio Sauli, of an old Genoese patrician family, is in Rome for the papal election and invites Orazio to Genoa. For Sauli, Orazio paints a *Penitent Magdalene*, a *Danaë*, a *Lot and His Daughters*, and "other works of great exquisiteness" (cat. nos. 35–37). (Soprani 1674, 316–18)	**1621**	*February 10* Inventory in Florence of household effects and studio materials for sale to Francisco Maringhi (see appendix 3). *March* In Rome, living on via del Corso with her husband, Pierantonio Stiattesi, her daughter Palmira, and servants. *November 17* Sublets a small apartment on via della Croce.
		1622	[Date on *Susanna and the Elders* (cat. 65).] Date on the reverse of the *Portrait of a Gonfaloniere* (cat. 66).

ORAZIO

1623 *April 2* Writes to Carlo Emanuele I, duke of Savoy, offering his services, and sends an *Annunciation* (cat. 43). Had already sent a *Lot and His Daughters* (cat. 42). (Baude de Vesme 1932, 319; Pizzorusso 73)

1624 *April 17* Carlo Emanuele I, duke of Savoy, writes to his son Vittorio Amedeo about 150 ducats that Orazio owes an innkeeper, stating that this sum should be paid if they want the artist to come to Turin and begin work. (Bava in Romano 1995, 248)
August 13 The Neapolitan painter Battista Caracciolo offers to prepare an estimate of the frescoes (destroyed) Orazio has just painted for Marc Antonio Doria's casino at San Pier d'Arena, near Genoa—a loggia to whose decoration Caracciolo had himself contributed. Orazio either is still in Genoa or has just left for France. (Pacelli-Bologna 1980, p. 27)
Arrives in Paris to work for Marie de' Medici.

1625 *May* The duke of Buckingham arrives in Paris for the proxy marriage of Marie de' Medici's daughter Henrietta Maria to Charles I; he acquires two works by Orazio (see cat. 45). Orazio is invited to London.

1626 *September/October* Arrives in London. On December 4, Amerigo Salvetti, the envoy of the grand duke of Tuscany, writes, "About two months ago there came here from France Signor Orazio Gentileschi, painter, whom I am given to understand, besides exercising his art, is also engaged in another matter of great importance, as he is often with the duke of Buckingham and also with the king." The duke of Buckingham outfits quarters for him at the cost of five hundred pounds. Orazio is seen in the company of noted members of the court. (Sainsbury 1859, 311–15; A. M. Crinò 1967, p. 532)

1627 *July 16* The Tuscan envoy in London, Amerigo Salvetti, writes to Florence to announce the imminent departure of Orazio's two sons Francesco and Giulio, who are to go to Genoa to purchase pictures for Charles I. They leave on August 20, but the purchase is later thwarted by Nicholas Lanier, the king's agent. (see Finaldi 1999, 35 n. 32)

1628 *January 31* Royal warrant granting Orazio an annuity of one hundred pounds, backdated to December 25, 1626. A fresh warrant is issued on January 31, 1630, for three hundred pounds. This sum is paid in three installments: April 20, 1630, November 12, 1630, February 4, 1631. (Crinò and Nicolson 1961, 145, and Wood 2001, 115, 125–26)

ARTEMISIA

Lent Living on via del Corso with her husband, her daughter Palmira, her brothers Giulio and Francesco, and servants.
June Finding a group of Spaniards on his via del Corso doorstep, apparently there to serenade his wife, Pierantonio is accused of having slashed one of them in the face.

1623 *Lent* Living on via del Corso with her daughter and servants. By this date Artemisia's husband has departed, and sometime thereafter she loses track of him.
[The Ludovisi inventory lists a *Susanna and the Elders* by Artemisia (Wood 1992, 522).]

1624 *February 27* A *Cupid and Psyche* by Artemisia is inventoried in the Patrizi collection at Rome.
Lent Living on via del Corso with her daughter and a servant.

1625 *March 17 or later* A *Saint Apollonia* painted by Artemisia on copper figures in an inventory of the Medici Villa Imperiale.
Lent Living on via del Corso with a daughter, Prudentia, and servants.
June 20 Sublets an apartment on via Rassella (via dei Serpenti); her home and studio remain on via del Corso.
July 1625–February 1626 Three paintings attributed to Artemisia—a *Christ and the Little Children* (fig. 132), a *David with a Harp*, and a *Penitent Magdalene* (cat. 68)—are acquired in Rome by the duke of Alcalá, Spanish ambassador extraordinary to the Holy See.
September 15 Appealing to the civil tribunal, Artemisia's servant Dianora Turca demands back pay in the amount of 30 scudi, of which she is awarded 20 (see October 18).
September 29 The artist witnesses as godmother the baptism of another Artemisia, daughter of a Luca from Siena and a Domenic from Zagarolo.
October 18 Date of Dianora Turca's claim that Artemisia still owes her 10 scudi for services rendered.
December 9 Enters into an agreement with her landlord concerning work to be done by him on her via del Corso residence.

1626 A *Mystic Marriage of Saint Catherine* thought to be by Artemisia is recorded by Cassiano dal Pozzo in the Madrid collection of the marqués de la Hinojosa.

1627 Date of the engraving by Jérôme David after Artemisia's *Portrait of the Engineer Antoine de Ville.*
Date of a pamphlet printed in Venice containing verses dedicated to three paintings—*Amoretto, Lucretia,* and *Susanna and the Elders*—by Artemisia.
Publication in Venice of the *Lettere di Antonio Colluraffi,* in which Artemisia's presence in the city is noted and she and her talent extolled by way of letters, Latin inscriptions, and madrigals.

1628 In Venice, where she receives a payment of 1,467 giulii, 14 baiocchi for a *Hercules and Omphale* commissioned by Philip IV of Spain through the intermediary of the conde de Oñate.

The painter-writer Joachim von Sandrart visits Orazio's London studio and sees a *Penitent Magdalene*, a *Rest on the Flight into Egypt*, and *Lot and His Daughters* (cat. 46).
August The duke of Buckingham, Orazio's primary supporter in London, is assassinated.
December 4 A pass is issued for Orazio's son Giulio to return to Italy. (Sainsbury 1859, 311 n. 37)

1629 A list is drawn up by the rival painter Balthazar Gerbier of the money Orazio has received from Charles I. The list mentions a *Magdalene*, a *Rest on the Flight into Egypt*, a *Christ at the Column*, and a *Lot and His Daughters* (see cat. nos. 45, 46, 49). (Sainsbury 1859, 314–15; and Finaldi 1999, 35 n. 31)
Gentileschi is called "his Ma[jesty]'s Picture Maker (Croft-Murray 1947, 90 n. 11)
January 29 Writes to Charles I about the hostilities between his son Giulio and Gerbier (see p. 226) (Sainsbury 1859b)
March Writes to the secretary of state, Lord Dorchester, about the trip Giulio and Francesco made to Italy on behalf of the king and accounting for payments received from the king between 1627 and 1629 (see appendix 4).
April 24 Writes to Lord Dorchester regarding the sums he has received and is owed (see appendix 4).

1630 Roger du Plessis de Liancourt, duke of La Roche-Guyon, pays 460 livres to Orazio for a painting of Diana (cat. 47). (Finaldi 1999, 36 n. 57)
October 13 Laments his financial condition to Lord Dorchester, the secretary of state (see appendix 4).

1631 *June 23* Warrant is issued to pay Orazio two hundred pounds for pictures delivered to Charles I. (Crinò and Nicolson 1961, 145)
July 28 The widow of the duke of Buckingham writes to Lord Dorchester that if Orazio receives his pay from the king, he will return to Italy, thus freeing up York House for her use. (Crinò and Nicolson 1961, 145)

1632 *June 14* Warrant is issued to pay Orazio four hundred pounds for his services. (Crinò and Nicolson 1961,145)

1633 *May 8* Letter of introduction from Sir John Coke, secretary of state, to Sir Arthur Hopton, the English ambassador in Madrid, for Orazio's son Francesco, who is accompanying Orazio's *Finding of Moses* (fig. 87) to Madrid to present the painting to Philip IV. (Harris 1967)
July 13 Writes to the grand duke of Tuscany, Ferdinand II, expressing his desire to return to Florence; sends a small painting as a sample of his work. (Crinò 1954, 203–204)
October 14 Balthazar Gerbier writes Charles I from Brussels that the queen mother, Marie de' Medici, and the infanta have admired Gentileschi's work (see appendix 4).
October 26 Sir Arthur Hopton, the English ambassador in Madrid, writes to Sir John Coke, reporting Philip IV's satisfaction with Orazio's *Finding of Moses*. (Harris 1967)
November 18 Philip IV authorizes payment of nine hundred ducats to Orazio for the *Finding of Moses*. (Bissell 1981, 106)

1633–34 An account for varnishing and gilding of picture frames at Greenwich mentions three pictures by Orazio: *Finding of Moses* (cat. 48), *Joseph and Potiphar's Wife* (fig. 88), and *Muses* (fig. 93); also a *Tarquin and Lucretia*, likely to be by Artemisia (Chettle 1937, 104).

1629 *July 1629–May 1631* A *Saint John the Baptist* and two paintings described as portraits of Artemisia are acquired by the duke of Alcalá, Spanish viceroy to Naples.

1630 Date on Capodimonte *Annunciation* (cat. 72).
August 24 Letter from Artemisia in Naples to Cassiano dal Pozzo in Rome, notifying him that she has received the measurements for a picture and that she will begin work on his commission after she completes "some works for the empress."
August 31 Letter from Artemisia to Cassiano dal Pozzo informing him again that he will have the portrait commissioned by him as soon as she finishes "some works for the empress."
December 21 Letter from Artemisia to Cassiano dal Pozzo reporting that she has returned to Naples and assuring him that the *Self-Portrait* he had commissioned will be dispatched to Rome.

1631 *August 21* Final 12 ducats paid to Artemisia of a 20-ducat fee for a *Saint Sebastian* for Giovanni d'Afflitto of Naples.
Autumn Visited in Naples by the German painter and writer Joachim von Sandrart, who sees a *David with the Head of Goliath* in her studio.

1632 Date on the *Clio, Muse of History* (cat. 75).

1634 *March 15 and 18* The English traveler Bullen Reymes, retainer of the duke of Buckingham, visits Artemisia and her daughter in their Neapolitan residence. Prudentia is said to be both a painter and a player of the spinet.

1635 *January 21* Letter from Artemisia to Cassiano dal Pozzo announcing that her brother Francesco is to arrive in Rome with a painting she has made which, through Cassiano's help, she wishes to present to Cardinal Antonio Barberini (January 25 and July 20, 1635).
January 25 Letter from Artemisia to Francesco I d'Este in Modena apprising him that she has sent her brother Francesco to Modena with pictures for the duke. She claims that her brother had been dispatched by Charles I to bring her to England but that she would prefer Francesco d'Este's patronage.
March 7 Letter from Francesco d'Este thanking Artemisia for her gift.
May 22 Letter from Artemisia to Francesco d'Este expressing her gratitude that the paintings had found favor. She entreats the duke to provide her with the means of serving him in person.
July 20 Letter from Artemisia in Naples to Ferdinand II de' Medici announcing the arrival in Florence of her brother with paintings for the grand duke. She also tries to guarantee patronage from the grand duke so that she can postpone her trip to England.
October 9 Letter from Artemisia in Naples to Galileo in Arcetri asking his help in determining whether the two large paintings she had sent to Florence had pleased the grand duke.
October (?) 20 Letter from Artemisia to Andrea Cioli in Florence asking if the two large pictures she had sent pleased the grand duke.
December 11 Letter from Artemisia thanking Andrea Cioli for his courtesies, and proclaiming her desire to send him a *Saint Catherine* by her hand and a painting by her daughter.

1636 *February 11* Letter from Artemisia to Andrea Cioli lamenting the "tumults of war" and the poor quality and high cost of life in Naples; again seeks employment in Florence.
April 1 Letter from Artemisia to Andrea Cioli asking his assistance in arranging the grand duke's patronage. Planning to journey to Pisa in May to sell some property there for money, to marry off a daughter; proposes to stop in Florence for a period of four months.
May 5 Receipt of 250 ducats as final payment for three paintings for Prince Karl Eusebius von Liechtenstein.
December 19 Transfer of 20 ducats from the bank account of Bernardino Belprato to Artemisia, as final payment of 60 ducats for a painting she is to deliver.

1637 *October 24* Letter from Artemisia to Cassiano dal Pozzo about her need for money for her daughter's marriage; asks whether or not her husband is still living.
November 24 Letter from Artemisia to Cassiano dal Pozzo identifying the pictures that she intends for Cardinals Francesco and Antonio Barberini as a *Christ and the Samaritan Woman* and a *Saint John the Baptist in the Desert*. Expresses her wish to return to Rome.
[*December 22* Inventory of Alessandro Biffi collection lists a *Madonna,* a *Lute Player,* an *Allegory of Painting* by Artemisia, and a *David* by Orazio (see cat. nos. 52, 63, 18) (Cannatà-Vicini 1992).]

1637–39 Three pictures by Artemisia are listed in the English royal collections: *Fame, Susanna and the Elders,* and *Tarquin and Lucretia.*

1638 [*Self-Portrait as a Lute Player* (cat. 57) and *Self-Portrait as an Amazon with Curved Sword and Helmet* are recorded in a Medici inventory of the Villa Medici at Artimino. (Papi 2000, 452)]
March A *David with the Head of Goliath* by Artemisia is inventoried in the collection of Marchese Vincenzo Giustiniani at Rome.
March 1 A *Judith Slaying Holofernes* is entered in a Medici inventory of the Palazzo Pitti.
March 3 Artemisia's *Judith and Her Maidservant* (cat. 60) is entered in a Medici inventory.

1639 *February 7* Orazio dies in London, "much mourned by his majesty." (Crinò and Nicolson 1961, 145)
July 2 Orazio's will is proved by his son Francesco. (Finaldi 1999, 33)

1639 *December 16* Letter from Artemisia in London to Francesco I d'Este in Modena telling the duke that her brother will arrive from England to present a painting to him.

1640　Document listing Artemisia's *Saints Proculus and Nicea* and *Saint Januarius in the Amphitheater* (cat. 79), and almost certainly her *Adoration of the Magi,* for the cathedral at Pozzuoli.
Date of the engraving by Jean Ganière after Artemisia's *Child Sleeping near a Skull.*
March 16 Letter from Francesco I d'Este in Modena to Artemisia in London, thanking her for the painting she has sent him.

1644　A painting by Artemisia described as "a woman with an Amore" is inventoried in the collection of Cardinal Antonio Barberini in Rome.

1646　*November 17* A *Judith* attributed to Artemisia, having been inherited by the Pio Monte della Misericordia, Naples, from the estate of D. Cesare di Gennaro, principe di San Martino, is evaluated.

1648　*September 5* Payment of 30 ducats to Artemisia in Naples made by Fabrizio Ruffo, prior of Bargnara, for a painting on which she is working.

1649　Five pictures by Artemisia are listed in the English royal collection: *Fame, Susanna and the Elders,* "A S^t laying his hand. on frutite," *Diana at Her Bath* (elsewhere identified as *Bathsheba*), and *Tarquin and Lucretia.* [Date on Brno *Susanna and the Elders* (cat. 83).]
A *Sacrifice of Isaac* and a *Saint Cecilia* appear under Artemisia's name in the Neapolitan collection of Vincenzo D'Andrea.
January 5 Payment of 160 ducats to Artemisia for a *Galatea* from Don Antonio Ruffo of Messina.
January 30 Letter from Artemisia in Naples to Don Antonio Ruffo in Messina for the *Galatea.* (Ruffo 1916, 48)
February 21 Letter from Ruffo to Artemisia containing 100 ducats as an advance for a *Diana at Her Bath.*
March 13 Letter from Artemisia to Ruffo reporting the receipt of 100 ducats and lamenting that the *Galatea* shipped in January had suffered from the sea journey. Adds that she will send Ruffo her *Self-Portrait* and a small picture by her daughter, whom she had married to a Knight of St. James. [She also notes that she is bankrupt and in need of work.]
June 5 Letter from Artemisia to Ruffo acknowledging his correspondence of May 24 and informing him that because of the indisposition of the model who was posing for it, the picture (identifiable as the *Diana at Her Bath*) was not yet finished. Notes she has made three paintings for Don Fabrizio Ruffo, a prior in Naples.
June 12 Letter from Artemisia to Don Antonio Ruffo requesting 50 ducats to help defray her high expenses for female nude models.
June 22 Two advances to Artemisia for the *Diana at Her Bath.*
July 24 Letter from Artemisia to Ruffo acknowledging receipt of the advance. Postpones delivery of the *Diana* to the end of the August.
August 5 Date of an accounting by Ruffo of expenses incurred in providing a shipping crate and a frame for Artemisia's *Galatea.*
August 7 Letter from Artemisia to Ruffo announcing receipt of his voucher and the imminent completion of the picture. She adds that she will show him "what a woman can do."

September 4 Letter from Artemisia to Ruffo explaining that she has not met the delivery deadline for the *Diana* because a change in the perspective had necessitated redoing two of the figures.
October 23 Letter from Artemisia to Ruffo expressing her mortification that he wished to cut by one-third her fee for the *Diana at Her Bath.*
November 13 Letter from Artemisia to Ruffo informing him that she had finished the *Diana at Her Bath* but could not let it go for less than the stipulated price. She comments: "You will find the spirit of Caesar in this soul of a woman."
A second letter is sent. In correspondence of October 26, Ruffo had informed the artist of a cavaliere in Messina who wanted works by her hand, specifically a *Judgment of Paris* and a *Galatea,* the latter to be different from the one for Don Antonio, and a preliminary drawing. Artemisia claims that "in none of my pictures is there the slightest repetition of invention, not even a single hand," and notes her resolve never again to submit drawings, since one for the bishop of Sant'Agata de' Goti representing souls in purgatory had been turned over to another painter to execute.
December Letter from Artemisia to Ruffo sending Christmas greetings while apprising him that if he wants the *Diana at Her Bath* he has to intervene, given the ill will between her and Don Antonio's nephew and intermediary in Naples, the prior Don Fabrizio Ruffo.

1650　*February 26* Advance of 25 ducats to Artemisia for the *Diana at Her Bath* in October 1649 is recorded in Don Antonio Ruffo's account book.
April 12 Artemisia receives a final payment of 80 ducats for the *Diana at Her Bath* from Don Flavio Ruffo in Naples acting on behalf of his brother Don Antonio.
April 30 Three notations in the account book of Ruffo note that Artemisia has been paid.
August 13 Letter from Artemisia to Ruffo expressing her gratitude that he has resumed communication with her and her hope of sending him a "little *Madonna* in small scale" (possibly cat. 84).

1651　*January 1* Letter from Artemisia to Ruffo informing him that she is still convalescing from an illness she contracted at Christmastime, and that she will send him the small *Madonna* on copper—now half-painted—when she is well. Reports she has in her studio two half-completed paintings as large as the *Galatea,* representing Andromeda Liberated by Perseus and Joseph and Potiphar's Wife, which she will finish by April for 90 scudi each, providing that Ruffo advances her 100 ducats.

1652　Date reported to have appeared on a *Susanna and the Elders* with Averardo de' Medici in Florence.

1653　Publication date in Venice of the *Cimiterio, epitafij, giocosi* by Giovanfrancesco Loredan and Pietro Michiele, which includes two posthumous epitaphs disrespectful of Artemisia.

Orazio Gentileschi

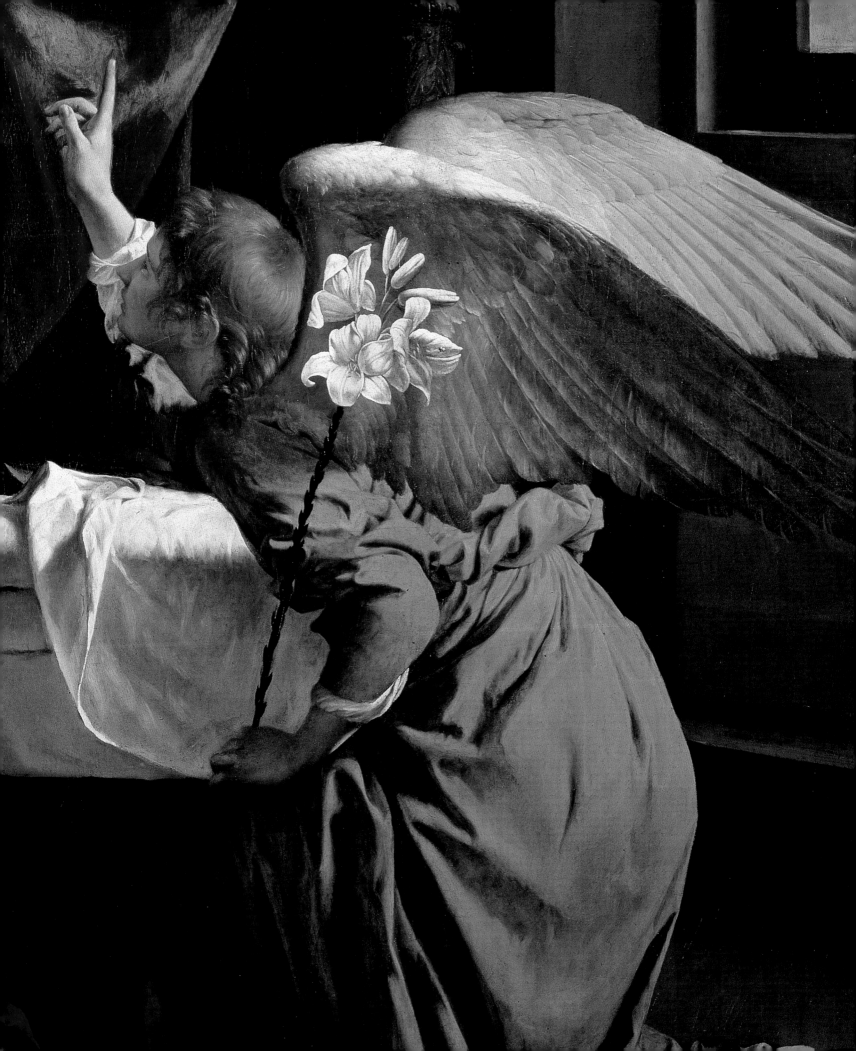

The Art of Orazio Gentileschi

KEITH CHRISTIANSEN

We possess two portraits of Orazio Gentileschi (1563–1639). As luck would have it, they date from two widely separated and crucial periods of his life. The first is from 1612, when Orazio was fifty years old. He had just completed work on two cycles of frescoes: one for an apartment in the grandiose palace of Pope Paul V (r. 1605–21) on the Quirinal hill (destroyed), the other for a garden loggia, or casino, for the pope's art-loving nephew, Cardinal Scipione Borghese (figs. 6, 7). These were collaborative enterprises, undertaken with the perspective specialist Agostino Tassi (1578–1644), and they should have crowned Orazio's decade-long effort to establish himself as one of the major painters in Rome, alongside artists such as the slightly older Cigoli (1559–1613) and the rising star of a younger generation, Guido Reni (1575–1642), both of whom were also employed by Scipione Borghese. In his 1674 biography, Raffaele Soprani specifically links Orazio's subsequent fame to his work for the Borghese. Yet this was a bittersweet moment, for while work on the projects proceeded, Tassi took advantage of his professional association with Orazio to quench an insatiable passion for the latter's daughter, Artemisia. After much frustration and scheming, he raped (or, in the legal terminology of the day, deflowered) her on May 3, 1611. Though he already had a wife, he convinced Artemisia to enter into a liaison that, he promised, would end in marriage—thus setting things aright. The affair came to a head when it was discovered, belatedly, by Orazio, who took Tassi to court, applying for justice to the same pope for whom he had been working.[1] It is in the context of the ensuing trial that the first, verbal sketch of the artist was made by a friend of Tassi's who was an innkeeper—conditioned, one imagines, to sizing up his clients. "Orazio is a man of fifty years, with a black beard that is beginning to turn a little white. He is of a good height and dresses in black."[2] To this thumbnail delineation

of his outward aspect, we may add a few tints of character. Carlo Saraceni (ca. 1579–1620), a fellow Caravaggista who had known Orazio for upward of ten years, described him as an honorable person ("persona molto honorata").[3] Then there is the testimony of the wife of Orazio's tailor, Costanza Ceuli, who had known the artist for fourteen years and lived next door to him on via della Croce—in the popular quarter of Rome between Santa Maria del Popolo and Piazza di Spagna. Costanza noted wryly that Orazio was truly a poor man, who spent grandly when he had money and did nothing when his pockets were empty ("quando non ne haveva faceva niente").[4] It is a genial enough image of an energetic, somewhat irresponsible man still lacking the financial rewards of success but dressed in their outward trappings. But we are well advised not to be too quick to color in these summary contours.

The second portrait is a drawn study made in London about twenty years later by Anthony van Dyck (1599–1641) as part of a series of illustrious men (fig. 1).[5] Orazio had arrived in the city in 1626, at the invitation of the minister of Charles I (r. 1625–49), George Villiers, duke of Buckingham, who provided the artist and his three sons with ample quarters and a studio in his house on the Strand. Orazio's position at court marked a pinnacle in his career. Five years earlier, he had accepted the invitation of the Genoese patrician Giovan Antonio Sauli to move from Rome to Genoa, only to be invited two and a half years later to accept a position at the court of Marie de' Medici (1573–1642), where he worked in her grandiose Luxembourg palace. The move to London followed the marriage of Charles I to Marie de' Medici's daughter, Henrietta Maria.

Van Dyck had met Orazio in Genoa and recorded two of the artist's compositions in his sketchbook (figs. 74, 94). The painters may well have established a cordial relationship, but there can be

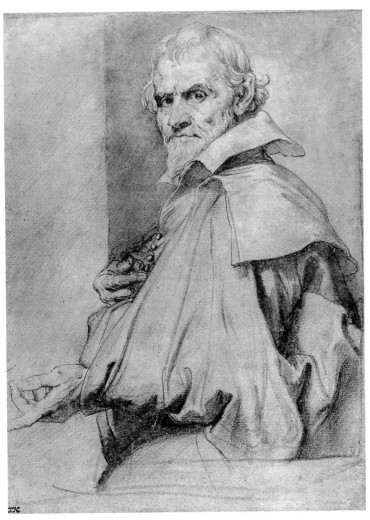

Figure 1. Anthony van Dyck (1599–1641), *Portrait of Orazio Gentileschi*. Black chalk with gray wash and pen and ink on paper. British Museum, London

no doubt that the aging artist felt himself outclassed by Van Dyck, whose rising position at the Caroline court would, in fact, relegate him to working for the queen (on this, see Finaldi and Wood, pp. 227–29). Van Dyck arrived in London in 1632; he was knighted, and a year later granted a retainer of £200 a year—twice that of Gentileschi. In Van Dyck's black-chalk portrait, we recognize the same distinctive features that had so struck the innkeeper in 1612: the beard—white rather than peppered with gray—the carriage, and the stature. There has, however, been a conspicuous alteration in social status. This is not someone living from hand to mouth, his pockets full one day and empty the next. He is dressed in the simple but elegant clothes of a court figure, with a large starched collar and well-tailored cloak. His attitude is that of a man of position and influence, his left eyebrow arched, one hand

extended in a rhetorical gesture of discourse. How different from the restless inhabitant of the rough-and-tumble neighborhood he lived in in Rome—from 1605 as a widower—and where he had frequented the popular taverns together with Caravaggio and his unruly claque. We know, in fact, that in London he rubbed shoulders with the nobility and with the king himself: the French ambassador in London, François de Bassompierre, noted Orazio's attendance at a state dinner, and the Florentine envoy suspected he was being employed on diplomatic missions.

Yet there is something churlish in his coarsely handsome face, and indeed we know that in London, as in Rome, Orazio did not get on with his fellow artists (admittedly, our view is colored by the testimony of his nemesis, Balthazar Gerbier, always on the lookout for anything he could use against the painter, whom he considered an interloper in his claims as royal artist, diplomat, and art adviser). Nor had his spending habits—so prominent in the memory of his Roman neighbor two decades earlier—improved: to respond to accusations of misuse of funds, Orazio was required to give an accounting of the large sums of money that had been advanced to him by the duke of Buckingham (this unfortunate habit of free spending was later exaggerated to almost criminal proportions in his scoundrel of a son Francesco).

Giovanni Baglione, in his unflattering biography, published in 1642, characterized Orazio's conduct as "more bestial than human" ("piu nel bestiale, che nel'humano egli dava"), noting that "he kept to his opinions, and with his satirical tongue offended everyone; let us hope that the good Lord forgives him his sins."[6] Baglione had belonged to a rival faction of artists in Rome and in 1603 had brought a libel suit against Caravaggio and three members of his inner circle, one of whom was Orazio. It was, in fact, Orazio who seems to have been the author of one of the libelously obscene verses directed at Baglione. At the trial Orazio played the innocent, just as, at the rape trial in 1612, he assumed the part of the offended and unjustly betrayed victim. But what did he expect from such friends?[7] (Tassi had a notorious reputation—above all, for sexual escapades.) The Florentine ambassador in Rome, Piero Guicciardini, in the assessment of Orazio that he sent back to Florence in 1615, echoed Baglione's low opinion of the artist's behavior,[8] and André Félibien recorded that in France Orazio's paintings "were rather well thought of, but as he had an utterly savage temperament ("d'une humeur tout à fait brutale") and was given to slander-mongering, he was not held in high esteem.[9]

There is a notable dichotomy between the coarse-seeming character of Gentileschi that emerges from these accounts and the refined work he produced. It is not a dichotomy that is easily explained, and it serves as a warning to anyone who seeks to read the painter's biography into his art. It is one thing for that apologist of classicism, Giovan Pietro Bellori, to have used Caravaggio's swarthy complexion and dark eyes and hair as a key to his brooding style, with its cellar light: this was a matter of Renaissance physiognomics. Or for Artemisia's more recent biographers to discern in the biblical female victims and heroines that are the subjects of her early paintings a self-projecting voice of protest (though we might question the distinctly late-twentieth-century accent of the voice these writers profess to hear).[10] But there is no obvious relationship between the coarse humor and demeaning, scatological language of Orazio's libelous poem about the work of Baglione and the poetry of the *Lute Player* in Washington (cat. 22) or the chaste, religious sentiment of the Turin *Annunciation* (cat. 43). These works seem to emanate from an expressive and refined imagination, of which there is little trace either in the proud but surly visage of Van Dyck's drawn portrait or in the various documents and writings that delineate Orazio's public biography.

Sixteenth- and seventeenth-century Italian writers were more open than we tend to be to the paradoxical relationship that sometimes exists between art and the public persona of its creator. They lived in a world of social tensions held together by hierarchies, a world in which individuals were skilled at constructing public masks and where appearances did not necessarily reflect reality. Van Dyck's portrait drawing of Orazio presents one such mask: Orazio Gentileschi as painter at the court of Charles I. The drawing reflects as much of his true character as the letter he addressed to Grand Duke Ferdinand II of Tuscany, in an attempt to solicit a position at the Florentine court. In the letter, Orazio adopts the conventional language expected of an artist, promoting himself as one who has always been in service to grand princes. He abases himself as unworthy of the grand duke's favor. He is "your most humble servant" ("suo humilissimo"), with only a "feeble talent" ("fiacco talento"). The picture he is sending the grand duke as an example of that talent is of little merit ("poco merito"), but Ferdinand will, he is certain, receive it as a sign of his devotion and because it is, after all, a product of the genius of one of his vassals ("quanto nasca dall'ingegno delli suoi vassali")—someone who had been born in Tuscany and proudly signed his name "Florentinus."[11]

If this letter reveals someone adept at negotiating the complicated social hierarchies on which his well-being depended, Gentileschi's art suggests regions of feeling and sensitivity that have left no written record and that were perhaps not much visible even to his colleagues and neighbors. His touching depictions of the Madonna and child (cat. nos. 8, 15) or of Saint Francis succored by an angel (cat. nos. 6, 21), his sparkling landscape settings (cat. 27), his radiant altarpieces showing miraculous visions (cat. nos. 25, 30), and his somber description of the Crucifixion (cat. 29) give indications of a capacity for tenderness and affection, a response to beauty—whether of nature, a young woman, or a helpless infant—and a sense of human tragedy and sorrow. If the subjects seem conventional, the terms of expression have a disarming directness, derived from their means of presentation. For Orazio's art is based on the Caravaggesque practice of painting directly from the model, and his models were the people he knew in his everyday life. It is through this intersection of life and art that, from time to time, his paintings seem to take on the character of a personal disclosure or confession.

GENTILESCHI, CARAVAGGIO, AND THE RIVALRIES OF PAINTING

Orazio's encounter with Caravaggio in the summer of 1600 was the central event of his life. Prior to the unveiling of Caravaggio's canvases showing the calling and martyrdom of Saint Matthew (fig. 4) in the French national church of San Luigi dei Francesi, which created a sensation by making the Lombard artist's work publicly visible for the first time, Orazio had painted in a style that was predicated on compromise and accommodation. His figures were types, his compositions conventional; his color was slack. There is a blandness, an anonymity, and a disturbing lack of conviction to his work of the 1590s that comes as a shock to those who know only his distinctive, post-Caravaggesque pictures. Small wonder that Guicciardini, in the report he sent back to Florence, pointedly omitted any mention of those paintings done before 1600, as though they were irrelevant to a proper appraisal of the artist's achievement (as, indeed, they are).[12]

The work of Caravaggio demanded a rethinking of the relationship between artist and model, the imagined and the real, the

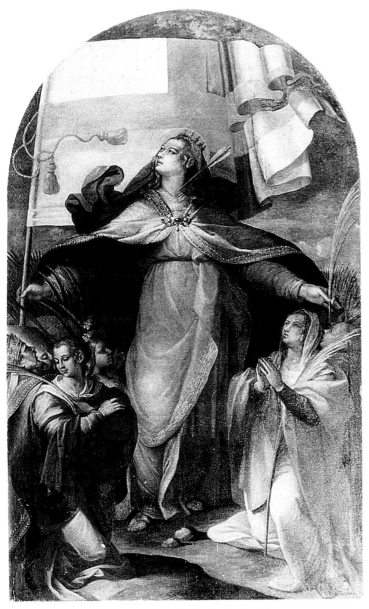

Figure 2. Orazio Gentileschi, *Triumph of Saint Ursula*. Oil on canvas. Benedictine Abbey, Farfa

painter and his artifact. In the critical language of the day, it opposed truth, or *il vero,* to verisimilitude *(verosimile),* by which ordinary experience was transposed into the exemplary and ideal.[13] It discarded the twin pillars of Renaissance painting, *invenzione* and *disegno,* by which imagination was prized over observation: "He claimed he imitated his models so closely that he never made a single brushstroke which he called his own, but said rather that it was nature's. Repudiating all other rules, he considered the highest achievement not to be bound to art," declared Bellori of Caravaggio.[14] It took Orazio the better part of a decade before he

dared to fully embrace this new dynamic. But when he did so, it was with a directness that none of Caravaggio's other followers could match. Indeed, as Longhi pointed out in 1916, in his seminal study of the artist, Orazio's work is actually more faithful to the model—more *vero*–than Caravaggio's, where the interpretive factor—the transformation of the everyday into the extraordinary and dramatic—is far greater.

Orazio arrived in Rome from his native Tuscany when he was still a boy, perhaps no more than thirteen. He lived with an uncle who was a captain of the guards in the Castel Sant'Angelo, taking from him his adopted name, Gentileschi (his family name was Lomi, which Artemisia used when she returned to Florence). We do not know from whom he received his training. Baglione states that his older brother, Aurelio Lomi (1556–1623), introduced him to the craft of painting, but this may be biographical invention. By the end of the 1580s, Orazio had managed to join the team of artists who, under Pope Sixtus V (r. 1585–90), decorated the Biblioteca Sistina in the Vatican and the nave walls of Santa Maria Maggiore. His contribution to the first is a matter of conjecture,[15] but for the great fifth-century Roman basilica he painted a pedestrian fresco of the Purification in the Temple that opens the cycle on the north wall. In 1596, he worked for the Benedictine order at San Paolo fuori le Mura, for which he provided an altarpiece of the Conversion of Saint Paul (destroyed by fire in 1823). Typically, Baglione says he obtained the commission by stealth, at the expense of a colleague. This, in turn, led to his commission to decorate two chapels at the ancient Benedictine abbey at Farfa, in the Sabine hills outside Rome (fig. 2).[16] The resulting frescoes and altarpieces, the products of collaboration, are of a qualitative level that can only be described as dismal, though it is in their lack of commitment to stylishness that their promise lies (see cat. 1).

Orazio did not lack work. Sometime after August 1597—possibly on the strength of his Tuscan birth—he was contracted to decorate a chapel for Filippo and Angelo Fiorenzuola, in San Giovanni dei Fiorentini, the church of the Florentine community in Rome. (He painted only the vault and entrance arch before abandoning or subcontracting the project.)[17] Then, virtually at the same time, he made a monumental figure of Saint Thomas in the transept of San Giovanni in Laterano[18]—part of Pope Clement VIII's (r. 1592–1605) vast scheme to decorate the basilica for the Jubilee celebrations of 1600—carried out four angels in the cupola of the Madonna dei Monti, and frescoed the tribune of the early medieval church of

San Nicola in Carcere, Rome, for Clement VIII's powerful nephew, Cardinal Pietro Aldobrandini (1572–1621). (The decoration in San Nicola is described in its cultural context in Zuccari, p. 42.)

By 1600, Orazio had carved out for himself a modest niche in the busy artistic world of Clementine Rome. His decision to become a follower of Caravaggio can only be termed unexpected and bold: he had a wife and four children and was thirty-seven—by far the oldest painter to associate himself with Caravaggio (by comparison, Orazio Borgianni was twenty-six in 1600, Carlo Saraceni about twenty-one, and Bartolomeo Manfredi—the key figure for the next generation of Caravaggesque painters—perhaps twenty). Moreover, because Caravaggesque painting was so little suited to fresco practice—to the kind of large-scale, decorative commissions that had, until then, sustained him—Orazio would have not only to transform his style but to refocus his career (though he continued to paint frescoes when suitable commissions came his way). All of which underscores the degree of his commitment to the new dynamic, with its emphasis on painting from the model.

An association with Caravaggio carried with it certain liabilities, as the Lombard artist had a notoriously volatile temperament and incited rivalry. (We know from the seventeenth-century biographer of Florentine artists, Filippo Baldinucci, that Cigoli allowed himself to get dragged to cheap trattorias with Caravaggio and his circle simply to avoid causing offense.)[19] Orazio, who shared studio props with Caravaggio, was immediately caught up in this bohemian life, in which a key figure was his near contemporary as well as future biographer, Giovanni Baglione (ca. 1566–1643). Baglione was an artist of far greater facility than Orazio and in the 1590s had risen to the top of his profession. His superficial brand of Caravaggism serves to throw Orazio's into clear relief.

At San Giovanni in Laterano, Orazio was assigned a single apostle, while Baglione painted one of the principal narrative scenes, carrying it out with great panache. He was clearly someone to watch, and his frescoes of the life of the Virgin in Santa Maria del Orto, in Trastevere (fig. 3), seem to have attracted the attention of Caravaggio himself. In his scene of the Presentation of the Virgin in the Temple, Baglione consigns the main subject to the background and fills the foreground with an enormous, plumed figure in contemporary dress—one very much like the dandies of Caravaggio's early paintings of fortune-tellers and cardsharps. The group of scantily clad beggars exemplifies the work of an ambitious artist who transforms an unpromising subject into a virtuoso display of his mastery of the nude. The fresco advertised the critical elements of *invenzione* and *varietà* (compositional invention and variety) by emphasizing *difficoltà* and *fantasia*. There can be little doubt that when, in his *Martyrdom of Saint Matthew* (fig. 4), Caravaggio inserted a group of nude male figures in the foreground, he was responding to precisely this sort of challenge. (Recent scholarship has identified the figures as neophytes. But while this may be so, the primary reason for including them was a desire on the part of Caravaggio to enter into the fray of artistic competition and, more specifically, to outdo a rival by the novelty of his dramatic lighting and the revolutionary naturalism of his figures.)

A competition was set in motion, one that involved not only artistic principles and reputation, but patrons. In 1601 or 1602, Caravaggio painted for Vincenzo Giustiniani a canvas depicting "a laughing Cupid who shows his contempt for the world, which lies at his feet in the guise of various instruments, crowns, scepters, and armor" (Gemäldegalerie, Berlin).[20] In direct competition with this picture—whose fame was celebrated by two madrigals written by Gaspare Murtola—Baglione painted a canvas showing Earthly Love subjected by Divine Love. He dedicated the picture to Cardinal Benedetto Giustiniani, the brother of Caravaggio's patron. Furthermore, at a public exhibition held on August 29, 1602, at San Giovanni Decollato to celebrate the feast day of John the Baptist, Baglione directed that his picture be hung opposite a painting by Gentileschi of the archangel Saint Michael (lost). Incensed at this obvious attempt to outclass him, Orazio confronted Baglione and criticized his picture for the incorrect manner in which he had depicted Divine Love—adult and in armor instead of young and nude. Baglione thereupon painted a second version. Both paintings found their way into Cardinal Giustiniani's collection (they are now in the Gemäldegalerie, Berlin, and the Galleria Nazionale d'Arte Antica, Rome), and Baglione was decorated by the prelate with a gold chain, thereby upstaging both Caravaggio and Orazio.

The culminating chapter of this rivalry came in 1603, when Baglione's enormous and coveted commission for an altarpiece, in the Gesù, of the Resurrection (destroyed, but known from a *modello* in the Louvre, Paris) was unveiled. The dramatic use of light and the dark and boldly sprawling seminude soldiers in the

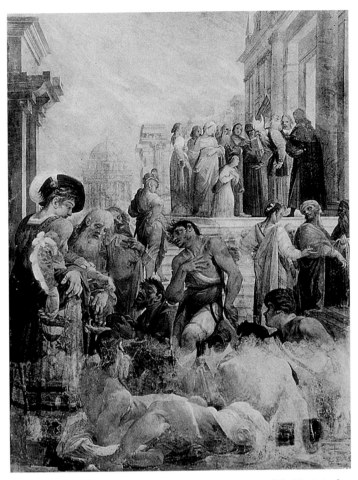

Figure 3. Giovanni Baglione (ca. 1566–1643), *Presentation of the Virgin in the Temple*. Fresco. Santa Maria del Orto, Rome

style—one of far greater modernity than those of either Borgianni or Saraceni. He was a slow, methodical worker, and his first experiments in a Caravaggesque idiom (cat. nos. 2, 3) show how painful the process of transformation was. Whether he could have become a successful popularizer of Caravaggism, in the manner of Bartolomeo Manfredi (bapt. 1582–1622), is doubtful. There is no evidence that he tried. Caravaggism was for him the means by which he made painting a vehicle of personal expression. It is this which makes Gentileschi's achievement so remarkable.

Unlike some of Caravaggio's followers, Orazio was also open to the more classicizing ideals promoted by Annibale Carracci (1557–1602) and his pupils. This is particularly evident in the pictures he carried out in the years immediately following Caravaggio's flight from Rome in May 1606 (see, especially, cat. nos. 12, 13). In March of that year, we in fact find him co-witnessing the will of the Mannerist sculptor Tommaso della Porta (1546–1606) together with Annibale Carracci and Annibale's pupil Giovan Antonio Solari (ca. 1581–1666). At the very least this document establishes an acquaintanceship beyond that of Caravaggio's circle and implies the personal relationships which stand behind the vein of Bolognese classicism that informs some of Gentileschi's most elegant compositions.

During Orazio's last years in Rome, around 1617–21, the physician and amateur art critic Giulio Mancini (1558–1630) described the outstanding artists of the day; Mancini placed Orazio not among Caravaggio's followers, but with those artists "who, possessing valor in their profession, have worked in their own manner and, in particular, without following in the footsteps of anyone else."[22] In other words, Orazio, having laboriously worked through the principles of Caravaggesque painting, went on to develop his own style, which Mancini singled out for its "good color and understanding" ("buon colorito e sapere"). These are not terms that say much today. Understanding, or "sapere," referred to a general mastery indicating knowledge about the art of painting. It is a term Mancini used to describe artists whose only trait in common was the sort of conspicuous display that connoisseurs ("gl'intendenti") could easily recognize. The second term, "buon colorito," meant, literally, a good sense of color.[23] However, it carried a reference to Venetian art and the implication of naturalism. In the entry for *colorito* in his *Vocabulario toscano dell'arte del disegno*, Baldinucci discusses the scientific relation of color to light—something that would be very apropos to Orazio's

foreground were recognizable allusions to and criticisms of Caravaggio's *Martyrdom of Saint Matthew*. A campaign of slander was launched against the work by Caravaggio and his cronies, leading to the libel suit noted earlier. Baglione, through it all, retained intact his Mannerist-based style. Caravaggism was, for him, merely a modish veneer, to be applied like makeup in accordance with the latest fashion. His real commitment was to the artistic establishment, and it is with some irony that, in the fall of 1606, we find him going to court to denounce two of Caravaggio's followers, Orazio Borgianni (1574–1616) and Carlo Saraceni (ca. 1579–1620), who had tried, unsuccessfully, to stage a takeover of the Accademia di San Luca and incited, into the bargain, a physical attack on Baglione, then president of the academy.[21]

Orazio's commitment to Caravaggio's revolutionary style was of a different order from Baglione's fashionable trappings. In it he sought a naturalistic foundation on which to build a personal art but which is probably not what Mancini had in mind. For him "buon colorito" stood in contrast to both Mannerist and Caravaggesque practice. The first emphasized washed-out, arbitrary colors. The second obtained striking effects by an unnaturalistically focused light. Guercino, Reni, Domenichino, and Passignano are all praised by Mancini for their "colorito." Reni's work, with its combination of compositional elegance and strength of color and its tendency to treat movement as a component of formal arrangement, was to provide an important example for Orazio (see cat. 12). Curiously, Mancini lets pass without comment Orazio's use of the model—his "osservanza del naturale." Yet this was the single factor that had transformed his work and on which his vision of painting was predicated.

ORAZIO'S STUDIO AND PAINTING FROM THE MODEL

Thanks to the testimony given at the rape trial in 1612–13, it is possible to sketch an image of what Orazio's studio was like in these crucial years. He moved three times between 1610 and 1613, but only the last move took him out of the popular neighborhood that lies between the church of Santa Maria del Popolo and the Piazza di Spagna, where he had lived for fifteen years. Until sometime after March 20, 1610, his house had been on what is today via del Babuino, next to the Greek church of San Atanasio. It had a room to the right as one entered, where he painted and met visitors; the private quarters on the left were kept scrupulously closed. The house on via Margutta, where he lived until April 1612,

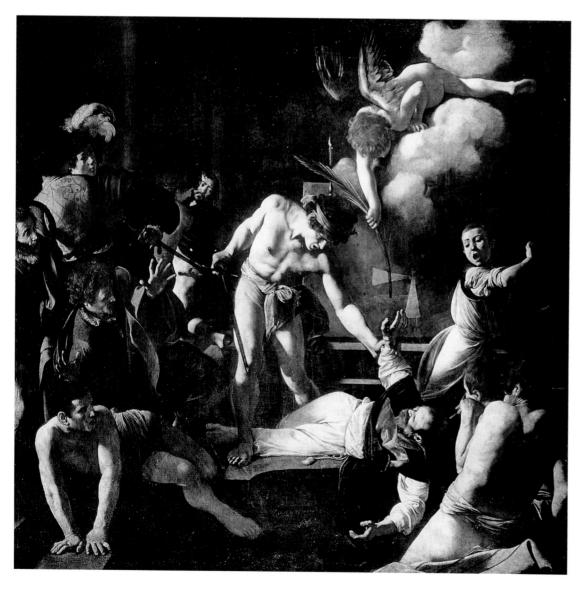

Figure 4. Michelangelo Merisi da Caravaggio (1571–1610), *Martyrdom of Saint Matthew*. Oil on canvas. San Luigi dei Francesi, Rome

when he moved to via della Croce, near the Piazza di Spagna, seems to have been larger, with a more elaborate layout. Visitors passed through a hall closed by a grille. There was a room in which laundry was done, a courtyard, and a double flight of stairs leading to the main quarters on the second floor. There were two rooms, the first of which was used as a kitchen/dining area, while the second, with two windows overlooking the street, served as Orazio's studio. The bedrooms on the floor above for Orazio, Artemisia, her three brothers, and, for a time, Orazio's nephew, were kept closed against a constant flow of visitors. Among these were Orazio's various hired models: a seventy-three-year-old pilgrim from Palermo named Giovanni Molli; Orazio's barber of twenty years, Bernardino Franchi; an apprentice named Francesco; and his tailor's wife, Costanza Ceuli, who would bring her children to be drawn. This assortment of neighborhood denizens presented quite a different cast of characters from the well-proportioned, athletic youths brought in as models at the academy. As might be expected, clients too paid visits: the agent of the duke of Mantua, the banker Settimio Olgiati (for whose chapel in Santa Maria della Pace Orazio provided the altarpiece; cat. 11), and some Theatine priests. There could be no greater contrast than that between these makeshift, crowded quarters and the spacious rooms and large studio the duke of Buckingham outfitted for Orazio and his three sons at York House, in London, sixteen years later. (It was there that the German painter and writer Joachim von Sandrart saw him at work on a number of canvases in 1628.)

Costanza Ceuli, who, as we have seen, lived next door to the Gentileschi household on via della Croce, seems to have spent a good deal of her day watching the activities of her artist-neighbor, though she never saw him paint. Orazio's oldest son, Francesco, ground colors and must have stretched and primed canvases as well. When, together with Agostino Tassi, Orazio was commissioned, in 1611, to decorate the Casino delle Muse for Scipione Borghese and an apartment in the Palazzo del Quirinale, he hired a former apprentice of Tassi's, Nicolò Bedino, to work for him. Costanza saw Nicolò in the courtyard drawing water from the well and grinding colors, but he also ran errands—shopping for meals, making the beds, and carrying the all-important cartoons required for the casino frescoes. According to Nicolò, Orazio worked on the cartoons at night and on feast days. When Orazio was away working, Artemisia instructed Nicolò in drawing.

Orazio must have been one of the very few artists who had observed Caravaggio working. As already noted, the two artists shared props—most famously a pair of wings and a Capuchin habit—and it stands to reason that Orazio must have seen how Caravaggio worked from the posed model. Just what was involved emerges from the testimony of Giovanni Molli, the pilgrim from Palermo whom Orazio employed to pose for a number of pictures, but most particularly for a full-length *Saint Jerome* (cat. 16). For this work, Molli stripped to the waist and assumed a position he could hold over an extended period of time. "He kept me in the house all during Lent, and three or four days a week I had to go to his house. Some days I would go and stay from morning to night, and I ate and drank in his house, and he paid me by the day, and I returned to my own house to sleep." During the times that Orazio's barber served as a model he came not once every week, as was his wont, but four or five times a day, "because many times he used me as a model."

The barber met Molli on some of his visits and gives a description of him that demonstrates how closely reality and imaginative reconstruction were made to intersect in the *Saint Jerome*: "Handsome in appearance, with a face like that of Saint Paul, bald-headed, hair turned white, with a fine thick beard that is as heavy on the cheeks as in the beard itself."

We might imagine the dark-haired youth in the *Executioner with the Head of Saint John the Baptist* (cat. 20) as Francesco Scarpellino, described by one witness at the trial as "an ugly type with long black hair, whom they said they used on occasion as a model for some paintings." The model for the *David Contemplating the Head of Goliath* (cat. 18), with his tan neck and hands, seems another of these characters—perhaps a porter. The short-haired, bearded, middle-aged model for Holofernes' head in the painting *Judith and Her Maidservant* in Oslo (cat. 13) also posed for the *David Slaying Goliath* in Dublin (cat. 12). Was this Orazio's barber? If so, then he also sat for Artemisia in her own *Judith Slaying Holofernes* (cat. 55)—this would have been before Orazio moved across the Tiber, in the summer of 1611.

Not surprisingly, we hear almost nothing about female models, though Orazio certainly employed them. In Britain, he listed both female and male models—"modelli tanto di femine quanto di huomini"—in the account of expenses he submitted to Sir Dudley Carleton, Lord Dorchester,[24] but a stigma was attached to any woman willing to submit herself to the prying scrutiny of an artist. The poor but honorable woman who modeled as the Madonna for Caravaggio found herself denounced to her mother by a suitor. (Typically, Caravaggio got even with the man by attacking him in Piazza Navona.)[25] While Costanza Ceuli was comfortable testifying that she had allowed her children to be drawn, she may have felt reluctant to confess to having herself posed. Yet a neighbor clearly sat for Orazio, nursing her baby, for the Bucharest *Madonna and Child* (cat. 15).

If posing clothed involved risks to a woman's reputation, what about posing nude? In her essay (pp. 262–81), Elizabeth Cropper makes an eloquent case for the shocking nature of Artemisia's self-presentation (if that is what it is) in the *Susanna and the Elders* of 1610 (cat. 51). What about the *Cleopatra* (cat. nos. 17, 53), the attribution of which has been much debated but which in the catalogue I argue was painted more or less contemporaneously by Orazio? This extraordinary picture—in which the female nude is treated with a boldness as shocking as that of Édouard Manet's *Olympia* of 1863—is key to our understanding of the way Caravaggesque painting from the model attacked the very roots of those idealizing conventions by which past and present, public and private, imagined and real were kept decorously apart. It is, therefore, of some interest whether seventeenth-century male artists in Rome painted from nude female models.[26] Certainly the rarity of the female nude in Caravaggesque painting might at first suggest that only artists with a classicizing bent, willing to base their depictions on Roman statues, could broach the theme. However, where sex can be easily bought—and the quarter where Orazio lived had a large population of prostitutes—female models cannot have been in short supply. During the trial the pigment dealer, Marc Antonio Coppino, brazenly asserted that Artemisa posed nude for her father.[27] Coppino was a witness for Tassi and probably part of the latter's plan at character assassination. Yet, the highly individualized features of the model for the *Cleopatra* recur in the richly attired woman holding a fan in Orazio's frescoes in the Casino delle Muse (frontispiece, p. 282). Based on its resemblance to a later engraving and portrait medal of Artemisia (fig. 95), that figure has long been identified as showing Orazio's daughter (see cat. 39). Whether or not Artemisia actually posed for the *Cleopatra*—and we might well doubt she would have done so—the fact that both father and daughter were producing paintings of naturalistic female nudes must have fueled the flames of circulating rumors. Following the trial, the

painting may well have become something of a firebrand and Orazio may have chosen not to market it in Rome, considering it first as a gift to the grand duke of Tuscany and eventually selling it, together with Artemisia's *Lucretia* (cat. 67), to a Genoese client, Pietro Gentile.[28]

In all respects, painting *dal naturale*—with a posed model—was a different proposition from the normal manner of working from drawings and the imagination, with only occasional reference to models. Annibale Carracci drew incessantly from the model, but the idea of painting from one over a period of some forty days would have seemed excessive and even counterproductive to the effects he sought of a perfected reality, and it is hardly surprising that Orazio maintained this practice only for a few years and only for single-figure compositions.[29] That during this time he also decorated the Casino delle Muse (fig. 6) for Scipione Borghese and managed to adapt this system of working from the model to fresco practice is remarkable. We must, I think, imagine highly elaborate cartoons of individual figures that were done from multiple sittings, the model posed on a table or other raised surface, so that Orazio could study the effects of the low viewing point. (He must have used the same method in painting the angel in the *Vision of Saint Cecilia;* cat. 9). Each figure was then inserted, using a modified fresco, or *mezzo fresco*, technique into the architectural setting Tassi had created (done in *buon fresco*).[30] It is a system completely at odds with the idealizing approach of Cigoli and Guido Reni in the two companion casinos in the Borghese garden. Reni, like Cigoli, worked out his composition in drawings and concentrated his efforts on effects of rhythm, movement, and the distribution of color across the whole expanse. By comparison, Orazio's fresco appears a piecemeal affair, and the arresting naturalism of the parts (fig. 7) hardly compensates for the loss in overall unity. The sheer beauty of Reni's *Aurora* left little room for Orazio's approach to decoration, and he soon moved away from the radical naturalism of the preceding years. In his subsequent works, there is a greater emphasis on formal presentation, with a creative tension between the artifice of the composition and the naturalistic treatment of the parts.

The root of the problem was well characterized by Mancini. "This school," he wrote, referring to Caravaggio and his followers, "succeeds well with a single figure, but in the composition of a narrative and in interpreting feelings, which requires imagination rather than observation, it does not seem to me that [these artists] succeed by portraying a model who is always before them, it being impossible to represent a story by putting in a room lighted from a single window a multitude of men, each one having to laugh or cry or feign walking and [at the same time] keep still in order to be copied. And so the figures, while they possess strength [in execution], lack motion and expression and grace."[31]

An echo of this verdict was sounded by Guicciardini, the Florentine ambassador in Rome, when he was asked his opinion about Orazio's work. "He's a man who lacks proper design ["non ha disegno"], and is unable to compose a narrative or to draw a single figure well. . . . His worth is in his careful, not to say diligent, execution ["diligenza"], . . . and in making a head or even a half figure, he seems to the eye to work well, since he imitates the model or object in front of him."[32] If the strength of painting from nature is illustrated by Orazio's *David Contemplating the Head of Goliath* (cat. 18), in which an individual figure is shown close up and cut off at the calf, the curiously static *Saint Michael and the Devil* (cat. 14) demonstrates its weakness. The picture reads like fragments of posing sessions pieced together, and it is not difficult to understand why Orazio should have concentrated his efforts on shallow, compact, friezelike compositions rather than those requiring figures to be disposed in a carefully articulated interior space. The one exception is the magnificent *Annunciation* at Turin (cat. 43), in which he achieves a perfect balance between space, figure, and action and creates one of the masterpieces of seventeenth-century painting.

Not surprisingly, we find the same compositional weaknesses in many of Artemisia's early paintings. Nowhere is this more evident than in her dramatic *Judith Slaying Holofernes* (cat. 55), a work that has elicited much discussion, little of which takes into account the representational problem that confronted Artemisia but that she conspicuously did not resolve. It is Orazio's washerwoman who informs us that Orazio (and presumably Artemisia) painted his posed models behind closed doors, evidently protective of the act of painting. Nevertheless, he was eager to show the results to visitors, who must invariably have commented on the resemblance of the painted figure to the model. In the case of the *Judith Slaying Holofernes,* it is clear that the composition is based not on an action staged by three figures, but a kind of patchwork of three models separately posed. Only this can explain the lack of spatial clarity, the disparities of scale (conspicuous, above all, in the oversized fist of Holofernes juxtaposed with

the head of the servant Abra), and the unwieldy knot of outstretched limbs, which X radiographs demonstrate caused the young artist special difficulties. Artemisia's later treatment of the subject, in Detroit (cat. 69), subordinates the *verismo* of the individual parts to a fluid, overall design and is the more successful work.

Orazio had received a conventional training, and he probably never entirely abandoned the use of drawings in favor of painting from life, though no drawings can be ascribed to him with certainty.[33] (Was it Manfredi's experiments in the style of Caravaggio that spurred Orazio's experiments in painting exclusively from the model—so crucial to the formation of Artemisia's working method?)[34] Thus, Orazio's increased use of drawings, and possibly cartoons, after 1612/13 would not be unexpected. He must also have made studies of heads, which he gathered together as a sort of repertory. Molli's apostolic features reappear years later in the frescoed, half-length figures of Saints Anthony Abbot and Jerome in the cathedral of Fabriano, and then again in the *Abraham and Isaac* painted in Genoa (fig. 63). For his *Vision of Saint Francesca Romana* (cat. 30), Orazio seems to have found two models—a girl of perhaps fourteen and a child of eight or nine months—whose features captivated him. Preparatory drawings seem to have been made for the painting, perhaps oil sketches as well (see cat. 31). (The practice of using oil studies of heads was not unknown in the early seicento and was a commonplace with Rubens.) In any event, the same two figures recur in an altarpiece of problematic attribution—the *Madonna of the Rosary,* in the Pinacoteca at Fabriano—and the features of the older girl seem also to have shaped those of the Magdalene at the foot of the cross in the *Crucifixion* for San Venanzio (cat. 29). A similarly featured figure reappears as the Virgin in the *Annunciation* Orazio sent to Carlo Emanuele I, duke of Savoy, in 1623 (cat. 43). It is this practice of re-using earlier studies that makes any chronology of Orazio's work based on the resemblance of models problematic; it also distinguishes his work from that of Caravaggio.

ORAZIO'S PATRONS IN ROME

As we have seen, the first decade of Orazio's activity centered on the collaborative production of large fresco cycles. His conversion to the style of Caravaggio in the years following the unveiling in 1600 of the canvases of the *Calling* and the *Martyrdom of Saint Matthew* entailed refocusing his career—not a simple task for someone who was thirty-seven years old. Like all Caravaggesque artists, Orazio became principally a painter of canvases, with only incidental fresco commissions. Private collectors now outnumbered sponsors of public, ecclesiastical projects. Not much attention has been paid to the changes in strategy this necessitated, and only now can we begin to chart the network of patronage that Gentileschi built up, patronage that would eventually take him to the courts of Marie de' Medici and Charles I.

Some of the commissions on which Orazio worked in the 1590s had been sponsored by Clement VIII, and they had brought him to the attention of the cardinal-nephew, Pietro Aldobrandini. It was for Aldobrandini's church San Nicola in Carcere that he painted, according to Baglione, figures of God the Father, putti, and a kneeling saint (destroyed), replacing the medieval decorations in the tribune. Aldobrandini also sat to Orazio for his portrait (lost), and through him the artist must have come into contact with other potential patrons, such as Duke Mario Farnese and the rich Sannesi brothers, Clemente and Jacopo. It was for a confraternity in the duke's fiefdom of Farnese that, around 1607–8, Orazio painted an altarpiece of Saint Michael combating the Devil (cat. 14).

The Sannesi were much favored by Clement VIII, who in 1604 raised Jacopo to the cardinalate.[35] They enjoyed the special protection of Clement's cardinal-nephew; indeed, Clemente Sannesi was Aldobrandini's Maestro di Camera. In the early-seventeenth century, the Sannesi were busy decorating their villa/casino in Borgo Santo Spirito. Giovanni Lanfranco (1589–1647) furnished it with frescoes around 1606–8, and for it, according to Passeri, Clemente Sannesi acquired numerous ancient statues, "spending prodigally on its decoration . . . and especially on paintings." The brothers owned two masterpieces by Caravaggio—the first versions of the *Crucifixion of Saint Peter* and the *Conversion of Saint Paul,* both of which had been intended for the Cerasi chapel in Santa Maria del Popolo but were rejected by the friars (only the *Conversion of Saint Paul* survives, in the Odescalchi collection, Rome).[36] They also owned a fine copy of Caravaggio's *Cardsharps*. The 1724 inventory of their last heir, Anna Maria Sannesi, lists three works by Gentileschi, a *Madonna and Child*, a *David with the Head of Goliath*, and a *Saint George*. These were clearly deluxe works: the first two were painted on panel, a support Orazio rarely used, and the third was on copper. If two of them may be identified with paintings in the exhibition (cat. nos. 8, 20), then

Orazio must have been in touch with the Sannesi between around 1607 and 1612—that is, during his most Caravaggesque phase.

The Sannesi were no less favored by Paul V than they had been by Clement VIII, and their interest in Orazio suggests that, after Clement's death in 1605, he continued to draw his patrons from people closely connected with the pope. Presumably, this explains how he managed to receive four commissions for major altarpieces outside Rome and one in the city between about 1605 and 1608. The earliest was for a painting of the *Madonna in Glory with the Holy Trinity* for a Capuchin church outside Turin (fig. 5). Although no documents have been traced, the commission almost certainly originated with Carlo Emanuele I, duke of Savoy. Carlo was a promoter of the Capuchin order and in 1581 purchased the spectacular site for the church. He probably placed the commission through his ambassador in Rome, who could well have sought papal advice.[37] Orazio's sympathies for the Capuchin order have never been investigated, but it is a singular fact that he painted a number of images of Saint Francis, both in Rome and in London, where Henrietta Maria was a strong supporter of the order.

Another altarpiece, the *Circumcision* (cat. 7), was commissioned for a Jesuit church in Ancona. The patron, Giovanni Nappi, was a member of a prominent Marchigian family, and his son Filippo was rector of the church. Perhaps in commissioning the altarpiece Giovanni sought to ingratiate himself with Paul V, an ardent supporter of the Jesuits.[38] Certainly, there is evidence that during these years Giovanni was trying to curry favor with the pope, with a view to improving his landholdings in Ferrara— since 1598 part of the Papal States. To do this, he assisted Scipione Borghese in obtaining some of the celebrated paintings by Dosso Dossi (ca. 1486–1541/42) still in the Este castle at Ferrara, using his kinsman in Rome, Francesco Nappi, as a go-between. Interestingly, Scipione Borghese's collecting activity also involved Paolo Savelli, who was to become Orazio's single most important patron.[39]

A third commission came from a prominent banker in Rome, Settimio Olgiati, who in 1607 commissioned the *Baptism of Christ* (cat. 11) for his chapel in Santa Maria della Pace.[40] Settimio's uncle Bernardo Olgiati had been papal treasurer under Clement VIII and in 1587 had commissioned the Cavaliere d'Arpino (1568–1640) to decorate the family burial chapel in the ninth-century church of Santa Prassede. To construct that chapel, an older one, dedicated to John the Baptist, was destroyed. The dedication of the

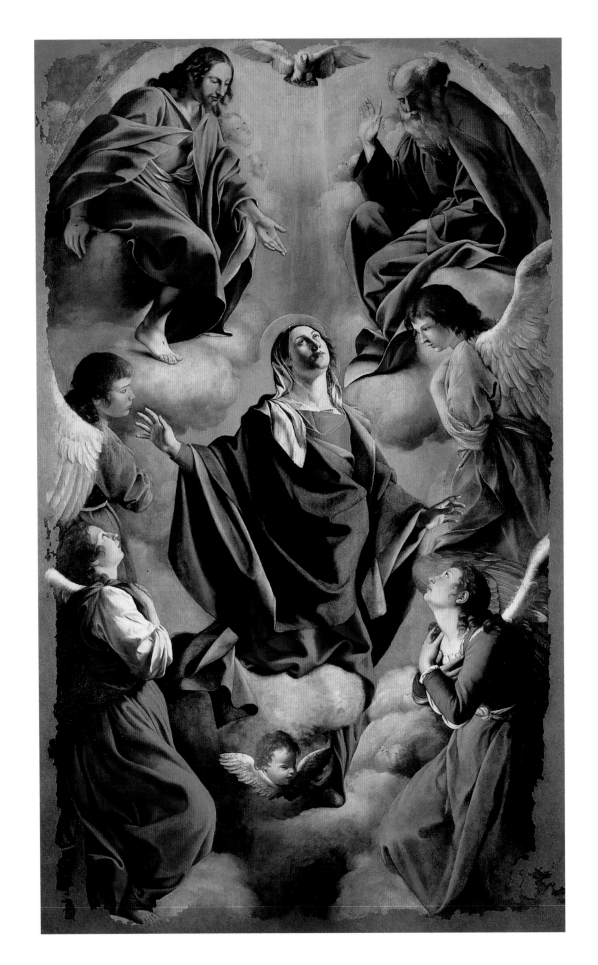

new chapel made amends for this destruction. Settimio appears to have been a man of taste. He hired the outstanding architect Carlo Maderno (1555/56–1629) to remodel his palace near the church of the Stimmate,[41] and according to Baglione, Onorio Longhi (1568–1619)—a companion of both Caravaggio and Orazio—designed the loggia for the Olgiati in Piazza Fiammetta. We get some idea of the kind of person we are dealing with from a notice in 1610 of Settimio's throwing a sumptuous banquet at his villa near the baths of Diocletian for the Spanish ambassador and his retinue. In 1612, it was the turn of Cardinals Montalto and del Monte.[42] Olgiati thus had contacts with the most cultured circles in Rome. He retained a keen interest in Orazio; he went to the artist's house on via Margutta to see his work in 1611, and in 1612 he visited Scipione Borghese's Casino delle Muse to view Gentileschi's frescoes then in progress.[43] Later sources mention two pictures by Orazio in the Olgiati collection: one of a saint and the other of the Madonna (described as hanging over a door). His commission of the *Baptism* provided Orazio a public forum in Rome.

The Olgiati were from Como, where they maintained a family chapel in the church of San Giovanni fuori le Mura, and it is possible that Settimio acted as intermediary in commissioning from Orazio the *Vision of Saint Cecilia* for the church of Saint Cecilia in Como (cat. 9).[44] The picture, installed by November 1607 (it is virtually contemporary with the *Baptism*), attracted the attention of no less a person than Cardinal Paolo Sfondrato, who visited the church shortly thereafter. Evidently, he expressed his opinion that Gentileschi, "with his valor walks in step with any of the more illustrious and famous painters in Rome." Given his patronage of Guido Reni, the remark takes on special resonance.

As we have seen, the opportunity to give a prominent, public demonstration of Gentileschi's talents came in 1611, when he was commissioned to carry out frescoes in the Palazzo del Quirinale of Paul V and in a garden casino belonging to Scipione Borghese (figs. 6, 7). The frescoes marked a new phase in his career, not simply for the wonderful attention given to pose, gesture, foreshortening, and light, but because they put him on equal footing with Cigoli and Reni. It may have been through Cigoli that

Orazio met Galileo Galilei (1564–1642), who was in Rome from the end of March to June 1611 to present his astronomical discoveries to the papal court. Cigoli was a close friend of the scientist and famously included Galileo's illustration of the surface of the moon in his depiction of the Immaculate Conception in the dome of the Pauline chapel in Santa Maria Maggiore.[45] We can, however, only speculate on whether Orazio's new interest in light and the naturalism of his landscapes might owe something to Galileo and his circle of friends, which—as Livia Carloni points out in her essay on Gentileschi's work in the Marches (p.124)—included the Fabrianese Francesco Stelluti.[46] In any event, both Orazio and Artemisia were later to appeal to Galileo for his support at the Florentine court. It remains unclear whether Scipione's patronage of Orazio extended beyond the frescoes in the casino; an eighteenth-century inventory of the Palazzo Borghese attributes seven pictures to him, but at least two are certainly incorrect.[47]

Scipione Borghese's patronage of Gentileschi clearly marked a watershed. It was possibly through him that Orazio was proposed to Pietro Campori, Scipione's secretary and majordomo, as the person best equipped to paint an altarpiece of the Magdalene for a small church in Fabriano (see cat. 24). This work may have served as Orazio's carte de visite for what became a highly profitable series of commissions in that Marchigian city (for an alternate view, see Carloni, pp. 121–23). But scarcely less important was the patronage of Paolo Savelli, a member of one of the old Roman baronial families.[48] Soprani is quite explicit about the importance of the Savelli in his generally well-informed 1674 biography of Gentileschi, stating that the artist first demonstrated his worth under Clement VIII and then acquired fame for his frescoes in the Palazzo del Quirinale and in the "delicious loggetta of Cardinal Borghese, and also in other paintings done for Prince Savelli and other notable men, for which his new manner of painting was admired not only in Rome but was sought after throughout Italy."[49]

A distinguished soldier, Prince Paolo Savelli (d. 1632) had accompanied Clement VIII to Ferrara in 1598, when the city was incorporated into the Papal States. He was sent to Hungary to assist Emperor Rudolf II in his battle against the Turks and, as a consequence, was promoted to governor of the papal armies in Bologna, Ferrara, and the Romagna by Paul V. In 1607, the pope raised the family's feudal holdings in Albano to a principality, whence Paolo's title. It was during this time that he was involved

Figure 5. Orazio Gentileschi, *Madonna in Glory with the Holy Trinity.* Oil on canvas. Museo Civico d'Arte Antica, formerly in Santa Maria al Monte dei Cappuccini, Turin

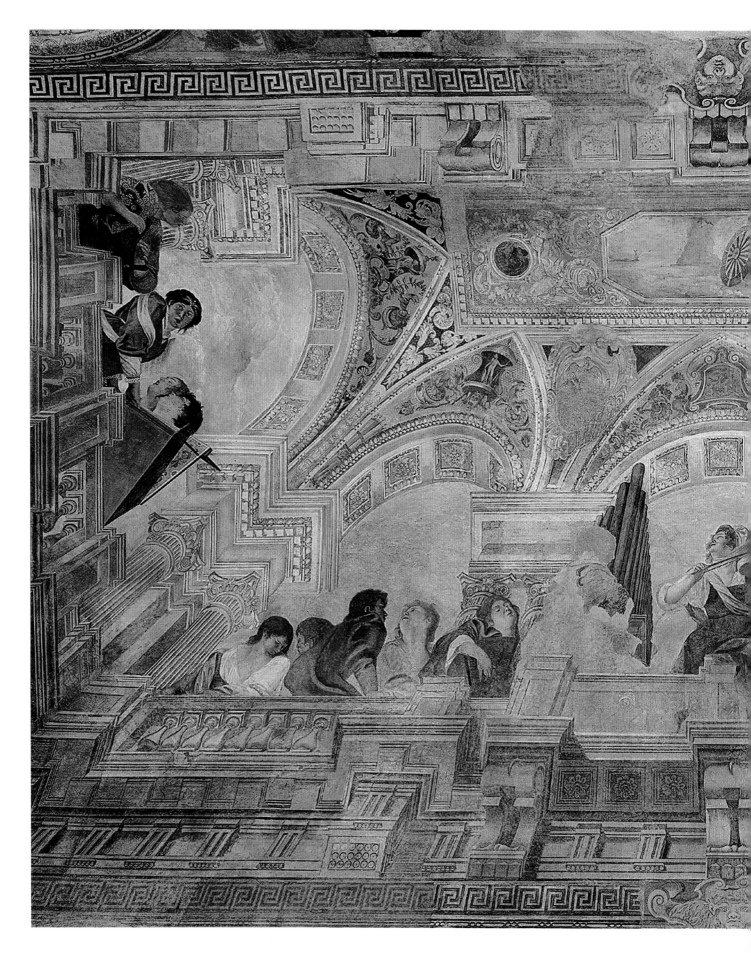

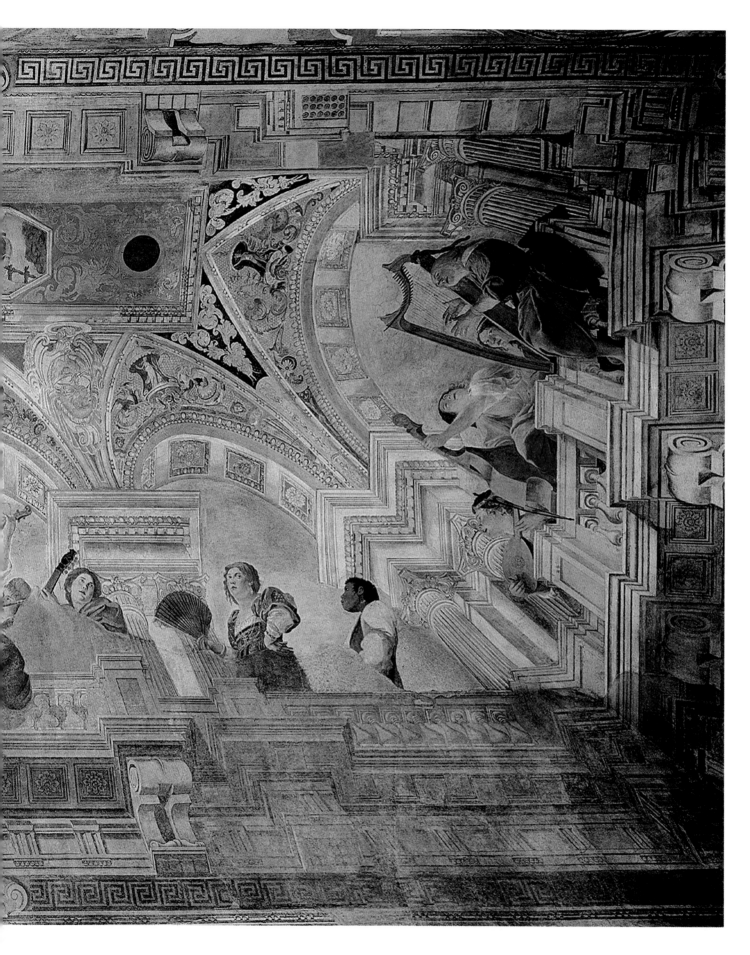

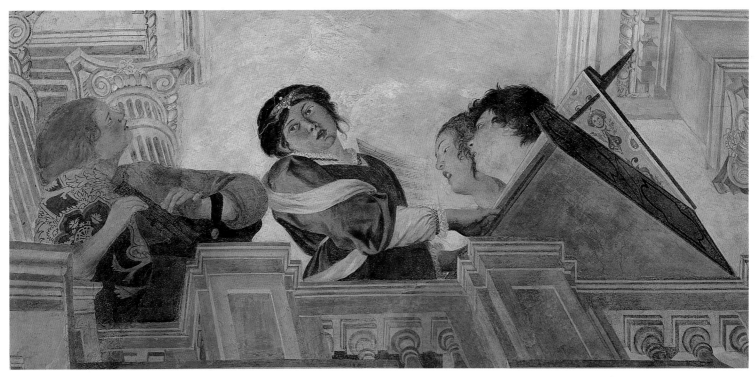

Pages 16–17: Figure 6. Orazio Gentileschi and Agostino Tassi (1578–1644), *A Musical Concert with Apollo and the Muses.* Fresco. Casino delle Muse, Palazzo Pallavicini-Rospigliosi, Rome

Figure 7. Detail of figure 6

with Scipione Borghese's schemes to acquire the works by Dosso Dossi in Ferrara. The climax of his political career came in 1620, when, as imperial ambassador to the pope, he made a magnificent ceremonial entrance into Rome with thirty-six carriages, "benissimo adornati."[50]

Paolo's brothers Federigo and Giulio also enjoyed distinguished careers. Federigo was his brother's coadjutor in Emilia and succeeded Paolo as field marshal of the Church. Like Paolo, he had profited from his time in Ferrara by purchasing paintings by Dosso Dossi, Garofalo (1481–1559), Scarsellino (ca. 1550–1620), and other Ferrarese and Venetian artists.[51] Giulio, destined for an ecclesiastical career, served as governor of Ancona from 1608 to 1610. Paul V elevated him to cardinal in 1615 and the following year appointed him bishop of Ancona. Traditionally, the Savelli had charge of the tribune of the Corte Savella, where the 1612 rape trial was held, and it is of some interest that we first hear of Orazio's association with the family the year after the case was settled, when at an October meeting at the Accademia di San Luca he is cited as in the employ of the Savelli and "outside Rome" ("fora di Roma").[52] Whether, as seems to me most likely,

he was working for the Savelli at one of their estates—Ariccia, for example—or whether he was on his way to Fabriano, possibly on the occasion of the transport of his painting of the Magdalene for the Università dei Cartai, cannot be ascertained (again, see Carloni's somewhat different analysis of the situation in her essay).[53] In 1614 and 1615, there are payments to him by the Savelli, and when Pietro Guicciardini wrote to Grand Duke Cosimo II of Tuscany in Florence, in March 1615, he specified that Orazio "is supported by and staying in the residence of Prince Savelli."[54] Guicciardini then added, "And if my Most Serene Master wishes, I know that the prince would most willingly send him, and the same Gentileschi would most willingly come. But concerning the excellence of his paintings, you have heard what I have to say." As we have seen, Guicciardini was no admirer of Orazio's work, and for this reason it is important to underscore that his opinion had been solicited because the artist's reputation as "one of the most excellent and famous painters to be found in Rome" had reached the ears of the grand duke.[55] Orazio's work for the Savelli capped his Roman career. Their patronage may be linked to the profitable employment he found in Fabriano, and it seems—as

Soprani implies—to have been Savelli's pictures that impressed Giovan Antonio Sauli when he came to Rome in 1621, following the election of Pope Gregory XV (r. 1621–23), and invited Orazio to come to Genoa.

GENTILESCHI, DOSSO DOSSI, AND VENETIAN PAINTING

What did Orazio paint for the Savelli, and what was the impact of his residence in their palace? First and foremost, Orazio owed to Savelli patronage the altarpiece of the stigmatization of Saint Francis for their chapel in San Silvestro in Capite (cat. 25)—one of his most individual and arresting compositions and only his second post-Caravaggesque public altarpiece in Rome. (Why, unlike his colleague Carlo Sarceni, Orazio received so few ecclesiastical commissions in Rome remains problematic.) But the bulk of the work, carried out for Paolo, consisted of gallery pictures for family palaces and villas. When the various inventories are collated, we find no fewer than twelve pictures, among which is the powerful *Christ Crowned with Thorns* (cat. 23) and small, precious works in an Elsheimer-like mode done on copper.[56] We do not know whether it was during the time Orazio was employed by the Savelli or immediately after that he worked in Fabriano (it cannot be ascertained how long his residence with them lasted). Nor is it at all clear whether Giulio's position as bishop of Ancona played a part in his commissions in the Marches (Fabriano was under the bishopric of Camerino, not Ancona).[57] However, it is during this time that Orazio's work acquires a new compositional refinement (Mancini's "sapere") and an unmatched handling of light and color ("buon colorito"), and we may well ask whether the Savelli' paintings by Dosso Dossi, Garofalo, and Scarsellino—not to mention those ascribed to Titian and Giorgione—played a part in this final transformation of Orazio's previous, Caravaggesque practice.[58]

Two Savelli commissions brought Gentileschi's work into direct—and probably intentional—competition with Dosso. One was a collaborative painting for a (lost) still life of fruits and flowers with three children—the only still life of which we have any record—which would have made an interesting comparison with the painting of birds and animals by Dosso listed in the Savelli inventory of 1610. (A similar collaborative work with two children is currently ascribed to Bartolomeo Cavarozzi [ca. 1590–1625] and an anonymous still-life painter).[59] The other was for a

sibyl (possibly cat. 33). The latter picture not only had a direct counterpart in a picture by Dosso—was it conceivably the marvelous painting in the Hermitage (fig. 8)?—but was accompanied by paintings of sibyls by Reni and Domenichino (see fig. 61). Then there was the *Adam and Eve* by Orazio—a subject difficult to imagine him treating but conceivably set in a landscape "alla veneziana." A listing in the inventories of a picture of "a figure who plays the lute, by Giorgione,"[60] brings to mind Orazio's *Lute Player* (cat. 22), about which we know only that it belonged to a Bolognese family, but which is deeply indebted to Venetian art and was perhaps painted during the time Orazio was a resident in the Savelli palace (the Savelli had close ties with Bologna). Paolo's patronage serves as a reminder that the character of Orazio's art depended on more than his contacts with artists in Rome; it was shaped as well by the taste of those for whom he worked.

In his seminal article on Orazio and Artemisia Gentileschi of 1916, Longhi reaffirmed his view that Caravaggio was the key figure of seventeenth-century European painting. He saw Orazio's place in this early history of modernism as a sort of middle term

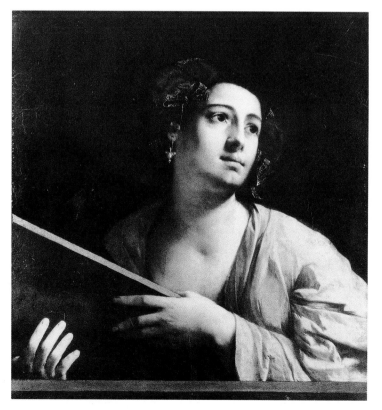

Figure 8. Dosso Dossi (ca. 1486–1541/42), *Sibyl*. Oil on canvas. The State Hermitage Museum, Saint Petersburg

between Caravaggio's early, Giorgionesque genre painting and the sunlit interiors of Johannes Vermeer's (1632–1675) scenes of domestic life.[61] Longhi emphasized the quotidian dimension of Orazio's paintings: his tendency, in a work such as the *Vision of Saint Cecilia* (cat. 9), to subordinate the religious subject matter and to "essentially realize a study of an interior in all its truthfulness as a calm, filtered, luminous container." "It is a fact," he declared, "that to find another case in which the pictorial necessities of giving truthful actuality to the setting brings an artist to such a strange, uncomfortable combination of a scene at once religious, mundane, and aristocratic, we would have to turn to Vermeer and his curious and perfectly Gentileschian *Allegory of Faith*" (Metropolitan Museum of Art, New York).[62]

This aspect of his art—what I have termed the intersection of life with art through his use of models—Orazio owed in large part to his encounter with Caravaggio. But Longhi then went on to point out that, in a work such as the *Vision of Saint Francesca Romana* (cat. 30), Orazio also became the first practitioner of what he christened "pittura di valori," by which he meant painting based, in the first place, on relationships of color, light, and form—the basis, as he saw it, of all of modern painting down to Claude Monet and Auguste Renoir. "Ordinarily I am not much predisposed, as so many others, to let photographs do the speaking!" teased Longhi rhetorically. "But in this case we are faced with such a clear and evident license for beauty that it is perhaps not worth the trouble to speak. Unless it is to say something not subtle but strong and resolute—as an affirmation. And that is that this work in Fabriano [where the *Saint Francesca Romana* altarpiece then was] is one of the first things to succeed on the basis of *valori* [values], instead of colors. Meaning that not since some hints in the work of [Lorenzo] Lotto and in Caravaggio's *Lute Player,* in the Liechtenstein Gallery, had one seen a work so complex, in which the loom of style, art's interweaving, was achieved not by the juxtaposition of areas of color, as in Venetian painting of the early cinquecento, but by a scaled relationship of quantities of light and color, quantities that, precisely because they are scaled, become qualities of art—*valori*."[63]

About Orazio's career, too little was known at the time Longhi wrote to indicate how and when the artist had attained this remarkable synthesis of light and color. In his search for antecedents, Longhi pointed to a picture then given to Caravaggio but which has since been recognized as one of Orazio's masterpieces—the Liechtenstein *Lute Player* (cat. 22), a work whose affinities with Giorgionesque painting as well as the early work of the Lombard master we have already noted. Longhi may have erred in his attribution, but he was surely correct to see Orazio as the greatest poet of light in seventeenth-century Italy. (Readers of the catalogue entries will note that I have taken as my guide to the dating of Orazio's paintings his early mastery of Caravaggesque lighting and his subsequent transformation of that heritage into something based on observation rather than artifice.) Is it too much to suggest that the Ferrarese and Venetian paintings in the collections of Scipione Borghese and, most particularly, the Savelli provided Gentileschi with the impetus to combine the dramatic, focused light of Caravaggesque painting with Venetian *colore* as the basis for a new kind of painting based on a marvelously nuanced response to *luce*?[64] This remarkable achievement is at the core of his art. What saves the gesticulating women of Pharaoh's court in the *Finding of Moses* (cat. 48) from rhetorical hollowness is a Veronesian sense of ceremonial splendor and an unmatched description of light playing across satin fabrics. It is easy to see why Longhi should have viewed this work as a precursor to Vermeer.

MARKETING SUCCESS

From a relatively early moment in Orazio's career as a Caravaggesque artist he began to market compositions, or *invenzioni*, in multiple versions. Among the earliest was a natural-seeming *Madonna and Child*, one version of which is in Bucharest (cat. 15). Variants of the picture are known from copies (fig. 47), as well as from a report written by Bartolommeo Pellini, the duke of Mantua's representative in Rome, to Giovanni Magno, secretary to Duke Vincenzo Gonzaga in Mantua. (It was Giovanni Magno who had viewed Caravaggio's *Death of the Virgin* [Louvre, Paris] with Peter Paul Rubens prior to its purchase by the duke.) "The child is no more than one month old," Pellini noted, "so one can see that naturalism is a very good thing."[65] Pellini's remarks testify to a real appreciation of Gentileschi's Caravaggesque naturalism and explain the demand for copies and variants.

A year later, Orazio seems to have replicated his striking image of Saint Jerome based on the Palermo pilgrim Giovanni Molli (cat. 16); a second version is known from photographs. The roughly contemporary *David Contemplating the Head of Goliath* (cat. 18) was repeated on a reduced scale, with another landscape setting and the giant's head placed differently (cat. 19). However, none of these repetitions is adequate preparation for the far more extensive recycling of compositions that followed Orazio's move to Genoa, Paris, and London: the *Lot and His Daughters* (cat. nos. 37, 42), the *Penitent Magdalene* (cat. 35 and fig. 26), the *Danaë* (cat. nos. 36, 41), the *Rest on the Flight into Egypt* (cat. nos. 34, 45). A replica of the *Lot and His Daughters* that Orazio had painted for his Genoese patron Giovan Antonio Sauli was sent to Carlo Emanuele, duke of Savoy, and it was conceivably a replica of Sauli's *Magdalene* that he sent to Marie de' Medici.

This activity indicates, on the one hand, the considerable demand for prized compositions by Orazio. On the other, it has sometimes been taken as a slackening of his inventive capacities. It is, therefore, well to remind ourselves that replicas were the direct product of collecting, as collectors have always preferred recognizable masterpieces to what is offbeat. Artists such as Bernardo Strozzi (1581–1644) had a virtual sideline in the production of replicas and variants of their most successful compositions— some of them autograph, others painted by workshop assistants. Even painters of the stature of Guercino (1591–1666) and Reni made replicas. To take only one example, Guercino's *Ecstasy of Saint Francis* (Louvre, Paris), dating to 1620, provided the prototype for two smaller, autograph variants (Gemäldegalerie, Dresden, and Muzeum Narodowe, Warsaw), one of which seems to have been owned by Cardinal Massimi, a collector of considerable standing. Giulio Mancini, usually so informative on artistic practice, does not deal with the matter of autograph replicas, but he believed that copies devalued the worth of an original, and we find him urging his brother not to allow copies to be made of their two paintings by Caravaggio and by Annibale Carracci. Yet such was his desire to own an example of a particularly admired composition by Caravaggio that he was forced to settle for a copy, negotiating with Cardinal del Monte to have one made.[66]

The great collector and connoisseur Vincenzo Giustiniani (1564–1637) said nothing about painters who replicated their own work, but he recognized that even copies reflected in varying degrees the excellence of the painters who made them.[67] Some copies were worse than the original, some indistinguishable, and some, he allowed, might even surpass it. The same can be said of Orazio's replicas and variants: usually the first, or prime, version is the freshest in execution and most responsive to observed phenomena, but this does not mean that a second version cannot

have its own characteristics—especially when it is painted many years later. In the case of the *Finding of Moses* (cat. 48), the second version (fig. 87), which was sent to Philip IV of Spain, is so decidedly superior to the first version that scholars perpetually reversed the relationship of the two pictures; X rays have now settled the matter.[68]

REPLICATION

In the 1637 catalogue of the collection of Charles I, Abraham van der Doort lists a *Rest on the Flight into Egypt* that was copied by Orazio.[69] An earlier version of this composition (by Orazio) belonged to the duke of Buckingham, and it is possible that the copy was taken directly from that work; this would have been simple to arrange. But how was a copy made of a painting that was not readily available? That had, in fact, been sold years earlier and was hundreds of miles away? From another entry in Van der Doort's catalogue, we learn of "a Booke in larg[e] folio in white vellam herein some 8 little drawings of Horatio Jentellesco."[70] Detailed drawings that record compositions are certainly one means by which Orazio could have produced variants, and the reduced version of the *David Contemplating the Head of Goliath* (cat. 19) demonstrates that he was adept at changing scale. But drawings such as these would hardly have enabled the easy production of replicas that retained the scale and the details of the original—down to the arrangement of drapery folds. For this, the most obvious expedient was the re-use of a cartoon made for, or a tracing taken from, the finished work. That Gentileschi used a mechanical means both for replicating and varying his designs— even when the original was readily available—can be demonstrated. (We know, incidentally, that Orazio supplied drawings for tapestries when in London, so the idea of creating designs for replication was not foreign to him.)[71]

Let us begin with the simplest scenario: the repetition of a composition that is identical in all but minor parts. This category applies to the two versions of Orazio's *Danaë* (cat. nos. 36, 41), both of which have been X rayed. That the picture painted for Giovan Antonio Sauli (cat. 36) is the prime version cannot be doubted. Quite apart from the sheer quality of execution (what Mancini termed the "osservanza del vivo quanto che la fierezza et risolutione della maniera")[72] visible to any viewer, the X ray reveals minor changes in contours and a creative method

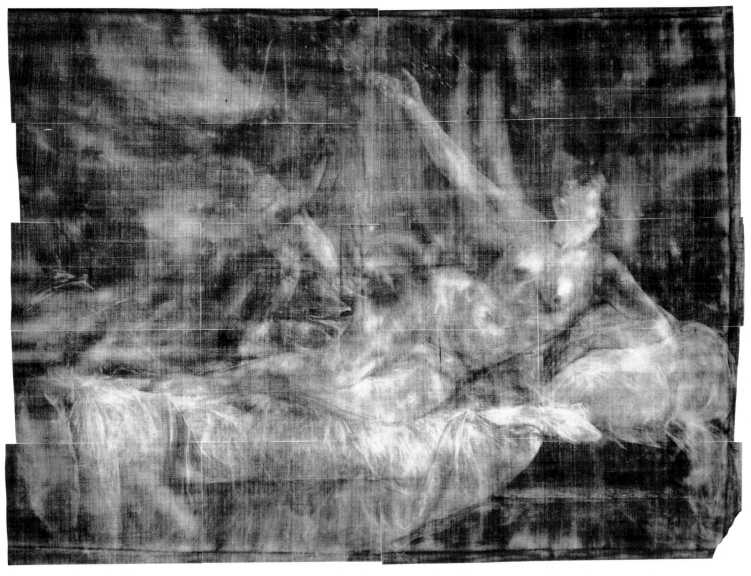

Figure 9. X radiograph of *Danaë* (cat. 36)

of working up the highlights (figs. 9, 10). By contrast, the X rays of the Cleveland version (fig. 11) show an approach in which the modeling no less than the contours is hard and predetermined by a carefully laid-in design. When a tracing of the ex-Sauli picture is superimposed over the Cleveland painting, there is a perfect match of part to part, though not of the whole. That is to say, the Cleveland painting was generated from a tracing or cartoon that was either in sections or was slightly shifted during the transfer process. Sections match up individually, but the tracing has to be shifted so that these sections align (for a detailed analysis, see cat. 41). We have notices of two *Danaës* in Genoese collections, and it

seems only reasonable to assume that the paintings in the exhibition are these two.

The same relationship characterizes the two versions of the *Judith and Her Maidservant* (cat. 39 and Pinacoteca Vaticana). Although no X ray of the Vatican painting was available, when a tracing of the prime version in Hartford was superimposed over the Vatican replica, the results yielded were exactly analogous to those obtained from the two *Danaës*: the one was clearly generated from the other using a mechanical means of transfer, and, again, there was a slight shifting from section to section.[73] In this case, it seems possible that the second version was for the most

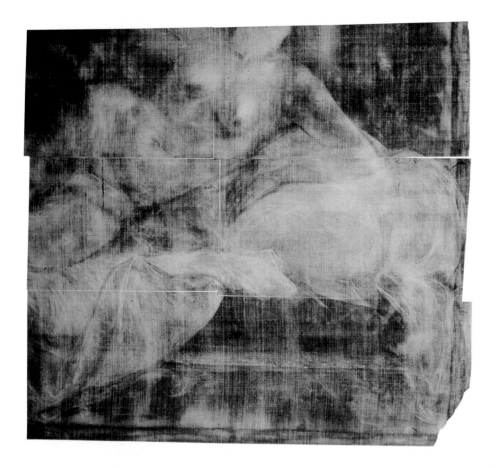

Figure 10. X radiograph of lower-right quadrant of figure 9

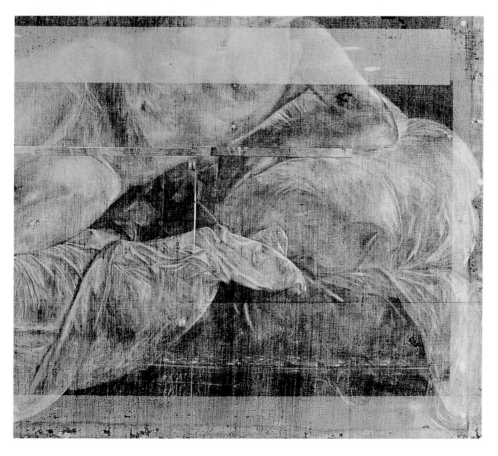

Figure 11. X radiograph of lower-right quadrant of *Danaë* (cat. 41)

Figure 12. X radiograph of *Lot and His Daughters* (cat. 37)

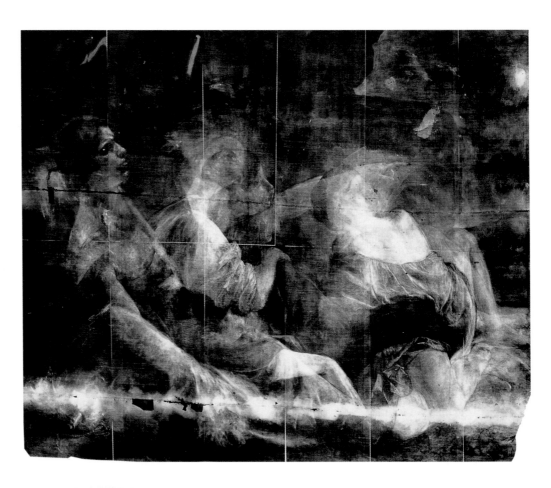

Figure 13. X radiograph of lower-right quadrant of figure 12

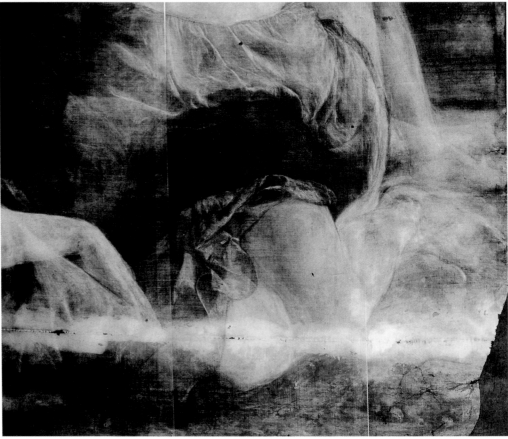

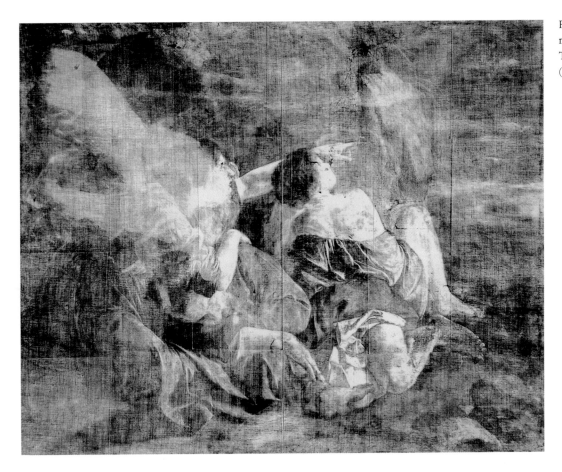

Figure 15. X radiograph of autograph replica of *Lot and His Daughters* in The National Gallery of Canada, Ottawa (cat. 42)

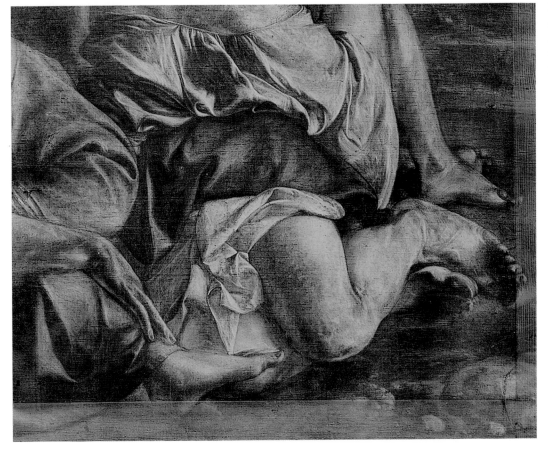

Figure 14. X radiograph of lower-right quadrant of workshop replica of *Lot and His Daughters* in the Staatliche Museen Preussischer Kulturbesitz, Gemäldegalerie, Berlin (fig. 72)

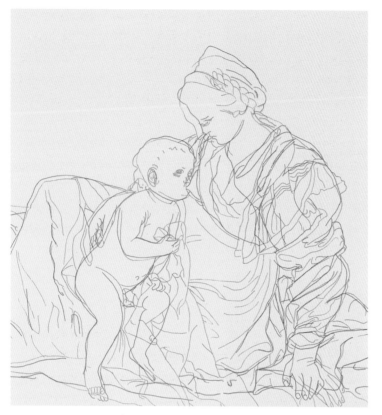

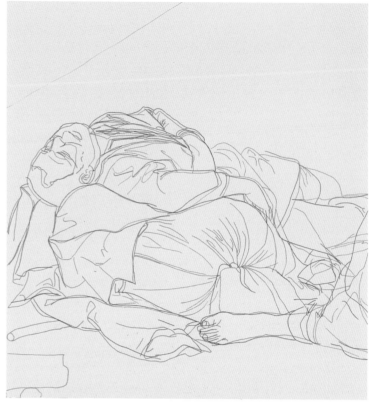

Figure 16. Superimposed tracings of the Virgin and Child from the two versions of the *Rest on the Flight into Egypt:* in Birmingham (cat. 34), shown in red, and in Vienna (cat. 45), shown in black. The Birmingham picture is earlier in date and based on direct studies from posed models, and must have provided the matrix for the design of the Vienna painting. The principal contours are in register, but the individualized faces of the Virgin and Child have been changed; the position of the child's right leg was raised, and that of the Virgin's right hand rotated. Only the right side of the tracings is in register, but as figure 17 shows, by shifting one of the tracings, the left side of the composition can also be brought into register.

Figure 17. Superimposed tracings of the figure of Joseph from the two versions of the *Rest on the Flight into Egypt:* in Birmingham (cat. 34), shown in red, and in Vienna (cat. 45), shown in black. The major contours for the figure of Joseph are in register, as is the extended foot of the Virgin. Note, however, that the Virgin's bent knee is now out of register—an indication of the way in which Gentileschi shifted the tracing/cartoon to adapt the composition to a different format.

part a workshop production, though this is a matter that is obviously subject to individual interpretation.

The process is repeated in the two versions of *Lot and His Daughters,* in the J. Paul Getty Museum (cat. 37) and the Gemäldegalerie, Berlin (fig. 72).[74] The X ray of the Getty picture—unquestionably that done for Giovan Antonio Sauli in Genoa—reveals considerable changes in the composition as well as, possibly, evidence of an abandoned composition (figs. 12, 13). A comparison with the X rays of the Berlin picture (fig. 14) together with superimposed tracings of both paintings definitively establishes their relationship: the Berlin version was laid in from a tracing of the Getty picture. As in the other examples already cited, this tracing—and that it was a tracing rather than a cartoon may be deduced from the simple fact that the changes in the Getty picture

revealed in the X ray are so extensive—was shifted in the course of laying in the design (in this case, alignment is obtained for each quadrant of the figure group). In the X ray of the Berlin painting, there is evidence of a hard contour such as one would expect from a mechanical transfer of a design. The execution of the Berlin painting is very much below Orazio's standards, and I have no doubt that we are dealing in this case with a workshop replica.

A tracing of the ex-Sauli/Getty picture was also used to produce the version of the composition now in Ottawa (cat. 42).[75] However, the X ray of that picture (fig. 15) shows a greater subtlety in the modeling, and there is every reason to accept this picture as an autograph work—probably the one Orazio sent to Carlo Emanuele in Turin.

This use of tracings to replicate and/or copy pictures is recorded by Vincenzo Giustiniani as well as by such compilers of artists' treatises as Richard Symonds (1617–1660).[76] It has, moreover, a long history, stretching back at least to the fifteenth century. The key point to be made here is that what must have been a widespread practice—both by copyists and by artists replicating their own work—also had a creative side.[77] This emerges most clearly in a comparison of a tracing taken from the *Rest on the Flight into Egypt* now in Birmingham (cat. 34) with one taken from the later version, in Vienna (cat. 45).[78] In this case, we are dealing not with a replica but with a revised version. We might have supposed that the composition of the Vienna picture was generated from a small record drawing, so different does it appear in the details. Yet the tracings (figs. 16, 17) reveal that the scale of the figures is virtually the same, and their silhouettes match up surprisingly well (always allowing for a slight shift in the position of the tracing). To take just one detail: the right arm of the Virgin is identically placed and the position of the hand merely shifted. The child—that part of the composition that has been most thoroughly rethought—remains quite close, with the head and right leg repositioned. It would seem that the composition of the Vienna painting represents a rethinking of the Birmingham picture, for which a tracing served as the point of departure. Whether the Vienna picture is the first revised composition is more difficult to ascertain. The X ray (fig. 18) reveals a hardness in the contours that certainly suggests a transferred composition, and the very existence of so many other versions (for which, see cat. 45) suggests the difficulties of reaching a definitive solution.

Curiously, the figures in the versions of the related composition in the Louvre and in a private collection in Mantua are slightly smaller in scale.[79] Yet, at least in the case of the version at Mantua (formerly in the J. Paul Getty Museum), there is evidence that, once again, a tracing may have been used (see figs. 19, 20). Here, it would seem that Orazio employed a tracing from the Vienna composition to obtain the upper silhouette of the Virgin and Child, and then slipped it upward to obtain the lower portion. The figure of Joseph was shifted to the right so that the bundle on which he rests disappears behind the Virgin's right leg. In the process, the proportions of the figures have been changed to fit a smaller picture field. X rays (fig. 21) reveal that throughout the composition minor changes and adjustments have been made, but in general the handling is harder and the result less satisfac-

tory than what is found in either the beautiful Vienna version, the slightly less fine picture in the Louvre, or that in Milan (compare figs. 22, 23, 24); this is even more true with the visible surface of the pictures. As this examination shows, Orazio used tracings in a creative fashion, and, in fact, any comparison between the various versions of this, his most repeated composition, reveals that he was constantly altering and refining it, rearranging the scarf around the shoulders of the Virgin, changing the color of her dress and the drapery on the ground. In effect, he created two variants, each of which became the matrix for other pictures. What may be one of the latest versions—a fragment showing only the Virgin and Child (fig. 25)—is also the most elegant.

GENTILESCHI'S FORMAL IMAGINATION

Orazio's use of tracings was both economical and creative, and it would be wrong to assume that simply because a composition was generated mechanically, it is necessarily inferior. Workshop intervention is best deduced from the picture's surface treatment, rather than from the sometimes ambivalent evidence of the X rays and tracings. Perhaps the most significant trait revealed by the tracings is Orazio's attachment to particular formal designs. I have remarked on this in the catalogue entries for the *Judith and Her Maidservant* in Hartford (cat. 39) and the *Young Woman Playing a Violin* (cat. 40), in which similar poses are used for different figures. Another figure with a similar pose appears in the X ray of the Getty *Lot and His Daughters* (fig. 12), suggesting that Orazio may have thought of beginning that picture by incorporating a favorite pose he had recorded in a tracing or drawing. His was a formal imagination, and, like Piero della Francesca almost two centuries earlier, he did not hesitate to re-use a pose or a figure, even at the risk of appearing to repeat himself.[80]

Tracings must have served as an aid to the young Artemisia as she learned her craft, and they became a staple in her own repetitions later in her career. They probably played as important a part in her artistic education in Orazio's house as his collection of prints, with its focus on designs derived from Raphael (that he had an extensive collection of etchings can be deduced from the compositional sources in his work). The resemblance of Artemisia's *Judith and Her Maidservant* in the Pitti (cat. 60) to two earlier compositions by Orazio (cat. 13 and fig. 46) may be explained by the intermediary of a tracing that she

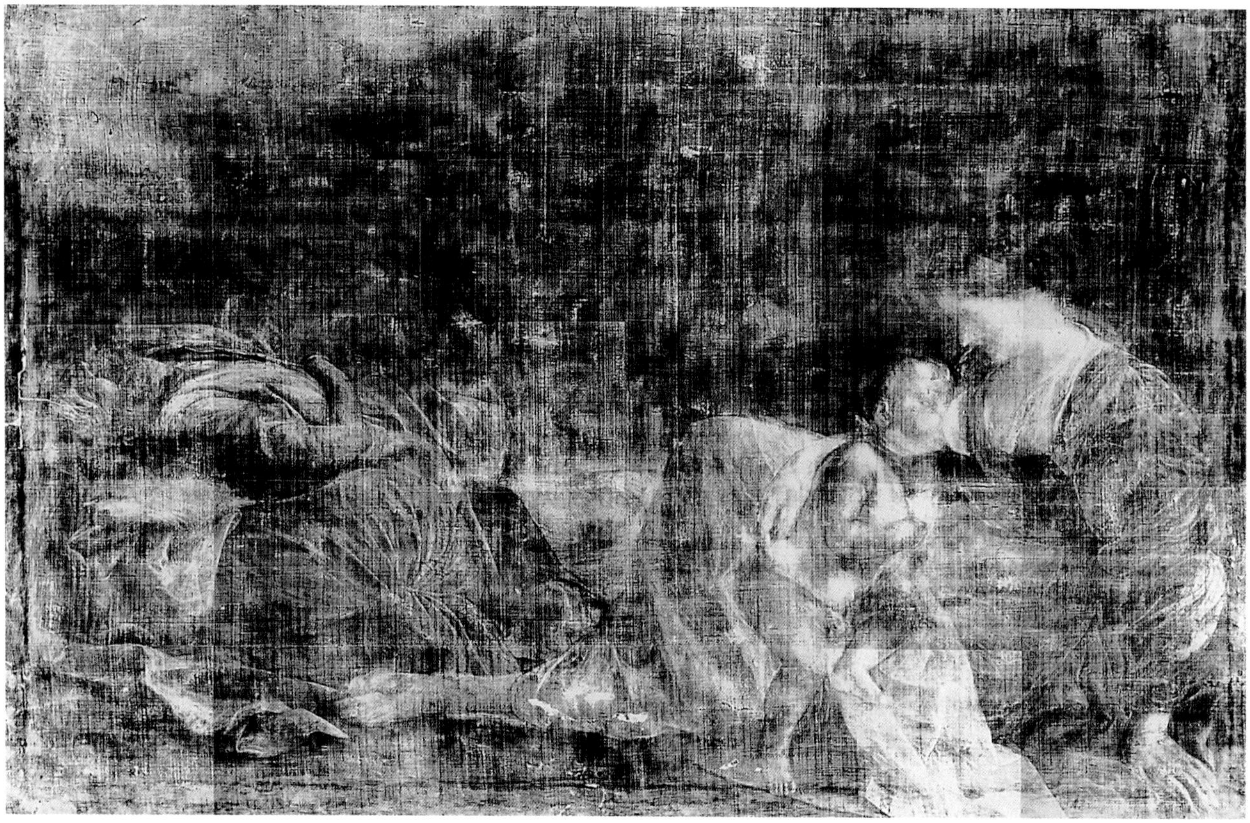

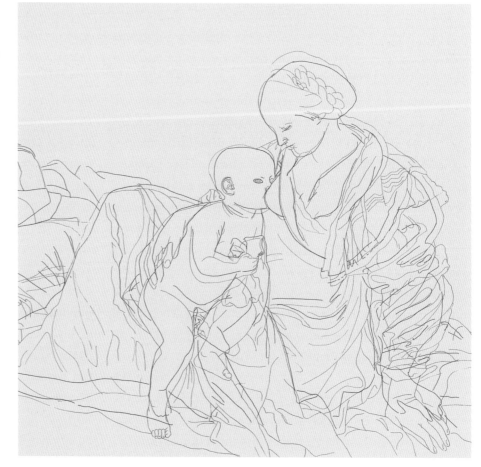

Figure 18. X radiograph of the *Rest on the Flight into Egypt* (cat. 45).

Figure 19. Superimposed tracings of the Virgin and Child from the versions of the *Rest on the Flight into Egypt:* in Mantua (see fig. 21), shown in red, and in Vienna (cat. 45), shown in black. The figure scale of the Mantua painting is smaller than that in the Vienna version. Nonetheless, the tracings suggest that Gentileschi generated the design from a tracing/cartoon of the Vienna version, shortening the child's legs and the Virgin's arm. This may have been done on the canvas by creatively shifting the cartoon. The X radiograph (fig. 21) demonstrates that Gentileschi made minor adjustments as he painted.

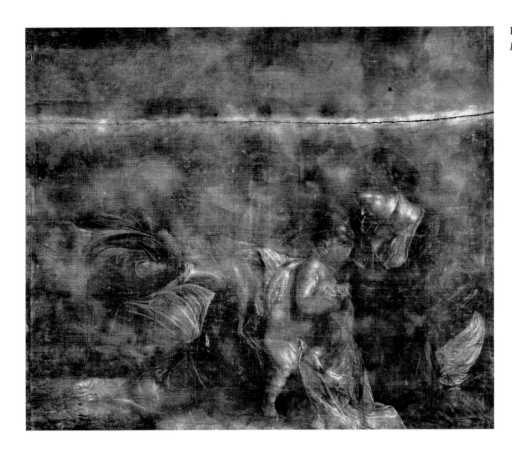

Figure 21. X radiograph of the *Rest on the Flight into Egypt*. Private collection, Mantua

Figure 20. Superimposed tracings of the figure of Joseph in the versions of the *Rest on the Flight into Egypt*: in Mantua, shown in red, and in Vienna (cat. 45), shown in black. The necessary adjustments for the reduction of the figure scale are evident. The Mantua picture was made by overlapping two parts of the original, Vienna, design; note how the Virgin's bent knee now cuts off Joseph's right knee and the bundle on which he sleeps. The tracing/cartoon must have been in two sections.

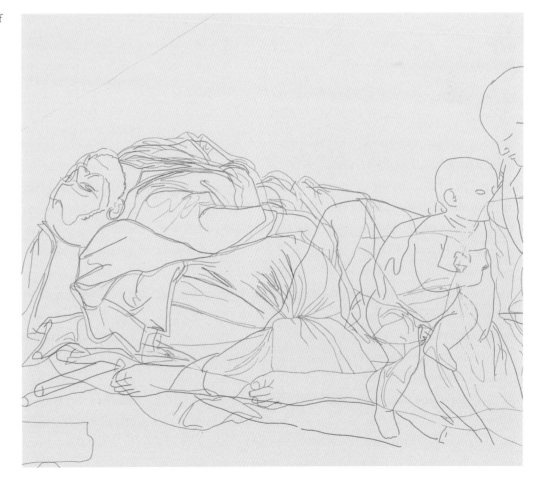

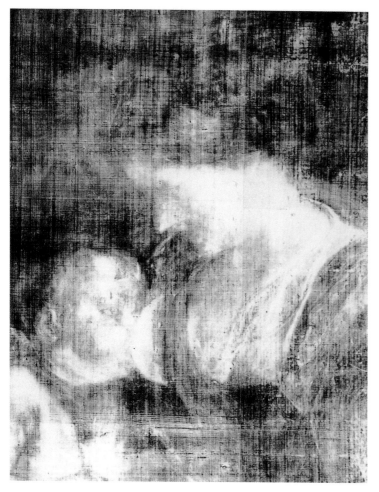

Figure 22. Detail of figure 18

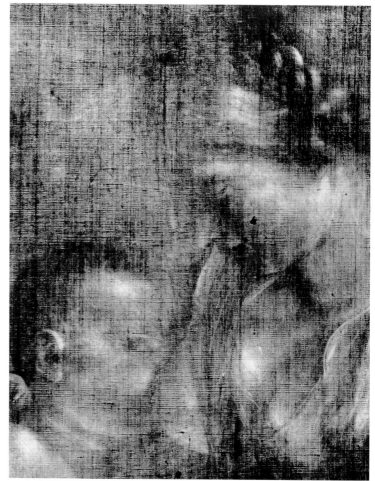

Figure 23. X radiograph of Virgin's head in the *Rest on the Flight into Egypt*. Musée du Louvre, Paris

adapted to her own purposes. The same may be true of her *Madonna and Child* in the Galleria Spada (cat. 52). Orazio himself was not beyond isolating a feature in a composition and using it as the point of departure for something else. The Virgin in the Fogg *Madonna with the Sleeping Christ Child* (cat. 28) could, with alterations, become a Saint Catherine (fig. 59). One wonders what use Francesco Gentileschi may have made of his father's tracings and, possibly, cartoons. Too lacking in talent to map out for himself an independent career, did he resort to pastiching his father's work?[81]

Perhaps the most interesting example of the nature of Orazio's fascination with formal designs occurs in the paired female figures of Danaë and the Magdalene that he painted around 1621–22 for Giovan Antonio Sauli (cat. nos. 35, 36). In the entries for these pictures, I suggest that the poses were intended to point up the contrast between the penitential, religious theme of the *Magdalene*

and the erotic, pagan theme of the *Danaë*. Just how closely related in his mind these two figures were is revealed by the X ray not of the ex-Sauli *Magdalene* (fig. 28), but of the version of the picture in Vienna (figs. 26, 27). X rays of that work, always considered—with good reason—the later of the two, reveal it to have, by far, the most significant and extensive changes. Indeed, based on the X ray alone, there would be every reason to believe this to be the prime version of the composition. Most astonishing is the fact that the figure was initially depicted nude. When a tracing of the Danaë is superimposed over the figure of the Magdalene (fig. 29), there can be no doubt that the one was generated from the other, with the position of the upper torso raised to enhance the different expressive content, but the outstretched right foot retained (this last detail was modified in the Sauli version).

What does this say about the dating of the Vienna painting? Does it, in fact, precede the Sauli version? Is it the picture Soprani

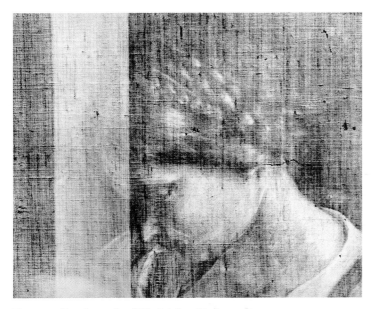

Figure 24. X radiograph of Virgin's head in figure 25

refers to as having been sent by Orazio from Genoa to Marie de' Medici and that she, in turn, gave to the duke of Buckingham (on these questions, see cat. 45)? Or does it reveal Orazio employing a tracing he had brought with him from Genoa to Paris as a point of departure for a fresh interpretation of an old composition?[82] Nothing would show less sensitivity to the character of Orazio's art—its "sapere" and its increasingly refined sense of "colorito"— than to force him into an intellectualized schema.[83]

GENTILESCHI AND THE BAROQUE

The interest in subtly varying a single formal design, so remarkably documented in a technical analysis of Orazio's paintings, is perhaps the distinguishing trait of his art—an art that can seem

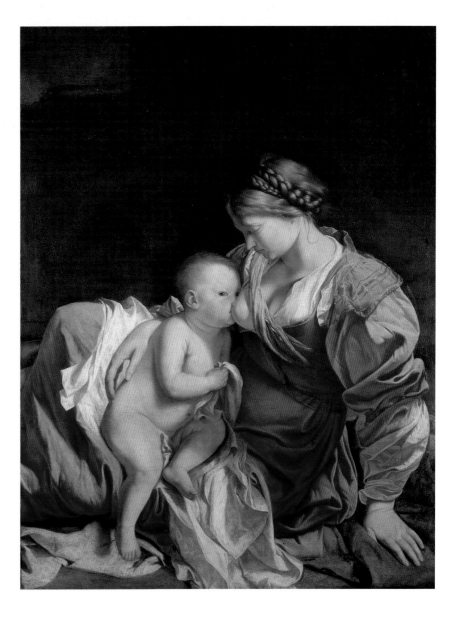

Figure 25. Fragment of the *Rest on the Flight into Egypt*. Formerly Finarte, Milan

Figure 26. Orazio Gentileschi, *Penitent Magdalene*. Oil on canvas. Kunsthistorisches Museum, Vienna

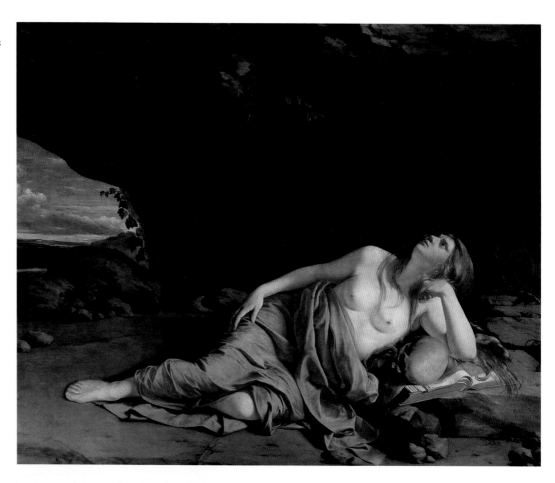

Figure 27. X radiograph of figure 26, showing how the figure was laid in nude

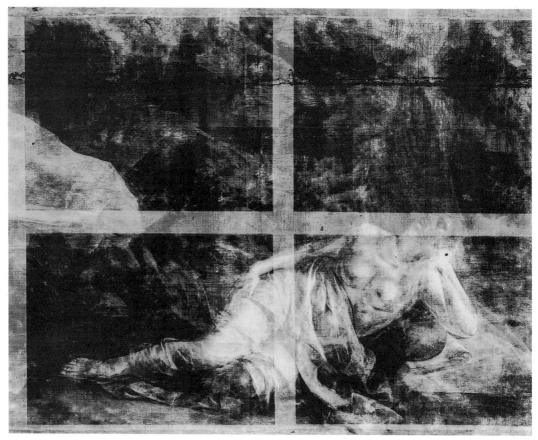

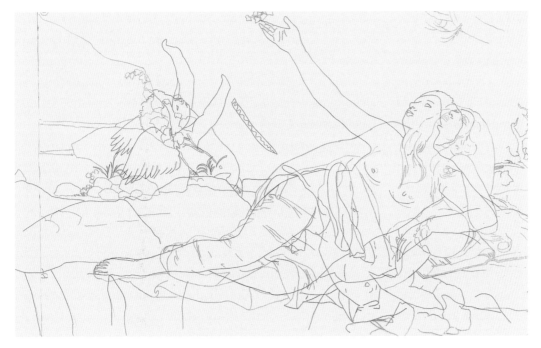

Figure 29. Superimposed tracings of the *Penitent Magdalene* in Vienna (fig. 26), shown in green, and the *Danaë* (cat. 36), shown in red. It is evident that the same cartoon/tracing was used to obtain the lower part of the torso and legs of the Vienna *Magdalene*. The upper torso and the position of the head, shoulders, and arms were altered to suit the different subjects and the required actions.

Figure 28. X radiograph of the *Penitent Magdalene* (cat. 35)

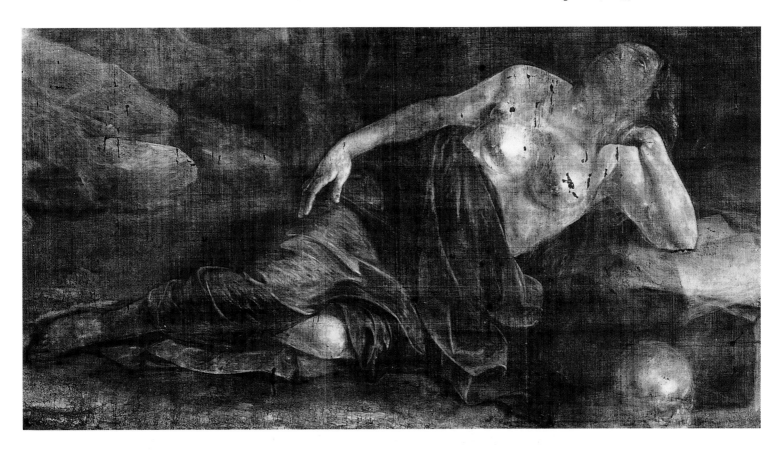

strangely out of step with its time even when it responds to those artists who so strongly shaped it. We have constantly to remind ourselves that Orazio was five years older than the Cavaliere d'Arpino (1568–1640), under whom he worked at San Giovanni in Laterano, and eight years older than Caravaggio. He belonged to the generation of Annibale Carracci, Cigoli, and Passignano—the generation of the reformers of Italian art. His fellow Caravaggisti, Orazio Borgianni and Carlo Saraceni, were younger by eleven and sixteen years, respectively; Reni, Domenichino, Adam Elsheimer, and Rubens all belonged to the next generation.

Although Rome was the seat of the Counter-Reformation, there was no reform movement in the arts comparable to those in Florence and Bologna that, in the 1580s, redirected artists to the study of nature and to the great masters of the High Renaissance. (Scipione Pulzone [1544–1598] is the closest equivalent in Rome to the outstanding figures in Florence and Bologna—Cigoli, Passignano, the Carracci.) Orazio's training was in every respect conservative. Watered-down Raphael was the currency of the day. His fascination with the purely formal elements of composition no less than the decorously pure sentiment of his religious paintings are the result of this training, while the modern guise in which they are presented has to do with his association with Caravaggio and his awareness of the most progressive trends in European painting.

He was on hand at the unveiling in 1600 of Caravaggio's paintings in San Luigi dei Francesi, and evidently looked with equal interest at Annibale's frescoes in the gallery of the Palazzo Farnese—those twin events that ushered in the new century and suddenly made everything Orazio and his contemporaries had done seem not simply inconsequential but irrelevant. He began work at the Palazzo del Quirinale just after Reni completed his frescoes of the life of the Virgin for the pope's private chapel—frescoes that established a new standard for beauty and devoutness. One wonders what the young Artemisia made of this spectacular cycle when she was taken to view the progress of her father's work. She was bound to compare Reni's celestial vision of music-making angels, so lavishly praised by the pope, with the more plebeian figures—for one of which she had possibly posed—that her father was painting in Cardinal Borghese's loggia, a five-minute walk away, and to reflect on the very different direction Orazio's art had taken. During the time he was painting those haunting altarpieces for the Marchigian town of Fabriano (cat. 30),

with their quality of domestic intimacy, Giovanni Lanfranco (1582–1647) and Carlo Saraceni were working together with Orazio's former partner, Agostino Tassi, in the Sala Regia of the Quirinale. Lanfranco's work established the basis for Baroque decoration, and it is not surprising that Orazio's bid to fresco the Benediction loggia at Saint Peter's was lost to Lanfranco.

Orazio was in Rome in 1608, when Rubens completed his grandiose paintings in the apse of the Oratorian church of Santa Maria in Vallicella, and he arrived in Genoa in 1621, a year after the installation in San Ambrogio of the Fleming's theatrical altarpiece showing miracles of Saint Ignatius of Loyola. In the catalogue I suggest that the latter work inspired Orazio to one of his greatest achievements, the hushed and precious Turin Annunciation (cat. 43). In Paris, he was on hand for the first installment of Rubens's stupendous cycle of the life of Marie de' Medici in the Palais de Luxembourg, and he had hardly begun work on his canvases for the ceiling of the Queen's House in Greenwich (fig. 85) before the arrival in London of Rubens's masterpieces for the ceiling of the Banqueting House, Whitehall (fig. 90). As we have seen, he met Van Dyck in Genoa and sat for him in London —with what mixed feelings we can only guess.

Despite these encounters, Orazio never embraced the all-conquering Baroque idiom, with its emphasis on expressivity and dynamic compositions or its love of the dramatic, as did Artemisia (who, after all, was of the same generation as Jusepe de Ribera, Simon Vouet, and Valentin de Boulogne). Nor did he remain completely unaffected. He expanded his art, notably creating his own formalized code for the rhetorical gestures that were at the heart of Baroque painting. Yet what could be less Baroque in effect than the *Joseph and Potiphar's Wife* that he painted in London around 1630–33 (fig. 88)?[84] In it, an erotic story of failed seduction is transformed into a still life of fabrics with incidental figures, the protagonists appearing to be the marvelous crimson curtain and richly tailored jacket that, with apparent regret, the well-dressed courtier seems to leave behind—like Saint Martin—to clothe a half-naked woman. Judged by the narrative standards of Rubens, Reni, or Domenichino, this picture is a travesty. But do not its perverse stillness and its air of detachment subvert the rhetorical language of the Baroque into something else? The action is subordinate to the act of description: "pittura di valori" has supplanted narration, and gesture is reduced to an emblem of a story pointedly not told.

Geography plays an important part in the way Orazio's art was perceived. Out of step with the trends in Rome and Genoa, his work takes on a strangely prescient quality in France, where his narrative reticence and elegant sense of design seem to look forward to aspects of classical painting (see Jean-Pierre Cuzin, pp. 208–12). In some of his religious pictures there is even a foretaste of the sacral naturalism of the early-nineteenth-century Nazarenes, and it is hardly surprising that a number of scholars have tried to demonstrate an antiquarian interest on Orazio's part in quattrocento art (see the discussion in cat. nos. 30, 43).[85]

The thorny issue of Orazio's possible "pan-European" influence has been discussed in detail by Bissell, in his indispensable 1981 monograph on the artist.[86] Orazio's position in the Italian seicento is perhaps even more difficult to define. He has occasionally been compared with Lorenzo Lotto (ca. 1480–1556), a compellingly original artist going his own way. However, Lotto's restless, psychologically probing art found its audience in the peripheral areas of Bergamo, Treviso, and the Marches, not in the cosmopolitan centers of Rome, Genoa, Paris, and London. No one has been more eloquent about the paradox Orazio's art poses than Sydney Freedberg, who, writing about the grandly elegant and hauntingly moving *Madonna with the Sleeping Christ Child* at the Fogg Art Museum (cat. 28), commented on how "Orazio passed beyond dependence on the art of Caravaggio into a powerful and highly personal style, for which the prior assimilation of Caravaggism was a threshold. There is, in the Fogg *Madonna*, a sudden growth to grandeur in the conception of form and theme, an absolute command of the image into unity." Orazio's light—what for Longhi was the artist's greatest contribution to European painting—Freedberg describes as "not just a deviation from Caravaggio's persistently classicizing model, but in a sense a development beyond it, towards a quality of baroqueness."[87] I have tried to suggest that, beyond the label we may decide to append to Orazio's paintings, they leave with us an indelible impression, as though we had encountered something both strange and familiar, at once remotely abstract in its formal language and hauntingly human in its quality of personal revelation: the youthful vigor of seicento naturalism in the hands of an old master of the Renaissance.

1. The trial has become so famous that it is pointless to try to cite the long bibliography dealing with it. An Italian transcription was published by Menzio 1981; Garrard (1989, 409–87) gives an English translation of the main portion. Cohen (2000) puts the trial in its proper historical context. Less well known parts are published here in appendix 1.

2. See appendix 1, under October 2, 1612: Luca fu Carlo Finocchi.

3. Ibid., under August 17, 1612.

4. Ibid., under October 21, 1612.

5. See Bray in London–Bilbao–Madrid 1999, 76. For a reappraisal of the years Gentileschi spent in London, see Wood 2000–2001.

6. Baglione (1642), 1935, 360.

7. Cavazzini (1998, 175) has noted that Orazio waited until he completed his work with Tassi before making his denouncement. She also tentatively suggests that he perhaps hoped to establish a continuing collaboration that would involve Artemisia.

8. See Crinò and Nicolson 1961, 144.

9. Félibien 1705, 237. It is always possible that Félibien's comments derive from Baglione's biography, especially given the similarity of the words *bestiale* and *brutale* to describe Orazio's character.

10. Pollock (1999, 98–103) is particularly eloquent on the problem of reading biography into Artemisia's paintings.

11. The letter was first published by Crinò 1954, 203–4.

12. For the report, see Crinò and Nicolson 1961, 144.

13. On this issue, see the observations of Dempsey 1993, 233–43.

14. Bellori (1672) 1976, 229–30.

15. See Zuccari 1992, 87 n. 41, for a recent survey of the problem.

16. Bissell (1981, 136) notes that in 1598 one of the payments was made in the name of the monastery at Farfa and of the monks of San Paolo. Cardinal Alessandro Montalto, the nephew of Sixtus V, was commendatory abbot of Farfa.

17. The documents are published by Germond (1993), who ascribed all the frescoes in the chapel to Orazio. I questioned this deduction: see Christiansen 1994. Since then, an early guidebook has been published by Dorati da Empoli (2001, 52, 54–55 n. 16) that ascribes the vault frescoes to Orazio. I have reexamined the chapel and find this attribution completely convincing. The fact that the guidebook makes no mention of the large frescoes on the lateral walls strongly suggests that they may not have been painted until after about 1615. Orazio must have abandoned the project or subcontracted it. A drawing related to one of the lateral frescoes is in the British Museum: see Turner 2000, 222–23. The frescoes resemble somewhat the work of Marzio Ganassini.

18. According to Baglione, Orazio painted the apostle Thaddeus "a man dritta vicino all'Organo." This should be the apostle to the right of the organ. Bissell (1981, 136–37) has, however, argued convincingly that the figure of Thaddeus is on the left. See also Freiberg 1995, 301. The question is whether Baglione is more likely to have misidentified the name of the apostle Gentileschi painted or the location of his contribution to the transept decorations, on which he also worked. The fact that the apostles to the left and to the right of the organ—one by Orazio, the other by Ricci—are so lacking in individual style says a great deal about Orazio's place in Roman painting at this date.

19. Baldinucci (1681) 1845–47, vol. 3, 277.

20. The picture is described in these terms in a 1638 inventory of the Giustiniani collection: see Salerno 1960, 135.

21. See Spezzaferro 1975, 53–55.

22. Mancini (1617–21) 1956–57, vol. 1, 110.

23. Baldinucci 1681, 17: "Colorito: Il colorire: fra i Pittori dicesi buon colorito, e cattivo colorito del tal Maestro; ed il tale à buon colorito, o cattivo colorito."

24. See Finaldi in London–Bilbao–Madrid 1999, 33. Spear (1997, 77) notes the study of the nude female model in the drawing academy of Bologna.

25. See Langdon 1998, 298–99.

26. The practice has been denied by Garrard (1989, 200, 532 n. 37) and Harris (1989, 9). The matter is sensibly discussed by Bissell (1999, 6). See also the comments of Cropper in her catalogue essay. Spear (1997, 77–94) discusses Reni's nudes and issues of viewer perception. It is worth noting that both Orazio and Artemisia later affirm their use of female models.

27. See appendix 1, under June 23, 1612.

28. Here I must record my view that the *Lucretia* dates from about 1611–12. Neither the technique nor the type of composition—with the figure cut off mid-calf in a fashion typical of Orazio's paintings at this period—seems to me to have anything to do with Artemisia's sophisticated work of the 1620s.

29. Malvasia ([1678] 1841, 346) recounts Annibale's description to Albani and Tacconi of how he had gone about creating the nude statues on the ceiling of the Farnese Gallery. His method, which was based on drawing rather than painting from the model, serves as a perfect foil for understanding the differences between the effects of verisimilitude sought in classical painting and the truth, or *vero*, that underlies Caravaggesque practice.

30. See Pedrocchi 2000, 62–65.

31. Mancini (1617–21) 1956–57, vol. 1, 108–9.

32. See Crinò and Nicolson 1961, 144. The letter was written from Rome on March 27, 1615. Guicciardini was not opposed to Caravaggesque painting: he purchased pictures by Gerrit van Honthorst, Bartolomeo Manfredi, and Cecco del Caravaggio for his own collection (the Cecco, painted to decorate his family chapel in Florence, he rejected). See Corti 1989, 108–46.

33. As noted above, at note 17, in the British Museum there is a fully developed compositional drawing, squared for enlargement, for one of the large, lateral scenes in the Fiorenzuola chapel in San Giovanni dei Fiorentini. The drawing was tentatively ascribed by Gere and Pouncey to Giovanni de' Vecchi, but in light of the documents published by Germond 1993, Turner (2000, 222–23) has recently reopened discussion of the drawing, which is superior to the actual frescoes.

34. We have no certain information about Manfredi's arrival in Rome, but it is usually thought to have been about 1605. We also know that he studied with Cristoforo Roncalli. Crucial to understanding his possible relationship with Orazio is the date of a work such as the the *Allegory of Four Seasons* at the Dayton Art Institute. Often dated to around 1610, it closely parallels Orazio's experiments at this time. And the *Allegory*, notably, is listed as a work by Gentileschi in an eighteenth-century inventory of the collection of Cardinal Alessandro Albani: "Un quadro in tela simile da Imperatore scarsa rappresentante le quattro staggioni, cioè la primavera con Ghirlanda di fiori, che sona il Liuto, e si abbraccia coll'Autunno, che tiene varj frutti, coll'Estate in forma di donna con spighe di grano, e l'Inverno in forma di Vecchio con berettone di pelle, di mano del Gentileschi…Lasciato a Sua Santità quando era Cardinale dalla bona memoria del Signor Abbate Passarini" (see *Quaderni sul neoclassico*, 5, 31). I do not believe the young Artemisia can have been the catalyst for Orazio's use of the model; a comparison of Orazio's *Madonna and Child* in Bucharest (cat. 15) with the related picture by Artemisia in the Galleria Spada (cat. 52) is enough to settle the direction of influence.

35. The Sannesi's patronage is discussed by Schleier in Florence 1983, 26–30, as well as by Le Pas de Sécheval 1993, 15–19.

36. Luigi Spezzaferro is currently reexamining the Cerasi commission and the issue of the rejected first versions of the pictures.

37. There is common agreement that it is to this work that Orazio referred in 1623, when he wrote the duke that he was sending an *Annunciation* (cat. 43), in recognition of the deep affection he had retained ever since he had served the duke as a young man ("l'antica mia servitù dedicatele fin da giovanetto"). On the original function of the picture, which was later used in the church of the Capuchins as a curtain for a statue, see Arena in Romano 1999, 83.

38. Clement VIII had not favored the Jesuits, who had become the focus of a political tug-of-war. They had been expelled from Venetian territories. The Spanish promoted the Dominicans. On September 4, 1606, Paul V confirmed his faith in the order with his statement *Quantum religio* and cut off debate about them on August 28, 1607. At the center of these issues was Cardinal Claudio Acquaviva, who had played a key role in commissioning Baglione's *Resurrection* for the Gesù in Rome and who likely played a part in the choice of Gentileschi for the Ancona altarpiece (cat. 7). See Carloni, pp. 118–19, in this publication.

39. For these complicated dealings, see esp. Venturi 1882, 16ff.; Marcon, Maddalo, and Marcolini 1983, 93–106; and Carloni in Fossombrone 1997, 22. Paolo Savelli emerges from the correspondence as a somewhat ambiguous figure, since he was advising the agent of Duke Cesare d'Este about Scipione Borghese's schemes.

40. Maniello 1994. On the Olgiati, see esp. Calvi 1884, vol. 3, 1–3.

41. See Hibbard 1971, 206.

42. Orbaan 1920, 177; Waźbiński 1994, vol. 2, 361.

43. See appendix 1, under fol. 433.

44. See Rovi 1992.

45. See Acanfora's (2000, 29–52) comments on Cigoli and Galileo.

46. On Galileo and Elsheimer, see Ottani Cavina 1976, 139–44.

47. See De Rinaldis 1936, 194–206.

48. For the Savelli, see especially Litta 1872, tavole VIII, IX, dispensa 167; and Moroni 1854, 301–4.

49. Soprani 1674, 316.

50. See Gigli 1958, 46, and, most particularly, Orbaan 1920, 32–33.

51. This is explicitly stated in his 1646 will: see Testa 1998, 348.

52. The notice, erroneously interpreted by Bissell (1981, 103), is transcribed by Gallo (1998, 314, 333–34).

53. It is worth noting that in 1620, when Paolo Savelli made his ceremonial entrance into Rome, he was met by, among others, Cardinal Campori, who, as we have seen, may have played a role in commissioning the *Magdalene;* see Orbaan 1920, 32.

54. For the payments, see Testa 1998, 349. Guicciardini's report is published by Crinò and Nicolson 1961, 144.

55. For the letter from the grand duke's secretary, Andrea Cioli, see Crinò 1960, 264. Cioli found Orazio's widespread reputation—"una voce quasi publica"—the more credible in that he knew firsthand the paintings of Artemisia, then in Florence.

56. That Paolo was Orazio's principal patron we learn from the 1646 will of Federico, where he specifies that the paintings by Guido Reni, Caravaggio, and Gentileschi were owned by his brother Paolo; see Testa 1998, 348. The Caravaggio is the *Denial of Saint Peter* in The Metropolitan Museum of Art. There are three inventories and several lists of pictures belonging to the Savelli: the 1610 inventory, published by Spezzaferro (1985, 71–72), is of the Monte Savello palace and does not mention artists' names; the 1631 inventory, also published by Spezzaferro (ibid., 72–73), is of the collection at the Palazzo di Ariccia, which Federico and Paolo took possession of only in 1605; a copy of a list compiled by Sig. Pio Domenico Gibellini and sent to Cardinal Fabrizio Savelli, the heir of Federico, is dated 1650 and is published by Testa 1998, 352; a 1650 list of pictures is given by Campori 1870, 161–66; and there is a 1659 inventory that I have transcribed: *Inventarii della robba del Card. Savelli Fabrizio* (Archivo di Stato di Roma, Sforza Cesarini 25). See also p. 128 n. 19. What follows are the pictures ascribed to Gentileschi that appear in these lists. 1-Un quadro del Gentileschi con tre ritratti cornice dorata [1631 inventory]; 2-Un quadro grande con diversi frutti e fiori del Gentileschi con tre putti cornice nera [1631 inventory]; 3-Un s. Fran.co del Gentileschi in cornice dorata [1631 inventory]; 4-Una tobia del Gentileschi in rame con cornice d'ebbano [1631 inventory]; 5-Un s.e Antonino da Padova del Gentileschi con il Christo, et quattro angili con cornice dorata [1631 inventory]; 6-Una d.a (una siblia) del Gentileschi cornice dorata [1631 inventory]; 7-Una Madonna grande con il putto sop.a un coscino del Gentileschi corn.ce dorata [1631 inventory]; Una Madonna col Bambino in braccio, alta p.mi 4 [89.36 cm] largo p.mi 3 [67.02 cm] del Gentileschi [1650]; un quadro della madonna col Bambino in braccio del Gentileschi con cornice negra rabescata d'oro [1659];

8-un Adamo et eva del Gentileschi [1610 inv., without attribution; 1631 inventory]; 9-Un christo penante con doi malandrini del Gentileschi cornice nera et oro [1650]; Coronazione di Christo 3 meze figure, del Gentileschi per traverso p.mi 6 [134.4 cm] in circa, D. 150 [1650]; 10-Un S. giovanni che beve del Gentileschi cornice nera et oro [1650]; 11-Una Giuditta del gentileschi cornice dorata; Giuditta con altra Donna, che taglia la testa ad Oloferne, alto p.mi 7 [156.38 cm] largo 5 [111.7 cm] del Gentilesci, D. 200 [1650]; 12-Un Santo in Ginochioni con un manigoldo in atto di tagliarli il collo, figure intiere alto p.mi 7 [156.38 cm] e 6 [134.04 cm] in circa, del Gentileschi, d. 200 [1650].

57. Pizzorusso (1987, 69–70) speculates on the importance of Giulio's position in Ancona, which, however, postdates Orazio's work there for the church of the Gesù, and Testa (1998, 350) suggests that Orazio transferred his activity to the Marches following Giulio's appointment as bishop of Ancona. It should be noted that, with the exception of the two fresco cycles in Fabriano, Orazio could easily have sent his paintings from Rome. On his activity in Fabriano, see Carloni, pp. 116–29.

58. Mancini mentions that Ferraù Fenzone transformed his color in Faenza, specifically comparing his paintings with the work of the Dossi. He particularly praises Scarsellino's work for its "assai buon colorito," calling the painter one of the finest artists in Italy and noting a "quadretto" by the artist of the *Magdalene* owned by the Savelli.

59. Sale, Sotheby's, New York, January 28, 2000, lot 132. The inventory notice in this publication (Carloni, p. 127 n. 19) establishes that Orazio's painting was collaborative.

60. Testa 1998, 348.

61. This position has been taken up in modified form by Nicolson (1958, 24–25) and by Bissell (1981, 68).

62. Longhi (1916) 1961, 236.

63. Ibid., 231.

64. Here it should be pointed out that Lanzi (1795–96, vol. 1, 234) seems also to have been struck by Orazio's "nuovo, e pressoche mai non veduto stile" in a painting of David and Goliath he saw in the Cambiaso collection in Genoa.

65. Luzio (1913) 1974, 61 n.

66. See Maccherini 1997, 74–76.

67. See Giustiniani 1981, 42.

68. See Weston-Lewis in London–Bilbao–Madrid 1999, 42–44.

69. See Millar 1958–60, 176, item 31.

70. Ibid., 126, item 49.

71. See London–Bilbao–Madrid 1999, 99.

72. Mancini (1617–21) 1956–57, vol. 1, 327. Mancini's text is perhaps the most eloquent testimony to the discriminating judgments of seventeenth-century amateurs.

73. I am deeply grateful to Andrea Rothe, of the conservation staff at The J. Paul Getty Museum, Los Angeles, for kindly performing this operation for me and documenting it in photographs.

74. My thanks to Gisela Helmkampf, at the Gemäldegalerie, for facilitating my examination of the Berlin picture and discussing the findings. She most generously provided the print of the X radiograph reproduced here.

75. Here I wish to thank Mark Leonard, at The J. Paul Getty Museum, who kindly passed on this information to me. He also helped to answer my numerous queries and made the tracing of the ex-Sauli *Danaë* when it was sent to the Getty for restoration.

76. See Beal (1984, 198–202), who gives a survey of copying techniques.

77. Here, I should note the article by Bauer and Colton (2000, 434–36), in which an attempt is made to ascribe to Caravaggio the practice investigated in these pages. I can only say that the article is, to my mind, based on a serious confusion between copies and autograph variants. I would also like to state my personal opinion that Caravaggio did not produce replicas of his work, though we can point to one case in which he used the copyist technique of a tracing as the starting point for a variant composition; see Christiansen 1988, 26–27. The article seems to me to show a curious disregard for the issue of quality, which is all-important in discussions of this kind.

78. For the tracing of the Birmingham painting, I am indebted to Gabriele Finaldi; for that of the Vienna paintings—both the *Rest on the Flight into Egypt* and the *Penitent Magdalene*—my debt is to Elke Oberthaler at the Kunsthistorisches Museum, Vienna, and to a student in a seminar I taught, Sandhya Jain.

79. I wish to thank Stephane Loire at the Louvre for kindly comparing tracings of both the Vienna painting and the Mantua painting with X rays of the Louvre's picture and for answering numerous queries. For the examination of the Mantua painting and a discussion of its technical features, I am indebted to Mario Amedeo Lazzari, who kindly furnished me with a detailed report of his findings as well as photographs of the X rays. I am indebted to Dorothy Mahon and Charlotte Hale at the Metropolitan Museum for discussing possible interpretations of this technical material.

80. I am here referring to Piero's well-known habit of reversing cartoons to create compositional echoes or to underscore thematic analogies—as in the identical heads of God the Father and Chosroes. This use of cartoons became a commonplace in the work of Perugino.

81. A prime candidate for this would be a *Madonna Adoring the Christ Child* in a private collection (Bissell 1981, 204 no. X-13). The Madonna is adapted from the Turin *Annunciation*, while the Vouet-like child is a feeble interpolation. Bissell and Strinati (2001) propose it as an autograph work, in part based on the X rays, but its flaccid execution makes this unlikely. Francesco may also have had a hand in the painting of the version of the Turin *Annunciation* in San Siro, Genoa.

82. The difficulty of this position seems to me to be the fact that the drapery of the figure in the Vienna painting so closely repeats the folds in the ex-Sauli picture. And, of course, there is the matter of its pendant, the *Rest on the Flight into Egypt*. In the end, I feel that on purely stylistic grounds these two pictures are more likely to have been painted in France than in Genoa. But so much in Orazio's chronology rests on supposition that the matter should be left open. See now, also, Wood 2000–2001.

83. We should perhaps modify the conclusions reached by Weston-Lewis in his analysis of the relationship of the two versions of the *Finding of Moses*. He excluded tracings as a means of transferring the design from the one picture to the other on the basis of a lack of total agreement in the size and details. As we have seen, Orazio was more creative in his use of tracings than Weston-Lewis's analysis allows.

84. On this picture and its installation in the Queen's House, see Weston-Lewis and Bray in London–Bilbao–Madrid 1999, 45, 72.

85. The most eloquent proponent of this is Bissell (1981, 32–38).

86. Ibid., 63–79. This remains a nebulous subject.

87. Freedberg 1976, 733.

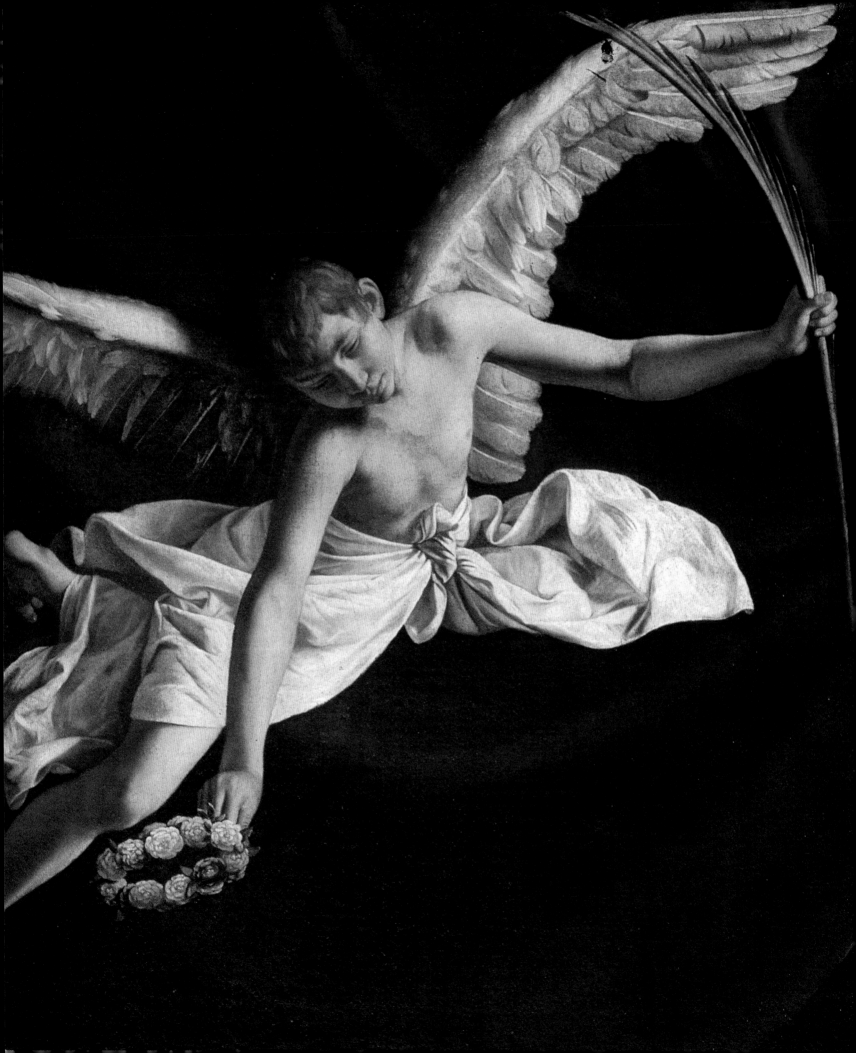

The Rome of Orazio Gentileschi

ALESSANDRO ZUCCARI

Rome "is the most cosmopolitan city in the world and one where they could care less if someone is a foreigner and from another country. On the other hand, the city is in part made up of foreigners and everyone feels at home here." Michel de Montaigne noted both the sophisticated and the familiar nature of the city in 1581, and this description most likely corresponds to the experience of many of the "foreign" artists who went to the papal city.[1] Among them was the Pisan painter Orazio Gentileschi, who arrived in Rome a few years before Montaigne; he too must have felt "at home" there, since he decided to make the city his place of residence for several decades. For a young artist, whether from another Italian city or from north of the Alps, Rome was an extraordinary place both because it provided an ideal location for him to finish his studies and because it offered ample opportunity for professional success and recognition.[2]

The pope at the time, Gregory XIII Boncompagni (r. 1572–85), favored artists from his native Bologna, commissioning them to decorate the new wing of the Vatican palace.[3] Yet artists from other regions—including those who, like Gentileschi, came from Tuscany—also found opportunities in Rome. Giovanni de' Vecchi, for example, oversaw the sophisticated and refined programs commissioned by Alessandro Farnese, the "Gran Cardinale," and Nicolò Circignani filled Jesuit churches with scenes of martyrdom.[4] Such painters as Antonio Tempesta (1555–1630) and Cristoforo Roncalli (1552–1626), who had just arrived in Rome, were hired to work on the pictorial cycles at the Vatican and the Oratory of the Crucifix.[5] Young talents who had not yet established their own reputations spent their time studying ancient art as well as works by the great masters of earlier generations, and as they waited for the chance to prove themselves independent masters, they took on marginal tasks. Such was the case with Gentileschi, who spent years establishing himself in the art world. Orazio arrived in

Rome between 1576 and 1578, but began to receive important commissions only a decade later, during the pontificate of Sixtus V Peretti (r. 1585–90), when he painted "in the lovely Vatican library and in other places."[6]

Thus Rome, a city receptive to artists of different cultural backgrounds, was a large artistic laboratory that encouraged the development and exchange of both old-fashioned and more current styles.[7] Sixtus V was especially active as a patron of architectural and decorative projects; his master plan for the city and the administrative reforms he sponsored made Rome a religious center and a modern capital where the art of painting thrived.[8] His activity also spurred a number of large pictorial cycles. These were promoted by the pope, the new religious orders—the Jesuits, Oratorians, and Theatines, for example[9]—and lay confraternities as well as by members of the Roman Curia and aristocracy who not only decorated their own palaces but financed a large number of altars, chapels, and oratories.

As Sixtus proceeded with his public-works projects, opening up more than six miles of new, straight streets, erecting ancient obelisks at key intersections, and restoring the Acqua Felice aqueduct, he was also mandating the decoration of buildings. Whole squadrons of fresco painters ascended scaffolding in the Sistine chapel at Santa Maria Maggiore, the Lateran loggia, the Scala Santa, the Vatican library, and the new papal palaces at the Lateran and on the Quirinal hill, their participation determined by a defined hierarchy of tasks and a logical distribution of assignments according to each artist's special skill.[10] Indeed, the increased value placed on individual specialties (narrative themes, landscapes, grotesques, and compositional motifs that look ahead to still-life painting) provided the basis upon which pictorial genres developed over the course of the seventeenth century. Sixtus's decorative projects were directed by two artists, Giovanni Guerra

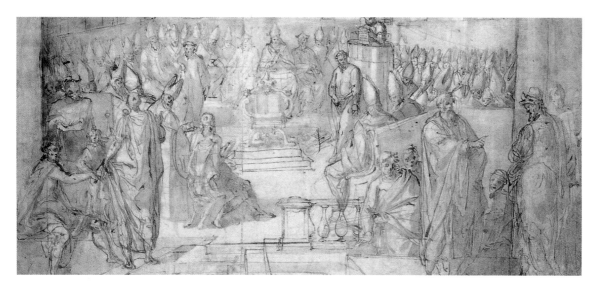

Figure 30. Cesare Nebbia (ca. 1536–1614), preparatory drawing for the *Nicene Council* (fig. 31). Pen and ink. Paul Prouté, Paris

(1544–1618) from Modena and Cesare Nebbia (ca. 1536–1614) from Orvieto. Guerra was an exponent of the sophisticated "international Mannerist" school and a versatile illustrator; he designed figurative and emblematic allegories and was in charge of distributing jobs among the artists who worked for the pope. Nebbia was a more measured artist and was influenced by the new, synthetic style of Girolamo Muziano (1532–1592). He was also responsible for all the historical-religious scenes executed in fresco. (It is with Nebbia that we find Orazio associated in the 1590s.)

While the content of every work was carefully monitored (each drawing was reviewed by the pope's team of learned advisers), artists did have a certain freedom, at least in terms of composition. The vast decorative cycles in the Vatican library (1588–89) are a good example (figs. 30, 31). There is no single style that unifies them; instead, they resemble a babel of languages, in which we find the confluence of a variety of regional schools as well as indications of the influence that Rome had on each artist who worked there.[11] Giovan Battista Ricci (ca. 1540–1627) of Novara and the Flemish painter Hendrick van den Broeck (ca. 1519–1597) stand out among the artists who came to work in the Vatican library with already established reputations in the art world. A far from secondary task was given to Orazio Gentileschi, who was probably responsible for the scene of the Third Lateran Council: one finds in it a style strongly rooted in Tuscan painting—lively but not yet mature, and deriving from his formative work with his brother Aurelio Lomi.[12] Among the crowd of as yet little-known artists painting there are the Emilian painter Ferraù Fenzone (1562–1645), Andrea Lilio (ca. 1570–after 1635) from the Marches,

and the Lombard Giovan Battista Pozzo (1561–1591), each of whom, in his own way, was working toward a revival of both the grand style of Raphael and a latent naturalism. Their very rapid success notwithstanding, these artists would never achieve Gentileschi's later international fame, when his style approached that of Caravaggio.

Sixtus V's large pictorial cycles indicate that he was most interested in the expeditious completion of his commissions, and thus he and his officials encouraged the practice of large numbers of artists working together but orchestrated according to their own specialties. They were less concerned with the quality of the resulting artistic creation. This situation also reflects the obsessive concern about the content of religious paintings according to the broad outlines of the Council of Trent, which were set forth in a variety of treatises (the first editions of Johannes Molanus and Gabriele Paleotti were published in 1570 and 1582, respectively) that attempted to codify the rules of a "correct" iconography according to the dictates of the Counter-Reformation.[13] These required that paintings be easily understood even by the uneducated and that images be purged of the "profane" and eccentric virtuoso passages which marked a Mannerist style, as well as of any iconography that was historically inaccurate. These rules combined the demands for an art that was both didactic and edifying with the need to respond to the often repeated criticisms leveled by Protestant reformers.[14] The theorists of the second half of the sixteenth century posited, furthermore, that in order to be a good painter it was not enough simply to imitate the great masters but that it was necessary "to follow nature" and to conform

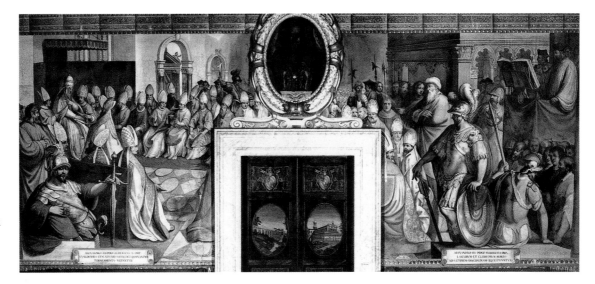

Figure 31. Hendrick van den Broeck
(ca. 1519–1597), *Nicene Council*.
Fresco. Biblioteca Apostolica,
Salone Sistino, Vatican

to "historical" truth; indeed, they were supporting the development of a new naturalism without being completely aware of it.

The interest during Sixtus's reign in painting that was both attentive to nature and bound by truth laid the foundation for the coming naturalism of the Carracci and the realism of Caravaggio. This was not so much the case, however, in the papal workshops, where, for example, the anatomical studies of the ironic Fenzone were an isolated instance and derived, perhaps, from the artist's sojourn at the Carracci Academy in Bologna. Instead, it was private commissions that encouraged the new tendencies in representation. The works of the three major protagonists of painting in the late sixteenth century—Federico Barocci (ca. 1535–1612), Scipione Pulzone (1561–1598), and Jacopo Zucchi (ca. 1541–1596)—stand as a good example of this diversity.[15] The first was a serene poet whose spiritual sensibility was mirrored in the personality of Saint Philip Neri (1515–1595). The second was a refined portraitist whom the Jesuits and Oratorians in particular valued for his faithful and solid "realism." The third—in his works for Ferdinando de' Medici and in the gallery of Orazio Rucellai—was a tormented and aristocratic interpreter of a mythical golden age. Although each painter took a different road in his art, they all contributed to preparing the ground for a new sensibility that no longer saw faith to nature as one possible component of painting but rather as its quintessential element. This attitude developed slowly, however, and it was only during the papacy of Clement VIII Aldobrandini (r. 1592–1605) that it fully flowered.

Ippolito Aldobrandini came to the papal throne in 1592 after a rapid succession of three popes in a little more than a year. He began his pontificate by announcing an Apostolic Visit to reform religious life, to revise divine offices, and to beautify the churches of Rome, all with an eye on the Jubilee of 1600.[16] Clement also worked, through deft negotiations, to increase the prestige of the papacy within the larger and complicated context of European affairs of state. Cardinal Bentivoglio noted that the pope had, in the short span of a few years, "achieved widespread fame through three events in particular. The first was to reconcile France and the Holy See. The second was to reconcile the two crowns [France and Spain]. And the third was to bring Ferrara back into the Papal States."[17] Having overcome Spanish domination of papal politics and reduced the fear of an unstoppable advance of the Turks, Clement created a sense that the Church had triumphed over Protestantism as well as heresy within the institution itself (Giordano Bruno was burned at the stake in Rome at the Campo de' Fiori in 1600). More important, perhaps, he also made the papacy once again an important player on the international stage. The notion of the Church Triumphant was reinforced by the conversion to Catholicism in 1593 of Henry IV of France (r. 1589–1610) and his reconciliation with Spain in 1598, the peaceful conquest of the duchy of Ferrara, and other successes (such as the conversion of a part of the Russian Orthodox Church to Rome through the Union of Brest). This idea was also destined to be celebrated in the arts.[18]

Unlike Sixtus V, Clement VIII did not concentrate on transforming the urban landscape; instead, he limited himself to finishing projects already under way, such as the Capitoline, Quirinal, and Vatican palaces, and the dome of Saint Peter's. It took the devastating flood of the Tiber in December 1598 to force

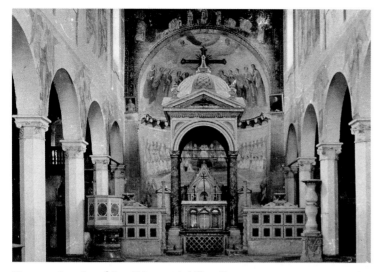

Figure 32. Interior of Santi Nereo e Achilleo, Rome

him to attend to streets, squares, bridges, and other damaged public works. His greatest interest, however, was in presenting a renovated splendor in the many churches of Rome, both inside and beyond its walls, to the pilgrims who would come for the Jubilee of 1600. This meant finishing and decorating new buildings and restoring old ones that languished in a state of deplorable ruin.[19] The investments required were huge and could not, furthermore, be supplied by the papal treasury. Instead, it was the confraternities, cardinals, and aristocrats, both old and new, who took on these extensive and expensive projects. Indeed, in these years the number of private commissions increased dramatically, intended not only to bring glory to the patron but also to reinforce the authority of the Roman Church and its teachings.[20]

These initiatives were further encouraged by the revival of interest in early Christianity and the cult of the martyrs, which was promoted by erudite historians dedicated to the study of ancient Christian sources, the Oratorian Cesare Baronio and other learned men, such as the Dominican Alfonso Chacon (see fig. 38) and Cardinal Federico Borromeo.[21] This fervent interest in the first centuries of Christianity was especially favored by the Oratorians of Philip Neri, who advocated a return to a purer spirituality and a direct faith even in popular ambients.[22] One consequence of this spirituality, encouraged by Saint Charles Borromeo and other influential people, was a concern for the poor and an emphasis on acts of charity; the impulse received its most exalted interpretation in the work of Caravaggio.[23]

This interest in the early Christian period also involved the systematic exploration of the catacombs by such talented scholars

as Antonio Bosio, who sought the "live image" of the apostolic Church.[24] This same sensibility encouraged a revaluation of the basilican form of churches and a desire to recover ancient frescoed and mosaic figural cycles among a group of cardinals who wanted to imitate the restorations of their colleagues Alessandro de' Medici and Cesare Baronio. Baronio's renovation of his titular church, Santi Nereo e Achilleo (fig. 32), provided a model of respect for ancient remains and a reverence for the relics of martyrs and early Christian iconography.[25] Gentileschi himself participated in a task of this sort: for Cardinal Pietro Aldobrandini he painted the apse of San Nicola in Carcere. Burzio has left a description of the destroyed frescoes that leads one to think that they were arranged in an archaic, symmetrical scheme: "Above, Our Lord surrounded by some angels who adored Him, and below, kneeling, Saints Nicholas, Mark, Marcellus, and Beatrice."[26]

Emblematic of this cultural climate is the general excitement created by the discovery in 1599 of the remains of Saint Cecilia in the church of Santa Cecilia, then being renovated under the supervision of Cardinal Paolo Emilio Sfondrato. The extensive restorations, which create a dialogue with the pre-existing medieval

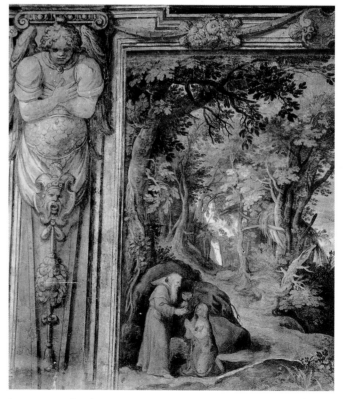

Figure 33. Paul Bril (1554–1626), *Saint Paul the Hermit*. Fresco. Santa Cecilia in Trastevere, capella del Bagno, Rome

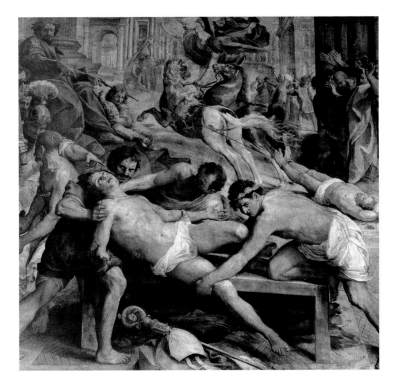

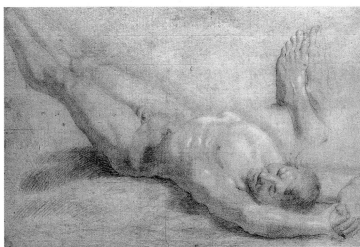

Figure 34. Giovanni Battista Pozzo (1561–1591), *Martyrdom of Saint Eleutherius.* Fresco. Chapel of Saint Lawrence, Santa Susanna, Rome

Figure 35. Giovanni Battista Pozzo, preparatory drawing for the *Martyrdom of Saint Eleutherius.* Galleria Marcello Aldelga, Rome

fabric of the building, included Paul Bril's (1554–1626) hermetic landscapes (fig. 33) and two canvases by the young Guido Reni (1575–1642) in the Martirio chapel, as well as Stefano Maderno's (1575–1636) sculpture of the body of Saint Cecilia on the high altar, placed in a sort of burial niche intended to suggest the tombs of the catacombs.[27] Particularly in the paintings by Reni and Francesco Vanni (1560/61–1610), there is evident a preference for a kind of protoclassicism that blended well with the archaic style of early Christian painting. As an ensemble, the interventions at Santa Cecilia reveal a plurality of tendencies that characterizes the art in the later years of Clement's pontificate.

This was not yet the case at Santa Prassede (1594–96), where Alessandro de' Medici—among the first cardinals to preserve the ancient arrangement of his titular church—commissioned a cycle of the Passion of Christ painted in a style typical of that during the pontificates of Gregory XIII and Sixtus V. However, Cardinal de' Medici's patronage of the arts was vast. Beyond his involvement in churches under his direct jurisdiction, he participated in the work undertaken at San Giovanni in Laterano and other important sites.[28] His preference for a classicism permeated with a historical sensibility is nowhere more evident than in the fresco he commissioned in the apse of Santa Maria in Trastevere in 1600 from the Florentine artist Agostino Ciampelli (1565–1630), who painted a sweet procession of angels carrying symbols of the

Virgin against a gold ground to match Pietro Cavallini's thirteenth-century mosaics above.[29]

Cardinal Domenico Pinelli's commission to decorate the nave of Santa Maria Maggiore around 1593 was more ambitious, although not entirely original. The large scenes from the life of the Virgin executed above the restored fifth-century mosaic cycle presented a difficult challenge for the artists who had been active under Sixtus V.[30] Lilio and Fenzone did their best to strengthen the dynamism and foreshortening of their figural representations; and the Bolognese artist Baldassarre Croce (1553/8–1628) tried to emulate the more poetic style of the new star in Clementine Rome, the Cavaliere d'Arpino (Giuseppe Cesari d'Arpino; 1568–1640). Ricci's traditional compositions are not unlike Gentileschi's still immature scene of the *Presentation of Christ in the Temple.*[31]

Cardinal Girolamo Rusticucci's campaign to decorate the church of Santa Susanna at the end of the sixteenth century offers an example of the abilities of Sixtus V's painters carried to their fullest extent. Nearly all the most important artists in Rome worked there for at least a brief period. Pozzo painted his masterwork in Camilla Peretti's chapel before his untimely death in 1591 (figs. 34, 35); Croce executed scenes from the story of Susanna in the nave and, together with Nebbia and Paris Nogari (ca. 1536–1601), worked in the presbytery.[32] These frescoes show a naturalistic tension that seems to open the door to Caravaggio's revolutionary

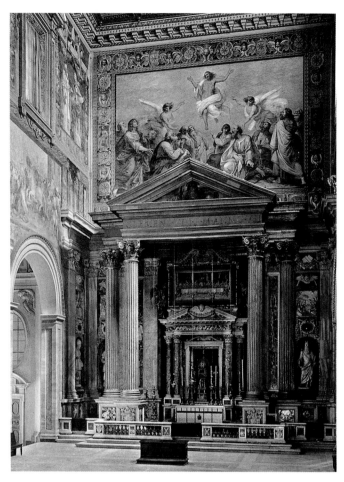

Figure 36. Cavaliere d'Arpino (1568–1640), *Ascension of Christ*. Fresco. San Giovanni in Laterano, Rome

style and makes it possible to talk about "a real relationship between Tommaso Laureti's powerful altarpiece the *Martyrdom of Saint Susanna*, painted in 1598, and the Contarelli chapel, which Caravaggio undertook in the Jubilee Year of 1600."[33]

The decoration of Santa Susanna provides but an indication of the changes that occurred in Rome in the space of a few years. Indeed, there was not simply an evolution of established styles but also a simultaneous and fruitful exploration of innovative avenues of representation. It was a period of extraordinary artistic production, and it involved perhaps even more artists than had worked during the pontificates of Leo X and Clement VII prior to the Sack of Rome, in 1527.[34] It is enough to note that in 1600, when Annibale Carracci (1560–1609) was finishing his work on the ceiling of the Farnese Gallery and Caravaggio was causing a sensation with his canvases for San Luigi dei Francesi (fig. 4), five first-rate artists were at work in Rome. The Cavaliere d'Arpino and the brothers Cherubino and Giovanni Alberti were occupied

with vast papal commissions. Federico Zuccari was finishing his very carefully thought-out decoration in the chapel of San Giacinto in Santa Sabina. And Cristoforo Roncalli was just beginning the mosaic decoration in the Clementina chapel in Saint Peter's and painting his masterpiece of classical monumentality, the *Death of Ananias and Sapphira*, now in Santa Maria degli Angeli.[35]

Immediately after, between 1601 and 1602, the future protagonists of European painting were to arrive in Rome. (The Venetian Carlo Saraceni had come to the city in 1598, and the German painter Adam Elsheimer in 1600.) These included the Emilian artists Francesco Albani, Domenichino, Giovanni Lanfranco, and Guido Reni; the Fleming Peter Paul Rubens, who joined his compatriots Paul Bril and Wenzel Cobergher; and Passignano, who became part of the large contingent of Tuscan artists that included Anastasio Fontebuoni, Andrea Commodi, and Antonio Tempesta. They were followed in 1604 by the Florentine Cigoli (fig. 102) and the Genovese Bernardo Castello, who came to execute two of the six enormous altarpieces for Saint Peter's, where Roncalli, Vanni, Passignano, and Giovanni Baglione were already at work on the other four.[36]

The number of Italian and foreign artists in Rome continued to grow over the succeeding years, attracted by the international art market and the great collectors of the time—the refined Cardinal del Monte, the rapacious Cardinal Borghese, and members of such families as the Aldobrandini, Farnese, Giustiniani, and Mattei.[37] Rome in the early seventeenth century saw a fortuitous conjunction of a taste for art and sumptuous lifestyles, "which in other periods had been restricted to only a few, especially cardinals and barons, and is now enjoyed by so many that it is truly a wonder."[38]

The oldest of the great masters in Rome was Federico Zuccari (1540/2–1609), who, in 1593, under the patronage of Cardinal Federico Borromeo, had reestablished the Accademia di San Luca. The academy's mission was, in part, to reaffirm the intellectual autonomy of painters and to defend their professional prerogatives. Zuccari did not receive any of the large papal commissions, and he spent most of his time on his theoretical writings and building his house on via Gregoriana, a sort of "Temple of the Virtues," which celebrated the artistic and familial dignity of its owner. At the time he finished his frescoes in Santa Sabina, he was writing his *L'idea de' pittori, scultori et architetti* (published in Turin in 1607), in which he proposed a close connection between metaphysical thought and the artistic process based on the concept of *disegno*.[39]

On the other hand, the Cavaliere d'Arpino and the Alberti brothers (Cherubino, 1553–1615; Giovanni, 1558–1601), from Borgo San Sepolcro, held official positions in the Roman art world. The latter two were especially sought after for the decorative system they created, with its extraordinary spatial effects and carefully calibrated architectural perspectives.[40] Clement VIII commissioned them to decorate rooms in the Palazzo Nuovo at the Vatican while they were still working on the ceiling of the Canons' sacristy at the Lateran; he later asked them to decorate the Aldobrandini chapel in Santa Maria sopra Minerva (for which he also wanted an altarpiece by Barocci). In the complex illusionism of the Sala Clementina (1596–1602), in which the painted architectural structure opens up to allow a view of the expanse of sky across the entire vault, the Alberti anticipate a perspective system that would be more fully developed in the Baroque period.[41]

The Cavaliere d'Arpino received the most prestigious commissions of this period. Entrusted with the frescoes in the Palazzo dei Conservatori as well as the cartoons for the mosaics on the interior of the dome at Saint Peter's, he also directed the decoration of the transept of San Giovanni in Laterano.[42] The Sala degli Orazi e Curiazi, a project he began in 1596, occupied him, on and off, until he was an old man. These scenes from the early history of Rome are masterpieces of narrative painting. Reflections of the work of Raphael in the Sala di Costantino gain poetic intonations— arcadian in the *Discovery of the She-Wolf* and epic in the two enormous battle scenes (against the Veii and Fidenae and between the Horatii and Curiatii). For the Jubilee, Arpino executed the iconic *Ascension of Christ* over the altar of the Sacrament in San Giovanni in Laterano (fig. 36), and he coordinated the efforts of a number of artists working on the *Scenes from the Life of Constantine*, including Cristoforo Roncalli (fig. 37) and Giovan Battista Ricci, who represented the extremes of innovation and tradition.[43] The result is a surprisingly unified decorative cycle. Nogari, Baglione, and the Cavaliere's brother Bernardino Cesari (1571–1622), as well as Orazio—who painted one of the imposing figures of the Apostles—fit between these two extremes.

The Cavaliere d'Arpino's workshop was, in the last decade of the sixteenth century, an important training ground for young artists. Even Caravaggio spent some time there shortly after he arrived in Rome. Arpino employed him "to paint flowers and fruit so well imitated that he showed that extraordinary beauty that everyone today admires."[44] This early period of Caravaggio's Roman career marked the beginning of his contribution to still-life painting, a genre brought to fruition by the Lombard painter in his *Basket of Fruit* (Pinacoteca Ambrosiana, Milan).[45] One of the centers of still-life painting in Rome was to be the academy of the aristocratic painter Giovanni Battista Crescenzi (1577–1635), who would be an artistic consultant to both Pope Paul V and King Philip IV of Spain.

The path to success for Caravaggio came in about 1595, when he joined the household of Cardinal del Monte, ambassador of the grand duke of Tuscany and a passionate student of art and science.[46] Just at the time that Caravaggio began to paint "with a vehemence of light and shadow," the artist obtained, through the offices of the cardinal, the commission to decorate the side walls of the Contarelli chapel in San Luigi dei Francesi (1599–1600). The

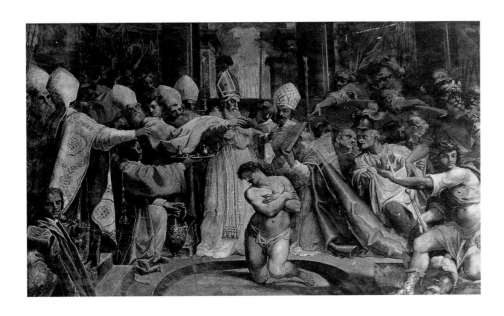

Figure 37. Cristoforo Roncalli (1552–1626), *Baptism of Constantine*. Fresco. San Giovanni in Laterano, Rome

real protagonist both in the quiet *Calling of Saint Matthew* and the tumultuous *Martyrdom of Saint Matthew* (fig. 4) is the powerful light that is a symbol of the grace of salvation as it bursts into the darkness of human existence.[47] This first public example of Caravaggio's exciting realism, which was both lauded and criticized, was followed by a number of masterpieces that hung in churches and private collections; together they mark an extraordinary turning point in style and taste. The impact of Caravaggio's work was disconcerting, "so much so that the painters of the day in Rome were taken by its novelty, and the young ones in particular flocked to him and praised him as the only imitator of nature, and, admiring his works as if they were miracles, competed with one another to follow his style."[48]

The Roman painter Giovanni Baglione (ca. 1566–1643), one of Caravaggio's rivals, was among the first to be influenced by the novelty of his style (fig. 39); he painted two lovely versions of *Sacred and Profane Love* (1602) for Cardinal Benedetto Giustiniani.[49] Nevertheless, these two pictures (one in Rome, the other in Berlin) could not compete with Caravaggio's recently completed *Amor Vincit Omnia* (Gemäldegalerie, Berlin), which its owner, Vincenzo Giustiniani, kept covered with a curtain so that it would not diminish the rest of the paintings in his collection.[50] Many painters followed Caravaggio's lead, although with varying results, and many were influenced by him, including Reni and Rubens. Among his Italian followers were Carlo Saraceni, Orazio Borgianni, Antiveduto Gramatica (fig. 120), Giovanni Serodine, and Bartolomeo Manfredi. Caravaggio's French imitators included Valentin de Boulogne and Nicolas Régnier, his Dutch followers Gerrit van Honthorst and Dirck van Baburen, and Jusepe de Ribera from Spain; these artists were in turn followed by a flood of painters working in a Caravaggesque manner, spreading it very quickly throughout Europe.[51] After having spent more than a decade trying to create his own style, Orazio too gradually became an adherent of his friend Caravaggio's revolutionary pictorial language. Nonetheless, as Giulio Mancini noted, Gentileschi should be placed with those artists "who have worked in their own manner and particularly without following in the footsteps of anyone."[52] In fact, his poetic naturalism and steely lighting reveal, among other things, a continual dialogue with the most refined products of "reformed" Tuscan painting.

The "school" of the Carracci brothers flourished in Rome alongside Caravaggio and his followers. Combining a lively naturalism with the ideal forms of a Raphaelesque classicism (fig. 43), it established another foundation for modern painting.[53] Leaving his cousin Ludovico in Bologna, Annibale Carracci, in 1595, had gone to Rome, where he was joined by his brother Agostino (1557–1602), to decorate the study of Cardinal Odoardo Farnese (1596–97) and then to paint the ceiling of the Farnese palace gallery (1598–1601). Annibale painted the vault of the gallery with "various emblems representing war and peace between sacred and profane love as described by Plato," in honor of the marriage between Ranuccio Farnese, duke of Parma, and the pope's niece Margherita Aldobrandini.[54] Mythological scenes were inserted into a fictive architectural framework that combines marvelously sculptural and naturalistic elements, medallions, and framed pictures that represent a joyful series of stories about the loves of the gods, culminating in the nuptial scene the *Triumph of Bacchus and Ariadne*.[55] Ingeniously inspired by Michelangelo's ceiling in the Sistine chapel, Carracci's vault is a festive counterpoint, and with its luminous colors and the naturalistic handling of fleshy figures and airy horizons, it points to the exuberant expressivity of the Baroque. The frescoes on the gallery walls (1602–3), which are connected thematically to the ceiling, were painted by Carracci's excellent students, including Domenichino and Lanfranco. These and the other Bolognese artists who came to Rome to study with Annibale and to work in his shop achieved what was almost a monopoly on all the large-scale fresco commissions in Roman villas, palaces, and churches in the first decades of the seventeenth century. (By contrast, Caravaggio's followers, like their master, painted mostly in oil.)[56]

The rich artistic heritage of Clement VIII's pontificate developed even further when Paul V Borghese (r. 1605–21) ascended the papal throne. It is at this time that the young Rubens was commissioned by the Oratorians to decorate the apse of the Chiesa Nuova (1606–8)—"the most beautiful and superb opportunity that there is in Rome."[57] These were also the years when the intelligent and open-minded policies of the powerful cardinal-nephew, Scipione Borghese, were predominant. Like the other great patrons of his time, Borghese knew how to choose the best painters both when he wanted to add to his collection and to decorate, so splendidly, the pavilions of his garden on the Quirinal hill (figs. 6, 7) and his famous villa at Porta Pinciana.[58]

After Caravaggio fled Rome in 1606 (he was accused of committing a murder during a street brawl), and following the deaths of Annibale Carracci and Federico Zuccari in 1609 and of Caravaggio himself in 1610, and the fading of the grand manner of the Cavaliere and Roncalli, the art world came slowly to be dominated by new players. The Bolognese artists, led first by Reni (fig. 49), who, in 1610, decorated the chapel of the Annunciation in the Palazzo del Quirinale,[59] emerged as the strongest artistic presence in Rome, although they were flanked by the great Florentine artists Cigoli (1559–1613) and Passignano (1559–1638)—who in 1610 received the lion's share of commissions for Paul V's project to decorate his chapel in Santa Maria Maggiore—and by the numerous followers of Caravaggio, including Gentileschi, who was to enjoy an enviable success.[60] The wealth and variety of artistic

expression was so great in Rome that a connoisseur of art such as Marchese Vincenzo Giustiniani could, in 1610, distinguish at least twelve modes or styles of painting in his *Discorso sopra la pittura* to classify the works of these diverse masters.[61] The first decade of the seventeenth century also witnessed great innovations in the music of Emilio de' Cavalieri (ca. 1550–1602) and Claudio Monteverdi (1567–1643).[62] And the new scientific method was marked by the founding, in 1603, of the Accademia dei Lincei, of which Galileo was a member. This vitality affirmed the possibility of a progressive blending of all fields of knowledge and the arts. Rome was a formidable arena, in which anyone might compete and which itself had much to offer.

1. Montaigne 1991, 211.
2. See Brussels–Rome 1995 for the important presence of Flemish painters in Rome in the sixteenth century.
3. Cornini, De Strobel, and Serlupi Crescenzi 1992, 151–67.
4. For Alessandro Farnese's patronage of the arts, see Robertson 1992.
5. For the work of these four and other Tuscan artists in Rome in the late sixteenth century, see Zuccari 2000, 137–66.
6. Baglione 1642, 359; Bissell 1981, 2.
7. For a general discussion of painting in the second half of the sixteenth century in Rome, see Freedberg 1975, 642–67, and Hall 1999, 189–214, 257–91.
8. For the reforms of Sixtus V and other aspects of his papacy, see Fagiolo and Madonna 1992; for an exhaustive discussion of the artistic production in Rome at that time, see Madonna in Rome 1993.
9. Haskell 1963, 63–72; Hibbard 1972, 29–49; Zuccari 1981b, 171–93.
10. Bevilacqua 1993, 35–46.
11. Zuccari 1992, 100, 139.
12. See Zuccari 1993, 71.
13. Prodi 1965, 123–88.
14. Scavizzi 1974, 171–212.
15. Zeri 1970, 82–97; Bologna 1975, 146–49; Morel 1999, 115–22.
16. Zuccari 1984, 9–13.
17. Bentivoglio 1807, 52.
18. For a general picture of Clement's pontificate, see Spezzaferro 1981, 185–200; for a comprehensive treatment of the period, see Puglisi 1998, 43–52.
19. See Abromson 1981 and Macioce 1990 for painting in Rome in the period of Clement VIII.
20. Spezzaferro 1981, 195.
21. Calvesi 1990, 294–95, 383–95; Jones 1992, 138–40, 152–62.
22. Zuccari 1995, 340–54.
23. Calvesi 1971, 123, 133–35.
24. Fiocchi Nicolai 2000, 105–30.
25. Zuccari 1981b, 171–93; Herz 1988, 590–620.
26. Zuccari 1984, 91.
27. Nava Cellini 1969, 18–41.
28. Zuccari 1984, 94–97, 109–26; Freiberg 1995, 38–41, 274, 285.
29. Prosperi Valenti Rodinò 1985, 519–21.
30. Barroero 1988, 224.
31. Zuccari 2000, 152; see ibid., fig.122, for Gentileschi's *Presentation of Christ in the Temple* after its recent restoration.

32. Strinati 1980, 26–28; Spezzaferro 1981, 234–36.
33. Strinati 2000, 61. For more general information on Laureti, see Spezzaferro 1981, 247–52.
34. Schleier 1989, 399–421; and, for the same period, see London–Rome 2001, esp. 16–41.
35. Chiappini di Sorio 1983, 112–13, 117–18.
36. Chappell and Kirwin 1974, 125–47.
37. For Cardinal del Monte's collection, see Frommel 1971, 5–55; for Scipione Borghese as a patron of the arts, see Coliva 2000, 16–24. For the Aldobrandini, Farnese, Giustiniani, and Mattei collections, see Cappelletti and Testa 1994; Parma–Munich–Naples 1995; Testa 2000; and Rome–Berlin 2001.
38. Paruta in Spezzaferro 1981, 186.
39. Strinati 1974, 104–11; Acidini Luchinat 1998–99, vol. 2, 234–36, 278–80.
40. Rome 1983, 7–12, and passim.
41. Macioce 1999, 133–41.
42. Rome 1973, 28–42.
43. Abromson 1981, 55–62; Freiberg 1995, 300–302.
44. Bellori 1976, 213.
45. See Rome 1995–96 for a recent acknowledgment of this argument.
46. Waźbiński 1994, 185–217, 409–91.
47. Calvesi 1990, 293–301.
48. Bellori 1976, 217.
49. Martinelli 1959, 82–96; Rome–Berlin 2001, 298–301.
50. Marini 1987, 459–61.
51. Nicolson 1979; Nicolson 1990.
52. Mancini (1617–21) 1956–57, vol. 1, 110–11; Marini 1981a, 385–87.
53. Bologna–Washington–New York 1986–87, 213–542.
54. Bellori 1976, 60.
55. Calvesi 1999, 127–31.
56. Schleier 1989, 435.
57. Letter from Rubens to Chieppo, published in Jaffé 1977, 88, 119.
58. Calvesi 1996, 13–42; Coliva 1998, 391–420.
59. Barroero 1988, 236–40; Ostrow 1996, 202–10. Cigoli painted the moon in the dome of the Pauline chapel according to Galileo's observations .
60. Pepper 1984b, 24–25, 224–25.
61. Giustiniani 1981, 41–45.
62. For these innovations in music and their relationship to the visual arts, see the essays by Strinati and Vodret and Macioce in Rome–Siena 2000–2001, 17–30, 95–104.

1.

Madonna and Child with Saints Sebastian and Francis

Oil on canvas, 30¾ × 31¼ in.
(78 × 79.5 cm)

Private collection, loan
arranged courtesy of
Matthiesen Fine Art Ltd.,
London

ca. 1597–1600

PROVENANCE: Private collection
(sale, Christie's, Rome,
December 4, 1984, lot 178,
attributed to Orazio Borgianni);
Matthiesen Fine Art Ltd.,
London (1985); private collection.

REFERENCES: London 1985,
36–38, no. 8; Schleier 1993, 196.

Sold in Rome in 1984 with an implausible attribution to Orazio Borgianni, the picture was ascribed to Orazio Gentileschi by Schleier and Todini and exhibited as such at Matthiesen Fine Art Ltd., London, in 1985. As possibly the earliest known easel painting by Orazio and his first devotional painting of the Madonna and Child, the picture is key to understanding the pre-Caravaggesque phase of his art.

A note of informal domesticity is struck by the seated pose and contemporary dress of the Virgin and the affectionate caress of the child, who extends his hands toward the veiled head of his mother. The latter motif was perhaps inspired by Raphael's much copied composition known as the *Madonna di Loreto* (Musée Condé, Chantilly), the original of which was acquired by Cardinal Paolo Emilio Sfondrato in 1591, and it reminds us of the importance Raphael had as a reference point for the generation of Mannerist painters with whom Orazio worked in the 1590s.[1] This attempt at a warmly human depiction is somewhat compromised by the incongruously formal attitudes of the two flanking saints. Especially the Saint Sebastian, on the left, reads as an insertion, and we are left to infer how his foreshortened right arm behind the Virgin's shoulder might connect to the arrow (his attribute of martyrdom) behind her head. As often happens in Orazio's early work, space has not been resolved. The insistently isocephalic composition seems distinctly archaic: the two saints would indeed be more at home behind a strictly frontal image of the Virgin, as might be found in medieval paintings. Is this effect coincidental, or is Orazio's composition motivated by the antiquarian interests espoused by the circle of the great Oratorian Cesare Baronio (1538–1607)—the kind of image, for example, that one finds in Baldassarre Croce's frescoed "icon" of Saint Gabinio between Saints Susanna and Felicità in the crypt of the church of Santa Susanna, Rome?

That the effect was intentional is suggested by the appearance of Sebastian: with a mustache and incipient beard instead of clean-shaven, as he is most frequently shown; decorously draped rather than nude; and with a single arrow piercing his neck. Interestingly, these features reappear—with the exception that the saint is fully bearded—in a medieval painting formerly in San Pietro in Vincoli that is recorded in a drawing (fig. 38) by the Dominican antiquarian Alfonso Chacon (1530–1599).[2] In the same church is a seventh-century mosaic showing the saint, aged and clothed, that was singled out by Baronio in his *Martyrologium romanum* (Rome, 1586) as a model contemporary artists should emulate.[3] Gentileschi's saint is young, not old, but there seems a real possibility that the archaizing touches were a response to an individual in Baronio's circle.

As might be expected from someone with Gentileschi's late-Mannerist training, the figures are

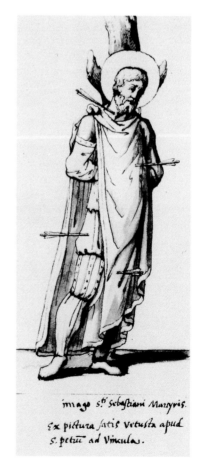

Figure 38. Alfonso Chacon (1530–1599), *Saint Sebastian*. Pen, ink on paper, and gray wash, after an icon in San Pietro in Vincoli. Biblioteca Apostolica Vaticana, Vat. lat. 5408, f. 24r, Vatican City

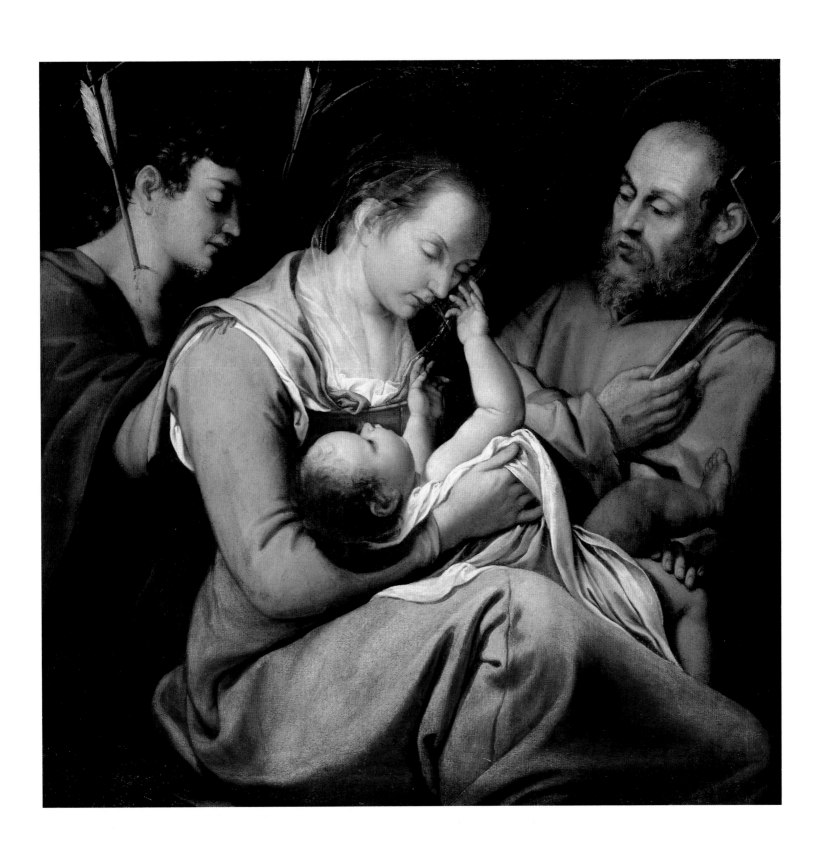

strikingly conventional in their generalized treatment and there is no hint of the use of posed models. But in the emphasis given to the coarse texture and sewn seam of the Virgin's dress, the coral-colored lace at the top of the sleeve, and the elegant description of Saint Francis's beard, there are clear signs of the direction Orazio's art will take under the aegis of Caravaggio.

Schleier has dated the picture to about 1601–2 and relates its style to Giovanni Baglione. My feeling is that the work may be even earlier. In the catalogue accompanying the Matthiesen exhibition, its style is compared with that of Gentileschi's work in the Benedictine abbey at Santa Maria, Farfa, contracted in February 1597 and completed two years later.[4] The style of the Farfa decorations is disparate, both because of Orazio's use of an équipe of assistants to speed work along and because at this date he adapted his style to circumstance. It is especially with the altarpiece of Saint Ursula, Farfa (fig. 2)— which is certainly autograph despite its rather disappointing quality and unappealing character—that the present picture bears comparison, the Saint Sebastian having the same morphological features as

some of the kneeling figures in that work. At the same time, the Madonna and Saint Francis have a bulk not unlike that of the enormous figure of an apostle that Orazio frescoed under the direction of the Cavaliere d'Arpino in the transept of San Giovanni in Laterano, Rome, as part of the decorations for the Jubilee year of 1600.[5] There is no hint of an awareness of the art of Caravaggio, with whom Orazio became associated about 1600. Paradoxically, the novelty of the picture resides not in an incipient naturalism but in its rejection of the stylishly Mannerist art of Cristoforo Roncalli and Arpino and its emphasis on plain—almost artless—figure types.

1. Sfondrato sold the picture to Scipione Borghese in 1608; the original is in the Musée Condé, Chantilly; see Gould in Chantilly 1979–80, 8–11.
2. *Vat. lat.* 5408, fol. 24r; see Herklotz 1985, figs. 16, 17, where the captions have inadvertently been reversed.
3. See Herklotz 1985, 69–72.
4. For a review of the documents and a proposal of the division of hands, see Bissell 1981, 135–37.
5. Which of two figures of apostles Gentileschi frescoed is not altogether clear; see p. 35 n. 18 in this publication.

2.

Saint Francis Supported by an Angel

Oil on canvas, 54⅞ × 39¾ in. (139.5 × 101 cm)

Private collection, New York

ca. 1600

New York, Saint Louis

PROVENANCE: Private collection, New York (from 1987).

REFERENCES: Nicolson 1979, 53; Nicolson 1990, 115, fig. 197; Schleier 1993.

In accordance with the renewed spirituality of the sixteenth century and, in particular, the reforming zeal of the Capuchin order (an independent branch of the Franciscans approved by Pope Paul III in 1536), the cult of Saint Francis enjoyed revived popularity.[1] The thirteenth-century saint became an exemplar of devotional practice, with emphasis placed on his conformity to Christ through his visionary and mystical experiences. He was now shown in ecstasy, consoled by an angel who either supports him or, flying aloft, plays a violin. Even in depictions of Saint Francis receiving the stigmata, one or more angels are frequently included. In her seminal study of 1969, Askew demonstrates that these images owe much to paintings of

the dead Christ supported by angels or of Christ in the Garden of Gethsemane consoled by an angel (as in Paolo Veronese's painting in the Brera, Milan, of about 1580). Among the earliest treatments of this new iconography is a lost altarpiece by Francesco Vanni reported to have been painted for the Capizucchi chapel in Santa Maria Maggiore, Rome, in 1592,[2] but unquestionably the most influential painting was Caravaggio's *Ecstasy of Saint Francis*, painted about 1594 (fig. 40). Rather than treat the stigmatization in its conventional form, as a dramatic miracle in which the saint, with arms outspread, is imprinted by a small seraph with the wounds of Christ, Caravaggio envisaged the event as a mystical occurrence—much as he was

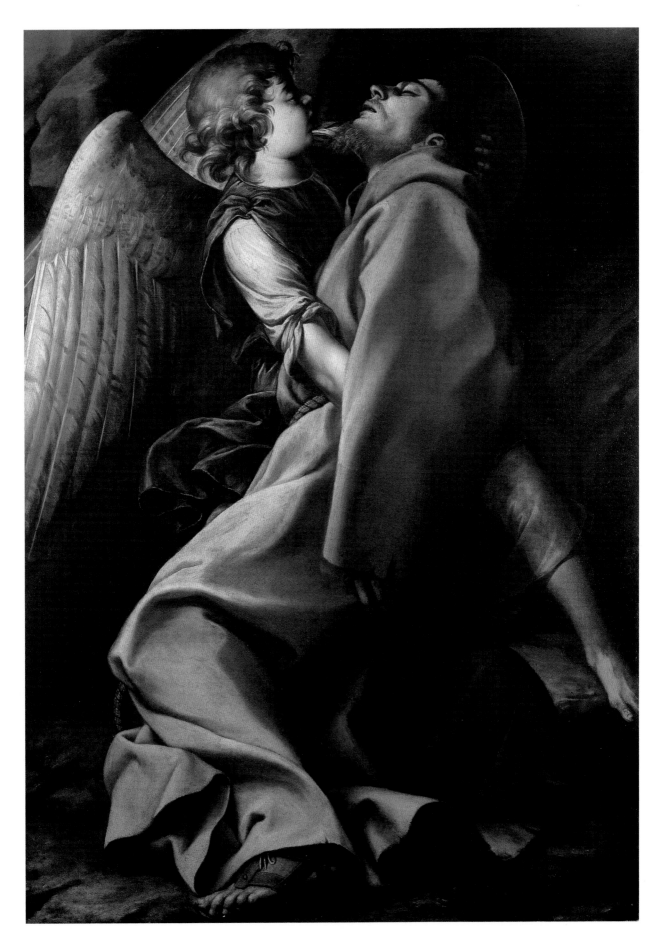

later to do in the Cerasi chapel (Santa Maria del Popolo, Rome) with the *Conversion of Saint Paul*.

Gentileschi treated the subject of Saint Francis consoled by an angel no less than four times (see cat. nos. 3, 6, 21). His growing ability to probe the theme and suggest the interior life of the saint is directly related to his grasp of one of the fundamental paradoxes of Caravaggesque painting: that far from being dependent on elaborate poses and expressive gestures, psychological intensity is actually increased by treating the figure in terms of still life and concentrating on the effect of real, physical presence. This, his earliest depiction, takes a first step in that direction. Saint Francis is shown full length, his body collapsing, his head cradled by a youthful angel, who looks intently at the blood-drained face. Perhaps not coincidentally, the saint's pose recalls that of the swooning Virgin at the foot of the cross; indeed, the Virgin's sorrow over Christ's Passion was associated by Saint Francis of Sales with the stigmatization of Saint Francis.[3]

The active pose of the angel is perhaps meant to offer a visual contrast—a contrapposto—to the limp body of the saint, but there is no denying that the splayed pose is both distracting and implausible. It would seem to derive by way of still unidentified intermediary sources from a sarcophagus relief of the abduction of the daughters of Leucippus (examples are in the Uffizi, Florence, and in the Vatican).[4] The strong, planar quality of the pose and the emphasis on fluttering, varicolored drapery are typically Mannerist. By contrast, the pose of Saint Francis seems to have been studied from a model, though Gentileschi has been content with a generalized description of the habit, elaborating the folds with a view to conventional standards of *bellezza*. Light, too, is treated referentially

rather than specifically described. It is worth comparing the delicately highlighted beard with that of the Saint Francis in the *Madonna and Child* (cat. 1). The fact that the saint is shown wearing sandals rather than barefoot probably indicates that the painting was not destined for a Capuchin establishment or a patron with Capuchin ties.

The picture must be slightly earlier than the *Stigmatization of Saint Francis* (cat. 3), in which the configuration of the drapery of the saint is closely similar but the poses of the figures and the treatment of light have been conceived along strictly Caravaggesque lines. Schleier has proposed dating the present painting to about 1601–3, and he has noted an affinity with the work of Giovanni Baglione. Like Bissell, I would place the picture earlier, and I would also note the importance of Cesare Nebbia as an influence.[5] It was in Gentileschi's four documented angels in the cupola of the Madonna dei Monti, Rome—a commission of 1599 that he shared with Nebbia—that he made the first move to shed his Mannerist chrysalis.[6] The angel can be compared with some of the sibyls at Farfa, and I do not believe the picture can be much later than that cycle of frescoes.

1. The classic study is Askew 1969. For a survey of Capuchin spirituality, see Petrocchi 1984, 195–201, 265–72.
2. Romagnoli 1976, vol. 8, 529.
3. Noted by Askew 1969, 290.
4. See Bober and Rubinstein 1991, 161 no. 126.
5. Bissell, in a lengthy analysis of March 25, 1989, originally suggested a date of about 1600–1601. In a letter of October 19, 2000, he has informed me that he is now inclined to place it about 1598–99—always allowing for the lack of firm points of reference.
6. See Barroero 1981.

3.

Stigmatization of Saint Francis

Oil on canvas, 64 × 45⅝ in.
(162.5 × 116 cm)

Private collection

ca. 1600–1601

Gentileschi here shows the moment after Saint Francis received the stigmata on Mount La Verna. A wooden cross is propped on a rocky ledge while, above, the rays of a miraculous light illuminate the figures. Tears course down the saint's cheeks, attesting to his sorrow for the suffering of Christ but also alluding, more generally, to what sixteenth- and seventeenth-century religious writers referred to as the gift of tears. In his treatise *Delli dolori di Christo Signor Nostro*, published in Bergamo in 1598, the Capuchin friar Mattia da Salò wrote of "sweet and bitter tears that, washing the face, leave the interior like fire."[1] Ignatius of Loyola distinguished three kinds of tears: those arising from the thoughts of one's own or other's sins, those arising—as here—from contemplation of the life of Christ, and those flowing from the love of divine persons.[2] Wings extended, an angel struggles visibly to support the saint's collapsing body. Francis's companion, Brother Leo, is normally included in representations of the stigmatization, but here the saint's steadfast gaze toward the rays of light and the presence of the stigmata on his hand and foot alone indicate the narrative moment.

Catalogue nos. 2 and 3 are closely related in theme and composition. It is indeed possible that Gentileschi laid in the initial pose of the figure of Saint Francis using a tracing from the other picture. Yet for all the similarity in the saint's pose and in the arrangement of his habit, there is a profound shift in mood and style. What in catalogue no. 2 is apprehended as an interior experience is here externalized, and the approach is far more descriptive. The way the angel, his leg bent and his head thrown back, grips the cord of the saint's habit with his left hand while with the right he supports Francis beneath his right arm suggests that Gentileschi studied the mechanics of the pose from a model. The same realistic intent is evident in the depiction of the coarse weave, patches, and tattered edges of the saint's habit (traits that associate the picture with the reforming zeal of the Capuchins), in the sheen and texture of

PROVENANCE: Private collection, Chile (sale, Sotheby's, New York, June 3, 1988, lot 72, as Roman school); Richard L. Feigen & Co., New York (1988–2000; exh., New York 1990b, no. 8); private collection.

REFERENCES: Nicolson 1990, 115; Papi in Florence 1991, 36; Schleier 1993, 196.

the angel's wings, and in the various plants. A dandelion (with one bloom and a flower gone to seed), clover, and a fig can be identified. The fig commonly refers to the Resurrection and is a motif underscoring the analogy of the Stigmatization with Christ's Passion.

There can be little doubt that Orazio was responding directly to the descriptive character of Caravaggio's painting of the same subject (fig. 40), then in the collection of the banker Ottavio Costa. But he has seen that early masterpiece through the lens of Caravaggio's more focused and dramatically lit paintings of about 1600–1601—not only the *Calling of Saint Matthew* and the *Martyrdom of Saint Matthew* (fig. 4), in the Contarelli chapel in San Luigi dei Francesi, Rome, but also the canvases in the Cerasi chapel in Santa Maria del Popolo. Only later was he to grasp the refined poetics of the Lombard painter's early work. Like many of his contemporaries, Gentileschi was overwhelmed by Caravaggio's first public commissions, which had an immediate and far-reaching impact. In 1601, just a year after the unveiling of the Contarelli canvases, Giovanni Baglione painted a *Saint Francis with Two Angels*, and it is with that picture (fig. 39)—Baglione's first and most impressive response to Caravaggio—that Orazio's picture should be compared.[3] Baglione's is a more successful work of art, seamlessly grafting onto an accomplished Mannerist style the dramatic lighting and realistic intent of Caravaggio's work. By comparison, Orazio's painting is awkward (the foreshortened face of the angel is especially unsuccessful) and even unappealing. The contradiction between the angel's agitated drapery, with its sharp colors, and the naturalistic rendering of the saint is unresolved. Yet Gentileschi's painting demonstrates a desire to press beyond Baglione's superficial Caravaggism and to treat Caravaggesque naturalism not as a veneer but as a basis of style. Here, that naturalism is restricted to details: the wings of the angel, the plants, the head of Saint Francis, all of which are treated in an almost overly emphatic way.

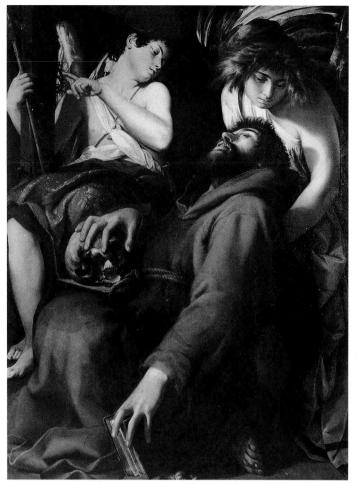

Figure 39. Giovanni Baglione (ca. 1566–1643), *Saint Francis with Two Angels*. Oil on canvas. Private collection

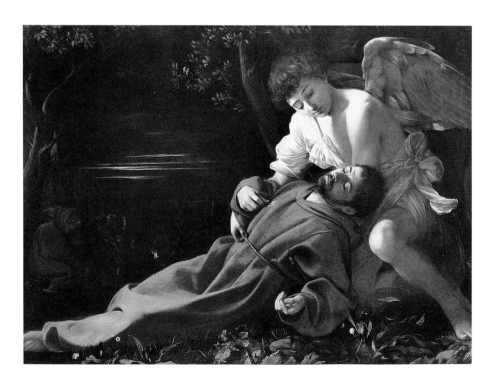

Figure 40. Michelangelo Merisi da Caravaggio (1571–1610), *Ecstasy of Saint Francis*. Oil on canvas. Wadsworth Atheneum Museum of Art, Hartford, The Ella Gallup Sumner and Mary Catlin Sumner Collection Fund

I see no reason why the painting should not be more or less contemporary with Baglione's. Certainly Papi's suggestion that the picture dates to as late as 1611 is unacceptable, for by that date Orazio was an artist of incomparable accomplishment. There is a temptation to identify the habit of Saint Francis and the wings of the angel with the props—"una veste da cappuccino" and "un par d'ale"—that Caravaggio borrowed from Gentileschi in 1603 (the former perhaps for Caravaggio's *Saint Francis in Meditation*, two versions of which are known [San Pietro, Carpineto Romano, and church of the Cappuccini, Rome]; the latter possibly already used in the *Love Triumphant* [Gemäldegalerie, Berlin]).

When the *Saint Francis* first appeared at auction in 1988, it was catalogued as "Roman School, circa 1610." Spike's attribution to Artemisia Gentileschi and an alternative one to Baglione are recorded. Nicolson points out its relationship to catalogue no. 2 but lists it with a question mark. The painting cannot be the one Clelia del Palaggio lent in 1703 to the annual exhibition held in San Salvatore in Lauro, Rome, since that *Saint Francis* measured approximately 132 centimeters.[4] The picture has not been cut (stretch marks are visible along the edges). Aside from abrasion in the angel's garments, especially in the darks, the picture is in good condition.

1. ". . . dolci et amare lagrime, le quali, bagnando il viso lasciano l'interiore tutto quanto fuoco" (Mattia da Salò 1598, 233, cited in Petrocchi 1984, 266).
2. Expressed in a letter written by Ignatius to Saint Francis Borgia, quoted in Meissner 1999, 559.
3. In a letter of October 19, 2000, Bissell underscores the comparison with Baglione's painting. He too sees this as a work of about 1601.
4. See Bissell 1981, 220–21, and De Marchi 1987, 176.

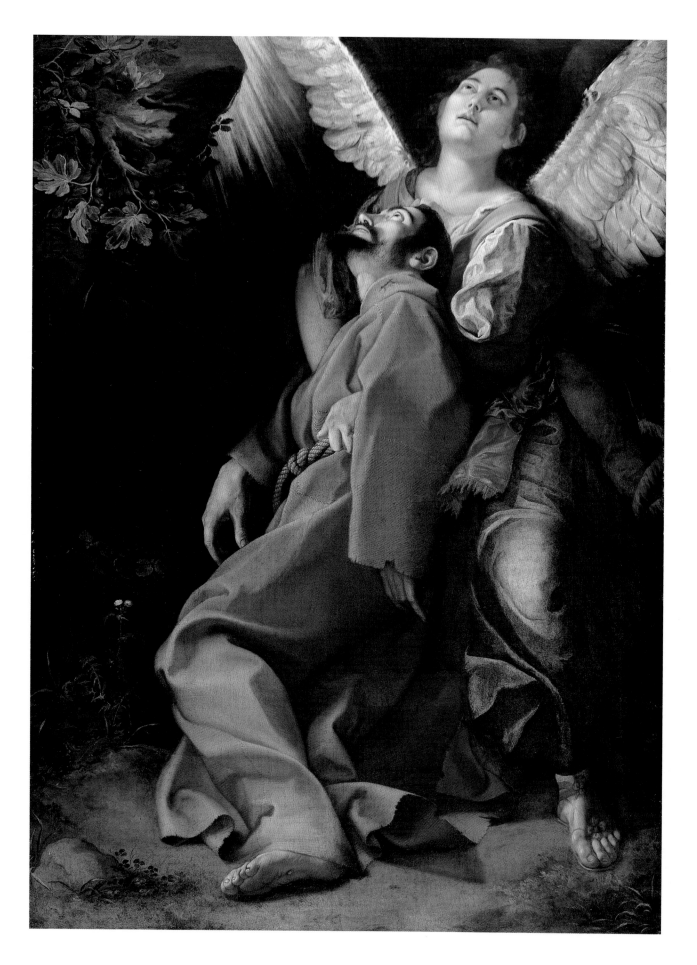

4.

FOLLOWER OF CARAVAGGIO, POSSIBLY ORAZIO GENTILESCHI

Madonna and Child

Oil on canvas, 51⅝ × 35⅞ in.
(131 × 91 cm)

Galleria Nazionale d'Arte
Antica, Palazzo Corsini,
Rome (inv. 261)

ca. 1603–5(?)

PROVENANCE: Cardinal
Lorenzo Corsini, Rome (before
1730); Corsini collection, Rome
(inv. 1750, no. 140, as by
Caravaggio); Prince Tommaso
Corsini, Palazzo Corsini, Rome
(until 1856; inv. 1808, as by
Caravaggio); Princes Tommaso
and Andrea Corsini, Rome
(1856–83; sold to the Italian
state in 1883); Galleria
Nazionale d'Arte Antica,
Palazzo Corsini, Rome.

RELATED PICTURES: Villa
Poggio Imperiale, Florence
(noted by Marangoni); private
collections, Rome and Bergamo
(cited by Longhi, 1916);
Sotheby's, New York, April 7,
1988, lot 192 (reduced at left,
bottom, and right).

REFERENCES: Burckhardt
1855, 1027; Longhi (1916) 1961,
230–31; Gamba 1922–23, 246;
Marangoni 1922–23, 220–21;
Longhi 1951, 26–27; Milan
1951, 36 no. 46; Longhi 1952, 31;
Mahon 1952, 19; Baumgart 1955,
111 no. 7; Wagner 1958, 228–29;
Berne Joffroy 1959, 162; Jullian
1961, 143–44; Kitson 1967, 91–92
no. 33; Moir 1967, 19 n. 27,
39 n. 70; Ottino della Chiesa
1967, 86 no. 9; Longhi (1968)
1999, 264; Cinotti in Dell'Acqua
and Cinotti 1971, 124, 193–94
n. 415; Marini 1974, 467–68

That there remain significant gaps in our knowledge about even Caravaggio's best followers is demonstrated by the problematic status of this alluringly intimate depiction of the Madonna and Child. In the eighteenth and nineteenth centuries, it was ascribed to the Lombard master,[1] and as such it was exhibited in the "Mostra del Caravaggio," held in Rome in 1914. This truly untenable attribution was rightly dismissed by Longhi (1916) in favor of one to Gentileschi, and it is Orazio who has gained the widest acceptance, having been taken up with various degrees of conviction by Gamba, Jullian, Baumgart, Ottino della Chiesa, Kitson, Marini, and Cinotti.[2] Surprisingly, Longhi (1951; 1952; 1968) later returned to Caravaggio and was followed in this by Berne Joffroy, Nicolson, and, briefly, Mahon. Marangoni proposes that the picture is a copy after a lost work by the Lombard master, and this opinion has also found a few supporters, most notably Bissell. When the picture was shown at the Artemisia exhibition held in Florence in 1991, Papi noted its problematic status, cataloguing it as Caravaggesque, about 1610. He cautiously introduced the name of Spadarino for consideration (I personally see no grounds for this speculation) but rightly emphasized the picture's Gentileschian character and did not exclude the possibility that it was by the young Artemisia, to whom Hermanin had ascribed it in the 1924 catalogue of the Corsini collection.[3]

As this brief survey makes clear, we are dealing with a picture of exceptional quality and individual character—one based on a close study of the work of Caravaggio but that in many respects approaches the aesthetic of Gentileschi. There is an echo—in the turn of the Virgin's head, the elegant line of her halo, the firm grasp of her right hand, the chipped stone block on which she sits, and the oversized infant—of Caravaggio's Madonna di Loreto (Sant'Agostino, Rome), a work of 1604–6. At the same time, the diffuse rather than strongly raking light, the densely modeled drapery, and the mood of tenderness recall Caravaggio's paintings of the previous decade—the Rest on the Flight into Egypt and the Penitent Magdalene (both Doria Pamphili, Rome). It is as though the artist had experienced the mature Caravaggio but was drawn ineluctably to an earlier moment. To a degree, this is the trajectory of Orazio's career up to about 1610–13. Bissell found the "rusticity" of the image troublesome but recognized the affinity with Gentileschi's later treatment of the theme in Bucharest (cat. 15). Another, earlier image (cat. 1) underscores the persistence of this trait in Orazio's devotional imagery. Equally, Caravaggio's only easel-sized painting of the Madonna and Child—the so-called Aquavella Holy Family, recently recovered—demonstrates how fundamentally foreign this sort of domesticity is to his art.[4]

The genrelike quality of the image was noted by viewers, as indicated by the entry in the 1808 Corsini inventory, which describes the Virgin as "dressed as a country maiden."[5] Similarly, Gamba singled out the "military greatcoat" (casacca alla moschettiera) worn by the child. It was Longhi (1951), with his tendency to read Caravaggio's work in terms of realism, who first described the Virgin as "weaning her child," whence the title Madonna dello svezzamento, by which the painting is sometimes known. But it is important to remember that the child's gesture is no mere genre motif. It occurs in several of Raphael's devotional paintings (Musée Condé, Chantilly; Gemäldegalerie, Berlin; National Gallery of Art, Washington, D.C.) and is meant to emphasize the Virgin's role as nurturer: she is, by implication, a "Madonna lactans."

The planar quality of the composition and the raspberry to olive-ochre palette suggest an artist who, like Gentileschi, was trained in a Mannerist mode. If this Madonna and Child is, in fact, by Orazio, as I am inclined to believe, it must predate circa 1605 and, like the Way to Calvary (cat. 5), it represents an extreme experiment in Caravaggesque imagery. (Berne Joffroy's comment on the picture was, "I don't believe Gentileschi was

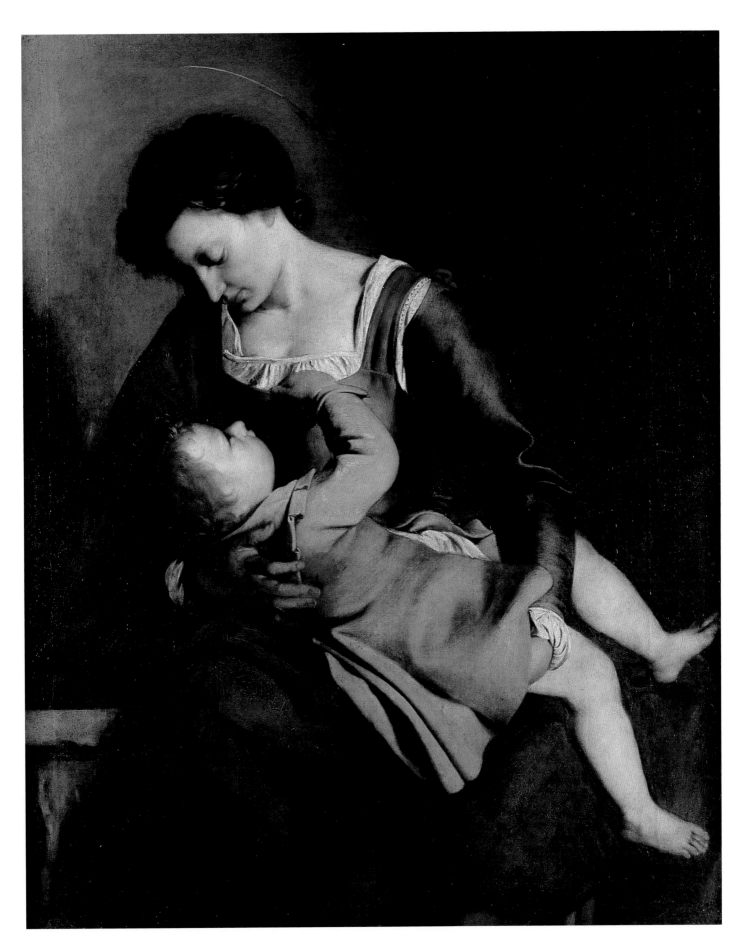

no. R-10; Nicolson 1979, 32;
Magnanimi 1980, 95, 104, nos. 7,
8; Bissell 1981, 144, 204 no. x-14;
Cinotti and Dell'Acqua 1983,
563 no. 83; Gash 1985, 255–56;
Nicolson 1990, 79; Papi in
Florence 1991, 90–93 no. 1.

ever this close to Caravaggio . . . that he ever understood as well the role of Caravaggesque light and
dark"—a position that today we might wish to modify.) If, on the other hand, it is dated later, it cannot
be by Orazio. Nor, I think, can it be by the young
Artemisia. Although her images of the Madonna and
Child certainly develop this domestic slant, there are
simply too few connections with the Spada *Madonna
and Child* (cat. 52).

1. For the inventory references, see Magnanimi 1980.
2. For a full account of the extensive bibliography, see Cinotti
and Dell'Acqua 1983, and Papi in Florence 1991, 90–93 no. 1.
3. The picture is reported to have been ascribed for a time to
Saraceni, though this attribution never had a following.
4. See Christiansen 1999.
5. Magnanimi 1980.

5.
Way to Calvary

Oil on canvas, 54½ × 68⅛ in.
(138.5 × 173 cm)

Kunsthistorisches Museum,
Vienna (inv. 1553)

ca. 1605–7

PROVENANCE: Cardinal
Alessandro Albani, Rome
(d. 1779; his estate, until 1800);
Kunsthistorisches Museum,
Vienna.

REFERENCES: Engerth 1881,
vol. 1, 318–19 no. 447; Glück and
Schaeffer 1907, 109; Voss 1912,
62; Longhi 1915, 66; Longhi
1943, 11–13; Longhi 1951, 28;
Longhi 1952, 24; Baumgart 1955,
113 no. 12; Berne Joffroy 1959,
97–98; Ottino della Chiesa 1967,
96 no. 48; Longhi (1968) 1999,
256; Fagiolo dell'Arco and
Marini 1970, 118; Cinotti in
Dell'Acqua and Cinotti 1971, 124;
Pepper 1971, 343 n. 47; Pepper
1972, 178 n. 4; Marini 1974, 467
no. R-9; Moir 1976, 119 no. 121,

The subject of this haunting picture derives not
from the Gospels, which are notably cryptic
about the *via crucis*, but from medieval devotional
literature. The thirteenth-century *Meditationes vitae
Christi* describes Christ's encounter with his mother,
his admonition to a group of women (based on
Luke 23:28), and his collapse beneath the weight of
the cross. The last event, which frequently includes
Veronica offering Christ a cloth on which his face will
be imprinted, is shown in depictions of the fifteen
Mysteries of the Rosary. All three incidents became
part of the devotion popularized by the Franciscans of
the Stations of the Cross, in which, in its final form,
Christ falls three times.[1] Gentileschi's picture differs
from the more elaborate representations of the subject found in altarpieces such as Raphael's *Spasimo di
Sicilia* (Prado, Madrid), of about 1516, and Federico
Zuccari's *Way to Calvary* (Olgiati chapel, Santa
Prassede, Rome), of 1595, in its reduction of the number of figures and its emphasis on the moving
exchange between Christ and the holy woman, most
likely Mary Magdalene. His approach, in which the
elaborate narrative drama of Renaissance practice is
transformed into a scene in which the action is frozen
and attention is concentrated on the protagonists,
captured in a moment of decision or revelation, derives
directly from Caravaggio's work of 1600–1603. Also
Caravaggesque is the choice of a half-length format

(actually, three-quarter length in the Gentileschi),
which increases the psychological concentration;
indeed, as in Caravaggio's most novel paintings, the
viewer has the impression of being a participant in
the event. I don't think there can be any doubt that
Gentileschi took inspiration from Sebastiano del

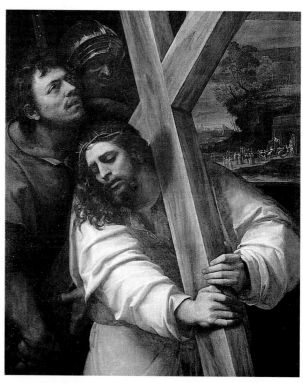

Figure 41. Sebastiano del Piombo (ca. 1485–1547), *Christ Bearing
the Cross.* Oil on canvas. Museo Nacional del Prado, Madrid

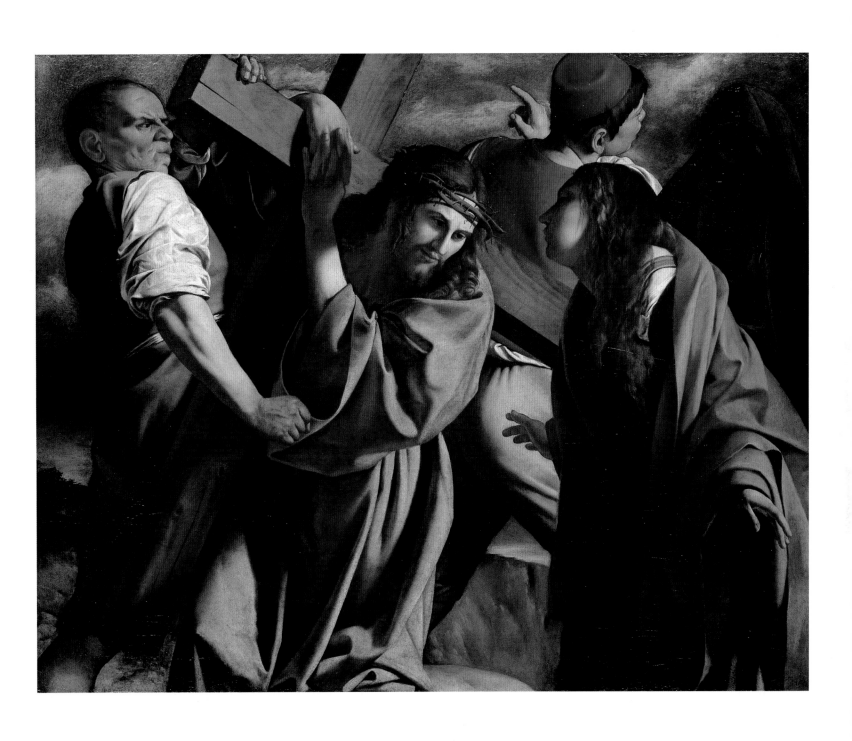

161 n. 287; Nicolson 1979, 52; Bissell 1981, 209 no. X-25; Cinotti 1983, 566 no. 90; Nicolson 1990, 114; Vienna 1991, 61; Bologna 1992, 348 no. 105; Bissell 1999, 201, 311, 346.

Piombo's powerful and enormously influential painting of Christ carrying the cross (fig. 41),[2] in which a half-length figure of Christ moves tragically but ineluctably toward the viewer (Orazio probably knew a copy of one of the three autograph variants).

Remarkably, only in the last thirty years has the *Way to Calvary* been recognized as a keystone in Orazio's career, marking his transformation into one of the most intelligent and personal followers of Caravaggio. Its early history is unknown, but it was among thirty-one paintings acquired by the Kunsthistorisches Museum in 1800 from the estate of Cardinal Alessandro Albani in Rome.[3] At the museum it was ascribed to the Bolognese painter Alessandro Tiarini until, in 1912, Voss argued that it was by a follower of Caravaggio active in Rome. In 1943, Longhi proposed that the picture was either by Caravaggio (in 1915, he had suggested Givanni Battista Caracciolo [1578–1635] as its author) or a copy of a lost work by the artist. Surprisingly, this improbable idea—the palette alone should have eliminated Caravaggio's name from consideration—enjoyed a certain critical fortune.[4] The value of Longhi's contribution lay not in the erroneous attribution (which strangely he continued to maintain), but in his acute characterization of the picture's style. The *Way to Calvary* could, he asserted, be associated with Caravaggio's *Martyrdom of Saint Matthew* in San Luigi dei Francesi, Rome (fig. 4), and belonged to a group of half-length compositions that were the products of an "intermezzo 'classicistico'" inspired by contact with Annibale Carracci.[5] Yet, with what now seems prescient qualifications, he remarked that the folds of Christ's drapery might be thought too self-consciously arranged for Caravaggio, "quasi Gentileschiane," and the head of Christ was perhaps "un po' troppo bella." But, he maintained, these were merely the indications on which Orazio and Caracciolo would build. That the picture is, in fact, by Orazio was first asserted by Pepper in 1971. This attribution has been accepted by Marini, Nicolson, Bissell, and Bologna,[6] and is the current designation at the Kunsthistorisches Museum.

The picture is closely related in style to Gentileschi's three great altarpieces—the *Circumcision*, the *Vision of Saint Cecilia*, and the *Baptism of Christ* (cat. nos. 7, 9, 11).

Marini places it somewhat later than the *Baptism*, which was contracted in March 1607, while Bissell (1981) notes similarities with the *Circumcision*, installed in the church of the Gesù in Ancona in June of that year but perhaps commissioned at Rome a year or two earlier. The background figure of a gesturing man wearing a striped turban in that work offers an analogy to the youth wearing a red cap in the *Way to Calvary*. However, in none of the three altarpieces does Orazio come so close to achieving the Caravaggesque effect of a tableau vivant—of figures in arrested movement. To an even greater degree than is found in the *Circumcision* and the *Vision of Saint Cecilia*, the composition of the *Way to Calvary* gives the impression of having been collaged together from individual studies.

Caravaggio's *Martyrdom of Saint Matthew* clearly provided the model for the interlocked figures, with Christ moving out of the picture plane and the youth in contemporary dress striding across the canvas. On the other hand, the open-armed gesture of the Magdalene must derive from Caravaggio's electrifying *Supper at Emmaus* (National Gallery, London). Typically, Gentileschi reduced the foreshortening to create a quieter, more meditative mood; the gesture is affective rather than demonstrative and does not break the picture plane. (The same decision to maintain the integrity of the picture plane, and thus the world of the pictorial fiction, is found in the *Vision of Saint Cecilia*.) The dense shadows and the pools of light are no less indebted to this and related works by Caravaggio, but the effect is very different: less dramatic and instantaneous, and the contradiction between the sharp, "cellar lighting" and the outdoor setting has not yet been resolved. (Note how Orazio uses a continuous cloud formation to bind the friezelike composition together.) The contrast between the grotesque face of Christ's tormentor and the shadowed visage of the Magdalene is not only a leitmotif of Caravaggesque painting but a device of classical painting. The emphasis on the noble aspect of Christ, shown with luxuriant locks of hair falling on his shoulder, points to Orazio's study of the art of Annibale Carracci, which was to be crucial to his mature style. Indeed, Gentileschi's concern for elegance and decorum marks the limits of his Caravaggism and looks to his future, highly personal achievement.

X radiographs show no significant compositional changes, and there are only minor pentimenti. The fingers of the Magdalene's left hand, for example, are painted over the sleeve and her hair over her blouse. Similarly, the fingers of Christ's tormentor are painted over the cross. The picture is generally in good condition but has suffered somewhat from an early harsh cleaning. This is especially apparent in the sky, which is underpainted in black. Christ's robe is notably faded; the highlights alone have retained their hue, because of the presence of lead white. The edges of the canvas, which is made up of three pieces stitched together, are intact.[7] The picture was cleaned for the exhibition.

1. For a concise history of the development of the theme, see Schiller 1971–72, vol. 2, 78–82.
2. Hirst 1981, 80–82, 133–36.
3. I have been unable to trace Orazio's picture in the published inventory of the Albani collection of 1798; see Albani 1980.
4. See Marini 1974 and Cinotti and Dell'Acqua 1983 for an account of the extensive bibliography Longhi's conjecture elicited.
5. This group comprised the *Supper at Emmaus* (National Gallery, London), the *Doubting Thomas* (Potsdam), the *Calling of the Disciples* (known from a copy at Hampton Court), and the *Holy Family* (the original on loan to the Metropolitan Museum; Longhi knew the composition from copies. See Christiansen 1999).
6. Bologna intriguingly compares the picture to a half-length composition of Saint Francis in the Johnson collection, a work he ascribes to Caravaggio but which I believe to be by Gentileschi and to date to about 1605.
7. The canvas consists of one large piece and a narrower, horizontal strip made up of two pieces. The large piece retains its selvage along the top and bottom edges. The narrower strip also has a selvage along the top edge. My thanks to Robert Wald.

6.

Saint Francis Supported by an Angel

Oil on canvas, 49 ⅝ × 38 ⅝ in. (126 × 98 cm)

Museo Nacional del Prado, Madrid

ca. 1607

Saint Francis is shown in a swoon, after having received the stigmata. The dark background and strips of white in the upper left are the only allusions to the night sky, recently illuminated by the saint's vision. Of Orazio's known depictions of the theme (cat. nos. 2, 3, 21), this one holds a special place by virtue of the atmosphere of hushed quiet. As in certain paintings by Francisco de Zurbarán—the *Saint Serapion* (Wadsworth Atheneum, Hartford), for example—spiritual drama is interpreted in terms akin to those of still-life painting, with a suppression of action or rhetorical gesture. The loving description of the angel's wings; the wounded hand and shadowed face of the saint (whose eyelids are slightly open to underscore a state of unconsciousness); the fall of light over the heavy folds of the Capuchin habit—these are Orazio's means of asserting poverty and humility as central to spiritual revelation, in conformity with Capuchin ideals. There are remnants of Orazio's Mannerist training in the choice of colors (especially the angel's orange-red-tinted tunic and golden puffed sleeves), in the S-like curve formed by the two figures, and in the bit of fluttering drapery to the left of Saint Francis (an emblem of spiritual stimulation, as well as of *bellezza*), but in all other respects this is an image of remarkable modernity.

Askew has emphasized the importance of Caravaggio's early *Ecstasy of Saint Francis* (fig. 40), painted for the Genoese banker Ottavio Costa. But the vertical format of the Prado canvas, with the

PROVENANCE: Museo Nacional del Prado, Madrid (cat. 1849–58, no. 810, cat. 1876, no. 96, as school of the Carracci; on deposit at the Museo de Gerona, 1882–1966); Museo Nacional del Prado.

REFERENCES: Pérez Sánchez 1965, 504; Askew 1969, 295, note; Madrid 1970, 278–79 no. 85; Milicua 1970, 6–7; Schleier 1970b, 342; Madrid 1972, addenda, 871 no. 3122; Previtali 1973, 360 n. 17; Röttgen in Rome 1973, 101; Seville 1973, no. 24; Moir 1976, 62, 122 n. 180 iv, 124; Nicolson 1979, 53; Bissell 1981, 141–42 no. 9, 144; Schleier in New York–Naples 1985, 148–50; Nicolson 1990, 115; Finaldi in London–Bilbao–Madrid 1999, 54; Mena Marqués in Segovia 2000, 201; London–Rome 2001, 269, 379.

figure shown cut off at the knees, relates it as well to a print by Francesco Vanni that in 1595 was copied by Agostino Carracci. Vanni shows the ecstatic Francis propped against a rocky bluff embracing a crucifix and consoled by a music-making angel. He does not draw the analogy with images of the dead Christ supported by one or more angels by which Orazio underscores the theme of Francis as a second Christ, transformed through spiritual revelation. Yet the intimacy and emotional tenor of Vanni's print must surely have been significant for him.

Orazio's compositional audacity is especially evident in the pronounced asymmetrical placement of the tightly knit figure group against a dark background relieved by the great expanse of the angel's wing. He used the same set of wings—obviously a studio prop—in his other depictions of Saint Francis (though with a change in the colors). He also lent them to Caravaggio. Yet nothing could be further from the agitated, ruffled wings in Caravaggio's *Love Triumphant* (Gemälde-galerie, Berlin). Orazio's approach is, by contrast, one of placid description.

The picture is usually thought to be slightly later than the *Saint Francis* in the Galleria Nazionale, Rome (cat. 21), but I believe that visitors to the exhibition will agree that these two works—never before shown together—are very different. As Schleier has noted, the closest stylistic analogies to the Prado picture are in the Ancona *Circumcision* (cat. 7), a work that was

installed in 1607. Indeed, it seems likely that Orazio employed the same model for one of the angels in the upper register of that work. The understated handling of light and shade in the Prado *Saint Francis* is also close to what is found in the *Circumcision*. Thanks to the documents relating to the Rome *Saint Francis*, both that painting and the Prado version can be seen to bracket the years of intense experimentation, 1609 to 1612, when Orazio made the Caravaggesque practice of working directly from the posed model (*dal naturale*) the centerpiece of his art.

Pérez Sánchez, the first to recognize the picture as a work by Gentileschi, has suggested identifying it with a *Saint Francis* ascribed to Domenichino that was among the paintings purchased by Philip V in 1722 from the collection of the Roman painter Carlo Maratta.[1] Although this identification has been widely followed, it cannot be sustained, and we thus have no information about when and how the picture entered the royal collections.[2]

1. See Pérez Sánchez 1965, 504, and Mena Marqués in Segovia 2000, 201. The inventory entry, republished by Bershad 1985, 75, reads: "un quadro d'un s. Fran.co che stà in deliquio con un angiolo che lo sostiene, figure al naturale le carnigioni sono del Domenichino, il resto è copiato."
2. Spear (1982, 281–82 no. 105) demonstrates that the entry refers to a painting Maratta obtained from Raspantino that is, in fact, a copy retouched by Domenichino. It is in the Palacio Riofrío, Segovia.

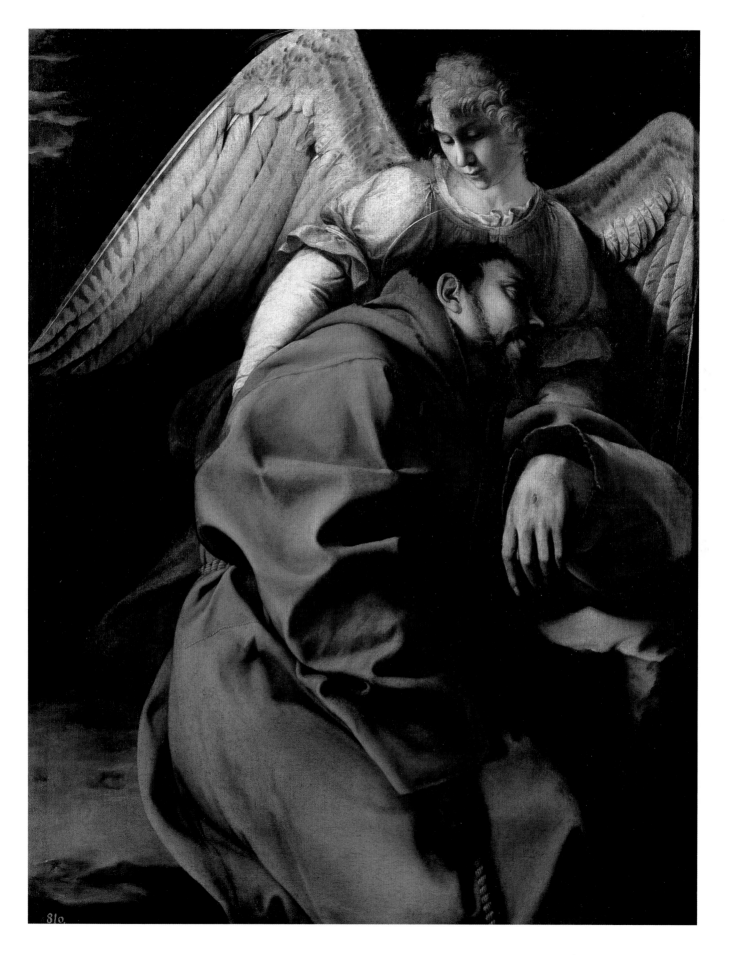

7.

Circumcision

Oil on canvas, 153½ × 99¼ in. (390 × 252 cm)

Church of the Gesù, Ancona (on deposit in the Pinacoteca Comunale)

ca. 1605–7

Rome, New York

PROVENANCE: Church of the Gesù, Ancona (on deposit in the Pinacoteca).

REFERENCES: Oretti 1777, vol. I, II (cited in Ancona 1985, 213); Maggiori 1821, 21, 66; Peruzzi 1845, 238, 240; Santoni 1884, 17; Voss 1925, 460; Mezzetti 1930, 551; Pevsner 1930, 274; Molajoli 1930–31, 100; Molajoli 1936, 34; Pirri 1952, 13; Bologna 1953, 44 n. 3; Zampetti in Urbino 1953, 35–36; Emiliani 1958a, 21; Emiliani 1958b, 40–42; Schleier 1962, 435; Moir 1967, vol. I, 38; Nicolson 1979, 52; Bissell 1981, 20–21, 144–45; Zampetti in Ancona 1985, 212–13; Pizzorusso 1987, 57–59; Nicolson 1990, 113; Zampetti 1990, 296–97; Carloni and Caldari in Fossombrone 1997, 22–23, 86; Costanzi 1999, 7.

The Feast of the Circumcision is celebrated on January 1, eight days after Christmas. It is the day Christ manifested his humanity by shedding blood for the first time, and it is the day he was given the name foretold by the angel: Jesus. Given its destination for the high altar of a Jesuit church dedicated to il Gesù, it is not surprising that Orazio has conceived the subject so as to emphasize the three meditations on the subject recommended by Ignatius of Loyola in his *Spiritual Exercises*. The first meditation is on the act of circumcising, which Orazio shows aligned with the vertical axis of the painting, with the turbaned priest performing his task, his instruments forming a beautiful still life, and the child, supported on a pillow, looking expectantly toward his mother. The second meditation—"His name was called Jesus, the name given him by the angel before he was conceived in the womb"—is indicated by the initials of Christ's name, IHS, that appear in a radiance, adored by cherubs. Above, God the Father, his head framed by a triangular halo standing for the Trinity, raises one hand toward an angel who, his left hand placed over his heart and his right extended toward Jesus' name, gazes tenderly at the child. This part of the composition recalls medieval altarpieces in which God charges Gabriel with the mission of the Annunciation. As for the third meditation, Saint Ignatius remarks, "They return the child to his mother, who felt compassion at the blood shed by her son." Mary is shown at the right, her hands joined devoutly as she looks lovingly at her son. To her right is Joseph, who was charged by the angel to name the child Jesus. Around this compact group, which includes a second priest and two acolytes, are additional figures—to the left, an old and a young man who, with demonstrative gestures, dispute the meaning of the event, and, to the right, an old and a young woman. The devout Simeon and the prophetess Anna, both of whom kept vigil in the Temple for the Messiah, may be intended. Simeon and Anna witnessed Christ at the time of the Virgin's Purification

(celebrated on February 2), but since in the Gospel of Saint Luke this event is recounted immediately after the Circumcision and has to do with the recognition of Christ's divinity, Orazio (or his adviser) may have included them to further enrich the theme of the Circumcision (Simeon and Anna are the focus of the second and third meditations on the Purification of the Virgin).

The circumstances surrounding the commissioning of the picture can now be established with a fair degree of certainty. Construction of the church of the Gesù in Ancona began on April 14, 1605, under the patronage of Giovanni Nappi. According to a document first published by Pirri in 1952 and reintroduced into the literature by Carloni, Nappi was also responsible for commissioning Orazio's altarpiece, which was installed on the Feast of Saint John the Baptist—June 24, 1607. Maggiori, quoting from a manuscript since destroyed, records that the price paid was the considerable sum of 303 scudi (Caravaggio received 400 scudi for the *Conversion of Saint Paul* and the *Crucifixion of Saint Peter* in the Cerasi chapel in Santa Maria del Popolo, and 270 scudi for the *Death of the Virgin* [Louvre, Paris]). Clearly, this was an important commission and testifies to Orazio's artistic stature in Rome.

The Nappi were highly respected figures in the Marches. Giovanni's son Filippo was rector of the Gesù, while his brother Monsignor Francesco Nappi resided in Rome; in 1615, Francesco was appointed governor of Camerino. The commission could have been placed through Cardinal Claudio Acquaviva, the general of the Jesuit order in Rome (he would also have advised Orazio on the theological issues of the subject).[1] With the election of Pope Paul V Borghese in 1605, Acquaviva had regained papal support, and the commission may well be related to the bull of September 1606 (*Quantum Religio*) reaffirming the pope's faith in the Jesuits. On the other hand, Francesco Nappi was in an ideal position to inform himself

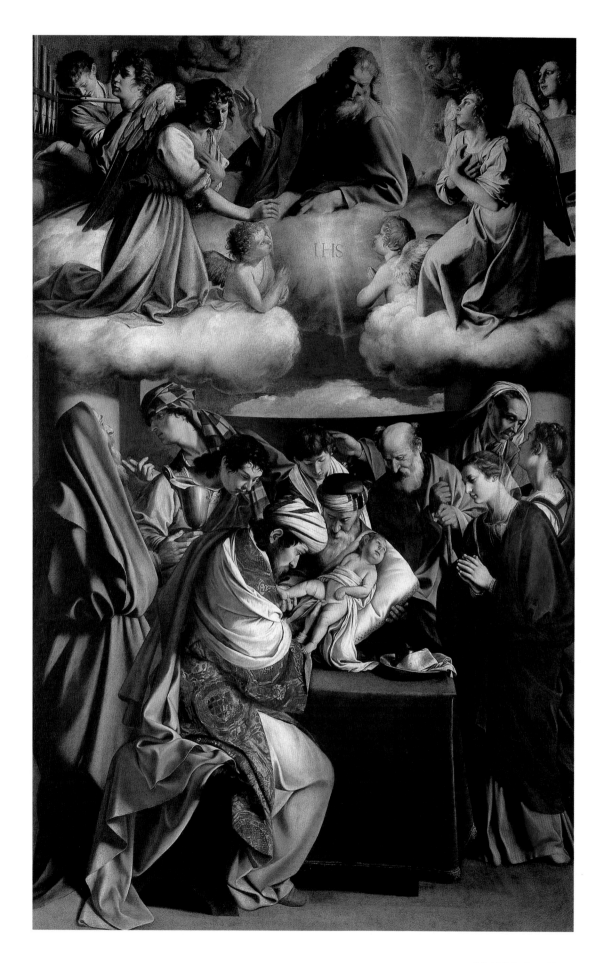

about the leading artists of the day. During 1607, Francesco lobbied Paul V on behalf of both his brother and Enzo Bentivoglio, who had agricultural investments in Ferrara. To facilitate matters, the Nappi involved themselves with Scipione Borghese's rapacious schemes to obtain paintings (see pp. 13, 15, 120–21). This activity also put them in touch with Paolo Savelli, who was associate to the vice legate to Ferrara (Scipione Borghese especially had his eyes on some cycles of paintings by Dosso Dossi in the castle of Ferrara).[2] Thus, Francesco Nappi was in contact with the two people who were to be Orazio's most important Roman patrons.[3] At the very least, this string of connections served to put Orazio at the center of the Roman scene.

In the *Circumcision,* Orazio makes a bold and remarkable move to adapt the populist realism of Caravaggio's art that had shocked so many critics and churchmen to the devotional requisites of traditional religious painting. It was an endeavor to which he would dedicate much of his career in Rome and to which we owe such extraordinary paintings as the *Vision of Saint Francesca Romana* (cat. 30) and the deeply moving *Crucifixion* (cat. 29). But the first successes in this vein are the trio of paintings documented to the years 1605–8: the *Circumcision,* the *Vision of Saint Cecilia* (cat. 9), and the *Baptism of Christ* (cat. 11). In each, Orazio experiments with a slightly different balance. In the *Saint Cecilia,* he stresses elegance in the figure types and an abstract, planar composition. In the *Baptism,* elegance is sacrificed to naturalistic effects and to an emphasis on believable figures taken from everyday life. In both cases, he is responding to the nature of the subject matter—the visionary aspect of the *Saint Cecilia;* the demonstration of Christ's humanity in the *Baptism.* Bissell has rightly remarked that "scholars have simply given insufficient attention to the connection between form and content in Orazio's art."

As we have seen, in the *Circumcision* Orazio seems to have responded to specifically Jesuit devotional practices, perhaps at the instigation of Cardinal Acquaviva. Caravaggio's focused lighting, used to achieve an effect of dramatic immediacy, is transformed by Orazio into a means of suggesting actual experience—a tempered

realism. The play of light on the neck, ear, and cheek of the woman at the far right is a tour de force of observation and signals the degree to which Orazio relied on the use of individual models to achieve this effect (the passage looks forward to the completely naturalistic style of the Bucharest *Madonna and Child* [cat. 15]). We recognize the same model who posed for Joseph in the God the Father and, possibly, in the figure of Simeon. The acolyte holding a silver vessel and the gesturing figure in a turban are, again, taken from the same model, and the two right-hand angels in the clouds seem to have the same features as the young woman at the far right. Within a few years, this practice of painting from the model was to become the focus of Orazio's art (cat. nos. 15–20), but here it is tempered by his desire to maintain a separation between the viewer/worshiper and the event depicted, so that the fiction, or poetic truth, of the religious story is retained (the Aristotelian distinction between poetic and historic truth, *verisimile* and *vero,* was very much a part of current artistic theory).[4]

By the same token, Orazio has been unable to fully free himself from late-Mannerist compositional formulas. The figural arrangement is almost pedantically symmetrical (as had been true of his fresco of the Presentation in the Temple in Santa Maria Maggiore of about 1593), and the horizontal division between the earthly and the heavenly realms is no less artificial. Giovanni Francesco Guerrieri's treatment of the subject for a church in Sassoferrato, painted in 1614–15 (fig. 55), reads as a critique on the claustrophobic, compressed, and old-fashioned composition of Orazio's altarpiece. The elaborately described costumes—something foreign to Caravaggio's work after about 1600—have affinities with the work of such Florentine artists as Andrea Commodi and Agostino Ciampelli, as noted by Pizzorusso.[5]

The transformation that Orazio has worked upon Caravaggio's realism is the more notable in view of those passages that are demonstrably inspired by the Lombard artist. The seated priest recalls the youth counting money in Caravaggio's *Calling of Saint Matthew* (Contarelli chapel, San Luigi dei Francesi)—the picture that first converted Orazio to a Caravaggesque style. The composition as a whole, with its row of figures behind the Christ child and the diagonal placement of the infant, seems to pay homage to the *Death of the Virgin*. Bellori later criticized those followers of Caravaggio who "never went into the light of the sun" but preferred "the brown air of a closed room."[6] More than any other artist, it was Gentileschi who adapted the artifice of Caravaggesque lighting to the open air.

Though less striking than the *Vision of Saint Cecilia*—the masterpiece of these years—the *Circumcision* is perhaps the most pregnant work of Orazio's first formulation of an independent Caravaggesque style. In it are the seeds for the simplicity and purity of expression that characterize his later religious paintings. It is also a work that had a formative impact on the young Artemisia—not for its exploration of a style at once real and devotional, but for the way it attempts to construct a narrative out of pieces of observed reality. Especially such figures as the angel playing the organ or the two men in heated argument—so like the conspiring elders in Artemisia's *Susanna* (cat. 51)—are fundamental to her conception of painting.

Following the remodeling of the Gesù by Luigi Vanvitelli, a semicircular lunette was added to the top of the altarpiece. This was removed when, under the

superintendency of Pietro Zampetti, the picture was restored after World War II.[7] Aside from local damage, clearly visible where the inpainting has been carried out in *tratteggio*, the picture is in good condition.

1. In 1605, Acquaviva promised the services of a Jesuit woodworker, Francesco Brunelli, to Filippo Nappi; see Pirri 1952, 13. For much of this information, I am indebted to a seminar paper by Claude Dickerson; see also Carloni's essay, pp. 117–21.
2. Pizzorusso (1987, 69) has investigated the Savelli's ties to the Marches. Giulio was governor of Ancona from 1608 to 1610.
3. For these complicated dealings, see especially Venturi 1882, 16 ff.; Marcon, Maddalo, and Marcolini in Ferrara 1983; and Carloni in Fossombrone 1997, 22. Paolo Savelli emerges from the correspondence as a somewhat ambivalent figure, since he was advising the agent of Duke Cesare d'Este about Scipione Borghese's schemes.
4. See, for example, Gilio da Fabriano in Barocchi 1960–62, vol. 2, 15–29, passim. Paleotti (in ibid., 364–70) touches on the matter in his discussion of *verisimile*. Of course, the key issue for the formulation of the classical-idealist point of view was Aristotle's distinction between those who imitated reality and those who improved on it. See the classic discussion by Mahon (1947) 1971, 124–43.
5. As Pizzorusso points out, the comparison with Commodi's *Consecration of the Church of the Santissimo Salvatore* (Cathedral, Cortona), which was painted in Rome beginning in 1603, is particularly striking. Ciampelli was, like Pomarancio and Giuseppe Valeriano, regularly employed by the Jesuits; see Hibbard in Wittkower and Jaffe 1972, 40–41.
6. Bellori (1672) 1976, 217.
7. See Urbino 1953, 35–36.

8.

Madonna and Child

Oil on wood, 36 × 28¾ in. (91.5 × 73 cm)

The Barbara Piasecka Johnson Foundation

ca. 1607

This touching, intimate depiction of the Madonna and Child must have been destined for a special patron. Its refined execution and rich use of color single it out as much as the panel support (it is one of only three works by Orazio on panel).[1] The yellow of the child's robe is particularly notable and recalls the uncharacteristically yellow dress reportedly worn by the Virgin in the lost *Madonna and Child* painted by Orazio for Vincenzo I Gonzaga, fourth duke of Mantua, in 1609 (see cat. 15). The figure types are close to those in Orazio's altarpiece of the Circumcision, installed on the high altar of the church of the Gesù in Ancona

in 1607 (cat. 77). Indeed, it is worth considering whether the same models were used. As in that work, the bulk of the figures is thwarted by an emphasis on surface pattern and by the minimal space that surrounds them. Orazio was never a painter of space, and his understanding of perspective seems to have been rudimentary; even in his most ambitious compositions, the figures are placed against a rocky mass, a clump of trees, a curtain, or a nondescript, dark background. Only through the study of artfully posed models viewed in a raking light was he able, like Caravaggio, to give his pictures what contemporaries would have called a sense of relief, or *relievo*. The most significant difference from the figures in the *Circumcision* is in the handling of light, which in the *Madonna and Child* is luminous and plays on the forms with a delicacy that more closely approximates observed reality. Indeed, the transparency of the shadows looks forward to Orazio's work of the next decade. (This delicacy in the handling of light and shadows, as much as the figure types, makes the attribution to Artemisia, advanced by Garrard, unconvincing.)

Throughout the first decade of the seventeenth century, Orazio's work shows a persistent conflict between his ingrained habits of painting *di maniera*—falling back on conventions of representation and composition—and the new, Caravaggesque practice of working from posed models *dal naturale*. Inevitably, it was in his more informal easel paintings that Orazio best resolved this dilemma. But if we compare the Johnson *Madonna and Child* with the work in Bucharest (cat. 15), it will be seen how much the painting owes to pictorial conventions as opposed to observed reality. The delicate placement of the Virgin's dimpled hands, her pensively lowered eyelids, the artful arrangement of the child's drapery so as to expose his genitals (a reference to Christ's human nature), and his wide-eyed stare—these are devices intended as devotional cues for the viewer and are far removed from the everyday world so successfully counterfeited in the Bucharest *Madonna*. The close cropping of the figures at once avoids any awkwardness Orazio may have encountered in elaborating their poses and enhances the effect of intimacy and informality.

Bissell has suggested that in conceiving this picture Orazio turned to quattrocento Florentine models, urged by his Tuscan heritage and a "nostalgia for what might have seemed to him a less complicated, more sincere age." In many ways this is an attractive suggestion, though less because of Orazio's Tuscan birth—he was, after all, trained in Rome and his experience of Florentine art was dependent on what he saw in the papal city—than because a number of Counter-Reformation writers, including Giovanni Andrea Gilio da Fabriano and Gabriele Paleotti, considered simplicity and purity more important than a demonstration of style and even went so far as to laud the purity of art

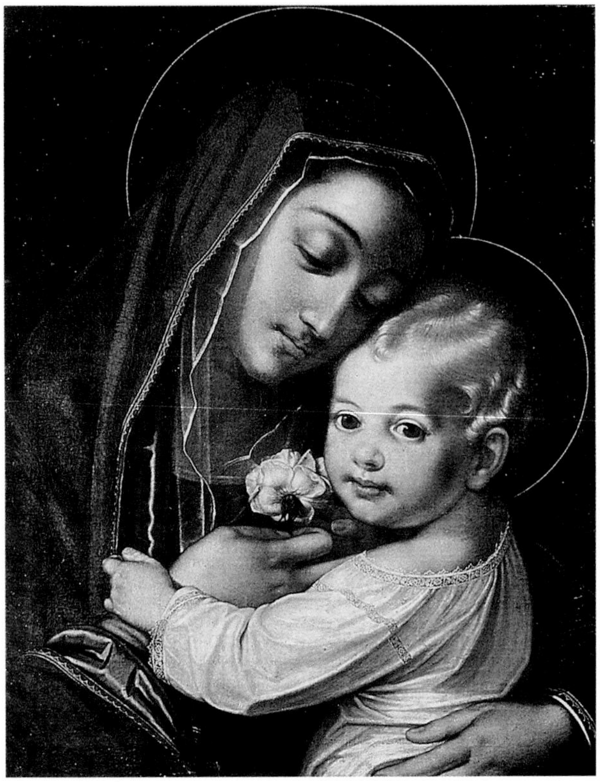

PROVENANCE: Possibly Marchese Clemente and Cardinal Giacomo Sannesi, Rome (until 1621); by descent, Anna Maria Sannesi, Rome (until 1724; postmortem inv. as by Gentileschi); Matthiesen Fine Art Ltd., London (1978–81); Barbara Piasecka Johnson Foundation, Princeton.

RELATED PICTURES: Vincenzo Bonello, Valletta, Malta (copy);[6] Finarte, Milan (copy).[7]

REFERENCES: Bissell 1981, 143–44 no. 12, 147; London 1981, 10–11 no. 1; Garrard 1989, 25–26, 32, 493 nn. 21, 22; Prohaska in Warsaw 1990, 180–83 no. 30; Bissell 1999, 326–27 no. X-18, 333.

Figure 42. Scipione Pulzone (1544–1598), *Madonna and Child*. Oil on canvas. Galleria Borghese, Rome

from before the time of Michelangelo.[2] By the 1590s, Scipione Pulzone had already explored a type of Madonna and Child composition (fig. 42) that combined Raphaelesque compositional models with a Northern emphasis on surface description to produce images possessing a sweet, and intentionally bland, domestic intimacy—what Zeri, in his groundbreaking book on Counter-Reformation art, terms "pittura senza tempo."[3] The degree to which this kind of image was fostered by Jesuit teachings remains ambiguous, but it is an important issue, since the Johnson painting is so closely related to Orazio's *Circumcision*, destined for a Jesuit church.[4] It is, in any event, to this tradition that Orazio's painting belongs, a tradition that is also reflected in the depiction of the Madonna and Child that Domenichino includes in his fresco at Grottaferrata showing Saint Nilo exorcising a possessed youth and that was to receive its definitive, seicento expression in the vast production of Sassoferrato. Given the demand for these images, it is hardly surprising that we know of two copies of the Johnson

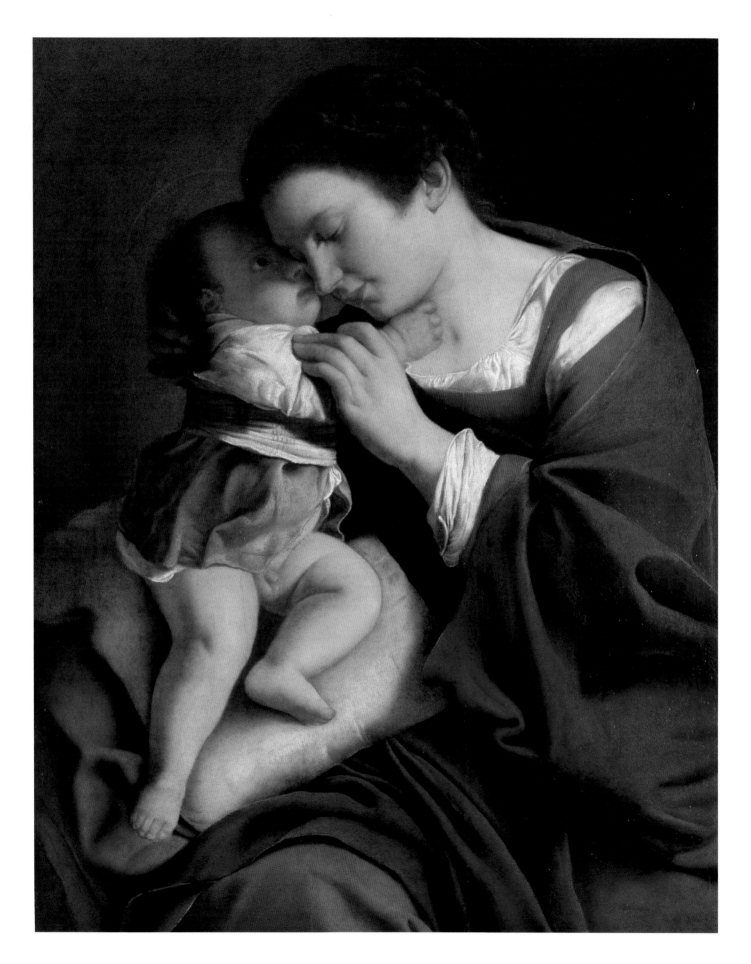

Madonna and Child (see under related pictures). It is important to emphasize that an image of this sort represents a specific moment in Orazio's career. In the Corsini *Madonna and Child* (cat. 4)—if indeed it is by Orazio—and the Bucharest *Madonna,* Orazio experiments with a more full-blooded Caravaggism, while in the later *Madonna with the Sleeping Christ Child* in Cambridge (cat. 28), he aims at the world of formal, Baroque artifice.

There is no certain record of the picture prior to 1978. However, a *Madonna and Child* by Orazio belonged to the Olgiati family in 1713 (it is listed as hanging over a door). In 1607, Settimio Olgiati commissioned from Orazio a *Baptism of Christ* (cat. 11) for his chapel in Santa Maria della Pace. His interest in Orazio's work continued until at least 1612, when he is known to have visited the artist's workshop and was taken to see the frescoes then under way in the casino of Scipione Borghese. The Savelli also owned a *Madonna and Child* by Orazio of similar dimensions (88 × 66 cm). Their patronage of Orazio from before 1613 is not known. Much the most fascinating possibility is a *Madonna and Child* listed in the postmortem inventory of Anna Maria Sannesi, the last heir of Cardinal Giacomo Sannesi (1551–1621). That picture was on panel and

measured 5 × 3 *palmi* (about 111 × 67 cm).[5] Cardinal Sannesi and his brother Clemente were major collectors in Rome and evidently owned three works by the artist: a *Madonna and Child,* a *David with the Head of Goliath* (see cat. 20), and a *Saint George,* the last on copper (see also p. 13).

1. The other two are cat. nos. 20 and 50.
2. See Gilio da Fabriano in Barocchi 1960–62, vol. 2, 55: "E mi pare che i pittori che furono avanti Michelagnolo più a la verità et a la devozione attendessero, che a la pompa." Elsewhere Gilio urges a return of art to "la sua purità primiera."
3. Zeri 1957, 76–77. For Pulzone's pictures in the Galleria Borghese, Rome, and San Carlo ai Catinari, Rome, see Vaudo 1976, 36.
4. Pulzone, of course, was intimately involved in the decoration of the Gesù in Rome and associated with the Jesuit painter Giuseppe Valeriano. Vaudo (1976, 39 n. 27) prints one of Pulzone's poems, in which, in a Michelangelesque vein, he laments blind affections and the inability to see his errors: "e non vede ne l'error." This type of sentiment certainly accords with his devotional paintings, which consciously avoid the "vanities" of style.
5. ASR, 39 notai Capitolini Joseph Paulinus Officio 13, vol. 502, f. 262: "Altro Quadro simile [in tavola] di pmi tre, e mezzo, e tre, con cornice nera filettata d'oro rappresentante la Madonna, ed il Bambino opera del Gentileschi." I owe this reference to Erich Schleier.
6. See Valletta 1949, 24, where it is ascribed to Artemisia.
7. See Bissell 1999, 327. Sold 1986, as school of Artemisia.

9.

Vision of Saint Cecilia

Oil on canvas, 137¾ × 85⅞ in. (350 × 218 cm)

Signed (on organ): HORATIVS GENTILESC[HVS] / FLORENTINVS FECIT

Pinacoteca di Brera, Milan (inv. 588)

ca. 1606–7

Rome, New York

According to Jacobus de Voragine's *Golden Legend* (ca. 1260), Cecilia, born of a noble Roman family, made a secret vow of chastity. This she confided to her pagan husband, Valerian, in their bridal chamber, saying that an angel of God kept watch over her. Only after he was baptized was Valerian granted the vision of the angel, who appeared bearing two garlands and telling of their future martyrdom (in the painting, symbolized by the palm held by the angel). The fragrance of the garlands caught the attention of Valerian's

brother Tibertius, who, after Cecilia's exhortations, was also converted. The organ on a table in the right background is Cecilia's emblem as patroness of music.

Pandakovic definitively established that the picture was painted for the high altar of Santa Cecilia, Como, a prestigious Augustinian convent that attracted daughters of leading aristocratic families. An inscription on the original frame, still in the church, reads: ANGELVS DOMINI / DESCENDIT DE COELO / ET LVMEN REFVLSIT IN / HABITACVLO (An angel of the Lord descended from

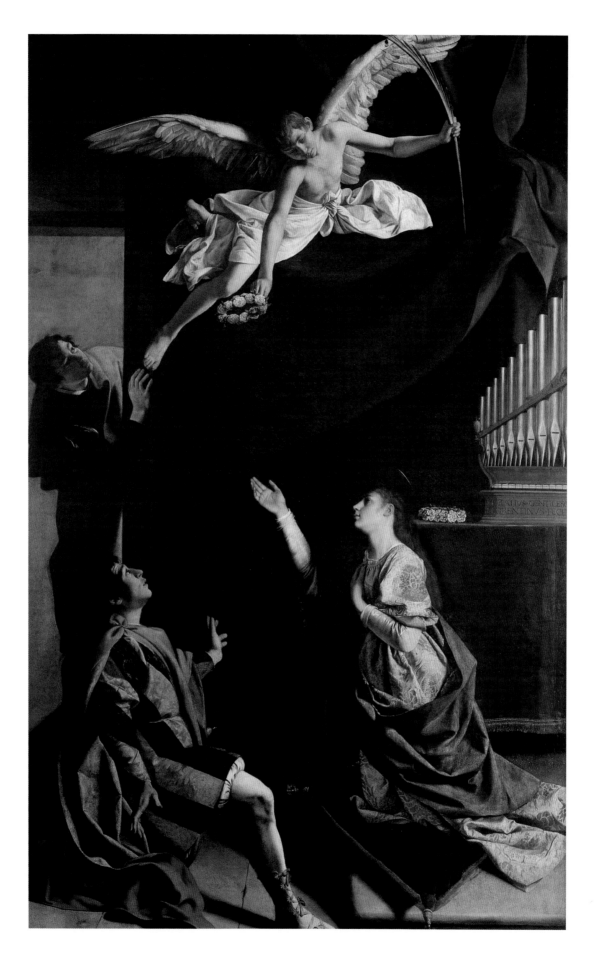

PROVENANCE: Church of Santa Cecilia, Como (by 1607–1798); Accademia di Belle Arte and Pinacoteca di Brera, Milan (from 1801).

REFERENCES: Longhi (1916) 1961, 235–36; Gamba 1922–23, 252; Voss 1925, 459; Wittkower 1958, 338 n. 2; Schleier 1962, 435–36; Pandakovic 1966, 161, 162 n. 15; Moir 1967, vol. 1, 74–75, 124–25, 134, 257, vol. 2, 77 no. 2; Bissell 1971, 278–79; Nicolson 1979, 53; Bissell 1981, 40–41, 170–72 no. 42; Nicolson 1990, 114; Papi 1992, 183; Rovi 1992, 107–9; Rovi in Pinacoteca di Brera 1992, 56–59, no. 22; Pescarmona in Gregori 1994, 46, 303.

heaven and light shone in the chamber). What remained uncertain was the date of the picture and, hence, an understanding of its stylistic traits. For a time, it was believed to date to the years 1617–20, when Orazio was in the Marches. Longhi placed it among Orazio's last Roman paintings, and Bissell (1981) argued for a date as late as 1621, suggesting the possibility that the picture was sent to Como from Genoa. While noting the strong Caravaggesque character of the painting—especially the spot-lighted figures—he found the blend of "the religious and the secular/aristocratic" similar to that in the Turin *Annunciation* (cat. 43). By contrast, Schleier insisted on the picture's Caravaggesque features and placed it prior to 1610. A firm basis for resolving this confusion emerged in 1992, when Rovi published the record of a visit to the church on November 25, 1607, by Cardinal Paolo Emilio Sfondrato, who had been invited by the nuns to perform Mass. In a lengthy description of the highly decorated altar is noted "a new picture by the Florentine Gentileschi, who, with his valor, walks in step with any of the more illustrious and famous painters in Rome." The characterization of the painting as "new" suggests that it had been installed only recently.[1]

With the critical perspective offered by this document, it is now possible to appreciate just how well the Brera altarpiece fits into Orazio's career in the years 1605–7. Its use of a focused (rather than dispersed) lighting with dense shadows, its quality of suspended action, and the dependence on a number of motifs seen in Caravaggio's work situate it in the same time frame as the Vienna *Way to Calvary* (cat. 5) and the Ancona *Circumcision* (cat. 7). So also do the muted colors: periwinkle to a saturated blue, deep green, coral, ochre, silver gray. There is none of the silken quality found in Orazio's work after about 1610. The flying angel, with his homely, twelve-year-old face and elegantly fluttering drapery, was clearly indebted to Caravaggio's *Calling of Saint Matthew,* completed in 1602 for the altar of the Contarelli chapel in San Luigi dei Francesi, while Valerian's outflung arms just as clearly derive from the Lombard painter's contemporaneous *Supper at Emmaus* (National Gallery, London). As he had done with the figure of the Magdalene in the *Way to Calvary,* Orazio lowers the

position of Valerian's right hand so as not to break through the picture plane—a detail that we may take as emblematic of his less assertive approach to Caravaggio's realism. Rovi believes that the magnificent green curtain which so effectively sets off the angel was inspired by the example of Caravaggio's *Death of the Virgin* (Louvre, Paris). As he remarks, the comparison serves to underscore Orazio's transformation of a dramatic motif (in Caravaggio's painting, the red cloth suspended from the ceiling serves as a canopy over the dead Virgin) into an elegant appointment— *arredo "borghese."*

What is remarkable is the way these Caravaggesque features have been incorporated into a late-Mannerist approach to composition that in certain respects recalls Orazio's work at the abbey of Farfa and at San Giovanni dei Fiorentini, Rome, where he decorated the vault of the Fiorenzuola chapel. For all his attention to the description of an interior, the room, with its steeply inclined floor, is curiously lacking in depth. The doorframe, table, floor, and the step on which Cecilia kneels serve as a geometric grid for the elegant collage of individual figures, whose studiously choreographed poses generate a surface pattern dominated by a large zigzag. The attitudes they strike are at once emblematically expressive and ornamental (Cecilia's outstretched hand, in a gesture denoting welcome or acceptance, reappears a decade and a half later in the *Danaë* [cat. 36]).

It took Orazio the better part of a decade to fully absorb the implications of Caravaggio's revolutionary naturalism; one need look no further than the *Madonna in Glory with the Holy Trinity* (fig. 5), of about 1605, to see how difficult he found the task of applying the practice of painting from the model to the execution of a complex, multifigure composition. Even Caravaggio's *Death of the Virgin* offered no real model for painting a complex interior space or of creating the visionary effect of the everyday infused by the divine (something Orazio was to make his specialty). The Brera altarpiece, like the Ancona *Circumcision* and the Santa Maria della Pace *Baptism of Christ* (cat. 11), belongs to a crucial, still experimental phase in Orazio's career, during which he sought by various strategies to balance his keen formal sense with Caravaggesque realism. In the *Saint Cecilia,* it is his formal sense that predominates, and it is this which led earlier scholars to relate its style to the sophisticated language of the late Roman and Marchigian paintings; in fact, though, nothing could be further removed from the naturalistic terms of the Turin *Annunciation* (cat. 43) in which the loving act of description transmutes familiar experience into something profoundly religious.

It is interesting to speculate on Cardinal Sfondrato's response to the altarpiece, as reflected in the comment that Orazio was able to keep step with the most celebrated masters of the day. The cardinal's titular church in Rome was Santa Cecilia in Trastevere, where in 1599 the body of the saint had been discovered. In 1601, he hired Guido Reni to decorate a commemorative chapel, the Cappella del Bagno, with, among other things, the very scene illustrated by Orazio, and five years later he commissioned from the artist a much admired devotional image of the saint (Norton Simon Museum, Pasadena). Reni's first work for Sfondrato was carried out in a neo-Raphaelesque style with references to early Christian art, as was popular in the circle of the great Oratorian church historian Cesare Baronio (to which Sfondrato belonged). However, his devotional image was painted in a reformed Caravaggesque style that was to exert a powerful influence on Orazio (see cat. 12). To a degree, the Brera altarpiece strikes an analogous balance between elegance and naturalism. Yet the concern for fabrics and costumes, the tempered naturalism, and the ornamental artifice of the composition recall aspects of late-sixteenth-century Roman and, more particularly, Florentine art rather than Reni's brand of Caravaggism, with its

more idealizing orientation. It is passages such as the angel—so obviously studied from a posed model—that reveal Orazio at his most modern. As Papi has rightly noted, such passages seem to forecast the aggressively realist art of the Spaniard Juan Bautista Maino (1581–1641), who was working in Rome during these years and who was, according to his early biographer, associated with Reni. The eccentrically foreshortened figure of Tibertius peering through the door evidently left an enduring impression on the young Artemisia, who introduced a similar figure in her painting *Susanna and the Elders* (cat. 51). He is indeed memorable and leads to one of the figures in Orazio's *Christ Crowned with Thorns* (cat. 23). In these ways the *Saint Cecilia* marks the threshold of Orazio's mature style.

Rovi speculates that perhaps Cardinal Sfondrato, the Como prelate Ulpiano Volpi, or Cardinal Tolomeo Gallio played a part in commissioning the altarpiece (Gallio died on February 4, 1607), which as a matter of course would have been painted in Rome and sent to Como. Another possibility is Settimio Olgiati, who in 1607 would commission the *Baptism of Christ* for his chapel in Santa Maria della Pace in Rome (cat. 11) and who continued to be interested in Orazio's work until at least 1612. The Olgiati hailed from Como, where they maintained a family chapel in the church of San Giovanni fuori le Mura. Settimio would have been an obvious conduit for someone in Como seeking to arrange for an altarpiece from a major Roman painter.

1. Rovi (in Pinacoteca di Brera 1992, 56) notes that in 1578 the congregation had been encouraged to commission a painting for the high altar but that by 1598 no action had been taken.

10.

Holy Family with the Infant Saint John the Baptist

Oil on copper, 22¼ × 16¾ in. (56.7 × 42.6 cm)

Inscribed (on reverse): 3 (?) 16 / G. Sassoferrato

Private collection

ca. 1607–8

New York

Unquestionably the most important recent addition to Gentileschi's oeuvre, this radiant and enchanting picture first came to public attention when it was sold at Sotheby's, London, on July 6, 2000 (lot 28). Its early history can be conjectured only on the basis of an old inscription on the support indicating that prior to its sale in Dublin, in 1912, it belonged to Viscount Powerscourt in County Wicklow, Ireland. In the Sotheby's sale catalogue, it was noted that the two members of the family most likely to have purchased it were Richard, the sixth viscount (1815–1844), who traveled to Italy and bought a number of Italian paintings, or his son Mervyn Wingfield, seventh viscount Powerscourt (1836–1904), who was also an avid collector. A further inscription on the reverse ascribes the painting to Sassoferrato, and, in fact, a *Holy Family* attributed to that artist was lent by the seventh viscount to the Irish Institution, Dublin, in 1858 and again in 1859.

The attribution to Sassoferrato (a pupil of Domenichino), while clearly incorrect, has the virtue of underscoring the classical character of the composition: the compact, pyramidal arrangement of the figures and the use of an anecdotal action as the expressive focus. Saint John has gently set aside his reed cross and offers the Christ child a nosegay of roses, usually associated with the Virgin. Beyond the obvious reference to High Renaissance models, there is an analogy with the work of Annibale Carracci and his revival of Raphaelesque classicism. During the first decade of the seventeenth century the Carracci pupils Francesco Albani, Domenichino, and Guido Reni all investigated similar, small-scale figurative compositions with a landscape setting, while about 1615–16 Giovanni Lanfranco made a free copy of one of Raphael's most celebrated images, the so-called *Madonna del Passeggio* (National Gallery of Scotland, Edinburgh), then owned by Pietro Aldobrandini.[1] A remarkably close analogy for the lively pose of the Christ child in Orazio's painting can be found, in reverse, in Carracci's *Madonna*

and Child with Saint Francis (fig. 43), which was painted in Rome about 1595–96. Interestingly, in 1606 Orazio and Annibale co-witnessed the will of the sculptor Tommaso della Porta and thus were evidently in touch with each other.

The Baptist was traditionally thought to be six months older than Christ and, according to the thirteenth-century *Meditationes vitae Christi*, met the Holy Family after the Purification of the Virgin and before the Flight into Egypt. Orazio has given him a beautifully articulated pose that combines an almost neoclassical clarity and expressive elegance with a muted naturalism that looks forward both to Sassoferrato and to Nazarene painting of the early nineteenth century. Descriptive details, such as Saint John's golden locks and ruddy cheeks, the chinked stone stairs and pitted plaster of the brick wall, and

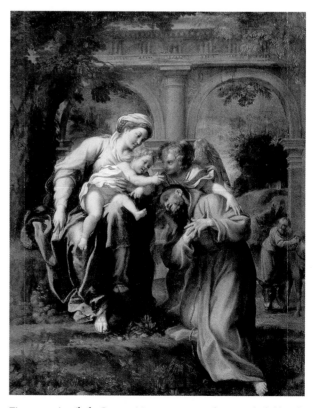

Figure 43. Annibale Carracci (1560–1609), *Madonna and Child with Saint Francis*. Oil on copper. National Gallery of Canada, Ottawa

PROVENANCE: Possibly Richard, sixth viscount Powerscourt, Powerscourt, County Wicklow, Ireland (until 1844); probably Mervyn Wingfield, seventh viscount Powerscourt (until 1904, as by Sassoferrato); (sale, Bennetts, Dublin, April 25, 1912, lot 33); private collection (sale, Sotheby's, London, July 6, 2000, lot 28, as by Orazio Gentileschi); private collection.

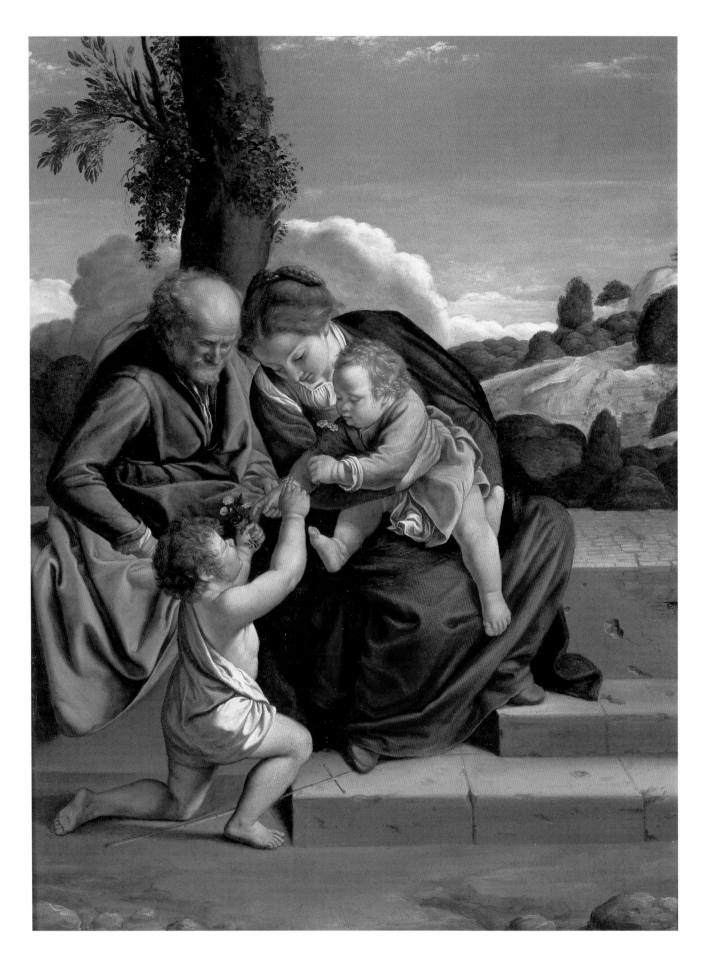

the plain clothes worn by Joseph and Mary, further enhance the interpretation of the scene as an extension of everyday life.

Given the absence of firm reference points, there is bound to be disagreement about the date of the picture and its relation to the three other paintings with landscape backgrounds in the exhibition (cat. nos. 19, 27, 38). The Sotheby's sale catalogue cites two contrasting views: one, put forward by Bissell, dates the painting to about 1605–10; the other, espoused by Schleier, sees it as a work of the second decade of the century and more or less contemporary with such pictures as the *Vision of Saint Francesca Romana* (cat. 30). A case can be made for either position, but I believe the balance of probability is that we are dealing here with Orazio's earliest surviving painting on copper and his first experiment in landscape. Not only does the figurative composition reflect Bolognese models in a more direct fashion than is found in his later paintings, but the landscape, with its stage-flat-like arrangement, formulaic clumps of trees, and generalized lighting, relates directly to the work of Carlo Saraceni around 1606–8, the date of the Venetian artist's four landscapes with subjects taken from Ovid (Capodimonte, Naples). Evidently painted for the Farnese family in Rome, Saraceni's landscapes are patterned directly on the example of Adam Elsheimer, whose work was to be so important to Orazio's landscape style.[2] Indeed, it may be that it was through Saraceni that Orazio first came in contact with the German artist (on this, see cat. 19).

In this catalogue, it is argued that the dating of Orazio's paintings with landscapes is best established by their reflection of the progressive innovations not only of Elsheimer and Saraceni, but of Goffredo Wals (see especially cat. 27). Orazio's mastery reaches a climax in the *Saint Christopher* (cat. 27), a tour de force of observation, with its astonishing atmospheric verity and attention to foliage (often dated to about 1610 but here placed about 1615–20). Over the years, his brushwork becomes more impressionistic and the shadows more transparent, animated by the play of reflected light, as demonstrated by the sparkling Burghley House *Madonna and Child in a Landscape* (cat. 38), of about 1621–22. By contrast, in the *Holy Family* the shadows are as deep as the colors are saturated, and there is an overall physical density to the composition that is especially characteristic of Orazio's work before about 1610. The closest analogy for this treatment is perhaps the Ancona *Circumcision* (cat. 7), in which the large, static forms of the figures are nonetheless animated by a beautiful study of light. In the *Holy Family,* an effect of heaviness is replaced by delicacy and luminosity. It is also worth mentioning the roughly contemporary Dublin *David Slaying Goliath* (cat. 12), in which we find a similar blend of Bolognese elegance (in this case derived, it would seem, from Guido Reni) and a naturalism based on the study of Caravaggio.

Despite the fundamental and striking differences between his various small-scale paintings with landscape backgrounds, we may note how, even in the *Saint Christopher,* Orazio consistently employs a background element to set off the figures in the foreground. There, it is a copse of trees arbitrarily enlarged; here, it is a cloud bank behind the heads of the Virgin and Saint Joseph. As sensitive as he was to developments in landscape painting and as responsive as he became to nature, Orazio remained principally a figurative artist, using landscape as a poetic adjunct.

1. See Weston-Lewis in Edinburgh 1994, 92.
2. See Ottani Cavina 1968, 13–22, for a discussion of the circle of artists around Elsheimer; see also New York–Naples 1985, 192–94.

II.

Baptism of Christ

Oil on canvas, 118⅛ × 94⅞ in.

(300 × 241 cm)

Santa Maria della Pace, Rome

1607

PROVENANCE: Santa Maria della Pace, Rome.

REFERENCES: Mancini (1617–21) 1956–57, vol. 1, 285; Celio (1638) 1967, 20; Baglione (1642) 1935, 359; Titi 1675, 253; Da Morrona (1789–93) 1812, vol. 2, 257; Longhi (1916) 1961, 225–26, 273; Voss 1925, 461; Orbaan 1927, 284; Brandi 1930, 339; Pevsner 1930, 257; Crinò 1960, 264; Crinò and Nicolson 1961, 144; Griseri 1961, 26–28; Chiarini 1962, 26–28; Moir 1967, 37–38; Nicolson 1979, 52; Barroero 1981, 169; Bissell 1981, 12, 14–17, 21, 139–140 no. 7; Nicolson 1990, 113; Papi in Florence 1991, 33–34; Maniello 1992, 155–160.

The painting was commissioned by Marchese Settimio Olgiati as part of the decorations for his chapel, dedicated to Saint John the Baptist, in the church of Santa Maria della Pace in Rome (for Olgiati, see pp. 13–15). From a document drawn up by the notary Gargario on November 19, 1612, we learn that Olgiati was ceded patronal rights to the chapel by the abbot Girolamo, prior of the Canons Regular of San Giovanni Laterano at Santa Maria della Pace.[1] Olgiati wished to replace an earlier image of Saint John ("Beati Giov. Battista imago in muro depicta stis modesta existebat nec manu eccell pictoris facta") with Orazio's *Baptism of Christ* both to express his veneration for Saint John and to make reparations for his family's destruction of an ancient oratory dedicated to the saint in the church of Santa Prassede, to make way for their own burial chapel. Through a representative, the marchese drew up a contract with the artist on March 23, 1607, stipulating with scrupulous precision the obligations of both parties. Orazio agreed to make "a painting of Saint John the Baptist when he baptizes Our Lord . . . in the church of the Madonna della Pace in Rome, in conformity with the height and width of said chapel . . . [and] to do it well and with fine colors . . . [with] the figures, that is, Christ, Saint John, God the Father, the Holy Spirit, with a glory of other angels and figures, designed in conformity with the drawing he has done . . . and to deliver it finished within six months of today."[2] For his part, the patron was to furnish the stretcher and canvas and the necessary ultramarine blue in addition to paying the agreed-upon price of 150 scudi, of which 60 were given as an advance. The discovery of this document has pushed the date of the painting forward to 1607 from the date of about 1600–1605 previously assigned on the basis of Giovanni Baglione's biographical account. It has also reignited discussion of this key phase of the artist's career, during which he sought to define his artistic identity.

It was in the early years of the century that Orazio began to give the first hints of his response to the dominant Mannerist style. The stimulus was provided by the paintings of Caravaggio in the Contarelli chapel of San Luigi dei Francesi and in Santa Maria del Popolo, which were the subject of much discussion and even scandal. As Bissell has noted, these works must have provoked a veritable crisis in Orazio's mind as he compared them with his own work of a few years earlier (in particular, the *Conversion of Saint Paul* in San Paolo fuori le Mura, Rome [destroyed]). Here, he seems to recant his former "unnatural" style, or *maniera*, and to adopt a more congenial, more "natural" manner. The *Baptism of Christ* seems to be the result of a synthesis between a traditional idiom and the Caravaggesque revolution; in it he has "already partly understood the open, lucid vision of the young Caravaggio."[3]

The compositional and iconographic scheme is traditional, despite the unusual placement of the Baptist on the left side. Marco Pino's painting in the oratory of San Giovanni Decollato, Rome, of about 1541, may be cited as a precedent. Although Orazio still employs multiple sources of illumination—three of them— the novelty of the picture resides in his identification of light as the *al naturale* means of conferring material density on the bodies. The angel at the left is particularly indicative of his use of a posed model, in the fashion of Caravaggio. Also noteworthy is the group of God the Father and the angels, who share physiognomic traits with the figures in the *Madonna in Glory* in Turin (fig. 5) and the *Circumcision* in Ancona (cat. 7). The golden radiance—symbolizing Paradise—with which they are lighted contrasts with the clear, cold terrestrial light. A sacred illumination emanating from the Holy Spirit, and directed downward by the hand of God, falls on Christ, underscoring the unity of the Trinity. The angel at the right is less successful than its companion, but it is also in

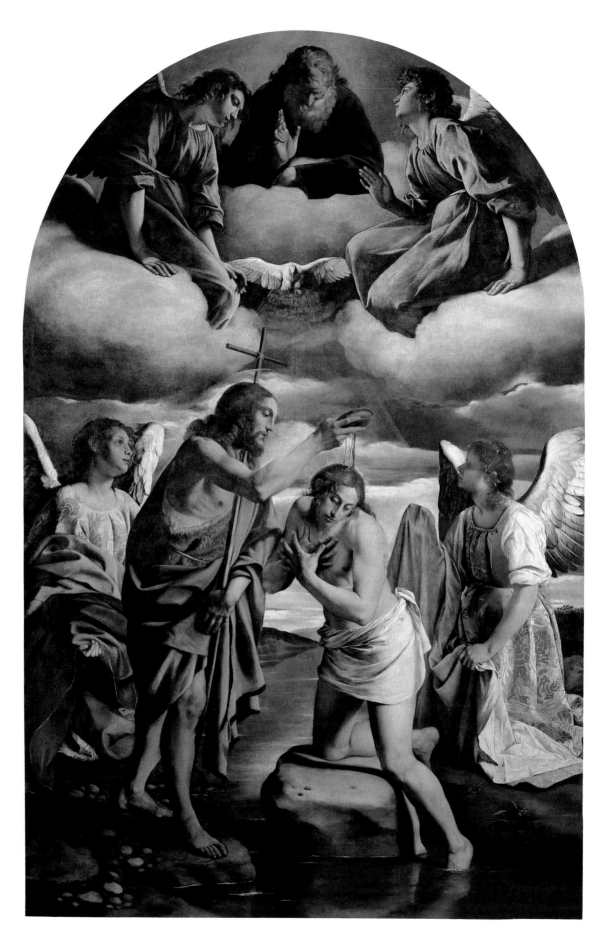

poorer condition; the face in particular has suffered. (When old repaints in the area around the left eye and forehead were removed, it was decided to employ glazes to reconstruct the missing parts in such a way that the reconstruction is visible on close inspection.)

In his 1642 biography of Orazio, Baglione remarks that "he similarly painted for the Olgiati a small chapel on the right side of the church of [Santa Maria della] Pace, where, above the altar, is shown Saint John the Baptist who baptizes Christ. And there is God the Father and angels, painted in oils with great love and diligence; the remaining stories of the saint were painted by him in fresco." On this basis the three small scenes on the vault of the chapel with stories from the life of the saint have been thought to be works by Orazio or his workshop. These modest frescoes, however, are by an assistant of Pietro da Cortona—someone who probably worked with the great painter-architect between 1656 and 1658, when Pietro directed a vast restoration project of the church financed by Pope Alexander VII Chigi. At this time, the Olgiati chapel was transferred from its original position beneath the octagonal crossing, becoming the third

rather than the first chapel, where a secondary entrance (referred to in the documents as the "porta piccola") was opened. The original position of the chapel is indicated in earlier plans of the crossing by Antonio da Sangallo the Younger, Jacopo Meleghino, and Francesco Torriani, as well as in the 1612 document mentioned above.

As part of the research on the chapel sponsored by the Soprintendenza per i Beni Artistici e Storici di Roma, the walls of the original site are being studied in the hope of finding some trace of Orazio's frescoes.

MPdO

1. Archivio di Stato di Roma, Trenta Notai, Capitolini Uff.9 b 94. I would like to thank Livia Carloni for calling my attention to this citation.
2. ". . . un quadro di San Giovanni Battista quando batteza Nostro Signore . . . nella chiesa della Madonna della Pace di Roma conforme alla grandezza et larghezza che è in d[et]ta cappella . . . di farlo bene con colori fini . . . le figure disegnate cioè Christo S Giovanni B, Dio Padre Spirito Santo con gloria di altri angeli et figure conforme al disegno fatto . . . e darlo finito fra sei mesi prossimi da oggi."
3. Chiarini 1962, 26.

12.

David Slaying Goliath

Oil on canvas, 73¼ × 53⅛ in. (186 × 135 cm)

National Gallery of Ireland, Dublin (inv. 980)

ca. 1607–9

Rome, New York

Having felled the giant Goliath with his slingshot, which lies in studied disarray in the foreground, the young David now uses the Philistine's sword to cut off his head (1 Sam. 17:50–51). The story is one of the most celebrated in the Old Testament and inspired a long line of distinguished paintings and sculpture. Key to Orazio's painting, which treats the story in narrative rather than emblematic terms—that is, David actively slaying Goliath rather than holding or contemplating his head—is Michelangelo's fresco for a lunette of the Sistine chapel (fig. 44). There the scene is paired with Judith and Holofernes, as it is again in the Della Rovere chapel in Trinità dei Monti, Rome, frescoed by Marco Pino and Pellegrino Tibaldi

in 1548–50. Both Old Testament scenes were commonly understood as symbolizing the triumph of godliness over corruption and of virtue over vice.

Orazio's remarkable depiction differs from other Michelangelo-inspired examples—for instance, Daniele da Volterra's painting in the château de Fontainebleau and Orazio Borgianni's in the Academia de San Fernando, Madrid—in adopting a vertical rather than horizontal format and in showing Goliath twisting around and raising his enormous hand to ward off David's blow. This device considerably increases the psychological tension, enabling the two opponents to make eye contact and further accentuating the differences in their size and physical strength. The motif of eye contact may have been inspired by Caravaggio's celebrated picture of Judith beheading Holofernes (Palazzo Barberini, Rome; fig. 109), in which the Assyrian general rolls back his eyes toward his murderer as she severs his head. Similarly, the idea of showing Goliath's body foreshortened along a diagonal with the head placed close to the picture plane may derive from Caravaggio's *Conversion of Saint Paul* (Santa Maria del Popolo, Rome). What cannot be doubted is that the pose and gesture of Goliath were important to Artemisia when she painted her *Judith Beheading Holofernes* (cat. 55). The shallow, tilted space suggests that Orazio's picture may have been conceived as an overdoor.

Yet to discuss this picture exclusively in terms of Caravaggesque realism scarcely does it justice, for in it two aesthetics compete for attention: Caravaggesque naturalism and a Mannerist-derived emphasis on the beauty of formal invention. The contrapposto attitude of David conveys a quality less of urgency than of studied *bellezza*. Garrard has identified the source of the pose as that of a figure of Orestes in a Roman

sarcophagus relief then in the collection of Marchese Vincenzo Giustiniani. This was a celebrated ancient sculpture that had influenced a large number of works of art. Indeed, by the early seventeenth century, the pose—extracted from its narrative context and developed in isolation for its inherent serpentine beauty—had become something of a topos. Titian had famously exploited it in his *Bacchus and Ariadne* (National Gallery, London), which in Gentileschi's day was in the Aldobrandini collection in Rome, as did Tiziano Aspetti in his figure of the giant for the entrance portal to the Libreria Marciana in Venice.[1] Michelangelo's *Apollo* (Bargello, Florence) and El Greco's figure of Christ in his various pictures of the Purification of the Temple belong to this same tradition. In the sarcophagus and in Titian's painting, the pose is dynamic and conveys movement. By contrast, in Orazio's painting the *serpentinata* features have been accentuated—the left foot raised, the right shoulder lowered, the left arm extended in balletic fashion. These changes are the more notable in that David's action is so akin to that of Orestes, who on the sarcophagus is shown

Figure 44. Marcantonio Raimondi (ca. 1470/82–1527/34?), *David Cutting off the Head of Goliath*. Engraving after Michelangelo's fresco in the Sistine chapel. The Metropolitan Museum of Art, New York

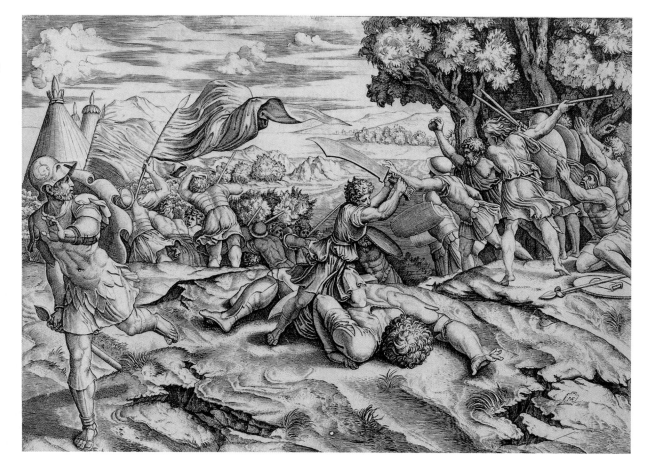

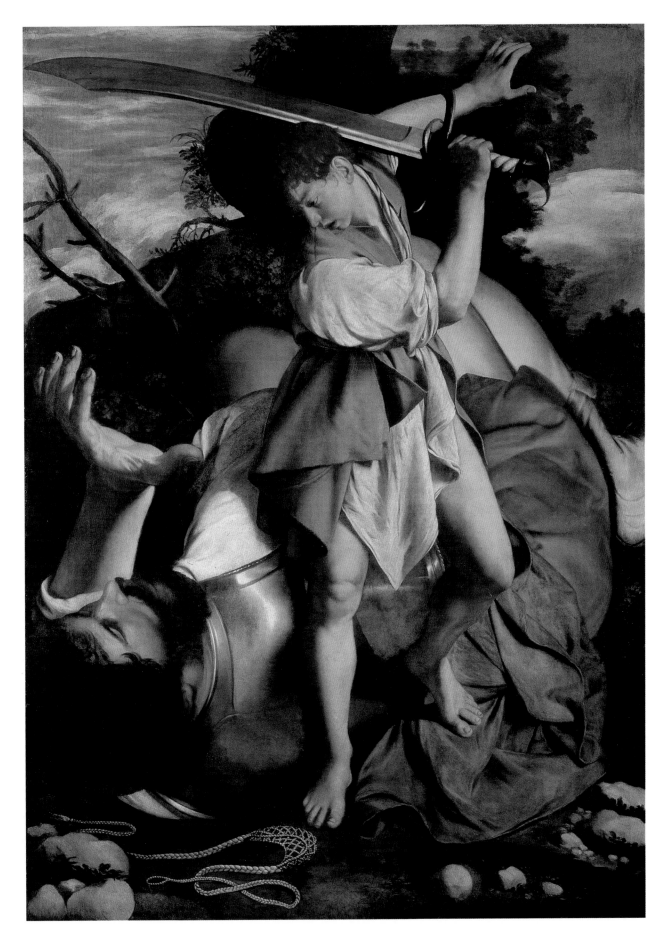

PROVENANCE: Confectioner's shop, Limehouse, East London (until 1935); Tomàs Harris, London (1935–36); National Gallery of Ireland, Dublin.

REFERENCES: Longhi 1943, 22; Milan 1951, 65 no. 107; Emiliani 1958b, 43; Wittkower 1958, 43; Schleier 1962, 435; Moir 1967, vol. 1, 70–71, vol. 2, 75 no. B.1; Pepper 1971, 337; Bissell 1981, 23–27, 146 no. 15, 148, 206; Garrard 1989, 16, 31, 184, 198; Nicolson 1990, 113; Papi in Florence 1991, 36, 59 n. 16, 110; Benedetti in Dublin 1992, no. 4; Schleier 1993, 196; Bissell 1999, 4–5, 12, 43, 193, 195–96, 201; Bray in London–Bilbao–Madrid 1999, 56 no. 2.

slaying Aegisthus. The impression is of an elegant statue that can be rotated in space, and it is worth noting that Orazio was friends with the Mannerist sculptor Tommaso della Porta, whose will he witnessed in 1606.

The issue of whether Gentileschi's point of departure was the sarcophagus rather than an intermediary source is of some interest. Did he intend the pose as an antiquarian allusion—a statement about classical *bellezza* rendered in naturalistic terms? Ought the picture be seen as part of the debate surrounding the emerging classical aesthetic? There is no written evidence that Gentileschi had a theoretical bent, and I am inclined to think that antiquarianism played no significant role in his art. However, it is surely not coincidental that in the years 1604–7 Guido Reni was experimenting with Caravaggesque realism in a similar fashion. In works such as Reni's *Crucifixion of Saint Peter* (Pinacoteca Vaticana, Rome), *David with the Head of Goliath* (fig. 49), and, perhaps most pertinently, the *Martyrdom of Saint Catherine* (Museo Diocesano, Albenga) and a *David Slaying Goliath* (Fondation Rau, Marseilles),[2] the realism of Caravaggio's art is recast in terms of *grazia*, *bellezza*, and decorum. Which is to say, Reni treated Caravaggism not as a pictorial revolution but as an alternative style whose elements were susceptible to personal interpretation and manipulation. His example may have been important to Orazio as the latter moved toward his own naturalistic *maniera*.

With the exception of Papi, who unconvincingly places the picture in the second decade of the century, scholars have dated the *David Slaying Goliath* to about 1605–8. Its style has been compared with that of the *Saint Michael and the Devil* (cat. 14) and the *David Contemplating the Head of Goliath* (cat. 18). The densely modeled shadows, without passages of reflected light, are characteristic of the three documented altarpieces of 1607, as well as of the *Way to Calvary* (cat. 5) and, especially, the Oslo *Judith and Her Maidservant* (cat. 13).

The picture was discovered in a confectioner's shop in East London in 1935. Nothing is known of its earlier provenance, and its tentative identification (most recently by Bray) with an overdoor in the Palazzo Cambiaso, Genoa, mentioned by Ratti, or with another painting mentioned by Ticozzi as in the Palazzo Doria, Genoa, cannot be demonstrated. The Cambiaso provenance is especially tantalizing.[3] The picture has lost some of its crispness due to abrasion; the blue of Goliath's cloak has altered.

1. Leandro Bassano portrays Tiziano Aspetti with a model of this statue; see Kryza-Gersch 1998.
2. In addition to Bologna–Los Angeles–Fort Worth 1988–89, 188–90, see Spear 1989b, 371 no. 16.
3. Ratti (1780) 1976, 264–65: "Un'altra pur sopraporta con Davidde trionfante di Golia, d'Orazio Gentileschi, è di migliori di questo artefice." Lanzi (1795–96, vol. 1, 233–34) described the same painting as follows: "Presso gli Ecc. Cambiasi è un Davide che sovrasta al morto Golia, così staccato dal fondo, con tinte sì vivide e sì ben contrapposte, che potria dare idea di un nuovo, a pressochè mai non veduto stile." This reference was associated by Gamba (1922–23, 256) with the Spada *David* (cat. 18). Bissell (1981, 146, 149) feels that these references are better applied to the Spada picture than to the Dublin *David*, but I confess I don't see why this should be so. The Cambiaso also owned a *Judith and Her Maidservant* and a *Woman Playing the Violin*, for which, see cat. nos. 39 and 40.

13.

Judith and Her Maidservant

Oil on canvas, 53 ½ × 63 in. (136 × 160 cm)

Nasjonalgalleriet, Oslo (NG.M.02073)

ca. 1608–9

The story of the Jewish widow Judith and her heroic act to save her people from the Assyrians is told in the Apocrypha. The city of Bethulia is on the verge of surrendering to the Assyrians when Judith proposes a subterfuge. Decked out in her finery, she and her servant Abra go unaccompanied to the enemy's camp, where she is seized and taken to their commander, Holofernes, whom she offers to help. Captivated by Judith's beauty, Holofernes invites her to feast in his tent at night. When he drinks himself into a stupor, Judith cuts off his head with his own sword and carries it back to Bethulia in triumph. The deed turns the tide of the battle.

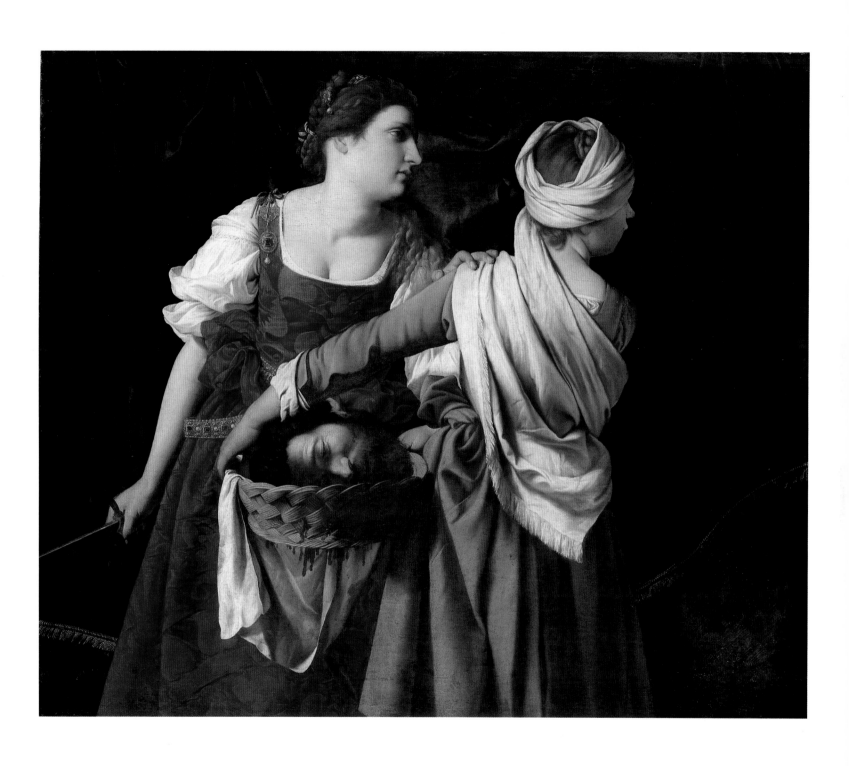

PROVENANCE: Scarpa collection, Motta di Livenza (sale, Giulio Sambon, Milan, November 14, 1895, lot 67, as by Caravaggio; evidently bought in and donated by Sambon to a sale benefiting war veterans arranged by the Syndicat de la Presse, Petit Palais, Paris, June 13–23, 1917, lot 46, as by Caravaggio); Wangs Kunst og Antikvitetshandel, Oslo (1917); Urban Jacob Rasmus Børresen, Oslo (1918–1943; his estate, 1943–45); Nasjonalgalleriet, Oslo.

RELATED PICTURE: Helsingen Kaupunginmuseo, Helsinki (copy; noted in Bissell 1999, 320).

REFERENCES: De Witt 1939, 51–53; Longhi 1943, 46 n. 38; Emiliani 1958b, 43; Moir 1967, vol. I, 71 n. 10; Borea in Florence 1970, 77; Oslo 1973, 346–47; Nicolson 1979, 51; Bissell 1981, 63–64, 155–56 no. 27; Gregori in Naples 1984–85, 147; Pepper 1984a, 316; Garrard 1989, 39–40, 497–98 n. 56; Nicolson 1990, 111; Palmer 1991, 28; Papi in Florence 1991, 96–99 no. 3; Spike 1991b, 733; Stolzenwald 1991, 22; Lerberg 1993, 182–90; Bissell 1999, 12, 13, 124, 198, 201–2, 311, 318–20 no. X-13; Boccardo 2000, 205.

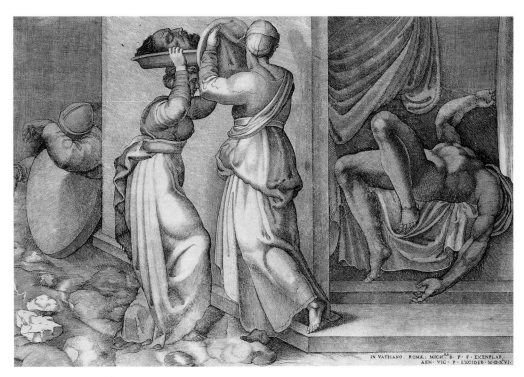

Figure 45. Enea Vico (1523–1567), *Judith and Her Maidservant*. Engraving after Michelangelo's fresco in the Sistine chapel. The Metropolitan Museum of Art, New York

Orazio depicts Judith and Abra leaving Holofernes' tent with the general's head packed in their food basket. (The Apocrypha mentions a meat sack rather than a basket, but in his Uffizi panel Botticelli shows Abra carrying the head in a basket and in the Sistine chapel, Michelangelo places it on a charger. Antiveduto Gramatica also shows a basket in his painting in the Nationalmuseum, Stockholm; fig. 120.) As the two women pause to glance back at the body of Holofernes, Judith places a reassuring hand on Abra's shoulder, while, grasping his sword, she stands ready to defend them in the enemy camp they must pass through.

Orazio's point of departure for this grand picture must have been Michelangelo's fresco in the Sistine chapel or one of the engravings after it (fig. 45).[1] Vasari had admired Michelangelo's scene for, among other things, the psychological slant he gave the story: "While putting her hands to the burden, [Judith] seeks to cover it, and, turning her head toward [Holofernes], who, having been killed while raising an arm and a leg, makes a noise in the tent, she shows by her attitude fear of the [military] camp and terror at the sight

of the dead body." Michelangelo's inclusion of Holofernes' corpse within a pavilion, a guard asleep outside, and his depiction of Judith performing an action were more in line with the Renaissance notion of a narrative—*un azione*—than is Orazio's painting. But Michelangelo's identification of the psychologically complex moment when the horrific deed has been accomplished but the escape not yet made served as the basis for Orazio's three treatments of the theme (cat. 39 and fig. 46).

In the Oslo picture, the effect is of a pause pervaded by reflection and stillness. Orazio employs the Caravaggesque device of arrested action not to create a sense of immediacy but as an occasion for lingering over details, almost as though he were painting a still life. In his hands even the drips of clotted blood and the stains on the towel acquire a macabre beauty. In a fashion typical of Baroque poetry—particularly that of Giambattista Marino—formal devices are employed as narrative strategies. The comradeship of the two women is underscored by their echoing profiles and the bunched folds of their dresses, while the contrast between Judith's rich, wine-colored silk brocade dress and Abra's simpler but no less elegantly colored costume reminds us of their very different social status. The comparison between the immaculately white scarf trailing over Abra's shoulder and the blood-stained towel hanging from the basket is a comment on the theme of purity and evil. And the repeated diagonals of the fringed hem of the tent, Abra's blue sleeve, the soft flesh of Judith's arm and shoulder, and the edge of the sword serve, like rhymes, to highlight the conflicts inherent in the story. This insistence on formal devices rather than dramatic gestures is very unlike Artemisia's approach to narrative, and it is surprising that several scholars have ascribed the picture to her. Perhaps the only feature it shares with Artemisia's work is the careful rendering of jewelry, as described in the Book of Judith (10:4): "And she put sandals upon her feet, and put about her her bracelets, and her chains, and her rings, and her earrings, and all her ornaments, and decked

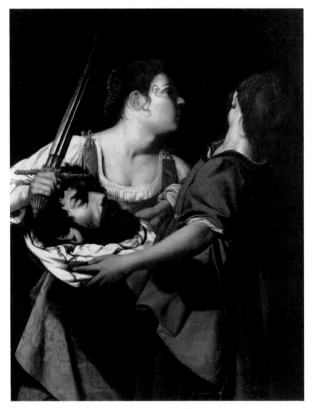

Figure 46. Orazio Gentileschi, *Judith and Her Maidservant with the Head of Holofernes*. Oil on canvas. Private collection

herself bravely, to allure the eyes of all men that should see her." Within Orazio's production, the Oslo picture marks a move away from his earlier, more tense interpretation of the theme (fig. 46), and it looks ahead to the Hartford painting (cat. 39), in which the psychological moment has been further abstracted from its narrative context.

Although Longhi's attribution of the picture to Orazio has been widely followed, Nicolson, Spike, and Palmer have all leaned toward an ascription to Artemisia, and Papi (who, however, like many others, had not seen the picture prior to its exhibition in Florence in 1991) does not exclude this possibility. By contrast, Garrard rejects the idea of Artemisia's authorship and accepts Orazio's because of what she sees as a "fussy confusion of drapery and detail" and a "dramatic disjunction between the figures' movements." Her characterization of Judith as "a languid, conventionally attractive female character who does not summon the energy required by the event" stems from her gendered approach to interpretation. While Garrard's description might be fine as an attempt to characterize Artemisia's response to her father's picture, as exemplified by her painting in the Pitti (cat. 60), it shows a total misunderstanding of the subtle poetry of Orazio's nondramatic art. No less dogmatic is her attempt to date the picture to about 1616, thereby making the Oslo painting dependent on Artemisia's canvas in Florence. The picture simply cannot have been painted that late.

In his monograph of 1981, Bissell proposes the identification of the picture with the painting by Orazio that was sequestered by the court during Artemisia's rape trial in 1612. A more likely candidate for that painting has since emerged (fig. 46), but Bissell continues to advocate a date of about 1611. It is my belief that the picture belongs to an earlier moment in Orazio's career. The focused light, still manifestly derived from the work of Caravaggio, does not set into play the brilliant reflections found, for example, in the Spada *David Contemplating the Head of Goliath* (cat. 18). It is a static light, which seems to fix the forms within the picture field rather than to suggest transient effects. The rich palette and fused modeling further emphasize physical weight and density.

Although Orazio has clearly based the composition on posed models, he has generalized their features so that they do not convey individual identity in the same way as the above-mentioned *David,* the Bucharest *Madonna and Child* (cat. 15), and the Turin *Saint Jerome* (cat. 16). An analogy to the arresting of the action and the aestheticizing of the dramatic moment seen in the Oslo painting can be found in the *David Slaying Goliath* (cat. 12). Like that work, the picture probably dates to about 1608–9.

1. The engraving by Giulio Bonasone dates to 1544–47; that of Enea Vico is dated 1546.

14.

Saint Michael and the Devil

Oil on canvas, 109½ × 75⅝ in. (278 × 192 cm)

Parish church of Santissimo Salvatore, Farnese (Viterbo)

ca. 1607–8

PROVENANCE: Chapel of the Sacrament, Santissimo Salvatore, Farnese (Viterbo).

REFERENCES: Schleier 1962, 432–35; Longhi 1963, 25, 27–28; Moir 1967, vol. 1, 30–31; Schleier 1970a, 172–73; Bissell 1974, 114–17 nn. 5–14; Nicolson 1979, 53; Bissell 1981, 26, 145–46 n. 14; Gregori and Schleier 1989, vol. 1, 420, 425; Nicolson 1990, 115; Papi in Florence 1991, 36; Röttgen 1992, 20; Germond 1993, 754; Arcangeli in Fossombrone 1997, 39, fig. 38; Papi in Salonika 1997, 190; Finaldi in London–Bilbao–Madrid 1999, 56.

Saint Michael the Archangel, the standard-bearer of the battalions of angels, expelled the devil from heaven to the depths of hell (Rev. 12:7–9). It is not known why the Confraternity of the Disciplinati— also known as the Flagellants—in Farnese chose this particular patron saint. The confraternity, by the middle of the sixteenth century, had already achieved a certain status, as well as a presence in the city's churches. The confraternity traced its roots to the medieval period and, like all the various groups of Disciplinati throughout central Italy, was founded as a pietistic society. In Farnese, which, with nearby Latera, was the seat in the sixteenth century of a collateral branch of the powerful Farnese family, the Disciplinati took on the more modern and charitable role of hospitalers.[1] They enjoyed the protection of Duke Mario Farnese, who must have been among the confraternity's most important members, since he had already acquired an altar for the Disciplinati in the renovated church of Santissimo Salvatore.[2] It was Schleier who first asked how and why a painting by Orazio Gentileschi came to grace an altar in a relatively small center, and how the confraternity would have gained access to such an élite figure in the art world. Schleier discovered the *Saint Michael and the Devil* when, following a notice by Bellori concerning a painting by Giovanni Lanfranco executed for the same church, he recognized this masterpiece by Gentileschi, about which he then published two important articles, in 1962 and 1970. Schleier also undertook a detailed reconstruction of the decorative phases of the church, the original interior of which had been obscured by an injudicious restoration in 1900–1901 under the direction of Don Pietro Benigni, the parish priest. In an attempt to prevent their theft, the paintings were removed from their frames and glued or nailed to the walls. In some cases, as with the Gentileschi, the paintings were given newly made-up edges, which also changed their original dimensions; these interventions have been reversed in a recent restoration.[3]

The former Castro diocese's records of the pastoral visits indicate that during the dukedom of Mario Farnese (he died in 1619), four altars—besides the altar with the lost picture by Lanfranco—were constructed at Santissimo Salvatore. Two altarpieces were executed by the Bolognese painter Antonio Panico: the *Rosary* for the chapel of the Confraternity of the Rosary, to which Mario's wife, Camilla Lupi di Soragna, belonged (the frescoes there were probably already under way in 1596), and the *Mass of Saint Bonaventure,* completed in 1603, for the chapel of the Confraternity of the Holy Sacrament and the Body of Christ. Another altar, dedicated to Saint Anthony Abbot, had a painting (now restored) that has been attributed to the circle of Palma il Giovane; the altarpiece was commissioned privately, by the doctor Antonio Abbati, though its execution was overseen by Duke Mario. Gentileschi's *Saint Michael* altarpiece was finished by May 31, 1608. Schleier correctly proposed this date as a terminus ad quem for the painting.[4]

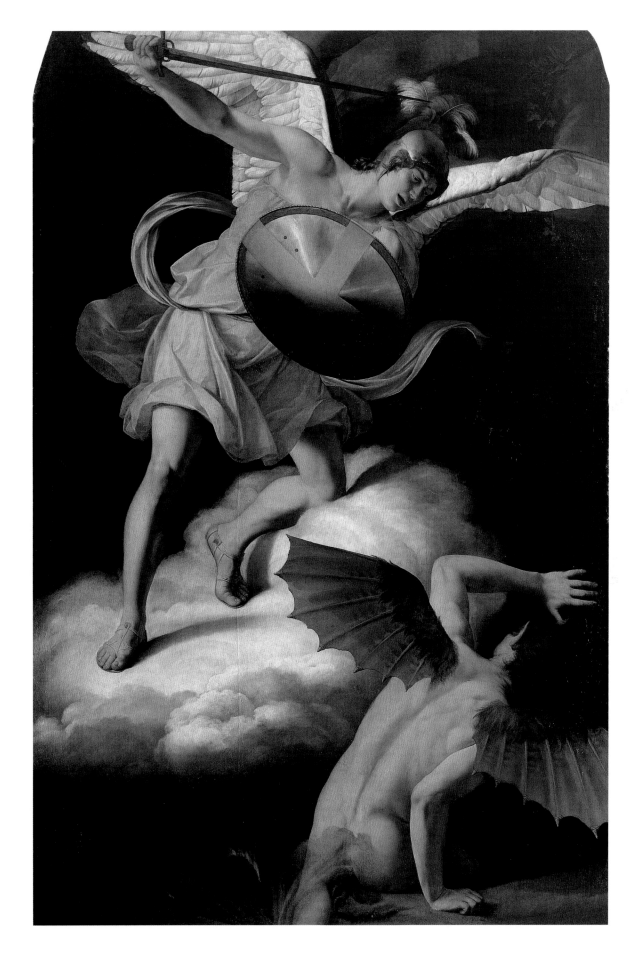

Little is known about Mario Farnese as a patron of the arts. He was a capable member of a collateral branch of the family, loyal first to Alessandro and then Ranuccio Farnese of Parma, a city where Mario also had a palace. His skills, which were very different from those of his brother, Ferrante, the bishop of Parma, led him to the post of lieutenant general of the papal armies. He also had close ties to the Aldobrandini family, in particular Cardinal Pietro, who was one of Gentileschi's patrons early in the century. Aldobrandini may well have suggested Orazio to Duke Mario as a candidate to execute the altarpiece for the Farnese.

Mario tried to improve the economy in his small duchy by creating a grain reserve, an aqueduct, and a printing shop, and as evidence of his piety he founded two Franciscan monasteries. In his political and military career, he steered a careful course between his allegiance to his family and his service to the Church. After living for several years in Parma, he purchased in 1606 the Palazzo Odescalchi (later Lancelloti) on the via Giulia in Rome. The duke was patron to several important artists; in Parma they included Francesco Mochi and the young Jusepe de Ribera (as attested in a letter from Ludovico Carracci to Ferrante Carlo), and in Rome he was in contact with Panico, Lanfranco, Antonio Carracci, and Orazio Gentileschi.[5]

In 1962, Schleier dated the *Saint Michael* to 1607–8. At the time, the dating was necessarily based primarily on style, on Schleier's recognition of the profound influence of Caravaggio; indeed, the gentle, measured light derives from the dreamy atmosphere of Caravaggio's early work, as does the lovely shaded, frowning face of the archangel. Certainly studied from life, the figure closely resembles that in the Dublin *David* (cat. 12) and the slightly earlier angel in the Brera, the *Vision of Saint Cecilia* (cat. 9). The affinity between the *Saint Michael* and the Brera altarpiece is especially evident in the rendering of the feathers of the wings and in the skillful contrasts in the shadows of the changeable whites; more broadly, the two works are characterized by the same softness in the skin and by the same treatment of the flesh tones and textiles. As always in Gentileschi's work, there is a

sense of his Mannerist inheritance directly below the surface, like an underground river. It does not, in itself, offer any evidence of the picture's date.[6] The painting is skillfully constructed on contrasts, most blatantly on that between a figurative style still indebted to Mannerism—as in the figure of Michael, which, with a somewhat forced pose, occupies all the available space, or as in the devil's profile—and the naturalistic rendering of the whole.

Other than a little-noticed suggestion by Longhi in 1963, the dating of the work has never been questioned. Documents recently discovered in the archive of the confraternity of the Gonfalone of Rome offer additional evidence that the painting was in fact in place at the time of the bishop's visit on May 31, 1608. These indicate that the Disciplinati of Farnese were first associated with the Roman Archconfraternity of the Gonfalone—the so-called Raccomandati della Madonna—not in 1616, as has been suggested, but on September 4, 1608, and again on May 19, 1610.[7] An association such as this, which could be repeated to allow the organization to receive a large number of indulgences,[8] undoubtedly signified an important change in status for the Farnese confraternity, one marked by the decision, made most likely by Mario Farnese himself, to commission an altarpiece from an important Roman artist. And, indeed, Saint Michael's shield bears the red cross of the Roman Raccomandati della Madonna; the motif also appears in the red and white feathers that decorate his small parade helmet.

Longhi had tried to suggest that the Farnese picture, despite its dimensions and apparent later date, was the same *Saint Michael* about which Orazio testified on September 14, 1603, during the libel suit brought against him by Giovanni Baglione. That work was painted by Orazio between 1601 and 1602 and exhibited in the cloister of San Giovanni Decollato in Rome. Longhi's hypothesis for the date is therefore unlikely, as the Farnese *Saint Michael* is much more evolved than Orazio's other paintings of that early date. However, it is interesting to note that the motif of the devil seen from the back is related to a figure in Baglione's *Divine Love Overcoming the World, the Flesh, and the Devil* (Gemäldegalerie, Berlin), which was, in part, the focus of the libel suit of 1603. It is possible that Baglione took this figure from a similar one in Orazio's 1601–2 *Saint Michael.*[9]

In the present painting, Saint Michael is shown standing on a large cloud as if he had just landed, his wings spread but not yet still, his blue cloth still fluttering in the breeze. X rays and infrared reflectographs show that the wings were repositioned along the axis of the shoulders to achieve this effect; originally, they were slightly folded. A sense of instability is also created by the position of the body, which is twisted with respect to the decidedly frontal position of the right leg and is bent to one side, following the example of the *Gladiator Battling a Lion,* an ancient sculpture that was in the Giustiniani collection. The archangel's unsheathed sword seems almost to measure the shallow depth of the dark ravine, barely enlivened by a rock and stunted shrubs. The large circle suggested by his body has its complement below in the curve of the devil's back. His face is hidden; only his ears, bent arms, satyr's tail, and huge bat's wings are visible. He sits precariously on a rocky outcropping; behind him flames burst from the depths of hell. Although there is weak illumination from above, the play of light on the plumage of the wings and especially the shadow of Saint Michael's legs on the clouds suggest a light source on the left, outside the picture—certainly the result of Caravaggio's influence. Other elements may be traced to Caravaggio's paintings in the Contarelli chapel: the fluttering drapery, for example, derived from the second version of the *Saint Matthew and the Angel,* and the devil's turned back, which recalls that of a figure in the *Martyrdom of Saint Matthew* (fig. 4).

The effects of light bring forth the subtle contrasts within the painting. The face, limbs, and shoulders of Saint Michael, for example, have a youthful solidity— one notes in particular the dirty nails of his feet, shod in almost impossible sandals—while his torso is almost incorporeal, enclosed in the folds of yellow material and then almost hidden by the ridiculously small shield he holds. The devil is formally linked to Michael by the point of his wings, and about him, too, there is a definite sense of corporeality—in the subtle indentation of the vertebrae along his back, in his obscured profile,

and in his hand reaching out to ward off the blow. Yet this corporeality is contradicted by the fantastical large dark wings, which seem abstracted from natural forms. This, then, is essentially a symbolic struggle between two supernatural beings, a struggle that remains suspended within the painting. The composition is deliberately theatrical, but Gentileschi uses the Caravaggesque light for his own ends. It is also likely, as is often noted, that in order to create this realm combining reality and the ideal, Gentileschi may have studied in some detail Guido Reni's Caravaggesque Roman works. The artist's masterly technique and formal achievement and the effort he expended on a work to be sent to a relatively unimportant venue remind us how little Gentileschi was concerned about the final destination of his works.   LC

1. See *Confraternite nell'Italia Centrale* 1993. Fiorani 1985 provides useful information on Roman confraternities and has an index of the archives of Roman confraternities.

2. Schleier 1970a, 172ff.; and recently, Andretta 1994, 44f. Don Luigi Egidi's manuscript, "Memorie rilevate dal libro vecchio della Confraternita de' Battuti di Farnese . . . L'anno del Signore 1808," is preserved in the Archivio Parrocchiale, Farnese, and the same archive has the statute of 1559.

3. This notice is in the Archivio Parrocchiale, Farnese; see also Schleier 1970a.

4. Schleier 1970a, 177, II, VI; compared again with the document in the Archivio della Diocesi di Acquapendente: Visite pastorali dell'ex Diocesi di Castro. Vescovo A. Caccia (1603–1608), fol. 68v, May 31, 1608, "Sequiter Altare S. Michaelis Arcangeli Societatis disciplinatorum pariter suis necessariis monitum. . . ."

5. Gallo 1998, 313.

6. Schleier 1962, 435.

7. Archivio Segreto Vaticano, Archivio del Gonfalone. See bb. 1232, 1334, 1235; b. 56 for the dates of the memberships: fol. 114v, September 8, 1608, and fol. 182v, May 19, 1610. In 1608 the prior was Agostino Rotondo. The earlier notarial acts of the notary Bonifacio Bottardi, who sanctioned the accords of August 18, 1608, and April 9, 1610, are unfortunately not preserved in folders 28 and 29 of this notary in the Archivio Notarile in the Archivio Statale, Viterbo.

8. Even Panico's picture *Mass of Saint Bonaventure,* which we know was in place in 1603, seems to have been executed through an association of the Confraternity of the Santissima Sacramento with the Roman Archconfraternity of the Santissima Sacramento di San Pietro (September 9, 1603).

9. See, most recently, Arcangeli in Fossombrone 1997, 39, and Danesi Squarzina in Rome–Berlin 2001, 298–99.

Restoration Report and Diagnostic Examination

M. Rossi Doria and
F. Matera; M. Cardinali,
M. B. de Ruggeri, and
C. Falcucci

The restoration, funded by the Italian government, was carried out in two phases in 1995. During the first phase the painting was detached from the inappropriate surface to which it had been attached in 1900–1901. At that time the canvas had been removed from its original stretcher (traces of which remained), cut irregularly along its edges (which had been secured with nails every 10 cm), reinforced, and glued on the wall over a layer of blue canvas. To give it a curved shape and to insert it into a frame made of cement, it had been trimmed along the upper corners, and a canvas lunette had been added, joined to the rest with plaster that projected over the original painted surface. The deformation and lifting of the canvas produced during these operations have now been eliminated by making incisions on the perimeters of the principal figures, for example, along the puffed sleeve on the right arm.

After being covered with Japanese tissue paper, the canvas was cut away from the wall with scalpels and blades, and any extraneous material attached to it was removed. The edges were reinforced with synthetic resins, a strip lining was added, and the whole was gently mounted on a wood stretcher constructed to the painting's presumed original dimensions. Subsequent procedures were more routine: the removal of old varnishes and retouching and the elimination of plaster. Losses to the canvas were reintegrated on a primed base; while losses along the edges were left exposed, fills in color were made where necessary. The painting's preparation was revealed to be a very thin combination of fine gesso, mild glue, and dark pigment.

Physical analyses of the painting were performed in 1998 with funding from the Italian government. The painting is made up of two pieces of linen canvas with a twill weave (also known as sailcloth), sewn together on the diagonal in the area of the shield and the hollow of the archangel's right arm. Although this type of canvas was not very popular in Rome in the 1600s, it was used by Reni, Poussin, and Guercino. The image in the X radiograph appears quite legible, particularly in the upper half, suggesting that the artist worked from a drawing. X radiographs indicate little use of overlapping layers in the background to create depth, and the unaided eye can see that the drapery does not overlap the flesh tones or the arms and the head over the wings. Infrared reflectography of many details reveals subtle underdrawing below the paint layer, where a brush was used to outline such parts as the devil's elbow and Saint Michael's right foot and chin. These traces, however, are not substantial enough to support a conclusion that an underdrawing exists for the entire composition. Moreover, the legibility of brushwork or drawing implement is limited by a lack of contrast between the paint layers and the dark primer ground.

The painter made small adjustments to refine the composition. Greatest attention was concentrated on the arrangement of the wings, which play an important role in the spatial definition. Saint Michael's right wing was initially lower and slightly folded. The change—making the wing echo the diagonal of the arm—was made as the artist laid in the design. In the X radiograph, the archangel's right wing is only partially legible as it passes beneath the arm. It is more visible in the reflectograph as a gray outline. The archangel's left wing also initially had a less foreshortened shape; in the X radiograph the feathers appear longer. The devil's left wing was adjusted when the painting of his back had been brought to a high degree of finish. In comparison to other fleshy areas, the devil's back is less easily penetrated by X radiographs, suggesting the presence of white lead. The upper edges of the wings were fixed at the outset, but their rounded feathers were replaced by the present bat-shaped forms. This adjustment, visible in infrared examination, was painted over the clouds. Other lesser adjustments include the expansion of the drapery over the right thigh and small reductions and extensions in the helmet, in the right arm, in the neck, in the left thigh, and along the contour of the devil's body. Analysis confirms that the paint was applied beginning with the dark areas, as is visible particularly in the flesh tones. The brushwork is smooth and blended. Anatomical details were clarified over the course of work with occasional modifications to the original sketch.

15.

Madonna and Child

Oil on canvas, 38¾ × 29½ in.
(98.5 × 75 cm)

Signed and dated (lower left,
on reverse of canvas):
HORATIUS GENTILESCHI
FACIEBAT 1609

Muzeul Național de Artă
al României, Bucharest
(362 / 8328)

1609

On October 24, 1609, Bartolomeo Pellini reported to Giovanni Magno, secretary to Duke Vincenzo Gonzaga in Mantua, on a picture of the Madonna and Child that Orazio was painting for the duke. "Four days ago, . . . [Gentileschi] came to invite me to go and see a picture he is making at your request. It is a seated Madonna, with the child in her arms, the child nude except for a little swaddling band that, girdling the body, covers a bit of it. And they look at each other with great affection, for all that the child is no more than one month old, but [the painting is] well executed and natural. The Madonna is dressed in yellow with a blue mantle that, although it has dropped, makes a lovely sight and adornment. She has a very beautiful face with no other ornament than the diadem, and her shoulders are uncovered and nude, so that the beauties with which nature has endowed her are visible. . . . In sum, [the picture] demonstrates that naturalism is a very good thing."[1] Were it not for the differences in the Madonna's clothing and the diadem she is reported as wearing, the correspondence with the Bucharest picture would be compelling.[2] Indeed, conservation work carried out at the J. Paul Getty Museum in 1990–91, following severe damage to the picture during the 1989 Romanian uprising, uncovered an inscription on the back of the original canvas with the date 1609.[3] We can only suppose that the duke's picture was a variant—perhaps somewhat prettified—of the Bucharest painting. This would be an early instance of Orazio's producing contemporaneous variants of a composition of real novelty (see fig. 47).

As Pellini's description suggests, in this case Orazio seems to have hired a woman from the parish of Santa Maria del Popolo, where he lived at the time, to bring her infant child to his studio to model for him. This is not surprising, for it has long been known that his barber modeled for him and that a pilgrim from Palermo posed for a *Saint Jerome* (cat. 16). Additionally,

another neighbor—Costanza Ceuli—testified that during the time Orazio lived on via del Babuino, she brought her children to his studio to model for him.[4] Is Costanza conceivably the model for this picture? In no earlier painting did a sense of artistic style, or *maniera*, yield so radically to what seventeenth-century critics saw as its polar opposite, truth to nature, *il naturale* or *il vero*.

There would seem to have been no effort on Orazio's part to make the woman's features conform to a notion of abstract beauty. Quite the contrary. Orazio emphasizes the bulk of her swollen breast just as he revels in the plainness of her braided coiffure. The coarse linen of her blouse interests him as much as the one-month-old child's wide-eyed stare and awkward limbs. It is apparent that the woman is seated on one of the low rush-seat chairs so common to homes of modest means. She has assumed a pose she could hold (and also one redolent of Raphaelesque precedent),[5] raising one leg, on which she rests her left arm, so as to position her child safely and comfortably. In works such as the *David Slaying Goliath* (cat. 12) and the Oslo *Judith and Her Maidservant* (cat. 13), which must precede the Bucharest *Madonna* by no more than a year or so, we feel the twin concepts of *grazia* and *bellezza*—ingrained by Orazio's Mannerist training and newly vital through the example of Guido Reni—modifying the experience of the studio toward an idea of art and style, *arte e maniera*. Here the opposite is the case, as Orazio transforms the grand artifice of Raphael's *Madonna della Sedia* (Palazzo Pitti, Florence) into a veristic scene of homely domesticity. Even Caravaggio, in his early *Gypsy Fortune-Teller* (Museo Capitolino, Rome) and *Penitent Magdalene* (fig. 126)—those works that Giovanni Battista Agucchi, the early proponent of classicism, saw as a refutation of high art—did not go as far as Orazio in asserting the ordinariness of experience over the imperatives of style. Giovan Pietro Bellori was later to decry the way

PROVENANCE: Felix Bamberg (ms. cat. 1879, no. 54); royal collection of Romania, Pelesh Castle, Sinaia (1879–1948); Muzeul Naţional de Artă al Românei, Bucharest.

RELATED PICTURES: Private collection, Prato d'Era (copy of Bucharest picture incorporating variations);[7] location unknown (fig. 47; copy of Bucharest picture incorporating a veil; sale, Christie's, London, March 4, 1927, lot 142).[8]

REFERENCES: Voss 1920a, 411; Voss 1925, 461; Longhi 1927, 114; Longhi 1943, 47; Emiliani 1958b, 20; Moir 1967, vol. 2, 78; Schleier 1971, 89; Teodosiu 1974, 23–24 no. 37; Nicolson 1979, 53; Bissell 1981, 146–47 no. 16, 158, 204; Nicolson 1990, 114.

young painters in Rome idolized Caravaggio, competing in their imitation of him by "undressing models and raising the light source without any longer paying attention to instruction and study, each readily finding in the streets and piazzas their master and subjects for copying from nature."[6] We can only speculate about the impetus behind this shift in Orazio's work—one that was to last until 1612, when he worked on the vault of Scipione Borghese's Casino delle Muse (fig. 6).

There can, I think, be no doubt that Artemisia's early painting at the Palazzo Spada (cat. 52) was based directly on the Bucharest *Madonna* or, conceivably, on the version sent to the duke of Mantua. However, any comparison of the two reveals that it is the father rather than the daughter who at this time was the more radical. Artemisia's picture, in the artful pose of the child, with his self-conscious gesture of affection, or the generalized treatment of the Virgin's face and bland description of the drapery, seems decidedly tentative and timid when compared with the extreme naturalism of her father's work. Was she, at this stage, not yet permitted to work directly from the model? By 1610, when she painted the *Susanna* (cat. 51)—almost certainly under Orazio's supervision and unquestionably in emulation of his work—this timidity has disappeared.

On all these counts the Bucharest *Madonna and Child* must be considered one of the key works in Orazio's oeuvre and one of the signal works of Caravaggesque naturalism. Perhaps only in Bartolomeo Manfredi's *Allegory of the Four Seasons* (Dayton Art Institute) do we find anything comparable.

1. See Luzio 1913, 61 n.
2. Bissell (1981) identifies the Bucharest picture with the Gonzaga painting.
3. The picture was punctured by bullets and shrapnel from behind, creating a 14 × 35.5 cm hole extending from the wrist of the

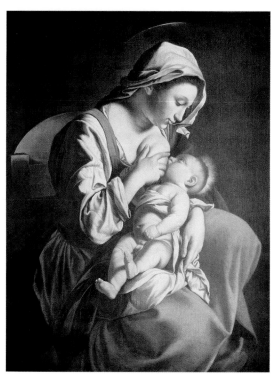

Figure 47. Copy after Orazio Gentileschi, *Madonna and Child*. Oil on canvas. Location unknown

Madonna's right hand to her lap and destroying the left foot and right leg of the child. These areas were reconstructed on the basis of photographs taken before the damage. At the same time, added strips at the top and sides were removed.

4. See appendix 1, under October 21, 1612.
5. Especially relevant are Marcantonio Raimondi's engraving of the Holy Family (Bartsch 60-I), and that of Agostino Carracci, fig. 106.
6. Bellori (1672) 1976, 219.
7. See Contini in Gregori and Schleier 1989, 329, 336 n. 20, where it is called an autograph work; see also Papi in Florence 1991, 137. I have not examined the picture, but the photograph does not inspire confidence. The Virgin wears a veil and the folds of her sleeve differ. It comes from the Oratorio di Pian de' Noci.
8. This may be the picture Longhi (1943, 47) cites as in the Heinemann collection in 1937. At the sale in 1927 it was ascribed to "Crespi." A photograph is on file at the Frick Art Reference Library; see fig. 47.

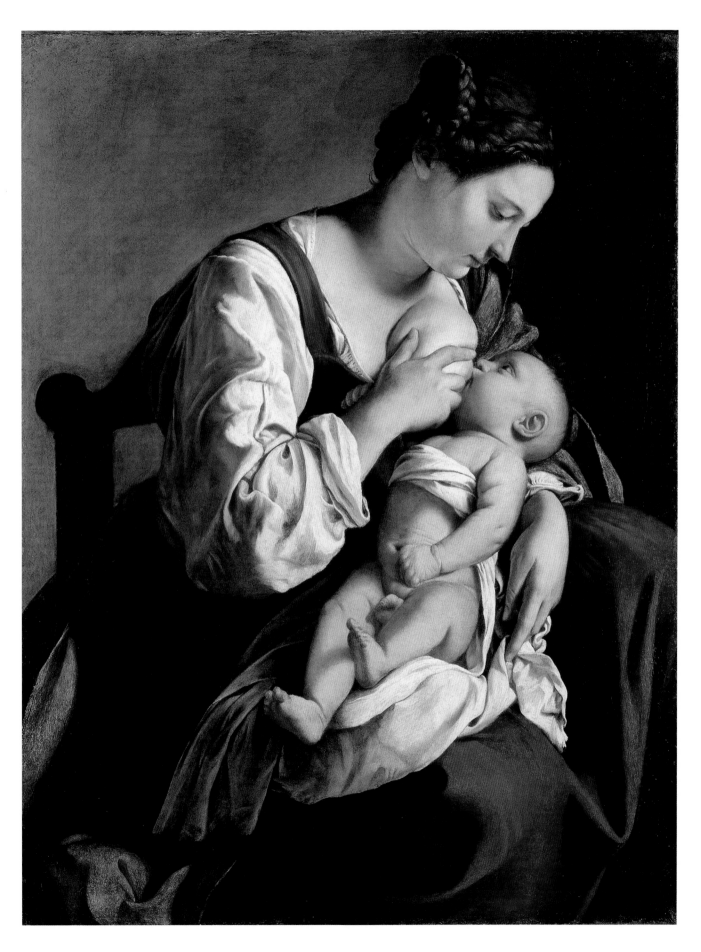

16.

Saint Jerome

Oil on canvas, 60¼ × 50⅜ in. (153 × 128 cm)

Museo Civico d'Arte Antica e Palazzo Madama, Turin (inv. 469)

1610/11

PROVENANCE: Private collection (sale, Finarte, Milan, 1966); Museo Civico d'Arte Antica e Palazzo Madama, Turin.

RELATED PICTURE: Private collection (a variant, thought by Longhi, on the basis of a photograph, to be autograph).[6]

REFERENCES: Moir 1967, vol. 1, 70–71, vol. 2, no. E.9; Mallè 1970a, 11; Mallè 1970b, vol. 2, 72–73; Bissell 1971, 289, 296 n. 43; Nicolson 1979, 53; Bissell 1981, 23, 65, 151 no. 21; Nicolson 1990, 115.

The fourth-century church father, ascetic, and translator of the Bible into Latin is shown in his retreat in the desert, practicing penitential devotions. The subject enjoyed enormous popularity from at least the fifteenth century and, together with depictions of Jerome writing or studying at his desk, was treated by virtually every Caravaggesque artist.

On July 27, 1612, Giovanni Pietro Molli, a pilgrim from Palermo, was summoned to testify at the rape trial of Artemisia. Depending on the way his testimony is interpreted, he had been employed by Orazio as a model during Lent of 1610 or 1611: "[The painter Signor Orazio Gentileschi used me] to portray a head similar to mine . . . and [also for] a full-length Saint Jerome he had me strip to the waist to make a Saint Jerome that resembled me."[1] Seventy-three at the time, Molli was described by Orazio's barber as "handsome in appearance, with a face like that of Saint Paul, bald-headed, with white hair, and with a fine, full beard that is as heavy on the cheeks as in the beard itself." Longhi connected this vivid testimony with a replica of the picture now in Turin, which became known to scholars only when it appeared on the art market in 1966. Bissell is surely correct in viewing the Turin painting as the prime version and hence the picture for which Molli posed. Not only does the physiognomic description match the figure precisely, but on grounds of style the picture can be dated to the period 1609–11, when Orazio often worked directly from a posed model, in emulation of Caravaggio.

As with the woman who posed for the Bucharest *Madonna and Child* (cat. 15), Molli assumed an attitude suitable to the subject but one that he could also maintain for protracted periods. His right arm is supported on what, in Orazio's studio, may have been a box or table, leaving the hand hanging limp. His left arm and hand, resting on a skull (emblem of mortality and sign of Jerome's meditation), help to steady the forward-leaning upper torso, while his gaze is directed upward; the beautifully described Christ on the cross

seems to turn his head toward the same area. The focused light falls not from the left, as Caravaggio preferred, but from the right, so that Jerome's face is enveloped in shadow. This device dissociates the light from any symbolic meaning but greatly enhances the expressive quality (Jerome's face is filled with kindness and humility). It also allows Orazio to explore the play of reflected light on the saint's body and to emphasize his physicality through the description of shadows. Those on the leg and arm are especially notable, but no less so is the way Christ's head on the crucifix casts a shadow on the cross and the cross casts a shadow on the rock on which it is propped.

A comparison with Caravaggio's *Saint Jerome Studying* (Galleria Borghese, Rome), which was painted for Scipione Borghese—a work Orazio must have known well—is telling. Caravaggio uses his incomparably bold painting technique and striking contrasts of light and dark to underscore the saint's immediacy and busy activity. The head, while it is marvelously characterized, does not have the appearance of a portrait. Orazio, on the other hand, creates a sense of stillness, and the individualized features confer the quality of an image taken from life—Jerome as an ordinary man. The method adopted here conforms to one described by the cultivated collector and critic Vincenzo Giustiniani: painting directly from nature, but with a knowledge of color and light (number eleven in his hierarchy of twelve).[2] Among the artists Giustiniani cites for their mastery of this technique are Rubens, Van Honthorst, and Ribera. None of these painters come as close as Orazio to the sensibility of a still-life painter, concentrating on the formal arrangement of objects, the rendering of their surfaces, and the effect of stillness. In keeping with this approach, Orazio has given equal emphasis to the skull, the book, the crucifix, and the plants (flowers in the lower left, ivy in the upper-right corner, and bare branches on the rocks, emblems of death and spiritual renewal).

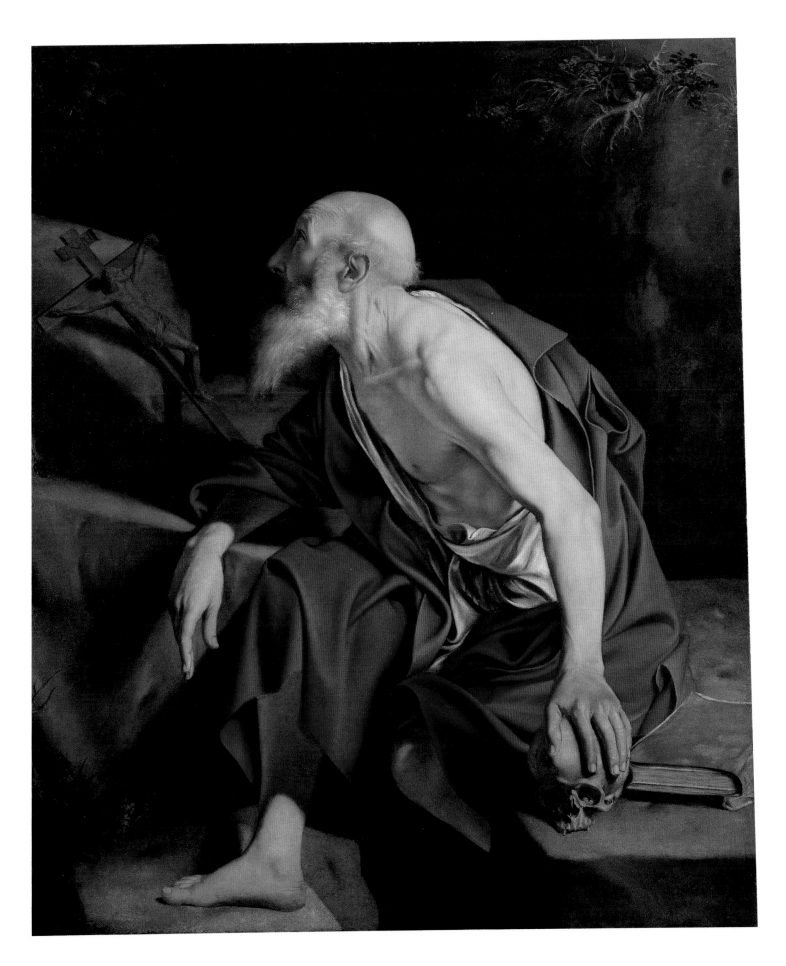

Molli's testimony reminds us what a long, drawn-out affair painting from a model—*dal naturale*—could be. During the forty days of Lent and for a few days after Easter, he would go to Orazio's house three or four times a week, sometimes staying from morning to evening and often sharing a meal with him. According to Molli, Orazio used his head for other pictures as well, and indeed the painter seems to have found in the pilgrim an ideal type for biblical figures. Saints Anthony Abbot and Jerome in Orazio's frescoed decoration in San Venanzio, Fabriano, and the Abraham in the *Sacrifice of Isaac* (fig. 63) appear to be based on a drawing or oil study of Molli's head, though no longer with the same emphasis on portraiture.[3] Molli's testimony is only a partial indication of Orazio's practice of making studies of figures that appealed to him. Additional evidence comes from a longtime neighbor who lived on the via della Croce, Costanza Ceuli, who brought her children to Orazio so that he could make drawn studies of them.[4] Such studies would have become part of his workshop material, and they explain why certain figure types recur at a remove of several years. For example, in Orazio's various depictions of Judith with the head of Holofernes, the features of the Assyrian commander are remarkably consistent and resemble, as well, those of John the Baptist in the Prado *Executioner with the Head of Saint John the Baptist* (cat. 20). In the case of the *Sacrifice of Isaac*, the tightly woven composition and brilliant effects of light, no less than the provenance from the Gentile collection in Genoa, point to a date of about 1622–23—more than a decade after the *Saint Jerome*.[5] Orazio's practice marks a significant departure from Caravaggio's use of a specific model for a number of contemporary canvases, but without making studies for later use. Here we are dealing with the creation of a repertory of figure types by means of drawings and, perhaps, oil sketches, something that permitted Orazio to move from Caravaggesque painting from posed models—perfectly exemplified in the *Saint Jerome*—to a reformed naturalism that stresses formal values over naturalistic effects: *verosimile* rather than *vero*.

Cusping is visible along the vertical edges and top of the canvas. The picture has suffered throughout from flaking losses, especially in the saint's left hand and the skull. The area of the shadows cast by the crucifix are badly worn. This does not, however, detract from the wonderfully solid painting of the figure. The hem of the red cloak is visible beneath the book, which was painted at a later date. This alone should establish the picture as the prime version. The picture was cleaned for the exhibition by Societá Rava e C.

1. In his testimony Molli states that he modeled during Lent of the previous year ("questa quadragesima prossima passata ha fatto l'anno"), that is, 1611; Orazio's barber gives the year as 1610 ("quadrigesima dell'anno 1610"). Key to resolving the matter is when exactly Orazio moved from via del Babuino to via Margutta, since Molli modeled in both houses and was able to describe them in detail. Easter fell on April 11 in 1610 and April 3 in 1611, so that the beginning of Lent fell in the first week of March in 1610 and the last week of February in 1611. Orazio is documented as living on via del Babuino on March 20, 1610; by February 16, 1611, he had moved to via Margutta, where he stayed until April 10, 1611. Tassi says that he helped Orazio beat up a would-be suitor of Artemisia's at the via del Babuino house in April (1610). Orazio's washerwoman, Margarita, testified on September 12, 1612, that Orazio had lived on via Margutta about two years earlier (that is, he would have moved in September 1610). By contrast, Tuzia, who lived across the street from Orazio on via Margutta, testified on March 2, 1612, that she had known Orazio about a year, which might suggest that he had not moved there much earlier (that is, shortly before February 16, 1611). No clear-cut answer emerges from these conflicting and fragmentary data. My thanks to Patrizia Cavazzini for pointing out the various conflicts.

2. See Giustiniani 1981, 43–44.

3. Bissell (1981, 172) notes the resemblance of Abraham to Saint Jerome. "Reminiscent" is the term he rightly used.

4. See appendix 1, under October 21, 1612.

5. The interwoven forms of the composition recall the work of Carracciolo, and it is worth asking whether this picture does not reflect the *Sacrifice of Isaac* that Orazio frescoed on the vault of a loggia for Marc Antonio Doria at Sampierdarena. Carracciolo had also worked there and proposed evaluating Gentileschi's contribution. See p. 167 in this publication.

6. The picture was published in Longhi 1943, 22, as in a private collection in Milan. Bissell (1981, 151–52) initially confused it with the painting in Turin, but the differently placed book clearly distinguishes the two.

17.

Cleopatra

Oil on canvas, 46½ × 71¼ in.
(118 × 181 cm)

Amedeo Morandotti, Milan

ca. 1610–12

This extraordinary image, possessing an almost shocking effect of carnality, stands at the heart of our understanding of Orazio's art and that of his daughter, Artemisia. It has been ascribed to each. The earliest notice is in Ratti's 1780 guidebook to Genoa, where the picture is listed in the collection of Pietro Maria III Gentile together with three other paintings as the work of Orazio. One of these, a *Lucretia* (cat. 67), is certainly by Artemisia. The other two, a *Sacrifice of Isaac* (fig. 63) and a *Judith and Her Maidservant* (cat. 39), are just as certainly the work of Orazio and were probably either commissioned or purchased from the artist by Pietro Maria I Gentile about 1622–23, when Orazio was living in Genoa.[1] Morassi was the first to ascribe the Morandotti picture to Artemisia. He was followed by most scholars, including Harris, Nicolson, Gregori, Garrard, Mann, and Contini and Papi. Indeed, there is now a presumption in Artemisia's favor. In her 1989 book Garrard, for one, believed it unnecessary to argue her authorship at length, remarking simply that the attribution to Artemisia of the *Lucretia* and the *Cleopatra* "can be sustained on both stylistic and expressive grounds." She conjectured that Artemisia visited Genoa in 1621, en route from Florence to Rome. At that time she would have painted the *Lucretia*. The *Cleopatra*, with its references to Roman sculpture (for which, see below), would have been painted shortly after her arrival in Rome in 1622 and sent back to Genoa.

Quite apart from the fact that there is no documentary evidence that Artemisia ever visited Genoa, two objections must be made to the prevailing view espoused by Garrard. The first is that the *Lucretia* and the *Cleopatra* are painted in completely different and, to my mind, incompatible styles—the one hard and schematic, the other luminous and richly descriptive. The second is that the style of the *Cleopatra* has very little in common with that of other works by Artemisia datable to the 1620s (here, the pertinent comparison would be with the Detroit *Judith and Her Maidservant*; cat. 69). Nor does it much resemble her early Roman works (among which I am inclined to include the *Lucretia*).

In his 1999 book Bissell reconsiders his own, earlier attribution of the picture to Artemisia and argues that it is, instead, a work by Orazio dating to the years 1610–11. This view had already been expressed by Schleier and Volpe (Schleier informs me that he has not changed his mind). It is also my view—though, I hasten to point out, not that of my colleague Judith Mann, who sustains the ascription to Artemisia (cat. 53). It is true that initially the unidealized nude might seem uncharacteristic for Orazio, especially when we think of his later *Danaë* (cat. 36). Gregori contrasts the "expressive concentration" of the *Cleopatra* to Orazio's normally "impassive detachment." Yet we have only to recall the *Madonna and Child* in Bucharest (cat. 15) and the *Saint Jerome* in Turin (cat. 16) to find analogies for this unadorned approach to naturalistic painting. What seems to me to speak most convincingly in favor of Orazio's authorship is the handling of the white linen sheet and red drapery, which are painted with a subtlety and rich variation for which I can find no ready comparison in Artemisia's work at any phase. (It is the much drier, more formulaic handling of the drapery in the small *Danaë* at Saint Louis [cat. 54], the composition of which derives from the *Cleopatra*, that argues for Artemisia's having painted that picture as a personal interpolation of her father's work.)

Garrard has written, insightfully: "There is in the figure a curious disjunction between general pose and specific anatomy, as if the artist had begun with a type and wound up with an individual." This perfectly characterizes Orazio's critical position in the crucial years 1609 to 1612. As with the *David* (cat. 18), so here the intention was to treat in naturalistic terms an artfully posed figure. In this case, the pose derives from the celebrated ancient statue in the Vatican (fig. 141), which today we know represents Ariadne but that in

PROVENANCE: Pietro Maria I Gentile, Palazzo Gentile, Genoa (until 1640/41); Gentile collection, Genoa (1640/41–1811/18; inv. 1811, as by Orazio Gentileschi); Palazzo Durazzo-Adorno (now Cattaneo-Adorno), Genoa (perhaps by 1818 and certainly by 1846–1967);[10] Antichità Rubinacci, Genoa (1967); Alessandro Morandotti, Rome (by 1971); Amedeo Morandotti, Milan.

REFERENCES: Ratti 1780, vol. 1, 119–20, 122; Gandolfi 1846, vol. 3, 294; Morassi in Genoa 1947, 101–3; Bissell 1968, 156–57; Schleier 1971, 89; Torriti 1971, 200, 202; Volpe 1972, 68; Harris in Los Angeles 1976–77, 120; Greer 1979, 195; Nicolson 1979, 50; Bissell 1981, 202 no. X-7; Gregori in Naples 1984–85, vol. 1, 147; Grabski 1985, 58; Pizzorusso 1987, 70–71; Garrard 1989, 19–20, 54–56, 244–73, 276–77; Harris 1989, 10; Nicolson 1990, 110; Contini in Florence 1991, 128, 149, 162; Papi in Florence 1991, 48–49, 61 nn. 57 and 64, 153, 210; Stolzenwald 1991, 34; Cropper 1992, 209; Merkel 1992, 350–51, 353; Mann 1996, 40, 43; Bissell 1999, 306–10 no. X-6; Boccardo 2000, 205, 212; Garrard 2001, 11, 27, 132 n. 7.

the sixteenth and seventeenth centuries was widely celebrated as a depiction of the dying Cleopatra (her armlet—or armilla—is an entwined snake).[2] Interestingly, under Pope Paul V the setting for the statue was remodeled, the new installation being commemorated by an inscription in 1613. The statue is draped, but there was a strong tradition for showing Cleopatra nude, as she is here, thereby striking a note of erotic physicality.[3] (One wonders if Orazio took some inspiration from Rubens's *Susanna and the Elders* in the Galleria Borghese, Rome, which was probably owned by Scipione Borghese, possibly already Orazio's patron at this time, and which similarly combines a pose that derives from an ancient statue with a sensually rendered figure.) In an even more polemical way than the *David*, the *Cleopatra* reignites the Caravaggesque opposition of an art based on ancient models and an art based on real life: of ideal beauty versus naturalism, *bellezza ideale* versus *il vero*.

Far from subscribing to the notion of artistic selection, the picture is almost portraitlike—whence the duality noted by Garrard. A resemblance between the Cleopatra and a lute player on the vault of the Casino delle Muse has been noted, but the closest likeness is actually from another portion of the casino frescoes showing a woman holding a fan (frontispiece, p. 282). The model for that figure is usually identified as the young Artemisia, and although I have elsewhere stated my reasons for treating this identification with caution (see cat. 39), the possibility that Artemisia posed nude for her father must be addressed. That she did so was evidently rumored in Rome. In any case, on June 23, 1612, Marco Antonio Coppino, a dealer in pigments, testified at the rape trial that Orazio did not want Artemisia to marry and that when he needed to paint a nude he had her undress and pose for him.[4] On the face of it, this seems an incredible accusation, and the tendency has been to dismiss it as slander (Coppino certainly belonged to Tassi's faction). Such a practice did indeed risk spoiling any marriage arrangement. But as Bissell points out, although Coppino's testimony cannot be accepted as fact, "it does hint"— I would say imply—"that the use of female nudes in male painters' Roman studios was not out of the question."[5] (That female models were employed by

artists has actually been denied by a number of modern scholars.)

In 1615 Niccolò Tassi, a neighbor and friend of Orazio's, wrote to Galileo describing, in a poem, a picture of Cleopatra that the artist had recently sent to Grand Duke Cosimo II de' Medici in Florence. Tassi's poem celebrating the picture makes the conventional points of Orazio's art bringing Cleopatra back to life and of beauty confronting death. As one might expect, the correspondence with the Morandotti painting is not clear; in fact, the asp is not shown biting Cleopatra's breast, as it was in the painting described by Tassi. But allowance must be made for literary license; at the very least, Tassi must have been referring to a variant of the composition. As both Pizzorusso and Bissell point out, the picture Tassi saw evidently never arrived in Florence (if it was ever sent). Or why, two months later, would Cosimo II's secretary, Andrea Cioli, inquire of the Tuscan ambassador in Rome about Gentileschi's abilities?

The following scenario seems possible. About 1610–12, Orazio painted a *Cleopatra*. It remained in his workshop, unsold. In 1615, he had his friend Tassi contact Galileo to announce its imminent presentation as a gift to Cosimo II as part of a move to secure a position at the Medici court (Artemisia was already well established in Florence). The effort backfired when the Tuscan ambassador in Rome, Pietro Guicciardini, sent to Florence a withering assessment of Gentileschi's abilities. The painting was eventually purchased by the Genoese patrician Pietro Gentile, together with a *Lucretia* by Artemisia.[6] What remains very much an open question is how Gentile came by the pictures. Was it through an agent in Rome? Or did Orazio conceivably take the picture with him when he moved to Genoa? No less significant is the matter of whether the pictures by Orazio and Artemisia in Gentile's collection were purchased to form part of an iconographic group of heroines. In 1638 Gentile also acquired, from Reni, a *Judith* (fig. 75), but in the 1811 inventory of the collection there is no indication of any particular focus or of a scheme for hanging the works beyond that of size. Gentile's motivations thus seem less programmatic than those of his compatriot Giovan Antonio Sauli (see pp. 172–73).

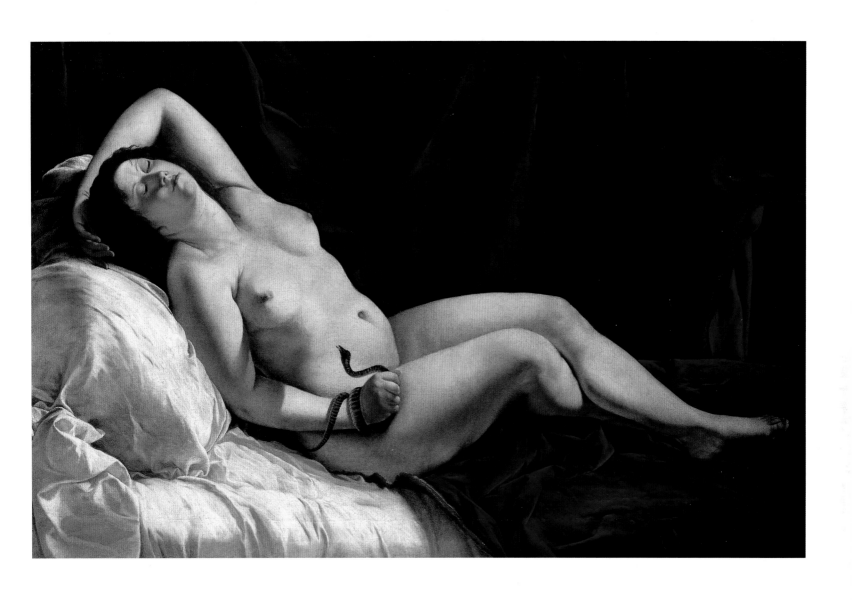

The visual and iconographic traditions that lie behind the *Cleopatra* have been well investigated by Brummer in his study of the Vatican statue that provided the compositional source.[7] His study, in turn, was the point of departure for Garrard's gendered reading of the picture. Garrard concludes with the following encapsulation of a complex argument: "The legendary, glamorous Cleopatra is seen as a homely young woman, a privileged mystic glimpse that we are given just as she reverts through apotheosis—theophany in reverse—to her fundamental and eternal identity as the goddess Isis."[8] My own feeling is that Orazio's painting is innocent of such erudite allusions. Rather, it takes its place in a long tradition of female nudes cast in mythological-historical guise (the most famous being Titian's *Danaë*, then in the Farnese collection). Its flagrant naturalism—perhaps matched only by that of Juseppe de Ribera's *Drunken Silenus* (Capodimonte, Naples), of 1626—was intended both as an artistic statement and as an erotic attraction. Tassi seems to have understood this. Addressing the figure of Cleopatra directly in his poem, he writes, "Happy is your lot. . . . You will bask in the gaze of the grand duke."[9]

The picture suffers from flattening during relining and from serious abrasion, especially in the body of the figure. The face and right hand are in reasonably good condition, as is the red drapery. The transparency of the shadows in the pillow and the variation of grays in the leg give the clearest indication of the quality (and authorship) of the picture. The snake is abraded and much repainted. At the time of its restoration, about 1975 (additional work was carried out for the exhibition), an added strip of canvas 27 centimeters wide was removed from the top of the composition. Bissell floats the possibility that this piece, perhaps folded over at one time, was original. He brings in as supporting evidence the relation of figure to picture field in the *Lucretia*, which, however, has also been enlarged (see cat. 67). Not only was the strip removed from the *Cleopatra* demonstrably added, so also, it would seem, was another strip attached to the top edge; the cusping along the top and bottom edges of the original canvas is clearly visible on the surface of the painting, which has perhaps been trimmed along the vertical edges. As noted by Boccardo, all the Gentileschis in the Gentile collection had their dimensions altered.

1. On Gentile, see Boccardo 2000.
2. See Brummer 1970, 154–84; and Haskell and Penny 1981, 184–87.
3. See Brummer 1970, 173–84. Garrard (1989, 247–59) has followed up on Brummer's analysis of the fluid traditions for showing Cleopatra, nymphs, and Venus.
4. Quoted by Lapierre 1998, 437. See appendix 1, under June 23, 1612.
5. Bissell 1999, 6.
6. Boccardo (2000, 206) raises the possibility that Gentile purchased the painting(s) by Artemisia from the duke of Alcalá, who is known to have admired Artemisia's work. However, the pictures in question are not listed in Alcalá's inventory.
7. Brummer 1970.
8. Garrard 1989, 272.
9. Bissell (1989, 309) gives a full transcription and translation of Tassi's poem.
10. The 1811 inventory of the Gentile collection was prepared with a view to its sale, and an anonymous guidebook of 1818 states that it had, indeed, been dispersed by that date. Gandolfi lists the *Cleopatra* in the Adorno collection in 1846; see Boccardo 2000, 209.

18.

David Contemplating the Head of Goliath

Oil on canvas, 68⅛ × 55⅞ in.
(173 × 142 cm)

Galleria Spada, Rome (inv. 155)

1610–12

New York

Following a tradition going back to Michelangelo, in his picture in Dublin (cat. 12) Orazio depicted David standing over the Philistine giant, cutting off his head, as related in 1 Samuel 17:50–51. Here, by contrast, the youth—older, more muscular, and wearing a shepherd's sheepskin rather than a jerkin—is shown after having completed the deed. Resting his foot on a stony outcrop, David contemplates Goliath's head lying tilted backward at his feet. In his left hand he holds the stone with which he felled the giant, while with the right he grasps a sword, emphasizing the humble means of his victory and the weapon the giant had wielded against him. David's victory was interpreted as a metaphor of virtue—an *exemplum virtutis*—and the picture has been conceived as a cue to a series of set responses: the physical beauty/goodness of the youth (described in the Bible as a handsome lad with ruddy cheeks and bright eyes) in victory over the ugliness/vanity/evil of Goliath, pride brought low by righteousness, and so forth. But beyond touching on these conventional moral contrasts, Gentileschi has endowed the picture with a psychological dimension that is less easy to specify, since David's pose is linked to no narrative or dramatic action.

Of Caravaggio's three depictions of David and Goliath—in the Prado, Madrid, the Galleria Borghese, Rome, and the Kunsthistorisches Museum, Vienna—Orazio's is closest in thematic moment to the Madrid painting (fig. 48), in which a prepubescent youth is shown quietly kneeling on the giant's corpse intently tying a string to his victim's hair so as to carry the head in triumphal procession.[1] Yet Caravaggio's depiction has a disturbing quality completely lacking in Orazio's. Goliath's fist is clenched and his open eyes stare wearily out at the viewer. Brute force humbled by innocence seems to be the moral thrust, and, as is usually the case with Caravaggio, the impression is of an arrested moment in time rather than of the transcription of a posed figure.

Orazio's primary source of inspiration was doubtless Guido Reni's splendid picture in the Louvre showing a teenage David leaning against a column as he contemplates his trophy, set atop a stone plinth (fig. 49). Yet any comparison between the two pictures underscores the degree to which Orazio has conceived his picture as a critical response—not an homage—to Reni's image, something that is even more evident in the full-length, reduced version in Berlin (cat. 19). Orazio's David is not the "nonchalant, haughty hero"[2] of Reni's canvas, well coiffed and sporting an elegant, feathered cap, his fur-lined cloak draped over the broken column (a parody of the dandy that appears in so many of Caravaggio's early paintings). To be sure, Orazio's hero is self-consciously posed, though not in emulation of an ancient statue of a faun. Instead, he is a youth from the neighborhood who has been provided with props and has assumed an artful pose in the studio; the giant's head—behind rather than alongside the youth—reads very much as an afterthought (an awkwardness corrected in the reduced replica). As with most Caravaggesque artists, Orazio emphasizes his use of a working-class model by painting the sun-colored neck and hands. The effect is surprisingly close to that of a nineteenth-century academy picture.

Orazio's point of departure for the Dublin *David* (cat. 12) had also been a work by Reni, but in the intervening years Reni's art had moved toward greater idealization. In the Dublin picture, Orazio had emulated the Bolognese's emphasis on *bellezza* and *maniera* within a Caravaggesque idiom. Here, the image is conceived in terms of *naturalezza* and *verità*. In effect, he has reopened Caravaggio's polemic with the classical aesthetics formulated by the art theorist Giovanni Battista Agucchi (1570–1632) and practiced by Domenichino. We have it from Carlo Cesare Malvasia that Caravaggio had threatened Reni for "stealing" his style. Orazio, having been momentarily attracted by Reni's bowdlerized Caravaggism, now distances himself by stressing the basis of his art in nature. It is a critical position Orazio staked out in more extreme terms in the Bucharest *Madonna and Child* (cat. 15), of 1609, and in the Turin *Saint Jerome* (cat. 16), of 1610–11, and there can be no doubt that the Spada *David* belongs to the same phase of his career. Where it differs from the Bucharest and Turin paintings is in the attempt to transpose Caravaggio's focused "cellar lighting" into a sunlit, outdoor setting. The result is not completely successful—the figure is still detached from the background—but in this work are the germs for the series of masterpieces Gentileschi was to produce over the course of the next decade. It need hardly be said that Artemisia's *Susanna and the Elders* (cat. 51), dated 1610, reflects these same critical issues and demonstrates the closeness of father and daughter at the moment of her artistic debut.

Ever since Longhi's groundbreaking article of 1916, the Spada *David* has occupied a central place in Gentileschi studies. Noting the unusual character of the landscape compared with those in other paintings

by Orazio, Longhi proposed that the work represented a collaboration between Orazio and Agostino Tassi, who returned to Rome in 1610 and of course worked with Orazio on the frescoes in Scipione Borghese's Casino delle Muse in 1611–12 (fig. 6). Since that time, various opinions have been voiced for and against the idea of a collaboration (significantly, neither Pugliatti nor Cavazzini, the leading experts on Tassi, accepts the attribution), but there has been almost universal consensus that the *David* dates to about 1610–11. Recently, however, Papi (in Salonika 1997) has rekindled Gamba's idea that this is a later work. He has moved the date of the picture to the end of the 1610s and raised the possibility of a collaboration with Giovanni Lanfranco. Both the date and the idea of a collaboration with Lanfranco depend on a comparison with Orazio's *Saint Cecilia* in Washington (cat. 31), which was apparently left unfinished when he went to Genoa, and was completed by Lanfranco. To my mind, the comparison is not very convincing. The *David* is unlikely to be later than about 1612. As to the notion of some sort of collaboration, I find it possible to convince myself both for and against it. I wonder if this is not a case in which an idea—here, ingeniously planted by Longhi—has not gathered a spurious art-historical credibility simply by being repeated. True enough, the landscape is not characteristic of Orazio's later work, but it is not incompatible with that of the earlier Dublin *David*, and, as pointed out by Schleier, the sky is typical of the artist. More important, it is one of Orazio's first attempts at a convincing outdoor setting, and perhaps we ought not to insist on the refined mastery of his later works.

Related to the issue of collaboration is the idea that the picture began as a smaller composition and was subsequently enlarged by Gentileschi to its present dimensions.[3] The origin of this conjecture is closely linked to the physical makeup of the canvas support, now put on firm footing thanks to X radiographs and infrared reflectography published by Lapucci. As it has come down to us, there is a large central section made up of two pieces of herringbone-weave canvas joined vertically, one having a tighter weave than the other. On all sides, strips of a plain-weave canvas have been stitched to the central section. Each piece was

PROVENANCE: Alessandro Biffi, Rome (until 1637; 1637 list of paintings, as by Orazio Gentileschi); Giovan Battista Veralli, Rome (1637–41); Maria Veralli Spada, Rome (by 1641/43–86); her husband, Orazio Spada, Palazzo Spada (1686–87); Spada collection, Rome (from 1687; inv. 1759, as by Poussin; Fidecommisso 1862, as by Caravaggio); Galleria Spada, Rome.

RELATED PICTURE: Di Castro, Rome (copy, without landscape, listed by Nicolson 1990); see cat. 19.

REFERENCES: Roisecco 1765, vol. 1, 627; Venturi 1910, 268–71; Voss 1911, 250–53; Longhi (1916) 1961, 236–37, 257, 278; Gamba 1922–23, 256; Voss 1925, 459–60; Longhi 1927, 112, 114; Drost 1933, 78–79; Buscaroli 1935, 328; Zeri 1954, 86–87 no. 175; Emiliani 1958b, 42; Waddingham 1961, 23 n. 13; Schleier 1962, 435; Moir 1967, vol. 1, 70–71, 76 n. 27, vol. 2, 75 no. B.2a; Rome 1968, 12–13 no. 7; Pepper 1971, 337; Pugliatti 1977, 10; Nicolson 1979, 52; Bissell 1981, 23–24, 26–27, 73, 146, 148–49 no. 18, 172, 206, 208; Schleier in New York–Naples 1985, 152–55; Nicolson 1990, 113; Vicini in Cannatà and Vicini 1992, 94, 103; Papi and Lapucci in Salonika 1997, 192–99, 199–201; Bissell 1999, 191, 195; Cavazzini, written opinion, 2000; Vicini 2000, 15–17; London–Rome 2001, 281.

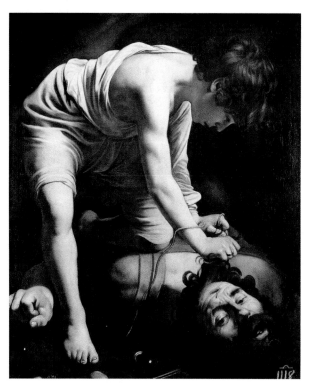

Figure 48. Michelangelo Merisi da Caravaggio (1571–1610), *David and Goliath*. Oil on canvas. Museo Nacional del Prado, Madrid

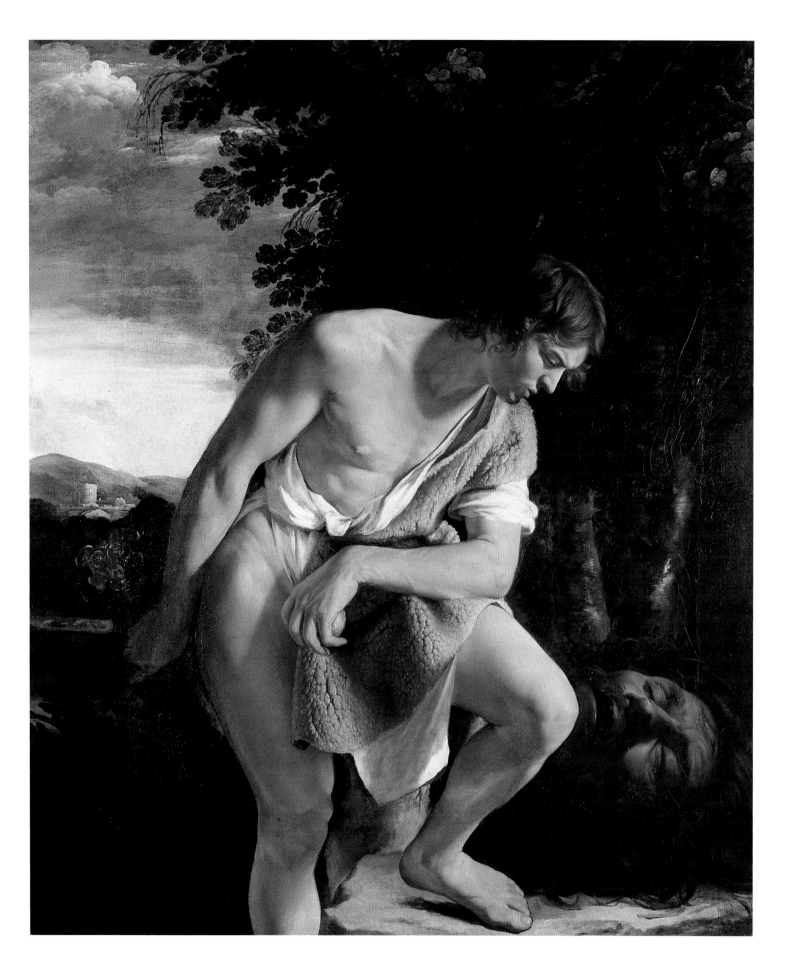

pregrounded—a procedure that is found in other works by Orazio (see cat. nos. 5, 28, 31, 39)—and a further, unifying ground was then applied, with particular care taken to mask the seams. It is the variety of canvases and preparations that is largely responsible for the different textures of the paint surface, but the picture was also damaged by heat during a radical treatment in the past. The X rays and infrared reflectography demonstrate that the paint film is continuous. It is possible that various areas, such as the torso, legs, and arms of David, were reworked, but by the same token, there are no major compositional changes. Indeed, the legs, arms, and head were painted in areas held in reserve (the pale, warm brown preparatory layer is particularly visible around the foot). The picture has been strongly cleaned, and certain passages—most notably the right hand holding the sword—have suffered. What cannot be determined is whether the picture was cut along the bottom— that is, that it may have shown David full length. All we can say with certainty is that its present dimensions are already recorded in 1758. On the basis of this analysis, I think we can rule out the possibility that Orazio conceived the picture as no larger than the central canvas and subsequently enlarged it.

Thanks to the archival work of Vicini, we now know that the first owner was Alessandro Biffi. In addition to the Gentileschi, four paintings by Artemisia (see cat. nos. 51, 57) and a work ascribed to Bartolomeo Manfredi were in his collection. The picture passed to the Veralli when Biffi was unable to meet the payment of a debt, and thence, by marriage, it became part of the Spada collection. Whether, as has been suggested, the "David trimphant over Goliath" seen by Ratti in 1780, in the Palazzo Cambiaso in Genoa, was a replica or a variant of this picture is pure conjecture; it seems more likely that it was an unrelated composition (see also cat. 12).[4]

1. The Prado picture has a complex critical history, and its attribution to Caravaggio is not universally accepted, though I consider his authorship unproblematic and would date it to about 1600–1602; see Gregori's fine analysis in New York–Naples 1985, 268–70. Bissell (1981, 206) very tentatively suggests Orazio as the possible author. Marini (in Gregori 1996, 135–39) published X radiographs that leave the status of the Prado picture as the prime version in no doubt: Goliath's head was originally shown as though screaming.
2. Spear 1997, 285.
3. Schleier (in New York–Naples 1985, 154) gives the most cogent analysis of this hypothesis.
4. Gamba (1922–23, 256) raised the possibility of identifying the Spada *David* with the Cambiaso painting. See also Bissell 1981, 149.

19.

David Contemplating the Head of Goliath

Oil on copper, 14 ½ × 11 ¼ in.
(36.7 × 28.7 cm)

Staatliche Museen
Preussischer Kulturbesitz,
Gemäldegalerie, Berlin (1723)

ca. 1611–12

New York, Saint Louis

PROVENANCE: Acquired by
the Kaiser Friedrich Museum,
Berlin, in 1914; Staatliche
Museen Preussischer
Kulturbesitz, Gemäldegalerie,
Berlin.

RELATED PICTURES: Private
collection, Berlin (contempo-
rary copy);[2] Herzog Anton
Ulrich-Museum,
Braunschweig (later copy);
Galleria dell' Arcivescovado,
Milan (copy with variations);[3]
see also cat. 18.

REFERENCES: Voss 1925, 459–
60; Longhi 1927, 112, 114; Drost
1933, 79; Longhi 1943, 22; Moir
1967, vol. 1, 70 n. 6, 76 n. 27,
vol. 2, 75 no. A.2b; Berlin 1975,
174 no. 1723; Nicolson 1979, 52;
Bissell 1981, 23–25, 149–50
no. 19, 172, 208; Schleier in
New York–Naples 1985,
152–55; Nicolson 1990, 113.

The history of this picture prior to 1914, when it was acquired by the Kaiser Friedrich Museum as a work by the German painter Adam Elsheimer, is not known (Voss was the first to ascribe it to Gentileschi). However, to judge from the three sur- viving copies, it enjoyed some fame. The painting— full length, as in Reni's depiction (fig. 49)—originated as a reduced variant of the picture in the Galleria Spada (cat. 18): sunnier, more exquisite, and with a land- scape that in its quality of atmosphere looks ahead to Orazio's later work. As Longhi (1927) states, the point of inspiration for this new landscape vision was the example of Elsheimer, who died in Rome in 1610. To this degree the old attribution of the picture to the German artist is understandable. Like so many of his contemporaries—Northerners as well as Italians—

Orazio was captivated by Elsheimer's miraculous small paintings and evidently adapted one of the artist's most celebrated compositions, a *Tobias and the Angel* (fig. 58), to a nighttime setting, showing the angel holding a torch.[1] Was it his association with Tassi, whose specialty was landscape painting and *quad- ratura*, that inspired Orazio's deepened appreciation of the work of Elsheimer? We know that in 1612, dur- ing the rape trial, Tassi wrote from prison to recom- mend Elsheimer's work to the Medici court in Florence, praising it as "the most rare thing in all the world." The parallel interests of Carlo Saraceni—another member of the Tassi–Gentileschi circle—should also be taken into account. (At the trial, Saraceni declared that he had known Orazio for eight to ten years, though they had not seen each other for the last two.) It is, then, the example of Elsheimer that enabled Orazio to reconceive the Spada canvas, using a rocky cliff bathed in light as a foil for the figure and opening up the left side to a convincing landscape view—one completely at odds in its naturalistic effect with the idealized land- scapes of Annibale Carracci and his pupils Francesco Albani and Domenichino. The shadows have not yet attained the transparency or the light the verity found in the exquisite *Saint Christopher* (cat. 27), and the cliff still has some of the character of a stage-flat silhou- ette, but the achievement is remarkable.

By comparison with the large canvas, there are a number of further compositional refinements. The ledge on which David's foot rests is lower, so that the foreshortening of the leg is less accentuated and Goliath's head can be placed differently and more convincingly. By having the head face downward, Orazio has also made the painting psychologically less disturbing and more reflective in mood; no longer do the two foes face each other. In all these ways, the Berlin picture improves on the larger canvas and fore- casts the new direction in Orazio's work, one empha- sizing formal clarity, a more refined sense of color and atmospheric unity, and delicacy of touch.

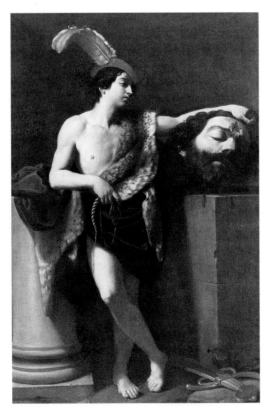

Figure 49. Guido Reni (1575–1642), *David with the Head of Goliath*. Oil on canvas. Musée du Louvre, Paris

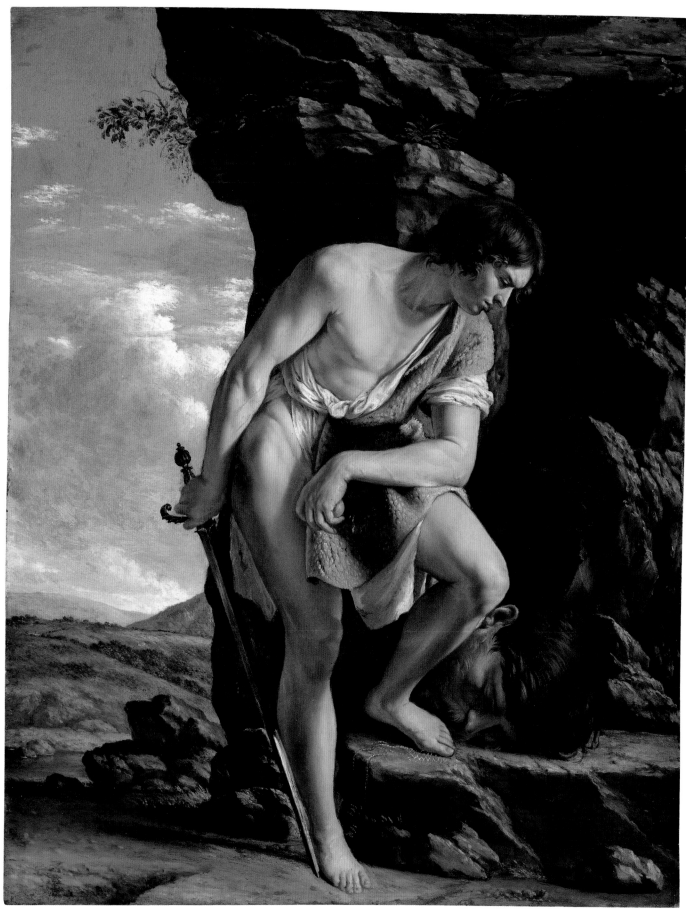

19

1. The picture is listed in a 1631 inventory of the Savelli collection as "Una tobia del Gentileschi in rame con cornice d'ebbano," and reappears in a 1692 Chigi inventory as "un Quadro in rame alto 2 [44.8 cm] e 1½ [33.53 cm], cornice d'ebano, con due figurine, una d'un Angelo, con una Torcia accesa in mano, con Paese, mano del Gentileschi." See Spezzaferro 1985, 72–73; and the Getty Provenance Index. Bissell (1981, 142, 221 no. L-62) identifies the subject of the Chigi picture as *Saint Francis's Vision of the Flaming Torch*, believing it a pendant to a *Christ Blessing Saint Francis* (formerly Marchese Incisa della Rocchetta) that is ascribed in the

inventory to Orazio Borgianni. The Chigi evidently purchased another Savelli picture, the *Christ Crowned with Thorns* (cat. 23). It is worth mentioning that by 1661 the Chigi had acquired the Savelli's estates at Ariccia.
2. See Schleier in New York–Naples 1985, 154.
3. For this picture, see Bissell 1981, 150, and Schleier in New York–Naples 1985, 154. The head of Goliath is differently placed, and there is no landscape background. Interestingly enough, it is paired with a reduced copy of Artemisia's *Judith and Holofernes* at Capodimonte.

20.

Executioner with the Head of Saint John the Baptist

Oil on panel, transferred to canvas, 32¼ × 24 in. (82 × 61 cm)

Signed (on the blade of the sword): HOR.S LOMI

Museo Nacional del Prado, Madrid

ca. 1612–13

PROVENANCE: Possibly Marchese Clemente and Cardinal Giacomo Sannesi (until 1621); by descent, Anna Maria Sannesi (until 1724; inv. as "David with the Head by Orazio Gentileschi"); Don Francisco Garcia Chico, Madrid (by 1849); Museo Nacional del Prado, Madrid (from 1969).

REFERENCES: Milicua 1970, 7; Schleier 1970b, 342; Bissell 1971, 294 n. 11; Madrid 1972, 871 no. 3188; Previtali 1973, 360 n. 17; Nicolson 1979, 53; Bissell 1981, 150–51 no. 20; Nicolson 1990, 115.

Surely one of Gentileschi's most arresting inventions, this picture can be traced with certainty only back to the early nineteenth century. There is, nonetheless, a possibility that it was acquired from Orazio by the Marchese Clemente Sannesi and his brother Cardinal Giacomo, as a painting of David with the head of Goliath, on panel and measuring 3½ × 3 *palmi* (78 × 67 cm), is listed in the 1724 postmortem inventory of their last heir, Anna Maria Sannesi.[1] This implies a misidentification of the subject, but so unusual is the interpretation that a misreading is not unlikely. A miniature copy is in the Academia de San Fernando, Madrid, the gift of Juan Montenegro (d. 1869), who became a member on May 8, 1827. At that time the Prado picture was still on its original panel—a support Orazio seldom used but that was conducive to delicacy and surface refinement (see cat. 8). An inscription on the reverse records both its transfer to canvas in 1849 and the owner at the time, Don Francisco Garcia Chico.[2] Within a year of its acquisition by the Prado, in 1969, the picture was published by Milicua and Schleier. The first expressed reservations about its ascription to Orazio, while the second was unsure whether it dated from the 1590s or the time of the Casino delle Muse frescoes (that is, 1612). Bissell, who knew the picture only from photographs,

also had doubts about the attribution and suggested that the signature was "redone by a restorer." It is hardly surprising, then, that this splendid work, so rich in descriptive detail and handling of light, has not received the attention it deserves. Although it has sustained some damage (there are repaints in the right cheek, in the jerkin and pink waistband, and in the sleeve), the quality is of the highest order. The emphasis on details such as the lips and teeth or the fleecy hat, the reflection of the cut neck on the executioner's sword blade, and the light playing through the lace holes of the leather jerkin fully explain why Orazio chose a panel support. The handling of light and the blonde tonality suggest a date around 1612—at the time of the casino frescoes.

Orazio's point of departure for this work was unquestionably Caravaggio's *David with the Head of Goliath* (Galleria Borghese, Rome), in which the young hero displays the head of the Philistine giant to the viewer. Caravaggio's novel composition was widely imitated, but never was it so singularly adapted, for the Prado picture shows not the Old Testament victor but a New Testament martyr. (It is unthinkable that David would be shown as this unkempt, uncouth youth, or that the giant's head would be depicted so small.) There are a number of sixteenth-century

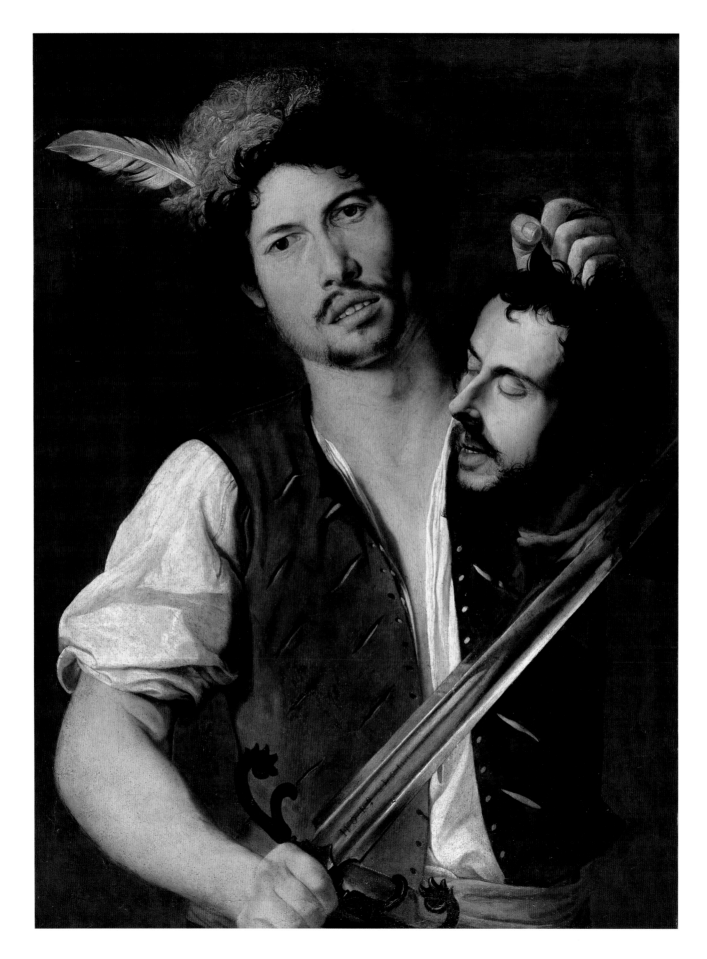

paintings—mostly Lombard—in which the story of the presentation of the head of John the Baptist to Salome is treated in abbreviated form by showing the executioner's hand suspending the head over a charger held by the young woman. In them, the head is displayed less as a trophy than as a relic, and the imagery is likely to be related to the cult of Saint John. But when the theme was again taken up in early-seventeenth-century Rome, it was for the dramatic, narrative possibilities the subject offered.[3] In none of these pictures, however, does the viewer assume the position of Salome being presented with the grisly reward for her fabled dance before King Herod, whose marriage to Salome's mother John the Baptist had condemned (Matt. 14:3–11). By adapting a composition associated with David and Goliath to John the Baptist, Orazio has shifted the role of the protagonist, who is now the victim rather than the victor, and introduced a new psychological dynamic. To anyone who thinks of Gentileschi as a painter lacking in expressive vigor, this painting stands as an eloquent refutation. Typically, however, the artist unsettles not through dramatic presentation but through descriptive analysis.

The characterization of the executioner could scarcely be more biting; he seems culled from the police records of seventeenth-century Rome and reminds one as well of the descriptions we have of one of Orazio's models, Francesco Scarpellino, whom a witness at the rape trial described as "an ugly type with long black hair whom they said they used as a model for some paintings on occasion." In his celebrated *David and Goliath* (Louvre, Paris; fig. 49), Guido Reni had shown David as a dandy, sporting a cap with a feather in it, thereby making a clever play on Caravaggesque realism. Orazio too uses a feathered cap, but in order to return Caravaggio's realism to the life of the streets

and the public executions held in the Campo dei Fiori.[4] Where Orazio departs from Caravaggio is in the relatively bright palette, the emphasis on descriptive detail, and the portraitlike quality of the youth.

Perhaps the most disturbing quality in the picture results from the way the executioner gazes directly at the viewer, untroubled by the object he holds. This is completely contrary to Orazio's usual preference for psychologically neutral, or at least nonaggressive, images. The approach is all the more notable when we recall that in Caravaggio's *David and Goliath,* the youthful hero contemplates his victim with an expression bordering on remorse. Orazio's idea seems to have grown out of his illusionistic frescoes in the Casino delle Muse, in which the figures look out at the viewer from behind a feigned balcony. But here the effect is startling and unexpected and underscores the degree to which the years 1609–12 define an experimental watershed for Orazio. Without his work at this moment, Artemisia's paintings would be unthinkable. The remarkable thing is that this should have happened to an artist when he was well into his forties.

1. Archivio di Stato di Roma, 39 notai Capitolini Joseph Paulinus Officio 13, vol. 502, fol. 259: "Altro quadro in tavola di pmi tre, e mezzo, e tre, con cornice nera filettata d'oro rappresentante David con testa in mano opera del Gentileschi." I owe this reference to Erich Schleier.

2. "Perteneciendo esta pintura a la selecta galeria del. Sr. D. Fran.co Garcia Chico, fué trasportada de tabla a lienzo en el mes de Nob.bre de 1849, por el laborioso primer forrador de Pinturas de S. M. en el Rl Museo D. Antonio Trillo; Habiendo sabido vencer las muchísimas dificultades que ofrecía esta arriesgadísima operación (por el estado en que se encontraba la tabla) en el corto espacio de veinte y dos dias." My thanks to Andrés Ubeda de los Cobos for kindly furnishing me with this information.

3. See, for example, the two pictures by Antiveduto Gramatica, one approximately contemporary with Orazio's painting, published by Papi 1995, nos. 6, 38.

4. Varriano (1999, 321–23, 327–28) has discussed the intersection between public executions and Caravaggio's imagery.

21.

Saint Francis with an Angel

Oil on canvas, 52⅜ × 38⅝ in. (133 × 98 cm)

Inscribed (lower right): ORATE PRO R.D. HORATIO GRIFFIO / HVIVS ORATORII ET CELLAE / FVNDATORE

Galleria Nazionale d'Arte Antica, Palazzo Barberini, Rome (inv. 1276)

ca. 1612

PROVENANCE: Orazio Griffio, Rome (until 1624?); Oratorio della Confraternità di San Girolamo della Carità, Rome; possibly Camillo del Palaggio, Rome (after 1631?);[6] Clelia del Palaggio, Rome (by 1703?);[7] Monte di Pietà, Rome (by 1857–1895; 1875 catalogue, no. 419, as school of the Caracci); Galleria Nazionale, Palazzo Corsini, Rome (from 1895); Galleria Nazionale d'Arte Antica, Palazzo Barberini, Rome.

REFERENCES: Longhi (1916) 1961, 226, 277; Venturi 1921, 152 no. 949; Gamba 1922–23, 246; Voss 1925, 461; Rome 1955, 12–13 no. 15; Faldi 1956, 5–7; Pérez Sánchez 1965, 504; Moir 1967, vol. 1, 29, 38 n. 67; Askew 1969, 295; Schleier 1970b, 342; Bissell 1971, 284–86; Röttgen in Rome 1973, 101; Moir 1976, 122 n. 180iii; Nicolson 1979, 53; Bissell 1981, 14–17, 19, 84 n. 23, 140–41 no. 8, 144; Mochi Onori and Vodret Adamo 1989, 76; Nicolson 1990, 115; Vodret in Hartford 1998, 71–74.

Of Orazio's four surviving depictions of Saint Francis succored by an angel (see cat. nos. 2, 3, 6), this one is in many ways the most sophisticated, eloquent in its formal language and meditative as a prayer. Particularly affective is the Bellini-like contrast between the touching, feminine-featured angel and the rustic saint, his flesh drained of color, who has collapsed to one side after having received the stigmata. (The similarity to a Pietà is obvious and underscores the mystical likeness of Francis to Christ, explored by Saint Francis of Sales, in his *Traité de l'amour de Dieu* of 1616.)[1] As in Orazio's picture in the Prado (cat. 6), so here the saint displays his left hand to the viewer for contemplation, but with a newfound elegance in the arrangement of the fingers and the play of the light over them. The wound is depicted as a nail piercing the saint's hand—as described in early Franciscan sources such as Saint Bonaventure's *Legenda maior* and the *Fioretti*: "And thus his hands and feet seemed nailed through the middle with nails, the heads whereof were in the palms of his hands . . . and the points emerged through the back."

One need only compare the beautiful contrapposto arrangement of the saint's legs or the sculptural folds in the sleeve of his habit to the same passages in the picture in the Prado to appreciate the increased effect of structural clarity, as though the figures had been conceived from the inside out. Orazio's keen sensitivity to texture and surface—the tailor's mastery of stuffs[2]— is not diminished (the worn edge of the saint's cowl is like a eulogy on poverty). But the use of dense shadows to create an impression of palpable physicality has been replaced by a new transparency. The light has a crystalline luminosity that works to define the forms and to suggest an ambient space. (This aspect has been much enhanced by the cleaning carried out in 1997.)

The picture can be seen both as the culmination of the period 1609–12, when Orazio worked primarily from the posed model, and as a new departure. As in those works (cat. nos. 15–20), so here he has hit upon a quasi-sculptural solution to the compositional challenge he faced—without, however, imitating a specific prototype. At the same time, in the picture Orazio has moved beyond the almost emphatic naturalism of the *Madonna and Child* in Bucharest (cat. 15) and the *Saint Jerome* in Turin (cat. 16) to strike a greater balance between the actuality of the posed model and an artistic idea. Although indebted to a work such as Caravaggio's *Saint Francis* (versions in the church of the Cappuccini, Rome, and in San Pietro, Carpineto Romano),[3] Orazio here employs his own personal amalgam of late-sixteenth-century formal concerns and Caravaggesque pictorial techniques. In his immediately preceding pictures, he asserts the verity of actual experience. In the *Saint Francis* he seems to abstract that experience, as though reconstructing a visual memory, whence the enhanced meditational mood.

Until recently, the painting was almost universally dated to the first years of the seventeenth century and considered somewhat earlier than the version in the Prado.[4] As has been repeatedly noted in this catalogue, our understanding of the first decade of Orazio's career has been transformed through a number of recent documentary discoveries. If, on the one hand, the Prado picture can now be dated with greater precision to about 1607—that is, contemporary with the *Circumcision* in Ancona (fig. 7)—as Vodret has shown, the painting in Rome (surely the later of the two) should be seen in relation to the man whose name is recorded in the inscription and the oratory he founded. The inscription reads: "Pray for Orazio Griffio, priest of God, and founder of this oratory and chapel."

Born in 1566, Griffio entered the papal chapel in 1591 and was ordained a priest in 1594. His interest in ecclesiastical music is documented through his association with the Congregazione dei Virtuosi di Roma (the nucleus of the future Accademia di Santa Cecilia) and with the papal choir, whose statutes he proposed reforming. Griffio's closest connection, however, was

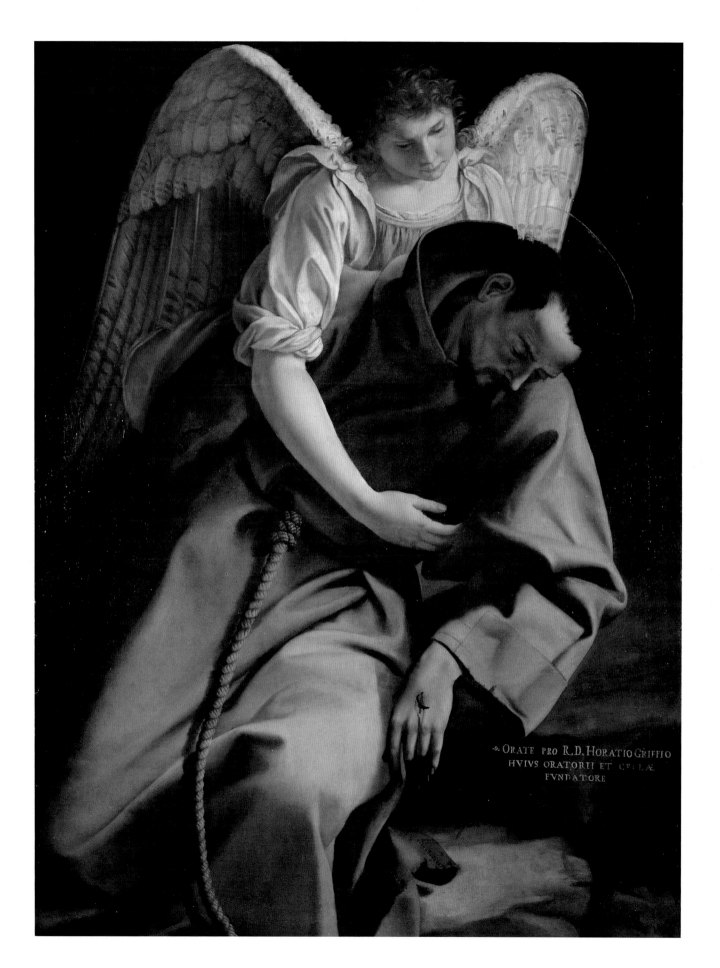

In the painting, the inscription reads:

ORATE PRO R.D. HORATIO GRIFFIO
HVIVS ORATORII ET CELLÆ
FVNDATORE

with the Confraterinty of San Girolamo della Carità, where Phillip Neri had founded his first oratory and lived for thirty-three years, from 1551 to 1583.[5] Griffio joined the Confraternity of San Girolamo in 1609 and was buried in the church in 1624. In 1610, he was nominated deputy of the congregation and in 1614 named superintendent of the new oratory built in 1612 adjacent to San Girolamo. In all likelihood, it is as founder of this oratory that Griffio is recorded in the inscription. The wording suggests that the picture hung in the oratory itself, which was badly damaged by fire in 1631 and had to be completely rebuilt (Francesco Barberini provided the lion's share of the funds). However, there is no mention of the picture in either the oratory or the church (one might have thought that Baglione would have cited it, since he mentions other works in the church). Griffio may well have commissioned the painting for himself and bequeathed it to the confraternity, which may have added the dedicatory inscription and installed it in the sacristy or in another, less public, ambient. Vodret has documented a strong personal attachment to Saint Francis by Griffio's uncles and cousin, but the congregation had historic associations with the Franciscan order (in 1524, under Clement VII, the buildings had been ceded to the confraternity by the Friars Minor).

Vodret has dated the picture to 1612–14, relating its commission to the building of the oratory. There are, indeed, close affinities between the luminous effect of the musicians in the frescoes of the Casino delle Muse, on which Orazio was working in 1611–12 (fig. 6) and the treatment of the angel, and a dating to about 1612 seems convincing on grounds of style.

Through the papal choir and the Confraternity of San Girolamo, Griffio knew Cardinals Francesco Maria del Monte and Pietro Aldobrandini. Del Monte was a major patron of Caravaggio's, and it is tempting to associate Griffio's choice of Orazio with this friendship (Del Monte sponsored a Mass in Griffio's memory)—except that Del Monte owned none of Orazio's works. Aldobrandini had commissioned a cycle of frescoes from Orazio for San Nicola in Carcere (1599–1600) and also had his portrait painted by him. In 1614, shortly after the installation of Domenichino's great altarpiece in San Girolamo, he is known to have attended the Feast of Saint Jerome at the church. There is also the fact that the Arciconfraternità was closely linked by duties and funding with the criminal courts, including the Corte Savella, where Artemisia's rape trial had been prosecuted in 1612. Perhaps we ought also to note that Griffio's family was from Varese, in Lombardy. Is there some connection between his commission to Orazio and to Settimio Olgiati, whose family hailed from Como and who continued to maintain an interest in the artist in the years 1611–12?

1. See Askew 1969, 290–94.

2. It was Longhi (1916) who called Orazio "il piu meraviglioso sarto e tessitore che mai abbia lavorato tra i pittori."

3. The autograph status of both paintings has been much discussed. See, most recently, Vodret in Bergamo 2000. I continue to favor the example in the Cappuccini.

4. See, for example, Pérez Sánchez, Schleier, and Bissell—the latter of whom, however, had not studied the Prado picture firsthand. It should be remembered that the terms of comparison have changed dramatically since the discovery of the documents relating to the Ancona *Circumcision*, the Santa Maria della Pace *Baptism*, and the Brera *Saint Cecilia* (cat. nos. 7, 9, 11).

5. For a brief history of the church and the institutions associated with it, see Papaldo 1978.

6. Vodret (in Rome 1999, 38) notes that Camillo del Palaggio was associated with the Confraternity of San Girolamo and suggests that he may have obtained the picture following the 1631 fire. This would explain how it came into the hands of Clelia del Palaggio (see note 7 below).

7. As Bissell (1981, 140–41) notes, in 1703 Clelia del Palaggio lent a picture of "S. fran.o in estasi in braccio ad un Angelo . . . dell'istesso Gentileschi" to San Salvatore in Lauro. The picture was a *tela imperatore* (i.e., about 132 cm in one direction) and could be this one; see De Marchi 1987, 176.

22.

Lute Player

Oil on canvas, 56½ × 50¾ in.
(143.5 × 129 cm)

National Gallery of Art,
Washington, D.C., Ailsa
Mellon Bruce Fund, 1962.8.1

ca. 1612–15

PROVENANCE: Girolamo
Cavazza, Bologna (until 1697);
Prince Johann Adam Andreas
von Liechtenstein, Vienna
(1697–1712; letter of purchase,
as by Gentileschi); Liechtenstein collection, Vienna and
Vaduz (1712–1962; cats. 1767, no.
452; 1789, no. 579; 1873, no. 61;
1885, no. 31; 1931, no. 31, as by
Caravaggio); National Gallery
of Art, Washington, D.C.

RELATED PICTURES: Private
collection, France (said by
Sterling to be a faithful replica,
possibly original);[6] Christie's,
London (sale, July 10, 1959,
lot 151; copy); country club,
New Orleans (according to
Moir, a good copy);[7] Finarte,
Milan (sale, June 10, 1987,
lot 108; a copy); Villa Lante,
Bagnaia (in 1964; according to
Bissell 1981, a copy); Akademie
der Bildenden Künste, Vienna
(a small eighteenth-century
copy on copper with a landscape background, destroyed
in World War II).[8]

It is indicative of the state of our knowledge of Gentileschi that we know so little about this picture, which in many ways epitomizes the poetics of his art. The first mention of it—as a work by Orazio—occurs in 1697, when, through the agency of Marcantonio Franceschini, it was purchased by Prince Johann Adam Andreas von Liechtenstein from the collection of the Bolognese merchant Girolamo Cavazza.[1] How Cavazza came by it—through the Savelli, who had interests in Emilia?—is unknown (he owned mainly paintings by Bolognese artists: Ludovico Carracci, Francesco Albani, Guido Reni, Guercino, Donato Creti, Elisabetta Sirani, and Marcantonio Franceschini). Scholars have assumed that it was painted in Rome and was widely known there, since, as Bissell has noted, a back-viewed figure in Pietro Paolini's *Concert* (formerly J. Paul Getty Museum, Los Angeles), dating to about 1620, seems to depend on it. Far more important for the history of genre painting is the inspiration Giuseppe Maria Crespi drew from the picture in the 1690s for his own *Lute Player* (Museum of Fine Arts, Boston). Indeed, Orazio's picture is the link between Caravaggio's early genre works in Rome—the *Musicians* (Metropolitan Museum of Art, New York), the *Lute Player* (Hermitage, Saint Petersburg, and private collection, New York)— and the new wave of naturalistic genre painting in northern Italy initiated by Crespi.

As with Caravaggio's two *Lute Players*, so with Orazio's painting we are faced with the problem— amply discussed by Bayer—of whether we are dealing with true genre or with allegory in the guise of an everyday scene. On the one hand, the scale of the picture and intent expression of the player suggest an allegory, perhaps a personification of music or harmony. (A depiction of Saint Cecilia can be ruled out.) Among the options Ripa offers for a depiction of Music is "a woman, who with both hands holds Apollo's lyre and at her feet has various musical instruments."[2] Orazio's painting might be seen as a modernized interpretation of this subject. (In his canvas in the Metropolitan Museum from a cycle of the Liberal Arts, Laurent de La Hyre chose to depict a woman playing a chitarrone with a similar array of musical instruments and a part-book on a table—but, it should be noted, with an organ and a nightingale, as also suggested by Ripa.) The woman's attentive listening suggests that she may be tuning the instrument, a necessary activity in any depiction of Music and one that would argue for her representation as Harmony. (In Caravaggio's *Musicians*, which is an allegory of Music, one of the figures tunes his lute.) On the other hand, the asymmetrical composition, with the figure placed to one side of the canvas while the other half is given over entirely to a still life of musical instruments, seems far too informal for an allegory. (It also serves as a reminder that Gentileschi is documented as having painted at least one still life, for which, see p. 128 n. 19.) Originally, this asymmetry was even more pronounced: a 10-centimeter strip of canvas attached to the right side of the picture is a later addition, while the left side has been trimmed.[3] The intentional crop- ping of the figure's feet further enhances the effect of informality. As De Grazia points out, the loosened bodice with a provocatively dangling cord strikes a distinctly lascivious note; love and music are invari- ably linked in Renaissance thought and poetry. Far from presenting "an idealization of the act of musical creation, a commentary on a beauty that transcends the ordinary,"[4] the painting may be seen as a solicita- tion to the (male) viewer, the musician's oblique posi- tion enhancing her seductive character. Unfortunately, the sheet music partially covered by the sitter's arm has been both damaged and reworked and has eluded identification. (In Caravaggio's *Lute Players*, the part- books contain amorous madrigals.)[5] Crespi's picture, which shows a disheveled woman tuning her lute with uncommon abandon, would seem to offer a commentary on this subtext to Orazio's masterpiece.

In the quagmire of Caravaggio studies in the early years of the twentieth century it was possible for

REFERENCES: Fanti 1767, 91 n. 452; Longhi (1916) 1961, 231; Gamba 1922–23, 262–66; Voss 1925, 459; Eigenberger 1927, 157; Longhi 1927, 112; Longhi 1943, 46 n. 38; Fröhlich-Bume 1954, 360; Sterling 1958, 118 n. 41; Neugass 1963, 16; Moir 1967, vol. 1, 75, vol. 2, 75 no. A.3; Moir 1969, 363–64; Bissell 1971, 275–76, 288–89; Freedberg 1976, 733; Nicolson 1979, 53; Shapley 1979, 201–3; Bissell 1981, 38–39, 65, 92–93 n. 16, 111, 158–59 no. 31; Garrard 1989, 28; Bayer in New York 1990b, 74; Nicolson 1990, 115; De Grazia and Garberson 1996, 96–101; Holmes in Bissell 1999, 179.

Longhi, in his groundbreaking article of 1916, to maintain the attribution to Caravaggio that Gentileschi's picture had acquired in the course of the eighteenth century. Gamba first ascribed it to Orazio, suggesting (largely because of its provenance from the Liechtenstein collection) that it may have been painted in France or England. Every other scholar has correctly dated it to the second decade of the seventeenth century, some closer to 1610 (Longhi, Shapley), others to 1620 (Moir), but most in the time frame 1610–15. I believe that, not unlike the *Saint Francis* (cat. 21), the picture marks that moment about 1613–15 when, following his work in the Casino delle Muse, Orazio moved away from the *verismo* of his paintings of 1609–12 and began working instead toward a more abstracted naturalism (not to be confused with the idealist approach of Bolognese artists, to whom, however, Orazio continued to turn for compositional ideas). Although Longhi ascribed the picture to Caravaggio, he saw the pivotal place it holds in Orazio's career, describing it as the stepping-stone to that mature style of painting based on a "scaled accord of luminosity in the colors (see pp. 19–20)."

Paradoxically, in this venture away from the mainstream of Caravaggism in Rome, Orazio looked for guidance to the early, Giorgionesque work of Caravaggio—works such as the *Penitent Magdalene* (fig. 126)—in which a Lombard naturalism is tempered by a Venetian softness (what Bellori describes as "Giorgione's frank manner, with tempered shadows"). In so doing, he helped to launch the vogue for Venetian painting, which was to dominate Roman art in the 1620s. (Was the catalyst his patronage by the Savelli, who owned a conspicuous group of paintings by Dosso Dossi?) Yet, if we compare Orazio's *Lute Player*

to Caravaggio's *Penitent Magdalene*, the sophistication and audacity of Orazio's picture, with its daring asymmetry, emerge clearly. Typically, the diagonal shaft of light in the upper-left corner does not merely indicate the source of illumination; it is part of the geometric grid that anchors the composition. The light here is more atmospheric than heretofore and marvelously subtle in the gradated shadows, but it does not yet possess that prismatic clarity we find beginning around 1615 (as exemplified in the *Saint Cecilia with an Angel*; cat. 31).

Fröhlich-Bume published a drawing, now in the National Gallery of Art, Washington, D.C. (inv. 1964.3.1), that she ascribed to Orazio and considered a first idea for the picture. As noted by Bissell, neither assertion is correct. (I do not believe the drawing is necessarily connected with the painting at all.)

1. See De Grazia and Garberson 1996, 97, 98 nn. 1, 2. Prior to De Grazia's publication the family name on the bill of sale was thought illegible. For the surviving correspondence between Franceschini and Prince Andreas, see Miller 1991, 209, 211, 212, 214–15, 220.
2. Ripa 1603, 166.
3. According to the technical report in De Grazia and Garberson 1996, 96. The original canvas would seem to have been trimmed only along the left edge.
4. Bissell 1981, 39.
5. The bibliography is summarized by Christiansen in New York 1990a, 42–44, 58–60.
6. If this is the picture measuring 125 × 155 cm of which a photograph (copyright Jean Weber) is in the Louvre's files, then it is no more than a copy.
7. This may be the same picture seen by Sterling and sold at Christie's; see Nicolson 1990 and De Grazia and Garberson 1996, where it is noted that the painting was purchased by the country club in 1959.
8. See Eigenberger 1927.

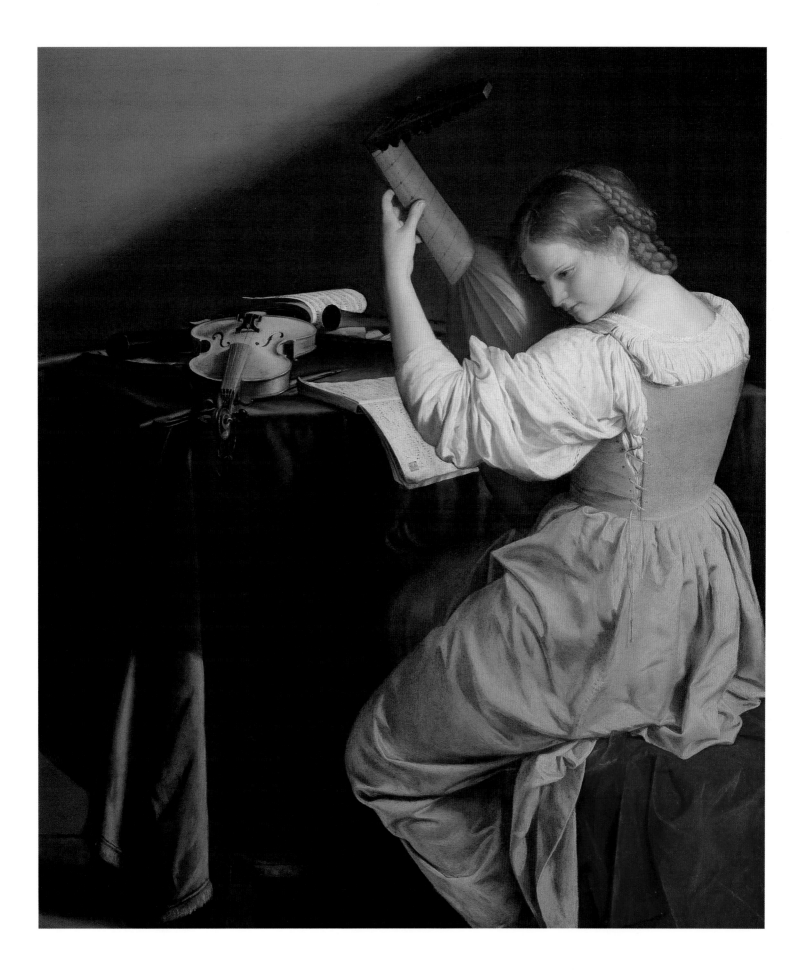

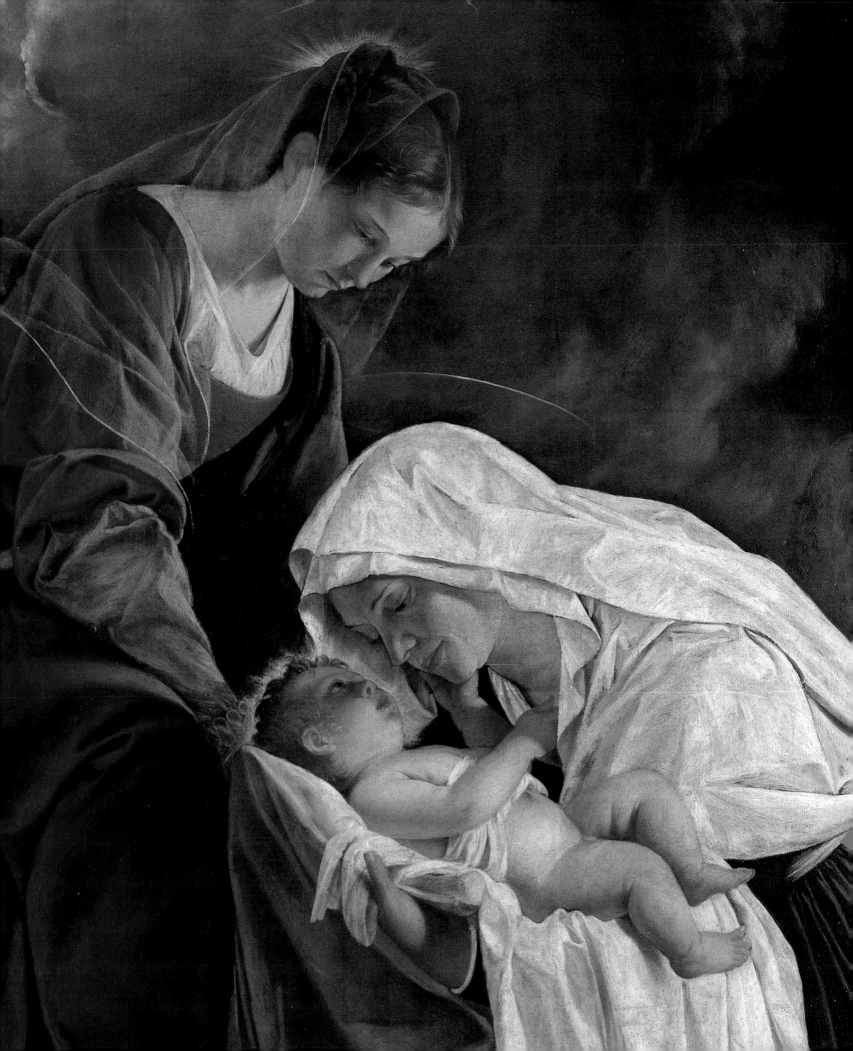

Orazio Gentileschi between Rome and the Marches

LIVIA CARLONI

Some of the most important and memorable works by Orazio Gentileschi are those he painted for the Marches, for the cities of Ancona and Fabriano. Ancona, which had lost its independence as a maritime republic as early as 1532,[1] was the most important city governed by the papacy in what was the most prosperous region of the Papal States. Although economic and cultural ties linked Rome to the whole region, the duchy of Urbino remained autonomous until its devolution to the papacy in 1631. The cultural interaction between the region and the central power in Rome is reflected in the fact that many artists left the Marches to work in Rome and, vice versa, that important works of art were sent to the Marches from Rome. These include Peter Paul Rubens's *Nativity* (1608) and Giovanni Lanfranco's *Pentecost* for the Oratorians in Fermo (Pinacoteca Civica, Fermo) and the altarpiece—either lost or perhaps never executed—commissioned from Caravaggio in 1604 for the Capuchins of Tolentino.[2] Moreover, in 1604 Guido Reni and Lionello Spada went to Loreto to negotiate terms for a fresco cycle in the new sacristy of the basilica of the Santa Casa (later to be carried out by Cristoforo Roncalli); Annibale Carracci had already made an altarpiece, the *Birth of the Virgin* (Louvre, Paris) for the same church.

Orazio's *Circumcision* (cat. 7), painted for the church of the Gesù in Ancona, must have been well received in the cosmopolitan and eastward-looking city, filled with Levantines, Turks, and Jews. Ancona, which had long been linked with Ragusa (now Dubrovnik) and the Dalmatian coast, had recently strengthened its identity as a maritime and trading city through the concession of tax exemptions, which were extended as well to resident foreigners by Pope Clement VIII Aldobrandini (r. 1592–1605). Gentileschi's "most noble painting the *Circumcision of Our Lord*" was triumphantly inaugurated in honor of the man who commissioned it, Giovanni Nappi, on June 24, 1607, the feast day of Saint John the Baptist, when, set in an elaborate wood frame carved by Francesco Brunelli, it was installed on the high altar of the nearly completed church atop the Guasco hill. A chronicle compiled by the fathers of the Collegio Romano and sent to Rome for printing constitutes the only documentary evidence of this event. It was noted by Pietro Pirri in an article published in 1952, but only recently has it been connected with the painting by the author of the present essay.[3]

The commission for the high altar of the new church was perhaps proposed by Claudio Acquaviva, the provost of the Jesuit Order in Rome. From his prior involvement with the church of San Vitale in Rome, we know that Acquaviva was very interested in Tuscan artists, and his opinion must have carried considerable weight. Orazio was, of course, Tuscan by birth and hardly a negligible figure. According to Alessandro Maggiori, he was paid 303 scudi,[4] which attests to the esteem in which he was held. It is not known if he ever went to Ancona to study the space or supervise the installation of the altarpiece, but such a trip would have been quite possible and may have been encouraged by the proximity of Ancona to Loreto, where the great Marian sanctuary, a pilgrimage destination even among artists, was undergoing renovations. (In 1602, Orazio had asked Baglione to bring him a souvenir Madonna from the shrine.) Ancona was hardly a city without artists or artistic attractions. Quite the contrary. Orazio may have been interested in Titian's (ca. 1485/90?–1576) *Crucifixion*, in the church of San Domenico (see p. 148), a short distance from the Gesù, or the fresco by Piero della Francesca (ca. 1415–1492) that, according to Giorgio Vasari, depicted the Marriage of the Virgin,[5] and which was still visible in the church of San Ciriaco in the late seicento.

The year 1607 was an enormously creative one for Gentileschi. Just before he delivered the Ancona altarpiece, a contract was drawn up in Rome, on March 23, between the painter and Settimio Olgiati, a banker from Como, for an altarpiece of the *Baptism of Christ* (cat. 11), for the church of Santa Maria della Pace in that city. And on November 25, Cardinal Paolo Emilio Sfondrato, in Como on a pastoral visit to the Augustinian monastery of Santa Cecilia, saw and greatly praised an altarpiece depicting the Vision of Saint Cecilia (cat. 9), described as "new."[6] Some years earlier, Orazio had been given an important commission for the Capuchins in Piedmont, an altarpiece of the Madonna in Glory (fig. 5), probably initially placed in the monastery in Rivoli and then transferred to the Turinese church of Santa Maria del Monte. The monastery had been financed directly by Carlo Emanuele, duke of Savoy, for whom Gentileschi later painted two pictures (cat. nos. 42, 43).[7]

The church of the Gesù in Ancona was part of an ecclesiastic complex that constituted the fourth institution established by the Jesuits in the Marches in the sixteenth century.[8] The rebuilding of the church, under way in 1604–5, and the commission of the *Circumcision* were financed by Giovanni Nappi,[9] a patrician of Ancona. Letters from those years among Father Acquaviva, Nappi, his Jesuit son Filippo, and the rectors of the Collegio are marked by great courteousness and collegiality.[10] The architect G. De Rosis came up with a relatively modest design with just three altars. In addition to Orazio's altarpiece, there was an *Assumption* on the left commissioned by Nappi's sister-in-law Camilla Trionfi and, on the right, a *Trinity Appearing to the Blessed Ignatius*, provided for by Marchesa Vittoria Malatesta Landriani. These two works were painted, respectively, by the Jesuit Michele Gisberti and by an artist in the circle of Agostino Tassi, perhaps Giovanni d'Ancona.[11] To judge from the other artists involved— all members of the Society of Jesus instructed to work "in our manner"—Nappi must have been directed by Acquaviva to employ Orazio, even though Orazio does not seem to have worked for the Jesuits in Rome. It is notable that the local painter Andrea Lilio (ca. 1570–after 1635), much favored by the Jesuits, was passed over, though he was active in his native city as well as in Rome, where he had worked alongside Orazio on the projects sponsored by Pope Sixtus V (r. 1585–90). Lilio's refined, flickering style is quite different from Orazio's more awkward manner, but he too, in his own way, reinterpreted the innovations of Caravaggio and other Roman artists, strengthening shadows and rendering figures with a certain clumsiness, without, however, sacrificing his

own innovative style. For some years, the Jesuits had favored Tuscan artists, such as Andrea Commodi (1560–1635) and Agostino Ciampelli (1560–1638), whose work, with its nobility and optical precision, corresponded to Jesuit spirituality, ever attentive to the accurate mental re-creation of historical and biblical events, in accordance with the precepts set forth in the *Spiritual Exercises* of Saint Ignatius of Loyola (1491–1556). This would have worked to Orazio's benefit.

Curiously, the strong Flemish component of the Ancona altarpiece has not been noted; rather the Flemish influence has been seen, instead, in Orazio's small paintings on copper, especially in the landscape elements, which are indebted to the manner of Adam Elsheimer (1578–1610). Yet the figure types in the *Circumcision* and their charged gestures seem, interestingly, to anticipate Gerrit van Honthorst (1592–1656). Connections with earlier Northern painters emerge as well: for example, with Wenzel Cobergher (1560?–1632), who was godfather to one of Orazio's sons.[12]

Although Giovanni Nappi had a son, Filippo, who studied at the Collegio Romano and was later rector at Ancona, we would be much mistaken if we were to consider him someone with a special devotion to the Jesuits. We must bear in mind that the founding of the Collegio as a center for advanced studies was an important cultural addition to the city. With the election of Pope Paul V Borghese (r. 1605–21), whom Nappi had met in 1605, when he was part of a delegation to Rome from Ancona,[13] the Society of Jesus once again acquired a position of importance. The strict policy regarding images, exemplified by the removal from Saint Peter's of Caravaggio's *Madonna dei Palafrenieri* (Galleria Borghese, Rome) and perhaps also the *Death of the Virgin* from Santa Maria della Scala (Louvre, Paris),[14] at the behest of Paul V, underscores the importance the papacy attached to the propriety of sacred images. Certainly, the Jesuits were always more carefully attuned to the religious and doctrinal significance of paintings and their effect on the faithful than to their beauty. When Caravaggio left Rome, Orazio was freed from his influence and designed for this Counter-Reformation order, for which Caravaggio had never worked, a decorous figurative scheme at once modern and antique. The division of the *Circumcision* into two realms—that of the eternal, above, and the worldly, below—is a typically sixteenth-century and un-Caravaggesque configuration. So also is the explicitly described light source (an expedient found again in the *Baptism of Christ*; cat. 11). Nappi may well have found it in his interest to comply with the wishes of the society, which again enjoyed papal favor. But protecting the Jesuits was also a way of ensuring for himself future papal favors for his economic interests in Ferrara, a city with which a number of people important to Gentileschi were associated.

In the region of Ferrara, recently acquired by the Church, Enzo Bentivoglio was actively promoting the construction of mills and the reclaiming of the swampy areas between the Po and the Tartaro rivers.[15] For this, in 1607, a lobbying effort was directed at the papal nephew, Cardinal Scipione Borghese, through Monsignor Francesco Nappi, a relative of Giovanni's. Above all, Francesco served as a go-between for Bentivoglio in furthering Scipione Borghese's passion for collecting works of art in Ferrara (see pp. 13, 15, 56).[16] Thus, the Nappi family must have had ties with Ferrara; it was certainly involved with the mills after papal approval was granted in 1609. The following year Giovanni Nappi died in Ferrara and his body was brought back to his church of the Gesù in Ancona.[17]

Orazio's patron Giovanni Nappi therefore moved among the highest ranks of the Jesuits and the papal world, assisted by Monsignor Francesco. His interests in Ferrara also linked him to Prince Paolo Savelli, another important collector and a protector of Orazio. In 1613, following the trial against Agostino Tassi for the rape of Artemisia, Orazio lodged with the prince and small payments to the artist from the Savelli are recorded in 1614 and 1615.[18] The many paintings executed by Gentileschi for Paolo Savelli, which are documented in inventories,[19] were spread over the second decade of the seicento and perhaps overlap with the artist's subsequent activity in Fabriano (on this see pp. 15–19).[20] Paolo Savelli (who was related to Caravaggio's patron Cardinal del Monte)[21] was in Ferrara when it became part of the papal states and accompanied Cardinal Aldobrandini to the city; in 1607, he too offered advice to Cardinal Borghese on the purchase of pictures.[22]

Given the number of important works carried out by Orazio for Fabriano—no fewer than five altarpieces and two fresco cycles—we must assume that he had a long and continuous activity there. A wealthy and prosperous town, with some 15,000 inhabitants and an equal number in the countryside, Fabriano returned to papal rule in 1610.[23] It was ruled by a prelate governor, distinct from the papal legate to the Marches, who, in 1612,[24] was Angelo Stufa, a Florentine. (Stufa, too, had ties with Ferrara.) There is no agreement regarding when this second period of Gentileschi's activity in the Marches began. My own feeling is that his absence from a convocation of the Accademia di San Luca in Rome in late October 1613, when he is cited as "fora di Roma," supports an early dating.

A first sojourn in Fabriano in 1613, to work on frescoes for the chapel of the Crucifixion in the church of San Venanzio (figs. 50–51), would not contradict the fact that, in 1614 and 1615, Orazio was active at the Palazzo Savelli in Rome, something we can deduce not only from the payments already referred to, but from two letters, one from Nicolò Tassi to Galileo and another from Pietro Guicciardini to Andrea Cioli, secretary to Cosimo II de' Medici.[25] Clearly he could have sent paintings to the Marches while working for the Savelli. However, much of his work in Fabriano must have been completed by January 1617, when he wrote to Giovanni de' Medici about the possibility of working at the ducal palace in Venice.[26] There is a consensus that his activity there ended in February 1619, when the Ferrarese cardinal, Bonifacio Bevilacqua, wrote to Francesco Maria II della Rovere, duke of Urbino, praising Orazio's efforts and asking if he might be considered for the decoration of the vault of the church of San Ubaldo, in Pesaro.[27] The duke's negative reply reflects the della Rovere family's resistance to Roman innovation and interference. Another sign that Orazio's activity in the Marches was winding down can be gleaned from a letter of July 24, 1619, that he wrote to the cardinals of the Reverenda Fabbrica di San Pietro, in Rome, humbly asking if he might be considered for the decorations for the Benediction loggia in Saint Peter's (the document is published in appendix 2).[28]

Cardinal Bevilacqua (who was interested in Orazio by 1619—perhaps earlier) was a lover of music, a supporter of the Accademia degli Intrepidi, a detractor of the unscrupulous Bentivoglio, and an enthusiastic supporter of artists patronized by Sixtus V, such as Lilio, Ferraù Fenzone, and Ventura Salimbeni. He was also a great friend of Federico Cesi and Cardinal del Monte.[29] Bevilacqua's fame as a collector was consolidated when he was legate in Umbria (by his own account, he had collected various works by Perugino [ca. 1450–1523] and left one of them to his nephew).[30] As early as 1609, he may have introduced Orazio to another passionate collector, Vincenzo I Gonzaga, fourth duke of Mantua, who commissioned from the artist a *Madonna and Child* (cat. 15). Gonzaga collected in inverse proportion to his wealth and without

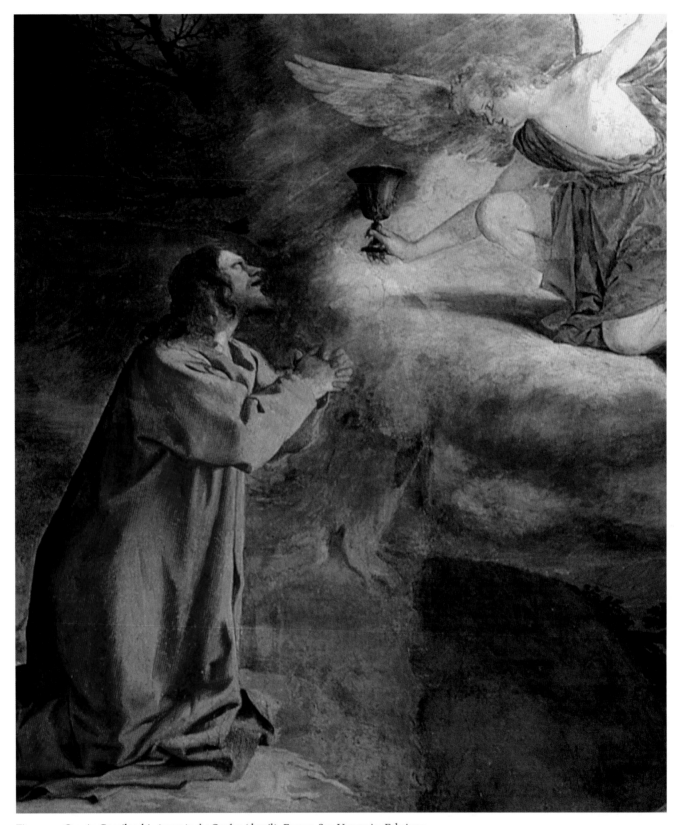

Figure 50. Orazio Gentileschi, *Agony in the Garden* (detail). Fresco. San Venanzio, Fabriano

any concern for the survival of his duchy, working through Roman channels to obtain works by living artists, such as Rubens, Domenico Fetti, Caravaggio, and Gentileschi. But he also wished to buy earlier paintings, and in 1605 asked Bevilacqua to act on his behalf in obtaining a Madonna by Perugino—at any cost.[31] Things did not go well, despite the intervention of Cesare Crispolti, a Perugian man of letters. Given the importance of the ties between his family and the Gonzaga, Bevilacqua could not afford to fail in this assignment, and eventually promised to send a Perugino from his own collection. Eventually, however, through these negotiations, he learned of the existence of another work by Perugino, a processional standard in Sant'Agostino in Fabriano (a fragment of which is now in Pittsburgh). A letter from Bevilacqua to Gonzaga states that he knew someone in Fabriano, Francesco Santacroce, who could investigate the availability of the painting, as he was a "prior and a person of authority in this area, and a very good friend of mine."[32] Santacroce appears to have been an important member of an old and aristocratic Fabriano family—a minor branch of a

Roman family related to the Borghese pope—residing in the neighborhood of Santa Maria in Publiculis. According to a seventeenth-century inventory, the family owned a work by Gentileschi.[33]

At the time Bevilacqua's letter was written, Santacroce was prior of Sant'Agostino, a position he would also hold with the chapter of the collegiate church of San Venanzio in Fabriano during the years of its renovation, from 1610 to 1614.[34] Because Fabriano did not have its own bishop—it was a dependency of the diocese of Camerino—San Venanzio was the most important religious institution in the city. To ensure that the municipality did not interfere with the administration of the church, from 1612 the office of prior was under the direct jurisdiction of the pope.[35] Santacroce may thus have acted as Cardinal Bevilacqua's intermediary in offering Gentileschi his first commission in Fabriano in its most important ecclesiastical building. At the very least, I find this argument more convincing than those advanced by Claudio Pizzorusso, who posits that Orazio's support came from Paolo Savelli's brother, Cardinal Giulio Savelli, who was governor of

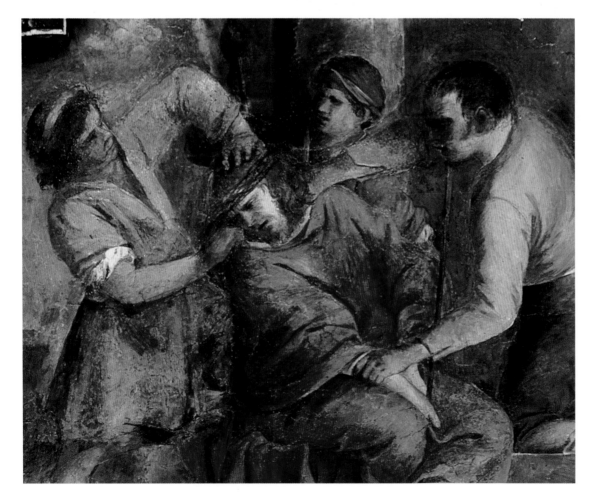

Figure 51. Orazio Gentileschi, *Crowning with Thorns* (detail). Fresco. San Venanzio, Fabriano

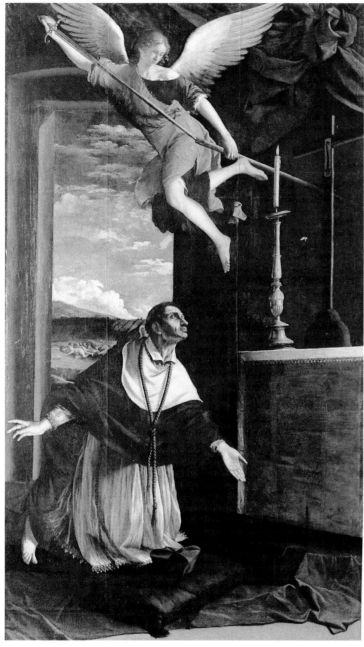

Figure 52. Giovanni Francesco Guerrieri (1589–1655/59) (and Orazio Gentileschi?), *Saint Charles Borromeo*. Oil on canvas. San Venanzio, Fabriano

was closely associated with the Borghese family and served as general preceptor (*primicerius*) of the Ospedale di Santo Spirito in Rome. He perhaps favored Orazio for the commission of the *Saint Mary Madgalene in Penitence* (cat. 24), which is datable to around 1615, when the members of the confraternity of the Università dei Cartai (which was devoted to the worship of the Magdalene and had a small church near the Ospedale) became associated with the archconfraternity at Rome.[38] However, the *Magdalene* is not necessarily the first of Gentileschi's paintings for Fabriano, although stylistically it resembles his work in the church of San Venanzio there.

Other people, too, may have acted as intermediaries in Rome. For example, there was Johannes Faber, the German doctor at Santo Spirito. A friend of Elsheimer and a collector of the artist's work,[39] Faber was an intimate of Prince Federico Cesi and of Cesi's most faithful and important collaborator, the Fabrianese Francesco Stelluti, who, with Cesi, was one of the four founders of the prestigious scientific society the Accademia dei Lincei.[40] Strange as it may seem, Stelluti—the most significant intellectual figure in Fabriano during these years—has never been considered in relation to Gentileschi's activity there. Unlike today, in the seventeenth century scientific and artistic circles were not mutually exclusive. Stelluti, for example, corresponded actively with Galileo (whose letters to Stelluti have unfortunately been lost). In the spring of 1611, Galileo arrived in Rome to be triumphantly inscribed in the Accademia dei Lincei, and it was then that he probably met Orazio. In 1615, Gentileschi's neighbor Nicolò Tassi wrote to Galileo, implying a special relationship with Orazio; the scientist was later an admirer of the work of Orazio's daughter, Artemisia.[41] Stelluti was himself a passionate student of art and science, a man of many talents and with a keen sense of discrimination. He was involved with the investigation of natural phenomena and he was adept at drawing, which early on proved useful in his relationship with Prince Cesi and the latter's in-depth research on plants and other scientific projects. As an officer of the Lincei, a post he held from 1611, Stelluti spent the years 1612 to 1618 in Fabriano, with brief visits to Naples, Rome, and Acquasparta. We know that in the summer of 1613 he wrote to Galileo from Fabriano about his observations with the telescope of the rings of Saturn.[42]

Stelluti also served as an intermediary between Rome and Fabriano in cultural matters, as, for example, in the commission to Antonio Viviani (1560–1620) for an *Annunciation* for the

Ancona from 1608 to 1610 and later bishop of the city, or from Giulio's successor as governor, Prospero Caffarelli, who was related to the Borghese family.[36]

What may be no less significant is the fact that the Savelli family, in the person of Bernardino (the father of Paolo and Giulio), had business contacts in Fabriano.[37] Of the people suggested by Pizzorusso who might also have been involved in securing work for Orazio, the most significant is Cardinal Pietro Campori, who

confraternity of the Gonfalone at the church of San Benedetto, during Viviani's stay in Rome from 1600 to 1601.[43] In Rome Viviani enjoyed the support of the Oratorian cardinal Cesare Baronio and may have been an expedient alternative to his teacher, Federico Barocci (ca. 1535–1612), who was often involved in other projects. Stelluti had a nephew at the Roman oratorio, and Orazio must also have moved in this circle, since, presumably in 1612,[44] he painted a *Saint Francis* for Orazio Griffi (cat. 21), who was associated with the Oratorian cofraternity of San Girolamo della Carità, and his brother Aurelio Lomi had ties to the Chiesa Nuova. Significantly, we find Viviani, a native of Urbino who had been employed alongside Orazio on Pope Sixtus V's projects in Rome, working in Fabriano in the chapel of San Flaviano in San Venanzio (his work was probably completed in 1616).[45]

When we remember that in 1613, acting through Prince Cesi, Cardinal Bevilacqua sought to obtain from Galileo his book on sunspots,[46] a frame of reference is created that includes the most advanced scientific culture of the seventeenth century. Clearly, Galileo's admiration for Gentileschi was not due solely to their common origins (like Galileo, Orazio was born in Pisa, though he always called himself a Florentine). Nor was it nurtured solely by the scientist's great open-mindedness. Rather, it must have derived from Galileo's recognition of the extraordinary visual precision, modernity, and elegance of the painter's work (this could also hold true for Stelluti). In the absence of firm documents, we can only speculate, but the Stelluti family tree shows that they were related to the Vallemani,[47] who seem to have been the patrons of the chapel of the Crucifixion that Orazio decorated in San Venanzio.[48]

There are several reasons for believing that it was this same Vallemani family that granted Orazio the commission. The Vallemani arms are coupled with those of the Benigni family in the stucco coat of arms above the entrance of the chapel, and, in a notary document dating to April 1620, the Confraternità del Suffragio obtained the bishop's consent to meet in the chapel ("in cappella siva Altari pro nomine il Santissima Crocifisso noncupato"), which is described as under the patronage of Camillo, Antonio, and other Vallemani family members. A list of the chapels in San Venanzio, attached to records of a pastoral visit in 1628, mentions "the third [chapel], of the Vallemani, dedicated to the Crucifixion."[49] The inconclusive documentation in the archives of the chapter house of San Venanzio and in notary

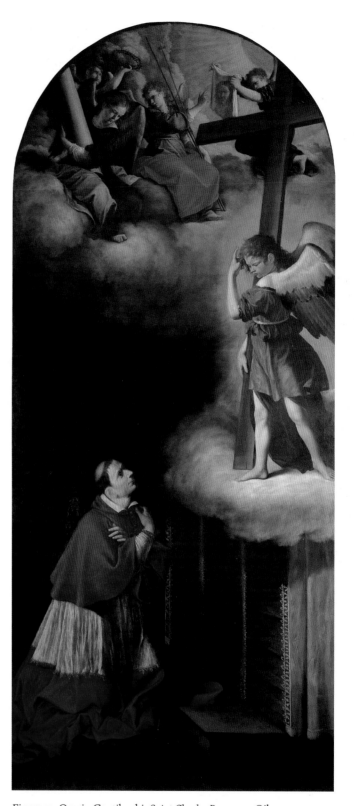

Figure 53. Orazio Gentileschi, *Saint Charles Borromeo*. Oil on canvas. San Benedetto, Fabriano

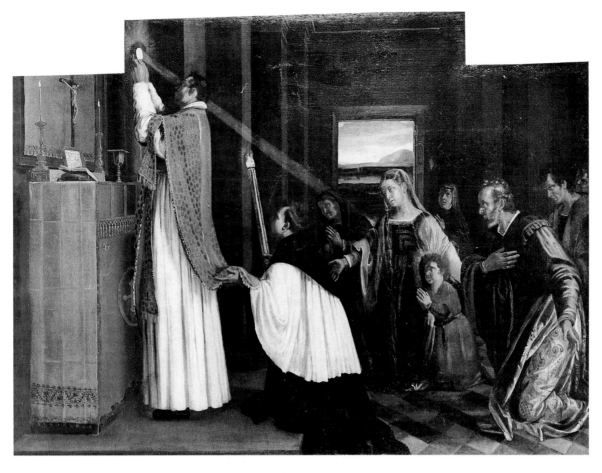

Figure 54. Giovanni Francesco Guerrieri (1589–1655/59), *Mass of Saint Nicholas.* Oil on canvas. Santa Maria del Ponte, Sassoferrato

documents leads me to believe that the Vallemani were patrons of the chapel long before the reconstruction of the church in 1607.[50] Thus, there was no need for a new concession of the chapel to the family, and a contract would simply have been drawn up with Orazio and the stucco worker (perhaps Francesco Selva;[51] these documents have not been found).

There may have been various reasons that led Orazio to leave Rome in 1613 for the Marches, where he executed works for the merchant class and the minor nobility, for both lay and religious confraternities (such as the Università dei Cartai and that of Saint Charles Borromeo or of the Most Holy Rosary), or for churches such as Santa Caterina or San Francesco (a lost fresco cycle). Projects in Fabriano may have been proposed by a well-placed figure and a friend, probably from Fabriano—such as Stelluti or Santacroce. Then too, Orazio was certainly aware that the scandal involving Artemisia—brought on by his denouncing of Tassi—had closed off the likelihood of official commissions in Rome or an auspicious return to Florence.

Two nearby and important churches were under renovation in Fabriano at this time. The ancient church of Santa Caterina,

formerly Silvestrine and then transferred to the Olivetans, was renovated by the Roman architect Giovanni Battista Cavagna between 1608 and 1613 (the year of his death). Cavagna was closely connected with Oratorian circles and was the architect of the church of San Pietro in Valle, Fano, and of the Santa Casa at Loreto.[52] In 1607, work also began on San Venanzio, based on the designs of Muzio Oddi (1569–1639). According to a memorial stone in the church, the building seems to have been completed in 1617.[53] The phases of the building of San Venanzio have been reconstructed by Andrea Emiliani and R. Ward Bissell, but some details still call for clarification. Work seems to have been carried out simultaneously in the chapels and the central nave,[54] and by late 1615 the church was "covered and nearly perfect." By June 18, 1610, and February 22, 1611, respectively, the large chapels in the transept were assigned to the confraternity of the Santissimo Sacramento e la Madonna, and to the Wool Merchants' Guild to be decorated by Giuseppe Bastiani (fl. 17th century).[55] In March 1613, the municipality committed a considerable sum to the enterprise.[56] That same year, the fifteenth-century choir acquired from the church of San Benedetto was installed,[57] a contract was

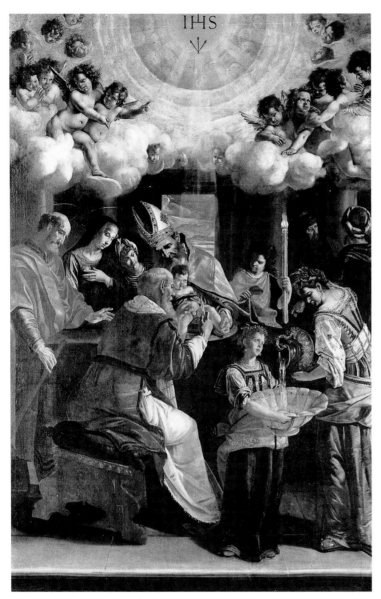

Figure 55. Giovanni Francesco Guerrieri (1589–1655/59), *Circumcision*. Oil on canvas. San Francesco, Sassoferrato

Francesco Guerrieri (1589–1655/59).[60] Both the attribution of this altarpiece and the date the chapel was assigned bear directly on our understanding of the adjacent chapel of the Crucifixion where Gentileschi worked. In the sacristy accounts is recorded an expenditure of 30 scudi in May of 1613 "to provide a painted frame for the picture of *Saint Charles* [Borromeo]":[61] a painting of Saint Charles was thus apparently in progress or perhaps completed and this would seem to be the work in the Calzettai chapel. However, the dedication of the chapel is first listed in the record of a pastoral visit of 1628, where the chapel is described as "of the Calzettai, dedicated to Saint Charles." (Thus, there is no basis to the claim that patronage of the chapel was transferred in 1619 to the Wool Merchants' Guild.)[62] Charles Borromeo (1538–1584) was often invoked against the plague. He had been canonized in 1610, and was an important figure for the city of Fabriano, supplanting Saint Emidio after the earthquake of 1612. On October 21 of that year the Consiglio di Credenza instituted a series of prayers and processions on the saint's feast day, to be held in San Venanzio.[63] Another confraternity dedicated to Saint Charles was granted a chapel in 1620, in the church of San Benedetto, where there is a painting by Gentileschi, *Saint Charles Borromeo* (fig. 53), most likely the last work painted by the artist for Fabriano.[64]

The *Saint Charles* in San Venanzio is fascinating for the way defects in the treatment of perspective[65] are combined with beautiful pictorial ideas, as in the depiction of the archangel Michael—to whom the city of Fabriano was dedicated[66]—as he places his sword back in its sheath, an allusion, perhaps, to the end of the city's most recent calamity. The gray floor, partially covered by a green cloth, and the sensitive hands of the saint are also striking. Roberto Longhi, Giampiero Donnini, and, more recently, Pietro Zampetti and Gianni Papi have suggested that Orazio may have laid out the composition in early 1613.[67] He might then have left the painting unfinished, pressured by having undertaken—and probably completing—the decoration for the chapel of the Crucifixion that same year. It is probable that the confraternity had the altarpiece installed in 1614 or 1615, after it had been significantly reworked by Guerrieri, prior to that artist's beginning his work in Rome at the Palazzo Borghese, in November 1615[68] (rather than in 1619, as Emiliani maintains).[69] During this time, Guerrieri was engaged in the execution of paintings in Fabriano, Serra San Quirico, and Sassoferrato (figs. 54, 55),[70] and was surely receptive to Gentileschi.[71] In the treatment of Saint

drawn up for the organ, and the sixteenth-century altarpiece by Battista Franco (il Semolei; 1498–1561) was installed on the high altar.[58] Also in 1613, nearly all the chapels of the left nave were assigned: that of the weavers, dedicated to Santa Barbara, that of the hosiers (Calzettai), and the chapel of the Crucifixion; the chapel of San Flaviano was completed in 1616.[59] By contrast, the chapels in the right nave appear to have been executed in the 1620s.

The second chapel to the left, that of Calzettai, was assigned on November 7, 1613, with the stipulation that it be decorated within four years. The altarpiece, of *Saint Charles Borromeo* (fig. 52), has been attributed by Emiliani to the Marchigian painter Giovanni

Charles's face, the painting closely resembles Guerrieri's own *Saint Charles and Saint Philip*, paid for in 1613 and discovered by Arcangeli in the Chiesa Nuova in Rome.[72] (From a payment for a painting for the confraternity of San Rocco in Fossombrone we know that Guerrieri was still in Rome in 1613.)[73] Guerrieri, who made frequent visits to Rome, was an original artist. He was rapidly developing his own style, one less crystalline and less refined than Orazio's, but more physical and more attuned to narration.

One of Orazio's secondary frescoes in the chapel of the Crucifixion, a single figure of Saint Anthony Abbot, may suggest that his patron was Antonio Vallemani. The other saints represented are Vincent Ferrer, perhaps Jerome, and Francis. Saint Francis, at the entrance to the chapel, seems to establish the usual parallel relationship between his life and the life of Christ. The principal frescoed scenes on the side walls depict the Taking of Christ and the Agony in the Garden (fig. 50). The altarpiece shows the *Crucifixion* (cat. 29). Work in the the chapel of the Crucifixion cannot, as Bissell proposes, be separated into two phases—an earlier one for the altar, and a later one for the frescoes, subsequent to a presumed trip to Tuscany, when Orazio was supposedly exposed to the work of Masaccio (1401–1428) and Piero della Francesca (ca. 1415–1492).[74] There is, in fact, no certainty at all about a trip to Tuscany: indeed, by all accounts Orazio was haunted by his separation from his native region. Clearly, the two large frescoes, which do not seem to the unaided eye to have been done in many *giornate*, preceded the altarpiece with the *Crucifixion*, which could certainly have been sent from Rome at a later time, but in any case does not differ from the frescoes stylistically so much as it does in terms of theme and technique. Even in the smaller frescoes of the vault, of the Flagellation and the Crowning with Thorns (fig. 51), the narrative is treated with a purity and simplicity seen both in the choice of colors, always contained, and in the compositions, of extraordinary clarity. The figures are aligned on the same plane against a shallow background defined by rock formations, mysterious and inhospitable. The scenes are pervaded by a melancholy, waning light or, in the case of the rupture of the dark clouds of the *Crucifixion*, with a sense of menacing cataclysm (Matt. 27:45–46). Far from the idealizing classicism of the type we see in Reni or Domenichino (1581–1641), and devoid of any facile effects of beauty, the cycle is characterized by a somber and meditative tone. The action unfolds almost without movement (even the violent gestures in the *Flagellation* are only

suggested), as Gentileschi evokes an internalized experience of the Passion.

It is not unlikely that Orazio's desire to work in a quiet and simple language as he began his commission in Fabriano was influenced by his knowledge of the town's earlier artistic heritage, still evident today despite many losses. There were the great trecento painters, such as Allegretto Nuzi (1316/20–1373/74), represented in San Venanzio itself, and the Master of Campodonico (fl. ca. 1346), who painted in the small church of the Magdalene for which Gentileschi provided the altarpiece. And there were the great quattrocento masters, Gentile da Fabriano (ca. 1385–1427) and Antonio da Fabriano (fl. 1451–89). But Orazio is not indebted solely to art from the past. In the somewhat static figures that return in the Malchus episode in the *Taking of Christ* and in the sleeping apostles in the *Agony in the Garden*, there is an unexpected echo of Caravaggio's *Christ in the Garden* (destroyed, formerly Kaiser Friedrich Museum, Berlin). And the angel that extends a chalice toward Christ is similar to the angels painted by Reni for the Oratory of Santa Silvia adjacent to San Gregorio Magno, Rome, one of the least classical works by the young Bolognese artist. In Orazio's *Magdalene* for the Università dei Cartai (cat. 24), for which a date of 1615 seems reasonable, we have a figure again shown in a simple pose, immersed in a setting defined by rocks, shrubbery, and light. This painting is remarkable for its luminous intensity and in the rendering of the Magdalene's tears and other details, particularly if seen in situ, where the image seems literally to invade the small, ancient church.

The *Vision of Saint Francesca Romana* (the so-called Rosei Altarpiece; cat. 30) is more difficult to place. Only scant contemporary documentation remains for the church of Santa Caterina, rebuilt by Cavagna for the Olivetans. We do not know whether the high altar was the original location for the painting, although we may assume this to have been the case, as the church was renovated again in the eighteenth century, at which time the painting was obviously cut down on the right. The episode depicted, from the life of Saint Francesca Romana, is one described in the saint's biography by Giovanni Mattiotti, and recorded in the 1608 chronicle of her life, compiled by the Jesuit Giulio Orsino at the time of her canonization.[75] Pizzorusso dates the picture to the period 1617–18, when Ippolito Borghese was father superior of the Olivetans.[76] According to documents preserved in Rome, in 1614 the superior general was Don Cesare Catani. Most important, from 1611 the

cardinal protector of the order was Paolo Emilio Sfondrato, the cardinal of Santa Cecilia in Rome, who had praised Orazio's altarpiece in Como some years earlier.[77] The painting is a masterpiece of static tranquility, built up with few colors and contrasting elements: a golden luminosity from which the young Madonna emerges, set off by the green curtain in the upper right; below, the sweet face of the Virgin is brought together with that of the child, realistic in its charmless features, and with that of Saint Francesca, no longer young, her incised features drawn, yet radiating the misleadingly youthful appearance that is sometimes encountered in those who have taken holy orders. A series of gray steps serves as a simple means of uniting the spiritual events unfolding in the picture with the day-to-day reality of a convent setting; they are, perhaps, the most inventive aspects of the composition and they constitute a true coup de théâtre in the suggestion of a proscenium.

In late 1614, Guerrieri carried out a commission for the *Circumcision* (fig. 55) in Sassoferrato, for the Confraternity of the Sacrament in San Francesco, committing to finish it by Christmas of 1615.[78] In Guerrieri's picture, but within a different context, there are steps similar to those found in the Rosei Altarpiece, bathed in the same crystalline gray light. Utterly different is the hint of a step we find in Caravaggio's *Madonna dei Pellegrini*, in Sant'Agostino, Rome. It is very possible that Guerrieri had more or less met his commitment to the confraternity, delivering the painting within

the year 1615, and that the agreement was made public because of a delay in payment. (At the end of 1615 he was expecting to begin a large project for the decoration of the Palazzo Borghese in Rome.) However, Guerrieri's delivery of the painting may have been made only in early 1616 (and, in fact, there is an unquestionable stylistic similarity with the canvases in the Palazzo Borghese). In either case, the painting contains an element of invention that betrays a personality much stronger than his own, namely, that of Gentileschi. The Rosei Altarpiece must therefore have preceded Guerrieri's *Circumcision,* dating Orazio's painting to about 1615. The conciseness of the expressive means and the play of whites and transparent shadows in the drapery that makes this painting so singularly rich imply the same elementary spiritual climate found in the *Magdalene* and the works in the chapel of the Crucifixion.

Orazio's other pictures for Fabriano can be dated to the end of his stay in the Marches, from 1619 to 1620. These, too, are important and, in their way, authoritative works, as seen in both the *Madonna of the Rosary* for Santa Lucia (or San Domenico) and the *Saint Charles* for the homonymous confraternity in San Benedetto, mentioned above.[79] Yet despite passages that are still lively—the almost choleric intrusion of the little angel above a somewhat weak Saint Charles and the sweetly archaicizing and self-quoting composition of the *Madonna of the Rosary*—much of the tension of the earlier works has been lost.

1. See Ancona 1982. The background provided by Zampetti 1990 is also useful.

2. See note 19 below.

3. Pirri 1952, 13; Carloni 1997, 22, 26 n. 31; the handwritten *Cronache Annue* are in the Archivium Romanum Societatis Jesu (hereafter, ARSJ), *Rom.* 129 I, *Romana Hist.,* 1605–1607, f. 153v, report of September 8, 1607.

4. Maggiori 1821, 66 n. 80.

5. On Piero della Francesca in the Marches, see Urbino 1992, 430.

6. Maniello 1994, 155–58; Rovi in Pinocoteca di Brera 1992, 56–60 no. 22; and Rovi 1992, 107.

7. Baudi di Vesme 1932, 319; from research in the Archivo di Stato, Turin, *Conti dé Tesorieri,* for the year 1604 it emerges that all ducal donations were made solely to the Capuchins of Rivoli, next to which, in the years 1605–7, the duke's castle was under construction. According to Isella and Lanza (1991, 84–85), the building of Santa Maria del Monte was suspended from 1596 to 1610, and Orazio's painting, which served as a screen at the high altar, thus could not have been made for the church but must have been transferred there from Rivoli.

8. Bösel 1985, vol. 2, 19–29; also see ARSJ, *Rom.,* 120, I, *Romana Fund. Collegia,* f. 61ff.; *Rom.* 128, II, f. 21; *FG.* 78 II, *Instrum.* c. 1577.

9. Saracini 1675, 403; Santini 1969, 290–91; Honorati 1990, 30; Albertini n.d., c. 254; Picchi Tancredi n.d., unpaged.

10. ARSJ, *Rom.* 15, I, and *Rom.* 15, II, *Epist. Gener.* 1601–109. In the letters of Acquaviva, however, no mention is made of Orazio's painting.

11. ARSJ, *Rom.* 129, I, *Romana Hist.,* 1605–1607, f. 153v, *Rom.* 130, II, *Romana Historia,* ff. 378v; Maggiori 1821, 66–67 n. 81; Cavazzini 1993, 318, 321, 323; and Cavazzini 1997, 411–12.

12. September 16, 1599: Hoogewerff 1938, 112. The artist had painted a work for the Chiesa Nuova, was in touch with Roncalli, and also had connections with Jacques Francart, F. von Casteele, Aert Mijtens, and Paul Bril; see Brussels–Rome 1995, 32–33, and Andrews 1977. Bril and Elsheimer were also artists protected by the Borghese and by Cardinal del Monte.

13. See Albertini n.d., f. 254. For Fillippo Nappi, see the ARSJ biographical entry; he was minister in Ancona in 1606 and rector from 1611 to 1614.

14. Calvesi 1990, 348–49; for Santa Maria della Scala, the cause of the removal may have been the Spanish Carmelite father Domenico di Gesù Maria, who was very close to and influential with the Borghese, as a comment by Mancini ([1617–21] 1956–57) would also lead us to believe.

15. See Fabris and Marcon, Maddalo, and Marcolini in Ferrara 1983, 41, 94.

16. Letters from 1607 and 1608 in Ferrara 1983, 94–103.

17. ARSJ, *Rom.* 130, I, f. 80.

18. Testa 1998, 349, January 1, 1614, and April 6, 1615, respectively; Gallo 1998, 312–15, 334. In the convocation at the Accademia di San Luca on October 24–25, 1613, regarding the next meeting scheduled for October 27, it was said that "Don Oratio Gentileschi is working at Monte [or Palazzo] Savello and is outside Rome."

19. Campori 1870, 162–66; Wiedmann 1979, 70; Testa 1998, 349–50, 352. In the Archivio di Stato di Roma (hereafter, ASR), Archivio Sforza-Cesarini, Parte I, b.1, fasc. "Nota dei quadri del Principe Savelli nel Pal. d'Ariccia," there is an "Inventario di quadri dell'Ecc.mo sig. Principe Savelli, quali erano della B.M. dell'Ecc.mo Principe suo padre riconosciuti da me Filippo Mignani," where there is listed: "One extremely large painting with portraits of the most Excellent Prince Abbot and Lady Donna Carlotta when they were children painted by Gentileschi, and a table of fruits and flowers by Gobbo in Rome," and "a painting made to hang above the door of three portraits made by Gentileschi and given to S.E. by those who are depicted in the painting." In this so-called Ariccia inventory, which would seem to have been made for Bernardino Savelli, there is no mention of other works by Gentileschi, which apparently passed to Fabrizio in 1646 (who sold many works to the Pamphili family in 1657). The children depicted must have been Paolo's three young children: Carlotta, Bernardino, and Fabrizio. Attached to the inventory, presumably dating to the mid-1600s, is a "list of paintings and prices" that includes Caravaggio, Reni, Guercino, and Titian, and paintings by artists from Ferrara. Bernardino was born in 1606, Carlotta Savelli in 1611 (ASR, Archivio Sforza-Cesarini, Parte I, b.1, fasc. "Nota dei quadri del Principe Savelli nel Pal. d'Ariccia," b.24). The two paintings, the one with the "triple portrait" and the one with the "three children," are mentioned briefly in the Ariccia inventory of 1631, published by Testa 1998, 349. The newly discovered inventory also mentions portraits of Zampeschi, since Battistina Savelli, whose married name was Zampeschi, was the aunt of Paolo Savelli. Within this context, it should be noted that the Capuchin church in Tolentino, where Caravaggio executed a painting in 1604 (now lost), had a female patron, specifically a Lady Laura, who was a member of this family and was related to the Savelli family; see Lopez in Ascoli Piceno 1992, 402, 408 no. 27. On the Savelli collection, see p. 36 n. 56 of Christiansen's essay.

20. In fact, the Braunschweig *Christ Crowned with Thorns* (see cat. 23) is compositionally very similar to the fresco in the chapel of San Venanzio in Fabriano, which has the same subject. Also see Finaldi in London–Bilbao–Madrid 1999, 64, no. 6, and Bissell 1981, 152–53, nos. 23, 24.

21. He was related to Del Monte through Isabella Savelli, marchesa of Monte Baroccio (an estate of the Del Monte family). It is known that the mathematician Guidobaldo, a brother of the cardinal, was a friend of Galileo. See Waźbiński 1994, vol. 1, 168 n. 131, 176.

22. See Marcon, Maddalo, and Marcolini in Ferrara 1983, 96, where it is noted that Paolo Savelli was a connoisseur as well as a collector of paintings; see the Savelli inventories cited in note 19 above.

23. See Castagnari 1986. The precise attribution of the paintings by Gentileschi appears in the early-eighteenth-century manuscript by Gilii and Guerrieri in the Biblioteca Communale of Fabriano (MS.29), as well as in Benigni (1728) 1924.

24. Weber 1994, 224.

25. Tassi's letter of January 17, in Pizzorusso 1987, 70, 74; and Waźbiński 1994, vol. 2, 490; the letters between Guicciardini and Cioli from the month of March 1615 are published in Crinò 1960 and Crinò and Nicolson 1961.

26. Crinò 1960, 264.

27. Gronau 1936, 273–74.

28. The brief document (see appendix 2) is in the archives of the Reverenda Fabbrica di San Pietro, Arm. 1, B14, N. 76. In tone, it contrasts strikingly with that of an analogous request from Lanfranco (N. 74, April 26), who proclaims that he is the best artist for the job, since he is a student of Annibale, and one from Pomarancio (N. 75, March 26), who is already convinced that he has the job, because he has the support of Cardinal Giustiniani. I am grateful to Dr. S. Turriziani for providing this information.

29. De Caro 1967, 786–88; also see Fioravanti Baraldi in Ferrara 1983, 178–82. The figure of the cardinal, which has been little examined, is tied closely to the Aldobrandini family (among Orazio's first patrons) and to the Savelli family

30. ASR, 30 Notai cap., uff. 18, L. Bonicontri, b. Testamenti 1627–1629, ff. 76ff., in the codicil to his will, dated April 5, 1627. Despite research carried out in Ferrara at the offices of the notary Giacomo Botti, for which I am indebted to Dr. M. Traina, it has not been possible to locate the cardinal's will, which would have clarified whether Bevilacqua was a collector of Orazio's work as well as his supporter. I myself would venture that this was the case, on the basis of the inventory of the Roman possessions of the cardinal, which must have been kept by the Mattei family, to whom Bevilacqua was related.

31. Braghirolli 1874, 52–60, 68.

32. Ibid., 59–60 (letter of December 21).

33. Pilati 1989, 142–43; Sassi 1952b, 3ff. For the painting by Orazio depicting Saint Ursula, belonging to the Santacroce family in Rome, see Sinisi 1963, 17 (inventory of Valerio Santacroce of 1670).

34. The dates are established by two notarile documents in the Archivio di Stato di Fabriano (hereafter ASFa), notarile document L. Venturini, vol. 29, August 20, 1610, c. 575r, and June 14, 1610, c. 375v; and documents from two pastoral visits to San Venanzio, February 8, 1611, and March 29–30, 1614, now in the Archivio della Curia Vescovile di Camerino (hereafter ACVCa), "Visite Pastorali di Monsignor Severini," vol. N. 1610–1621, f. 48ff.

35. Sassi 1952b, 18.

36. Pizzorusso 1987, 69–70, 73.

37. ASR, Archivio Sforza-Cesarini, Parte I, b.22, fasc. 42. According to this document, there was a legal action with the Reverenda Camera Apostolica that continued until the 1630s, which involved the heirs of Bernardino Savelli, including Paolo, and was related to a company the father owned with, among others, Nicola Marri in Fabriano, contractors for the building introduced by Sixtus V for the development of the Wool Merchants' and Light Wool Merchants' Guild; for more on the Wool Merchants' Guild and its importance to Fabriano, see Zonghi 1990.

38. Pizzorusso 1987, 72. The official deed of association with the archconfraternity is in the ASR, Ospedale di Santo Spirito, *Aggregazioni*, b. 1301, f. 15: "Confraternitas seus Societas Cartariorum in ecclesia Sanctae Mariae Magdalenae quae membrum est Archihospitalis preteriti S. Spiritus in Saxia de urbe di Roma extra terram Fabriani . . . petit et obtinuit dictam Societatem Archihospitalis . . . uniri et aggregari," solicitor for Fabriano, appointed by Bishop E. Pieruccio Pierucci.

39. Andrews 1977, 22; see Rome 2000, 37–41.

40. Alessandrini et al. 1986 and Solinas in Rome 2000, 94–97, are essential publications on Stelluti.

41. See note 25 above.

42. Stelluti to Galileo, August 17, 1613, written from Fabriano; see Alessandrini et al. 1986, particularly the biography; Mezzanotte in ibid., 217ff.; and Gabrieli 1996, 379. Stelluti's explorations with the telescope in the summers of 1617 and 1618 are documented. We know that Galileo's passion for the telescope was taken up by artists with whom he was acquainted, such as Cigoli. It is not unlikely that the indication of the curvature of the earth represented on the horizon of Orazio's *Crucifixion*, in San Venanzio, derives from astronomical studies undertaken with Stelluti himself, or from direct contacts with Roman scientific circles.

43. Sassi 1952b, 60–61.

44. Vodret in Rome 1999, 38, 40 no. 7.

45. Donnini 1981, 20–22; Molajoli 1990, 90; in the Archivio del Capitolo di San Venanzio (henceforth ACSV), "Repertorium decretorum capit. Ab anno 1612 usque ad 1683," fol. 16v.

46. Gabrieli 1996, 400–401 n. 289, of November 30, 1613.

47. See Alessandrini et al. 1986, partially reproduced as pl. 9; during this period there was also a homonymous member of the Lincei who was one of the priors of San Venanzio. Antonio Vallemani married Dorotea Stelluti, Pier Paolo Vallemani

married Livia Stelluti, and Michele Vallemani married another member of Stelluti clan; Joanna Stelluti perhaps married Marco Vallemani.

48. Sassi (1951, 68 n. 1) calls it the Vallemani-Benigni chapel. For more on the chapel, see Bissell 1981, 159–63 no. 32, with bibliography.

49. In the archives of the Marchese Carlo Lalli Benigni Olivieri Carbelli, there is a family tree dating to 1710 in which one sees the subsequent passage of the chapel to the Benigni family through the branch of Marchese Venanzio Vallemani, who married a certain Erminia Benigni (d. 1643). The relationship through marriage of the Vallemani family with the Stelluti family is indicated there through a P. Aloisio Vallemani, who married Eufrasia Stelluti. The document cited is dated April 10, 1620, and is found in the ASFa, notarile G. A. Manari, vol. 16, ff. 125v; ACVCa, pastoral visits, "Visitatio Terrae Fabriani, 1592–1628," vol. K., attached to the visit of June 21, 1628, f. 462r. For more on the Vallemani, see also Pilati 1989, 159–61, 205, and Zonghi 1990, 105, according to whom the heads of the Wool Merchants' Guild, in 1617–18, were Battista Stelluti and Giuseppe Vallemani; Sassi 1989, 229.

50. This can be deduced from the family's strong interest in the church, attested to by the fact that Antonio Vallemani, as early as August 20, 1610, had shifted an income of three hundred scudi from San Luca to San Venanzio, a loan "pro fabrica"; see ASFa, notarile L. Venturini, vol. 29, fols. 574v–575v, and ACSV, Instrum. Liber II, fols. 29r–30r; Antonio, as an appointee of the Papermakers' Guild, appears again in a document of June 13, 1620, listed between two Stelluti brothers—Costanzo and Michele—and the aforementioned guild, which was committed to the decoration of the first chapel on the right in San Venanzio, see ACSV, Instrum., II, ff. 196r,v; on September 3, 1614, Pietro Paolo Vallemani (who died by 1616 and was the father of Camillo and Geronimo) gave money to the sacristy for the celebration of masses for the dead; see ASFa, notarile document G. A. Manari, vol. 11, f. 227v and ff. Another appointee of the Wool Merchants' Guild was a certain Rainaldo, who appears in the deed granting the transept chapel to the Wool Merchants' Guild, dated February 22, 1611.

51. Molajoli 1990, 100, where the name of Francesco Selva is mentioned in relation to the stucco work for the chapel of Santissimo Sacramento.

52. Sassi 1954, 4ff.; Sassi 1926, 10–11; Venditti 1979, 560–63; Biblioteca Comunale Archivio Storico di Fabriano, ms. carte Graziosi, III, f. 99v, where the date of 1608 is noted, as well as the cost of ten thousand scudi.

53. See Emiliani in San Severino Marche–Bologna 1988, 57–58, and Bissell 1981, 160–61.

54. Bissell 1981, 161.

55. Pilati 1991, 15, 132; the relevant documents are in ACSV, Instrum., II, ff. 26r,v, and fols. 31v–32v, and in the ASFa, notarile L. Venturini, vol. 29, fols. 375v–377r, and vol. 30, fols. 128v, 129v; Lopez in Ascoli Piceno 1992, 40 no. 44, 406.

56. Bibl. Com. and Arch. St. di Fabriano. Sez. Cancelleria, vol. Reformat. 1611–1613, vol. 77, fol. 169v: March 23, 1613; see Emiliani 1958b, 46, 55 n. 7.

57. Sassi 1932, 143–47, and ACSV, vol. Sacrestia, 1610–1910, "Spese che si fanno per la sacrestia di San Venanzio per l'anno 1613," fol. 2r, expenses of 17 scudi.

58. ACSV, vol. Sacrestia, 1610–1910, "Spese che si fanno per la sacrestia di San Venanzio per l'anno 1613," fols. 3v, 4r, 9r, and ACSV, Repertorio Decret. Cap., 1612–1633, fol. 13v: July 28, 1613, assignment of the chapel of the High Altar to F. Lotti; the contract for the organ is in ASFa, notarile document L. Venturini, vol. 33, fols. 3303r and fols. of September 17, 1613.

59. ACSV, Repertorio Decret. Cap., 1612–1633, f.16v (Santa Barbara); ASFa, notarile G. A. Manari, vol. 12, fols. 192v and fols., of June 27, 1616, then the chapel of the Calzolai by B. Lauri. The correct date for the granting of the chapel of the Calzettai has been re-established by Bissell 1981, 161; see ACSV, Instrum., II, fol. 65r,v, and ASFa, notarile L. Venturini, vol. 33, fols. 554v–555v.

60. Emiliani 1958b, 47; Emiliani in San Severino Marche–Bologna 1988, 51–52; Emiliani 1991, 23–24 no. 18.

61. ACSV, vol. Sacrestia, 1610–1910, "Spese che si fanno per la sacrestia di San Venanzio per l'anno 1613," fol. 2r.

62. ACVCa, pastoral visits, Vitatio 1628, vol. K., f. 462r; a document from 1619 appears to have been misunderstood by Emiliani (1958b, 46), and repeated by Bissell (1981, 161).

63. Sassi 1939, 8–11, cited by Bissell 1981, 160.

64. Bissell 1981, 170 no. 41, and Sassi 1932, 150; Zampetti in Ancona 1985, 66–67 no. 67.

65. As noted earlier in Molajoli 1930–31, 105.

66. Sassi 1926–27, 105.

67. Longhi, as noted in Emiliani 1958b, 47; Donnini 1981, 19; Zampetti in Ancona 1985, 219–20 no. 68; and Zampetti in Fossombrone 1997, 60 no. V; Papi 1991, 148. Bissell (1981, 207 no. X20), however, rejects any relationship with Orazio and attributes the painting to Guerrieri.

68. Fumagalli in Fossombrone 1997, 29; the first payment at Palazzo Borghese is dated November 28, 1615.

69. See note 61 above for the basis of the erroneous conviction that the chapel of the Cartai was transferred to the Wool Merchants' Guild in 1619.

70. Carloni in Fossombrone 1997, 19ff.

71. An opinion that has recently been shared by Zampetti (1990, 299–300) and Contini (in Fossombrone 1997, 8).

72. Arcangeli in Rome 1995, 537–38 no. 97.

73. Emiliani 1991, 8 n. 5.

74. Bissell 1981, 31–34.

75. See Picasso 1984, pl. 6.

76. Pizzorusso 1987, 73.

77. ASR, Congregazioni religiose maschili, Benedettini olivetaini, "S. Maria Nova," b. 1, f. 122. There is a folder of documents in Rome pertaining to the convent of Fabriano from the mid-1600s (busta 3548). Between 1611 and 1618 the father superior of Fabriano was a certain Clemente; see Fabriano 1982, 81.

78. Carloni in Fossombrone 1997, 23, 27 n. 34; see also Emiliani 1991, 47–48 n. 35.

79. Sassi 1928–29, 108ff.; Sassi 1932, 150; see also Arcangeli in Ancona 1981, 527–28 n. 165, and Zampetti in Ancona 1985, 216–17 n. 67.

23.

Christic Crowned with Thorns

Oil on canvas, 47 × 58 ½ in.
(119.5 × 148.5 cm)

Herzog Anton Ulrich-Museum,
Braunschweig (inv. 805)

ca. 1613–15

New York

PROVENANCE: Probably Paolo
Savelli, Rome and Ariccia
(d. 1632); probably Federigo
Savelli, Palazzo Savelli, Ariccia,
and Palazzo Montesavello,
Rome (1632–49); probably
Cardinal Fabrizio Savelli,
Palazzo Montesavello, Rome
(by 1650; inv. 1650, as by
Gentileschi); probably Cardinal
Flavio Chigi, Palazzo a Piazza
SS. Apostoli, Rome (after 1650–
93; inv. 1692); Cardinal Joseph
Fesch, Rome (d. 1839; inv. 1841,
no. 2856); private collection,
Rome (until 1867); private col-
lection, England (from 1867);
Thomas Agnew and Sons, Ltd.,
London (1977); Herzog Anton
Ulrich-Museum, Braunschweig.

RELATED PICTURES: Lizza-
Bassi collection, Varese (possibly an autograph replica);[5]
private collection (copy; sale,
Finarte, Milan, December 3,
1992, lot 31).

REFERENCES: Campori 1870,
162; Klessmann 1978, 106;
Wrede 1978, 56; Nicolson 1979,
52; Bissell 1981, 152–53 no. 24,
201; Klessmann 1985, 383–84;
Schleier in New York–Naples
1985, 155–57; Utrecht–Braunschweig 1986–87, 265; Nicolson
1990, 114; Papi in Florence 1991,
38, 95, 102; Schleier 1993, 196,
199–200.

The Braunschweig *Christ Crowned with Thorns* is among Orazio's most memorable paintings, a work in which the violent contrasts of Caravaggio's dramatically charged canvas in the Kunsthistorisches Museum, Vienna—painted around 1603–4 for Vincenzo Giustiniani and certainly known to Orazio[1]—are frozen into a design of consummate sophistication. The effect is not so much of an arrested action, or the isolated frame of a narrative sequence, as of a tableau vivant: figures posed to simulate an action. This quality, so prominent in Caravaggio's paintings of the 1590s, was much censured by seventeenth-century critics, who strongly believed that a narrative should include indicators of time and continuity. They correctly saw the source of the problem in the practice of painting directly from the model. Caravaggio's late work demonstrates the degree to which he labored to overcome this perceived limitation.[2] Paradoxically, whereas in Caravaggio's mature Roman paintings it

is the harshly focused light that seems to arrest the action, mercilessly transfixing the notionally active poses of the figures in a timeless space, in Orazio's painting it is the figures that are still while the light sets up an animated play of transparent shadows and reflections. The sheer beauty of Orazio's effects of light and shadow and his emphasis on such purely formal devices as the carefully arranged folds of the drapery and the planar abstraction of the composition— an X amplified by a splendid interplay of diagonals and interlocking curves—might be thought of as a Caravaggesque equivalent to the idealistic style of Guido Reni. Something similar was already present in the Oslo *Judith and Her Maidservant* (cat. 13), but here the result is even more compelling because of the nature of the subject— and the sheer technical mastery.

This is not to say that the picture has no narrative interest. Quite the contrary. The action of the figure

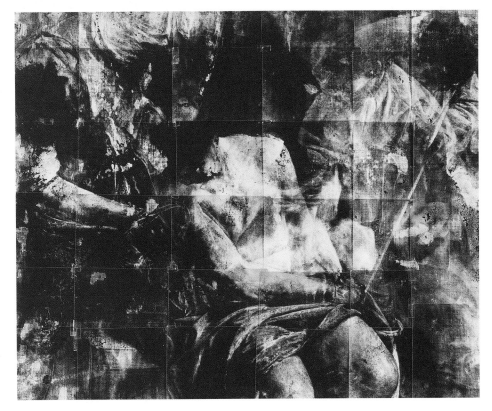

Figure 56. X radiograph of cat. 23

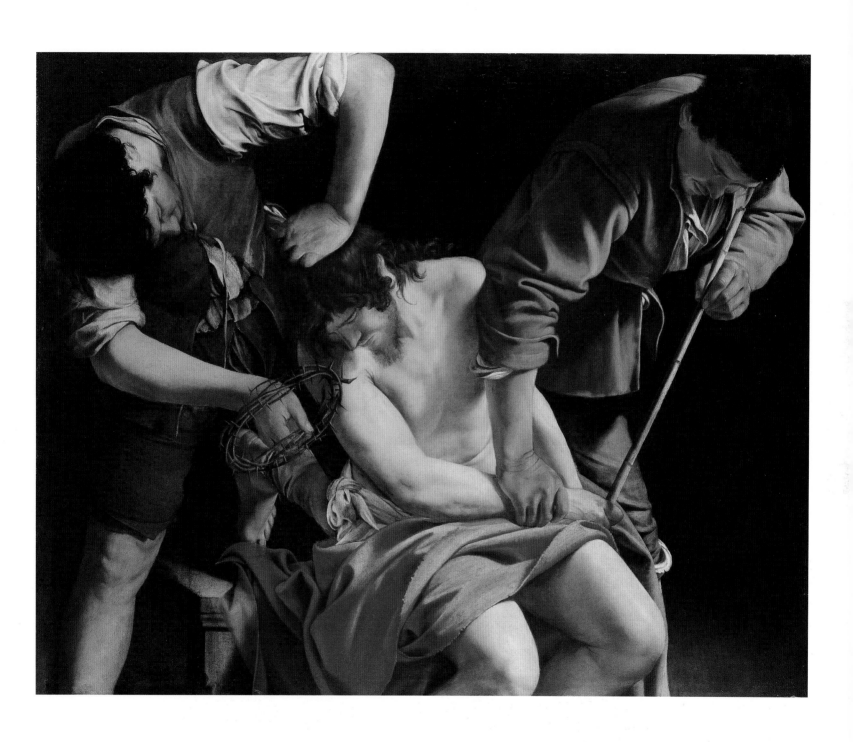

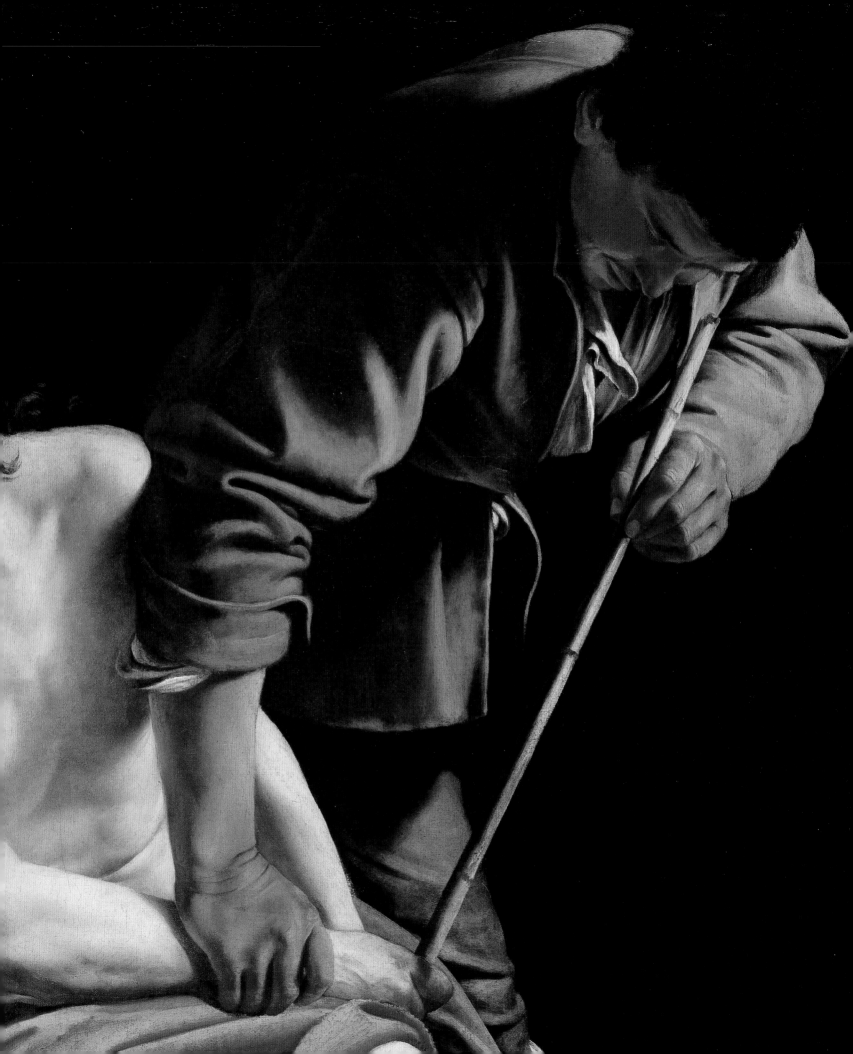

on the left, who jerks Christ's head back as he taunts him with the crown of thorns, is incomparably vivid, and the attention to the unlaced jerkin and pants, exposing his undergarments, provides a biting comment. The way the figure on the right roughly grips Christ's wrist to make him hold a mock scepter demonstrates just how familiar Orazio was with the psychology of torture. By comparison, the figures in Caravaggio's painting in Vienna seem almost archetypal. Caravaggio's canvas was not, of course, Orazio's sole point of reference. The elegance of the design and the unusual palette—brown, salmon, and green blue—suggest his awareness of the younger generation of Caravaggisti. But most important for his conception was the small, late etching by Annibale Carracci of the same subject (the possibility of this work as a source for Gentileschi is noted by Bissell). It is from this etching that Orazio took the contrapposto attitude of Christ and the actions of his two tormentors. Initially, the similarity was even closer, for X radiographs show that the right-hand figure originally moved toward Christ rather than away from him (fig. 56). This solution was adopted by Orazio for his frescoed decoration in the church of San Venanzio in Fabriano, which was painted after about 1613/15 (fig. 51).[3] Where Orazio departs most signally from Annibale's print is in dispensing with the armor for the left-hand figure (he perhaps found the image of the gauntlet-clad hand seizing Christ's hair too chilling) and in playing down the expressions by the use of foreshortening and lighting (Annibale's figures are truly brutes and bring into play the classical notion of heightened contrasts). When Orazio treated the theme later, in Genoa and London (see cat. 49), it was in a more demonstrative vein and without the quality of compressed energy or brilliant use of light.

The Braunschweig picture first came to public attention in 1977. Previously, the composition was known through what Schleier has demonstrated to be a replica. That work, published by Longhi in 1943 and included by him in the Caravaggio exhibition held in Milan in 1951, has most frequently been dated to shortly after 1610. This dating has been carried over to the Braunschweig painting as well, Bissell expanding the time frame to about 1610–15. It is my belief that the elegance of the composition and the brilliant treatment of light, with transparent shadows, indicate a date toward 1615. Far from epitomizing Orazio's most intensely Caravaggesque moment—exemplified by the *Way to Calvary* (cat. 5)—it marks his personal reinterpretation of the work of the artist he had befriended in the early years of the century, a reinterpretation emphasizing formal values derived, in part, from Bolognese models. The dating proposed here finds additional support from the reference to a "Crowning with thorns, 3 half-length figures, by Gentileschi, about 6 *palmi* in width," mentioned in two inventories of the Savelli collection in 1650. What is almost certainly the same work reappears in a 1693 inventory of the Chigi collection.[4] And indeed, Orazio was working for Paolo Savelli—unquestionably his principal Roman patron—from at least 1613.

Cusping around the perimeter of the canvas demonstrates that the audaciously tight cropping of the figures was intentional. Numerous pentimenti show Orazio constantly modifying details to obtain the right effect: the contours of Christ's right arm show changes; his red robe rises up to cover the toes of the torturer at the left; the right arm of the torturer at the right was altered. The hand holding the crown of thorns has been severely damaged, and indications of the *abbozzo* are visible in the sleeve of the right-hand torturer's right arm, as they are in the shadow of Christ's right arm.

1. The authorship of the Vienna *Christ Crowned with Thorns* has long been disputed. However, it is now established that it was purchased from the Giustiniani collection and is thus the painting cited by Bellori (1672) 1976, 222. See Rome–Berlin 2001, 288. A date of about 1603–4 seemed the most plausible when the work was shown at the Caravaggio exhibition in 1985 and has been adopted by Mina Gregori (in Florence 1991, 238–39).
2. The most famous criticism of the problems of creating a narrative from posed models is Mancini's; see pp. 11–12 in this publication.
3. In the 1613 roll of the Accademia di San Luca, Orazio is listed as "outside Rome." This is the earliest probable date for the frescoes in the chapel; see cat. 29 and pp. 124–25 in this publicaiton.
4. This is one of two works acquired by the Chigi from the Savelli. The other was a *Tobias and the Angel*; see cat. 27.
5. See Schleier (in New York–Naples 1985, 155–57), who analyzes the changes in the color scheme and composition.

24.

Saint Mary Magdalene in Penitence

Oil on canvas, 86⅝ × 61⅞ in. (220 × 157 cm)

Santa Maria Maddalena, Fabriano

ca. 1615

The life of Mary Magdalene—that paradigm of the converted sinner—culminates in a wilderness near Marseilles, where the former prostitute, who had washed Christ's feet with myrrh mingled with tears and dried them with her hair, took refuge in order to devote herself to penitence and reflection on heavenly things. In a desolate cave she spent the last thirty years of her life, borne aloft each day by angels to hear celestial music—her sole source of nourishment. In the Middle Ages, Mary Magdalene was often depicted as the consummate ascetic, her ravaged features veiled by her abundant hair. The Renaissance preferred her young and beautiful, to point up what she had renounced (fig. 68). Orazio's picture is conventional in showing the saint tearfully contemplating a crucifix, the jar of perfume with which she washed Christ's feet and anointed his body near her, and a book and skull (emblem of mortality) atop the stone that functions as a prie-dieu.

Painted for a small church dedicated to the Magdalene, this picture is usually considered the first of Orazio's commissions for the Marchigian town of Fabriano (but see Carloni, pp. 121–26). Emiliani, in his seminal article on Orazio's work in the Marches, dates the picture to about 1611—possibly a bit earlier—based on a signed and dated work by Giovanni Francesco Guerrieri (Cassa di Risparmio, Fano) that he believed was a derivation (in fact, the resemblance is generic rather than specific). Bissell has dated the painting to about 1605, which now seems too early, but he perceptively notes that "the rich play of mood-creating light is more fully realized than in any of Orazio's previous works, and the loving, even excessive attention to the details of the setting reveals the influence of the German painter Adam Elsheimer as it anticipates certain more mature pictures." Most interesting is Pizzorusso's suggestion of a date about 1615, based on a reconstruction of the circumstances surrounding the painting's commission.[1]

Situated outside the walls of the city, the small church or oratory of Santa Maria Maddalena functioned as the chapel of a hospital that was a dependency of the great Ospedale di Santo Spirito in Rome. Since 1557, it had also been the seat of the celebrated and powerful Università dei Cartai (the guild of paper makers in Fabriano), which had made Mary Magdalene its protector.[2] It would have been normal practice for the hospital or guild officials to seek a painter for the principal altarpiece of their church through the Roman institution with which they were associated. Between 1609 and 1617, Pietro Campori held the position of general preceptor (*primicerio*) of the Ordine degli ospedalieri di Santo Spirito; he was commendatore of Santo Spirito in 1616.[3] He would have had administrative charge of both the Roman hospital and its dependencies. Campori was a close associate of Paul V's, by whom he was made a cardinal in 1616. He had been the private secretary and then the majordomo for Scipione Borghese and would, in consequence, have known of Orazio's work in Scipione's casino and in the Palazzo del Quirinale. Moreover, in July 1611 Orazio had moved from the area between Santa Maria del Popolo and the Piazza di Spagna to Borgo Santo Spirito, on the other side of the Tiber and in the immediate neighborhood of the hospital. There was, then, ample opportunity for Campori to have established contact with him. Pizzorusso has reasonably conjectured that the commission was placed through Campori in 1615, when the Università dei Cartai officially affiliated itself with the Arciconfraternità di Santo Spirito. Commenting on this scenario, Carloni has suggested that 1615 might be taken as a *terminus ad quem* for the commissioning of the altarpiece, which could have been undertaken in anticipation of this formal affiliation. If this is so, the date of 1613, when Orazio is listed in the roll of the Accademia di San Luca as "outside Rome" ("fora de Roma"), assumes importance, though in truth there is no compelling reason that a picture of this sort should not have

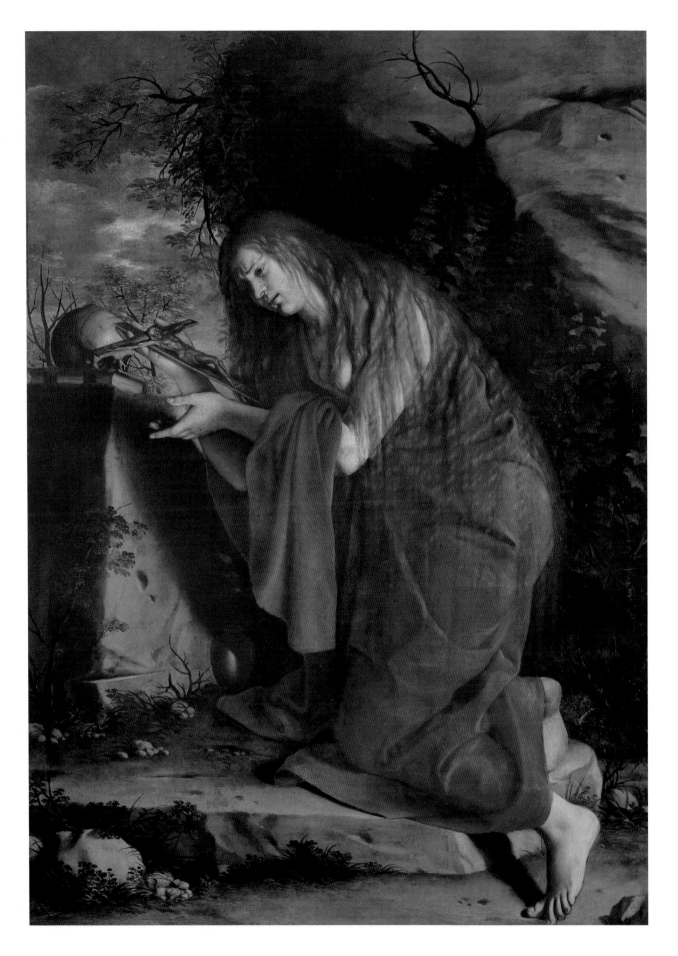

been commissioned and painted in Rome and sent to Fabriano. (The only works requiring Orazio's presence in the Marchigian city were the frescoes he undertook in the chapel of the Crucifixion in San Venanzio and those cited in an eighteenth-century manuscript as in a chapel in San Francesco, since destroyed.)[4]

The rigorously devotional aspect of the picture somewhat compromises direct stylistic comparisons with Orazio's other canvases, for the visual language of his altarpieces was in many respects strikingly different and more conservative than that of his paintings destined for private collectors. Still, the silvery lighting and striking still-life details do suggest a work from the middle of the second decade rather than earlier (taken in isolation, the crucifix, skull, and book seen against the trees might be thought to date from the nineteenth century). Pizzorusso rightly emphasizes the relationship of the landscape setting to that of the San Silvestro *Saint Francis* (cat. 25). Nowhere is the nature of Orazio's religious painting more conspicuous than in the attention he has lavished on the mass of silken hair, the furrowed brow, and the tears coursing down the saint's cheeks. These belong to a Counter-Reformation semiotics of penitence, to which Orazio gives brilliant visual expression: "Never, since life was lived, were received / From India or the Atlas pearls or gold / More beautiful than the tears of her fair eyes / Or the gold of her waving, outspread tresses"; "I lived blindly, but now unto you I open / My eyes filled with tears, my Sun, my God, / For your beams illuminate me and cause me to see / That the sweets of yesteryear were but poisons," in the words of two sacred sonnets set to music by Girolamo Frescobaldi (1583–1643).[5]

It is worth noting that in Fabriano, the Counter-Reformation writer Giovanni Andrea Gilio had initiated a tradition of composing poems about an image of Mary Magdalene painted by Gentile da Fabriano.[6] Yet, over and beyond the Counter-Reformation language of penitence, there is the matter of Orazio's personal response to the theme. Artemisia had had to defend herself against accusations of being a whore, and the 1612 trial had unquestionably taken a psychological toll on both father and daughter. Is the resemblance of the Fabriano Magdalene to Artemisia—or at least to those images thought to be like her—intentional?[7] And ought we to attach significance to the fact that the figure of Christ on the cross, so tenderly held in one hand and eloquently addressed with the other, turns its head away from the saint's pleading face (in the *Saint Jerome* [cat. 16], by contrast, it shares in the penitent's vision)?

1. Pizzorusso 1987, 72–73, and Pizzorusso in Fossombrone 1997, 58.
2. Molajoli 1990, 131.
3. On Campori, see especially Becker 1974 and De Angelis 1950, appendix.
4. See Emiliani 1958b, 57, and Carloni, pp. 124–25 in this publication.
5. "A pie della gran Croce," from the *Primo libro d'arie musicali,* and "Dove, dove sparir," from the *Secondo libro d'arie musicali,* both published in Florence in 1630. I have taken these from a Harmonia Mundi recording, *Canta la Maddalena* (2000).
6. For the sonnets, see Sassi 1923–24, 273–82.
7. Here, I am thinking not only of the woman with a fan who appears in Orazio's frescoes in the casino (frontispiece, p. 282), but even more of Artemisia's depictions of Susanna (cat. 51), Judith (cat. 55), and Lucretia (cat. 67). If the *Cleopatra* (cat. nos. 17, 53) is indeed by Orazio and depicts Artemisia, the issue of Orazio's response to a subject like that of the penitent Magdalene becomes even more complex. I do not wish to suggest that a biographical reading of this picture is key to understanding it, only that its expressive character may have a personal, biographical dimension—which is hardly contrary to the way Baroque images were intended to work upon the viewer's imagination.

PROVENANCE: Santa Maria Maddalena, Fabriano.

REFERENCES: Benigni (1728) 1924, 101; Marcoaldi 1873, 94 no. 52; Longhi 1927, 114; Molajoli 1930–31, 106 n. 4; Molajoli 1936, 128; Emiliani 1958a, 68; Emiliani 1958b, 43–44; Schleier 1962, 435; Moir 1967, vol. 1, 70–71, vol. 2, 77 no. E.10a; Aliberti Gaudioso in Urbino 1968, 90–92; Nicolson 1979, 53; Bissell 1981, 143; Zampetti in Ancona 1985, 213–15; Pizzorusso 1987, 59–61, 72; Molajoli 1990, 131; Nicolson 1990, 115; Zampetti 1990, 307 n. 21; Arcangeli and Pizzorusso in Fossombrone 1997, 41 n. 17, and 58–59; Bissell 1999, 190–91, 326, 346; Garrard 2001, 41–42.

25.

Saint Francis Receiving the Stigmata

Oil on canvas, 112¼ × 68⅛ in. (284 × 173 cm)

Ministero dell'Interno, Direzione Generale per gli Affari dei Culti, Rome

ca. 1616–20

PROVENANCE: Savelli di Palombara Chapel, San Silvestro in Capite, Rome.

RELATED PICTURE: See cat. 26.

REFERENCES: Giacchetti 1629, 59, 69; Baglione 1642, 360; Titi 1675, 213; Carletti 1795, 41; Federici 1899, 30; Longhi (1916) 1961, 228, 277; Voss 1925, 458, 461; Toesca 1960b, 286 n. 8; Schleier 1962, 435; Gaynor and Toesca 1963, 85–86; Moir 1967, vol. 1, 38 n. 68, 61 n. 150, vol. 2, 77 no. E.8b; Nicolson 1979, 53; Bissell 1981, 32, 35–36, 38, 163–64 no. 33; Strinati in Rome 1982–83, 93 no. 85; Pizzorusso 1987, 61; Nicolson 1990, 115; Contini 1996, 97–98.

Saint Francis is shown gazing in rapture at an unseen vision, his arms flung out in wonder as he turns from his devotional reading, his body describing an elegant arc against the jagged edge of the rocky grotto on Mount La Verna, where, before sunrise on September 14, 1224, he received the stigmata. A miraculous light illuminates his face, his hands and extended foot—marked by the stigmata—and the curving folds of his habit. The painting is one of Orazio's most arresting compositions and his only Roman altarpiece to earn the praise of Baglione, who remarked, "In the church of San Silvestro, a monastery of virgins, is admired the second chapel on the right, above the altar of which is Saint Francis receiving the stigmata, a very good figure, colored in oil." So far as we know, Orazio had received only two other commissions for altarpieces in Rome. One, of 1596, showed the conversion of Saint Paul, and by 1615 seemed so little worthy of note that Pietro Guicciardini overlooked it in his letter to the secretary of Grand Duke Cosimo II de' Medici, in which he gave a damning description of Orazio's reputation. (The altarpiece was destroyed by fire in 1823.) The other is the *Baptism of Christ*, commissioned by Settimio Olgiati in 1607 (cat. 11). This paucity of public commissions in Rome must be one of the reasons Orazio repeatedly sought employment elsewhere and ultimately moved to Genoa. It also accounts for the extraordinary care that went into this altarpiece.

Although not a large church by Roman standards, San Silvestro in Capite possesses a number of important relics and is one of the twenty principal abbeys in the city. Through the sponsorship of the Colonna family it had, in 1285, become home to a congregation of Poor Clares of the Franciscan order. Between 1596 and 1601, it was completely remodeled under the direction of Cardinal Dietrichstein. Orazio's altarpiece was part of this redecoration. The chapel in which it is located, the second on the right, was under the patronage of the Savelli di Palombara (recorded in a

plaque in the pavement).[1] Paolo Savelli, Orazio's chief patron from 1613, belonged to the Palombara branch of the Savelli and, like the rest of the family, was a supporter of the Franciscans: he and his wife, Caterina, founded a convent of Poor Clares in Albano, where she is buried, and from 1306 the Savelli maintained a chapel in Santa Maria in Aracoeli, where many members of the family are buried. Although there are no known documents that can be associated with the picture, the commission surely came from a member of the Savelli family, possibly Paolo himself.[2]

Since Guicciardini does not mention the altarpiece in his notorious letter of 1615, it was, as Bissell has noted, certainly installed after that date (Voss had dated it to 1600 and Longhi to 1612 or earlier). My own feeling is that the picture may well date to several years after 1616—that it follows the *Magdalene* at Fabriano (cat. 24), which documents now place at about 1615, and is roughly contemporary with the Santa Francesca Romana altarpiece at Urbino (cat. 30).

The picture is unusual in its depiction of Saint Francis in a semi- or quasi-kneeling pose. Contini identifies Orazio's source in a fresco of the Annunciation by the Lombard Giovan Battista Pozzo in Santa Maria Maggiore, Rome. This is a fresco that Orazio surely knew, since he had worked in the basilica a few years after Pozzo, but we may well wonder that Pozzo's work, conceived in a reformed Mannerist style, should have exerted any appeal at this date. For this reason it is important to underscore the fact that Pozzo's conception of the scene is dependent on two designs of the Annunciation by Michelangelo, one (Uffizi, Florence) showing the Virgin standing at a prie-dieu, the other (Pierpont Morgan Library, New York), seated. In the latter, the Virgin rests one arm on a table while, turning, she raises the other toward the angel in a gesture of surprise. The drawings were widely copied and became enormously influential, and it is hardly surprising that both Pozzo and Orazio should have turned to them

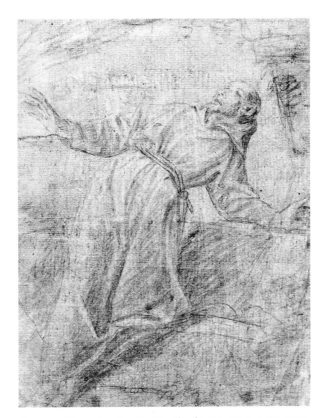

Figure 57. Copy after Orazio Gentileschi, *Saint Francis Receiving the Stigmata*. Red chalk and lead white on reddish paper. Location unknown

for inspiration. The thematic analogy between the Annunciation to the Virgin and the appearance of the seraph to Saint Francis may have led Orazio to these pictorial sources, but what he extracted from them was the use of a formal device—a contrapposto attitude—to signify spiritual revelation. By eliminating the seraph, he emphasizes the event as a mystical experience—of the saint inwardly transformed by love.[3]

In his brilliant exploitation of a nocturnal setting and divine illumination, it is possible that Orazio also responded to the innovative works of the Dutch Caravaggisti, above all of Gerrit van Honthorst. Indeed, there is a half-length Saint Francis tentatively ascribed to Van Honthorst (Cassa di Risparmio di Calabria e Lucania, Cosenza) that may have a bearing on the *Saint Francis* and serves as a link between

Orazio's picture and Caravaggio's much copied half-length *Magdalene in Ecstasy*, painted for the Colonna estates after the artist fled Rome in 1606 (the picture is known through copies).[4] In the abstract beauty of the pose Orazio has given to Saint Francis, there is something analogous to what his fellow Tuscan Francesco Mochi was doing in sculpture: a balance between *maniera* and what, in Gentileschi's work, was now only a residual attachment to Caravaggesque naturalism. (A comparison between Mochi's work and Gentileschi's has been made in the literature, but it is only at this stage of Orazio's career that it is truly meaningful.)[5] Orazio's is an elegant, reformed Caravaggism, utterly different from the Caravaggesque, low-life genre scenes that were so popular among collectors.

A small replica of the altarpiece (cat. 26) is said to have been owned by the Colonna family, which had strong attachments to the church of San Silvestro and was related to the Savelli (Andrea Palombara married Caterina Colonna in 1470; their arms decorate the dado in the chapel). A drawing that shows the figure of Saint Francis (fig. 57) was sold at Finarte, Milan (April 21–22, 1975, lot 177), where it was attributed to Orazio Gentileschi. The proportions of the figure are awkward, the draftsmanship crude, and the likelihood is that the drawing is a copy after the painting. However, Orazio must have carefully composed the composition through preparatory drawings like it. In this, too, he had abandoned his allegiance to Caravaggesque naturalism, with its emphasis on painting directly from the model.

In 1961, the repainted addition of a seraph was removed. As best as I can tell, the canvas has not been cut: cusping marks are visible on all sides.

1. See Forcella 1877, 84.
2. The attempt of Toesca (1960b, 286 n. 8) and Moir (1967, 38 n. 6) to associate this painting with the payment for a canvas made in 1609 must be rejected. On this, see Bissell 1981.
3. See Askew 1969, 286.
4. For the picture ascribed to Van Honthorst, see Papi 1999, 141–42.
5. See, for example, Borea 1966, n.p.

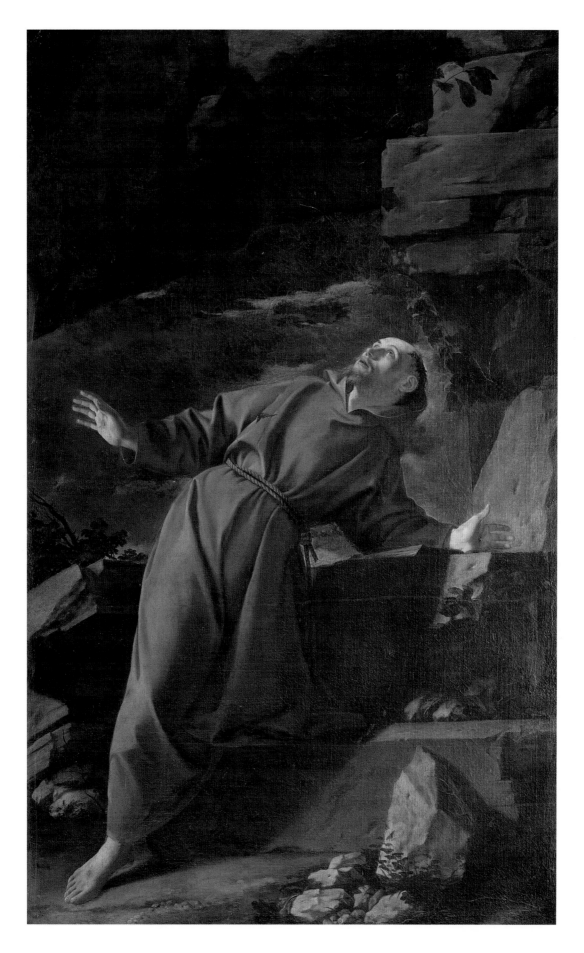

26.

Saint Francis Receiving the Stigmata

Oil on canvas, 30⅜ × 22 in.
(77 × 60 cm)

Private collection, loan
arranged courtesy of the
Matthiesen Gallery, London

ca. 1616–20

New York, Saint Louis

PROVENANCE: Galleria
Colonna, Rome (?); private collection, Switzerland; Matthiesen
Fine Art Ltd., London, 1984–87;
private collection (from 1987).

REFERENCES: Chiarini 1962,
26–29; Gaynor and Toesca 1963,
86; Moir 1967, vol. 1, 39, passim,
vol. 2, 77 no. E.8a; Nicolson
1979, 53; Bissell 1981, 164–65
no. 34; Strinati in Rome 1982–83,
93; London 1985, 68 no. 18;
Nicolson 1990, 115.

This beautiful *Saint Francis Receiving the Stigmata* bears much the same relationship to the San Silvestro in Capite altarpiece (cat. 25) as does the Berlin *David Contemplating the Head of Goliath* (cat. 18) to its prototype in the Galleria Spada (cat. 19). Aside from the different angle of the head and details such as the knotting of the cord and the tear in the habit where the saint received the stigmata, the figure is virtually the same. The setting, however, has been expanded and completely rethought to give the subject a more lyrical tone. Dawn colors the sky blue; the light is more pale; the rock formations have been reconceived so as to frame the saint and suggest a more hospitable environment; a different assortment of plants grows from the crevices and contrasts with the branches of dead shrubs; and behind the saint is a view of a flat, distant landscape. These changes bring the style of the picture closer to the *Saint Mary Magdalene in Penitence* in Fabriano (cat. 24). One further change makes clear the subtlety of Orazio's art: the viewing point has been raised, since the picture was not meant to be seen from the low vantage point of the altarpiece.

Chiarini has written that the Colonna family owned a small replica of the San Silvestro altarpiece. This cannot be confirmed; no picture similar to the one catalogued here is mentioned in the various seventeenth- and eighteenth-century Colonna inventories. In the 1756 inventory, there is listed in the collection of Caterina Salviati Colonna a half-length figure of Saint Francis "in the manner of Gentileschi."[1] Its measurement is given as 5 *palmi* (111.7 cm), including the frame, so it cannot be the picture shown here. On the other hand, the Colonna were closely associated with the church of San Silvestro, so it would not be surprising if they ordered a small version of Orazio's altarpiece. That it is a *modello* for the altarpiece seems highly unlikely in view of its fine facture.[2]

The picture has suffered from some abrasion and hence lacks the sharpness of the *David* and the *Saint Christopher* (cat. 27), which are on copper rather than canvas.[3] But it is no less delicate in its treatment and fully justifies Pietro Guicciardini's report to Cosimo II de' Medici's secretary that "in these [paintings on] alabaster and on other, small works, [Orazio Gentileschi] has diligently made some charming little pictures."[4]

1. Safarik 1996, 608 no. 36.
2. For this suggestion, see London 1985, 68.
3. Moir mistakenly published the *Saint Francis* as on copper.
4. See Crinò and Nicolson 1961, 144.

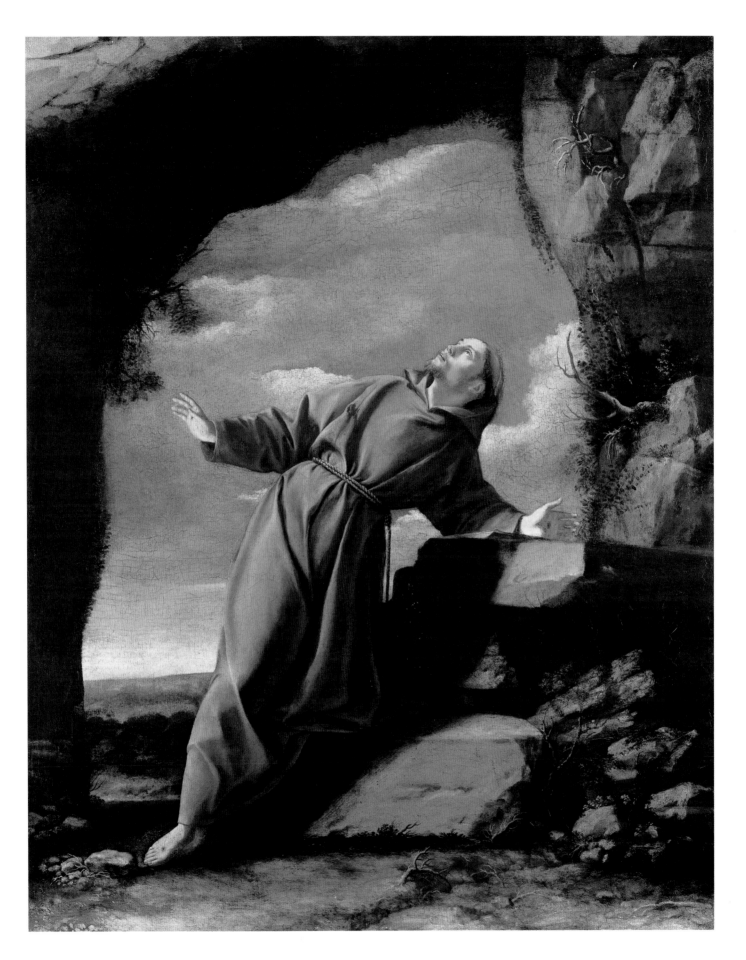

27.

Saint Christopher

Oil on copper, 8¼ × 11 in. (21 × 28 cm)

Staatliche Museen Preussischer Kulturbesitz, Gemäldegalerie, Berlin (inv. 1707)

ca. 1615–20

Rome, New York

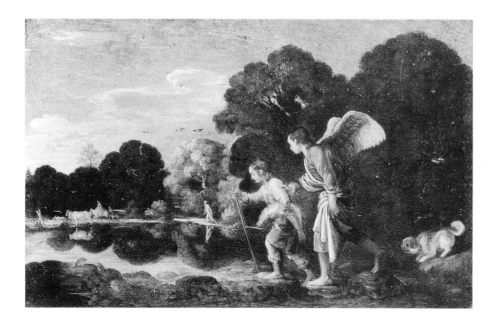

Figure 58. Adam Elsheimer (1578–1610), *Tobias and the Angel*. Oil on copper. Historisches Museum, Frankfurt am Main

We know nothing about the early history of this evocative depiction of the patron saint of travelers, whose Christian duty it was to ferry people over a treacherous river. (The child he bears is Christ, who one night appeared and requested this service; the saint nearly drowned from his weight.) The picture entered the Staatliche Gemäldegalerie as a work of the German painter Adam Elsheimer and was still accepted as such in Drost's 1933 monograph—six years after Longhi had put forward Orazio's name. So striking is the attention to light and atmosphere and the reflections in the icy water that another Elsheimer scholar, Weizsäcker, went so far as to attribute the work to the nineteenth-century Austrian landscape painter Ferdinand Georg Waldmüller (whose name had already been mentioned by Wilhelm von Bode and Frimmel in 1913)! Although there has been a consensus that the *Saint Christopher* is indeed by Orazio (see especially Schleier's detailed analysis in 1985), Bissell (1981) maintained that the picture must be by a landscape artist, probably German, from the circle of Elsheimer and Carlo Saraceni.

Elsheimer's importance for shaping Orazio's notion of landscape painting has been noted earlier (cat. 19).

More generally, his example may have inspired Orazio to experiment with the enamel-like brilliance that copper supports encourage. As remarked by Harris, here the connection is less with Elsheimer's *Saint Christopher* (Hermitage, Saint Petersburg), which is a vertical composition with a nocturnal setting, than with his *Tobias and the Angel* (fig. 58). In that work the two foreground figures are seen against distant trees that recede along a shoreline and are reflected in the still water. In certain respects, Orazio's picture is composed in a more artificial fashion, but it is more acute in its description of light and atmosphere and, ultimately, more naturalistic in feeling. The almost arbitrary fashion in which the trees on the opposite shore, their leaves glistening in the light, are increased in scale so as to set off the figures is indicative of a figurative artist's experimenting with an expanded landscape setting. Essentially, this effect is achieved in the small *David Contemplating the Head of Goliath* (cat. 58), where a rocky bluff is used for the same purpose. Yet whereas in the *David* the impression is of a studio-lit figure superimposed against a landscape backdrop, here a plein air, constantly shifting light unites landscape and figure and confers an effect of transience. It is the quality of a moment in time that accounts for the extraordinary modernity of the picture. In this respect, Orazio has surpassed his model.

Elsheimer was, of course, only one of several key figures in the development of landscape painting in the first decade of the century. His insistence on observation and optical verity had its counterpart in the structured, idealizing landscapes of Annibale Carracci and Domenichino. These two traditions reached a culmination in the years 1605–10, which saw the creation of Saraceni's four landscapes with mythological themes (Capodimonte, Naples), a series of brilliant, small-scale landscapes by Domenichino (for example, the *Landscape with Saint Jerome*, in the Glasgow Art Gallery), and the series of lunette-shaped pictures

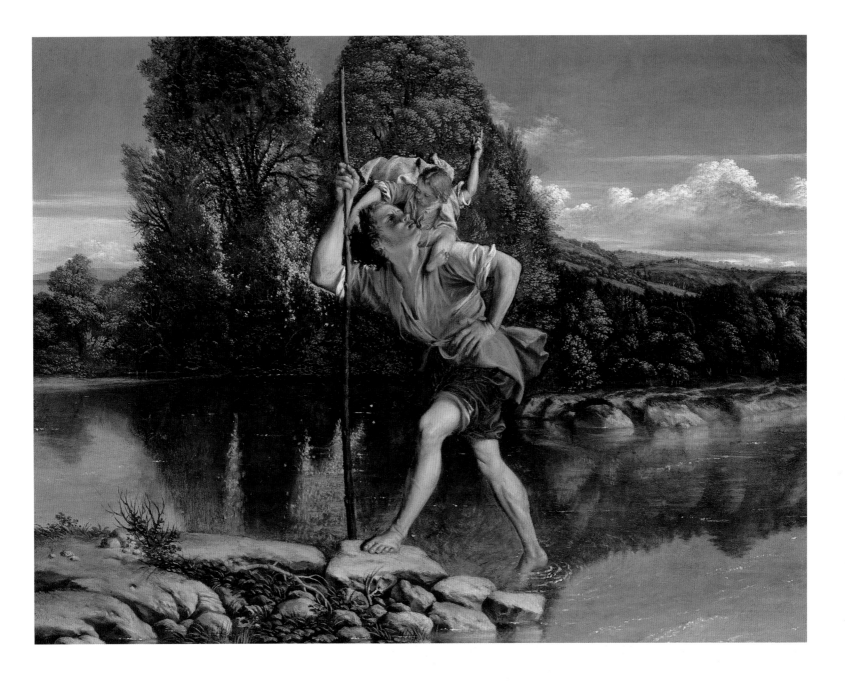

designed by Annibale Carracci for the private chapel of Pietro Aldobrandini (Doria Pamphili, Rome).

Another force in the development of landscape painting was the studio of Agostino Tassi, with whom Orazio worked in 1611–12. Saraceni had been in close touch with Tassi, and Giovanni Lanfranco collaborated with both in the Sala Regia of the Palazzo del Quirinale. The latter's marvelous landscape compositions for the Camerino degli Eremiti in the Casino Farnese (surviving canvases in the Capodimonte, Naples) may owe something to Tassi's influence, though their style is highly personal. In 1616 the German

painter Goffredo Wals, perhaps the most individual landscape artist after Elsheimer, also worked with Agostino.[1] It is with the naturalistic vision of Wals, with its sensitivity to light and its simple division between foreground, middle ground, and background, that Orazio's landscape bears closest comparison (Wals's *Rest on the Flight into Egypt*, in the National Museum of Western Art, Tokyo, which is dated 1619, is especially pertinent).

Orazio's participation in this moment of intense activity has received surprisingly little comment, since he remained first and foremost a figurative painter. Did

PROVENANCE: Balthasar von Hausschen, Vienna (inv. 1838, no. 84); possibly Feillers (according to an inscription on the back of the painting); Joseph Winter, Vienna (d. 1862); his daughter Auguste, Baronesse Stummer von Tavarnok, Vienna (from 1862); by descent, Baron Stummer von Tavarnok, Berlin (until 1913); Staatliche Museen Preussischer Kulturbesitz, Gemäldegalerie, Berlin.

REFERENCES: Frimmel 1913, 45–46; Longhi 1927, 112, 114; Voss 1929, 24–26; Drost 1933, 76–79; Milan 1951, 65 no. 105; Weizsäcker 1952, 71–74; Moir 1967, vol. 1, 39, 58, 76 n. 27, vol. 2, 77 no. E.5; Ottani Cavina 1968, 16–17; Bissell 1971, 287 n. 33; Waddingham 1972, 611 n. 56; Salerno 1977–80, vol. 1, 132–33; Schleier in Berlin 1978, 173–74 no. 1707; Nicolson 1979, 53; Bissell 1981, 207–8 no. x-21; Harris in New York 1985, 203; Schleier in New York–Naples 1985, 150–52; Nicolson 1990, 114; London–Rome 2001, 31.

the impetus for this development also owe something to his trip(s) to Fabriano beginning, it would seem, in 1613? The landscape in the *Saint Christopher* is certainly more evocative of the Marches than of the Roman campagna (see also cat. 24). The picture can be seen to anticipate the remarkable backgrounds that give a topographical dimension to the *Lot and His Daughters* (cat. 37) and the *Finding of Moses* (cat. 48). Regarding the latter, Weston-Lewis suggests that the river seen in the distance is the Thames.[2] This observation is crucial to understanding Orazio's frame of mind in his approach to landscape painting: not the Carracci-sanctioned notion of a perfected nature, but a Northern/Caravaggesque emphasis on direct observation. In 1927, Longhi alluded to the special place Orazio holds, when he remarked that if the Berlin *David* were shown together with the Vienna *Magdalene* (fig. 26), the two versions of *Lot and His Daughters* (cat. nos. 37, 42), the *Magdalene* in Fabriano (cat. 24), and the *Rest on the Flight into Egypt*, "they would create a superb introduction to the most subtle Dutch landscape painting of the middle of the seventeenth century." Might we see, in this instistence on observation and interest in light, a reflection of Orazio's contact with Galileo as well as, possibly, Galileo's Fabrianese correspondent, Francesco Stelluti?[3]

The small, informal format of the *Saint Christopher* seems to have encouraged Orazio to experiment, much as it did Saraceni and Lanfranco, but we should not make the mistake of thinking this was a unique work in his oeuvre. A Savelli inventory of 1631 lists a "Tobias by Gentileschi, on copper, with an ebony frame" ("Una tobia del Gentileschi in rame con cornice d'ebbano"), which was surely another essay in Elsheimer's landscape style; the *Tobias* must be the same picture described in the 1692 inventory of the Chigi collection as a nocturne "with a landscape."[4]

As the above comments suggest, although the *Saint Christopher* has been generally dated to about 1610—roughly contemporary with the *David* (cat. 19)—I prefer a date around 1615–20. Within Orazio's oeuvre, the picture seems to me to form a group with the *Rest on the Flight into Egypt* in Birmingham (cat. 34) and the *Madonna with the Sleeping Christ Child* in Cambridge (cat. 28). In their full mastery of a sharp yet atmospheric lighting—whether in an indoor or outdoor setting—and their keen feeling for surface description, these works belong to Gentileschi's final years in Rome, prior to his departure for Genoa. There was really nothing quite like them in contemporary Roman painting.

1. On Wals, see Repp 1985 and Röthlisberger 1995, 9–14.
2. Weston-Lewis in London–Bilbao–Madrid 1999, 44.
3. On the relationship of Galileo to Elsheimer, see Ottani Cavina 1976; for Stelluti, see Carloni, pp. 123–24 in this publication.
4. The Chigi inventory reads: "un Quadro in rame alto 2 (44,68 cm), e 1½ (33, 53 cm), cornice d'ebano, con due figurine, una d'un Angelo, con una Torcia accesa in mano, con Paese, mano del Gentileschi."

28.

Madonna with the Sleeping Christ Child

Oil on canvas, 39⅛ × 33½ in. (99.5 × 85 cm)

Fogg Art Museum, Harvard University Art Museums, Cambridge, Mass.; Gift of William A. Coolidge in memory of Lady Marian Bateman (1976.10)

ca. 1615–16

The *Madonna with the Sleeping Christ Child* is unquestionably Orazio's masterpiece of devotional painting. In it he represents a theme famously treated in the early sixteenth century by Raphael and Sebastiano del Piombo, in which the Virgin draws a transparent veil over her infant. In Raphael's much copied *Madonna di Loreto* (Musée Condé, Chantilly), the child is awake and reaches toward the Madonna (this work, then in the collection of Cardinal Sfondrato, had provided a point of departure for Orazio's earliest

devotional painting; cat. 1). In the two versions of Sebastiano's *Madonna del velo* (Capodimonte, Naples; Národni Galerie, Prague), he is asleep on a ledge, and the action of the Virgin acquires the sacramental significance of wrapping the dead Christ for burial. Orazio has greatly enriched the associative aspects of the theme by showing the child lying across the Virgin's lap, as in a Pietà, and the Virgin using her own veil to cover him. The child holds an apricot, which appears to be an erudite correction for the

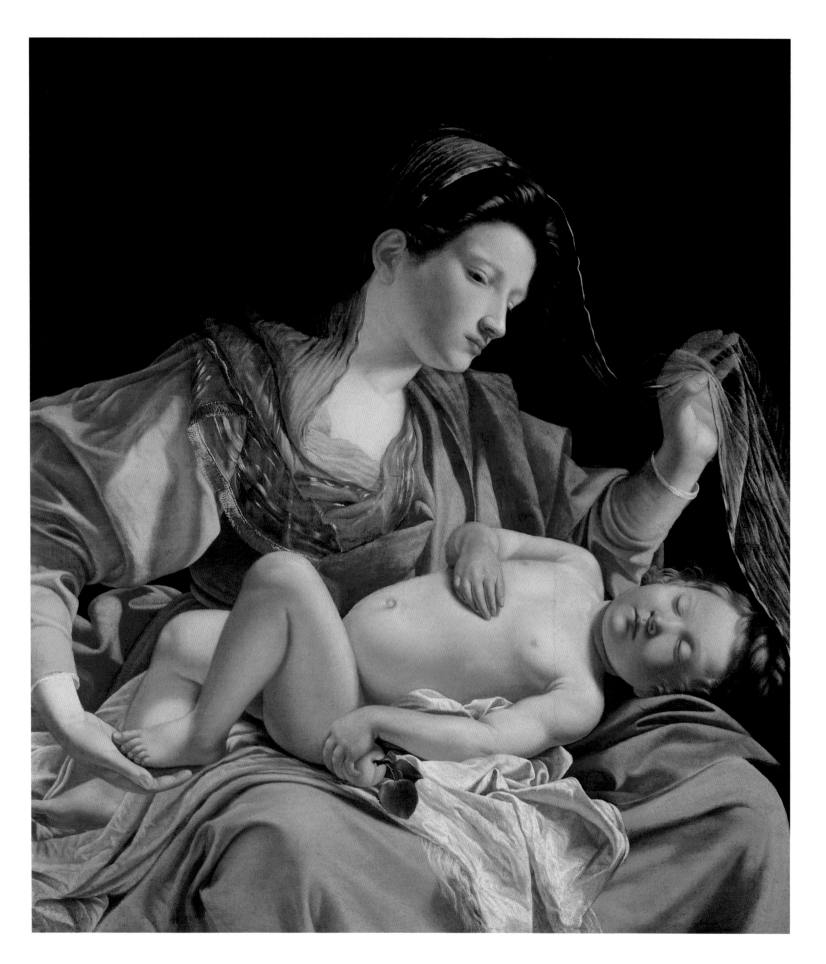

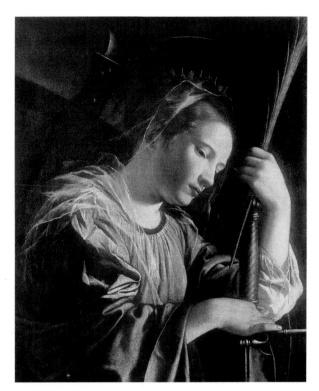

Figure 59. Orazio Gentileschi, *Saint Catherine of Alexandria*. Oil on canvas. Location unknown

PROVENANCE: Private collection, Milan (until 1931); Conte Alessandro Contini-Bonacossi, Florence (after 1931); Thomas Agnew and Sons, Ltd., London (until 1976); Fogg Art Museum, Harvard University Art Museums, Cambridge, Mass.

REFERENCES: Porcella 1931, 5–6; Longhi 1935, 5; Longhi 1943, 22, 46 n. 37; Moir 1967, vol. 1, 39, 57–58, 61, 65, vol. 2, 76 no. C.3; Freedberg 1976, 732–35; Moir 1976, 133 n. 222 vii; Nicolson 1979, 53; Bissell 1981, 38–39, 147, 158 no. 30, 165; Nicolson 1990, 114; Schleier 1993, 196; Giffi Ponzi 1994, 53–54; De Grazia and Garberson 1996, 104; Holmes in Bissell 1999, 178–79.

more common apple of Original Sin. In an unsurpassed analysis of the picture, Freedberg encapsulates its dense meaning as follows: "The body of Christ, in a sleep that foretells His offering in sacrifice, is revealed beneath the humeral veil upon his shroud, the cloth laid on an altar which is the broad lap of Mary Virgin, who is Mother Church." He is no less eloquent in characterizing the stylistic moment of the picture and its salient features: "With the Fogg *Madonna* and its chronological companions Orazio passed beyond dependence on the art of Caravaggio into a powerful and highly personal style, for which the prior assimilation of Caravaggism was a threshold. . . . The image combines majesty with seeming truth of actual existence, and grandeur with the closeness and particularity of a scene of genre."

Where, in my estimation, Freedberg errs is in assigning the painting a date of about 1610, as previously suggested by Longhi, who, however, had mistakenly identified the picture with a *Madonna a sedere con il bambino in braccio*, which Gentileschi painted for Duke Vincenzo Gonzaga in 1609–10. That work must have been a version of—or at least similar to—the

Madonna and Child in Bucharest (cat. 15). A greater difference between two works that treat the same theme is difficult to imagine: one an essay in *verismo*, in which sacred history is envisaged in terms of the everyday; the other a grandly articulated, formal statement, in which gesture, expression, and costume assert a realm beyond that of ordinary experience.[1] Bissell has argued for a date in the mid teens, which seems to me the more likely.

In his analysis, Freedberg draws analogies with the *David Contemplating the Head of Goliath* in the Galleria Spada (cat. 18)—a work that demonstrates a concern for formal pose but is altogether more naturalistic—and, more specifically, with the *Judith and Her Maidservant* in Hartford (cat. 39), a picture that was probably painted about 1621–24, when Orazio was in Genoa. Recently, Giffi Ponzi has suggested that the Fogg painting, too, is a Genoese work. It is, however, difficult to believe that a picture of this originality and beauty would not have been noted by our primary sources on Genoese painting, Soprani and Ratti, or listed in the inventory of one of Orazio's Genoese patrons. It is my feeling that the monumental effect of the Fogg *Madonna*—due as much to the structural clarity of the folds of the drapery as to the close cropping of the image—marks it as a Roman work, an argument supported by the fact that the *Madonna and Child* in the Cini Foundation, Monselice, by an anonymous Roman artist clearly derives from Orazio's painting. A number of Madonna and Child compositions by Orazio are listed in seventeenth- and eighteenth-century Roman inventories. One was owned by the Olgiati family, another—"una Madonna grande col Putto"—was owned by Ippolita Ludovisi, principessa di Piombino, and a third was listed in 1650 as part of the Savelli collection.[2] Whether any of these was the Fogg picture cannot be determined.

Longhi referred to the Fogg painting as "almost a Bronzino turned Caravaggesque," and this perfectly describes Orazio's newfound equipoise between his pre-Caravaggesque, Mannerist training and his experience of the art of the great Lombard. The black background is suggestive of slate—the support Sebastiano had chosen for his *Madonna del velo*, and which was enjoying renewed popularity in Rome following the arrival in 1614 of Alessandro Turchi, Pasquale Ottino, and Marcantonio Bassetti.

As Freedberg observes, there is "not just a deviation from Caravaggio's persistently classicizing model, but in a sense a development beyond it, towards a quality of baroqueness." Orazio can hardly have been unaware of the new directions signaled by Domenichino's cycle of frescoes devoted to the life of Saint Cecilia in San Luigi dei Francesi, of 1611–14, or of Giovanni Lanfranco's canvases in the Buongiovanni chapel of Sant'Agostino, of 1616, all of which posit a new dynamic between the actively posed figures and the space they inhabit. It is the Fogg *Madonna*, with its cold, somewhat abstract beauty—"dalla bellezza gelida e lontana," as Giffi Ponzi writes—that sets the stage for Orazio's achievement in Genoa. For this reason, it is worth noting that the sheer veil with gold stripes, gold edging, and a gold fringe would become one of his favorite props, recurring in the *Danaë* (cat. 36), the Turin *Annunciation* (cat. 43), the *Public Felicity* (cat. 44), and in various versions of the *Rest on the Flight into Egypt* (cat. 45).

After 1615, Gentileschi articulates a new relationship between art and nature. Drawing rather than painting from life seems to inform the abstracting tendency in his work. Of course, drawing from a posed model was hardly novel. What is new is the way Orazio brings this practice into line with his experience of Caravaggio. Building a repertory of carefully observed heads and hands enabled him to concentrate on formal relationships while maintaining a naturalistic effect. None of these drawings have survived, and the practice must be deduced from the habit he developed of recycling the heads of female models in a number of paintings. A *Saint Catherine of Alexandria* (fig. 59), for instance, repeats the features and angled placement of the Madonna in the Fogg painting and must have been taken from the same drawing (for other examples of this practice, see pp. 20–21).[3]

The picture is painted on three pieces of canvas. There is marked cusping on all sides, and the picture retains its original dimensions.[4]

1. It should be noted that Freedberg does not mention the Bucharest *Madonna and Child* and was uncertain about the attribution of the *Saint Jerome* published by Longhi (see cat. 16). Knowledge of these works would have transformed his analysis.

2. For these pictures, see Bissell 1981, 218, and De Marchi 1987, 150, 281. The Savelli painting measured 4 × 3 *palmi*, or about 88 × 66 cm. Measurements in seventeenth-century inventories are notoriously imprecise: the measurements of the *Saint Cecilia* in Washington (cat. 31) are given as 3 × 5 *palmi*, whereas it measures 87.5 × 108 cm.

3. See Schleier 2000, 169–70.

4. First reported by De Grazia and Garberson (1996, 104). I am less sure about the main canvas having been prestretched and primed, as I saw no dramatic evidence of cusping along the seam of the main canvas, which runs vertically to the right of the Virgin's head, top to bottom. Extra gesso was applied to fill the seams.

29.

Crucifixion

Oil on canvas, 12 ft. 7/8 in. × 6 ft. 10 5/8 in. (368 × 210 cm)

Cathedral of San Venanzio, Fabriano

ca. 1613–18

New York, Saint Louis

Despite the severe damage this painting has suffered, it remains one of Orazio's most impressive works—striking for the archaic simplicity of its composition, the tragic nobility of the figures, and the expressive use of light. Behind Christ, his head bowed in death, the clouds have parted to reveal a heavenly radiance, as though in response to the earthquake that, we are told in the Gospel account, released "many bodies of the saints which slept" (Matt. 27:52). A yellow-tinted evening sky brightens the horizon beyond the crest of Golgotha (Mark 15:42), while the figures of Mary, John, and Mary Magdalene (John 19:25–26), still shrouded in the darkness that, from the sixth to the ninth hour, enveloped the land (Matt. 27:45; Mark 15:33), are illuminated by a shaft of light falling from outside the picture. The gestures of

Mary and John, often contrasted in depictions of the Crucifixion, here mirror each other, though the beloved disciple looks up at Christ while the Virgin looks downward, solemnly averting her gaze. Mary Magdalene's ritualistic embrace of the cross takes on special poignancy, as her face is not juxtaposed with Christ's feet but is pressed against the bare wood; the elevation of Christ on the cross heightens the effect of abandonment. (The conventional juxtaposition of the Magdalene's head with Christ's feet alludes to her having washed his feet and dried them with her hair as an act of atonement.) Nothing could be further from the emotionalism of Federico Barocci's great altarpiece for the cathedral of Genoa, dated 1596, on the one hand, or the rhetorical eloquence of Guido Reni's 1619 *Crucifixion* for the Capuchins in Bologna (Pinacoteca Nazionale, Bologna), on the other. As Voss notes, the most relevant analogy for the stark composition is Scipione Pulzone's *Crucifixion* in the Chiesa Nuova in Rome—a work that Orazio must have known well and that exemplifies the devotional concerns of the Counter-Reformation.[1] The figure of Saint John in Pulzone's picture, shown from the back with arms outflung, his drapery falling in sharply modeled folds, derives from the dramatic *Crucifixion* that Titian painted for the church of San Domenico in Ancona, and there is a strong possibility that Titian's picture, much admired by Vasari, also provided a reference point for Orazio.

Whatever his pictorial sources, Orazio has re-created the Crucifixion not as a dramatic event but as a meditation—"a prolonged pause, full of the silence of spiritual events," in the words of Emiliani.[2] It is this effect of stilled quiet that sets the picture apart from so much Baroque imagery and suggests an archaizing intention that has reminded some viewers of fifteenth-century painting.

Our understanding of the visual language of the *Crucifixion* is tied up with the frescoed decorations of the chapel for which it serves as an altarpiece: the fourth on the left in the cathedral of San Venanzio in Fabriano. Orazio frescoed the walls and vault with scenes of Christ's Passion (figs. 50, 51). There are no documents that relate directly to the chapel, but a general time frame for the frescoes and altarpiece has been established by Emiliani and Bissell. Prior to 1601, the Urbino architect Muzio Oddi was preparing designs for the modernization of the medieval building. The project was approved in 1607, and by 1615 there is a notice that the roof was finished and the church nearly completed; a dedicatory inscription on the interior facade records the date 1617. Four years earlier, on November 7, 1613, the Arte dei Calzettai (or hosiers' guild) was assigned the second chapel on the left, dedicated to Saint Charles Borromeo, and was charged with commissioning an altarpiece and installing it within four years. This action was linked to severe earthquakes the preceding year, during which the saint's aid was invoked and an annual procession in his honor instituted.[3] Presumably, Orazio was commissioned to decorate the chapel of the Crucifixion sometime after 1613/15; he may have completed it about 1617, though this really is no more than conjecture. Carloni suggests that Francesco Stelluti may have played a role in promoting Orazio to the Vallemani family, who she convincingly argues were the patrons of the chapel (see pp. 123–24).

A persistent theme in the critical literature on Orazio's frescoes concerns the possible influence on them of fifteenth-century Florentine painting. Mezzetti, in 1930, wrote of "recollections of ancient Florentine elegance," while Voss, writing in 1960, drew analogies between Orazio's frescoes and those of Piero della Francesca and Masaccio. Building on these observations, Bissell has suggested a trip to Florence in 1616, when Orazio's name is cited in the register recording Artemisia's matriculation in the Accademia del Disegno.[4] (However, in 1633 Orazio declared that he had not been to Florence for fifty-five years.) In both the frescoes and the *Crucifixion*, Gentileschi's art shows a distinctively reductive approach to composition, but I remain unconvinced that this is the result of his study of quattrocento Florentine art. There seem to me to be more pertinent late-sixteenth-century and Caravaggesque models that Orazio could have drawn on, as well as the engravings of Dürer, which Voss argues he also studied (as did many artists throughout the sixteenth and seventeenth centuries). The key issue here is Orazio's development of a Counter-Reformation narrative style that draws in equal

PROVENANCE: Chapel of the Crucifixion, cathedral of San Venanzio, Fabriano.

REFERENCES: Benigni (1728) 1924, 96; Marcoaldi 1873, 95 no. 56; Voss 1925, 460–61; Mezzetti 1930, 546; Molajoli 1936, 94–95; Molajoli, Serra, and Rotondi 1936, 78; Emiliani 1958b, 51–52; Voss 1960–61, 99–107; Moir 1967, vol. 1, 72–74, vol. 2, 76 no. c.4; Nicolson 1979, 52; Bissell 1981, 159–62 no. 32a; Nicolson 1990, 114; Zampetti 1990, 297–98.

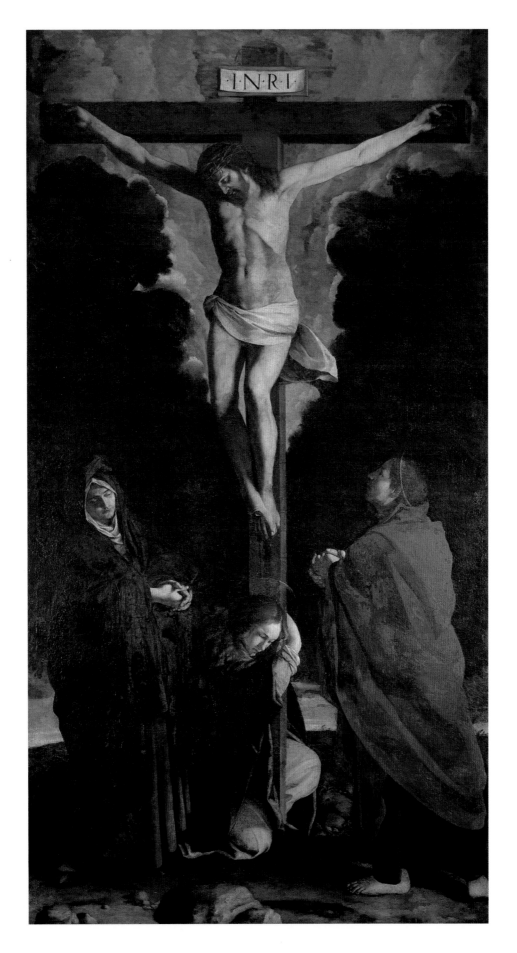

measure on Caravaggesque realism and Bolognese classicism and reflects as well his training in Rome in the 1580s and his essentially conservative approach to spatial composition. Domenichino's contemporary frescoes in the Nolfi chapel in the cathedral of Fano, painted in 1618–19, show a similar archaistic tendency—"a distinctively simple style, a mood more tranquil in its neo-Renaissance, plain piety than had existed before," observes Spear.[5] This analogy raises the possibility that both artists accommodated their styles to suit what they may have viewed as a more conservative clientele—though the variety of artists commissioned to do work for the Marches seems rather to testify to a remarkable openness. It would, in any case, be wrong to underestimate the fundamental modernity of the work Orazio produced for San Venanzio.

In the fresco of the Agony in the Garden, the foreground is audaciously set by the cutoff figures of three sleeping apostles—the kind of Baroque device we might expect of Lanfranco (for example, his *Agony in the Garden,* in San Giovanni dei Fiorentini, Rome, painted about 1622–23), except that Orazio does not use extreme foreshortenings or illusionistic effects. The composition of the *Crowning with Thorns* is intimately bound up with the great canvas at Braunschweig (cat. 23), which no one would characterize as "archaistic." The truly innovative and modern aspect of both the frescoes and the *Crucifixion* resides in Orazio's handling of light, a light that has a crystalline purity and confers on the figures a quality of physical presence that is key to their devotional affect. The play of the light and shadow on the face and clasped hands

of the Virgin at once affirms her actuality and bestows on her the statuesque immobility of a cult object. The model for this achievement was obviously Caravaggio's *Madonna di Loreto*, in the church of Sant'Agostino, except that Orazio's figure conveys greater vulnerability and a less heroic humanity, retaining the quality of a real individual. As commented on elsewhere (cat. nos. 30, 31), the young woman who posed for the Magdalene was also used by Orazio for other pictures. The primary differences between the frescoes and the altarpiece result from the media employed and the effects Orazio sought: a quality of largeness and sculptural solidity in the altarpiece, with saturated colors and dramatic contrasts of light; elegance of design and diffused lightness and transparency in the frescoes. These features seem to me to suggest a date for the chapel decorations—for both the frescoes and the altarpiece—of about 1613–18. The picture has been restored with the generous support of Abramo Galassi.

1. See the evocative and insightful description in Zeri 1957, 80–81.
2. Emiliani 1958b, 51: "Un prolungato tempo di posa, colmo di silenziosi eventi spirituali, par dominare la scena."
3. The resulting altarpiece is by Giovanni Francesco Guerrieri, though it includes a strikingly Gentileschian flying angel that has led to the plausible suggestion that Orazio may have received the commission and begun but not finished the altarpiece. On this see, most recently, Zampetti in Fossombrone 1997, 60, and Carloni, p. 125 in this publication.
4. For a discussion of the different opinions that have been voiced regarding Orazio's name in Artemisia's matriculation in the Accademia in Florence, see Bissell 1999, 399–400 n. 24.
5. Spear 1982, 61.

30.

Vision of Saint Francesca Romana

Oil on canvas, 106¼ × 61⅞ in.
(270 × 157 cm)

Galleria Nazionale delle
Marche, Urbino

ca. 1614/1618–20

Although she was canonized by Paul V only in 1608 (she was beatified in 1460), Saint Francesca Romana (1384–1440) had long been the object of a cult, having founded an association of noblewomen, who in 1433 formed the Oblate Congregation of Tor de' Specchi at the foot of the Capitoline, in Rome.

Within just a few years of her death, a series of panels recording scenes from her life—especially her many visions—was painted, probably for the Roman Olivetan church of Santa Maria Nuova, and a couple of decades later the old church of Tor de' Specchi was decorated with a similar cycle of frescoes. The vision

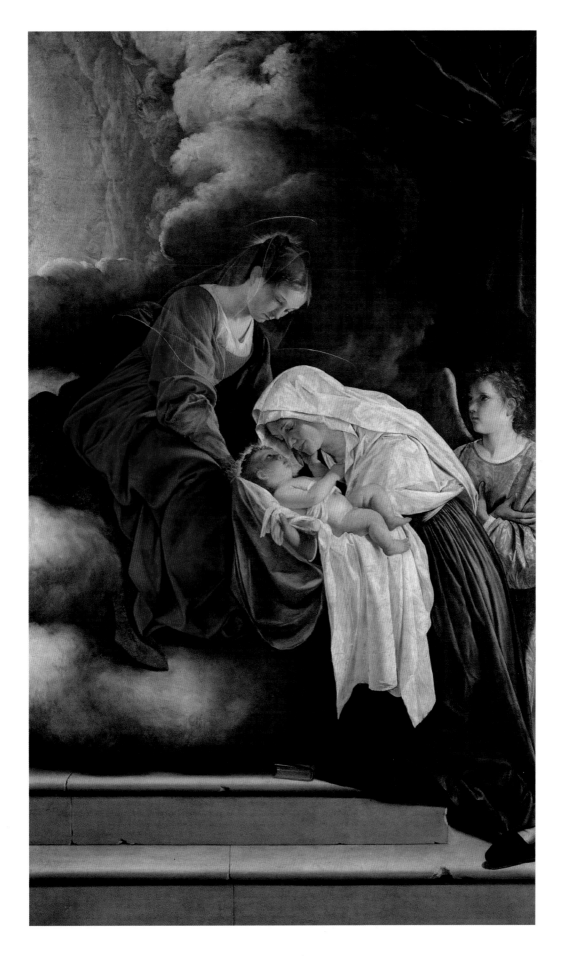

Orazio depicts, in which the Virgin has granted the saint the privilege of holding the infant Christ, is shown in both cycles and is also recounted, in five different episodes of her life, in a contemporary biography.[1] The inscription beneath the fresco that depicts this scene reads, "How the blessed Francesca, being in a beatific vision as she so often was, saw the eternal God in the arms of the glorious Virgin his mother and how he deigned to come into her arms." This type of mystical experience, with its combination of the physical and the visionary, was especially congruent with seventeenth-century spirituality. The angel who appears with Francesca Romana is her guardian angel, who, according to hagiographic sources, accompanied her as a divine favor.

The altarpiece, among Orazio's most beautiful, comes from the Olivetan church of Santa Caterina Martire in Fabriano, where it is mentioned in early-eighteenth-century guides. The church was extensively restored between 1590 and 1620, and Orazio's altarpiece was doubtless part of the renovation. This would point to a date toward the end of his activity in the Marches, as Gamba and Longhi recognized on the basis of style in their groundbreaking essays of 1922–23 and 1927 (both, however, misidentified the saint as Clare). By contrast, Carloni argues for a date prior to 1615 (see pp. 126–27). How much time Orazio actually spent in Fabriano remains a matter of speculation; his last probable trip to the Marches was in 1619, when Cardinal Bevilacqua put his name forward to fresco the tribune of the church of Sant'Ubaldo in Pesaro. Of course, the altarpiece could well have been painted in Rome as late as about 1620 and then sent to Fabriano.

As with Orazio's other Marchigian commissions—most particularly his frescoed decorations for a chapel in San Venanzio, Fabriano—the simplicity of the composition and emphasis on detailed description have elicited speculation about the possible influence of Florentine art, either that of Santi di Tito (Gamba) or that of fifteenth-century painting (Bissell). Echoes of the Marchigian work of Lorenzo Lotto have also been noted (see especially Emiliani). There is something to be said for each of these suggestions, insofar as they attempt to address the special visual language

Orazio employs to convey that quality of the everyday pervaded by the divine. What needs to be stressed is that this visual language is closely bound up with Counter-Reformation attitudes toward religious art that Orazio surely learned in Rome in the 1580s and that must have been even more pertinent in Fabriano, the hometown of Giovanni Andrea Gilio da Fabriano (d. 1584), one of the most conservative critics of artistic practice.[2] Gilio's dialogue on the abuses in art, which appeared in 1564, puts forward the twin principles of faithfulness to the historical—that is, biblical or hagiographic—source and the sense of decorum, or appropriateness. Despite many of his extreme positions—especially his famous diatribe against Michelangelo's *Last Judgment* in the Sistine chapel—his notion that good painting should inspire feelings of "chastity, purity, and reverence for religion" in the beholder had widespread resonance and is clearly pertinent to Orazio's altarpiece.[3]

Gilio urged artists to return their craft to its first purity ("la sua purità primiera") and to strive for truth and beauty by painting simply and purely ("farlo semplice e puro, perché mescolarlo col poetico e finto altro non è che un difformare il vero et il bello").[4] These were not hollow phrases, for he wrote a laudatory poem about a representation of Mary Magdalene by the celebrated early Renaissance painter Gentile da Fabriano.[5] Gilio's legacy may have been particularly strong in Fabriano, but we have only to think of certain works by Guido Reni (his 1628–29 *Annunciation* at Ascoli Piceno, for example), Guercino (the *Madonna of the Rosary* in the church of San Marco, Osimo, to pick one of his numerous Marchigian commissions), or Sassoferrato—that proto-Nazarene pupil of Domenichino's—to realize the strength of this current in seicento painting and, most important, its basis in Raphaelesque classicism. In the case of Orazio's *Vision of Saint Francesca Romana* there is the added fact that the iconography is based not simply on a literary text but on fifteenth-century images accessible to him. On all these counts, this altarpiece may be said to encapsulate the various strands that run through all his religious commissions in the Marches.

The composition, with the seated Virgin appearing to the kneeling saint from a bank of clouds, was fairly

PROVENANCE: Church of Santa Caterina Martire, Fabriano (until about 1798); Abbot Silvestro Marcellini, Fabriano (1798–1821); Carlo Rosei, Fabriano; Agabiti Rosei (by 1936); Galleria Nazionale delle Marche, Urbino.

RELATED PICTURE: *Head of Saint Francesca Romana* (copy; formerly Milan, Bonomi collection).[9]

REFERENCES: Benigni (1728) 1924, 98; Marcoaldi 1873, 94 n. 53; Longhi (1916) 1961, 231–32; Gamba 1922–23, 256; Voss 1925, 461; Longhi 1927, 114 n. 1; Molajoli 1936, 132; Emiliani 1958b, 52–53; Moir 1967, vol. 1, 72–73, passim, vol. 2, 76 no. c.5; Nicolson 1979, 53; Bissell 1981, 35–37, 40, 70, 76, 165–66 no. 36, 167–69, 208; Zampetti in Ancona 1985, 216–17; Pizzorusso 1987, 73; Nicolson 1990, 114; Zampetti in Sassoferrato 1990, 25; De Grazia and Schleier 1994, 68, 73.

common. It was, for example, the way Domenichino showed the Virgin appearing to Saints Nilius and Bartholomew in his fresco at the abbey of Grottaferrata, and the way he depicted the Virgin appearing to Saint Anthony, who holds the Christ child, in a small painting in the Musée de Toul.[6] The Domenichinos are of interest because of their domestic simplicity. Where Orazio differs most significantly from the rudimentary classicism of Domenichino is in his treatment of the event as an actual occurrence—*vero* rather than *verisimile*—as experienced by the saint herself (here, again, we note the pertinence of Gilio's ideals).

A curtain has been drawn back. The steps—their nicks and joins emphatically described—about the picture plane, establishing a shallow stage. The simple, cloglike slippers and prayer book of Francesca Romana, like her matronly features, create the impression of the everyday world interrupted by a visionary experience. Behind the vaporous clouds that fill the room and support the Virgin is a glimpse of the golden light of the heavenly hosts (a device Raphael had famously used in his *Sistine Madonna*, then in the church of San Sisto, Piacenza). This diaphanous, angelic radiance, like the depiction of the child as an eight-month-old baby, is a precise realization of the relevant passage in Giovanni Mattiotti's fifteenth-century biography of the saint: "Post haec ductus fuit in aliam maiorem lucem, in qua plures angelici spiritus existebant . . . In qua quidem luce celestis Regina, Filium Dei et suum in bracchiis tenens quantum ad humanitatem parvulum fere in etate octo mensium, stabat."[7] The genius of Orazio is to have drawn a contrast between this divine radiance and the very real, sharp light that falls across the figures in the foreground, creating a magical play of shadows on the faces of the saint and the infant Christ, who raises one hand affectionately. As Longhi wrote in 1916, "Not since some hints were given in the work of Lotto . . . had one seen a work so complex, in which the framework of style, the cohesion

of art, is established not by the juxtaposition of areas of color, as in Venetian painting of the early cinquecento, but through scaled relations of luminosity in the colors."[8] This new kind of pictorial unity—"pittura di valori"—Longhi saw as the basis of modern painting. We might say that in this work, Caravaggesque realism has acquired a devotional, as well as aesthetic, character.

The Virgin has the beauty not of the Queen of Heaven but of an ordinary young woman. The model must have captivated Orazio, since he used her for the Magdalene at the foot of the cross in the *Crucifixion* he painted for the cathedral of Fabriano (cat. 29) and for the *Saint Cecilia with an Angel* (cat. 31). Even in the Virgin in the *Annunciation* he sent from Genoa to Carlo Emanuele I, duke of Savoy (cat. 43), there seems to be an echo of this entrancing young woman.

Pizzorusso has noted that between 1616 and 1618, the abbot general of the Olivetans, Ippolito Borghese, was a member of the Sienese branch of the Borghese family. The order's protector was Scipione Borghese, cardinal-nephew to Paul V Borghese. Given the devotion of the pope to the saint, the commission to Orazio may have come through his former patrons in Rome, although by this time he was certainly a well-known figure in Fabriano. This circumstantial evidence would seem to support a date for the altarpiece around 1618. Carloni, however, has argued for a date prior to 1615, based on the motif of the steps in an altarpiece by Guerrieri that was finished in that year (fig. 55). She notes that from 1611, the cardinal-protector of the Olivetans was Sfondrato (see p. 126).

1. See Rossi 1907, 8, and Kaftal 1948, 54.
2. On Gilio, see Di Monte 2000, 751–54.
3. Gilio in Barocchi 1960–62, vol. 2, 79.
4. Ibid., 38–39.
5. See Sassi 1923–24, 275.
6. See Spear 1982, 164 no. 35ix, 229 no. 77.
7. Vision XIII: see Romagnoli 1994, 439.
8. Longhi (1916) 1961, 231.
9. See Bissell 1981, 208 no. X-23.

31.

Saint Cecilia with an Angel

Oil on canvas, 34⅝ × 42½ in. (87.8 × 108.1 cm)

National Gallery of Art, Washington, D.C., Samuel H. Kress Collection (1961.9.73)

ca. 1618–21

From 1621 onward, Orazio frequently repeated his most successful compositions, often, it would seem, with the aid of a tracing from the prime version (see pp. 20–30) and taking only a limited part in their realization. He also used portions of one work as a point of departure for others. This occurs in the Fogg *Madonna with the Sleeping Christ Child* (cat. 28), where the figure of the Virgin was recycled as a Saint Catherine, and in the *Judith and Her Maidservant*, in which the head of Judith served as a model for that of a female musician (cat. nos. 39, 40). Far from being merely a shorthand working method, the process underscores Orazio's interest in the variation of formal solutions. The closely related paintings in Washington and in Perugia (cat. 32) pose just such a problem, not only because similar figures appear in each painting, but because these figures clearly derive from Orazio's altarpiece, the *Vision of Saint Francesca Romana* (cat. 30). The exhibition of all three works together ought to clarify issues of attribution as well as of Gentileschi's

working habits, some of which are raised in a detailed article by De Grazia and Schleier that discusses the Perugia and Washington paintings.

Although the pictures at Washington and Perugia are closely related, they differ in motif, interpretation, and execution. In the Washington painting the patron saint of music, Saint Cecilia, plays an organ, while in the Perugia painting she plays a spinet. In the one a youthful angel holds the music for the saint, while in the other the angel appears to follow her performance or sing in accompaniment. In one, it is the presence of the angel alone which attests that the image is indeed of Saint Cecilia and not merely of a young woman practicing (a conflation of sacred and profane typical of Orazio). In the other, the saint has a halo and wears her traditional attribute, a garland of roses. The presence of the garland and halo on the Perugia Saint Cecilia is probably explained by the picture's destination, a Franciscan convent in Todi (where it was discovered in 1972 by Francesco Santi); the picture presumably

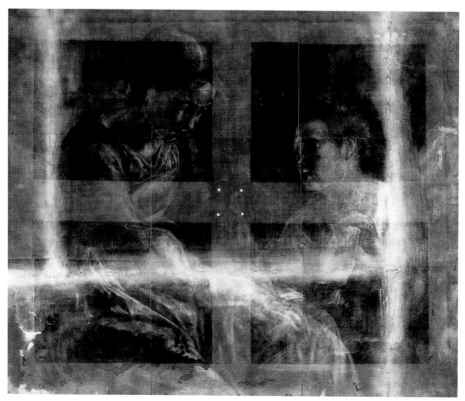

Figure 60. X radiograph of cat. 31

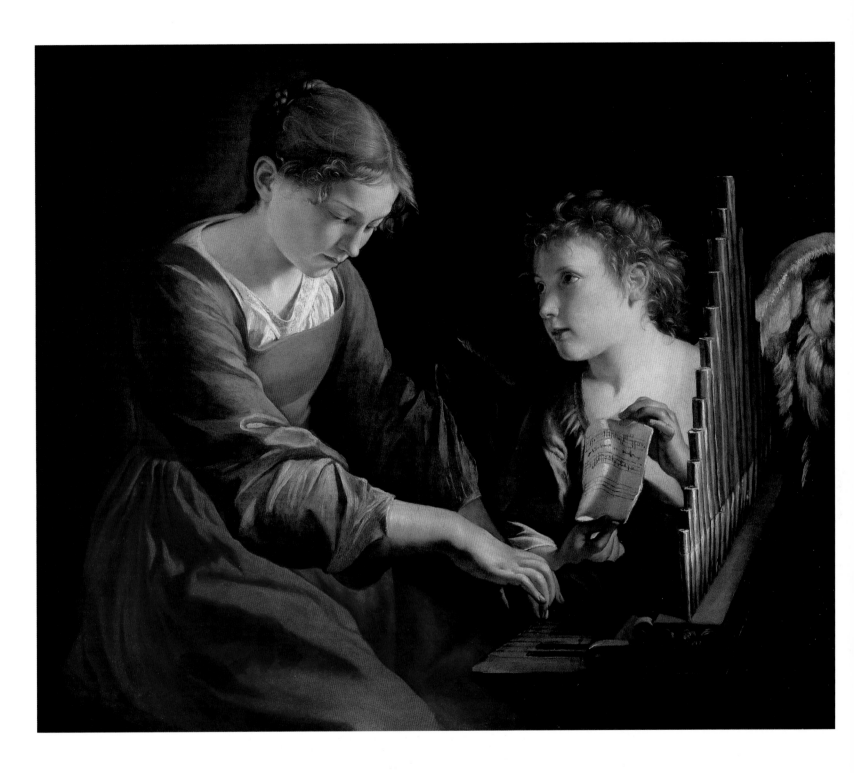

PROVENANCE: Natale Rondanini?, Rome (d. 1627); Alessandro Rondanini, Rome (1627–39); his wife, Felice Zacchia Rondanini, Rome (1639–67; inv. 1662, as by Orazio Gentileschi and Giovanni Lanfranco); Alessandro Rondanini, Rome (1667–40; exh. 1694 and 1710, San Salvatore in Lauro; inv. 1741, as by Gentileschi and Lanfranco); by inheritance to the Del Bufalo della Valle Cancellieri family, Rome; Marchese Paolo del Bufalo della Valle, Rome (by 1840); by inheritance to Monsignor Federico Fioretti, Rome (by 1944); Vitale Bloch, The Netherlands (before 1951–52); The Samuel H. Kress Foundation, New York (1952); National Gallery of Art, Washington, D.C.

RELATED PICTURES: Cat. 32; Mrs. Randolph Berens (copy; sale, Sotheby's, London, July 25, 1924).[5]

REFERENCES: Hermanin 1944, 45–46; Milan 1951, 64 no. 107; Emiliani 1958b, 43; Salerno 1965, 280; Moir 1967, vol. 1, 70–72, vol. 2, 76 no. E.1; Shapley 1973, 83; Santi 1976, 43–44; Nicolson 1979, 53; Shapley 1979, 199–200; Bissell 1981, 39–40, 165, 166–67 no. 37; Nicolson 1990, 114; De Grazia and Schleier 1994, 73–78; Negro in Negro and Pirondini 1995, 182; De Grazia and Garberson 1996, 103–12.

belonged to one of the nuns (it is still in its original frame). By contrast, the Washington painting is first mentioned in a 1662 inventory of the collection of Felice Zacchia Rondanini in Rome and was probably acquired by Felice's father-in-law, Natale Rondanini, who was a member of the Congregazione di Santa Cecilia.

In the Rondanini inventory of 1662, it is noted that the heads of the figures in the Washington picture were painted by Gentileschi, while the rest of the painting was by Giovanni Lanfranco, a favorite artist of Natale Rondanini's.[1] X radiographs and a technical analysis undertaken at the National Gallery of Art, Washington, confirm that Orazio left the painting unfinished. He completed the heads and busts of both figures and also painted Saint Cecilia's bodice and skirt. The sleeves of Cecilia's dress, the drapery over her left leg, the sheet of music, the drapery, and the wings of the angel, the hands of both figures, and the organ were painted by Lanfranco, sometimes covering up or modifying portions already painted or begun by Orazio.[2] It is likely that Lanfranco did this around 1620–21, perhaps after Orazio had left for Genoa, and at more or less the same time that he carried out an independent picture of the same subject and about the same size for Natale Rondanini (Bob Jones University Museum and Art Gallery, Greenville, South Carolina). Interestingly, this was not the only unfinished painting by Orazio owned by Rondanini; he also acquired the earliest version of Orazio's *Judith and Her Maidservant* (fig. 46).

The X rays reveal that prior to Lanfranco's completion of the Washington picture, Saint Cecilia's right arm was positioned lower and at a sharper angle (whether Orazio also painted the hands is uncertain). This made it more similar not only to the composition in Perugia but, more important, to the figure of the Madonna in the Santa Francesca Romana altarpiece. Indeed, there can be little doubt that the two figures in both pictures trace their origin to that altarpiece.

De Grazia and Schleier have both suggested that after completing the altarpiece, Orazio blocked out and partially painted the two figures in the Washington canvas. The Perugia painting, which De Grazia does not believe to be autograph, would have been done with reference to the Washington painting for the general composition, and to the altarpiece for the position of the angel's wing, the color of his costume, and the motif of the rolled-up sleeve of Saint Cecilia. I would like to suggest, more simply, that a combination of tracings and drawings may have been used for both, which is why they relate in slightly different ways to the altarpiece and to each other.[3] For example, the puffy-faced angel in the Perugia painting is closer to its counterpart in the altarpiece than it is to the angel in the Washington version, while it is the Saint Cecilia in the Washington painting that is closest to the figure in the altarpiece. A second altarpiece painted for a church in Fabriano, the *Madonna of the Rosary*, recycles the same heads. It has been proposed that that work is a pastiche. But done under Orazio's supervision or independently?

There is no question that the Washington picture is in every respect superior to that in Perugia. Indeed, in the handling of light—sharp, focused, and with a wonderful effect of transparency—the Washington picture is in every way equal to the Saint Francesca Romana altarpiece. One might even posit that it is the Washington painting that conveys more fully the firsthand study of a posed model, right down to the treatment of the bodice of the saint's dress. By comparison, the altarpiece has a more abstracted quality. Did the Washington picture perhaps originate as a study of the models for the altarpiece, and was it subsequently transformed into a *Saint Cecilia with an Angel*? The problem here is drawing a line between Orazio's tendency to combine the worlds of genre and sacred painting and his means of achieving a naturalistic effect. In any event, as Schleier has pointed out, the Perugia *Saint Cecilia* should not automatically be demoted to a workshop variant or a pastiche by another artist. It is certainly not by the Marchigian Giovanni Francesco Guerrieri, as proposed by Bissell (who, however, was unaware that large portions of what he considers Orazio's version are by Lanfranco). There are minor pentimenti (for example, in the wings), and the brushwork of the original blocking in (the *abbozzo*) is visible in the saint's left arm. Definitive judgment should be postponed until the exhibition. A reasonable date for both pictures would be about 1618–21. As is often the case with Orazio's easel-sized pictures, the Washington *Saint Cecilia* is painted on four separate pieces of plain-weave fabric sewn together. The center piece was prestretched and probably pregrounded.[4]

1. "Un quadro Longo Palmi cinque, alto tre con una Santa Cecilia conle Teste di m[an]i del Gentileschi, il resto di Gio:Lanfranchi con cornice intagliata et indorata nella Galeria del. S.r Card.le." First published by Salerno 1965, 280, the transcription has been corrected and republished by De Grazia and Schleier 1994, 73, and again in De Grazia and Garberson 1996, 103, where a detailed discussion of the painting can be found.

2. For a full report, see De Grazia and Garberson 1996, 104.

3. Related to this issue is the proposal by Pizzorusso (1987, 61–63) that another altarpiece in Fabriano, the *Madonna of the Rosary*, is not by Orazio but is a pastiche of elements, some deriving from the Saint Francesca Romana altarpiece. Regardless of its autograph status, the *Madonna of the Rosary* testifies to the same sorts of issues raised by the paintings under discussion. A figure in a painting formerly in the Wittgens collection derives from the figure of Santa Francesca Romana; see Bissell 1981, 208. To judge from the reproduction, this is only a copy.

4. See De Grazia and Garberson 1996, 103.

5. See ibid., 111 n. 49.

32.

Saint Cecilia with an Angel

Oil on canvas, 35⅜ × 41 in. (90 × 105 cm)

Galleria Nazionale dell'Umbria, Perugia

ca. 1618–21

See cat. 31.

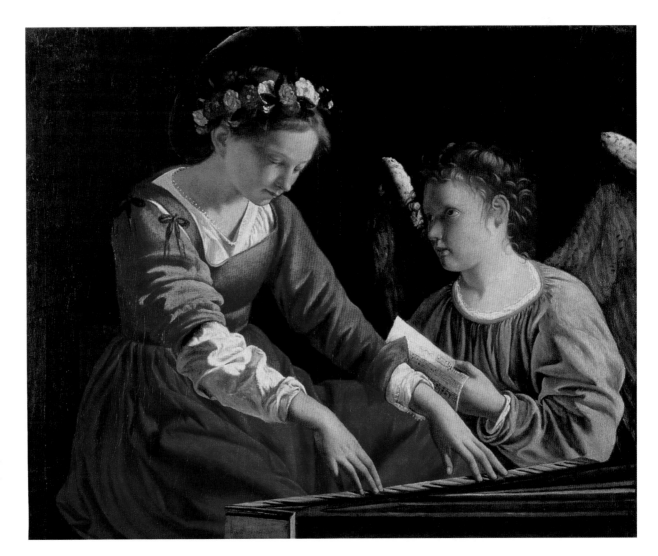

PROVENANCE: Monastero di San Francesco, Todi (until 1976); Galleria Nazionale dell' Umbria, Perugia.

REFERENCES: Santi 1976, 43–44; Bissell 1981, 167; De Grazia and Schleier 1994, 73–78; De Grazia and Garberson 1996, 106–8; Castrichini et al. 1999, 205–9.

33.

Sibyl

Oil on canvas, 31 ½ × 28 ⅜ in. (80 × 72 cm)

The Museum of Fine Arts, Houston, The Samuel H. Kress Collection (inv. 61.74)

ca. 1618–21

PROVENANCE: Private collection, England (sale, Christie's, June 22, 1951, lot 88, as by Artemisia Gentileschi, to J. Tooth); David Koester, New York; Samuel H. Kress Foundation, New York (1952); The Museum of Fine Arts, Houston.

RELATED PICTURE: Paris (copy; Hôtel-Drouot, sale, March 31, 1995, lot 60).

REFERENCES: Houston 1953, pl. 18; Moir 1967, vol. 1, 75 n. 22, vol. 2, 75 no. A.1; Providence 1968, no. 4; Cleveland 1971, 102–3 no. 31; Shapley 1973, 83–84; Nicolson 1979, 52; Bissell 1981, 187 no. 60; Houston 1981, 48 no. 88; Nicolson 1990, 112.

This engaging composition, in which the sibyl turns to address the viewer, her partly shadowed face animated by the play of reflected light, is something of an anomaly in Orazio's oeuvre. Rarely do his sitters seek to engage the viewer directly. Perhaps only in the Prado *Executioner with the Head of Saint John the Baptist* (cat. 20) does one do so in a fashion comparable to the Houston *Sibyl*. Otherwise, it is only an occasional, incidental glance that breaks the lyrical mood which Orazio prefers: a music-making angel in the upper left gazing out of the *Circumcision* in the church of the Gesù, Ancona, or the nursing Christ child in the various versions of the *Rest on the Flight into Egypt* (cat. nos. 34, 35). It is to the earliest version of the latter composition—the one in Birmingham—that the *Sibyl* seems to me closest in style, both for the treatment of light and for the gen-

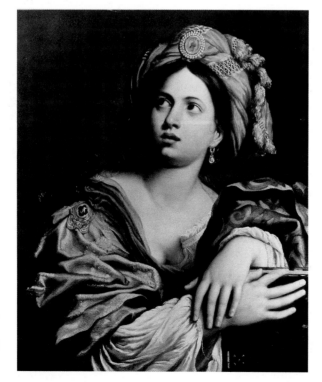

Figure 61. Domenichino (1581–1641), *"Persian" Sibyl*. Oil on canvas. Wallace Collection, London

eral tonality. (I am not able to agree with Bissell's dating of the picture to after 1620 and see no connection with Orazio's English-period paintings.)

The richly articulated pose may owe something to the sibyls of both Michelangelo (the turning figure in the *Libyan Sibyl* in the Sistine chapel) and Raphael (the figures in Santa Maria della Pace, Rome), but the key comparison is with Domenichino, who in 1616–17 painted a *Sibyl* for Scipione Borghese (Galleria Borghese, Rome). In that work there is a like emphasis on rich fabrics and an even more elaborate play in the hands, similarly paired on the right side of the composition.[1] The comparison is of more than passing interest, since, according to a 1631 inventory, the Savelli also owned a *Sibyl* by Domenichino that was evidently displayed together with Orazio's and another by Guido Reni. Although the Savelli *Sibyls* cannot be certainly identified with existing pictures by these two artists, it seems possible that Orazio's was designed to form part of a series and that the formal beauty of the pose was intended to meet the challenge of the works of the two leading Bolognese painters (fig. 61).[2] The 1631 inventory also lists, in addition to these three *Sibyls*, one by Dosso Dossi (fig. 8). Could this conceivably be the painting now in the Hermitage?[3] If so, the picture, with its brilliant—one might say proto-Gentileschian—description of silken fabrics, must have been important to the Venetianizing trend in Orazio's work after about 1613, when he is first documented working for the Savelli family.

The pose of Orazio's sibyl has a contemporary counterpart in Angelo Caroselli's comical figure of Vanity (Galleria Nazionale d'Arte Antica, Palazzo Barberini, Rome), shown as a plebeian girl with an unforgettably toothy smile.[4] Compared with Caroselli's somewhat cheeky interpretation of Caravaggesque naturalism, Orazio's seems, indeed, elevated and poetic, if still at great remove from the classicizing style of Domenichino.

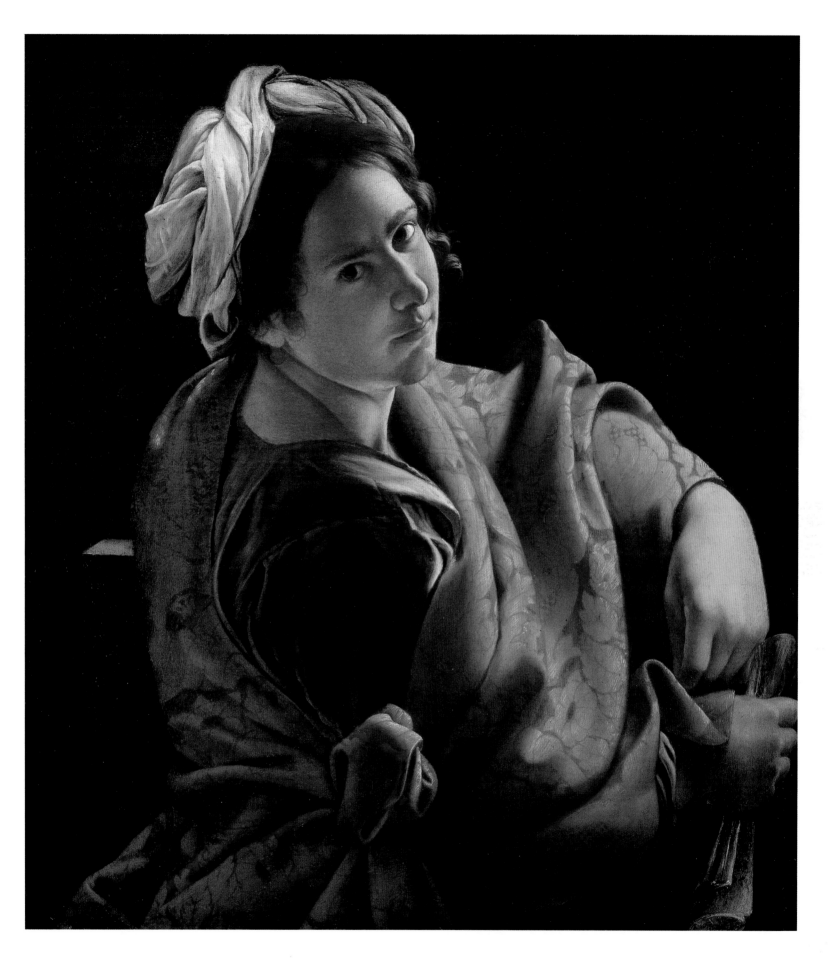

1. For Domenichino's *Sibyl*, see Rome 1996–97, 422 no. 25.

2. For the 1631 inventory, see Spezzaferro 1985, 72. It is perhaps worth noting that the Hermitage Dosso measures 69 × 64 cm. Of the four known *Sibyls* by Domenichino, only that in the Wallace Collection, London, has compatible measurements: 80 × 72 cm. The *Sibyl* by Reni in the Mahon collection measures 74 × 58 cm. Thus, there are paintings by each of these artists that would be appropriate companions to Orazio's. The Mahon *Sibyl*, however,

is listed in a 1637 inventory of the collection of Carlo de' Medici and is unlikely to be the Savelli picture (it is also a work of the 1630s). The picture in the Wallace Collection cannot be traced prior to the eighteenth century.

3. See Lucco in Ferrara–New York–Los Angeles 1998–99, 184–87. The picture entered the Hermitage in 1814.

4. For the most recent opinions of this work, see Rome 1999, 78 no. 26.

34·

Rest on the Flight into Egypt

Oil on canvas, 69½ × 86¼ in. (176.6 × 219 cm)

City Museum and Art Gallery, Birmingham (P. 5 47)

ca. 1620–22

PROVENANCE: Pietro Massei, Lucca (d. 1695; postmortem inv., as by Guercino);[4] his daughter Bianca Teresa Massei Bonvisi (1695–1713; sale, 1713, as by Guercino); Stefano Conti, Lucca (1713–39; in his ms. cat. as by Guercino); by descent, Marchese Cesare Boccella, Lucca (until about 1830); Carlo Ludovico II di Borbone, duke of Lucca (ca. 1830–41; 1840 cat., no. 15, as by Simone Cantarini da Pesaro; sale, Phillips, London, June 5, 1841, lot 38, as by Simone Cantarini da Pesaro); Talbot collection, Margam Castle (from 1841); Miss Emily Talbot, Margam Castle (until 1941; sale, Christie's, London, October 29, 1941, lot 376, as by Artemisia Gentileschi); H.R.H. the duke and duchess of Kent (1941–47; sale, Christie's, London, March 14, 1947, lot 35, as by Orazio Gentileschi); City Museum and Art Gallery, Birmingham.

One of Orazio's most ambitious as well as masterful multifigure compositions, the Birmingham *Rest on the Flight into Egypt* engendered a series of variants—at least five—over the course of the third decade of the century (see cat. 45). One or another of these variants had an enduring effect on French artists, from Jacques Blanchard and the Le Nain to Laurent de La Hyre (see pp. 210–12). Yet none of the versions attain the beauty of the Birmingham picture. It is, therefore, difficult to understand how Longhi could have questioned whether the picture was entirely the work of Orazio and how both Voss and Bissell—perhaps relying on black-and-white photographs rather than a clear recollection of the paintings—could consider the variants superior. As will be clear to visitors to the exhibition, the more tightly edited composition of the Vienna painting (cat. 45)—to my mind the finest of the variants—is no compensation for the loss of airiness, tonal beauty, and warm humanity that make the Birmingham *Rest on the Flight* one of Orazio's masterpieces. As so often with Orazio, his primary source of inspiration was a print after Raphael, the so-called *Virgin with the Long Thigh* (fig. 62). There we find the reclining Virgin with her child in front of a brick wall, the stepped shape of which echoes her pose. The print includes a cradle, the infant Saint John the Baptist, and the adoring figure of Joseph. These, together with the architectural

backdrop, Orazio jettisoned in favor of a more reductive and, it should be emphasized, natural-seeming grouping. His composition is more planar and the effect is of independent motifs drawn from life and, quite literally, collaged together.

As is the case with his finest achievements, the picture combines a subtle instinct for formal arrangement with a keen response to observed phenomena. The stepped profile of the plastered Roman brick wall anchors the simple geometry of the composition (the raised portion of the wall bisects it almost exactly), while the angled placement of the figures, one overlapping the other, and the foreshortened leg of Joseph define the space. Within that structure Orazio puts into play his love of surface variation: the donkey's matted fur and the cottony clouds; the sheen of the Virgin's lavender gray dress and the woolen surface of Joseph's coral-colored coat and orange cloak; the texture of crumbling brick and pitted plaster. The compositional procedures are the same ones that Orazio employs in the *Lot and His Daughters* painted for Giovan Antonio Sauli (cat. 37). Although the figurative arrangement in that picture is more tightly structured and the rocky backdrop opens at the right to admit a distant landscape vista, the two paintings share a like balance of light, form, and surface and must be fairly close in date, suggesting the possibility that the *Rest on the Flight into Egypt* is a Genoese rather than a late

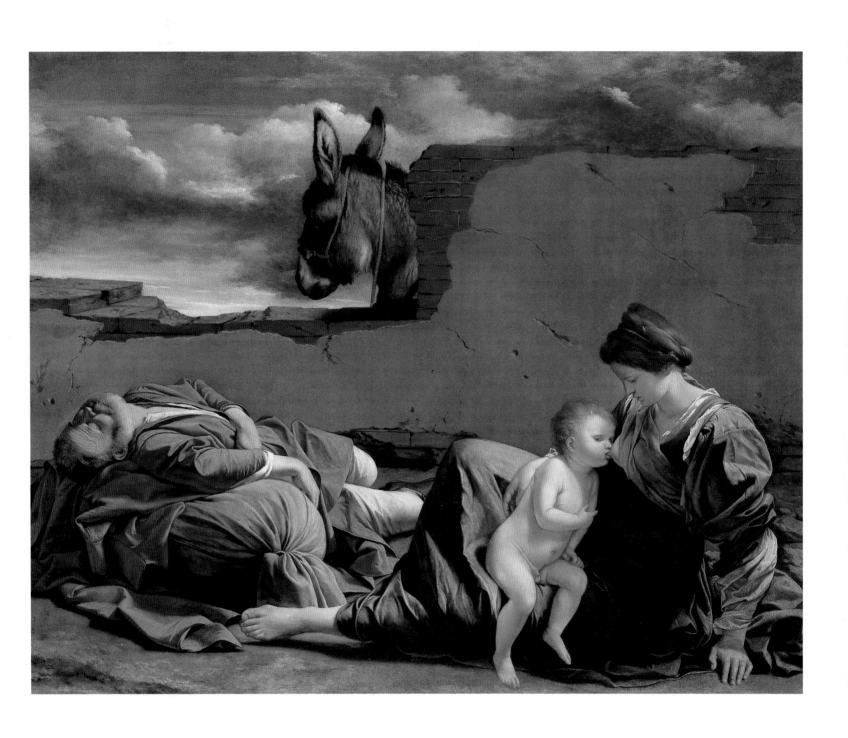

RELATED PICTURE: See
cat. 45.

REFERENCES: Longhi in Milan
1951, 67 no. 113; Sutton 1959, 88;
Voss 1959, 163–64; Birmingham
1960, 59–60; London 1960,
27, 143–45 no. 376; Moir 1967,
vol. 1, 76 n. 23, vol. 2, 76 no. D.5c;
Fredericksen 1972, 45–46;
Nicolson 1979, 52; Bissell 1981,
39–40, 48, 167–68 no. 38, 169, 184,
187; Nicolson 1990, 113; Marcolini
1996, 69–75; Bissell 1999, 49, 229;
Finaldi in London–Bilbao–
Madrid 1999, 58–59 no. 3.

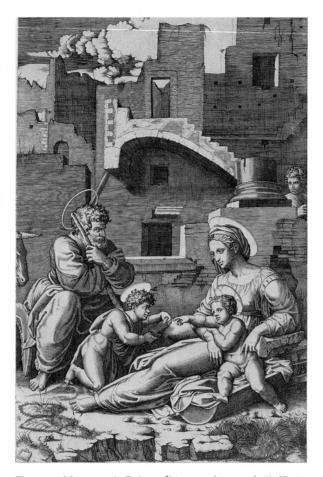

Figure 62. Marcantonio Raimondi (ca. 1470/82–1527/34?), *Virgin with the Long Thigh*. Engraving after Raphael. The Metropolitan Museum of Art, New York

Roman work (this would stretch somewhat Bissell's time frame of about 1615–20).

Given the bilateral nature of the composition, it is hardly surprising that two of the surviving variants show only the Virgin and child (although these are almost certainly cut-down fragments of the full composition). In the exquisite Burghley House *Madonna and Child* (cat. 38), Orazio himself was to develop the right side of the picture into an independent composition. The idea of contrasting the maternal care of the young Virgin for her child with the aged Joseph's fatigue and of irreverently linking him with the donkey has a long history. As had Caravaggio more than two decades before in his *Rest on the Flight into Egypt* (Doria Pamphili, Rome), Orazio seized on this tradition

as an opportunity to create a study of contrasts: of gender, age, type, and activity. This, too, is an aspect we encounter in Orazio's work only toward the end of his long activity in Rome, and it is worth noting that the model for Joseph resembles the model used for the Sauli *Lot*.

The earliest notice of the picture is in the 1695 postmortem inventory of the collection of the rich Lucchese merchant Pietro Massei. There it is ascribed to Guercino—a not far-fetched idea, given the similarity of Orazio's approach to that of Guercino in the late 1630s and 1640s.[1] Bearing in mind the greater naturalism of Orazio's picture and his continued reliance on the posed model, it is nonetheless remarkable how apt Calvi's description of these works by Guercino seems: "His manner of composing was very judicious and governed by a certain ingenuous simplicity; by devoting himself to this and by concentrating both on the real world and on the nature of objects, he often ended up by discovering original details that he knew how to choose and dispose wisely, and to embellish with pleasing accessories. And always, perhaps even more in his late style, he used such delicious, clear, and natural hues, which led to a magical enchantment."[2] It is not known when or where Pietro Massei acquired the picture. The incorrect attribution points to a second- or thirdhand purchase. Although Bissell tentatively suggests that this Tuscan provenance might indicate a Florentine origin and a date of 1616, when he believes Orazio was in Florence,[3] it is difficult to draw any conclusion from Massei's ownership. The picture might just as easily have been purchased in Rome or Genoa.

1. The classic treatment of this is that of Mahon in Bologna 1968, 160–64, and Bologna and other cities 1991–92, 217–19.
2. Calvi 1808, 39; translation in Bologna and other cities 1991–92, 253 n. 18.
3. On the interpretation of the very ambiguous documentary evidence, see Pizzorusso 1987, 72 n. 53, and the discussion in Bissell 1999, 399–400 n. 24.
4. For the early provenance of the picture, see Marcolini 1996, 69–70.

Opposite: Detail of the *Rest on the Flight into Egypt* (cat. 34)

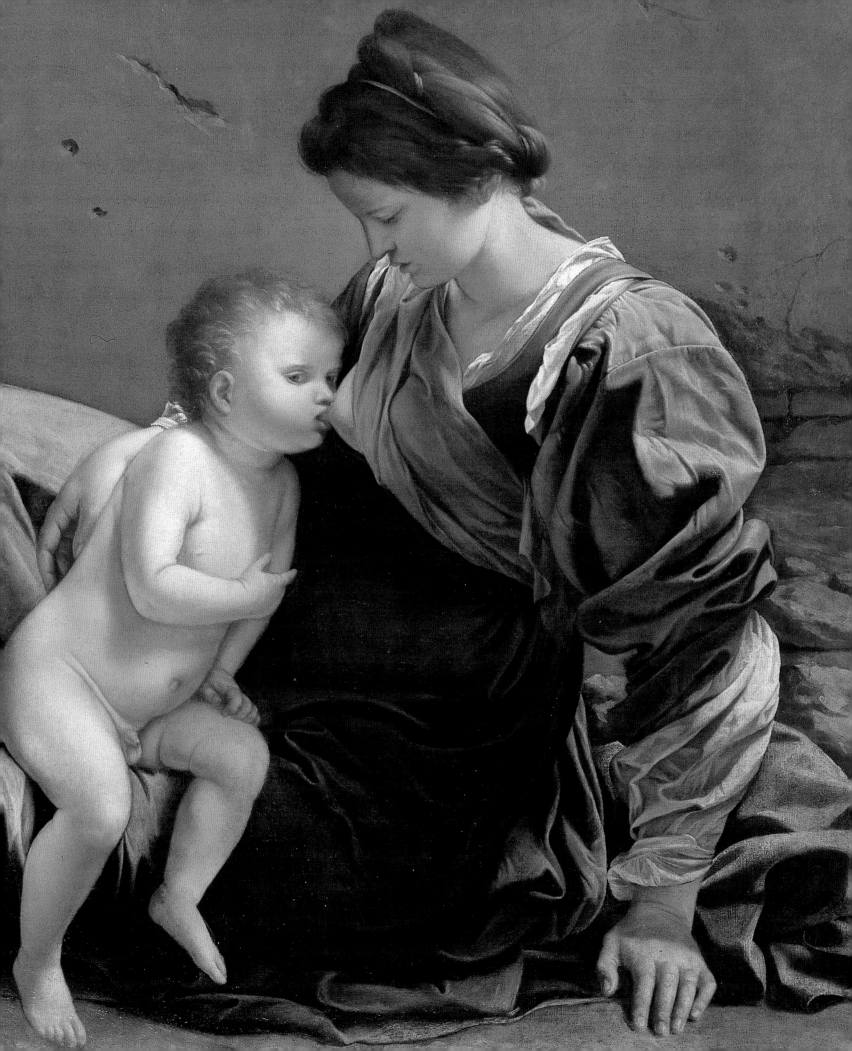

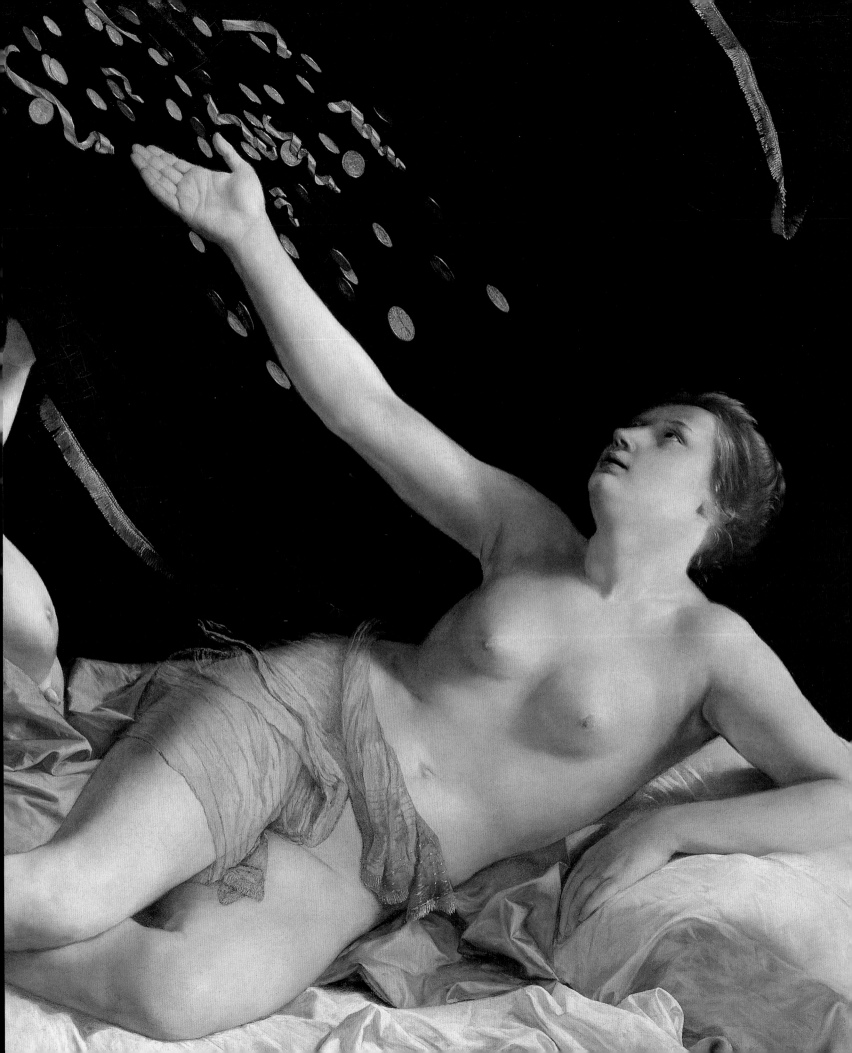

Orazio Gentileschi in Genoa

MARY NEWCOME

The artistic importance of Genoa has usually been thought of in terms of its having been a rich maritime city where the Flemish painters Peter Paul Rubens (1577–1640) and Anthony van Dyck (1599–1641) worked and where two of its streets, via Balbi and via Garibaldi, are still lined with magnificent palaces built in the sixteenth and seventeenth centuries. The presence of both Rubens and Van Dyck in Genoa and the surge of architectural development came about as the result of Andrea Doria's establishing Genoa as a republic in 1528. Under his leadership, Genoa became the leading banking and commercial center of the Spanish Hapsburg empire in northern and central Europe, the Mediterranean, and the New World. This development re-energized the social and political structure of Genoa, and the Genoese began to use their abundant financial resources to reshape their city. Frugality was abandoned as the wealthy competed with one another to have well-designed, stately palaces and churches filled with paintings, sculpture, and lavish furnishings. With the help of this expansive and ambitious patronage, Genoa was idealized as a New Athens and became known as "La Superba."

At the beginning of the seventeenth century, there was a local art school under the leadership of Giovanni Battista Paggi. The work of many non-Genoese artists also found a conspicuous place in the city. Federico Barocci's (ca. 1535–1612) sentimentally exquisite *Christ on the Cross Adored by Saints* for the Senarega chapel in the cathedral of San Lorenzo arrived from Urbino in 1596; Guido Reni's (1575–1642) *Assumption of the Virgin*, commissioned by Cardinal Stefano Durazzo for his family chapel in the Gesù, was sent to Genoa in 1617; and Rubens's *Circumcision*, commissioned from the artist when he was in Genoa by Nicolò Pallavicino for the high altar in the Gesù, was installed for the Feast of the Circumcision on January 1, 1606. Pallavicino also

commissioned Rubens to paint another altarpiece, the *Miracle of Saint Ignatius,* for his family chapel in the Gesù. Completed in Antwerp in 1619, the picture arrived in Genoa the following year.

Rubens had first visited Genoa in 1603 and was much attracted to the city, where both he and his work were appreciated by collectors. Although he painted several mythologies for Giovanni Vincenzo Imperiali, his main occupation was painting portraits. Through them, outsiders became aware of a city filled with wealthy patrons, such as Paolo Agostino Spinola and his wife, who sat for Rubens in 1606. Rubens also made outsiders aware of the special quality of Genoa's new buildings: after returning to Antwerp, he published a book of engravings (1621) showing the plans and elevations of the city's palaces.

Orazio Gentileschi became part of this remarkably diverse, international setting when he was invited to the city by the Genoese nobleman Giovan Antonio Sauli (or Saoli). Assured of employment, Gentileschi arrived from Rome in February 1621. Given the eagerness of the Genoese to collect art and his own forwardness, one has to wonder why he had not come sooner, especially since his erstwhile partner, Agostino Tassi (1578–1644), had been to Genoa in 1605,[1] and his brother Aurelio Lomi (1556–1622) had lived and worked in the city from 1597 to 1604. Lomi, in contrast to Orazio, was an extremely prolific painter and draftsman. Two of his paintings, the *Last Judgment* and the *Resurrection of Christ,* were commissioned by the Sauli for their basilica of Santa Maria in Carignano;[2] and the date of 1603, a year after the structure was completed to the designs of Galeazzo Alessi (1512–1572), suggests they were perhaps the very first pictures to be installed in the church. Admittedly, these pictures are quite different from the sensual, predominantly single-figure compositions Gentileschi would paint for Giovan Antonio Sauli; perhaps they reflect the taste of his uncle Anton Maria Sauli, who was archbishop of

Genoa from 1585 to 1591 and who was made a cardinal by Pope Sixtus V in 1587. However, they establish that Sauli patronage of the Lomi / Gentileschi family was long-standing, and they give a different slant to Soprani's account in his 1679 biography that Sauli was so impressed by Gentileschi's work in Rome that he persuaded the artist to accompany him back to Genoa.

With Sauli's promise of patronage, Gentileschi probably did his first work in Genoa for him. According again to Soprani,[3] for Sauli the artist painted a *Magdalene* (cat. 35), a *Danaë* (cat. 36), a *Lot and His Daughters* (cat. 37), and "altre tavole di molta esquisitezza."[4] Among these "other pictures" by Gentileschi may be the tender image of the *Madonna and Child* (cat. 38), since a copy of it bears an inscription on the back of its frame stating that in 1867 it was given to Brignole de Ferrari di Galliera by Maria Sauli in memory of her mother, Maria de Ferrari Sauli (Palazzo Rosso, Brignole Sale, Genoa).[5] The poetic sensuality of these paintings must have reflected the taste of Orazio's patron, for although Benedict Nicolson has remarked that "Sauli remains too shadowy a personality for any deductions to be drawn about his artistic inclinations,"[6] in his 1780 guidebook to the city, Ratti listed paintings in Domenico Sauli's palace that were similar in character and subject.[7]

Our knowledge of Genoese collections is based in large part on Ratti's guidebook. To judge by what it itemizes as belonging to the Sauli family, they were not major collectors, although the Sauli's palace on via San Lorenzo, where their major pieces were housed, had many of its rooms frescoed by the leading local artists active in the late seventeenth and the early eighteenth century, including Domenico Piola, Paolo Gerolamo Piola, and Lorenzo de Ferrari. Rather, the Sauli family's importance in promoting the arts in Genoa was in acquiring for its basilica (whose position on a hill dramatically frames the city on one side, just as the lighthouse does on the other) paintings and sculpture by local and foreign artists: Giulio Cesare Procaccini from Milan, Guercino from Cento, Carlo Maratta from Rome, and Pierre Puget from Toulon.

Gentileschi's direct contact with another patron, Pietro Maria Gentile, is less clear, but Ratti records at least four paintings attributed to the artist in the family's palace: a *Cleopatra*, a *Judith*, a *Lucretia* (now ascribed to Artemisia), and a *Sacrifice of Isaac* (cat. nos. 17, 53, 39, 67, and fig. 63). Listed by Ratti as in the Palazzo Pietro Gentile on Piazza Bianchi, they were transferred to the Palazzo Cattaneo-Adorno before 1846.[8] Judging from the *Catalogo di quadri vendibili in Genova* (dated September 11, 1640),[9] Ratti's list, and an 1811 inventory of the collection,[10] Gentile was an avid collector, acquiring paintings by Rubens, Reni (fig. 75), and Giovanni Lanfranco (1582–1647), as well as by local artists.[11]

Pietro Gentile may not have acquired all his paintings ascribed to Orazio directly from the artist; recently, Boccardo has suggested that Gentile bought the *Lucretia* in the sale in Genoa in 1637 of the collection of the duke of Alcalá.[12] The matter remains very problematic, but Gentile's *Cleopatra,* thought on grounds of style to date from before Orazio's arrival in Genoa, could also have been purchased through sale. As it anticipates the *Magdalene* and the *Danaë* that Orazio painted for Sauli, one wonders if it played a part in their genesis, or if Gentile saw Sauli's paintings and then bought the *Cleopatra* (see also p. 98).

Ratti's 1780 guidebook also cites paintings by Gentileschi in the collection of Carlo Cambiaso: "S. Sebastian, cui le Matrone Romane cavan le frecce," "David trionfante di Golia," "Giuditta," "mezza figura di femmina che suona il violino."[13] Cambiaso's interest in collecting art[14] is obvious from Ratti's long list of items, and what is special about him is that he put his collection (either inherited or formed by him) into a palace that was not his but instead belonged to the Brignole Sale family, who had restored it in 1711. Whether all the paintings listed in the palace in 1780 actually belonged to Cambiaso is unclear, but the agreement on the part of the Brignole Sale family to have Cambiaso as a renter and the fact that Cambiaso's example was followed by two other collectors (Carlo Dongi and Giacomo Pierano,[15] who kept their paintings in the palace), imply that the Brignole Sale family already had plans for using the palace as a museum (now known as the Palazzo Bianco).[16] Unfortunately, the Gentileschi paintings did not stay in the palace. In 1805, Andrew Wilson purchased the half-length figure of a woman playing the violin (cat. 40), and the suspicion arises that much of the collection was dispersed shortly after Ratti's listing. Lost is any record of the picture *Saint Sebastian Tended by Women,*[17] but, thanks to Orazio's practice of repeating compositions, we perhaps know what the *David Triumphing over Goliath* (see cat. 12) and the *Judith* (see cat. 39) looked like.

Among other lost paintings by Gentileschi that are recorded in Genoese collections are the *Virgin with a Sleeping Putto / Christ Child* in the Palazzo Paolo Spinola;[18] a half-length figure of Saint Francis acquired by Ridolfo I Brignole Sale in 1678;[19] a *Danaë* in the collection of Camillo Gavotti in 1679 (possibly the picture now in the Cleveland Museum of Art; see cat. 41); a *Portrait of a Woman*, showing a figure with a feather or pen in her hand, also said to be a self-portrait by Artemisia, in the Palazzo Giacomo Balbi,[20] which may be the same composition as the *Saint Catherine* in the Palazzo Negrone;[21] and a painting of an unidentified subject in the Palazzo de Fornari in 1780.[22] Lost also are his frescoes in the now destroyed "delizioso casino" located on the grounds of the palace of Marc Antonio Doria in Sampierdarena, outside Genoa.[23] This is probably the same casino for which in August 1605 Marc Antonio (brother of the collector Giovanni Carlo Doria) tried, unsuccessfully, to engage Caravaggio to fresco "la loggia" (this is usually interpreted as the casino).[24] In 1618, Caravaggio's Neapolitan follower Battistello Caracciolo began work in the casino[25] and one of the two ceilings was perhaps by him.[26] But the project must have been left unfinished. There remains the question of why the family did not ask Simon Vouet (1590–1649), then in the employ of Giovanni Carlo, to complete the frescoes when he visited the Doria villa in Sampierdarena in September 1621 to paint their portraits.[27] Had Gentileschi already been commissioned to carry out the task?

As Orazio had enjoyed considerable success in frescoing Scipione Borghese's casino with Tassi in Rome in 1611–12, it is perhaps understandable that Doria chose him. However, instead of the contemporary figures shown standing behind a fictive balustrade that decorates the vault of the Borghese casino (fig. 6), Doria had the artist fresco Old Testament subjects. It is impossible to know exactly what the frescoes looked like. By the time Ratti described them in 1768, one of the vaults, showing Saint Jerome trumpeting the Last Judgment, was already in shambles, and by the late eighteenth century the casino was destroyed. Nonetheless, we can gain some sense of the complexity of the decoration of one ceiling from Ratti's rather lengthy description.[28] Using the old-fashioned system of *quadri riportati*, whereby an independent composition is embedded into a decorative scheme, the artist frescoed the *Sacrifice of Isaac* in the center of one vault and surrounded it with four stories of Jacob (the Benediction of Jacob, Esau Selling His Birthright, the Dream of Jacob, and Jacob Wrestling with the Angel). Lunettes showed additional biblical scenes (Moses Parting the Red Sea, Job Afflicted, Tobias Raised from the Dead, the Curing of Tobias, and so forth), as well as depictions of Old Testament figures (Moses, Aaron, Joshua,

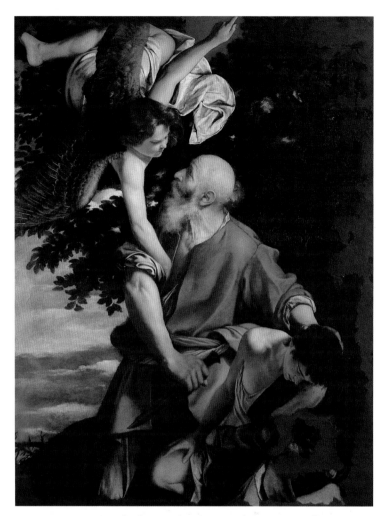

Figure 63. Orazio Gentileschi, *Sacrifice of Isaac*. Oil on canvas. Galleria Nazionale di Palazzo Spinola, Genoa

Jonah, David, Judith, Job, and Samson). Sibyls adorned the corners.[29] The casino frescoes were Gentileschi's most ambitious undertaking, and they may have been finished only in 1624, since in a letter to Marc Antonio Doria dated August 13, 1624, Caracciolo offered to do the estimate. To have designed at least nine different scenes in a decorative ensemble far exceeded Gentileschi's earlier work in San Venanzio in Fabriano, where he frescoed four scenes on the walls of a chapel (figs. 50, 51). With the sole exception of the *Sacrifice of Isaac*, he did not repeat any of the subjects on canvas. For this complicated project, Orazio's main assistant was probably his son Francesco (1597–ca. 1665). During the years 1621–24, Francesco helped him in the studio and was also his courier, taking an *Annunciation* to the duke of Savoy in Turin in 1623 as a follow-up to Orazio's *Lot and His Daughters*—gifts aimed at securing a position at the court of Carlo Emanuele (cat. nos. 42, 43). A son

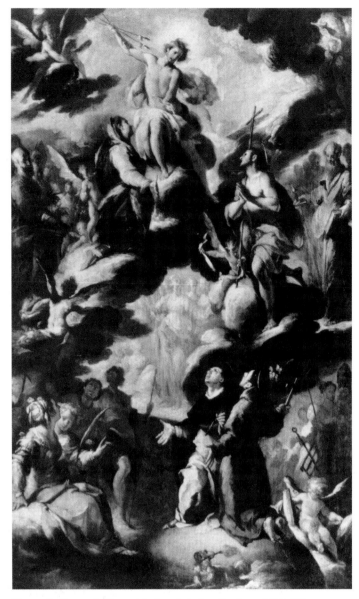

Figure 64. Bernardo Strozzi (1581–1644), *Paradise* (a *modello*). Oil on canvas. Accademia Ligustica, Genoa

his frescoes in three rooms on the piano nobile and in four rooms on the ground floor of Marc Antonio Doria's palace in Sampierdarena (now known as the Palazzo Bagnara).[33] Here, too, the subjects were biblical: the Sacrifice of Isaac, Tobias and the Angel, and the Dream of Joseph. The choice offers a striking contrast to the mythological and historical scenes that were being frescoed around 1621 in other palaces in Sampierdarena, such as those by Bernardo Strozzi in the Palazzo Centurione, and those by Giovanni Carlone in the Villa Spinola di San Pietro. Ansaldo's repetition of some of the subjects treated by Orazio emphasizes not only the role of a patron in dictating the themes but also Doria's desire to unify the decoration in his palace with his garden casino. The repetition also implies that the story of the Sacrifice of Isaac had a special significance for Doria, since it formed the center medallion in Gentileschi's ceiling and was the center medallion in two rooms on the piano nobile of the palace, one frescoed by Calvi, the other by Ansaldo.

For many reasons, patronage was at its peak during the years of Gentileschi's stay. Fresco decoration was undergoing a revival led by a trio of painters (Domenico Fiasella and Bernardo Castello and his son-in-law Giovanni Carlone) who had worked in Rome in the 1610s. All three must have known Gentileschi in Rome, and his casino frescoes of 1611–12 may have inspired Carlone's frescoed frieze in the Palazzo Lomellini Patrone, in Genoa. Painted about 1621, it shows figures in contemporary dress standing on balconies.[34] In the same period, the vault in the apse of the cathedral of San Lorenzo was frescoed (in 1622) by Lazzaro Tavarone. For Giovanni Stefano Doria, Strozzi frescoed a *Paradise* in the apse of San Domenico (ca. 1620–21; fig. 64), and for the Centurione family palaces in Genoa and Sampierdarena he painted decorative medallions on the ceilings (ca. 1621–25). The activity of Genoese artists and their patrons also involved the northern colony of artists who ably transcribed some of the narrative images in these panoramic frescoes into highly intricate silver objects.[35]

Gentileschi arrived in Genoa the same year Van Dyck came from Antwerp, in November 1621, to stay with Cornelis and Lucas de Wael. Called upon to paint fashionable portraits of the Genoese nobility who remembered what Rubens had done for them, Van Dyck succeeded in promoting his sitters, their city, and himself. (He returned to Antwerp in the winter of 1627.) Van Dyck's subject matter, although completely different from Gentileschi's, perhaps increased the desire on the part of the nobility to have

was born to Francesco in 1623, and when his father left for France in 1624 (after having sent a picture to Marie de' Medici), Francesco stayed on with his family. One gets the impression that much of his activity was based on enhancing family matters.[30] If this was, in fact, the case, then it seems only appropriate that, from 1628 to 1641, Francesco would have chosen to live in the seaside suburb of Sampierdarena, where he could meet and be seen by the wealthy Genoese nobility.[31] Francesco's brother Giulio, listed as "un procuratore per affairi" in 1630, lived in the city until at least 1656.[32]

While Orazio was working in the casino, the Genoese painter Giovan Andrea Ansaldo (1584–1638) was using a similar layout for

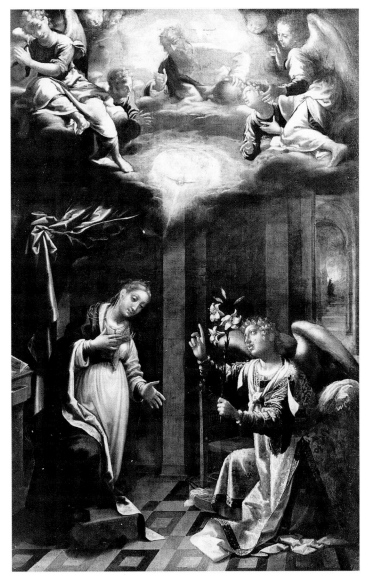

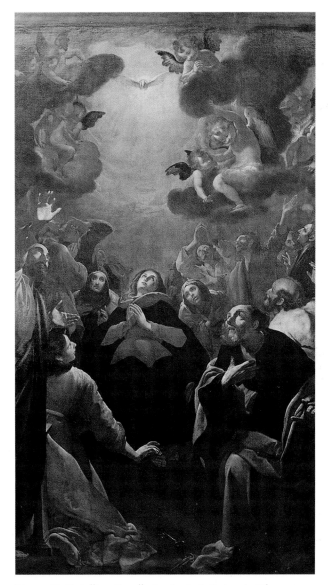

Figure 65. Aurelio Lomi (1556–1622), *Annunciation*. Oil on canvas. Santa Maria Maddalena, Genoa

Figure 66. Castellino Castello (1576–1649), *Pentecost*. Oil on canvas. San Matteo, Lagueglia

elegant pictures—which in turn may have inspired Orazio to make his figures even more refined during this period. Van Dyck recorded Orazio's *Judith* (cat. 39) in his Italian sketchbook (fig. 74). As both artists worked for the Doria (as they did, later, for Charles I), their paths must have crossed a number of times in Genoa.

Gentileschi responded to his Genoese patrons by adjusting his painting style as well as by taking on new subjects; several times his paintings repeat subjects previously painted in Liguria by his brother Aurelio Lomi. The differences between the brothers' work are easily seen by comparing Lomi's *Annunciation* (fig. 65), commissioned in 1603 by the Spinola family, with Gentileschi's (cat. 43). Stylistically, they have little in common. Lomi may have taught

Orazio to paint, and he shared Orazio's skill and interest in describing draperies with sharp accents of light, but his figures were never Caravaggesque and remained tubular, while Gentileschi's naturalistically conceived figures became increasingly refined.

Unfortunately, Gentileschi's refinement and compositional layout, apparent especially in his paintings in Genoese collections, had no great impact on local artists. One has only to look at the tall, demure figure of the Virgin standing against a dark background in the *Annunciation* to realize that it is unlike any other treatment of the subject in Genoa. Unique also is the compact cluster of large, foreshortened figures who fill the foreground, pointing toward a distant landscape, in his *Lot and His Daughters*

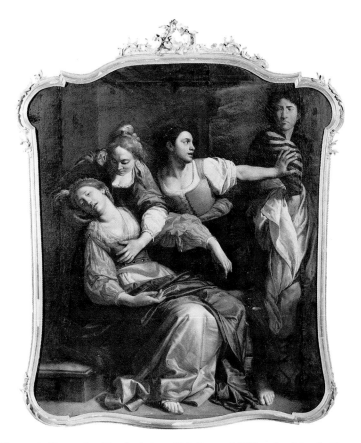

Figure 67. Domenico Fiasella (1589–1669), *Pompey's Widow Receiving the News of His Death*. Oil on canvas. Formerly Cattaneo Adorno collection, Genoa

(cat. 37). His reclining female figures (cat. nos. 35, 36) have an elegance that makes the Magdalenes painted by Bernardo Castello look heavy and rustic. Strozzi painted the subject of Judith, as did Luciano Borzone, but their canvases lack the Caravaggesque substance of Gentileschi's. Nor can his compositions of half-length female figures bathed in a strong, raking light be related to anything known in Genoese painting, although in the 1620s Genoese artists used dramatic lighting effects to model their figures. This is true of Paggi in his *Last Communion of Saint Jerome* (San Francesco da Paolo, Genoa), dated 1620, and of his student Castellino Castello (who is said to have painted Van Dyck's portrait) in his *Pentecost* (San Matteo, Lagueglia; fig. 66), dated 1623. These light effects were probably not the result of Gentileschi's influence. Nor did they derive from Caravaggio's *Martyrdom of Saint Ursula*, commissioned by Marc Antonio Doria (Banca di Napoli). They were a sign of the times: a reference to the local example of Luca Cambiaso, as well as a reaction to the few Caravaggesque paintings that could be seen in Genoa, among them Gerrit van Honthorst's *Christ Crowning Saint Teresa* (Santa Anna). Of the local

artists, only Ansaldo is known to have enjoyed patronage from Gentileschi's patrons Marc Antonio Doria and Pietro Gentile (for example, his frescoes in the Palazzo Gentile-Bickey in Cornigliano of ca. 1625).[36] This may be why Ansaldo's frescoes sometimes have crisply defined, colorful figures remotely resembling the manner of Gentileschi.

However, Gentileschi's legacy—such as it is—remained mainly in the hands of Domenico Fiasella (1589–1669), who had been a pupil of Lomi and Paggi before going to Rome. In Rome, from 1607 to 1615, Fiasella absorbed a knowledge of Caravaggio's followers and those of the Carracci, painted for the Giustiniani, and worked with Domenico Cresti (il Passignano) and the Cavaliere d'Arpino. Considered by Federico Alizeri "the best naturalist of our school,"[37] Fiasella produced paintings that, like those of Orazio, are characterized by their static compositions. Similarities between his work and Orazio's can be seen in the intricate twisting drapery folds, the strong whites, the skillful modeling, and the variety of color tonalities of his paintings of the 1620s (*Martyrdom of Saint Barbara,* 1622, San Marco al Molo, Genoa; *Saint Ursula with the Holy Family,* 1624, San Quirico parish church; and *Pompey's Widow Receiving the News of His Death*, fig. 67). The connections between the two artists, both personal and stylistic, were further advanced in Genoa when Orazio's son Francesco (four years younger than Artemisia) studied with Fiasella. In so doing, Francesco would have been working with the painter whose style most closely resembled that of his father. This does not help identify Francesco's work, and without documentation one can only suggest that he may have been responsible for making replicas of his father's paintings and that some of the paintings and frescoes traditionally given to Fiasella but not quite typical of his work may be by Francesco, particularly those done in Sampierdarena, where he lived until 1641. Two paintings (location unknown) have been given to Francesco,[38] and the *Man Playing a Guitar* (Carige collection, Genoa), monogrammed on the guitar F. G., has tentatively been attributed to him.[39]

In summary, Gentileschi left very little record of his presence in Genoa besides his paintings. Although we might think his style memorable enough to be imitated, few tried. In contrast, he benefited substantially from his stay in the city. He arrived when patronage in La Superba was at its height, and it was patronage that forced him to expand his subject matter, to refine his painting style, and to increase his productivity.

1. Belloni 1988, 13–15.

2. Ciardi, Galassi, and Carofano 1989, nos. 37, 38.

3. Soprani 1674, 317–18.

4. Ratti, in updating Soprani in 1768, left out this last phrase; Ratti 1768, 452.

5. Ponzi 1994, 51–71.

6. Nicolson 1985, 12.

7. Ratti 1780, 112.

8. Ibid., 119–22. With the exception of the *Judith* (see cat. 39), which is perhaps the picture listed in an 1811 inventory as by Valentin (see Boccardo 2000, 212).

9. Campori 1870, 140–42; Boccardo 2000, 211 n. 30.

10. Boccardo 2000, 205–13. The "Gentilischi" paintings listed in the December 2, 1811, inventory are:

    Quadro di Orazio Gentileschi che rappresenta Cleopatra colla vipera, palmi 6 altezza, 7 larghezza, stima 1000

    Detto di Orazio Gentileschi rappresentante Lucrezia Romana, palmi 5½ altezza, 4½ larghezza, stima 150 [now attributed to Artemisia]

    Detto del Gentileschi rappresentante Esau che vende la Primogenitura a Giacobbe, 7 altezza, 9½ larghezza, stima 300 [ascribed by Ratti (1780, 122) to Fiasella]

    Detto di Scuola Veneta rappresentante il Sacrifizio di Abramo, palmi 7 altezza, 9½ larghezza, stima 150

    Caravaggio rappresentante la coronazione di Spine di N.Sig., 7 altezza, 9½ larghezza, stima 1000 [Boccardo 2000, 213, as by Gentileschi?].

11. Gentileschi's *Sacrifice of Isaac* is listed (as Venetian school) at the end of the 1811 Gentile inventory together with three other paintings of the same size: *Rebecca Giving Drink to the Servant of Abraham,* by Giovanni Andrea de Ferrari (perhaps the painting in the Zerbone collection, October 1994); *Hercules,* by Reni (identified as *Samson Wrestling the Lion,* private collection); and the *Crowning with Thorns,* by Caravaggio, suggested by Boccardo (2000, 213 n. 17) as possibly the composition by Gentileschi that Van Dyck recorded in his Italian sketchbook. Unfortunately, its size (175 × 237 cm) does not correspond with either of the known versions. Boccardo further suggests that Gentile could have been responsible for commissioning the *Annunciation* for San Siro, since the Grimaldi-Ceba chapel was not finished until 1639. Although the identical dimensions of the five paintings (three of which have had attributions to Gentileschi) might indicate they were done as a series, it is quite possible these paintings were acquired at different times and perhaps made to fit into prescribed stucco frames on the wall by 1811. The Gentile *Sacrifice of Isaac* could thus be the same picture listed in the collection of Giovanni Luca Doria in 1678. See Belloni 1973, 63.

12. Boccardo 2000, 206.

13. Ratti 1780, 264–65.

14. Gardner 1998, 176.

15. Torriti 1971, 273.

16. The palace remained in the family until Maria Brignole Sale de Ferrari bequeathed it, together with a number of paintings, to the city in 1884. The museum was opened to the public in 1892 to celebrate the anniversary of the discovery of America by Columbus—ten years after the family had given the family residence across the street (now called the Palazzo Rosso) to the city.

17. A painting of the subject was recorded as being in the Palazzo Reale in Turin; Bissell 1981, 221 no. L-67.

18. Poleggi and Poleggi 1974, 173, as a pendant to an oval Christ carrying the cross by Strozzi.

19. Tagliaferro 1995, 158.

20. Pesenti in Genoa 1992, 194.

21. Bissell 1981, 220 no. L-56.

22. Ibid., 224.

23. Ratti 1768, 452.

24. Pesenti in Genoa 1992, 108.

25. A document dated December 12, 1618, records payments for a fresco begun for M. A. Doria by Caracciolo; see Bissell 1981, 222.

26. Da Morrona 1787–93, vol. 2 (1792).

27. Vouet wrote in a letter of September 4, 1621, that he was going with Signori Doria to their country residence in Sampierdarena, where they want him to paint their portraits; see Crelly 1962, 29.

28. Ratti 1768, 452–53.

29. See Genoa 1992, 45, 107.

30. Letters note (Bissell 1981, 113–14) that Francesco bought art in Italy for King Charles I in 1627–28, presented Orazio's *Finding of Moses* (fig. 87) to Philip IV in Madrid in 1633, and acted as business manager in Italy for his sister in 1635 (see ibid.).

31. Francesco's household included his wife, two children, his wife's mother and her daughter, recorded on December 29, 1635, as living "nel quartiero del Mercato e Ponte: Francesco Gentileschi pittore 36 anni; Geronima moglie 34 anni; figli: G.B. anni 12; Maria Prudenzia anni 7, ivi battezzata il 13 agosto 1628; Battina Giane suocera 60 anni, Anna Maria di detta Battina 26 anni (Chiesa di S. Martino e di S. M. della Cella in Sampierdarena, registro B.M.D. 1602–1626, carta 563 verso, famiglia num. 23)." See Alfonso 1976, 45.

    Francesco stayed at least until 1641, the year when the death of his son Giovanni Battista, on October 25, is listed in the records of the church of San Martino della Cella in Sampierdarena.

32. The earliest record of Giulio's existence is on May 10, 1630, when Giulio Gentileschi di Orazio, "civis Romae," was named "un procuratore per affari." His problematic business affairs were cited in testaments of July 9, 1638, and January 3, 1648, the latter concerning a transaction on April 4, 1645, that remained unpaid.

    With five children, Giulio's household was considerably larger than Francesco's. He stayed in Genoa, where he is last listed on February 7, 1656: "Giulio Gentileschi fu Orazio; Barbara moglie, figlia di Marcello Marana, figli: Orazio, Laura Maria, Gio. Carlo, Maria Maddelena, Giobatt (Chiesa di N. S. delle Vigne, stato delle Anime del 7–2–1656)." See Alfonso 1976, 45–46.

33. Ciliento and Boggero 1983, 187–90.

34. Poleggi 1995.

35. For example, the basin and ewer for the Lomellini, dated 1619 (Ashmolean Museum, Oxford); the basin and ewer for the Grimaldi, after designs by Lazzaro Tavarone and made by GAB/Giovanni Aelbosca Belga, dated 1621 and 1622 (Victoria and Albert Museum, London); the basin for the Giustiniani, after designs by Bernardo Strozzi, ca. 1620–25 (J. Paul Getty Museum, Los Angeles); see Frankfurt am Main 1992, nos. 150–52.

36. Di Fabio 1988, 85–97.

37. Alizeri 1846–47, 344.

38. Bissell 1981, 114.

39. Pesenti in Genoa 1992, 80, ill. (with bibliography).

The Sauli Paintings, cat. nos. 35–37

In his 1674 biographical notice on Orazio, Raffaele Soprani recounts how, as part of the Genoese delegation sent to Rome in 1621 to honor the newly elected pope, Gregory XV, Giovan Antonio Sauli became so enamored with Orazio's paintings that he invited the artist to Genoa. (The Sauli were an old and prominent Genoese family; Giovan Antonio's kinsman Anton Maria was archbishop of the city and, from 1585, cardinal; he had been one of the papal candidates.) For Sauli, Orazio painted "a penitent Magdalene, a Lot fleeing his burning city with his two daughters, [and] a Danaë with Jupiter [appearing] in a shower of gold, and other paintings of great exquisiteness." Soprani suggests that Orazio's success in Genoa was the direct result of these three paintings, and we should not be surprised that multiple versions survive for each. It was a version of the *Lot* that Orazio sent to the duke of Savoy in 1622 to solicit a court appointment (cat. 42).

Sauli's pictures remained together well into the eighteenth century. According to Ratti, in 1780 they were installed in the same room in the palace of Domenico Sauli. Ratti particularly admired the *Lot and His Daughters*, which he described as "one of the best and best-preserved paintings by this master."[1] Yet, by 1792 Da Morrona could locate only the *Danaë*. And after this date all trace of the pictures is lost until the twentieth century, when there appeared in Arenzano, near Genoa, versions of all three compositions.[2] These were acquired by the London dealer Thomas Grange and have since been sold (the *Magdalene* and the *Danaë* are cat. nos. 35, 36; the *Lot* is in the Thyssen-Bornemisza Collection, Madrid).

There is a presumption that the three ex-Grange pictures are those Orazio painted for Sauli and, indeed, two of them—the *Penitent Magdalene* and the *Danaë*—are unquestionably autograph versions of the highest quality. X radiographs of the *Danaë* reveal major compositional changes, and pentimenti in the *Magdalene* attest to its high status. The Thyssen *Lot*, however, which is lackluster in tone, has the characteristics of a workshop replica or even of a later copy.[3] It is smaller in both size and scale than the other two paintings and can hardly be the picture Ratti praised so highly. Fortunately, a far more likely candidate reappeared in 1997 (cat. 37). This version can be traced back only to the early twentieth century, when it was in a Genoese collection. Exported to England between 1925 and 1928, it remained with the same family until its acquisition by the J. Paul Getty Museum. Not only do X rays establish that this is the prime version of the composition, it is also one of Orazio's most beautiful and, in the words of Ratti, among his best-preserved paintings, possibly even retaining traces of the original varnish.[4] The lower corners of the *Lot*, like those of the *Magdalene*, have been cut diagonally; all four corners of the *Danaë* have been cut, though more on the bottom than the top. Because this feature, probably done to adapt the pictures for new frames, can be found in none of the other versions of any of the compositions, it is convincing evidence that these are indeed the three Sauli paintings. They are reunited here for the first time since the eighteenth century.

The fact that Soprani mentions the three pictures together and that Ratti says they were in the same room raises the issue of whether the pictures were in some way intended as a group. All the canvases have been trimmed, but they must have been about the same height; the *Lot* and the *Magdalene* were evidently also of matching width.[5] Each painting has as its protagonist a female—or, in the case of the *Lot*, two females. Ubiquitous though each of the subjects is in the seventeenth century, the combination strikes an unusual note and is unlikely to be casual. Far from being a cycle of Old Testament, New Testament, or mythological themes, they offer a compendium: the subject of one is taken from classical mythology, another from the New Testament, and the remaining one from the Old Testament. It might also be argued that one is erotic, the other (Lot's seduction by his daughters) moral in tone, while the third is distinctly devotional, or that they all have to do with themes involving women. But beyond these factors we may note that one is a complex, multifigure narrative composition, while in the other two a reclining female figure is used to convey contrasting subjects: the Magdalene seeking divine illumination through penitential exercises and Danaë experiencing physical union with Jupiter. In one the figure is modestly draped, while in the other she is provocatively veiled; in one the setting is an isolated cave, in the other a richly appointed bedroom. These analogies and contrasts seem to call attention to the parameters of Orazio's poetic language and to emphasize the importance of variation within a rigorously restricted formal vocabulary. It is in this sense that Soprani may well have been right that this group of pictures established the artist's fame and served as a notice to other potential patrons.

These three large and impressive canvases were the most celebrated of Sauli's pictures by Orazio, but Soprani also mentions "other paintings of great exquisiteness." Among these may have been the small copper *Madonna and Child in a Landscape* now at Burghley House (cat. 38). But here we are on extremely shaky ground. When, in 1768, Ratti put out a revised edition of Soprani's *Lives*, he eliminated any mention of additional paintings in the Sauli collection. Had Giovan Antonio's heirs already begun to sell off his remarkable group of paintings by Orazio—a smaller collection than that owned by the artist's principal Roman patron, Paolo Savelli, but certainly equal in quality and interest?

Bissell laments the tendency in Orazio's Genoese paintings toward an aristocratic refinement—a final severing of the Caravaggesque basis of his Roman production. And he believes that Orazio's contacts with Genoese noble families and the increasing importance of private commissions both contributed to an art in which "it appeared uncertain whether the figures . . . were living out human experiences or acting out roles." My own sense is that, on the one hand, Orazio's renewed contact in Genoa with the paintings of Rubens, as well as with those of Van Dyck, had a greater impact on his art than the taste of his patrons and that, on the other, the increased emphasis in his work on surface effects and formal arrangement was part of a general trend in Italian painting. Regardless, the seeds for these qualities were sown in Rome, and in many respects the Genoese paintings represent the climax of that continuous dialogue between naturalism and *maniera* that is at the core of his art.

1. Ratti was the editor of a 1768 edition of Soprani, and there he singled out the *Danaë* as the finest.
2. In 1906, Suida recorded a version of the Magdalene in the collection of Marchese Pierino Nerotti, whose family owned a villa at Arenzano.
3. Not only do the colors have a hard, steely quality, but the picture seems to have been carefully drawn in and painted section by section. This is particularly clear in the case of Lot, where the brown preparation is visible around the figure as well as between the color divisions. The wine flask and drinking cup have no texture, the shadows no transparency, and the grass is painted in mechanically.
4. See Leonard, Khandekar, and Carr 2001, 7–10.
5. The *Magdalene* has been examined in the Metropolitan's conservation studio. The canvas has been trimmed on all sides; painted canvas has been turned over the top and sides of the stretcher for tacking. It is not possible to establish precisely how much has been lost.

35.

Penitent Magdalene

Oil on canvas, 58⅞ × 72 in. (149.5 × 183 cm)

Private collection

1622–23

New York

PROVENANCE: Giovan Antonio Sauli, Genoa (from 1621); Palazzo Sauli, Genoa (until at least 1780); Marchese Pierino Negrotti, Genoa (by 1906); Marchesa Carlotta Cattaneo-Adorno, Arenzano, near Genoa (until 1975); Thomas P. Grange, London (from 1975); his wife (until 1999); private collection.

RELATED PICTURES: Kunsthistorisches Museum, Vienna (variant);[15] Richard L. Feigen, New York (variant);[16] Pinacoteca, Lucca (copy);[17] Musée des Beaux-Arts, Dijon (copy with a traditional attribution to Jean Tassel);[18] private collection, Madrid (said by Pérez Sánchez to be a copy of the Vienna version).[19]

REFERENCES: Soprani 1674, 317; Ratti 1768, 452; Ratti 1780, 112; Suida 1906, 156; Voss 1925, 460; Nicolson 1979, 53; Bissell 1981, 173–74 no. 46, 177–78, 182; Nicolson 1985, 11–14; Nicolson 1990, 115; Bissell 1999, 50, 229; Leonard, Khandekar, and Carr 2001, 5–6; Matthiesen 2001, 162.

It was Correggio who first painted the full-length Magdalene reclining in a landscape.[1] But it is Titian's half-length depiction in the Galleria Palatina, Palazzo Pitti, Florence (fig. 68), and its later variants that best elucidate the religious psychology that underlies Orazio's *Penitent Magdalene*, painted for Giovan Antonio Sauli.[2] Titian's painting was unquestionably the most celebrated and influential devotional image of the saint, and the one that exemplifies the very different cued responses of sixteenth- and seventeenth-century, as opposed to modern, viewers. In it Mary Magdalene is shown nude, sensually robust, her gaze directed heavenward, her luxuriant hair gathered up by her hands in a gesture that recalls a Venus *pudica* but leaves her breasts exposed. Ridolfi believed that Titian based his figure on an antique statue. Certainly his image, like Orazio's, plays on the convention of the beautiful female nude derived from ancient sculpture. Titian later varied this composition, showing the figure draped, standing before a rocky outcrop and a distant landscape. Tears—the emblem of contrition and penance—course down the saint's cheeks. An open

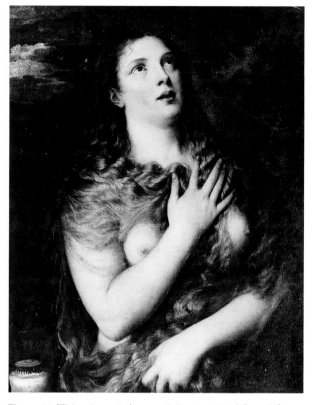

Figure 68. Titian (ca. 1485/90–1576), *Penitent Magdalene*. Oil on canvas. Galleria Palatina, Palazzo Pitti, Florence

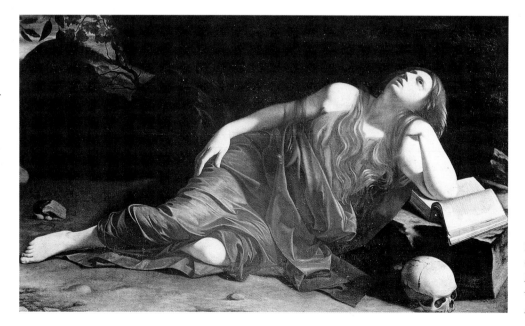

Figure 69. Jean Tassel (?) (ca. 1608–1667), *Penitent Magdalene*. Oil on canvas. Musée des Beaux-Arts, Dijon

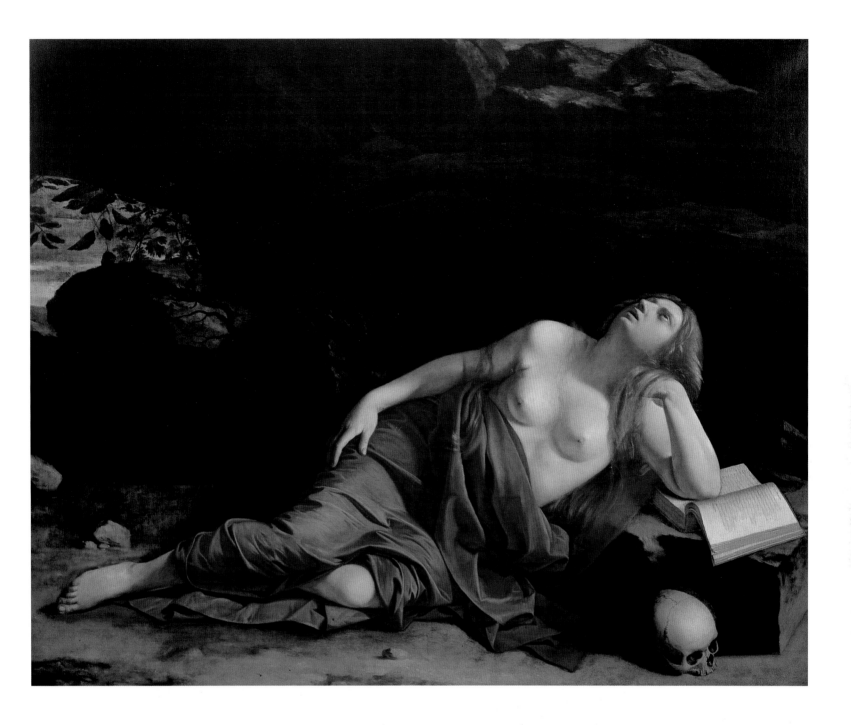

Bible is propped on a skull to one side while on the other is an ointment jar, symbolic of the perfumes she used to bathe Christ's feet and brought to anoint his body following the Crucifixion.

To modern eyes, the Pitti prototype and its variants are provocatively ambiguous images—devotional pretense seeming barely to mask overt eroticism. Many later critics have found Titian's depictions lacking in religious decorum. In their groundbreaking mono-

graph of 1881 on the artist, Crowe and Cavalcaselle declare, "It is clear that Titian had no other purpose in view than to represent a handsome girl," and more recently another scholar has questioned how many sixteenth-century viewers responded to the image in a spiritually edifying fashion.[3] This modern attitude seems prefigured in Cardinal Gabriele Paleotti's 1582 *Discorso intorno alle imagini sacre e profane,* in which the Counter-Reformation churchman condemned the practice of depicting mistresses in the guise of the Magdalene.[4] However, it is a matter of record that sophisticated sixteenth- and seventeenth-century viewers responded to the many versions and copies of Titian's *Magdalene* as a devotionally efficacious image, at once beautiful and devout. Of the version sent to Philip II, king of Spain, Vasari writes, "Raising her head, with her eyes fixed on heaven, she reveals remorse in the redness of the eyes, and in her tears [she shows] repentance for her sins: wherefore the picture greatly moves all who look at it, and, what is more, although she is very beautiful, it does not inspire lust but compassion."[5] A copy of the Pitti picture was owned by Paleotti's fellow churchman Federico Borromeo, who noted that Titian showed the saint "consumed with grief and love but nevertheless full of life. In order to express all this the painter represents [the Magdalene] in the flower of youth, going perhaps against the evangelical story."[6] Borromeo's response touches on the mainspring of the painting, what we might call a poetics of contrapposto. Revealingly, in 1531 Federico Gonzaga had asked Titian to paint him a Magdalene "as beautiful and as tearful as possible."[7] (The picture was intended as a gift to that paragon of piety Vittoria Colonna, who was hardly interested in sublimated erotica.) Virtually every religious poem about the Magdalene written in the seventeenth century plays on the twin themes of the saint's beauty and the redeeming power of her tears, almost inevitably compared to precious pearls. Richard Crashaw's "Saint Mary Magdalene, or The Weeper" (stanza 14), exemplifies the genre: "Well does the May that lies / Smiling in thy cheeks, confess / The April in thine eyes. / Mutual sweetness they express. / No April e'er lent kinder showers, / Nor May return'd more faithful flowers." Titian sought not to depict the ascetic Magdalene but to evoke both aspects of the saint's life: as a prostitute redeemed through contrition and as the personification of sensual beauty transfigured through penitence. Without Titian's painting and the responses it inspired, we would be ill equipped to understand a whole series of seventeenth-century depictions of the Magdalene by artists as diverse as Guido Reni, Simon Vouet, Rubens, Bernini— and Gentileschi.

Orazio must have decided on a reclining Magdalene as a thematic counterpoint to the *Danaë* (cat. 36)—the one an encomium to sensual love, the other, "with her eyes fixed on heaven," to divine love. As in Guido Reni's full-length *Penitent Magdalene* painted for the Barberini (Galleria Nazionale d'Arte Antica, Rome)— shown seated rather than recumbent—the devotional effect on the viewer is achieved not by any overt expressivity but with a pose of great formal beauty.[8] It was through penance and the renunciation of her life of sin that the inner purity of the Magdalene's soul was made manifest, and in Orazio's painting the Magdalene—her beauty given added poignancy by the presence of the skull (a conventional emblem of *vanitas*)—literally turns her head away from earthly matters and, inspired by the text she has been reading, sorrowfully gazes upward. Through an opening in the cave the sky can be seen. The Magdalene's head is propped on her arm—a pose denoting contemplation, used by both Reni and Vouet, among others. The figure's hair has suffered from abrasion; originally, the highlighted golden tresses against the nude torso suggested yet another devotional meditation, since the Magdalene is shown scorning those attributes most admired in beautiful women.[9]

That the picture catalogued here is the one owned by Sauli cannot be doubted (see p. 30). That it is also the prime version is another matter (see pp. 172–73). The contour of the skull was moved to the left, but X radiographs (fig. 28) demonstrate that the figure was laid in with no significant adjustments. The landscape, by contrast, is painted very loosely, and it further develops Orazio's sense of atmospheric effects seen initially in his small paintings on copper. The picture is darker in tonality than its companion pictures and, like the *Danaë*, sets the figure against an almost black background. The resulting quality, first explored in the Fogg *Madonna with the Sleeping Christ Child* (cat. 28), is of exceptional elegance. Because the painting is less well preserved than the *Lot and His Daughters* (cat. 37), the face does not appear as crisply drawn and the sheen on the drapery and hair lacks an equal brilliance. This is, nevertheless, a stunning picture. The *Penitent Magdalene* must be contemporary with Sauli's other paintings. The success of the composition is indicated by two variants (Kunsthistorisches Museum, Vienna [fig. 26], and Richard L. Feigen, New York), as well as copies (see under related pictures).

Bissell suggests the possibility that the picture was painted in Rome and given to Sauli or that it was based on a still earlier version—perhaps the picture now in the Pinacoteca, Lucca.[10] The painting in Lucca seems, however, to be no more than a copy of the Sauli picture, though with differences in the landscape. Its primary interest is the additional testimony it provides to the fame of the Sauli picture, since it was given to the Pinacoteca in 1847, by Leopold II of Tuscany. To my mind, there is not much reason to believe a lost Roman prototype ever existed. It is true that a *Magdalene* ascribed to Orazio is listed in 1700 as in the Palazzo Borghese, but what kind of composition this was—half-length, full-length?—is unknown, and the reliability of the attribution is problematic at best.[11] An engraving by Claude Mellan, who was active in Rome between 1624 and 1636, has been presumed to reflect his knowledge of Orazio's composition, and Bissell has adduced it as further proof for the existence of a lost Roman prototype.[12] However, the relationship does not seem to me sufficiently close to presuppose a dependence on Orazio's painting.[13] And can we be sure that Mellan did not see the Sauli painting in Genoa, en route to Rome, or a version sent to Paris?[14] The latter possibility is suggested by a copy ascribed to Jean Tassel (fig. 69) that certainly does derive from the Sauli picture or a closely related version. It has a provenance from the Convent des Lazaristes, near Dijon (appropriately, given the destination of the picture, the saint's breasts have been covered with drapery and abundant hair). With this provenance, it seems more likely that the copy was painted in France rather than in Rome and that it derives from a version of Orazio's picture which was sent to Paris (see p. 213 n. 23).

1. For Correggio's much copied composition, formerly in the Gemäldegalerie, Dresden, see Gould 1976, 279–80. Correggio's composition was known widely and was, for example, crucial to Giovanni Lanfranco's picture in the Alte Pinakothek, Munich.

2. See Aikema 1994, and Goffen 1997, 171–92. Goffen reviews the various literary responses noted below, and the reader is referred to her for a fuller discussion. My one reservation about Aikema's groundbreaking article is his assertion that the Counter-

Reformation so changed attitudes that Titian's image became incomprehensible. I believe that the evidence suggests that many seventeenth-century artists—including Gentileschi—understood exactly what Titian was about and constructed their images along the same lines.

3. Mormando in Boston 1999, 117. There is some confusion in many of these discussions between the general censure of nudity in religious art by sixteenth-century reformers and the specific iconography of the Penitent Magdalene, in which nudity is at the very core of the picture's meaning. See, for example, Brown in London–Rome 2001, 286–88. Of course, for some beholders nudity was always associated with arousal.

4. Paleotti in Barocchi 1960–62, vol. 2, 266 and 367.

5. Vasari (1568) 1878–85, vol. 7, 454.

6. See Quint 1974, 230.

7. Crowe and Cavalcaselle 1881, vol. 1, 451.

8. For an interesting, psycho-sexual discussion of Reni's depictions of the Magdalene, see Spear 1997, 163–80.

9. Aikema 1994, 48 n. 4, quotes from F. Luigini da Udine's *Il libro della bella donna*, in which "crini d'oro" and breasts "simili a due rotondi dolci pomi" are praised. The illustration for Penitence in Philip Galle's *Prosopographia* is a young woman with bared breasts who holds a scourge in one hand.

10. Bissell 1981, 174, and Bissell 1999, 229.

11. See Sterling (1958, 117), who notes that in the same inventory a picture by Lelio Orsi was also erroneously ascribed to Orazio. The *Magdalene* appears in no other Borghese inventories. This seems to me very shaky evidence on which to build a thesis.

12. For Mellan's print, see Thuillier 1960, 92; Brejon de Lavergnée 1979; and Rome 1989–90, 254–56.

13. Another picture has been introduced into this discussion by Bissell 1999, 228–30, a *Penitent Magdalene*, in a collection in Naples, which has been ascribed to Artemisia. I know the picture only from reproduction, but it does not appear to me to be by Artemisia. Its relation to Orazio's composition strikes me as generic.

14. Da Morrona (1792) 1812, 476, asserted that Orazio sent a picture to Marie de' Medici to solicit her patronage, but he does not mention a subject. The basis of his statement is not known, but see p. 203 in this publication.

15. For this splendid, fully autograph picture, see Bissell 1981, 108–9, 182–83; Finaldi in London–Bilbao–Madrid 1999, 17; and cat. 45. It belonged to the duke of Buckingham and is inventoried at York House in 1635. It may, however, have been painted in France (or even Genoa), since it is known that Gentileschi sent the duke two canvases prior to his arrival in London. There is record of a payment for a Magdalene in the accounts drawn up in 1629 by Balthazar Gerbier, who acted on behalf of the duke. In the Vienna version, the right foot of the Magdalene is extended in a more horizontal position than in the Sauli painting and the skull sits on the open book, which is rotated ninety degrees; the cave and the landscape are completely different. When a tracing from the Sauli picture is laid over the Vienna painting, there is a part-to-part match, except for the foot. See p. 30 in this publication. Clearly, a tracing or cartoon was used to lay in the composition.

16. See, again, Bissell 1981, 181–82. The provenance of this picture cannot be firmly established before 1805, when it was bought in Paris by the seventh earl of Elgin. To my eyes, it is the latest of the known versions (see Bissell for a contrary view) and could conceivably

be the picture Sandrart saw in Orazio's London studio in 1628 being painted for Charles I. However, the matter is far from clear.

17. For the Lucca picture, see, in addition to Bissell 1981, Florence 1986, 197, and Borella and Giusti Maccari 1993, 269. The picture has all the earmarks of a copy: overly emphatic definition and exaggerated contrasts of light and dark.

18. See Ronot 1990, 285, and the essay by Jean-Pierre Cuzin in this publication, p. 213 n. 23.

19. See Pérez-Sánchez 1965, 503; and Bissell 1981, 183. Pérez-Sánchez has kindly informed me that the whereabouts of the picture, which he knew only from a photograph made during the Spanish civil war, are not known.

36.

Danaë

Oil on canvas, 62¾ × 89¼ in. (159.4 × 226.7 cm)

Richard L. Feigen, New York

1621–23

New York

PROVENANCE: Giovan Antonio Sauli, Genoa (from 1621/22); Palazzo Sauli, Genoa (as late as 1792); Marchesa Carlotta Cattaneo-Adorno, Arenzano, near Genoa (1975); Thomas P. Grange, London (1975–79); Richard L. Feigen, New York.

RELATED PICTURES: See cat. 41.

REFERENCES: Soprani 1674, 317; Ratti 1768, 452; Ratti 1780, 112; Da Morrona (1792) 1812, 475; Suida 1906, 156; Voss 1925, 460; Bissell 1969, 20, 30–31; Nicolson 1979, 51–52; Bissell 1981, 45–46, 49, 174, 176–77 no. 49, 178; Mann 1985, 383–87; Nicolson 1985, 11–12, 16, 21; Garrard 1989, 242; Nicolson 1990, 112; Genoa 1997, 160; Bissell 1999, 6, 7, 49, 50, 312; Leonard, Khandekar, and Carr 2001, 5–7, 10; Matthiesen 2001, 162.

The *Danaë* is one of Orazio's most brilliant creations—arresting in its formal beauty and dazzling in its depiction of light playing across the varied surfaces of satin, linen, and gilt metal. Only in the *Annunciation* in Turin (cat. 43), painted for Carlo Emanuele I, duke of Savoy, in 1622–23, did Orazio produce a work of comparable descriptive richness and splendor, although in that work the effect is of quiet intimacy rather than bravura display.

Danaë is shown reclining on a bed, locked in the secret chamber to which her father, King Acrisius of Argos, had confined her so that she would never meet a man and bear the son whose hand would deprive him of his life. Jupiter, who had seen and fallen in love with her, appears in a shower of gold coins and shavings (the latter detail is unprecedented in depictions of the subject and, so far as one can establish, an invention without literary source).[1] Cupid, his genitals suggestively exposed between the crisp folds of the coverlet, draws back the curtain as the god enters the closed room and Danaë extends one hand in a rhetorical gesture signifying her acceptance or solicitation (Guercino gives a similar gesture to Potiphar's wife as she tries to seduce Joseph, in his painting of 1649 in the National Gallery, Washington, and Orazio used it for his altarpiece in the Brera, Milan, in which Saint Cecilia receives her crown of roses from an angel). As pointed out by Bissell, her pose has been adapted from a *Danaë* designed by Annibale Carracci (destroyed; formerly Bridgewater House, London), in which, however, the extended hand is used to push back the curtain while Cupid kneels beside the bed, drawing an arrow from his quiver.

The closeness of Danaë's pose to that of the figure in the companion *Magdalene* (cat. 35) has the effect of pointing up the contrast between two kinds of union—spiritual and sexual.[2] Although the subject is an erotic one, Orazio's protagonist is a far cry from the Danaës of Correggio's and Titian's canvases (or, indeed, from his own *Cleopatra*; cat. 17). Orazio was familiar with Titian's celebrated painting in the Farnese collection, Rome, which Vasari describes appositely as "a nude woman portrayed as Danaë."[3] As with Guido Reni's and Guercino's heroines, Orazio's Danaë is curiously chaste. The contrast with Artemisia's earlier, small rendition (cat. 54)— an image of sexual greed, emphasized by the coins in the princess's lap and those she holds tightly in her fist—could not be greater. (In Orazio's picture the coins, which bear the images of Jupiter and thunderbolts, fall not in her lap but toward her face.) The real frisson in Orazio's picture comes from the way Danaë's ivory-skinned body is set off by the icy sheen of the citron-colored satin coverlet.

The comparison with Reni's work may extend beyond a modest approach to depicting the female nude. Reni's great *Assumption of the Virgin,* installed in the Gesù in Genoa in 1617–18, with its striking use of pale-colored fabrics in the upper register and its composition constructed on the basis of echoing diagonals, cannot have failed to impress Orazio. But perhaps even more important for the new emphasis in his work on the sheen of fabrics—apart from the fact that Genoa was a major center of textile production—was the arrival in 1620 of Rubens's spectacular altarpiece

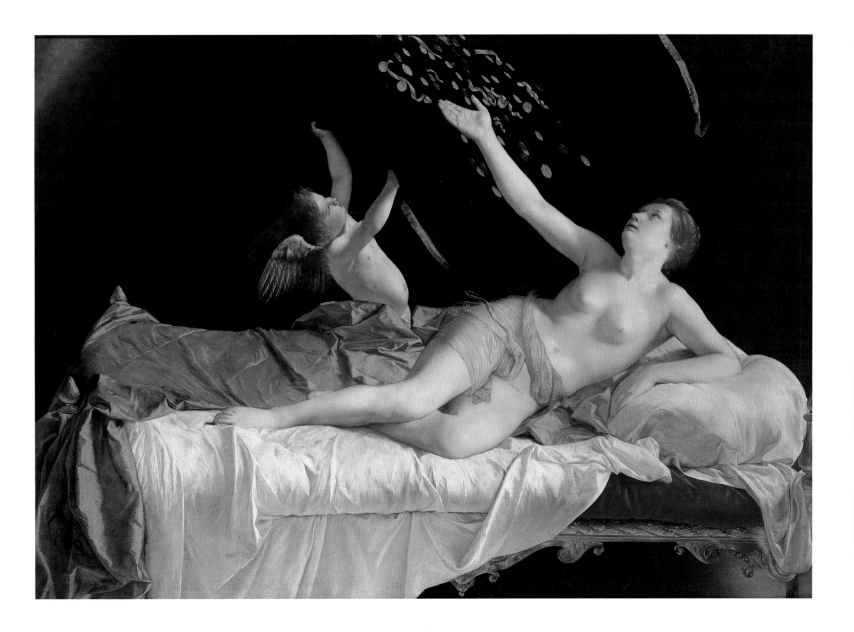

showing a miracle of Saint Ignatius of Loyola. Installed in the transept of the Gesù opposite Reni's *Assumption*, this picture must have struck Orazio as unsurpassed in its depiction of costumes: the eye-catching magenta silk dress worn by the mother in the center of the composition, the gold-threaded chasuble worn by Saint Ignatius, and the red curtain of the baldachin over the saint (a motif Orazio was to use to great advantage in his *Annunciation* sent to Turin in 1623). Rubens enjoyed great prestige in Genoa, where during his Italian sojourn he had painted a number of aristocratic portraits, and although the Fleming's restless, spatially complex compositions were well beyond Orazio's abilities, it would be surprising if

the Pisan did not respond in some way to his art. It should, moreover, be remembered that one of Orazio's Genoese patrons, Pietro Gentile, owned a *modello* for the Gesù altarpiece (see cat. 39). Then there is the factor of Van Dyck, who arrived in Genoa for a three-month stay in November 1621, returning to the city for several months every year from 1623 until 1627. What Orazio's work shares with Van Dyck's is an emphasis on refinement and elegance rather than drama and expressivity. Might we not see Danaë's citron coverlet as Gentileschi's answer to, for example, the shimmering red robe in Van Dyck's portrait of Agostino Pallavicino (J. Paul Getty Museum, Los Angeles): an attempt to match the virtuosity of the

Flemish master on his own terms? On one of his later visits to Genoa, Van Dyck sketched two of Orazio's compositions (cat. nos. 74, 94), but in the *Danaë* it is perhaps Van Dyck who has spurred the Italian to greater heights.[4]

Garrard draws an analogy between Rembrandt's and Orazio's treatment of the theme, going so far as to suggest that the Dutchman knew the Italian's painting. Given the location of the picture in Genoa, this can be ruled out.

1. The primary sources for the story of Danaë are Ovid's *Metamorphoses* and Boccaccio's *De genealogia deorum gentilium*. In the *Genealogia*, Boccaccio recounts how Jupiter became enamored of the princess and transformed himself into a shower of gold that seeped through the tiles of the roof and dripped onto Danaë's lap. The same account is given by Comes and is also found in Michel de Marolles, *Tableaux du Temple des Muses* of 1655. It is as a shower of gold that Jupiter appears in Correggio's depiction. Horace, however, speaks of *pretium* (money), and this is what the coins in Titian's, Tintoretto's, and Orazio's pictures convey.

2. A medieval tradition saw Danaë's impregnation by Jupiter as an analogue to the Virgin birth of Christ, but another tradition, going back to Augustine, saw her as an antitype to the Virgin and an emblem of immodesty and sexual licentiousness—someone paid in gold for her services. On this, see Settis 1985. Whether Orazio was aware of either tradition may be doubted, but the pairing is suggestive.

3. Perhaps, significantly, a version or copy of Titian's canvas was in the Doria collection in Genoa. See Genoa 1997, 214.

4. Gamba (1922–23, 246) interprets the influence as running in the opposite direction.

37.
Lot and His Daughters

Oil on canvas, 59¾ × 74½ in. (151.8 × 189.2 cm)

The J. Paul Getty Museum, Los Angeles (98.PA.10)

ca. 1621–22

PROVENANCE: Giovan Antonio Sauli, Genoa (from ca. 1621–22); Palazzo Sauli, Genoa (sold after 1780); Teophilatus (d. 1910) collection, Genoa; Margaret Pole, her villa at Diano Marina, near Impèria (until 1925/28) and England (from 1925/28); by descent, Jean Milne, Hertfordshire (d. 1986); her niece (1986–98); Johnny van Haeflten, London (1998); The J. Paul Getty Museum, Los Angeles.

RELATED PICTURES: Gemäldegalerie, Berlin (workshop variant);[2] National Gallery of Canada, Ottawa (variant);[3] Thyssen-Bornemisza Collection, Madrid (reduced copy of the Getty picture);[4] Castello di Carrù, near Turin (copy related to Ottawa version);[5] private

The third (though probably not the latest) in the triad of paintings Orazio carried out for Giovan Antonio Sauli and the one that most attracted Soprani, our primary source for the commission, shows Lot, the nephew of the Old Testament patriarch Abraham, asleep in the lap of one of his daughters. She leans over him, pointing into the distance—toward, one supposes, the burning city of Sodom and their mother, who was transformed into a pillar of salt for disobeying God and looking back at the sinful city, which the sisters had fled in the wake of its destruction. Father and daughters, we are told in Genesis 19:30–38, took refuge in a cave and there the daughters, fearful that the human race had been extinguished and that they would find no husband with whom to bear children, got their father drunk and slept with him.

The story of Lot and His Daughters was often taken as a warning against drunkenness. Lot was also an old man made a fool by love. The daughters were sometimes interpreted as examples of pride or carnal desire—despite the fact that some biblical commentators had excused their actions because they were based not on desire but on fear of extinction.[1] The story was seldom illustrated before the sixteenth century;

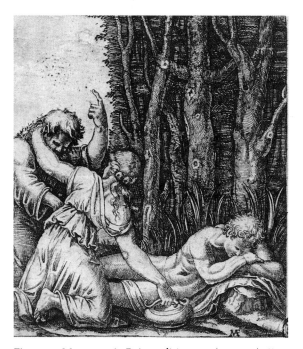

Figure 70. Marcantonio Raimondi (ca. 1470/82–1527/34?), *Man Sleeping at the Edge of a Wood*. Engraving. The Metropolitan Museum of Art, New York

in the seventeenth it became enormously popular and we find it included in cycles of paintings with biblical themes, such as the three canvases Guercino painted for Cardinal Ludovisi in 1617. These showed Lot and

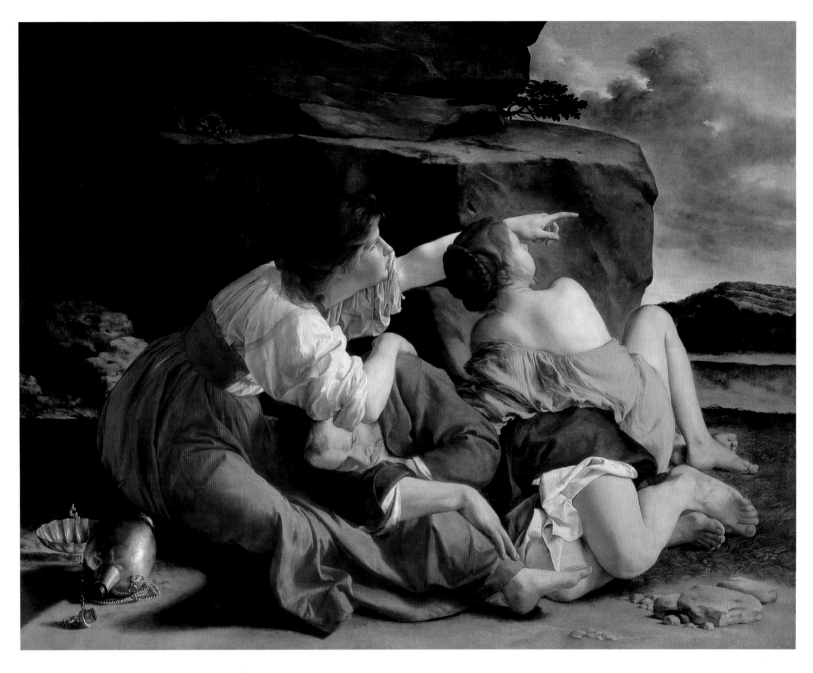

collection, Rome (copy of the
Ottawa version);[6] Burghley
House, Stamford (reduced
copy of a lost picture);[7] Musée
de l'Assistance Publique, Paris
(copy of lost picture).[8]

REFERENCES: Soprani 1674,
317; Ratti 1768, 452; Ratti 1780,
112; Bissell 1969, 30, no. 1;
Bissell 1981, 174–75; Laskin
and Pantazzi 1987, 114;
Leonard, Khandekar, and
Carr 2001, 4–10.

His Daughters, Susanna and the Elders, and the
Prodigal Son. The theme is also sometimes included
in cycles relating to celebrated or notorious females
(*femmes fortes*). In the late 1620s, Claude Mellan made
a number of engravings, not all of his own design, on
precisely this sort of theme—Judith and Holofernes,
Samson and Delilah (fig. 79), Herodiae, Caritas
Romana, Lot and His Daughters. As in Guercino's
paintings, Mellan shows Lot being plied with drink
by his daughters, and the Latin inscription carries
the admonition "What good was it to flee those flames
if a harsher fire inflames chaste breasts with an

incestuous torch?" ("Quid flammas fugisse iuvat; si
saevior ignis / Incesta accendit pectora casta face?")
This is precisely the sort of moralistic conceit we
would expect to be attached to the subject.

Orazio's painting departs from such depictions by
showing Lot asleep, having emptied the discarded flask
of wine, while his daughters, one of whom is obviously disheveled, discuss their fate. The daughters are
hardly the revelers so often encountered, but there is
no question that they are the protagonists. Lot is a
passive presence, the spent object of his daughters'
schemes. In this resides the psychological fascination

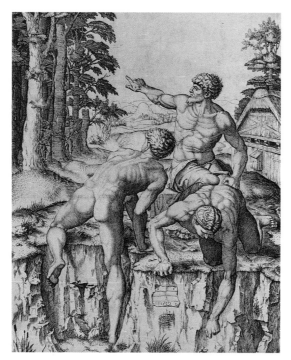

Figure 71. Marcantonio Raimondi (ca. 1470/82–1527/34?), *Climbers*. Engraving after Michelangelo. The Metropolitan Museum of Art, New York

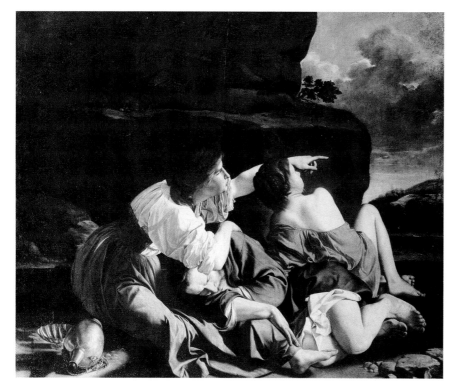

Figure 72. Orazio Gentileschi, *Lot and His Daughters*. Oil on canvas. Gemäldegalerie, Staatliche Museen zu Berlin

of a picture that is conspicuously lacking in conventional narrative action. As in the Hartford *Judith and Her Maidservant* (cat. 39), the effect is of a tableau vivant. The psychological dimension emerges from formal juxtapositions: the exposed legs of Lot and those of his daughter, paired suggestively as mirror images (X radiographs show that Orazio significantly altered the position of the daughter's legs to achieve this effect; see fig. 13); Lot's right hand on the leg of the daughter in whose lap he rests his head; the prominent, phallic spout of the emptied flask of wine. The use of demonstrative gestures—which becomes almost pedagogical in his later depiction of the subject for Queen Henrietta Maria (cat. 46)—must reflect Orazio's awareness of such artists as Giovanni Lanfranco and, especially, Simon Vouet, whose *Birth of the Virgin* was installed in San Francesco a Ripa, Rome, not long before Orazio left for Genoa. (Has there ever been more activity generated by the mere passing of a piece of linen from one person to another?) But in conceiving this composition Orazio may also have turned to his collection of prints, in particular to Marcantonio Raimondi's engravings of a man sleeping at the edge of a wood (fig. 70), with its combination of a sleeping male figure and an emphatic pointing gesture, and the so-called *Climbers* (fig. 71), based on Michelangelo's cartoon for the *Battle of Cascina*. In Orazio's painting, the emphasis is on elegance of design (not least the splendid triad of rose, blue, and citron set off by white) and refinement of execution—the keynotes of his Genoese paintings.

The Getty *Lot* was known from a photograph taken in the early years of the twentieth century, but the picture came to public attention only in 1997. Its whereabouts were unknown to Bissell, who mistakenly put forward as the Sauli painting what I believe to be no more than a copy, now in the Thyssen-Bornemisza Collection, Madrid. X rays of the Getty picture (fig. 12) show significant changes (these are published and discussed at length by Leonard, Khandekar, and Carr). What is not clear is whether Orazio painted the composition over a previously used canvas. Beneath the daughter at the left is a figure shown leaning back, in an attitude of abandon. Is this a first idea for the *Lot*, or possibly the remnants of an unfinished composition? The scale is different from that in the completed picture and the style of the figure—so far as can be judged—does not look particularly Gentileschian. A companion figure was depicted in close proximity, turning back and glancing upward—very much like the *Young Woman Playing a Violin* (cat. 40). This figure suggests Gentileschi's habit of recycling in other compositions poses he had already used.

In 1622, Orazio, in an effort to procure a position at court, sent a version of the Sauli picture to Carlo Emanuele, duke of Savoy (he refers to this in a letter of April 2, 1623). The picture is usually identified with the version of the composition in Berlin (fig. 72), which was painted by Orazio's workshop using a tracing of the Sauli picture (see pp. 22–26). In his 1674 biography, Soprani writes that Orazio also sent pictures to Marie de' Medici in France. This statement was picked up by Da Morrona, who notes that *a* picture was sent to Marie de' Medici. No subject is mentioned, but the version of the *Lot* now in Ottawa (cat. 42) has occasionally been identified with that picture. However, a copy of the Ottawa picture has been noted in a Savoy castle, the Castello di Carrù, and it now appears likely that the Ottawa rather than the Berlin version was sent to Carlo Emanuele (see note 2, below). It does not attain the quality of the Getty picture and was produced with the aid of a tracing, but like the Cleveland *Danaë* (cat. 41), it appears to be an autograph replica.

1. For a history of the various interpretations attached to the story, see Kind 1967.

2. See Bissell 1981, 175–76. Ever since it was published by Oertel (1971, 237–42), this version, which comes from the nineteenth-century collection of José Madrazo in Madrid, has often been identified with the painting sent by Orazio to Carlo Emanuele I, duke of Savoy, in 1622. Also in the Madrazo collection was a version of Orazio's *Rest on the Flight into Egypt* that, it was asserted in the 1856 catalogue, was a gift of Carlo Emanuele's son Cardinal Maurizio of Savoy to the marquis of Leganés, who was Spanish governor of Milan from 1635 until 1641. (Cardinal Maurizio's brother Vittorio Amedeo I, who succeeded Carlo Emanuele as ruler of Savoy, died in 1637, and Maurizio relinquished his cardinal's hat in 1642, when he married Ludovica di Savoia.) Both pictures are listed in Leganés's inventories of 1642 and 1655, without attribution but with the cardinal of Savoy provenance noted for the *Rest on the Flight*. Whether the *Lot* was a Savoy picture and whether either painting belonged to Carlo Emanuele is speculative, although pictures from the duke's collection are known to have been used as diplomatic gifts. Carlo Emanuele's *Lot*

can be traced in successive Savoy inventories of 1631, 1635, and one drawn up before 1646; no *Rest on the Flight* by Gentileschi is mentioned in any of these. On balance it therefore seems more likely that Cardinal Maurizio owned his own versions of Orazio's pictures. There is a copy, moreover, of the *Lot* composition in the Carrù, near Turin, that repeats the Ottawa picture (see note 3 below); see Bava in Romano 1995, 246 n. 158. In the 1856 catalogue of José Madrazo, the *Lot* is described as depicting in the background the burning city of Sodom; this was shown on an additional strip of the Berlin picture that has since been removed.

3. The most thorough treatment of this picture is in Laskin and Pantazzi 1987, 113–16. The picture, invariably accepted as autograph, was at one time thought to be the *Lot* sent by Orazio to the duke of Savoy in 1622; see Bissell 1969. It has a provenance from the collection of the duke of Orléans, where it is recorded after 1737. Curiously, the illustration in the 1808 catalogue of the Orléans collection (by Couché) shows not the Ottawa picture but a version now in the Musée de l'Assistance Publique, Paris, which includes in the background the burning city of Sodom. Evidently, Couché did not have a drawing of the Orléans picture, which had been sold in 1790, and took his design from another available version (see note 8 below). In the Ottawa painting and the copy of it in a Roman private collection, the face of the daughter on the left, beautifully foreshortened in the Sauli picture, is viewed—rather unsuccessfully—in strict profile. Bissell (1981, 180–81) suggested, very hypothetically, that this picture was sent by Orazio from Genoa to Marie de' Medici, but the existence of a copy in the Castello di Carrù, near Turin, makes it probable that the Ottawa—not the Berlin—picture was sent by Orazio to Carlo Emanuele; see Bava in Romano 1995, 246 n. 158, and note 2 above.

4. See Bissell (1981, 174–75), who incorrectly confuses this with the picture now in the J. Paul Getty Museum. Its provenance prior to the early twentieth century is not known.

5. See Bava in Romano 1995, 246 n. 158.

6. See Marini (1981, 179), who ascribes it to Orazio and his workshop. To judge from the reproduction, the quality does not attain this level.

7. See Bissell 1969, 31 no. 3. This small picture (48.5 × 60.5 cm, on panel) records a composition identical to one engraved in the 1808 catalogue of the Orléans collection (see note 8, below). Bissell notes that, as with the *Madonna and Child* (cat. 38), the *Lot* was given to the ninth earl of Exeter in 1774 by Pope Clement XIV. I am informed by John Culverhouse, curator at Burghley House, and by John Somerville, that this is incorrect. It seems to me worth considering the possibility that the Burghley House picture, which was ascribed in early guidebooks to Velázquez and then (even more surprisingly) to Mantegna, is identical to the painting sold at Le Brun in Paris on April 11, 1791. That work, also ascribed to Velázquez, was described as "un petit tableau du grand dans la coll. du Palais d'Orléans. Bois. H. 9 pouces L. 12½ pouces" (about 24 × 33 cm). In a copy of the ninth earl's 1753 *Abécédario* he made a note opposite the entry for Velázquez (p. 141): "Lot & his 2 daughters by d[itt]o in the Orleans pallace in Paris. d[itt]o by d[itt]o in the Royal Collection at Turin. d[itt]o by d[itt]o but smaller at Burghley."

8. This is evidently the picture reproduced by Couché in the 1808 *Galerie du Palais Royal*. Couché began his engravings for this

publication in 1786, four years prior to the dispersal of the Orléans collection. The Revolution occasioned delays, and although Couché based his engravings on previously made drawings, in this case he seems, exceptionally, to have copied the version in the Musée de l'Assistance Publique rather than the actual Orléans painting, which is now in Ottawa and does not include the detail of the burning of Sodom in the background. It should be noted

that both the Paris copy and the small Burghley House copy (for which, see note 7 above) show the same composition and background—except that there is more landscape in the Burghley House painting. Presumably the Paris picture has been cut down. The picture suffers from flaking. I have not been able to examine the original, but have studied photographs procured by Stéphane Loire at the Louvre.

38.

Madonna and Child in a Landscape

Oil on copper, 11⅜ × 8½ in. (28.8 × 21.5 cm)

Burghley House, Stamford

ca. 1621–22

New York, Saint Louis

PROVENANCE: Probably the Jesuit order in Rome (by 1771, as by Castiglione); Clement XIV, Rome (until 1774); the ninth earl of Exeter (1774–93); the earls of Exeter (first recorded in Burghley House in 1797).

RELATED PICTURE: Palazzo Rosso, Genoa (slightly reduced copy).

REFERENCES: Burghley House 1797, 78–79; Waagen 1854, vol. 3, 405; London 1960, 24 no. 23; Nicolson 1960, 76–77; Oertel 1960, 95; Crinò and Nicolson 1961, 145 n. 15; Pérez Sánchez 1965, 502; Moir 1967, vol. 1, 39 n. 69, vol. 2, 76 no. c.4; Nicolson 1979, 52; Bissell 1981, 165, 167, 168 no. 39, 208; Nicolson 1990, 113; Giffi Ponzi 1994, 51–66; Brigstocke and Somerville in Pittsburgh 1995, 82–83 no. 21; London–Bilbao–Madrid 1999, 60–61 no. 4.

This exquisite picture was a gift of Pope Clement XIV (r. 1769–74) to the ninth earl of Exeter in 1774.[1] At the time, it was thought to be by the Genoese painter Giovanni Benedetto Castiglione; this attribution is recorded in an inscription on the back of the painting: "Del Fo. Gio. Benedetto Castiglione da Comp[ani]a di Gesù Genovese" (by Father Giovanni Benedetto Castiglione of the Genoese Society of Jesus). Interestingly, three years earlier the art dealer James Byres had attempted to acquire for the earl a small picture attributed to Castiglione from the Jesuits in Rome. He reported that "the Jesuits will not part with their little picture by Castiglione . . . [for] it is the only thing they have of that Father's work."[2] Clement signed a papal brief dissolving the Jesuits on July 21, 1773, and it is possible that the small picture passed into his possession at this time. That the two are the same work is suggested by the confusion between the seventeenth-century Genoese painter Giovanni Benedetto Castiglione (1609–1664) and the eighteenth-century Jesuit lay brother-painter Giuseppe Castiglione (1688–1766). While we can only speculate about how the picture came into the possession of either the Jesuits or the pope, an indication of its first owner is provided by a second version now in the Palazzo Rosso, Genoa. The interest of that picture, which Giffi Ponzi published as an autograph replica of the Burghley House copper but which I believe to be no more than a copy,[3] is that it has an inscription stating that it belonged to the Sauli family.

In his mention of the series of paintings Orazio carried out for Giovan Antonio Sauli, Soprani notes, in addition to the *Danaë* (cat. 36), the *Penitent Magdalene*

(cat. 35), and the *Lot and His Daughters* (cat. 37), "other paintings of great exquisiteness."[4] This description certainly applies to the Burghley House copper. Did Giovan Antonio's heirs make a gift of the painting to the Jesuit order, replacing it with a copy? The attribution to Castiglione, which has no stylistic basis, must derive from the picture's Genoese provenance. Castiglione, of course, was also a master of the miniature format, and the poetic beauty of the distant blue trees and the sky colored by the setting sun may have contributed to the erroneous attribution. In this picture, Orazio seems to have passed from the Elsheimerian, proto-Nazarene purity of the landscape of the *Saint Christopher* (cat. 27) into a more modern, plein-air vision. The picture is redolent with recollections of Rome. The brick wall with its chipped surface and crumbling plaster is typically Roman, and the figures recall, on a more intimate scale, the large *Rest on the Flight into Egypt* (cat. 34). In no other work does Orazio communicate a like sense of the fragility of life and the poignancy of the passage of time at day's end. Bissell dates the work to about 1615–20. As this entry suggests, I am inclined to think it a Genoese picture, of about 1621–22.

1. The details are found in Pittsburgh 1995, 82.
2. Ibid.
3. I have examined the picture on two occasions, the second time with Mary Newcome and Erich Schleier, and we were all of the mind that it is not conceivably by Orazio. The modeling throughout is hard and metallic. There is no quality of vibration to the light. The brickwork is dull, and the ivy leaves without life. While I would not want to eliminate the possibility of the picture's being a workshop replica, I think it more likely a later copy.
4. Soprani 1674, 316–17.

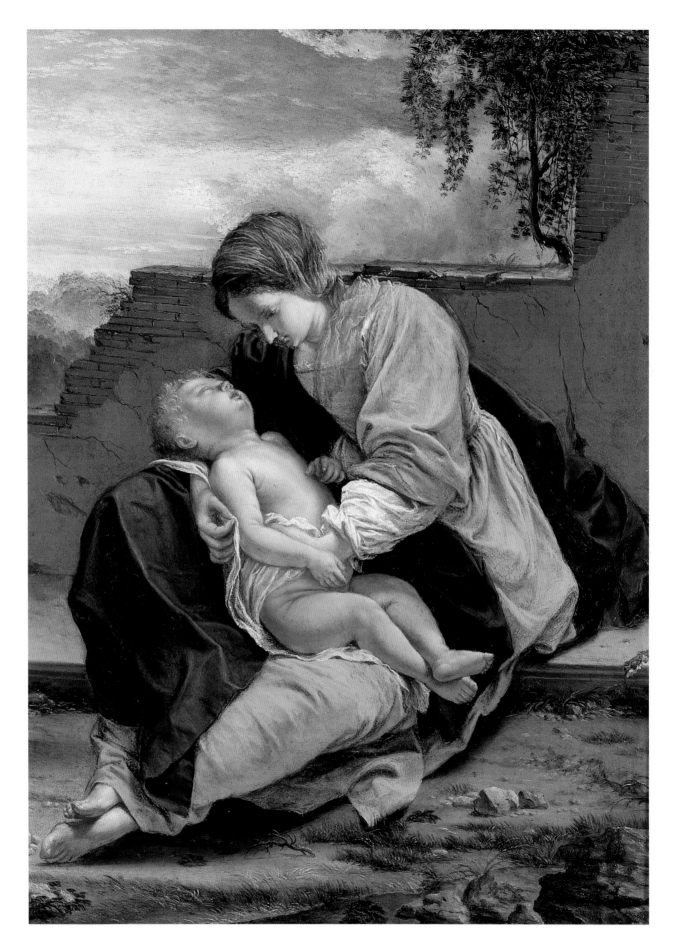

39.

Judith and Her Maidservant with the Head of Holofernes

Oil on canvas, 53¾ × 62⅝ in.
(136.5 × 159 cm)

Wadsworth Atheneum
Museum of Art, Hartford,
Conn., The Ella Gallup Sumner
and Mary Catlin Sumner
Collection Fund (1949.52)

ca. 1621–24

Of Orazio's depictions of the theme of Judith and Her Maidservant, the one in Hartford is the most refined and compelling. As in an earlier treatment in Oslo (cat. 13), the two women, united by their common task, are shown after Judith has beheaded the drunken Assyrian general and before they have made their successful escape to Bethulia. A noise has caused them to turn their heads, Abra glancing furtively backward, and Judith upward, as though seeking divine guidance. The moment is seized upon by Orazio as an occasion to describe the differences between the two women and their responses.[1]

Isolated against a plain black background, they appear almost excised from their setting and context (the black background must refer to the night); it is the viewer who must make the narrative connections. The contrasts of dress and character so brilliantly alluded to in the Oslo painting are here even more pointed.

The highborn Judith, inspired by God and dedicated to a sacred mission, is blonde, blue-eyed, and richly attired. Abra has a more swarthy complexion, she is brown-haired, and there is an incipient mustache on her anxious face. Even in the shared action of carrying Holofernes' head, whose beautifully painted, pale features exert a repellent fascination, the strong yet delicate and manicured hands of Judith contrast with the thicker hands and dirty nails of Abra. In operatic terms—and the staged effect of this picture is undeniable—Judith is the soprano to Abra's dusky contralto. There is an interesting analogy with Federico della Valle's handling of the characters in his drama *Iudit*, written about 1600 and published in Milan in 1627. In one scene, Della Valle has the two women pause in the valley of Bethulia, where they have gone to pray. Abra confides her doubts and fears to Judith: "I confess my fear . . . but often my soul, trembling,

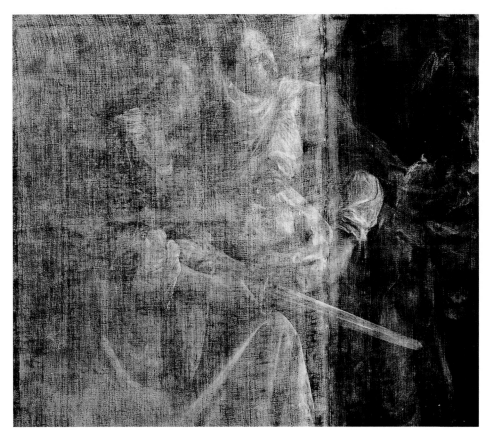

Figure 73. X radiograph of
cat. 39, without added strips

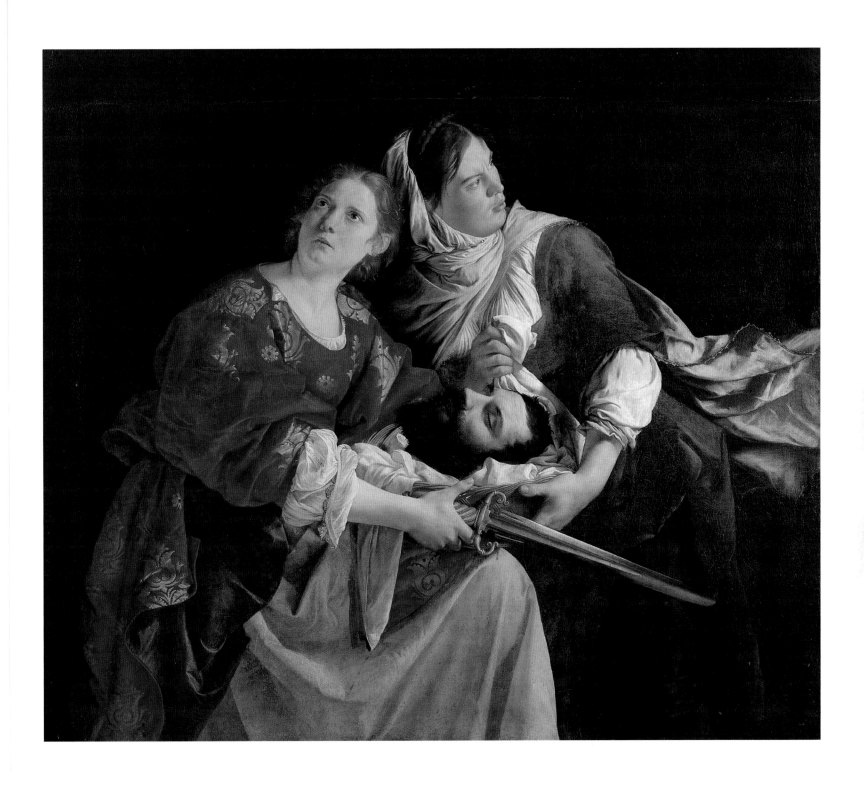

Judith as actively putting Holofernes' head into a sack. His picture was, interestingly, paired with a depiction of Jacob being shown the bloodstained coat of his son Joseph.

5. This is argued in Bissell 1981, 154, 157.

6. This was proposed by Redig de Campos when, in 1939, he published the Vatican picture. At that time the Hartford painting was still unknown. Redig de Campos has been followed by Emiliani (1958b, 43) and by Garrard.

7. On these, see Levey 1962; Loire 1998, 164; and Bissell 1999, 38–39.

8. See Adriani 1940, 77.

9. Ratti 1780, 119, 265. Brusco (1781, 35–36) notes only those in the Gentile collection. Ratti mentions the picture in the Cambiaso collection simply as a *Judith*, while both he and Brusco describe the Gentile painting as a *Judith and Her Maidservant*. Bissell (1981) mistakenly believes the references to a *Judith* in the Gentile collection were actually to a painting by Reni. In fact, the Gentile owned a *Judith* by each artist; see Boccardo 2000.

10. On Pietro Gentile's collection, see Boccardo 2000. It is unclear whether the *Sacrifice of Isaac* is the same picture listed in an inventory of 1678 in the collection of Gio Luca Doria; see Belloni 1973, 63; and Genoa 1992, 195–96. If it is, then it was acquired from the Doria by one of Pietro Maria Gentile's heirs. The other possibility is that Doria and Gentile owned versions of the same composition.

11. In 1803–5, several pictures from the Gentile collection were acquired by the rival Scottish painter-dealers Andrew Wilson and James Irvine; see Buchanan 1824, vol. 2, 103, 129, 135; Brigstocke 1982; and Boccardo 2000. They seem not to have been interested in Orazio's *Judith*, which is listed in the Gentile inventory of 1811 (though, curiously, as a work by Valentin). The picture must have been sold prior to 1818, when a guidebook remarks that the Gentile collection was dispersed. Unlike the three companion Gentileschis, it was not purchased by the marchese Adorno, since it is not mentioned in Gandolfi's guidebook of 1846 or in Alizeri's of 1846–47. All that is known of the Vatican replica is that it was a gift to Pope Pius XI by Agnese De Angelis Gammarelli.

12. See Boccardo 2000.

13. Alizeri (1846–47, 432) states that when they were displayed in the Palazzo Adorno, both the Gentileschis and the Renis were hung on one wall.

14. Boccardo (2000, 211 n. 34) remarks on the difficulties posed in identifying works listed in the 1811 inventory with surviving paintings, as added strips have often since been removed and the dimensions changed. In the case of the works ascribed to Gentileschi, the additions to the *Lucretia* were removed after 1967, while one strip was removed from the *Cleopatra*, leaving two others. The latter case serves as a reminder that the 1811 dimensions may include more than one set of additions.

40.

Young Woman Playing a Violin

Oil on canvas, 32¾ × 38½ in. (83.2 × 97.8 cm)

The Detroit Institute of Arts, Gift of Mrs. Edsel B. Ford (68.47)

ca. 1621–24

New York, Saint Louis

In his guidebook to Genoa of 1780, Carlo Giuseppe Ratti described a painting by Orazio in the collection of Carlo Cambiaso showing a "half-length figure of a woman playing the violin." Cambiaso owned three other works ascribed to the artist—a *Judith and Her Maidservant* (see cat. 39), a *David and Goliath* (see cat. 12), and a *Saint Sebastian*; whether he inherited the collection or assembled it has not been established.[1] In 1805, the *Young Woman Playing a Violin* was sold by the Cambiaso to the Scottish painter-dealer Andrew Wilson, who put it up for auction in London two years later.[2] In the sale catalogue it is described as "St. Cecilia; a beautiful clear and animated picture, with all the force of Caravaggio, without his sombre tints. —The figure completely alive. From the Cambiaso Palace."[3]

Although these two references date to over a century and a half after the painting was made, they encapsulate the issue of whether it was intended to be read as a genre or as a religious work. (Unlike the *Lute Player* [cat. 22], there really are not enough musical paraphernalia to suggest that it is an allegory of music.) In his canvases of Saint Cecilia now in Washington and Perugia (cat. nos. 31, 32), Orazio had given a genrelike slant to a religious subject, showing the saint as a young woman in contemporary dress intently playing the organ, the instrument most closely associated with the patron saint of music. An angel holding a sheet of music securely identifies the subject. Here, there is no attribute, and we are left with a work that allows—even encourages—simultaneous or layered readings as a secular and a religious work. Analogies

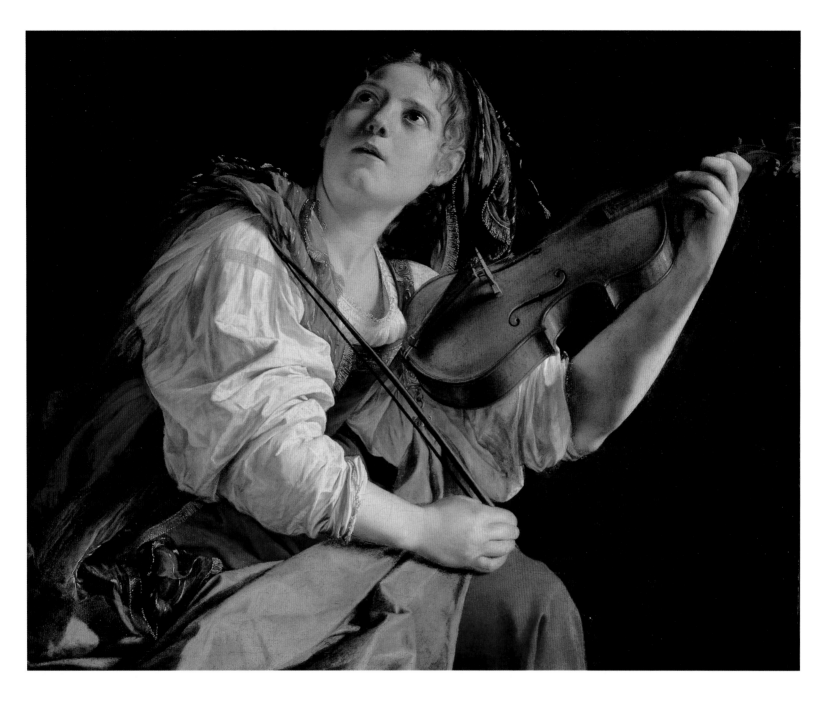

for this sort of ambiguity—an ambiguity that serves to enrich the viewer's experience—can be found in the work of other artists, such as Bernardo Strozzi[4] and Artemisia, whose *Lute Player* in the Galleria Spada was identified as a *Saint Cecilia* in 1637 (obviously because of the rapt expression rather than the instrument she plays; see cat. 63). Indicative of Orazio's ultimate source for this approach is Ottaviano Parravicino's characterization of Caravaggio's art as in a style halfway between the sacred and the profane ("in quel mezzo fra il devoto, et profano").[5] Where

Orazio's painting differs most significantly from a work such as Caravaggio's *Penitent Magdalene* (fig. 126), which Bellori read as a genre scene in the guise of a religious painting,[6] is in its recourse to a well-understood and standard repertory of gesture.

Since the time of Raphael and his landmark depictions of Saint Catherine (National Gallery, London) and Saint Cecilia (Pinacoteca Nazionale, Bologna), the contrapposto attitude, with the head turned upward, in a direction opposite that of the body, was used to contrast divine inspiration, or heavenly aid, to earthly

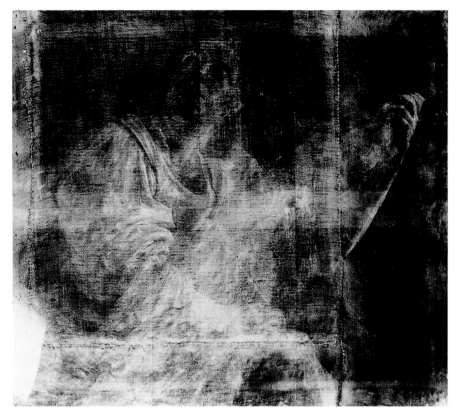

Figure 76. X radiograph of cat. 40

PROVENANCE: Carlo
Cambiaso, Palazzo Brignole,
Genoa (by 1780–1805); Andrew
Wilson (1805–7; sale, Peter
Cox, London, May 6, 1807, lot 7,
as by Gentileschi); Thomas
Trevor Hampden, second vis-
count, Hampden (from 1807);
W. A. Coats, Esq.; Major J. A.
Coats and Thomas H. Coats,
Levernholme, Nitshill, and
Renfrewshire (sale, Christie's,
London, April 12, 1935, lot 83, as
by Vermeer); Bennett; Anthony
Rau; Arthur Appleby, London;
Wildenstein, New York; gift of
Mrs. Edsel B. Ford, Detroit
Institute of Arts, 1968.

RELATED PICTURES:
R. Monaco, Rome (copy or
workshop replica with addition
of open part-book on a table
in lower right);[10] Piero Corsini
(variant composition of Saint
Mary Magdalene).[11]

REFERENCES: Ratti 1780,
vol. 1, 265; Longhi 1943, 47 n. 38;
Bissell 1967, 71–77; Pepper 1969,
28–35; Bissell 1971, 276; Volpe
1972, 67; Nicolson 1979, 53;
Bissell 1981, 24–27, 35, 38, 67, 78,
153, 156 no. 28, 166; Brigstocke
1982, 8, 447, 449, 489; Garrard
1989, 28, 493 n. 24; Nicolson
1990, 115; Mahoney in Cadogan
1991, 150; Papi in Florence 1991,
102; Giffi Ponzi 1994, 52–53; De
Grazia and Garberson 1996,
97, 104; Bissell 1999, 189, 194,
321–22, 328.

activities. This pose became a visual cliché in Baroque art. Yet, precisely because of its ubiquity, it allowed artists to play on its meaning by varying secondary features.[7] As a Saint Cecilia, Orazio's image could be read in terms similar to those Bellori ascribed to Reni's depiction, painted for Cardinal Sfondrato (Norton Simon Museum, Pasadena): "Then that man had [Reni] paint a half-length figure of the same saint, bowing the violin, turning her head and her eyes toward harmony."[8] However, whereas Reni strove for a standard devotional affect through modest dress and pious expression and attitude, Orazio emphasizes human warmth and spontaneity, thereby suggesting a private musical performance that has been momentarily interrupted.

As has been remarked by a number of scholars, the same figure in an analogous pose appears in the Hartford *Judith and Her Maidservant* (cat. 39). The fact that in the Cambiaso collection the Hartford picture (or the replica of it in the Vatican) was exhibited along-side the *Young Woman Playing a Violin* suggests that this sort of variation on a formal pose (what amounts to a rhetorical figure) was understood and appreciated by

collectors. Nonetheless, the paintings can hardly have been made as pendants; the Detroit picture, unlike the Hartford *Judith*, is seen from a low viewing point and may have been conceived as an overdoor.

The picture has always, and correctly, been consid-ered contemporary with the Hartford *Judith and Her Maidservant*. As with that work, I prefer a date of about 1621–24—during Orazio's Genoese period—to the one of about 1610–12, which is frequently accepted. The brilliant handling of the white blouse and general effect of transparency are, to my mind, hallmarks of the later moment, as is the elegance of design. The Detroit picture is of exceptional quality. X radiographs (fig. 76) reveal a painting freely worked up (though with no significant changes). Like the *Judith*, it is painted on a canvas support made up of prestretched and evi-dently pregrounded pieces (four in all).[9]

1. Mahoney (in Cadogan 1991, 150) tentatively identifies Carlo Cambiaso with one of the brothers of Doge Michelangelo Cambiaso (1738–1813).
2. On Andrew Wilson and the record of his payment for the pic-ture, see Brigstocke 1982.

3. Graves's *Art Sales*, vol. 1 (1918), 351, seems to have originated the idea that the picture in the Cambiaso collection was ascribed to Artemisia. The 1807 sale catalogue ascribes it to Gentileschi, which conventionally meant Orazio.

4. In his paintings of a woman playing a violin, Strozzi sometimes includes a martyr's palm branch and/or an angel to identify her as Saint Cecilia and sometimes he does not, thus leaving the matter (intentionally?) ambiguous. See Mortari 1995, nos. 126–30, 282–85, 363.

5. See discussion in Calvesi 1990, 196–200.

6. Bellori 1672, 215. For the archclassicist Bellori, this was a defective approach and revealed an overly strong dependence on nature.

7. Few things elucidate the adaptability of these stock poses as does a picture from Orazio's workshop showing Mary Magdalene. The figure was clearly taken directly from the Detroit picture, with the hands rearranged so as to rest on a skull. See *Important Old Master Paintings* (Piero Corsini, Inc.), 1986, no. 18.

8. Bellori 1672, 495.

9. The central piece is of a herringbone weave; the added pieces on the sides and bottom—of unequal width—are of a modified plain weave. The central piece shows stretch marks along the bottom seam; the pieces on the left side and bottom seem to have been pregrounded. A misunderstanding of this procedure—common in Orazio's work—is responsible for Garrard's notion that the model was originally shown with her hands in her lap and transformed into a musician only later.

10. Photograph from Heim Gallery, on file at the Detroit Institute of Arts. See Nicolson 1990, 115.

11. Exhibited in Corsini's New York gallery in 1986.

41.

Danaë

Oil on canvas, 63¾ × 90 in. (162 × 228.5 cm)

The Cleveland Museum of Art, Leonard C. Hanna Jr. Fund (1971.101)

ca. 1622–23

When the Cleveland *Danaë* appeared on the art market in 1971, it was identified as the lost work painted about 1621–22 for Giovan Antonio Sauli. "An exciting addition" is how one critic (Pepper) responded to its inclusion in the landmark exhibition *Caravaggio and His Followers*, held in Cleveland that year. Yet it is worth noting that Volpe, one reviewer of the show, felt that the style of the painting pointed to its being a later work, perhaps done in France. The picture is, in fact, an extremely fine, probably autograph replica of the Sauli canvas (cat. 36), and the strong impression it made when seen in isolation serves as a reminder of why there was such a demand for copies and variant compositions of Orazio's best work and how poorly, by and large, these replicas hold up to the prime version when direct comparison is possible. This is the first time the Sauli and the Cleveland pictures have been shown together, but those who have had the opportunity of studying the two pictures on successive days will find it difficult to subscribe to Bissell's observation that "more often than not autograph replicas in Gentileschi's oeuvre represent improvements upon his initial conception." This is rarely true (but see cat. 45). Gone is the effect of transparency, the coloristic brilliance, and the dazzling rendition of light playing on silk and gilt metal. In the Cleveland painting, there is a leaden quality that borders on dullness. Some of this effect must be ascribed to the very process by which the picture was made.

There can be no question that a template, probably in the form of a tracing, was used to lay in the design on the brown ground. This process is discussed elsewhere in the catalogue (see pp. 21–22), but the differences between the two pictures are worth describing in some detail, since in many ways the Cleveland picture can be taken as a paradigm (in the best sense of the word, since the quality of the picture is so much finer than is the norm among paintings produced in Orazio's workshop).

There is not complete conformity between the two pictures. Rather, when a tracing of the Sauli picture is laid over the Cleveland painting (as I was able to do in December 2000), the correspondences prove to be part to part. For example, the lower part of Danaë's torso and legs in both pictures align closely, but when her breast, left arm, and hand align, her head is out of register with the tracing, being slightly higher in the Cleveland painting, and her right hand is farther extended. A shift in the tracing brings the features of the face into almost perfect alignment (except for the

PROVENANCE: Probably
Q. Camillo Gavotti, Genoa
(by 1679);[4] possibly Lord
Sunderland, England (before
1752); private collection, England;
Hazlitt Gallery, London (1971);
Cleveland Museum of Art.

RELATED PICTURE: See
cat. 36.

REFERENCES: Spear in
Cleveland 1971, 103–5; Pepper
1972, 170; Volpe 1972, 67–68;
Lurie 1975, 75–81; Nicolson
1979, 52; Bissell 1981, 45–46, 49,
177–78 no. 50; Garrard 1989, 56,
200, 242, 244, 271; Nicolson
1990, 112; Mann 1996, 40–41;
Barnes in Genoa 1997, 160;
Bissell 1999, 312.

lips). The position of Cupid is the same in both paintings, but he has a broader torso and his arms are marginally thicker in the Cleveland painting. His head and genitals, however, align with the tracing. In a similar fashion, while the main folds of the satin coverlet match, the silhouette of the white sheet, where it is raised to expose the red mattress, is wider in the Cleveland version. The bed frame does not align completely; the bedposts are broader and the artichoke-shaped finials have an added row of petals, giving them a rather unfortunate, flatter shape. The coins and gold shavings are placed differently in the Cleveland painting and were not transposed from a tracing. The differences between the tracing of the Sauli picture and the composition of the Cleveland painting can be accounted for by a combination of slippage, carelessness (the tracing was perhaps in sections anyway), and intentional adjustments, but that they are the result of a mechanical transfer process cannot be doubted. In X radiographs (fig. 11) the contours of Danaë's arms, torso, and legs can be seen to be as sharp as one would expect from tracing a design. Similarly, there is a clean division between the satin coverlet and the white sheet, as well as in the arrangement of their folds. Even to the naked eye, the signs of working from a predetermined design are evident, for the shapes of the various figures were clearly held in reserve (the brown ground is especially visible around Cupid). In contrast to the Sauli picture, where Orazio has constantly adjusted contours and shapes, in the Cleveland painting everything has been prefixed. For example, the right-hand bedpost does not overlap the bedsheet, and the white bedsheet was not painted over the red mattress. And there is none of the variation in brushstrokes found in the Sauli picture. The general effect of dullness is due less to abrasion than to thinness in the application of the paint (the ground was sometimes left exposed in shaded areas).[1] Over time, the transitions between light and shade have become harder and an overall darkening (or "sinking") has taken place.

Orazio's object in the Cleveland picture was to produce a replica, but, as was usual in such works, changes were introduced. Bissell notes the "pained" expression of the Cleveland Danaë, but more important is the change in the curtain from green to bluish and of the satin coverlet from citron to dull olive, with an almost total loss of those electrifying effects of sheen. Is the work autograph? On balance, I believe the answer is yes. The matter will certainly be debated during the exhibition, but it is important to remember that a conclusion based only on a comparison of the two works is misleading. A proper evaluation would require comparison with other cases in which Orazio replicated a composition—works that have not been included in the exhibition because of their inferior (what I deem to be workshop) status. Among these is the Berlin *Lot* that was, it has been thought—incorrectly—sent by Orazio to Carlo Emanuele I, duke of Savoy, as a demonstration of his abilities. The picture gave a good idea of his *invenzione* but not of his technical abilities, since the painting was mainly a workshop production. The following year, he made a more assertive attempt to acquire a place at the Savoy court in Turin, sending to Carlo Emanuele the prime version of an *Annunciation*—an incomparable display of his *arte*—while the inferior replica (workshop, in my opinion) was delivered to the church of San Siro in Genoa (see cat. 43). Surprisingly, the San Siro *Annunciation* is widely accepted as a fine autograph work and has even been accorded precedence over the Turin picture.[2] It provides a meter for evaluating the quality and the date of the Cleveland *Danaë*, with which it shares a general leaden effect.

A *Danaë* by Orazio is listed in the 1679 inventory of Camillo Gavotti in Genoa, and between 1742 and 1752 George Vertue recorded a "Gentilesco. a Danaë" belonging to Lord Sunderland.[3] Bissell has suggested that these might refer to the same picture. Certainly the style of the Cleveland painting suggests a Genoese rather than an English-period picture.

1. This was already noted in a conservation report the Cleveland Museum made in 1978, after the Feigen picture had appeared.
2. See the evaluation of Pesenti in Genoa 1992, 194.
3. Vertue 1940–42, 55–56. For the Gavotti inventory, see Belloni 1973, 64.
4. It measured 15 or 16 × 8 *palmi*. A Genoese *palmo* is equivalent to 25 cm: thus 375 × 200 cm. Whether this included the frame cannot be said.

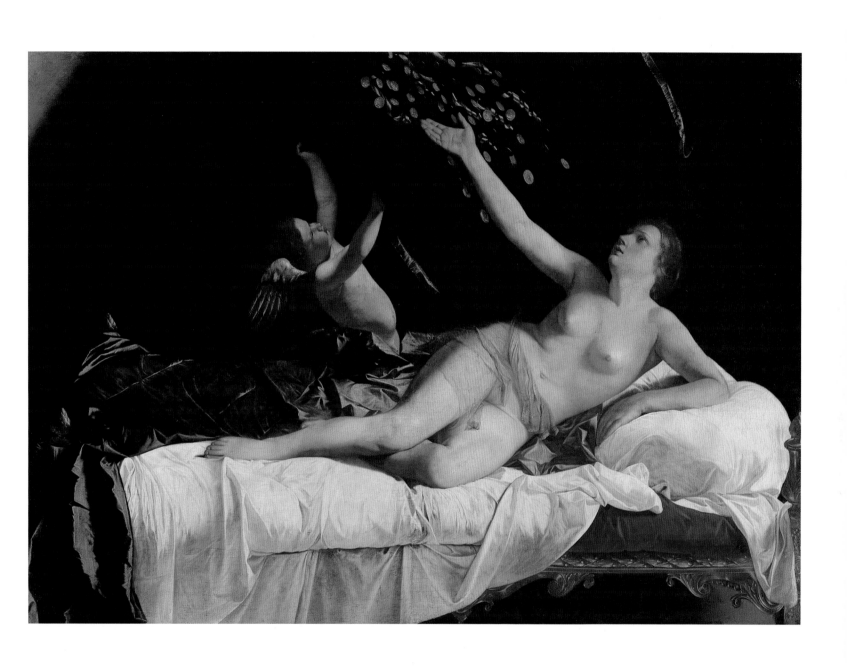

42.

Lot and His Daughters

Oil on canvas, 62 × 77 in.
(157.5 × 195.6 cm)

The National Gallery of
Canada, Ottawa (inv. 14811)

1622

PROVENANCE: Probably Carlo
Emanuele I, duke of Savoy,
Turin (1622–30; inv. 1631, as by
Gentileschi); probably the
dukes of Savoy (from 1630;
inv. 1636, as by Gentileschi; inv.,
before 1646, as by Gentileschi);
Louis, duke of Orléans, Palais
Royal, Paris (after 1737–52; inv.
1752, as by G. Canlassi [i.e.,
Guido Cagnacci]); Orléans
collection (1752–90; inv. 1785,
as by Caravaggio); Walkners,
Brussels (1790); M. Laborde
de Mereville; (exh. with ex-
Orléans collection at Pall
Mall in 1798, no. 166, as by
Velázquez); Henry Hope,
London (1798–1816; sold,
Christie's, London, June 29,
1816, lot 34, as by Velázquez);
Croome (anonymous sale,
Stanley's, London, June 12,
1832, no. 88, as by Gentileschi);
John Rushout, 2nd Lord
Northwick, Thirlestane House,
Cheltenham (until 1859; sale,
Philips, Thirlestane House,
August 9, 1859, as by Velázquez;
bought in by his nephew
George, 3rd Lord Northwick);
George, 3rd Lord Northwick,
Northwick Park (1859–87); by
descent to Capt. Edward
George Spencer-Churchill
(until 1964; sale, Christie's,
London, May 28, 1965, lot 22,
as by Gentileschi); National
Gallery of Canada, Ottawa.

REFERENCES: Couché 1808,
vol. 2, pl. 87; Barry 1809, 97;
Buchanan 1824, vol. 1, 146;
Waagen 1854, vol. 2, 498, vol. 3,
204; Stryienski 1913, 176; Gamba
1922–23, 262; Voss 1925, 115, 460;
Longhi 1943, 23; Sterling 1958,
117; Pérez Sánchez 1965, 503;
Moir 1967, 76 no. 7, 78; Bissell
1969, 16–33; Schleier 1970b, 342;
Bissell 1971, 294 n. 18; Spear in
Cleveland 1971, 30; Nicolson
1979, 52; Bissell 1981, 44–46, 52,
76, 176, 180–81 no. 53, 182, 203;
Laskin and Pantazzi 1987, 113–16;
Galante in Abrate 1989, 171–74;
Nicolson 1990, 112; Bava in
Romano 1995, 246 n. 158.

This is the finest variant of the work Orazio painted for Giovan Antonio Sauli and the most likely candidate for the picture he gave to Carlo Emanuele I, duke of Savoy, in 1622, in an attempt to secure a position at the court in Turin. Orazio refers to a picture of this subject in a letter that accompanied the *Annunciation* (cat. 43), which he sent to the duke in April of the following year: "I have always maintained a lively affection for you, and for that reason I sent you the painting by my hand of the Flight of Lot, and having heard from my son [Francesco] how it pleased Your Highness and, being honored beyond my merit by those sentiments . . . I have been encouraged to send you another [picture], larger and better than the first, which is [of] the most holy Annunciation."

The means of production of the Ottawa picture and its relationship to the ex-Sauli painting and the inferior version in Berlin are discussed on pages 22–26. Here, it is enough to note the revised cave setting and more extensive landscape, as well as the somewhat pedestrian profile view of the face of the daughter on the right (which has sustained damage). In 1989, Galante Garrone published a copy of the picture (fig. 77) in the Savoy castle at Carrù, near Turin, and this copy provides the strongest evidence that the Ottawa version was sent to Carlo Emanuele. It would now appear that Carlo's son Cardinal Maurizio of Savoy owned the workshop replica in Berlin, which he gave to the marquis of Leganés when the latter was the Spanish governor of Milan between 1635 and 1641. (He also owned and gave to the marquis a version of the *Rest on the Flight into Egypt*; see cat. 45). For the confusing evidence relating to the early provenance of the various versions of the *Lot* pictures and their bibliography, see catalogue no. 37.

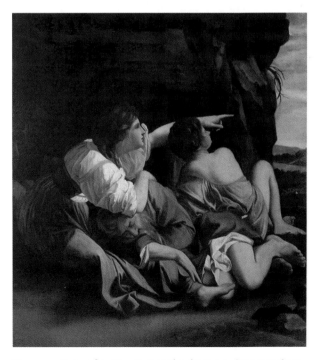

Figure 77. Copy after Orazio Gentileschi, *Lot and His Daughters*. Oil on canvas. Castello di Carrù, Cuneo (Italy)

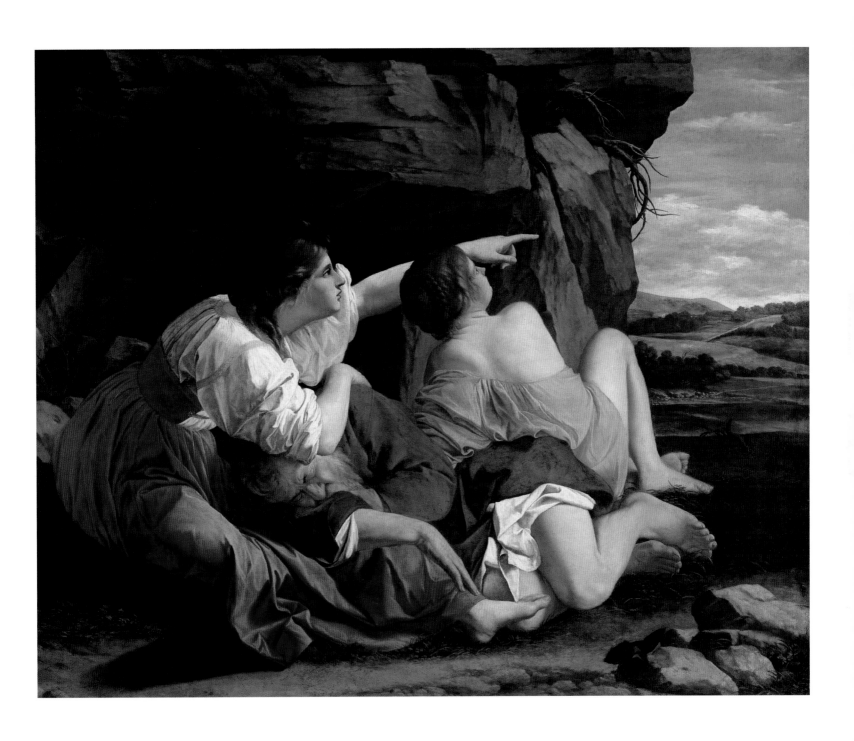

43.

Annunciation

Oil on canvas, 112 5/8 × 77 1/8 in. (286 × 196 cm)

Galleria Sabauda, Turin

1623

Rome, New York

PROVENANCE: Carlo Emanuele I, duke of Savoy (from 1623; listed in the castle chapel, inv. 1631 and 1635, as by Gentileschi); the dukes of Savoy, Turin (taken to Paris under Napoléon from 1799 to 1815–16); Galleria Sabauda, Turin.

RELATED PICTURE: San Siro, Genoa (a smaller workshop replica with variations).[11]

REFERENCES: D'Azeglio 1836–46, vol. 1, 15, 24, 80 n. 102; Campori 1870, 103; Baudi di Vesme 49 n. 369; Longhi (1916) 1961, 241–42; Voss 1925, 459; Baudi di Vesme 1932, 319–20; Griseri 1961, 27–28; Moir 1967, vol. 1, 75, 197 n. 4, 256–57 n. 10, vol. 2, 76 no. c.1; Nicolson 1979, 52; Bissell 1981, 42–43, 66, 89 n. 11, 169, 171, 179–80 no. 52, 204; Nicolson 1990, 114; Bava in Romano 1995, 62, 248; Arena in Romano 1999, 85.

Orazio had been in Genoa for two years when, on April 2, 1623, he sent to Carlo Emanuele I, duke of Savoy, this extraordinary painting of the Annunciation. It was accompanied by his son Francesco with a letter in which Orazio noted that the previous year he had given the duke a painting of Lot and His Daughters which, he understood, had been much admired. "And so, animated by such exalted favor, I have been encouraged to send you another [picture], larger and better than the first, which is [of] the most holy Annunciation, so that Your Highness may better judge the point at which my art has arrived." The *Lot and His Daughters* was a replica of the picture Orazio had painted for Giovan Antonio Sauli (cat. 42). That he did not send an original composition of the highest quality suggests that the first gift was intended merely to test the waters of the duke's interest. Having received a positive response, he then followed up the gift with a work of truly exceptional character: one that he must have known would appeal to the duke's religious fervor. A lackluster variant was instead painted for the church of San Siro in Genoa, a clear sign that Orazio's ambitions were to leave Genoa and gain employment at one of the courts of Europe. He seems also to have sent a painting to Marie de' Medici at about the same time (according to his seventeenth-century biographer Soprani), and it was to France that he eventually moved.

Curiously, there is no record of Orazio's having received any compensation for the picture, which was installed in the chapel adjacent to the duke's apartments in the Savoy castle. Indeed, until recently there was no evidence that he received any employment at the Savoy court in Turin. However, we now know that on April 17, 1624, Carlo Emanuele wrote his son, urging him to see to the payment of 150 ducats owed by Gentileschi to an innkeeper in order to ensure that Orazio would begin the task he had been contracted to carry out.[1] Presumably, Orazio had already been in Turin to discuss this matter with the duke. Whether

this has anything to do with a *Rest on the Flight into Egypt* that Carlo Emanuele's son Cardinal Maurizio of Savoy later gave to the marquis of Leganés is impossible to say (see cat. 45), though it seems unlikely that the duke's "task" would have been no more than the repetition of an already existing composition.

The character of the *Annunciation* has provoked much comment. Longhi's bizarre description of it as "superb human nonsense . . . a woman of the aristocracy who listens attentively to the words of a young gentleman in her bedroom" seems very wide of the mark—a singular lapse of his normally acute critical faculties. Others—most notably Bissell—have found the combination of refinement, grace, and dignity reminiscent of Florentine art—of Donatello and Filippo Lippi in the fifteenth century and of Santi di Tito in the late sixteenth.[2] In so doing, he pinpointed the outstanding feature of the painting: its seemingly archaic conception.

Gentileschi's interpretation of the subject, with the Virgin standing in a carefully described bedchamber, her left arm modestly grasping the hem of her cloak, her right hand raised in a gesture that might be interpreted alternatively as reflection or as dutiful submission at the message conveyed by the angel Gabriel, shown kneeling before her and holding a lily, is reminiscent of a whole series of fifteenth-century Florentine paintings.[3] Orazio may have stopped in Florence en route from Rome to Genoa in 1621, though when he wrote to the grand duke of Tuscany from London in 1633 he declared that he had not been there for fifty-five years. Regardless of whether he made such a trip, there would still be the matter of the motivation behind his purported interest in earlier Florentine art. As was the case with Orazio's Marchigian paintings (see cat. nos. 29, 30), the answer would seem to be bound up with his Counter-Reformation perspective on religious painting.

What the *Annunciation* testifies to is an acute interest in a specifically devotional style of painting. We

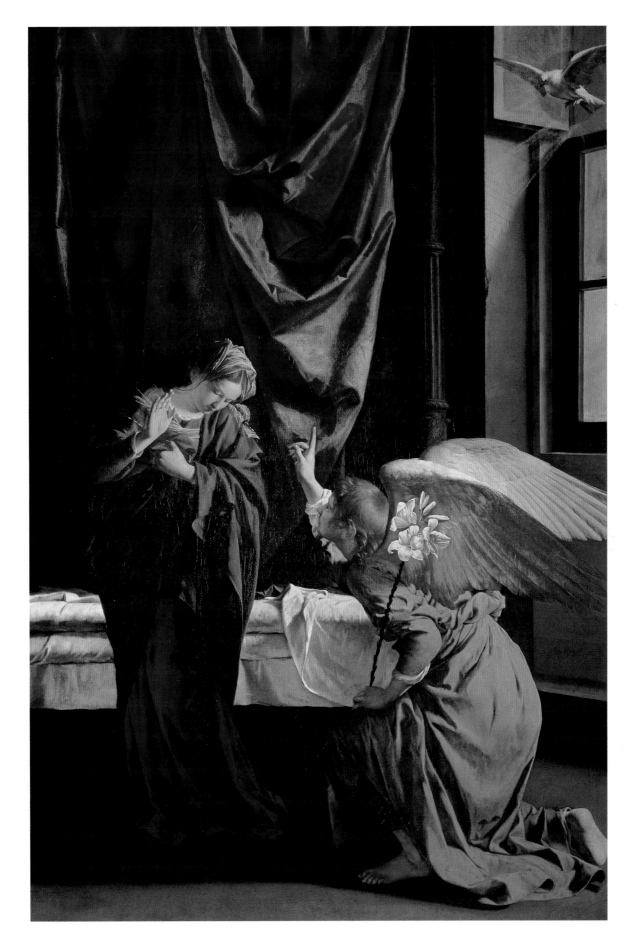

may deduce that this was a real issue at the end of the sixteenth and beginning of the seventeenth century not only from the writings of ecclesiastical theorists such as Gilio da Fabriano and Gabriele Paleotti, but from the work of various artists as well. There is, for example, Ludovico Carracci's *Annunciation* (Pinacoteca Nazionale, Bologna), painted about 1584, with its reminiscences of the work of Francesco Francia. Malvasia records the esteem Guido Reni felt for his Bolognese compatriots of the fourteenth and fifteenth centuries, who, he declared, "knew how to represent a holiness, a modesty, a purity, a gravity, that any modern painter, despite all his studies and powers would not know how to express."[4] Even the archclassicist Giovan Pietro Bellori seems to have appreciated Reni's desire to recapture a purity of expression. In his encomium of Reni's altarpiece of the Annunciation in the chapel of Paul V in the Quirinal palace—a work that Orazio knew well—he describes the angel as "humbling himself before the Virgin, bending a knee [while the Virgin], the obedient servant of the Lord, folds her arms, lowers her gaze, and receives the Holy Spirit that infuses her. The more her beauty shines, the greater is the humility of her face, which, in looking at the ground, partakes of the heavenly."[5] We might almost think this description was written with Orazio's painting in mind, were it not for the fact that Reni's response to the problem of a devotional style was, in fact, diametrically opposed to Orazio's. In Reni's painting, everyday reality is transformed by the artist's imagination into an ideal, timeless realm. The ethereal beauty of his Virgin, with that much admired "dolce aria di testa," is at the opposite pole to that of Orazio's Virgin, in which we recognize the same young woman who modeled for the *Vision of Saint Francesca Romana* (cat. 30) and who wears on her head the artist's favorite sheer scarf banded in gold. Reni's example reminds us that an interest in earlier art did not necessarily result in a retrospective style.

It is worth noting that in 1603, Orazio's brother Aurelio Lomi painted an *Annunciation* for the Genoese church of Santa Maria Maddalena that has some of the domestic traits—though none of the aesthetic merits—of Orazio's painting (see fig. 65).[6] More pertinent, perhaps, is the example of that paradigmatic Counter-Reformation painter Scipione Pulzone, who in 1587 painted an *Annunciation* for a Dominican church in Gaeta (Capodimonte, Naples). Although based on a brilliant composition by Titian, Pulzone's painting has a distinctly archaic flavor—one emphasizing devoutness over artistic demonstration ("verso un significato non 'honesto' e 'devoto', ma onestissimo e devotissimo," in the words of Zeri).[7] This Pulzone accomplished by tempering expressivity and by emphasizing a meticulous attention to surface description. The rudimentary synthesis of a Raphaelesque classicism with Flemish realism that stands at the core of his work is, to a degree, what Orazio also attempts, though with an inspired sensibility and breadth of experience for which Pulzone's art can have offered no real model. Whether Orazio found inspiration in some of the early Netherlandish paintings that existed in abundance in Genoa is difficult to say, but the way in which the radiance that surrounds the dove of the Holy Spirit as it flies through the open window (its panes evidently of oiled parchment rather than glass) contrasts with the soft daylight of the room certainly recalls such works.[8] So, too, does the passage of light over the white linen sheets, like a sermon on the purity of the Virgin. He had achieved a similar effect of the natural world miraculously invaded by the divine in the *Vision of Saint Francesca Romana*.

Yet Orazio, for all his emphasis on the description of the event as though taking place in a real-life setting, was no less eager to respond to the challenge in Genoa offered by Rubens's overwhelming genius, for there can, I think, be little doubt that the stunning red curtain behind the Virgin—its folds animated by the light falling through the window—is Orazio's answer to the dazzling curtain Rubens uses to theatrical effect in his altarpiece showing a miracle of Saint Ignatius in the church of the Gesù. What we end up with, then, is a work that, motivated by the Counter-Reformation concerns for a devotionally effective art, transposes the terms of quattrocento painting into those of post-Caravaggesque realism. This was, in short, a work perfectly suited to Carlo Emanuele, who took an active part in his various artistic projects, wrote religious poetry, and showed a marked appreciation for Caravaggesque painting.[9] Almost twenty years earlier, Orazio had painted an altarpiece (fig. 5) for a Capuchin church founded by the duke—a fact to which he alludes in the letter that accompanied the *Annunciation*[10]—and he must have been keenly aware of the character and tastes of the person he was dealing with.

The Turin *Annunciation* is Orazio's finest achievement as a religious artist and one of the masterpieces of seventeenth-century painting. That it, and not the related picture, in San Siro, Genoa, is the prime version is attested, in the first place, by its sublime quality, which is even more evident since its cleaning in 1982. There are also a number of subtle alterations and visible pentimenti: a piece of lavender drapery was painted over the angel's right heel; there are refinements in the contour of the angel's citron drapery and in the fold hanging from the left knee; the shape of a higher or differently placed step can be seen below the window. Although the San Siro version was thought by Bissell to precede the Turin painting, it lacks Orazio's response to the play of light. Its color is drab and its execution hard, and Orazio is unlikely to have had a hand in its realization.

1. Bava in Romano 1995, 248.
2. Chiarini (1962, 28) makes the most comprehensive case for the importance of Santi di Tito, though whether we have to do with a parallel culture or influence remains problematic.
3. On the various mental states of the Virgin at the time of the Annunciation, see Baxandall (1972) 1988, 49–56.
4. Malvasia (1678) 1841, vol. 1, 34.
5. Bellori (1672) 1976, 502.
6. For a discussion of the relation of Aurelio's art to Counter-Reformation ideas with his *Annunciation,* see Ciardi, Galassi, and Carofano 1989, 29–32, 220–21.
7. Zeri 1957, 73.
8. It is worth noting that in 1506, Gerard David painted an elaborate polyptych for Vincenzo Sauli, an ancestor of Giovan Antonio Sauli, for the abbey of San Gerolamo della Cervara, near Genoa; see Ainsworth in New York 1998–99, 296–301.
9. For an overview of Carlo Emanuele's collecting, see Bava in Romano 1995, 212–52. For Caravaggesque paintings in the Savoy collections, see Arena in Romano 1999, 82–95.
10. In the letter, Orazio states that he has no other ambition than "to show Your Highness my ancient servitude that I have dedicated to you since my youth." This has usually been taken as a reference to a commission, of which the Cappuccini *Madonna in Glory with the Holy Trinity* is the most plausible—indeed, the only—candidate. The picture was used as a shutter or curtain for an altar constructed in 1636. Initially, it must have been intended as an altarpiece; see Arena in Romano 1999, 83.
11. Bissell 1981, 178–79, and, most recently, in Genoa 1997, 162.

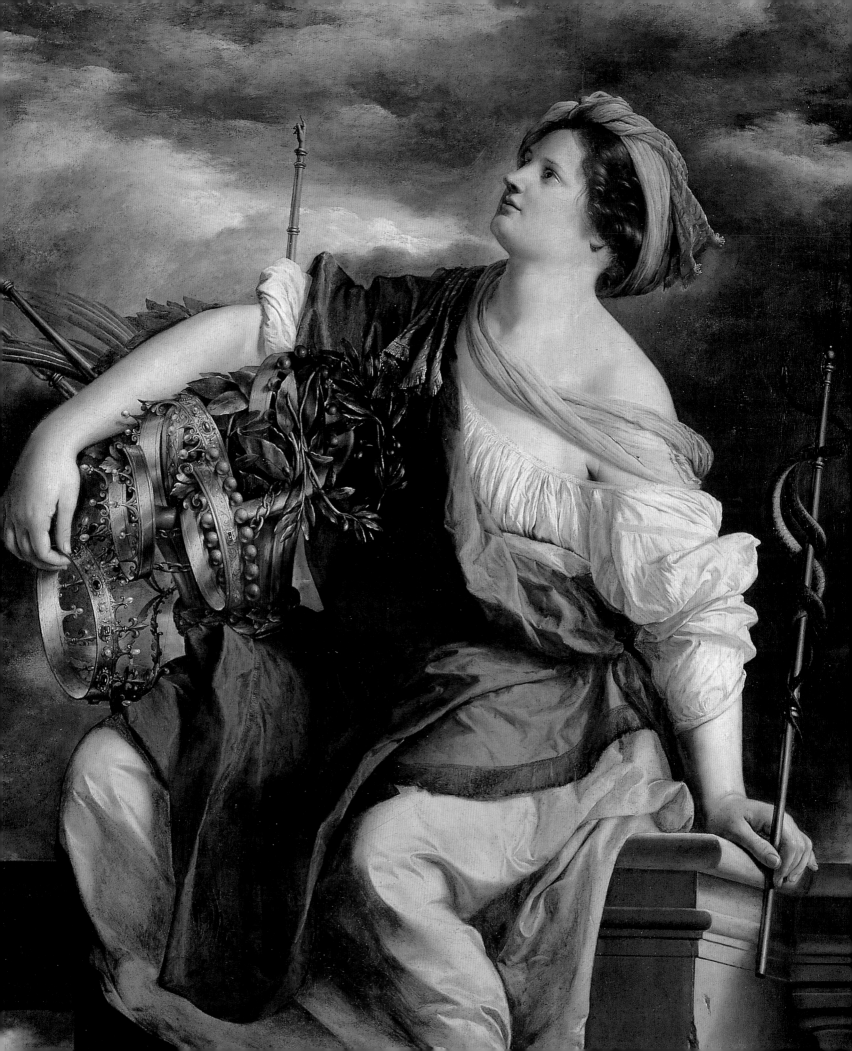

Gentileschi and France, Gentileschi and the French

JEAN-PIERRE CUZIN

Little is known about the approximately two years that Orazio Gentileschi spent in France or about what he may have painted there, and we can only guess at what his role and influence may have been. Under these circumstances, it may appear presumptuous—even after more than forty years have passed—to attempt to expand upon Charles Sterling's article "Gentileschi in France," which was published in 1958, given that the information he provides remains reliable and the insights he offers remain pertinent.[1]

Let us review some of the biographical data that has been discussed elsewhere in this volume, much of which has become clearer since Sterling's article appeared. Gentileschi seems to have left Genoa for France in the summer or autumn of 1624 to place himself in the service of the queen mother, Marie de' Medici (1573–1642). How long did he stay? Joachim von Sandrart (1606–1688) writes that he did not stay long, as he was unhappy there. But, in fact, we know that he remained for two years, since he arrived in London, at the invitation of the duke of Buckingham, in September or October 1626. Raffaele Soprani, the Genoese historiographer, whose work was published posthumously in 1674, tells us that Orazio had sent a painting to Marie de' Medici from Genoa and that it pleased her a great deal. Perhaps, Sterling adds, Gentileschi's Florentine origin also appealed to the queen, reminding her of her own family. Which work (one canvas or several?) was sent from Genoa? A *Rest on the Flight into Egypt*? A *Mary Magdalene*? Was this picture—or one of them—related to those later given to George Villiers, duke of Buckingham? We do not know. What we do know is that it belonged either to Cardinal Richelieu or to Marie de' Medici and that it was, in all likelihood, a picture of one of these subjects (see cat. 45).[2]

Why this relatively brief stay? Perhaps, in fact, the artist was not happy in France; very likely, he did not receive the commissions he was hoping for. In any case, it seems probable that Gentileschi's departure for London was related to the marriage of Henrietta Maria, the daughter of Marie de' Medici and sister of Louis XIII, to Charles I. In May 1625, the duke of Buckingham—the king's chief minister—was in Paris to accompany the future sovereign to her new country, and he may have met Gentileschi at that time. Balthazar Gerbier, Buckingham's artistic adviser and more or less his agent, may have recommended the painter to him, and it is very possible that Gentileschi accompanied François de Bassompierre, France's new special ambassador to London, who assumed his post in late September 1626. In their essay (pp. 223–24), Gabriele Finaldi and Jeremy Wood assume, probably correctly, that the painter's entry into service at the English court was part of a series of diplomatic agreements between Buckingham and Bassompierre.[3] In any event, in 1633, in a letter to Ferdinand II de' Medici, grand duke of Tuscany, Orazio indicates that it was with the agreement of the queen mother that he left for England. Whether he was pleased or resigned we will never know.

Thus, we can only conjecture about the work—or works—that Gentileschi sent to Marie de' Medici, and which convinced her to call the painter to Paris. The results of his Parisian stay seem meager; we know of only one painting that was certainly executed there: the *Public Felicity* (cat. 44), painted for the Palais du Luxembourg and today in the Louvre. Originally attributed to Jean Monier, it was identified by Sterling in 1958.[4] The painting, monumental in its beautiful *di sotto in sù* effect, with a clear-toned blue, white, and yellow color scheme, was obviously executed by a painter hoping to obtain major commissions by convincing patrons of his "decorative" skills. The figure's apprehensive expression has not been adequately noted. She holds to herself, almost protectively, a kind of jumble of crowns and scepters, together with a cornucopia, and she looks upward as though

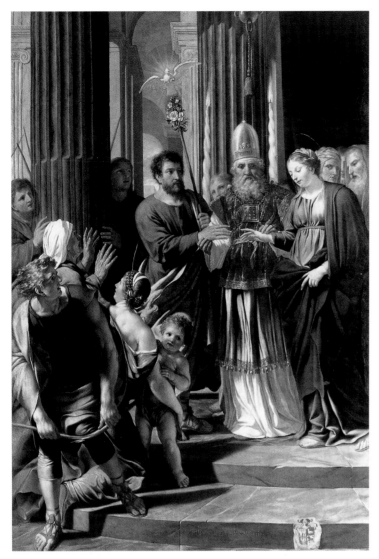

Figure 78. Michel I Corneille (1603–1664), *Marriage of the Virgin*. Oil on canvas. Private collection

fearful of something above. The cloudy sky, so often rendered by Gentileschi, is particularly dark and menacing as in none of his other pictures. The caduceus that she holds in her left hand is an emblem of peace (in Peter Paul Rubens's *Conclusion of Peace* [Louvre, Paris] it is the attribute of Mercury, who brandishes a similar object while entering the Temple of Peace), but the snakes, as they writhe about it, seem to allude to the dangers that threaten the kingdom. Orazio undoubtedly wished to treat the theme not only of public felicity, but of public felicity tested by dangers and vicissitudes. Is this an allusion, as in the last episodes of Rubens's "saga," to the misfortunes of Marie de' Medici, who was enmeshed in a dispute with her son? Or to broader threats to the peace and prosperity of the land? Indeed, we should

perhaps title the painting, with its decidedly nontriumphant figure, *Public Felicity Threatened* rather than, as Sterling did, *Public Felicity Triumphant over Dangers*. The choice of the latter title, in its reference to the theme of the painting, could have come only from Marie de' Medici and her advisers. In any case—although we have no direct commentary to support this view—to judge by the absence of subsequent commissions and the fact that everyone so quickly forgot that Orazio was its creator, we are obliged to conclude that the picture was not well received.

I have said that the *Public Felicity* is the only painting that was certainly executed in France. *Diana the Huntress* (cat. 47) is a picture that has also been thought to have been made there. It is now known to be a work executed in London, thanks to a document discovered by Laurence Lépine, which states that the painting was paid for in 1630 by Roger du Plessis de Liancourt, duke of La Roche-Guyon, Louis XIII's special ambassador to Charles I.[5] This point merits careful attention, since the *Diana* seems to have had a direct influence in France and is, even more perhaps than the *Public Felicity*, in perfect harmony with the spirit of Parisian painting (if that expression does indeed have any meaning). At least, it is in perfect harmony with the spirit of Parisian painting in the years 1630 to 1640, a spirit believed to have been inspired by Gentileschi. Are we to imagine that there was a first version of the *Diana* painted in France, of which the Liancourt painting would be a repetition executed four or five years later, and that this first version was the source of the French copies? The hypothesis of two versions is not untenable, as Orazio was a painter who did not hesitate to repeat his compositions, at the request, no doubt, of his patrons. But we must rather assume that the canvas, installed in the Liancourt mansion on the rue de Seine, was admired upon its arrival and quickly imitated by French painters. Arguments based on sources other than the rediscovered document convince us that the *Diana*—despite the difficulty we have in proving it—is a product of the English period. The color harmonies, with their delicate shot greens, are very different from the more clear-toned blues, yellows, and whites of the *Public Felicity*, and the complex, pivoting pose of the figure—seen from the back—which pushes the limits of anatomical verisimilitude, is similar to that of Joseph in *Joseph and Potiphar's Wife*, at Hampton Court (fig. 88), made in England about 1632. As Finaldi and Wood remark, it is also similar to the attitude of one of the Muses in *Apollo and the Muses* (fig. 93), also painted in England, before 1630.[6] In his catalogue entry for the *Diana* (cat. 47), Keith Christiansen has noted how intimately in harmony that painting is with French sensibilities, evoking the painters of Fontainebleau and Jean Goujon's (ca. 1510–ca. 1565) *Nymphs* for the Fountain of the Innocents.[7] In the *Public Felicity,* the fluid and complex arrangement of both the nude and draped parts of the body in a narrow, vertical format brings to mind many figures of the school of Fontainebleau; let us recall that *Diana the Huntress,*[8] originally narrower than it is today, could have decorated a fireplace mantel—as did perhaps Gentileschi's canvas.[9]

How to describe the painters' Paris at the time Gentileschi arrived, in the fall of 1624? The most popular studios were probably those of Georges Lallemant and Quentin Varin—both younger than Gentileschi. Did he see Lallemant's *Pietà* (1620), on an altar of the church of Saint-Nicolas-des-Champs? Or Varin's *Wedding at Cana*, on the high altar of the church of Saint-Gervais (Musée des Beaux-Arts, Rennes), probably painted only a short time before? Did he see the canvases of Martin Fréminet, who was a few years younger (he died in 1619)? Louis Finson's *Circumcision* (ca. 1615), on the high altar of Saint-Martin-des-Champs? Or, on the high altar of Saint-Leu-Saint-Gilles, the *Last Supper* (1618; Louvre, Paris) by Frans Pourbus, who had died two years earlier in Paris, after spending twelve years in the capital? Gentileschi may have found the *Last Supper* quite striking. It was quickly to become famous—it is reputed to have been admired by Nicolas Poussin himself—and, in the eighteenth century, was still cited in guides to the capital as "one of the marvels of Paris." The picture's somewhat weighty realism, its sharp and chiseled forms, even its austerity move decidedly away from the late-Mannerist style of Lallemant, Varin, and Fréminet. Pourbus's taste for rendering materials, with very specific fabrics, in a perhaps too insistent manner, may have fascinated Orazio, who was sensitive to such effects. Other religious compositions painted by Pourbus in Paris must also have interested the artist: the *Annunciation* (1619) and the *Saint Francis Receiving the Stigmata* (1620) for the convent of the Jacobins on the rue Saint-Honoré (Musée des Beaux-Arts, Nancy, and Louvre, Paris)—or the *Vic Family Virgin* (ca. 1616?), which has remained at Saint-Nicolas-des-Champs, with its complex Italianism and naturalist set pieces. Let us recall that Pourbus, born in Antwerp six years after Orazio, was closely connected to Marie de' Medici and did many portraits of her. Marie's sister Eleonora was duchess of Mantua, and Pourbus worked in Mantua

for the Gonzaga beginning in 1600. Thanks to their intervention, he went to Innsbruck, Turin, and Paris, where, in 1606, he made portraits of Marie de' Medici and her son the dauphin, the future Louis XIII (r. 1609–43). After 1610, Pourbus returned definitively to Paris as painter to the queen; in 1618, he became a French citizen. Pourbus lived at the Louvre, and he died in the French capital. His art represented the most "advanced" Parisian painting of the day. Let us say, to simplify matters, that Orazio found a Parisian mode of painting that was at times attached to the last moments of Mannerism, at times tempered by a strained naturalism, and, on the whole, somewhat Northern in its tradition.

The activity centered on the Palais du Luxembourg presents a completely different view. Is it possible to define a taste peculiar

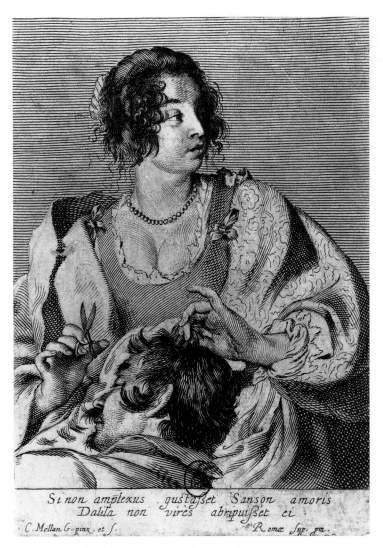

Figure 79. Claude Mellan (1598–1688), *Samson and Delilah*. Engraving. Bibliothèque Nationale de France, Paris

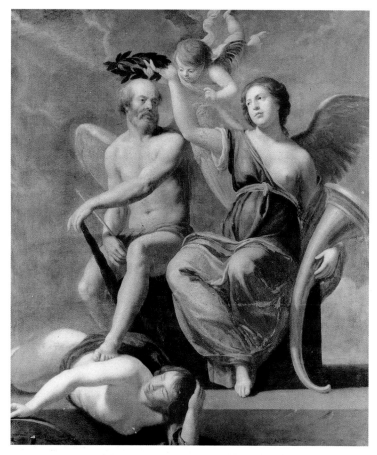

Figure 80. Jean Monier (1600–1656), *Allegory*. Oil on canvas. Musée de Château de Blois

to Marie de' Medici and to characterize her artistic patronage? Certainly, it is not an easy task. Antoine Schnapper, who has recently taken it on, has told of the queen's (Florentine) fondness for tables embellished with hardstone marquetry and, more generally, for precious objects.[10] I have spoken of her attraction to the works of Pourbus, but this seems to have been limited to his work as a portraitist—which is hardly surprising, given that the sovereign liked portraits very much. The undertaking of the Luxembourg palace and its painted décor are, of course, what mattered, and the connections to the queen's native country, especially through the familial ties to the court of Mantua, were of major significance.[11]

This is not the place to focus on the history and importance of the commission Rubens received from Marie de' Medici for the gallery of twenty-four paintings devoted to her life, or to analyze their iconographic richness. Let us, instead, look again at the Italian context of that enterprise, entrusted to an artist who had been given a variety of commissions by the Gonzaga and who

was acclaimed for having spent eight years in Italy. The paintings (today in the Louvre, Paris) were installed at the Palais du Luxembourg in 1625, and unveiled at the festivities for the marriage of Henrietta Maria to Charles I. Orazio could not have failed to see and study them; this is what he was up against.

Another series of paintings at the palace was also significant. This time, it was a gift to the sovereign. In 1624, Ferdinando Gonzaga, sixth duke of Mantua, in order to obtain the title of Highness, and on the advice of Giustiano Priandi, his ambassador to Paris, sent to Marie de' Medici a series of ten paintings by Giovanni Baglione, *Apollo and the Nine Muses* (on deposit at the Musée d'Arras; the *Melpomene* is lost). These had been commissioned a few years earlier by the duke and executed in Rome in 1620.[12] In a letter to the court of Mantua, Priandi had emphasized quite pointedly that to please the sovereign, the figures had to be "eccellenti e non del tutto ignude ne troppo lascive" (excellent, with no nudity, and not too lascivious). This gives an idea, if not of the queen's tastes, then at least of her bias. The paintings, in a somewhat gentle Caravaggesque style, elegant and a little loosely painted, were very much admired by the courtiers, some of whom judged Baglione superior to Rubens.

The third and last series of paintings was commissioned by Marie de' Medici in 1623 as decoration for the Cabinet Doré. The ten large canvases were executed by artists active in Florence, and their subjects, most of which alluded to marriages of the Medici, were chosen by the queen at the beginning of the following year. Seven of the ten—those by Jacopo Ligozzi, Giovanni Bilivert, Jacopo da Empoli, Francesco Bianchi Buonavita, Passignano, Marucelli, and Anastasio Fontebuoni—still survive in a private collection; three of the canvases—by Vignali, Ligozzi, and Zanobi Rosi—are lost.[13] The paintings arrived in Paris only in December 1627. This great undertaking, dedicated to the glory of the Medici family and carried out by many of the finest Florentine painters of the day, was an affirmation by Marie of her origins in her (very Florentine) palace in Paris, built by Salomon de Brosse as a tribute to the Palazzo Pitti.

The queen's patronage was not, however, limited to works for the Luxembourg palace. Indeed, she bestowed works of art on several religious institutions, notably the Carmelite convent on the rue Saint Jacques, which she founded in 1603 and for which she commissioned Guido Reni's (1575–1642) *Annunciation*, now in the Louvre. This was the first large painting by that artist to have

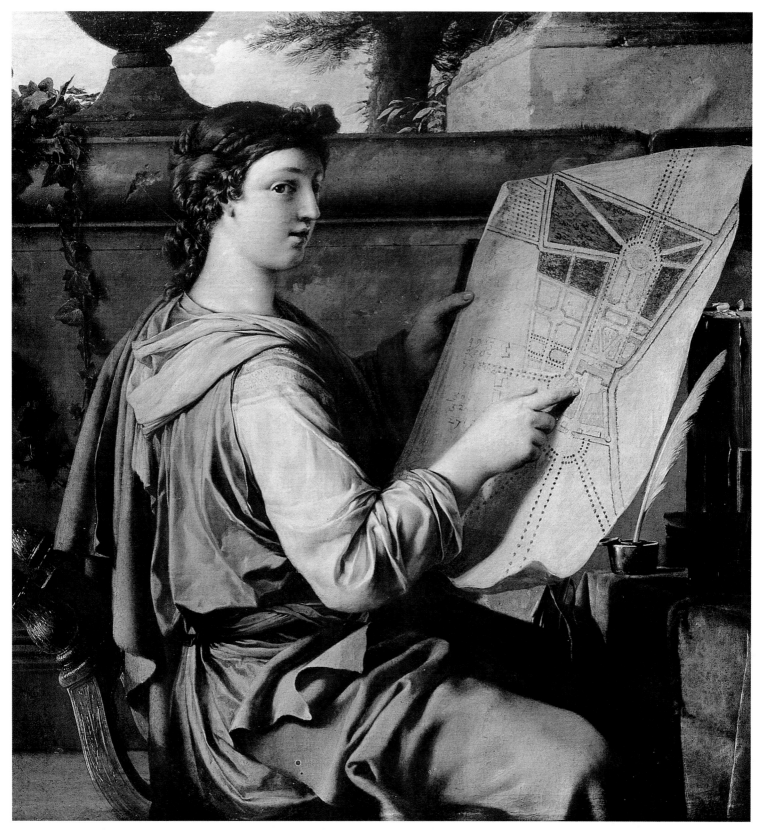

Figure 81. Laurent de La Hyre (1605–1656), *Allegory of Arithmetic*. Oil on canvas. Hannema-de Stuers Foundation, Heino, The Netherlands

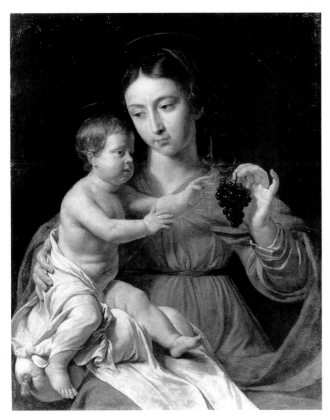

Figure 82. Philippe de Champaigne (1602–1674), *Madonna and Child*. Oil on canvas. Musée Baron Gérard, Bayeux

come to France; it appears to have been contracted in 1624. Reni deliberated over it a long time, and it did not arrive in Paris until early 1629.[14] It was almost certainly upon receiving the *Annunciation* that Marie de' Medici decided to ask Reni to Paris to decorate one of the galleries at the palace. The invitation, as we know, went unheeded. There had earlier been a plan to have the Cavaliere d'Arpino (1568–1640) undertake the task, but this was abandoned because of the painter's advanced age. Guercino (1591–1666) was subsequently approached, also to no avail.

The influence of Giovanni Baglione (ca. 1566–1643) on the development of French art is certainly negligible (though he perhaps exerted some on Mathieu Le Nain, with his taste for figures in feathers, for musical instruments, and for very clear-toned reds and blues). The mark left by Rubens was considerable, but it was not felt until the end of the seventeenth and the beginning of the eighteenth century. What role could Gentileschi's paintings have played in France? It remains a matter of conjecture, since, with one exception, we are not sure which canvases he painted there, or which may have been there during his stay and subsequently.

Nevertheless, historians of French painting have always considered his role to be a major one.

Did Simon Vouet (1590–1649) have a sympathy with Gentileschi? That he did can be argued, but, beyond a shared taste for ample forms and sharp, clear-toned colors, their worlds are irreducibly different. I also remain unconvinced by the arguments that link the half-length female figures painted by Vouet in Rome to those by Orazio, since the work of Orazio's daughter, Artemisia, could have contributed to this connection. In the same vein, the similarities between the *Public Felicity* and Vouet's *Allegory of Wealth* (Louvre, Paris) do not seem particularly notable.[15] Nevertheless, in the rich and diverse visual material accumulated by Vouet during his travels, the memory of one Gentileschi or another, whether the father's or the daughter's, seen in Genoa or elsewhere, may have been a contributing factor in his artistic development. Some paintings by close followers of Vouet are not dissimilar to Gentileschi's in manner. A half-length *Jael* (present location unknown), for example, was obviously made within the master's immediate orbit—either in the final years in Rome or in Paris shortly after 1627[16]—with its authoritative sense of volume and subtle rendering of white fabric.

At present, no one is bold enough to state definitively that Vouet's return to the French capital in 1627 constituted the sole event that set a new course for Parisian painting, one that reflected the painter's lyrical, largely decorative vision, marked by bright colors and a broad technique. It has been said often enough that Vouet's visual language at the end of his stay in Italy was complex, marked by Giovanni Lanfranco (1582–1647) and by the time spent in Venice, Genoa, and Naples. It was a long way from his experience of Caravaggio, even if that experience was harmoniously integrated to support a healthy naturalism. Had they been painted in Paris, Vouet's canvases from the beginning of his stay in Rome, such as the *Fortune-Teller* in the Palazzo Barberini, Rome, or the painting of the same subject in the National Gallery of Canada, Ottawa, might have determined or reinforced completely different currents. They are intimately Caravaggesque and in close harmony with the French tradition of gesture and mime, which derive from the theater. Vouet's role in Parisian art as a whole, beginning about 1630, is quite evident, and there is a style specific to Vouet—that of the master's studio and family—to which Michel Dorigny, Charles Poerson, Eustache Le Sueur, and the young Charles Le Brun were connected: the physical types, the color schemes, the sense of monumentality, and the taste for decoration all are, with subtle variations, similar, and in every way far removed from Caravaggism.

Sometimes, however, artists closely associated with Vouet appear to have also been in tune with Gentileschi. What is striking in his work—the tranquil weightiness of figures in vivid colors and immobilized in a bright light, with blues and yellows tempered by whites—is very similar to what one finds in the work of Michel I Corneille (1603–1664), a nephew and student of Vouet, whose style can be distinguished from that of his master by the attentive and careful rendering of realist set pieces, by an occasional ungainliness, and often by a taste for white, citron yellow, bright blue drapery, and milky carnations. As an example, let us cite the large *Marriage of the Virgin*, recently on the art market (fig. 78).[17]

Claude Mellan (1598–1688) also deserves a few words. "Gentileschiano del bulino" (Gentileschian with the burin), said Roberto Longhi, drawing attention to the stylistic affinity between the engraver from Abbeville (fig. 79) and the painter from Pisa. The clear, almost transparent, craft of the engraver, who captures figures that are sharply depicted in the light, instantly intelligible, stands as an equivalent to the painting style of Gentileschi, whether the engravings are executed after Vouet, after Poussin, or after his own creations. In certain cases, Mellan's work is directly Gentileschian: his *Saint Mary Magdalene in Penitence* is often cited as an example. The preparatory drawing for the engraving still survives (Musée Boucher de Perthes, Abbeville). The drawing, made around 1629, according to Jacques Thuillier, was obviously influenced by Gentileschi's canvas of the same subject (Kunsthistorisches Museum, Vienna; fig. 26).[18]

Other, more modest artists, not in the circle of Vouet, must also be mentioned. Foremost among them is Jean Monier (or Mosnier; 1600–1656), a painter from Blois, who, in spite of himself, has helped to expand our knowledge of Gentileschi's activities in France. As noted earlier, the *Public Felicity* was for a long time attributed to Monier, until correctly identified by Sterling. In his article, Sterling explains how the picture may have been confused with a work by a painter who also worked at the Palais de Luxembourg and who appears, according to testimony given in 1682, to have served as Gentileschi's replacement when he left for London and when Monier was returning from Rome.[19] Monier's participation in the decoration of the palace is still unclear, and it is not certain which passages perhaps executed by him remain.[20]

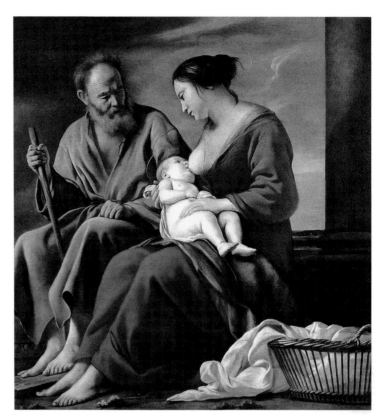

Figure 83. Louis Le Nain (ca. 1600–1648), *Holy Family*. Oil on canvas. Private collection

The works that are generally attributed to Monier, especially the beautiful series of mythological subjects at the château de Cheverny, the *Allegory* in the museum of the château de Blois (fig. 80) originally installed at Cheverny, and the decoration for the château de Chenailles (now in the Toledo Museum of Art), are restrained in expression and similar to those of Gentileschi in the depiction of massive figures seen *di sotto in sù*, elegant and with a quality of pleasing quietude.[21] No one has ever challenged the claim that Monier was responsible for a copy executed after Gentileschi's *Diana*. That painting depicts only the upper body. It was published by Sterling in 1964 and assigned to Monier.[22] But Sterling noted its stylistic similarities to the mythological compositions at Cheverny before the original by Gentileschi had been identified. I wonder now how convincing that explanation is, and whether the argument does not too easily lend itself to making the work conform to documents that link the two artists. The attribution of the copy of the *Diana* to Monier, though certainly not impossible, must remain hypothetical.[23]

It is interesting to link to Gentileschi the name of another painter of the same generation, still relatively unknown: Nicolas

Prévost (1604–1670), who was rescued from oblivion by the work of John E. Schloder on the decoration at the château de Richelieu, with which the artist's name remains linked.[24] Prévost, a student of Varin, was chosen by Cardinal Richelieu in the 1630s to decorate his sumptuous château in Poitou. If we are to judge by the few elements of that decoration which can be identified, he would appear to have practiced a complex, rather eclectic art, reminiscent of Jacques Stella, Lubin Baugin, and Laurent de La Hyre. Prévost was strongly influenced by classical statuary filtered through the sensibility of the school of Fontainebleau, a sensibility reflected in the series *Strong Women* (private collection), which are among the relics of the château de Richelieu. The *Kiss of Justice and Peace* (now in the Musée de Richelieu), which once decorated the mantel in the queen's antechamber, displays a manner fairly close to that of La Hyre, somewhat stilted and with a certain naïveté, but in which, despite the choice of warm colors, there are obvious echoes of Gentileschi's art.[25]

With Laurent de La Hyre, Philippe de Champaigne, and the Le Nain brothers, we must imagine artists of a very high stature, all active in Paris, none of whom made the trip to Italy (was this by chance?), and who were, to varying degrees, profoundly marked by Gentileschi. La Hyre (1605–1656), whose first works (ca. 1623–24?) can be placed within the tradition of the second school of Fontainebleau, with elongated, fluid forms, a softness in the modeling of the figures, and foliage that is unnaturalistic and fancifully decorative, certainly cast an envious eye toward Gentileschi, as Sterling has aptly pointed out.[26] La Hyre was between eighteen and twenty years old at the time of Gentileschi's stay in Paris, certainly the determining moment, when his work displayed a new concern for monumentality with heavy sculptural forms, a more defined modeling in strong light, and an interest in the analysis of "bits of reality," which led him to describe in fine detail the tactile surfaces of rocks and plants and trees, and the soft fur of animals. The connection to Gentileschi, particularly to the *Public Felicity*, is very evident. Chipped stones, worn rocks, and abandoned buildings are a constant in La Hyre, as are volumetric forms seen in almost palpable changing light that brings them into strong relief. With the victory of Christianity over Greco-Roman paganism their underlying theme, La Hyre's paintings are a meditation on the passage of time. Similarly, split and fissured stones are part of Gentileschi's vocabulary—the balustrade in the *Public Felicity*, the broken steps in the *Vision of Saint Francesca Romana* (cat. 30),

and the heavily indented rocks in the *Saint Francis Receiving the Stigmata* in Rome (cat. 25). The last painting (and its smaller version; cat. 26)—its Italian lyricism and feeling expressed in the execution of the plants and in the saint's robe and cord—seems almost a La Hyre "avant la lettre."[27] Gentileschi's luminous colors, his whites and pale grays, his mastery of color relationships—yellows, blues, lilacs—that are both audacious and refined, exerted a lasting influence, as did his forms, which served as the prototype for La Hyre's classical and sculptural female figures. His series of the Liberal Arts, now dispersed (Musée des Beaux-Arts, Orléans; Metropolitan Museum of Art, New York; Hannema-de Stuers Foundation, Heino [fig. 81]; National Gallery, London; and private collection, New York),[28] is a good indication that the Gentileschian manner, of figures with vast polychromatic drapery and beautiful still-life details in the spirit of the *Public Felicity*, was not lost on him.

Philippe de Champaigne (1602–1674), who was slightly older than La Hyre and, like him, did not go to Italy, may have known Gentileschi personally. Shortly after Champaigne's arrival in Paris from Brussels in 1621, he worked, between 1622 and 1626, under the direction of Nicolas Duchesne on landscapes for the Palais du Luxembourg. After his return to Brussels in 1627, he was called back by Marie de' Medici to succeed Duchesne, with the title of painter ordinary to the queen; he lived at the palace. Champaigne settled in Paris in January 1628, before marrying Duchesne's daughter in November of the same year. His first years in Paris thus seem to gravitate toward the Palais du Luxembourg, and there is no doubt that he saw and carefully studied Gentileschi's *Public Felicity*. As an example of the Italian painter's mark on Champaigne, R. Ward Bissell offers *Anne of Austria as Minerva* (formerly Henri Rouart, Paris), the attribution of which is not certain.[29] But it is clear that many elements in Champaigne's work are Gentileschian, once allowances are made for his Flemish temperament (fig. 82): the perfect and pronounced definition of forms in space; their sculptural weight, even massiveness; the careful description of materials, in a cold, precise light; the taste for bright, gay colors, which almost contradicts the naturalism of the figures; and the yellow, pale blue, and rose color schemes.

The influence of Gentileschi on La Hyre and Champaigne has to do with tactility in the rendering of materials and, in a certain sense, with light and color. On the Le Nain brothers (Antoine, ca. 1600–1648; Louis, ca. 1600–1648; Mathieu, ca. 1607–1677), the influence

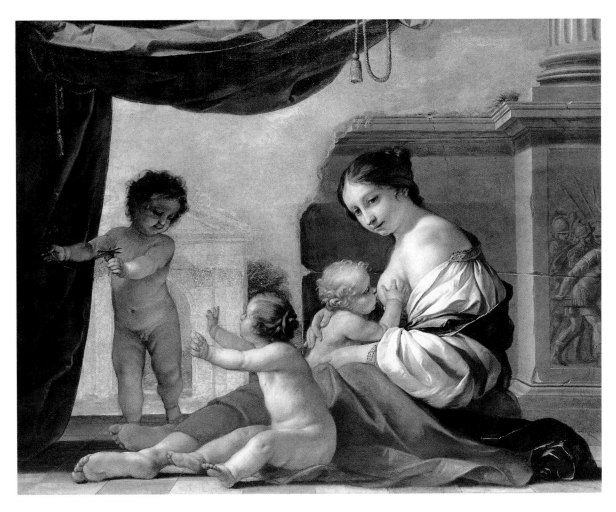

Figure 84. Jacques Blanchard (1600–1638), *Allegory of Charity*. Oil on canvas. Toledo Museum of Art. Purchased with funds from the Libbey Endowment, Gift of Edward Drummond Libbey

is more profound; indeed, we can discern a real spiritual kinship. Here, the execution itself and the color schemes are very different from those of the Italian painter. But the somber figures, the patches of soft light, and the discretion of feeling, with facial expressions turned inward, are all similar. Bissell has very aptly analyzed these elements. The figures in Gentileschi's depictions of the Rest on the Flight into Egypt (cat. nos. 34, 45), their quality of measured realism, their restrained elegance, and even the gentle melancholy that emanates from them, have often been compared with several figures by the Le Nain, as have many female faces, almost childlike, with slightly puffy cheeks, tangled blonde hair, and a closed, almost obstinate expression. The combination of refined, aristocratic elegance with working-class simplicity seen in the paintings of the Le Nain brothers—the *Magdalene* (formerly Vitale Bloch), the *Holy Family* (fig. 83), and their most ambitious altar paintings, the *Saint Michael and the Virgin*, in the Église Saint-Pierre in Nevers, and the *Birth of the Virgin*, in Notre-

Dame de Paris—are also evocative of the Italian painter. Let us recall as well the often-reproduced figure with lowered eyes from *The Adoration of the Shepherds* in the Louvre, the *Small Card Players* from the queen's collection in England, and the strangely grave and chastely immodest figure in the *Victory*, also in the Louvre. These reflect Gentileschi at his most intimate, his most tender: the Gentileschi of the *Saint Francesca Romana* (cat. 30), the *Saint Cecilia* (cat. 31), and the various paintings of the Rest on the Flight into Egypt that the works of the Le Nain brothers most resemble. The Birmingham version (cat. 34), with the magnificent idea of the ass's head silhouetted against the sky, is in perfect harmony with the poetics of the Le Nain—would that they had seen the painting.

I can only point to these similarities, making note of the fragility of an argument that rests solely on personal feeling. How can we fail to observe that the startling *Public Felicity*, the only undisputed "French" Gentileschi, really is not much in tune with the honest realism and earth colors of the Le Nain brothers?

We must remain cautious, as it is possible that the similarities were casual ones. Are not the Le Nain angels, in their resemblance to the witty, generous, and rebellious Parisian urchin Gavroche in Victor Hugo's *Les misérables,* the brothers of those in the Spanish artist Juan Bautista Maino's two versions of the *Adoration of the Shepherds* (Prado, Madrid, and Hermitage, Saint Petersburg), which were painted earlier and far from Paris?

The Gentileschian mark on the Parisian painters can be found in diluted form in the work of other artists, in particular Jacques Blanchard (1600–1638). Blanchard's two *Magdalenes* (both lost, but of which engravings exist) are reminiscent of *Magdalenes* by Gentileschi (see cat. 35 and fig. 26), as are his beautiful, ample figures—often young women surrounded by naked children, a Charity, a Virgin and Child. The admirable large *Charity* in Toledo (fig. 84) and the one at the Courtauld Institute Galleries in London (the latter, a fragment, is dated 1637) are good examples. Here and there, Gentileschi's influence can be found, always in painters unfamiliar with the Vouet current. An anonymous *Adoration of the Shepherds* of surprisingly high quality (Museo de Bellas Artes, Bilbao), with its small figures that bring to mind both Champaigne and the Le Nain brothers, is a good indication that in Paris at mid-century (if this is, in fact, the date that should be assigned to the work) the impact of Gentileschi remained a vital one. In the center of the painting, a half-kneeling shepherdess in profile seems an echo of the Italian painter, with the blue and white fabric subtly defined by a strong lateral light.[30]

It would thus appear that, unlike Marie de' Medici, who preferred Pourbus and Rubens and did not encourage Gentileschi to remain in France, the Parisian painters—at least those not directly in the orbit of Vouet—favored the Italian artist. Gentileschi introduced them to an echo of Caravaggism that was felt more strongly than that transmitted by Vouet and was truly in harmony with the country (if not peasant) tenor of their work. Should one speak of painters working after nature, as opposed to "decorators"? The distinction might be simplistic, but it is fitting.

We arrive, inevitably, at the question of the role of Caravaggio's followers among French painters. It is a commonplace to say that Caravaggism had no effect on Parisian painting, and, in fact, the most obvious examples of Caravaggism in France are found in the southwest, the central regions, the Midi, Burgundy, and—though this region had not yet been annexed by France—Lorraine. The pictures were often, but not necessarily, executed by painters who had spent time in Italy, and are examples of tenebrism, to use the Spanish term, and sometimes of nocturnes illuminated by candlelight. But the work of the Le Nain brothers eludes such a simplistic view; both the *Nativity with a Torch* (private collection, formerly Farkas) and the *Denial of Saint Peter,* which has recently resurfaced (art market, Paris) reflect a powerful and total Caravaggism, and they were certainly painted in Paris. And although such paintings were unusual in the capital, a Parisian Caravaggism did exist. Gentileschi's Caravaggesque contribution to Parisian painting, which stands apart, was a determining factor—even if it is difficult to say which of his paintings were seen by French artists—because his work found fertile ground in the capital, given the realist taste of the Northern painters. The power of Gentileschi's paintings, their compelling, almost tactile naturalism executed in brilliant, sunny colors, was enormous. As a result of his short stay, there emerged a truly Parisian "Gentileschianism"—sometimes with a classical bent, sometimes with a more naturalistic tone—to which we owe a few of the most refined inflections of French painting.

I would like to express my warm thanks to my colleagues in the department of painting at the Musée du Louvre, Jacques Foucart, Sylvain Laveissière, and Stéphane Loire, for their assistance.

1. Sterling 1958, 112–20.

2. Bissell 1981, 47–49.

3. See Finaldi's excellent "Orazio Gentileschi at the Court of Charles I," in London–Bilbao–Madrid 1999, 10–11.

4. Sterling 1958, 114, fig. 1.

5. Finaldi 1999, 24, 36 n. 57. See Sterling (1964), who argues that the work was executed in France, and Bissell (1981, 194; no. 69, fig. 134), who claims it was painted in England in the mid-1630s. On the painting, see Arnauld Brejon de Lavergnée in Paris–Milan 1988–89, no. 77; Sarrazin 1994, 196–97 no. 145; and Alain Mérot in Dijon–Le Mans 1998–99, no. 1.

6. Finaldi 1999, 22–24, fig. 11.

7. See the entry on the *Diana* (cat. 47) in this publication.

8. "Ecole de Fontainebleau," mid-sixteenth century, inv. 455; Compin and Roquebert 1986, vol. 4, 293.

9. A beautiful and faithful copy of the *Diana* (fig. 92) of somewhat smaller dimensions, in the Musée de la Chasse et de la Nature, Paris (156.4 x 92 cm; inv. 66,131; acquired in 1966), which appears to be by a French hand, dates, in my opinion, to the second half of the eighteenth century. It is notable in having its four corners notched at right angles, as in the *Public Felicity*. One would have to verify whether the corners of the painting in Nantes have been added, which could suggest that the picture was intended for the decoration of a fireplace mantel. My thanks to Claude d'Anthenaise, director of the Musée de la Chasse et de la Nature, for the information he so generously provided.

10. Schnapper 1994, 53, 125–33; see also Marrow 1982.

11. See Schnapper 1994 and Paris 1991.

12. See Schnapper 1994, 129, and Brejon de Lavergnée in Paris–Milan 1988–89, 121–26, nos. 11–19. See also Askew 1978, 273–95, figs. 14–22, and Borea 1980, 315–18, figs. 2–7.

13. The seven paintings came up for public sale at Sotheby's, London, on April 21, 1993, lots 27–30.

14. Loire 1996, 273–77.

15. Bissell 1981, 77–78.

16. Oil on canvas, 95.5 x 72 cm. The painting was previously in the Pardo gallery in Paris (October 1980), attributed to Simon Vouet.

17. Oil on canvas, 260 x 173 cm; Heim Gallery, London, summer 1974, then Paris art market; *Old Master Paintings from the Lagerfeld Collection*, sale, Christie's, New York, May 23, 2000, lot 37.

18. See Rome 1989–90, esp. no. 64 (by Barbara Brejon de Lavergnée).

19. Sterling 1964, 219.

20. See the (now dated) article, Blancher-Le Bourhis 1939, 204–15, and Bissell 1981, 75.

21. Unfortunately, Marie-Paul Durand's (1980) thesis for the École du Louvre remains unpublished.

22. Sterling 1964, 219, fig. 4 (formerly K. Stern collection, New York; 96 x 93 cm). The painting came up for sale at Finarte, Rome, on November 26, 1992, lot 130, color ill.

23. Similarly, I wonder whether we ought not to question the still-accepted attribution of the *Magdalene in Penitence* after Gentileschi in the Musée de Dijon (fig. 69) to Jean Tassel (Sterling 1958, 117 n. 27), which does not rest on very reliable stylistic criteria. The canvas, seized from the convent of the Lazarists in Dijon during the Revolution, was attributed to Tassel by F. Devosge (see Guillaume 1980, 150–51, ill.), perhaps because there were several works by that painter in the region. The picture may be a copy by another Frenchman (or an Italian?) of the version in Lucca and London (Bissell 1981, nos. 45, 46, figs. 96, 97) with variants, "for modesty," of hair and fabric covering the chest. It would not be prudent to say whether it is a copy of the *Magdalene* that Gentileschi purportedly sent to Marie de' Medici from Genoa, but the variants might lead us to believe so, especially if the queen's prudishness is taken into consideration. In that case, it would be a copy of a *Magdalene* that is now lost.

24. Schloder 1982, 59–60. A series of six paintings stored by the Louvre at the Musée de Vendôme (*Faith and Hope*, *Strength*, *Truth*, inv. 8575 bis; *Charity*, *Justice*, and *Temperance*) is attributed to Prévost by Eric Moinet; see the exhibition "Les maîtres retrouvés," Musée des Beaux-Arts, Orléans, summer 2000, catalogue not yet published.

25. For a good color reproduction, see Meaux 1997–98, 131.

26. Sterling 1958, 199; Bissell 1981, 77.

27. Bissell 1981, nos. 33, 34, figs. 79–81.

28. Grenoble–Rennes–Bordeaux 1989–90, 292–302, nos. 255–64.

29. Bissell 1981, 77 n. 90, 97; Sterling 1958, 116, fig. 7.

30. Museo de Bellas Artes, Bilbao, bequest of Don Laureano de Jado, 1927, inv. 69.378, 92.5 × 105 cm. I am indebted to Xavier Bray, to whom I express my warm thanks, for so generously providing information about this painting.

44.

Public Felicity

Oil on canvas, 105½ × 66⅞ in.
(268 × 170 cm)

Musée du Louvre, Département
des peintures, Paris (inv. 6809)

1624–26

PROVENANCE: Marie de'
Medici, queen's antechamber,
Palais de Luxembourg, Paris
(1625/26–31); by inheritance,
Gaston d'Orléans, Palais de
Luxembourg (1646–60; procès-
verbal of 1645, without attribution); Orléans collection, Palais
de Luxembourg (1660–94; inv.
of Paillet, 1687–93, as by Jean
Monier); Royal Collection
(from 1694; inv. of Bailly, 1709–
10, no. 206, as by Monier);
Musée du Louvre, Paris (lent
to Foreign Affairs Office for
the French ambassador, Berlin,
1904/5–8, and to the Ancienne
Légation, Vienna, 1908–about
1939).

REFERENCES: Bailly and
Engerand (1709–10) 1899, 572
no. 206; Blancher-Le Bourhis
1939, 207, 213–15; Sterling 1958,
113–17; Blunt 1970, 112; Nicolson
1979, 52; Bissell 1981, 48, 75, 78,
181 no. 54, 187, 193; Marrow 1982,
27, 69–71; Brejon de Lavergnée
in Paris–Milan 1988–89, 226–28;
Nicolson 1990, 112; Schnapper
1990, 425; Béguin and Baudouin-
Matuszek in Paris 1991, 35, 265;
Baudouin-Matuszek 1992,
290–92.

This magnificent allegorical painting is Orazio's only surviving work that can be associated with the decorative enterprises of Marie de' Medici, who had invited the artist to Paris (he made the trip from Genoa in the summer or early fall of 1624 and remained until the fall of 1626). It formed part of the decorations of the Palais de Luxembourg, where it decorated the queen's antechamber, situated between the two pavilions of the west wing—the only wing the queen succeeded in decorating before her exile from France in 1631.[1] An official inventory made in 1645 gives the fullest description of the room: "The following antechamber also has parquet floors and a wainscoting five feet high against the walls, doorframes, a revêtement on the mantle over the fireplace with a picture representing Felicity, a ceiling with nine paintings in compartments, the whole ornamented with architecture and sculpture, and embellished with gold and blue."[2] The nine ceiling compartments showed Minerva flanked by allegorical figures alluding to peace and prosperity, and putti. Presumably the revêtement over the fireplace was carved wood, as in the adjacent room, and the molding surrounding the canvas had cutout corners. Orazio clearly took the high placement and architectural features of the room into consideration, since the balcony on which Felicity sits is seen from below and to the right—the view the queen would have had as she entered the room from her private apartments. The room was lit by two windows opposite the fireplace, and Orazio seems to combine in the picture two sources of light: one that coincides with the sky and lights the balustrade and the caduceus from behind; the other, more dispersed, that lights the figure from the right and may be intended to suggest illumination from the windows of the room.

In his widely influential handbook of iconography, Cesare Ripa describes Public Felicity in the following terms: "A woman seated on a regal throne. In her right hand she holds a caduceus, in her left a cornucopia filled with fruits and garlanded with flowers.

Felicity is a repose of the spirit . . . for which reason she is depicted seated, with the caduceus as a sign of peace and wisdom. The cornucopia holds the fruits of labor without which felicity cannot be attained. . . . The flowers indicate happiness, from which contentment can never be severed. The caduceus also signifies virtue, and the cornucopia riches, because happy are those who have so many temporal goods that they can provide for the necessities of the body, and so virtuous that they can lighten the needs of the soul."[3] Ripa's description obviously provided Orazio's point of departure, but the artist has suppressed some aspects of the allegory and added others to subtly shift its meaning. Gone are the fruits and flowers, replaced by laurels and palm fronds, scepters, and metal crowns. In his seminal article, in which the picture is reintroduced to modern scholarship as the work of Orazio, Sterling notes that the crowns and scepters are taken from Ripa's allegory of Europe, who, "with the finger of her left hand indicates reigns, diverse crowns, scepters, garlands, and similar things, since the major and most powerful princes of the world are in Europe." The crown of France is identifiable by the fleurs-de-lis; the others are ducal. With the two scepters is seen the hand of Justice, an attribute of the French monarchs. By contrast, the white blouse and yellow dress derive from Ripa's description of *Felicità breve*, or temporal Felicity ("A woman dressed in white and yellow with a gold crown on her head"). The laurel crowns and palms shown together—visible above the figure's right arm—are attributes of *Felicità eterna*, and signify that eternal felicity cannot be attained without tribulations. Ripa's figure of eternal Felicity is shown nude, but she too raises her eyes heavenward, since "she is not subject to the rapid course of the stars and the changeable movements of time." What this adds up to is a highly personalized allegory that Sterling rightly sees as referring to the vicissitudes of Marie de' Medici's life following the assassination of Henry IV in 1610. Conspiracies,

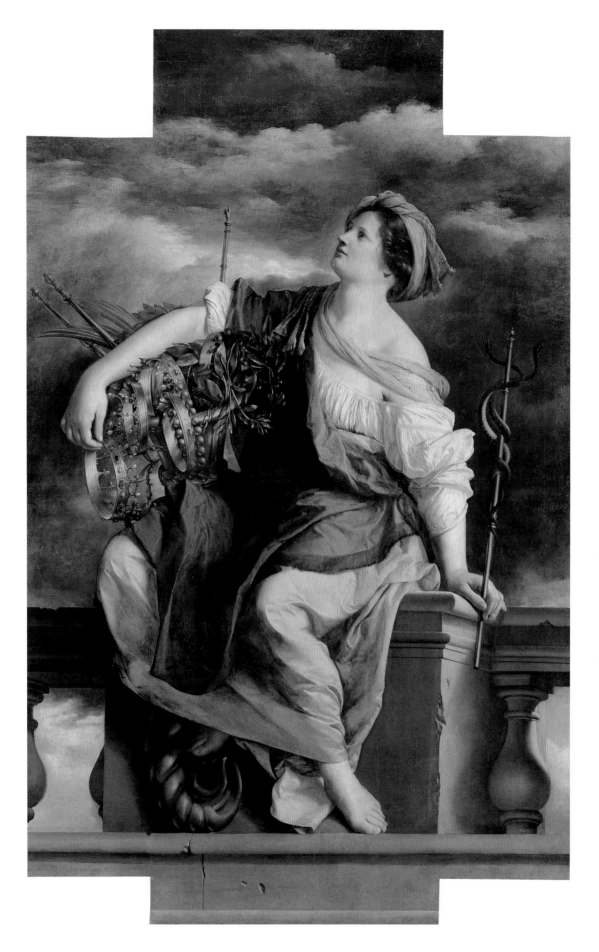

the hostility of the Protestants, and problems with her son leading to her exile at Blois in 1617 are among the tribulations borne by the queen. The message of Orazio's allegory is that these tribulations, so memorably commemorated in Rubens's cycle of the life of Marie de' Medici (installed in the Palais de Luxembourg in 1625), are the basis of true felicity. The dark storm clouds are shown parting, and a soft light—unmistakably that of the Île-de-France—plays over the figure. The comforting augury of the picture was to prove illusory: Marie de' Medici was exiled again in 1631 and died in Cologne after residing in Flanders and England.

The allegorical paraphernalia of Orazio's picture are used throughout the paintings in the palace and are a staple of Rubens's cycle. The caduceus entwined by two live serpents is carried by Mercury in Rubens's *Flight of Marie de' Medici from Blois,* and the cornucopia with crowns, scepters, a palm, and the hand of Justice recurs in Rubens's *Birth of Marie de' Medici*, where it is carried by the *Genius natalis*. The queen holds the hand of Justice in Rubens's *Marie de' Medici as the Patroness of the Fine Arts*. The queen's bedroom contained an oval painting with a similar allegorical figure of a female dressed in blue and yellow holding a cornucopia and caduceus, and two putti with a laurel crown at her feet. As Sterling remarks, the imagery was ubiquitous.

The commission offered a unique and daunting challenge. Rubens's series of canvases celebrating the life of Marie de' Medici, designed to decorate the long western gallery, was contracted in 1622. Nine of the canvases arrived in May 1623 and were, understandably, much admired. The following year, a series of Apollo and the nine Muses by Orazio's old nemesis, Giovanni Baglione, arrived for another room, a gift from the duke of Mantua.[4] They too garnered praise. Surprisingly, some courtiers—obviously more accustomed to the Mannerist decorations at the château de Fontainebleau than to the new Baroque idiom—preferred them to Rubens's canvases. (Ironically, in his early-eighteenth-century inventory, Bailly describes Baglione's canvases as done in the manner of Gentileschi, though in his *Felicity* Orazio defines a position at the opposite pole to that of Baglione's elegant but highly mannered figures.) Orazio must have been aware that in 1623 an attempt had been made to lure Guido Reni to Paris

(a second invitation was extended in 1629). Reni's early masterpiece *David with the Head of Goliath* (fig. 49) was destined to be placed in the Cabinet des Muses. In the *Public Felicity*, Orazio seems to have carefully staked out his position. Quite clearly incapable of competing with the facility, virtuosity, and narrative invention of Rubens, he strove for an effect of grand monumentality. The brilliant effects of light playing on silk and metal that are the hallmarks of Orazio's Genoese paintings are here played down, but his powers of description are everywhere in evidence (note his favorite gold-banded, sheer scarf on the figure's head and shoulders).

It is unclear what sort of success the picture enjoyed. On the one hand, the overall effect of an elevated realism must have been important for the younger generation of French painters, particularly Philippe de Champaigne, who was already in the employ of the queen and succeeded Nicolas Duchesne as first painter in 1628. On the other, Orazio's authorship had been forgotten by the late seventeenth century, and there is no clear evidence that he was engaged to do other decorations in the palace. Just a few years later, in 1629, Reni refused the invitation to come to Paris, in part because he had heard that Gentileschi had not found the court sympathetic.[5] Félibien records that Gentileschi's work was well thought of, but that his bad temper—"tout-à-fait brutale"—brought him into bad repute.[6] All of which throws light on Orazio's eagerness to move to London. Was the picture complete and installed by May 1625, when the duke of Buckingham attended the proxy wedding of Henrietta Maria? He was entertained at the Palais de Luxembourg, "which, for the first time, was seen decorated with very rich hangings and a quantity of royal ornaments of a greater splendor than any king or queen has ever seen in this reign."[7] In any event, Buckingham soon received two pictures from Orazio and extended the invitation to come to London.

1. For the location of the antechamber within the western apartments of the palace, see Baudouin-Matuszek 1992, 292.
2. The procès-verbal is reprinted in Paris 1991, 265.
3. Ripa (1611) 1976, 167.
4. For this series, see Paris–Milan 1988–89, 121–26. Marie de' Medici had solicited gifts from all her relations in Italy to help furnish

the palace. In return for Baglione's muses Cardinal Ferdinando Gonzaga, Marie's nephew, hoped to obtain the title *Altezza* for Prince Vincenzo II Gonzaga.

5. On July 7, 1629, Cardinal Spada wrote to Francesco Barberini laying out the case for Reni's refusal. Among the reasons given he notes, "forse anco vien spaventato da qualcuno con l'esempio del Pittor Gentilesco, e col mettergli innanzi quei pericoli ch'in paese straniero possono sovrastargli da l'invidia, e da l'emulazione d'altri pictori. . . ." See Dirani 1982, 86.

6. Félibien (1666–88) 1705, vol. 3, 237.

7. The quote is from a letter of the Florentine ambassador, Giovanni Battista Gondi, to Florence; see Marrow 1982, 107 doc. 39.

45.

Rest on the Flight into Egypt

Oil on canvas, 54½ × 85 in. (138.5 × 216 cm)

Signed (lower left): HORA-TIVS / GENTILESHVS / FECIT

Kunsthistorisches Museum, Vienna (inv. 180)

ca. 1625–26

PROVENANCE: George Villiers, duke of Buckingham, York House, London (1625/26–28); Richard Grenville, second duke of Buckingham (1628–48; possibly inv. 1635, with no attribution; sold, Antwerp, 1648/49; cat. 1649, as by Gentileschi); Archduke Leopold Wilhelm, for his brother Kaiser Ferdinand III (1648–57); imperial collections, Prague and Vienna (from 1657; inv. 1718, no. 188, as by Gentileschi; moved from Prague to Vienna in 1772); Kunsthistorisches Museum, Vienna.

No *invenzione* of Orazio's enjoyed greater popularity than the Birmingham *Rest on the Flight into Egypt* (cat. 34). A replica or variant of it seems to have been made by Orazio when he was in Genoa and was subsequently owned by Cardinal Maurizio of Savoy.[1] Other variants belonged to the duke of Buckingham, to Charles I and his queen, Henrietta Maria, and to Louis XIV. At least six variants can be traced today, of which three show only the Virgin and child (fig 25). Of these, pride of place belongs to the Vienna painting, which can be associated with a group of Orazio's pictures owned by George Villiers, first duke of Buckingham. The duke was responsible for Orazio's move from Paris to London in the fall of 1626, providing quarters for the artist at York House on the Strand, and he must have met Orazio on the occasion of his mission to France in May 1625 for the proxy marriage of Henrietta Maria, daughter of Marie de' Medici, to Charles I of England. The Vienna picture can be identified with the "Virgin M[ary] & Chr[i]st & St. Joseph sleeping" recorded in the sale catalogue of the duke of Buckingham's collection, drawn up in 1649 by Brian Fairfax.[2] The inventory lists as well "a Magdalene lying in a grotto," which is unquestionably the companion picture, also in Vienna. Commenting on this inventory about 1731–36, George Vertue noted that "most of these pictures were in the Times of the Civil Warrs carried over to Antwerp, their [*sic*] sold [to raise money] and furnisht several of [the] greatest famous gallerys abroad."[3] The pictures were purchased from the second duke of Buckingham by Archduke Leopold Wilhelm, who was governor of the Netherlands from 1647 to 1656. They are not, however, mentioned in the 1659 inventory of his collection and were, presumably, sent to his brother Kaiser Ferdinand III; both pictures are listed in 1718 in the imperial collections in Prague and can be traced continuously thereafter.[4]

What remains uncertain is whether either (or both) of these pictures were sent to the duke of Buckingham from France or painted after Orazio's arrival in London. Following Buckingham's assassination in 1628, Orazio's poor relationship with the duke's painter–art adviser Balthazar Gerbier came to a head, and the artist was required to account for the moneys he had received from Buckingham and the king. In a letter of April 1629 he mentions having received an unspecified sum of money for "pictures sent to [the duke of Buckingham] from Paris."[5] In his tally of expenses, Gerbier left blank the sum of money Orazio "had by Milords . . . for two pictures he sent from France, the one having bin the Cardinals [i.e., Cardinal Richelieu, Marie de' Medici's first minister]."[6] Later in the same account is an entry of £50 for a *Magdalene* Orazio "hath sent,"

RELATED PICTURES:
Formerly J. Paul Getty Museum,
Los Angeles (variant of the
Vienna picture, but smaller in
scale, with the colors of the
Louvre version and the figures
moved closer together);[13]
Chudleigh Collection, Lawell
House, Ugbrooke Park (copy of
the Vienna picture);[14] art market, Amsterdam (sale, Christie's,
Rome, December 4, 1991, lot 72;
replica of the right side of the
Vienna painting, but with the
Virgin's hand differently positioned);[15] formerly Canessa
Gallery, Rome (variant of the
right side of the Vienna painting, with sky and foliage in the
upper left);[16] Musée du Louvre,
Paris (autograph variant, later
in date and smaller in scale
than the Vienna painting, introducing new variations in the
drapery and showing the sky in
the upper left, with Joseph in
blue and the Virgin wearing a
rose-colored dress);[17] private
collection, Italy (sale, Finarte,
Milan, 1971; a fragmentary
autograph variant of the right
side of the Louvre picture).[18]

REFERENCES: Vertue (1713–56)
1935–36, 68; Fairfax 1758, 14;
Mechel 1784, 41, 49; Engerth
1884, 157; Köpl 1889, CL no. 223;
Davies 1907, 380; Glück and
Schaeffer 1907, 84; Longhi
(1916) 1961, 243, 275 n. 42, 276;
Cammel 1939, 345–47; Hess
1952, 163; Vienna 1954, 20; Voss
1959, 163–64; Moir 1967, vol. I,
75–76; Fredericksen 1972, 45–46;
Nicolson 1979, 52; Bissell 1981,
48–49, 76, 159, 167, 182, 183–84
no. 57, 186, 209; Nicolson 1990,
113; Marcolini 1996, 72–73;
Wood 2000–2001, 111–12.

followed by entries for a "Maghdelen with Joseph," a "Christ at the Pillare" (see cat. 49), and "the picture he hath maide in Englant of Lott, that wich the King hath" (that is, cat. 46).[7] The "Maghdelen with Joseph" seems probably a confusion with "Mary and Joseph" (that is, the *Rest on the Flight into Egypt*).[8] Were these the pictures that the duke of Buckingham had heard the king of France and either Cardinal Richelieu or Marie de' Medici were contemplating giving to him even before he made his trip to Paris in May 1625?[9] There is no way of being certain, although it seems strange that Buckingham would have awarded Orazio for gifts made not by him but by the French court. Much more plausible is that, unhappy at the court of France, Orazio sent one or more paintings to the duke of Buckingham to solicit a position at the Caroline court. Nevertheless, the possibility that the pictures were the French gifts adds yet another wrinkle to our understanding of the "genealogy" of the Vienna picture, since in 1674 Soprani, our primary source for Orazio's activity in Genoa, states that the artist sent pictures to Marie de' Medici in an effort to secure an appointment in Paris. Thus, a continuous, if highly conjectural, trail leads from the two paintings eventually owned by the duke of Buckingham to Genoa, where both compositions had been treated by Orazio.

Like Bissell, I would be disinclined to accept a date earlier than about 1625–26 for the Vienna *Rest on the Flight into Egypt*. In that painting, Orazio has made the crucial move from the brilliant, light-infused world of his Italian paintings to the more controlled modulation of his trans-Alpine style, with its emphasis on elegance and detailed refinement—traits that were specifically geared to appeal to courtly taste. The way in which the more individualized, homespun Virgin of the Birmingham picture—surely based on a posed model—has been replaced by the more generalized figure in the Vienna variant, with her well-coiffed hair and elegant dress, speaks volumes about Orazio's ability to modulate his style to meet the circumstances. The sheer gold-banded scarf that made its debut in the Fogg *Madonna with the Sleeping Christ Child* (cat. 28) and would have been completely out of place in the Birmingham painting is perfectly at home around

the ivory shoulders and bust of the Vienna Virgin; it becomes a standard prop thereafter. Needless to say, the rustic donkey has been suppressed and does not appear even in those versions that retain the cutout in the wall.

When he left Genoa, Orazio seems to have taken with him tracings (or cartoons) of his most successful Genoese compositions with a view to replicating or revising them (on this practice, see pp. 20–27). When a tracing of the Sauli *Magdalene* (cat. 35) is superimposed over the Vienna version, the figures match up perfectly. A tracing of the Birmingham painting superimposed over its Vienna counterpart does not yield such tidy results, but there is an agreement in the size and placement of the two main figures and an approximate agreement in their silhouettes. There can be little doubt that a mechanical transfer was the first stage in revising the Birmingham composition. Interestingly, an X ray of the Vienna painting (fig. 18) reveals an emphasis on contours and outlines probably resulting from the use of a cartoon or pattern. We might imagine that such a cartoon was based on a tracing of the Birmingham picture and subsequently transferred to the canvas. At the same time, however, the X ray reveals no mechanical approach to the actual process of painting: this is a fully autograph work of high quality. Orazio first considered showing the Christ child gazing toward his mother rather than the viewer.

When he visited Orazio's studio in 1628, the German painter-biographer Joachim von Sandrart saw a *Penitent Magdalene* and a "Mary sitting on the ground, the Christ child drinking from her breast, the old Joseph however lying to the rear and resting his head on a sack."[10] The *Penitent Magdalene* was for Charles I, and there is a presumption that the *Rest on the Flight* was also a royal commission. Both compositions must have been variants of those owned by the duke of Buckingham. Around 1637–39, Abraham van der Doort recorded "An other peece. Of our Ladie Christ and Joseph Being coppied by oracio Jentillesco." Levey suggests that this is the painting that hung in the queen's second bedchamber at Whitehall.[11] One of these pictures may be the version in the Louvre, which is thought to have belonged to Charles I. It

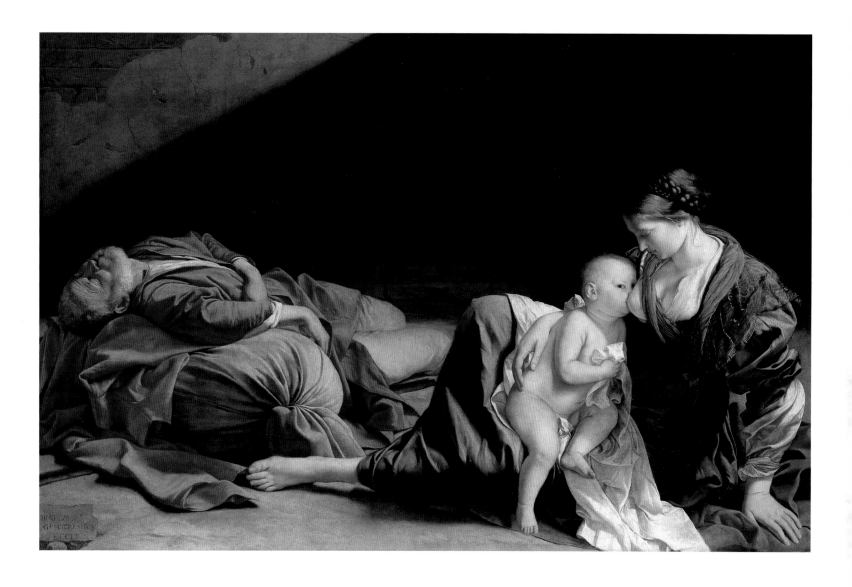

differs in a number of details from the Vienna painting. The sky is reintroduced in the upper left, the scarf around the Virgin's shoulder and the drapery on the ground are rearranged, plants and a rock are added, Joseph's right leg is differently foreshortened, and the color system is altered: the Virgin wears a rose-colored dress and Joseph is in blue. These changes seem to me to denote the special status of the picture and, not surprisingly, it too was replicated. Its presence in the collection of Louis XIV made it, rather than the *Public Felicity* (cat. 44), the touchstone of Orazio's art in France; it is the only picture by Orazio that Félibien refers to in his *Entretiens*.[12]

The existence of these multiple versions complicates any attempt to sort out the chronology and provenance of the various paintings. Some of the versions show only the Virgin and child. They may be fragments of the whole composition or they may reveal Orazio's cannibalizing his own invention for motives of profit. Certainly the use of a cartoon made it simple to rearrange and adjust the component parts of the image. Although two primary models—that at Vienna and that at Paris—for the composition can be individualized, it is probably foolhardy to attempt a chronological sequence for the surviving paintings; variation of details should be expected. In the version formerly in the J. Paul Getty Museum, Los Angeles, the figure of Joseph is moved closer to the Virgin (her knee cuts across his right hand), while in one of the fragments the scarf of the Virgin is newly rearranged. In some versions, the thumb of the Virgin's left hand is hidden by a fold of drapery. In others, the angle from which it is shown is altered. It seems only reasonable to suspect workshop participation in some of the surviving paintings, though they must be judged on a case-by-case basis. They testify to Orazio's willingness to repeat himself, and to the fact that in the face of stiff competition in England, Orazio continued to draw patronage.

1. This can be deduced from a 1642 inventory of the collection of the marquis of Leganés (Spanish governor of Milan from 1635 to 1641), in which the picture, albeit without attribution, appears together with a version of the *Lot and His Daughters* (for this picture, see cat. 37, under related pictures, Berlin). The *Rest on the Flight* was stated to have been a gift from "el cardenal de saboya." It can be traced until 1856, when it was inventoried in the Madrazo collection. It measured 176 × 253 cm. See Bissell 1981, 220 no. L-53.

2. As Bissell suggests, the picture may be the "great piece of Our Lady, Christ, and Joseph" listed, without attribution, in a 1635 inventory of the paintings in the duke of Buckingham's house. That work hung in the king's bedchamber. A *Magdalene* by "Gentilisco" hung in the drawing room. See Davies 1907, 380.

3. Vertue 1935–36, 68.

4. See Köpl 1889, cxxxiv.

5. The letter is printed in Sainsbury 1859b, 313, and appendix 3 in this publication.

6. Ibid., 314–15.

7. Ibid., 315.

8. Bissell (1981, 109, 183) believes it more likely that the *Magdalene and Joseph* was a confusion with *Joseph and Potiphar's Wife*. Both are two-figure compositions, but one would have expected that the *Joseph and Potiphar's Wife* now at Hampton Court would have been assigned the same value as the *Lot and His Daughters* (cat. 46), which is closer in size and was valued by Gerbier at £100 rather than £80.

9. Betcherman (1970, 254) cites the command issued by Buckingham to the English ambassador in Paris to hurry matters along. See, most recently, Wood 2000–2001, 111–17.

10. Sandrart (1675) 1925, 166.

11. Levey 1964, 13. Bissell (1981, 185) attempts to reconstruct a plausible history for this picture, which would have been sent to France with the exiled queen and returned to England following her death in 1669. Van der Doort's reference was published by Millar (1960, 176) and is reprinted in London–Bilbao–Madrid 1999, 99.

12. Félibien (1666–88) 1705, vol. 3, 237: "Vous pouvez voir un Tableaux de [Gentileschi] dans la Chambre du roi."

13. Bissell 1981, 186–87. Sale, Christie's, New York, May 21, 1992, lot 12; this version is in a private collection in Mantua. Fredericksen (1972, 45) traced the picture back to Richard Grenville, second duke of Buckingham. The scale of the figures is smaller than in the Vienna painting. There are a number of pentimenti and indications of an earlier, unrelated composition. The picture has suffered from abrasion and the execution is quite tight. The hand of the Virgin is fully exposed.

14. I know this picture only from a 1977 photograph on file at the Courtauld Institute of Art and the Frick Art Reference Library. The dimensions given are 56 × 72 inches, or 142.2 × 182.9 cm. It appears to be a rather mediocre copy.

15. This picture, measuring 107 × 101.5 cm., was formerly with A. Seligman & Co. It has suffered from harsh cleaning in the past and is much damaged along the lower border, especially in the white drapery trailing on the ground and in the Virgin's hand. It is clearly inferior to the Vienna painting.

16. See Bissell 1981, 184. The dimensions are 140 × 108 cm. This picture was sold at Parke-Bernet, New York, March 13, 1957, lot 15. The picture must be badly damaged and repainted along the bottom, for there are substantial differences between the two photographs.

17. For the provenance, see Bissell 1981, 184–85 no. 58, and Brejon de Lavergnée 1987, 317–18. The picture was acquired from Everard Jabach in 1671 for Louis XIV. There is no definitive proof that it belonged to Charles I, but the circumstantial evidence makes it likely. Brejon de Lavergnée notes that another version/replica of the *Rest on the Flight* belonged to the Parisian dealer Perruchot (Nicolas Estienne), who died in 1660. The Louvre picture was reported in the Bailly inventory of 1709 as having been "réduit à l'ovale" (it then measured 172 × 234 cm as opposed to the 205 × 222 cm given in the Le Brun inventory of 1683; its current dimensions are 157 × 225 cm). Although Bissell is disinclined to believe this, X rays have demonstrated that the canvas, enlarged by additions to the top, bottom, and right side, was mounted on an oval stretcher: nail holes are still visible in the corners. Subsequently, the additions on the bottom and right side were removed. The original canvas measures 132 × 225 cm; there is cusping along the sides and bottom and only the top has been trimmed by perhaps 5 to 7 cm. The strip of canvas 25 cm wide at the top is an addition. My thanks to Stéphane Loire and to Elizabeth Ravaud at the Louvre for this information. Although I find this a rather disappointing picture—the modeling is dull and the treatment of light uninspired—the X rays reveal a fine execution and the picture must be autograph.

18. The painting (fig. 25) measures 137.5 × 106 cm. As in the Louvre picture, the Virgin wears a rose-colored dress. It shows greater variation in arrangement of the drapery beneath the Christ child and in the scarf around the Virgin's shoulder than any of the other versions. As in the Louvre picture, the brick wall drops to reveal a view of the sky. I know it only from a transparency, but the quality appears to be high.

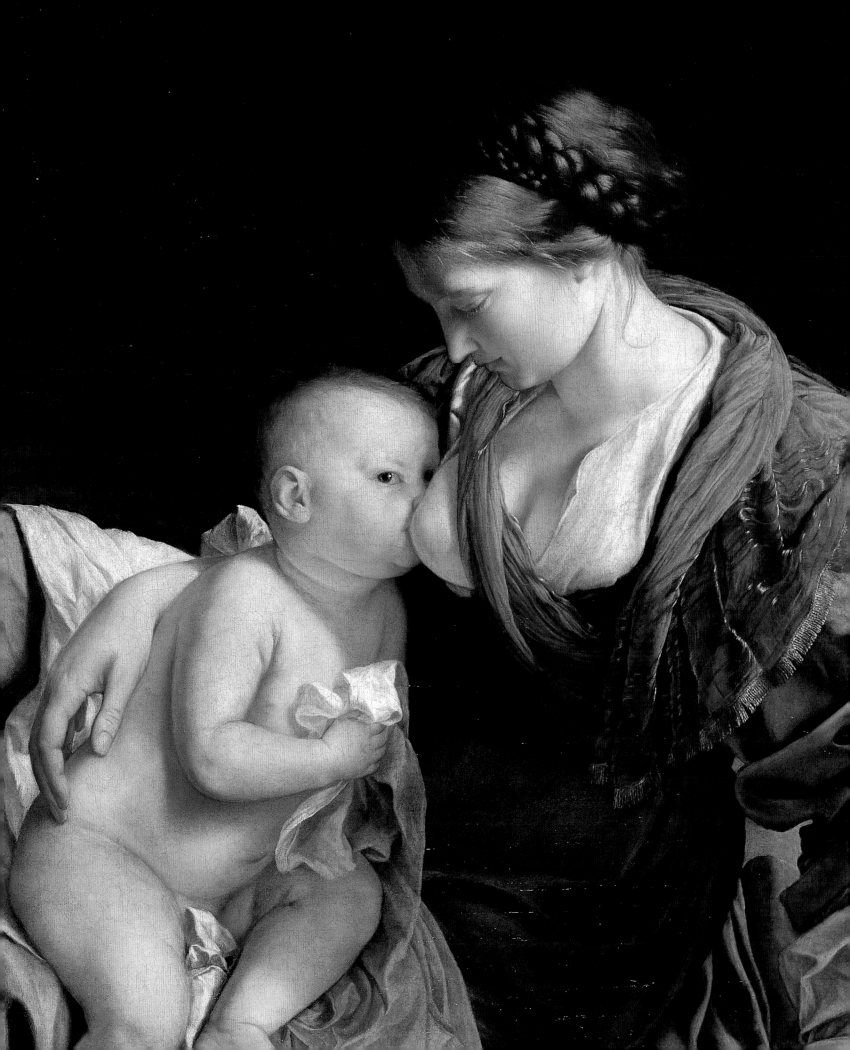

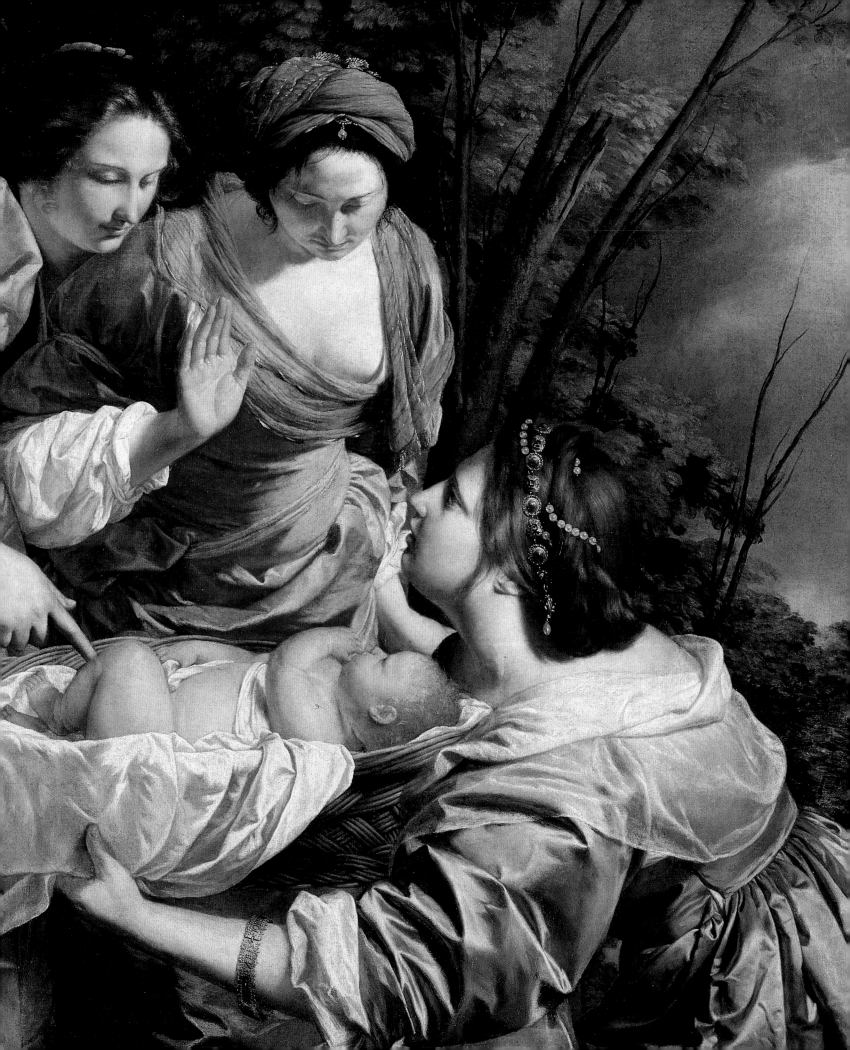

Orazio Gentileschi at the Court of Charles I

GABRIELE FINALDI AND JEREMY WOOD

When Orazio Gentileschi arrived in London from Paris, in the autumn of 1626, he was nearly sixty-three years old.[1] The prospect of honorable employment at the court of the newly crowned Charles I (r. 1625–49), who had a genuine understanding of and interest in painting, was highly attractive. Unlike Guercino (1591–1666), who had also been invited to settle at court, Orazio was clearly undeterred by the bad weather and felt no scruples about having to consort with heretics.[2] In the event, the king did not show much interest in his work and Orazio eventually became, to all intents and purposes, painter to Queen Henrietta Maria. The reputation of Gentileschi's work in England has suffered on account of the great fashion in the earlier art-historical literature for all things Caravaggesque, but by the mid-1620s, Orazio was no longer a Caravaggesque painter, and his work needs to be understood in terms of Stuart court patronage and the international taste for art in The Hague, Brussels, Paris, Madrid, and London.

Orazio's output during his twelve-year stay in England is surprisingly small, amounting to perhaps little more than two dozen pictures. From the inventory of Charles I's collection, drawn up in the late 1630s by the keeper, Abraham van der Doort, and from the lists of the king's goods made after Charles's execution in 1649, we know that there were eleven easel paintings by Gentileschi in the royal collection, in addition to the nine ceiling canvases in the Queen's House in Greenwich (fig. 85).[3] Despite the presence in London of several wealthy aristocrats who spent conspicuously on works of art, he painted for only one of them: George Villiers, first duke of Buckingham (1592–1628).

It was, in fact, Buckingham who had recruited Gentileschi to work in London. He had met the artist during his visit to Paris for the proxy marriage of Charles I and Princess Henrietta Maria, sister of Louis XIII, in 1625.[4] Buckingham was the favorite of Charles I,

his trusted minister and reportedly "the best-made man in the world,"[5] who created something of a sensation at the French court. Although it has been said that Orazio believed Henrietta Maria "would want a Catholic painter in England,"[6] it is unlikely he would have moved to London without the generous patronage of the duke, which he doubtless saw as a means of obtaining the favor of the king. A letter of April 24, 1629, from Orazio to the secretary of state, Sir Dudley Carleton, the viscount Dorchester (1573–1632), makes it clear that nearly all the money received by him up to that date had come from Buckingham, although some had been provided by the king and given to the duke for the artist.[7] If Gentileschi had been brought to London to serve either the king or the queen, it would have been unthinkable for him to have joined the duke's household and to have worked for him first, which is indeed what happened.

Orazio's presence in England is first reported in a diary entry of the maréchal de Bassompierre, the French ambassador extraordinary to Charles I. Bassompierre, in whose train Orazio may have traveled, went to London in September 1626 to negotiate the delicate matter of the composition of the Catholic household of Queen Henrietta Maria.[8] He recorded that on the evening of November 21, he hosted a dinner for Buckingham that was attended by Gentileschi, in addition to several prominent courtiers.[9] Two weeks later, on December 4, 1626, Amerigo Salvetti, the envoy in London of Ferdinand II of Tuscany, wrote to the secretary of the grand duke: "About two months ago there came here from France Signor Orazio Gentileschi, painter, who I am given to understand, besides exercising his art, is also engaged in another matter of great importance, as he is often with the Duke of Buckingham and also with the King."[10] Salvetti speculated that Gentileschi was involved in secret negotiations with the arch-duchess Isabella, governor of the Spanish Netherlands, aimed at

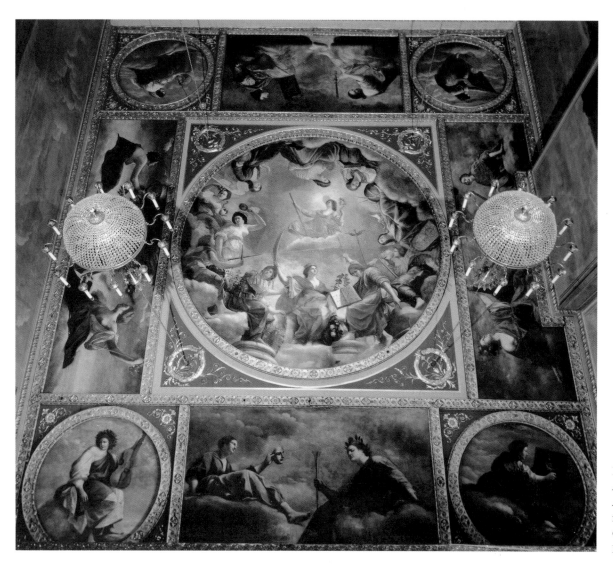

Figure 85. Orazio Gentileschi, *An Allegory of Peace and the Arts.* Oil on canvas. Ceiling from the Queen's House, Greenwich, now installed at Marlborough House, London

securing an accommodation between England and Spain, which were then at war.

It was not unusual in the first half of the seventeenth century for painters to act as diplomatic agents. The nature of their profession brought them in contact with powerful and influential figures at court and provided excellent cover for foreign journeys. The gift of works of art formed an increasingly important part of diplomatic relations during this period. Peter Paul Rubens (1577–1640), the best known of the artist-diplomats, played a significant role in preparing the ground for the exchange of ambassadors between England and Spain in 1630. That said, what we know of Gentileschi's character—he was difficult, arrogant, and vindictive—suggests that he might not have been the most suitable person to tread delicately through the minefield of international relations in the early years of Charles's reign. At present, no evidence that

confirms Salvetti's suspicions of Gentileschi's diplomatic activity has been forthcoming.

Gentileschi's arrival in London was preceded by the dispatch of two pictures to Buckingham, a *Penitent Magdalene* (fig. 26) and a *Rest on the Flight into Egypt* (cat. 45). These announced the artist's skills as a painter of large figure compositions, proficient in Catholic devotional subjects. The reasons why such an artist was recruited by Buckingham are far from clear, except that his newly rebuilt mansion in London, York House on the Strand, required decoration, and Orazio was soon commissioned to paint a large circular canvas for the ceiling of the "saloon" depicting "Apollo lying alone upon a cloud, and Nine Muses underneath it, each of them playing to him on a Several Instrument."[11] The destruction of this important work inevitably distorts our understanding of the painter's debut in London.

Gentileschi was accommodated with his three sons, Francesco, Giulio, and Marco, all in their twenties, at the duke's mansion as a member of the household. His living quarters were generously furnished to the tune of £500 (not £4000, as has usually been stated),[12] and the painter was assigned a "great upper room" as his studio.[13] All this confirms that the artist was seen, to begin with at least, as a great catch.

The first intimation that the Gentileschi family might be more trouble than they were worth occurred soon after their arrival in London. Charles I decided to employ two of Gentileschi's sons, Giulio and Francesco, as art agents, Orazio being too old to travel long distances. On August 20, 1627, the two young men set out for Genoa in order to purchase the collection of a certain Filippo San Micheli (otherwise unknown to us). They appear to have arrived in Milan, where they apparently expected to meet Nicholas Lanier (1588–1666), the English art dealer and Master of the King's Musick, who was then absorbed in the purchase of the collection of the duke of Mantua for Charles I and was, as might be expected, in Venice, where he was negotiating with the dealer Daniel Nys.[14]

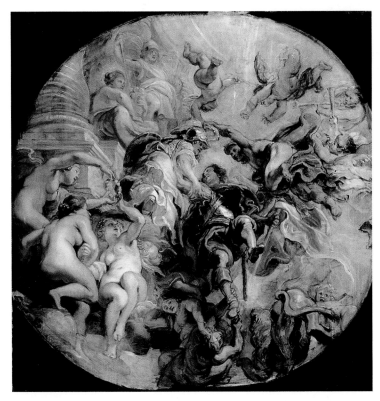

Figure 86. Peter Paul Rubens (1577–1640), *Minerva and Mercury Conduct the Duke of Buckingham to the Temple of Virtue.* Oil on wood. The National Gallery, London

There then followed a farce in which the brothers raced across northern Italy, consuming the money given to them for the purchase of works of art in the process, and Giulio took the opportunity to have an extended holiday with some relatives in Pisa. In an undated letter to the king, probably written in March 1629, Orazio composed one of the lengthy and detailed pieces of self-justification at which he excelled, attempting to cast Lanier's conduct in as bad a light as possible.[15]

At York House, Gentileschi found himself living in close proximity to Balthazar Gerbier (1592–1663/67), Buckingham's trusted factotum, political agent, keeper of his collection, and an artist in his own right.[16] It is worth reconstructing the brilliant but also precarious world that Orazio had now entered. Between 1624 and 1625, Gerbier had supervised major alterations to this mansion, which were said to have disconcerted the English architect Inigo Jones (1573–1652).[17] The Tudor buildings of York House were transformed by Gerbier into a battlemented block with an open arcade and projecting pedimented wings, and the interior incorporated a marble fireplace and gateway valued at £400, which had been given to Buckingham by Dudley Carleton (later Lord Dorchester).[18] Carleton, who had had much experience dealing with artists while ambassador in Venice (1610–16) and The Hague (1616–26), became secretary of state in 1628, and Gentileschi was to turn to him on several occasions during the next few years. York House contained an astonishing collection of pictures, which had been assembled by Gerbier from the collection of Charles de Cröy, duke of Aarschot, in 1619,[19] and during his travels in Italy of 1621.[20] Buckingham's last major acquisition was a collection of paintings and antique sculptures bought from Rubens, which was dispatched to York House on May 19 and September 18, 1627,[21] not long after Gentileschi's arrival. Orazio was therefore surrounded not only by great Italian pictures by Titian (ca. 1485/90–1576) and Paolo Veronese (1528–1588), among others, but by many recent works by Rubens, who had also been commissioned to paint two large canvases for York House when he met Buckingham in Paris in 1625. These were a large ceiling painting, the *Minerva and Mercury Conduct the Duke of Buckingham to the Temple of Virtue* (fig. 86), and the *Equestrian Portrait of the Duke of Buckingham*, both destroyed but known from preparatory oil sketches.[22] If Gentileschi had felt outclassed in Paris by the arrival of Rubens's great cycle of paintings for Marie de' Medici, the work of his Flemish rival followed him to London, and before long the artist

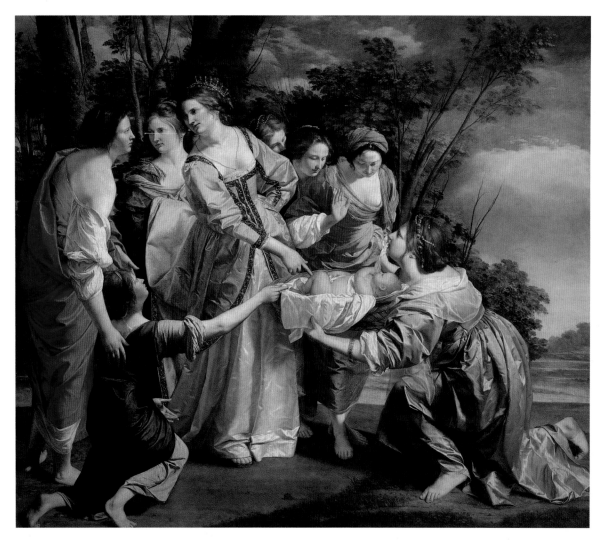

Figure 87. Orazio Gentileschi, *Finding of Moses*. Oil on canvas. Museo Nacional del Prado, Madrid

himself arrived, staying in England from May 1629 to February 1630, residing with Gentileschi's archenemy, Gerbier.[23] Professional rivalry—as well as art patronage—provides a key to understanding Gentileschi's checkered career in London.

Gentileschi had a short temper, and it did not take long for him to be at loggerheads with Gerbier. The assassination of Buckingham on August 23, 1628, only exacerbated their conflict. Both found themselves without a patron and had to turn to the king for favor. On January 29, 1629, Orazio wrote to Charles I complaining of persecution by Gerbier.[24] The "first distaste" between the two men apparently arose when Orazio refused to endorse the quality of some works of art in which he had been offered a cut by Gerbier. More seriously, he had then refused to approve Gerbier's choice of purchases for the collection at York House, challenging his competence as an art agent. Gerbier

responded by having two of Gentileschi's sons, Francesco and Marco, arrested for debt. On January 19, the third brother, Giulio, met Gerbier in the Strand and, "strooke him once or twise with his swoorde in the Scaberd over the heade," before making his escape. The enraged Gerbier then waylaid Marco, who "defended himself as well as hee coulde," but both brothers were subsequently imprisoned for their violent behavior, and Gentileschi may quickly have realized that he had miscalculated in his choice of enemy.

With Buckingham dead, the king took the widowed duchess and her family under his protection and shouldered responsibility for her husband's debts and his monument in Westminster Abbey.[25] But there were limits to his patience, and Gerbier, who was far more experienced at court than Gentileschi, was able to position himself more skillfully. Gerbier understood the need to demonstrate his devotion to the crown by becoming a British national (he was a Protestant, born in Middleburg, Zeeland) and by taking the oaths of Allegiance and Supremacy,[26] steps that would have been impossible for Gentileschi, who as a Catholic recognized the pope's spiritual sovereignty. In 1631, Gerbier was rewarded by being appointed diplomatic agent in the southern (Spanish) Netherlands, with generally disastrous results—even by the standards of Charles I's ambassadors—except in matters to do with art. A letter from Gerbier to the king, written in Brussels in 1633, indicates that Gerbier was still in touch with Gentileschi; he mentions grudgingly that the painter wanted the king to know that the archduchess Isabella and Queen Marie de' Medici, who was then in exile from France, had admired a work by Orazio, presumably in Paris.[27]

In 1628, perhaps before completing the York House ceiling, Gentileschi painted the large *Lot and His Daughters* for the king (cat. 46).[28] Charles had accepted some responsibility for Gentileschi even before Buckingham's death; in 1627, he is referred to in a document as "his Ma[jesty]'s Picture Maker" (although this may not have been an official title),[29] and a pension of £100 was awarded to him by Privy Seal Warrant on January 31, 1627/28.[30] No payments were made, however, and a new warrant authorizing the pension was drawn up on January 31, 1629/30.[31] Nevertheless, as was often the case, payment was slow to arrive, and Orazio was soon in need of money. A letter of October 13, 1630, published here for the first time, reveals him writing to Lord Secretary Dorchester at great speed and clearly under pressure. Orazio was desperate to get Dorchester's help in obtaining money owed him under the Privy Seal from the lord treasurer, Sir Richard Weston, earl of Portland. It was perhaps mere coincidence that after Buckingham's death, Gerbier had attached himself to Weston and was currently engaged on rebuilding his house, Putney Park at Roehampton, southwest of London.[32] The letter also reveals that Gentileschi wanted Dorchester to provide a passport for two men with whom he had recently been to Windsor, so that they could take goods to Paris without being hindered by customs officials. It is tempting (although purely speculative at this stage) to assume that they may have been intending to take Orazio's *Diana the Huntress* (cat. 47) to France to deliver it to Roger du Plessis de Liancourt, duke of La Roche-Guyon, who had very recently been in London as a French envoy, and who is recorded as having made a payment of 460 livres for the picture in 1630.[33] Sir John Finet

(1571–1641), master of ceremonies to Charles I, recorded that "no ambassador nor stranger of quality (excepting one French marquis)" was present at the Saint George's Day Feast at Windsor on September 5.[34] If he was referring to Liancourt—which seems likely, as there were few other visiting noblemen from France around this time—this perhaps would explain why Orazio was at Windsor with some Frenchmen.

It has been claimed that the paintings of Gentileschi's English period reflect Charles I's taste in art and that they are close in spirit to the work of the Caroline poets, to the extent that the artist has even been called a "Cavalier painter."[35] In fact, all these assumptions must be challenged.[36] Orazio was an isolated figure at the Caroline court. The king seems to have taken little interest in his work following Buckingham's death, and only one work by Gentileschi, at Whitehall, the damaged panel painting *Head of a Woman,* now in the Snider collection (cat. 50),[37] is described as "bought by your Majesty" in the detailed catalogue compiled by Abraham van der Doort.[38] As early as 1631, the widowed duchess of Buckingham had reported that "the King hath noe great use of him,"[39] and by 1633 Gentileschi had determined to leave London, writing to the grand duke of Tuscany in the hope of obtaining employment "for what little remains of my life."[40] Orazio's second version of the *Finding of Moses* (fig. 87), undoubtedly his late masterpiece, was taken to Madrid in 1633 by his son Francesco and presented to Philip IV with a view to obtaining his support for the artist's return to Florence.[41]

Gentileschi's isolated position among the group of foreign artists in London needs to be understood. There was only one other Italian artist in London, the one-eyed sculptor Francesco Fanelli, and few other Catholics, although after his arrival in 1632, Anthony van Dyck (1599–1641) was a very prominent exception. These were far outnumbered by Protestant artists from the Netherlands, and, in a moment of paranoia, Orazio wrote to Charles I that "all the Dutchmen had combyned togeather to weary mee, and make me leave the Kingdome."[42] The annuities provided by the crown for these artists give some idea of Gentileschi's ranking within this group.[43] His pension of £100 put him on the same level as Gerrit van Honthorst (1592–1656), a distinguished artist from Utrecht who had also been recruited by Buckingham but stayed in London only from April or May to December 1628,[44] and Frantz Clein (1582–1658), a German painter and printmaker much needed to design tapestries for the factory

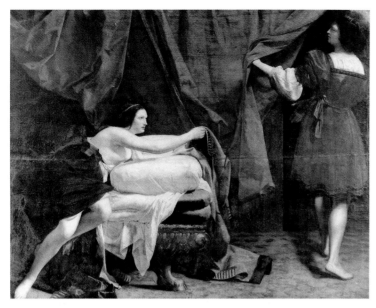

Figure 88. Orazio Gentileschi, *Joseph and Potiphar's Wife*. Oil on canvas. Royal Collection, Hampton Court

at Mortlake. Van Dyck was given a significantly higher pension of £200 in 1633,[45] clearly intended to set him above all the other artists at court, apart from the French medalist Nicolas Briot (ca. 1579–1646), who probably had been recruited in Paris at the same time as Gentileschi and who received a substantial £250 in December 1628.[46]

Left without Buckingham's protection, isolated from other artists working in London, and with the king having apparently lost what had probably been only a mild interest in his work, Gentileschi shifted the focus of his activities to the *petite cour* of Henrietta Maria at Somerset House. This was, in any case, perhaps a more congenial arena. He would have known Henrietta Maria in Paris, where he had served her mother, Marie de' Medici. The queen, like the painter, was part Florentine; she was Catholic, surrounded by Catholic courtiers and attended by Franciscan Capuchins, a religious order for which Orazio felt some affinity. Although no payments made directly to Gentileschi are recorded in the ledgers of the queen's treasurer, Sir Richard Wynn,[47] there are substantial payments made to the artist in the early 1630s, under the Privy Seal, for pictures that must have been intended for her.[48]

In 1629, Henrietta Maria was granted Greenwich Palace and Park as part of her jointure, and the following year she set about completing there the construction of the Palladian villa, known

as the Queen's House, that Inigo Jones had begun in the 1610s for Anne of Denmark. By 1635, the building was finished and the decoration of the interior could begin. Gentileschi was to play a central role in the adornment of Henrietta Maria's "House of Delight" close to the Thames.[49] As early as 1633–34, the building accounts for Greenwich show that Orazio's *Finding of Moses* (cat. 48) and *Joseph and Potiphar's Wife* (fig. 88) were given new frames, probably in preparation for hanging in the Queen's House.[50] Henrietta Maria was making a concerted effort in the mid-1630s to gather for herself works that had been painted by Orazio. A version of the *Rest on the Flight into Egypt* was recorded by Van der Doort as having been "given to the Queen" (presumably by the king), and by 1637 the *Lot and His Daughters* of 1628 had been been removed to Greenwich Palace from Whitehall, doubtless at the queen's request, and was soon to be found in the Queen's House.[51] It was surely Henrietta Maria herself who entrusted to Orazio the decoration of the ceiling of the Great Hall in the Queen's House (fig. 85). Thus by 1639, the year of his death, the building had become the repository of about half of Orazio's English oeuvre, including as it did the nine canvases making up the ceiling of the Great Hall and three large history pictures. It was Orazio's stately images of a serene and elegant humanity that the queen wanted to surround herself with in her Italianate retreat at Greenwich.

Refinement and artificiality are the currency of Gentileschi's late style, a style that cannot be classified as either Catholic or Protestant, but one that is aristocratic and international, practiced equally by Gerrit van Honthorst at The Hague and by Simon Vouet (1590–1649) in Paris.[52] Orazio's English paintings were designed to suit the aesthetic taste of a sophisticated and cosmopolitan court. They are luminous and high-key works, painted in saturated colors and with a smooth finish. They are peopled by figures with porcelain skin, enveloped in rich draperies and fabrics. The affectedly laconic gestures and the studied dishevelment of the Egyptian princess's ladies-in-waiting in the two versions of the *Finding of Moses* (cat. 48 and fig. 87) mirror ideals of courtly beauty and aristocratic deportment. Orazio had abandoned Caravaggesque lighting over the course of the 1620s in favor of a more even illumination; although his works remained highly staged, they were less obviously dramatic. He responded knowingly to the history pictures of the sixteenth-century Venetian painters so coveted by Charles I and the clique of noble collectors

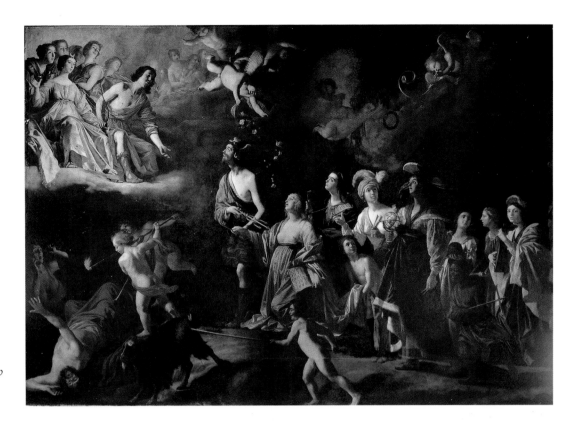

Figure 89. Gerrit van Honthorst (1592–1656), *Mercury Presenting the Liberal Arts to Apollo and Diana*. Oil on canvas. Royal Collection, Hampton Court

in London, particularly in the *Finding of Moses* pictures, which contain echoes of several paintings by Veronese then in the king's collection. It may be appropriate to criticize Gentileschi's late works because of their lack of psychological depth, but to do so is to misinterpret his aesthetic aims.

The iconography of the Queen's House ceiling, executed between 1635 and late 1638 (and now installed in a much damaged and much repainted state at Marlborough House, in central London), was almost certainly conceived by Orazio in collaboration with Inigo Jones.[53] Around the figure of Peace, on the large central canvas, are ranged the Liberal Arts, Victory, and Fortune; and in the other compartments on the ceiling, the nine Muses and personifications of Painting, Sculpture, Architecture, and Music.[54] The theme of the paintings, that under the reign of Peace the arts flourish, constitutes a leitmotif of Caroline imagery. It is articulated in *Albion's Triumph,* Aurelian Townshend's masque of 1632 in which the personification of Peace descended onto the stage in a cloud machine designed by Jones, and also in James Shirley's *Triumph of Peace,* which was performed before the king and queen in February 1634. Van Honthorst's enormous canvas *Mercury Presenting the Liberal Arts to Apollo and Diana* (fig. 89), painted some years earlier, shows

a similar subject: Mercury (with the likeness of Buckingham) leads a procession of the Liberal Arts to pay homage to Apollo and Diana, who bear the likenesses of Charles and Henrietta Maria.[55]

The general impression of the ceiling in its pristine state must have been richly decorative, with its use of intense local color and soft lighting effects. There remain individual passages of great beauty in the draperies and in the still-life details, for example in the panel with the muses Urania, Calliope, and Melpomene.[56] However, even allowing for the sorry state of the canvases, it would be difficult to argue that the ceiling represents the triumphant culmination of Gentileschi's career. The differences between this ceiling and the recently installed canvases by Rubens in the Banqueting House at Whitehall Palace showing allegories of the rule of James I could hardly have been more marked (fig. 90). The dynamism of Rubens's figures contrasts sharply with the static and imperious women who garland the Queen's House ceiling, while the brilliance of Rubens's handling of the allegorical subjects makes Gentileschi's treatment seem relatively unsophisticated. It could be argued that the two ceilings reflect the essentially divergent tastes of the king and queen, the one preferring a bold, forceful, and energetic form of painting, the

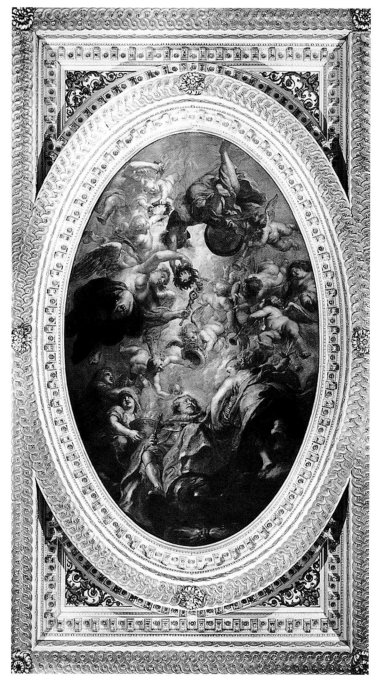

Figure 90. Peter Paul Rubens (1577–1640), *Apotheosis of James I*. Oil on canvas. Central detail of the Banqueting House ceiling at Whitehall, London

was almost certainly finished and installed by October 1638,[58] and she is first recorded in London toward the end of 1639 (although works by her were in Charles I's collection some years earlier, perhaps brought from Italy by Orazio or by one of her brothers), it is extremely unlikely that she had any role at all. Orazio's collaborator in the execution of the ceiling canvases (and he must have received some help) is much more likely to have been his son Francesco, who was also a painter.[59]

In January 1639, Orazio was already suffering from the illness from which he would die.[60] On February 11, 1639, the same Amerigo Salvetti who had announced the artist's arrival in England a dozen years earlier wrote to the Medici in Florence: "Four days ago the famous painter Gentileschi died, much lamented by His Majesty and by every other admirer of his virtue."[61] Because the artist was Tuscan, he had every reason to emphasize how much the king mourned his passing. The queen most certainly did, and so too perhaps did Van Dyck, who had made an impressive portrait drawing of Orazio for inclusion in his Iconographia, the series of engravings of famous artists (fig. 1).

The Stuart court has been described as favoring art that was escapist and "brittle," encouraging an illusory "sense of security and isolation."[62] This point of view has led to Orazio's work in England being too lightly dismissed in the earlier literature. Like any court painter, he had to please his patrons, and political realism in art was the last thing required by the royal families of Europe. Orazio's work for Charles I was international not only in terms of its pictorial style but also in its courtly iconography. The world that Gentileschi had been a part of was to dissolve very rapidly within a few years of his own death. Following the king's execution in 1649, his paintings were acquired by royal creditors, and several left England almost immediately. There was really no opportunity for an artistic legacy to be established in Britain, although Robert Streeter's painted ceiling in the Sheldonian Theatre in Oxford, showing the *Triumph of Religion, the Arts, and Sciences* and executed in 1668–69,[63] suggests the influence of the Queen's House ceiling. Gentileschi was granted the honor of burial in the Queen's Chapel at Somerset House. The altarpiece there was a large *Crucifixion* by Rubens.[64] This was the small, final irony of Gentileschi's London career.

other a refined, reticent, and archaizing style. Charles's aesthetic preference explains why he could never muster great enthusiasm for Orazio's art.

It is usually stated that the painter's daughter, Artemisia, played a part in the execution of the ceiling.[57] But since the ceiling

1. The most extensive treatments of Gentileschi's English career are Bissell 1981, Finaldi 1999, and Wood 2000–2001, 103–28. See also Hess (1952) 1967; Levey 1991; Weston-Lewis 1997; and Weston-Lewis in London–Bilbao–Madrid 1999.

2. For Guercino's invitation to London, see Malvasia 1678, 366. According to the Italian sources, Charles tried to lure several Italian painters to London, including Guido Reni, Albani, and Angelo Caroselli.

3. See London–Bilbao–Madrid 1999, app. 1, 99–100.

4. For the visit, see Lockyer 1981, 233–42.

5. According to a member of Anne of Austria's household; ibid., 236.

6. Bissell 1981, 51.

7. Sainsbury 1859b, 313–14. The original Italian text is London, Public Records Office (hereafter PRO), State Papers (SP) 16/141/35.

8. For the instructions Bassompierre received from Cardinal Richelieu, see Avenel 1856, 241–55.

9. Bassompierre 1837, quoted in Finaldi 1999, 34 n. 4.

10. Skrine 1887, 97; Crinò 1967, 533.

11. Croft-Murray 1962, 202; Bissell 1981, 214–15, no. L-2; Finaldi 1999, 35 n. 29.

12. A document hostile to Orazio, datable to early 1629, "The Sommes of monnys Gentilesco hath recaeved" (London, PRO, SP 16/141, fols. 120v and 121r), written by Balthazar Gerbier and intended to show that the artist had produced very little for a huge cash outlay, has been interpreted to suggest that the furnishing of his house cost £4000. See Sainsbury 1859b, 311; Sainsbury 1859a, 121; Bissell 1981, 51; and Finaldi 1999, 17. This would have been an astonishing sum, sufficient at this date to build a moderate-sized country house. The figure of £4000 is in fact a subtotal and the actual cost was £500. This is discussed in more detail in Wood 2000–2001, 118.

13. Croft-Murray 1947, 90 n. 11; McEvansoneya 1987, 33.

14. For Lanier in Italy, see Wilson 1994, 83–164.

15. Sainsbury 1859b, 311–13. The original Italian of the letter is transcribed in appendix 2 in this volume.

16. See Betcherman 1970, 250–59.

17. Goodman 1839, vol. 2, 360.

18. See Lockyer 1981, 215, and McEvansoneya 1987, 31.

19. McEvansoneya 1987, 29.

20. Philip 1957, 155–56.

21. Muller 1989, 78.

22. These are in the National Gallery, London, and the Kimbell Art Museum, Fort Worth, respectively; see Held 1980, 390–95, nos. 291, 292.

23. Gerbier called himself "innkeeper" to Rubens; Sainsbury 1859a, 144. For the financial arrangements, see London, PRO, Privy Seal Books (Auditors), E 403/2565; Exchequer of Receipt, Warrants for Issues, E 403/153, part 3, numbered 82.

24. London, PRO, SP 16/133, fols. 44r–45r, published by Sainsbury 1859a, 121–22. The quotations in this paragraph are retranscribed from the original document.

25. See Lockyer 1981, 460–61.

26. For the reception given to the bill of naturalization, see *Calendar of State Papers, Domestic, 1628–1629*, 1859, 183.

27. The relevant part of the letter is transcribed in appendix 4 in this publication. It is not clear which work he might be referring to. We are grateful to David Howarth for this reference.

28. Described by Gerbier in the "Sommes of monnys" document referred to in note 12 above, as "that wich the king hath" (fol. 121r); see Sainsbury 1859b, 315. For Van der Doort's description of this work when removed to Greenwich, see Millar 1958–60, 194.

29. The document (which is extremely difficult to read) is entitled "Inquisition as to the possessions of Balthazar Gerbier, an alien, at Buckingham House" (London, PRO, E178/5973), and mentions Gentileschi only in passing. It was first referred to in Croft-Murray 1947, 90 n. 11.

30. Published with the correct date by Crinò and Nicolson 1961, 145. See Wood 2000–2001, 125, app 2, doc. 1.

31. Bissell (1981, 105) cites the earlier document but gives it the later date, as found in Sainsbury 1859b, 315, without realizing that the warrant was reissued. See Wood 2000–2001, 116.

32. See Alexander 1975, 169.

33. See Lépine 1984; see also Schnapper 1994, 161 (who says, however, that the picture was painted in France), and Finaldi 1999, 36 n. 57.

34. Finet 1987, 90.

35. Bissell 1981, 50–62.

36. As regards Cavalier poetry, there is no evidence that Gentileschi took any notice of it, and, given his reluctance to master the English language, it is doubtful if he could have understood it.

37. See Bissell 1981, 193–94 no. 68.

38. Literally "boeht bij ju M," in Van der Doort's words; Millar 1958–60, 38.

39. Letter of July 28, 1631, London, PRO, SP 16/197/45, published in Crinò and Nicolson 1961, 145.

40. Crinò 1954, 203–4.

41. Bonfait in Rome 1994–95, 208, and Weston-Lewis in London–Bilbao–Madrid 1999, 49.

42. Sainsbury 1859a, 121.

43. This issue is discussed at greater length in Wood 2000–2001, 116–18.

44. See Millar 1954, 36.

45. Carpenter 1844, 65.

46. Backdated to 1626; see Symonds 1913, 363–65. Our thanks to Mark Jones for this reference.

47. The full set of accounts for the 1630s is preserved in the Wynnstay manuscripts, National Library of Wales, Aberystwyth, 174–86.

48. For a summary of these payments, see Bissell 1981, 105–6.

49. For the history of the Queen's House, see Chettle 1937 and Bold 2000. The description of the building as a "House of Delight" dates from 1659; Chettle 1937, 35.

50. Chettle 1937, 104.

51. Millar 1958–60, 176, 194.

52. Interestingly, both these painters, like Gentileschi himself, had had an intensely Caravaggesque phase earlier in their careers.

53. For the dating of the ceiling, based on the building accounts for Greenwich, see Finaldi 1999, 30–32.

54. For a discussion of the identity of the personifications on the ceiling, see Bissell 1981, 195–98 no. 70, and Finaldi 1999, 27–30.

55. White 1982, 53–56 no. 74.

56. Finaldi 1999, fig. 18.

57. Hess (1952) 1967, 254; Bissell 1981, 61, 91 n. 47; Garrard 1989, 112–21. Roberto Contini sounded an appropriate note of caution on the attribution of some of the figures to Artemisia in Florence 1991, 75. More recently Artemisia's presumed involvement has been reiterated, although with no new evidence advanced, in Bissell 1999, 87, 271–72.

58. Finaldi 1999, 32.

59. For Francesco's activities, see Bissell 1981, app. 4, 113–17, and Finaldi 1999, 35 n. 35, with further references.

60. For Gentileschi's will, published in Finaldi 1999, 33, see appendix 4 in this publication.

61. Translated from Crinò 1960, 258.

62. Whinney and Millar 1957, 6.

63. Croft-Murray 1962, 44–45, 227, figs. 87, 88.

64. Loomie 1996, 680–82.

46.

Lot and His Daughters

Oil on canvas, 89 × 111 in.
(226 × 282 cm)

Signed (indistinctly, on rock at
right of standing daughter):
HORA.VS / GIENTIL.VS

Museo de Bellas Artes, Bilbao
(69/101)

1628

PROVENANCE: Charles I,
Whitehall Palace, London;
Greenwich Palace; Queen's
House, Greenwich (1628–49;
Van der Doort inv. 1637–39; inv.
1649–51, no. 2, as by Gentileschi;
Commonwealth sale, London,
October 23, 1651); William
Latham and his fourth divi-
dend, London (1649–54); Don
Alonso de Cárdenas, Spanish
ambassador in London, for
Don Luis de Haro y Gusmán,
marqués de Heliche, first min-
ister to Philip IV, Madrid (1654–
61; list of purchases of May 25,
1654, as by Gentileschi);[9] his
son, Don Gaspar de Haro y
Gusmán, marqués de Eliche
and del Carpio (1661–87; 1689
post-mortem inv., no. 5, as by
Gentileschi);[10] his daughter,
Doña Catalina de Haro y
Gusmán, Madrid (from 1687);
Carpio-Alba Collection,
Madrid; duke of Alba, Madrid
(until after 1911; 1911 cat.); Don
Luis de Ardanaz (until 1924);
Museo de Bellas Artes, Bilboa.

This ambitious painting is perhaps the pivotal
royal commission to Orazio. It was seen in his
studio by the German painter-biographer Joachim
von Sandrart, who accompanied the Dutch painter
Gerrit van Honthorst to London in 1628, and the following year it was listed by Balthazar Gerbier in his
account of disbursements made to Gentileschi by the
king and the duke of Buckingham, whom Gerbier
had served as art adviser.[1] Sandrart describes it as "Lot
sleeping on the lap of his daughter, the other daughter looking back on her father's activity, a wondrous
work, incapable of improvement."[2] Sandrart and
Gerbier also mention a *Magdalene* and a *Rest on the
Flight into Egypt*, but while these were unquestionably
variants of compositions Orazio had created in Italy,
the *Lot* bears no relation to the painting he had done
in Genoa six or seven years earlier for Giovan Antonio
Sauli (see cat. 37). Initially hung at Whitehall, it
was moved to the queen's withdrawing chamber in
Greenwich Palace, and thence to the Queen's House,
Greenwich, where it was probably installed in the
Great Hall opposite the *Finding of Moses* (cat. 48).[3]
Arguably, it was this picture that led to Orazio's other
major commissions from the king and queen.

In his earlier treatment of the theme for Sauli,
Orazio had created a compact, tightly interlocked
group of figures that fills the foreground and is set
against the strong rectilinear forms of a cliff, thus
making a virtue of his weak command of spatial
effects. The landscape is reduced to a distant vista at
the right. Here, by contrast, the figures are far more
loosely grouped in an ample picture field, their actions
related more by gesture and glance than by arrangement within the composition. The episode takes place
in a cave, which is opened to the sky at the left and to
a distant landscape on the right. Details such as the
placement of Lot's hand on the leg of his daughter or
the position of the open wine flask, which in the Sauli
painting were charged with eroticism, here become
incidental. In both paintings, Lot is shown in a state

of drink- and sex-induced exhaustion while the two
daughters actively discuss their fate. However, whereas
in one a mood of anxious excitement prevails, in the
other there is a coquettish chattiness as one daughter
insistently defends their incestuous act by indicating
the burning city in the background and the minuscule
figure of Lot's wife turned to a pillar of salt. In short,
the story has acquired the trappings of a courtly
moral drama: two women led to perform a sinful act
in order to perpetuate the human race.[4]

No less indicative of the very different direction
Orazio's art took in England is the emphasis on the
richly colored silk fabrics, especially notable in the
raspberry and blue of Lot's coat, and on such still-life
details as the exquisitely painted vine with grapes.
Quite apart from Orazio's difficulty in creating a convincing space for the figures, there is about this work
a shift in focus, as though it had been painted at close

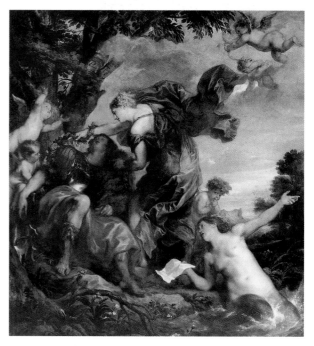

Figure 91. Anthony van Dyck (1599–1641), *Rinaldo and Armida*.
Oil on canvas. The Baltimore Museum of Art, Jacob Epstein
Collection

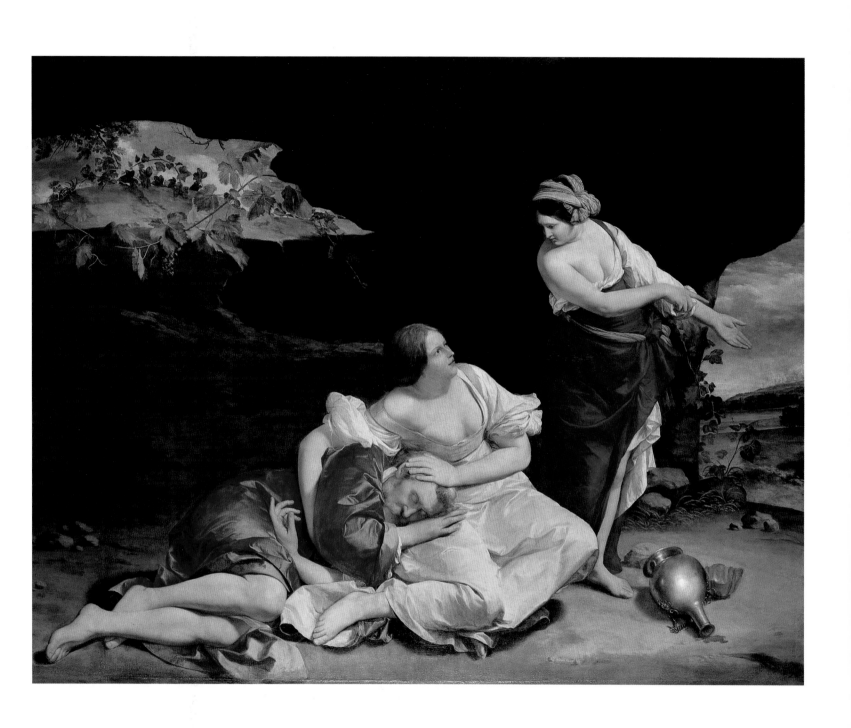

REFERENCES: Sandrart (1675) 1925, 166; Vertue (notebook, 1716) 1931–32, 131; Sainsbury 1859b, 315; Barcia 1911, 250; Chettle 1937, 36; Hess 1952, 162; Millar 1958–60, 194, 235; Pérez Sánchez 1965, 502–3; Moir 1967, vol. 1, 75 n. 24, vol. 2, 76 no. B.4a; Bissell 1969, 26–27, 31–32; Millar 1970–72, 137 no. 2; Seville 1973, no. 23; Nicolson 1974, 608; Bissell 1981, 51–53, 188 no. 61; Burke 1984, vol. 2, 153, 167; Nicolson 1985, 20–25; Nicolson 1990, 113; Bilbao 1991; Burke and Cherry 1997, vol. 1, 837, no. 116; Weston-Lewis 1997, 30–31; Finaldi, Weston-Lewis, and Sánchez-Lassa de los Santos in London–Bilbao–Madrid 1999, 27, 45–47, 66, 79–97; Wood 2000–2001, 120, 122.

range: compositional strength has been sacrificed to beauty of detail. Because of the emphasis on surface refinement, the loss of glazes (for example, in the lemon yellow dress of the seated daughter) is particularly unfortunate. Originally, the figures must have registered like brilliantly glazed enamels against a dark background. Today, the most satisfying area is in the upper left, where the grapes, ivy leaves, and bare branch viewed against the blue sky reveal the subtle effects Orazio strove to achieve throughout the picture.[5]

What were the driving forces behind this distinctive shift in Orazio's work? Elsewhere (cat. 49), I have commented on the use of demonstrative gesture, something that was to characterize all of Orazio's royal commissions. It is, however, important to recognize that the pictures he painted in England are by no means uniform in style. The fastidious concern for detail at the expense of compositional unity in the *Lot* gives way to a grandeur of statement in the *Finding of Moses* (cat. 48), where stunning surface effects combine with a splendid, friezelike composition. If, in the latter, the impetus seems to be Venetian art—particularly Veronese—perhaps here we ought to see Orazio's responding to the challenge posed by the presence in London of Van Honthorst (whose earlier, Caravaggesque work Orazio had known in Rome). As early as 1620, the Dutch artist had attracted the attention of Sir Dudley Carleton, who sent to the earl of Arundel a mythological painting of Aeneas fleeing Troy (untraced) that earned praise from that most perspicacious of English collectors for its masterly use of pose and its Caravaggesque coloring, "wch is nowe soe much esteemed in Rome."[6] It is difficult to imagine more fertile ground for Orazio to build on, and his movement toward a blonde tonality and a reduction of light-dark contrasts becomes all the more significant. Van Honthorst himself had moved in a similar direction, particularly in his mythological paintings and his portraits. The duke of Buckingham acquired from Van Honthorst a genre picture and a mythology (of Venus and two satyrs, no longer traceable), and then

twice sat for the artist (fig. 89). As already noted, in 1628—when Orazio was at work on the *Lot*—the Dutchman arrived in London (sometime after April 5).[7] To see the *Lot* as Orazio's attempt to assert his place at the court of Charles I seems to me the most sympathetic way of appreciating its peculiar character and avoiding the overly simplistic verdict of a decline in his creative abilities—something that his two splendid paintings of the *Finding of Moses* disprove.

X radiographs of the picture show no major changes to the composition. The technique is direct, and the brushwork is nowhere labored. However, the contours are remarkably sharp and to the naked eye there is what appears to be a line around the yellow dress and protruding right foot of the seated daughter that suggests the careful planning that went into the work. Whether or not Orazio developed a full-scale cartoon for the composition cannot be said, but at the very least he must have made a number of preliminary drawings and carefully worked it out on the canvas. There is a published report of its restoration in 1991.[8]

1. For Gerbier's list, see Sainsbury 1859b, 315, and Bissell 1981, 108.
2. Sandrart (1675) 1925, 166: "nict geringer war ein in seiner Tochter Schoss schlaffender Loth, dessen andere Tochter auf ihres Vatters Action umsehend, verwunderlich und unfähig einiger Bässerung ausgebildet."
3. See Van der Doort's inventory in Millar 1960, 194. See Weston-Lewis in London–Bilbao–Madrid 1999, 45–49, for a discussion of the arrangement of pictures at the Queen's House.
4. See Kind 1967 for a survey of the exegetical literature on the theme. Weston-Lewis (in London–Bilbao–Madrid 1999, 51 n. 39) tentatively suggests that the picture could have been read by the court in terms of dynastic succession.
5. There are scattered losses, perhaps most importantly in the face and bosom of the seated daughter. Her head and Lot's eyes have lost definition. Throughout the picture there is a loss of sharpness.
6. Sainsbury 1859b, 291.
7. On Van Honthorst and the Caroline court, see the fine summary of White 1982, xxiii–xxvii.
8. See Bilbao 1991 and Sánchez-Lassa de los Santos in London–Bilbao–Madrid 1999.
9. See Burke 1984, vol. 2, 153, 167, and Burke and Cherry 1997, vol. 1, 153–70, for the Carpio family in general.
10. Burke and Cherry 1997, vol. 1, 837 no. 116.

47.

Diana the Huntress

Oil on canvas, 84⅝ × 53⅛ in. (215 × 135 cm)

Musée des Beaux-Arts, Nantes (inv. 6735)

1630

PROVENANCE: Roger du Plessis de Liancourt, duke of La Roche-Guyon, Paris (1630–74; inv. 1674, as by Gentileschi); François, duke of La Rochefoucault, Paris (until 1728; inv. 1728, as by Gentileschi); Gentil de Chavagnac collection (until 1854; sold, Paris, June 20, 1854, no. 17); Count Toinet de La Turmelière, château de la Turmelière (until 1945); given by him to the city of Ancenis (1945–65); Musée des Beaux-Arts, Nantes.

RELATED PICTURES: Formerly Kurt Stern, New York (copy of upper portion of figure, ascribed by Sterling to Monier);[7] Musée de la Chasse, Paris (copy; fig. 92).[8]

REFERENCES: Rambaud 1964, 562; Sterling 1964, 217–20; Previtali 1973, 359; Nicolson 1979, 51; Bissell 1981, 53–58, 76, 98 n. 99, 194 no. 69; Brejon de Lavergnée in Nantes 1983, 22–23 no. A; Nicolson 1985, 22, 25; Brejon de Lavergnée in Paris–Milan 1988–89, 226–28 no. 77; Brejon de Lavergnée and Volle 1988, 161; Nicolson 1990, 112; Béguin in Paris 1991, 35; Sykes 1991, 335; Sarrazin 1994, 196–97 no. 145; Merot in Dijon–Le Mans 1998–99, 32, 58; Finaldi in London–Bilbao–Madrid 1999, 24, 36 n. 57.

Surely one of the most poetic pictures of Gentileschi's post-Italian years, *Diana the Huntress* was purchased in 1630 by Roger du Plessis de Liancourt, duc de La Roche-Guyon, for 460 livres.[1] Liancourt was in London at the time as French ambassador extraordinary to mark the birth of Prince Charles and cemented his relations with the English court by a series of gifts, exchanges, and sales. The most important gift was a painting of John the Baptist by Leonardo da Vinci (Louvre, Paris), for which the duke received in return a *Madonna* by Titian that had belonged to John Donne.[2] He also gave the king some novel pictures "in the manner as they doe make turkey carpetts worke" (that is, woven images with a nap), and he sold him several works.[3] The acquisition of the *Diana* should be seen as part of this ambassadorial exchange (it is unclear whether it was purchased from the artist or through the crown).

The painting was installed in Liancourt's splendid Parisian house on the rue de Seine, not far from the Palais de Luxembourg, where it is described in a 1674 postmortem inventory as, "In the antechamber near to the green room, a large painting above the fireplace showing a Diana by Gentileschi."[4] Diana is depicted as the goddess of the hunt, a subject frequently associated with the French monarchy, especially under Henry II (r. 1547–59). Indeed, it is difficult to believe that Orazio did not consciously have in mind the sixteenth-century decorations of Rosso Fiorentino, Primaticcio, and Nicolò dell'Abate at the château de Fontainebleau when he painted this wonderfully elegant figure. Charles I's French queen, Henrietta Maria, was also portrayed, at Hampton Court, as the virgin goddess in Gerrit van Honthorst's immense and elaborate allegory, which dates to 1628 (fig. 89), and Sykes has shown how important this imagery was to her. It is possible that Orazio's painting was initially conceived for the queen and diverted to Liancourt.[5]

The contrapposto pose sets off the goddess's face, bare shoulder, and legs with her windswept, ash-blonde hair and lime-colored drapery and is further enhanced by the turned head of the collared dog. A delicate crescent moon—Diana's emblem—can be seen directly above her head, an echo to the hunting horn. The planarity of the design, anchored by the curves of the great bow, makes this an image more in keeping with French than with English taste, a worthy successor to the great works of the French Renaissance sculptor Jean Goujon.

Superficially, the style of the picture seems consonant with the new court manner then holding sway in Paris under Simon Vouet, who had transformed himself from the Caravaggesque artist Orazio had known in Rome to an advocate of decorative classicism.[6] Yet by comparison, Gentileschi's figure, for all the Mannerist elegance of the pose, remains rooted in reality, and in fact we know that in his English period he continued to employ models—both male and female—for his paintings. Sterling and Merot have emphasized the importance a work like this may have had for the Le Nain, Laurent de La Hyre, and Philippe de Champaigne and the classical style of painting—"l'atticisme parisien"—that dominated French art between about 1640 and 1660.

Understandably, when, in 1964, Sterling brought the picture to public attention, he assumed it was painted during the two years Orazio worked for Marie de' Medici. His opinion has been followed by other French scholars, although the 1630 payment from Liancourt is strong evidence that the picture was painted in London. As Bissell notes, the pose of the figure is related to that of one of the Muses in a painting of Apollo and the nine Muses that was far enough advanced in 1630 to attract the attention of Rubens (fig. 93). It is even closer to the figure of Joseph in Orazio's large canvas *Joseph and Potiphar's Wife*, destined for the Queen's House at Greenwich (fig. 88).

Compositionally, then, the picture is typical of Orazio's English work. Yet the style has less to do with the finicky, overly detailed *Lot and His Daughters*

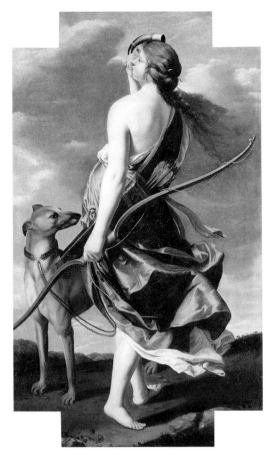

Figure 92. Copy after Orazio Gentileschi, *Diana the Huntress*. Oil on canvas. Musée de la Chasse et de la Nature, Paris

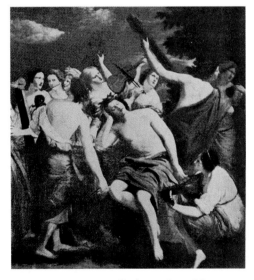

Figure 93. Orazio Gentileschi, *Apollo and the Muses*. Oil on canvas. Formerly Lily Lawlor Collection, New York

of 1628 (cat. 46) or with the enamel-like, pearly beauty of the two versions of the *Finding of Moses* (cat. 48 and fig. 87) than it does with the noble forms of *Public Felicity* (cat. 44) of 1624–26, painted for Marie de' Medici. In those works destined for Henrietta Maria, one senses Orazio's vying with Van Honthorst, who, at Hampton Court, was granted an annual pension of £100 before leaving. With the *Diana*, Orazio seems to be consciously modulating his style to suit the tastes of his French patron. And he was right to do so, since the picture was evidently much admired in France; at least two copies exist (fig. 92).

1. *"Autre despence extraordinaire . . . premièrement une diane de Gentilesques 460 livres,"* see Finaldi in London–Bilbao–Madrid 1999, 36 n. 47. The information comes from an unpublished thesis by Laurence Lépine.

2. See Haskell in MacGregor 1989, 216. The Leonardo is listed in Van der Doort's catalogue of the collection of Charles I; see Millar 1958–60, 89 item 71.

3. Millar 1958–60, 91 item 79, 125 item 42, 156 item 28, 157 item 4.

4. See Paris–Milan 1988–89, 226–28. John Evelyn visited the house in 1644 and has left an admiring description; see Evelyn 1873, 240–42. The 1728 inventory of the collection is published in Rambaud 1964, 561–63.

5. See White 1982, 53–56. It is not certain whether the picture was commissioned by Charles I or the duke of Buckingham. By the seventeenth century, this sort of allegorical portraiture was ubiquitous in the various courts. Elizabeth, queen of Bohemia, the sister of Charles I, had her children portrayed in similar guise by Van Honthorst (the picture is also at Hampton Court).

6. Orazio's awareness of Vouet's art remains an elusive issue. In his *Entretiens* Félibien notes that Vouet sent a number of paintings to Charles I, one of which may have been the *Diana* at Hampton Court, and he painted a ceiling for a royal residence (destroyed). The *Diana* is dated 1637; the ceiling seems also to date to the later 1630s.

7. Attributed by Sterling (1964, 218) to Monier. See also Bissell 1981, 194.

8. The picture (fig. 92) was called to my attention by Stéphane Loire. The corners are cut out, in the manner of Orazio's *Public Felicity* (cat. 44), suggesting that this picture too was set over a fireplace.

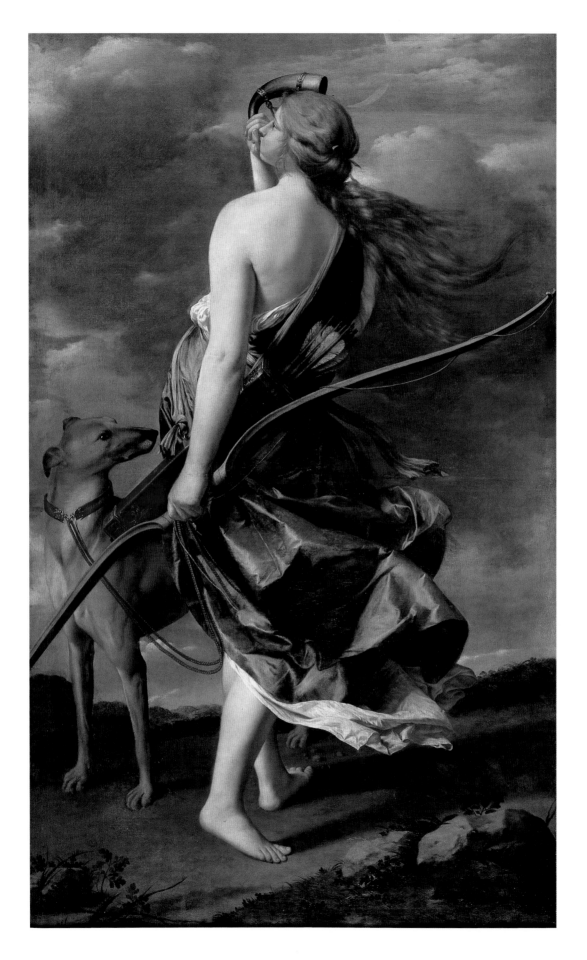

48.

Finding of Moses

Oil on canvas, 101⅛ × 118½ in.
(257 × 301 cm)

Private collection

ca. 1630–33

PROVENANCE: Royal collection, Greenwich Palace and the Queen's House, Greenwich (by 1633–34; inv. 1649, as by Gentileschi); William Latham and his fourth dividend (October 23, 1651); Emanuel de Critz, Austin Friars, London);[10] Philip Sydney, Lord Lisle, Sheen (until September 8, 1660, when ceded to the crown; Sydney inv., as by Gentileschi);[11] Henrietta Maria, château de Colombes (1661–69; postmortem inv. 1669, without attribution); her daughter Henriette Anne, Palais Royal, Paris (1669–70; postmortem inv. 1671, as by Ribera); her husband, Philippe I, duke of Orléans, Palais Royal, Paris (1671–1701; postmortem inv. 1701, as by Velázquez); the Orléans collection, Palais Royal, Paris (1701–92; inv. 1727 and cat. 1737, as by Velázquez); the earl of Carlisle, the earl of Bridgewater, and the earl of Gower (sale, London, December 1798; reserved for the fifth earl of Carlisle); the fifth earl of Carlisle, Castle Howard, Yorkshire (1798–1825); the earls of Carlisle, Castle Howard (until 1995; sale, Sotheby's, London, December 6, 1995, lot 61A); private collection.

Orazio's royal commissions culminated in two sumptuous canvases showing the Old Testament story of the Finding of Moses (Exod. 2:2–10), one for Charles I, the other for Philip IV of Spain (fig. 87). Both canvases are first mentioned in 1633–34 but are likely to have been begun and possibly even completed earlier. On May 8, 1633, Charles I's secretary of state wrote to the British ambassador in Madrid asking him to assist Orazio's son Francesco in presenting Philip IV with a picture "his father hath made, and w[i]th his Ma[jes]ties [i.e., Charles I's] good liking and permission dedicated and now sent unto that kinge."[1] Pleased with the picture, on November 18, Philip IV authorized the payment of 900 ducats to the artist. As for Charles I's version, in 1633–34 there are payments in the accounts for Greenwich for preparing frames for three paintings by Orazio—a *Joseph and Potiphar's Wife* (fig. 88), an *Apollo and the Muses*,[2] and the *Finding of Moses* (referred to as "Pharoes Daughter")—as well as a *Tarquin and Lucretia* by Artemisia.[3] Probably by the late 1630s, the *Finding of Moses* was installed in the Great Hall of the Queen's House, Greenwich, opposite the *Lot and His Daughters* (cat. 46) and below a ceiling with nine inset canvases painted by Orazio showing an allegory of Peace and the Arts (Marlborough House, London; fig. 85).[4] Following the execution of Charles I in 1649, the *Finding of Moses* was given in lieu of payment of debts to the woolen draper William Latham and his fourth dividend; it was eventually repossessed by the crown and in 1661 taken by the dowager queen, Henrietta Maria, to her château at Colombes in France.[5]

According to the Old Testament, the infant Moses was placed in a basket and concealed among the bulrushes so that he would not be a victim of Pharaoh's edict that all newborn sons of the Hebrews be killed. His sister hid herself and watched as Pharaoh's daughter came to the river with her maids to bathe. Catching sight of the mysterious basket, they opened it and, finding the child inside, took him back to

court. In Orazio's picture the princess, dressed in a sumptuous yellow satin dress with pearls and gems embroidered along the neckline and cuffs, points to the infant as she enlists the help of the woman at the left to take charge of his care (the woman is none other than Moses' mother, fetched by his sister). The maid who had fished the basket from the river wears a loose-hanging white shift, while two of her companions gesticulate toward the river where the infant was found. (The landscape has a distinctly English character and may, as Weston-Lewis argues, be intended as a view of the river Thames.) The picture has the quality of a pageant, and its air of unreality has been associated with the masques and poetry of the Caroline court.[6] Yet, in point of fact, the clothes do not bear much resemblance to the fanciful costumes designed by Inigo Jones. Nor do they reproduce court dress, with its abundance of lace bodices, collars, and cuffs. Rather, the analogy is with the allegorizing portraits by Van Dyck and the grand manner of Rubens. As with them, Orazio's model was Veronese.

The royal collection included a number of works by or attributed to Veronese, including a small *Finding of Moses* that may have been the picture now in the Prado.[7] Yet for all its costumed elegance, Orazio's painting differs from Veronesan practice in three crucial respects. The figure grouping is compact and friezelike rather than open and loosely linked. In this the artist has rediscovered the essentially figurative basis of his art that is so conspicuously absent from the dispersed design of the *Lot and His Daughters*. The male servants and dwarfs that play such eye-catching roles in Veronese's art find no place in Orazio's composition, with its all-female cast. (Does this shift signify that the commission came not from the king but from Henrietta Maria and that a gendered reading is implied?) And finally, gestures play a dominant— even distracting—role. Moses' mother responds affectionately toward her daughter Miriam, who in turn points to the child as she gazes at the princess.

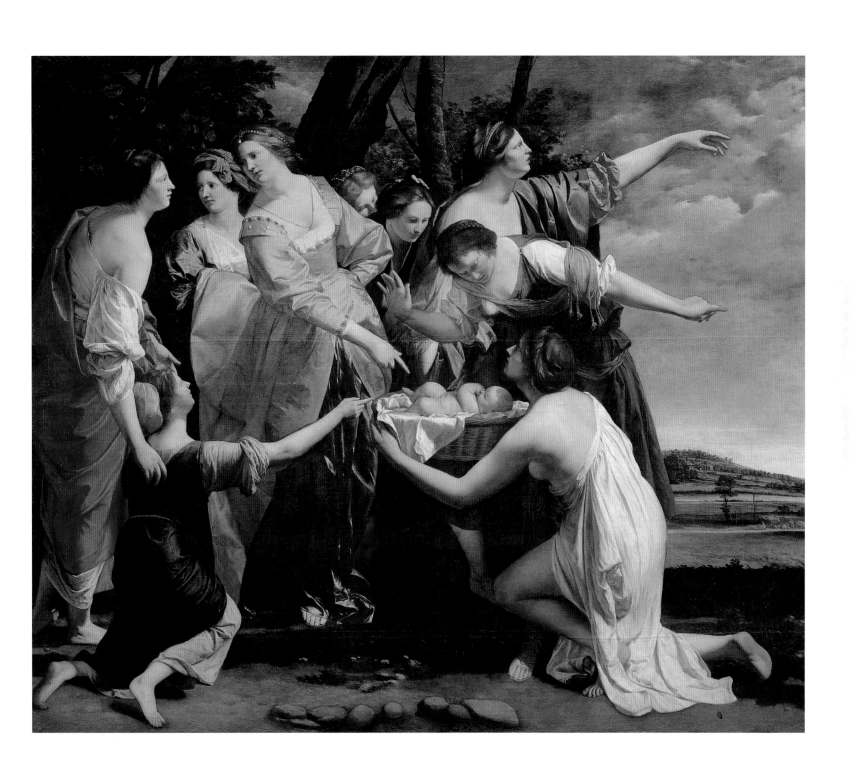

RELATED PICTURES: Museo Nacional del Prado, Madrid (autograph variant for Philip IV); formerly Salzer, Los Angeles (reduced copy of London painting; sale, Christie's, New York, October 5, 1995, lot 60).

REFERENCES: Dubois de Saint Gelais 1737, 116–17; Couché 1808, vol. 1, pl. 86; Buchanan 1824, 146 no. 2; Stryienski 1913, 176; Longhi (1916) 1961, 247; Voss 1925, 461; Vertue 1935–36, 131; Chettle 1937, 104; London 1938, 72 no. 285; Hess 1952, 163; Sterling 1958, 118 n. 37; Pérez Sánchez 1965, 502; Harris 1967, 86, 89 nn. 5, 6; Millar 1970–72, 137 no. 1; Nicolson 1979, 52; Bissell 1981, 53, 60, 189–90, 191–92 no. 66; Beal 1984, 309; Nicolson 1990, 113; Christie 1997, 36–37; Weston-Lewis 1997, 27–35; Maddicott 1998, 120–22; Finaldi, Weston-Lewis, and Sánchez-Lassa de los Santos in London–Bilbao–Madrid 1999, 27, 29, 39–52, 68, 79–97; Wood 2000–2001, 106, 120–22.

Pharaoh's daughter strikes a pose of aristocratic command as she addresses Moses' mother. One of the maids expresses delighted surprise with one hand while with the other she indicates the river in the background. This is a picture that attempts to recount the story via pose and gesture—what was known as the *affetti*—and it does so in a far more successful way than either the *Mocking of Christ* (cat. 49) or the *Lot and His Daughters*.

It is precisely this focus on gesture that disappears (or is toned down) in the Prado version, painted by Orazio as a gift for Philip IV. In that work, moreover, the description of costly costumes is carried one step further. Pharaoh's daughter wears a crown, one of the maids wears a turban with a pendant pearl (the turban is made of Orazio's favorite gold-banded scarf), and the scantily clad figure who in the London picture has fetched the basket from the river is in the Prado painting decked out in a sumptuous silvery blue dress with a string of pearls worked into her elaborately coiffed hair.[8] To modern taste, the Prado version is the more satisfying work—it has, indeed, often been seen as Orazio's late masterpiece. Yet surely these very differences underscore the special character of the pictures Orazio painted for the English court and suggest that behind the histrionic posturing there was the desire not simply to accommodate British taste or to give the picture a topographical gloss by calling attention to the relationship of the landscape in the picture with the real view of the Thames visible through the windows of the Queen's House.[9] The object was to introduce an expressive element based on the rhetorical models of Cicero and Quintilian.

However, if the use of expressive gesture was his intent, the result was something quite different. The gestures have a formal rather than an expressive effect—take, for example, the scissors-like arrangement of the paired pointing hands of the two maids. Because of the artificiality of their arrangement, they can seem distracting or simply vacuous. The rhetorical basis of much Baroque painting is not what appeals to modern audiences, and it is hardly surprising that these late works by Orazio should be undervalued.

Until recently, the Prado *Finding of Moses* was considered the earlier of the two versions, but

Weston-Lewis has demonstrated through a technical analysis that the London picture was painted first—or, at any rate, it was begun before the Prado version. He did not discuss the change in tonality between the two, but when the pictures were displayed together in London, in 1999, it became apparent that the Prado version introduces a silvery quality that recalls not simply the work of Veronese but that of Van Dyck, who arrived in London in 1632, but whose great masterpiece of Venetian style, the *Rinaldo and Armida* (Baltimore Museum of Art), was painted for Charles I in 1629 and sent to him from Antwerp (fig. 91). Orazio could not hope to match the dynamism of Van Dyck's art (indeed, he probably did not wish to), but in the *Finding of Moses* he shows himself responsive to new ideas and trends. We may regret the loss of the realistic, Caravaggesque vigor of his Roman works and the sheer brilliance of his Genoese pictures, but it is wrong to write off the English paintings as a sad decline of an aging, out-of-touch artist (in 1633 he was seventy years old).

In what is by far the most thorough discussion of the paintings that decorated the Queen's House, Weston-Lewis has suggested that the picture ought to be read in terms of the queen's tastes and interests. The Old Testament subject may have carried dynastic allusions, since a long-standing tradition traced the origins of the House of Stuart to Pharaoh's daughter (interestingly, the earliest reference to the picture cites the subject as Pharaoh's daughter and does not mention Moses). He also notes that Henrietta Maria was the sister of Isabella of Bourbon, the Spanish queen; might this have been a factor in Orazio's decision to send a like-subject picture to the king of Spain? For both queens, the fact that the composition focused on a newborn male child (the princess points to his genitals) who would become the leader of his people would certainly have given the picture a special significance. The heir to the British throne was, in fact, born on May 29, 1630—not long before work on the picture is likely to have begun.

1. Harris 1967, 89; Trapier 1967, 242.
2. The identification of the *Apollo and the Muses*—identified simply as the "Muses" in the payment—has been debated. Finaldi (in

London–Bilbao–Madrid 1999, 27) suggests that it was not a painting by Gentileschi but one by Tintoretto that appears in a later inventory of the pictures in Greenwich Palace. Given the date of the document, I find this suggestion unconvincing and think it more likely that the picture is the one that belonged to the Lily Lawlor collection in New York (fig. 93). See Bissell 1981, 190.

3. Chettle 1937, 104.

4. On the arrangement of the room, see Weston-Lewis in London– Bilbao–Madrid 1999, 45. In 1629, Charles I transferred ownership of Greenwich Palace to the queen. The basic fabric of the Queen's House was completed in 1635, but four years later the interior was still not finished. The first record of the pictures in the house is in 1649.

5. Maddicott (1998) has clarified the history of the picture following the execution of Charles I.

6. See the case made by Bissell 1981, 55–58.

7. The painting is described in Van der Doort's inventory as "conteyning some 11 little intire figures." It was on a thin panel painted on both sides (the other side was supposedly by Bassano and showed the Nativity). The Prado picture, which is upright and measures 50 × 43 cm includes eleven figures. A replica is in the National Gallery of Art, Washington, D.C. See Wood 2000–2001, 106.

8. It seems to me that the Prado picture lends itself better to the analysis by Weston-Lewis in London–Bilbao–Madrid 1999, 47: "The courtly refinement of Gentileschi's canvas, with its extremely elongated and emotionally neutral figures and its opulent costumes, must have mirrored perfectly the tastes of the Queen and her circle of précieux."

9. This is the suggestion of Weston-Lewis in ibid. 1999, 44–46.

10. It was seen there by the writer Richard Symonds; see Beal 1984, 309.

11. On this and other sources for the early history of the picture, see Owen 1966, 502, and Maddicott 1998.

49.
Mocking of Christ

Oil on canvas, 49 × 62¾ in. (124.5 × 159.5 cm)

Matthiesen Gallery, London

ca. 1628/30–35

New York, Saint Louis

PROVENANCE: Possibly King Charles I, Somerset House, London (by 1629–49; sale, October 23, 1651); possibly Edmund Harrison, London (from 1651); Meuron collection, Lucerne (until 1963; sold, Galerie Fischer, Lucerne, December 3–7, 1963, lot 1115); private collection, London).

RELATED PICTURE: Formerly Andrea Busiri-Vici, Rome (copy).[8]

Among Gentileschi's greatest works in a Caravaggesque vein is the *Christ Crowned with Thorns* in Braunschweig (cat. 23), and it should come as no surprise that on at least three other occasions he treated the theme. The first was in a frescoed compartment of a chapel in the cathedral of Fabriano (fig. 51). The second was in a picture done in Genoa and recorded by Van Dyck in a sketchbook used during his Italian sojourn from 1622 to 1627 (fig. 94). Inscribed "Gentileschi," the drawing is paired with a Virgin mourning the dead Christ derived from a painting by Titian. The third was a picture evidently done in England that is recorded in the "Inventories and Valuations of the King's Goods" drawn up after the execution of Charles I in 1649. The entry reads: "129 Christ betweene 2 Jews. Done by gentilesco."[1] The picture cannot be traced after its "sale" to one of the king's creditors, the embroiderer Edmund Harrison, on October 23, 1651.[2] It may be the "Christ at the Pillare" listed in Balthazar Gerbier's 1629 account of disbursements made to Orazio by the duke of Buckingham and the king (the designation of Christ at the pillar or column normally implies a Flagellation, but it could

also apply to a Mocking of Christ, despite the absence of a column).[3]

What bearing these notices have on the present painting is not altogether clear, for although Van Dyck's sketch is similar to the present painting, there are significant differences. In the drawing, Christ stands more erect, with his hands bound in front of him, and his rod is held at a downward angle. Greater space separates him from the tormentor at the right, who also stands more erect and whose arm is extended horizontally. The figure on the left is viewed at an angle from the back, rather than from the front. His face is in profile, and with his right hand he presses against Christ's shoulder. Because of these differences Bissell classifies the present painting as a variation, possibly by a Northern master, based on a lost original by Orazio. Schleier, by contrast, sustains Orazio's authorship of the picture, which he considers a variant of the composition recorded by Van Dyck but also done during the artist's Genoese period (1621–24). Finaldi includes the picture as a work possibly from Orazio's English period.

In point of fact, the somewhat small-featured figures, their slightly awkward, angular movements,

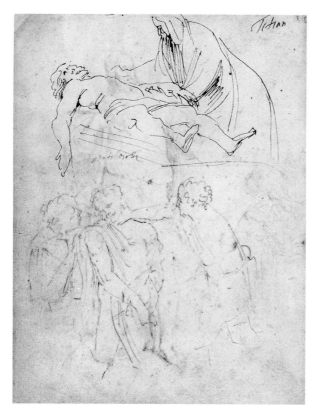

Figure 94. Anthony van Dyck (1599–1641), folio 23v from the *Italian Sketchbook,* with drawing of Orazio Gentileschi's *Mocking of Christ.* Pen and ink on paper. The British Museum, London

REFERENCES: Pijoán 1957, 15 fig. 19; Moir 1976, 147 n. 245.xii; Nicolson 1979, 54; Bissell 1981, 201 no. X-4, 216 no. L-13; Nicolson 1990, 116; Schleier 1993, 194–200; Finaldi in London–Bilbao–Madrid 1999, 64–65 no. 6; Brown in London 2001a, 234–41.

and the emphasis on finely wrought (almost finicky) surface details find their closest analogy in the *Joseph and Potiphar's Wife* Orazio painted prior to 1633 for the Queen's House in Greenwich (fig. 88). If we accept that the description "Christ between two Jews," in the 1649 inventory, is a confusion between the event actually shown—Christ's mocking by Roman soldiers, when he is clothed in scarlet and crowned with thorns (Matt. 27:27–30)—and Christ taunted before the high priest Caiaphas (Matt. 26:67), then there is good reason to identify this as the picture recorded in the collection of Charles I.

In the Braunschweig *Christ Crowned with Thorns,* the lost painting sketched by Van Dyck, and the *Mocking of Christ* we have an incomparable record of the transformation in Orazio's art from the terms of Caravaggesque realistic drama to those of a highly crafted morality play. No longer are we urged to participate empathetically with Christ, to experience his ordeal as a physically real event. Rather, we are

presented with a lesson whose points are made through carefully calculated gestures and figure types. The figure on the left raises his left hand in a gesture Domenichino also used in his 1609 fresco of the martyrdom of Saint Andrew in San Gregorio Magno, Rome, and that Bellori interpreted as "menacing."[4] The right-hand figure grasps Christ around the neck, pressing his thumb into his cheek. Christ's elegant pose is meant to establish a meaningful contrast to those of his two torturers and is further set off by the rich patterning of folds in the drapery. By these means, he is singled out for contemplation as "a man of sorrows, and acquainted with grief" (Isa. 53:3). The picture thus serves as a gloss on its biblical source in a way that is foreign to the Braunschweig picture. At the same time, the lighting is less dramatic and details are treated with a refinement that borders on preciosity— the pitted wall, for example, and the drops of blood coursing down Christ's face.

It is, of course, true that some of the traits of the *Mocking of Christ*—the tendency toward abstraction and frozen action, a love of surface refinement— were already present in his earlier work. A demonstrative type of gesture appears in the Sauli *Lot and His Daughters* (cat. 37). Yet, there is nothing in Orazio's Roman or Genoese paintings that prepares one for the self-conscious use of gesture we find in the pictures he painted in London, gestures that led Levey to castigate the works as "costume-drama almost absurdly lacking in real significance."[5] Modern taste so strongly favors Caravaggesque realism that we have forcibly to remind ourselves that the trajectory of European art after about 1625/30 was toward art as emblematic exposition rather than realistic presentation. Interestingly, some of the same traits we find in Orazio's art can also be observed in Guercino's paintings of the second half of the 1620s. (Guercino, of course, had been the first choice of Charles I for a position at court; Orazio was invited only after Guercino refused.) Fortunately, with Guercino, there is a body of contemporary written evidence to guide us toward an appreciation of the goals he set himself. We lack this sort of literary evidence for Gentileschi and are, in consequence, left to wonder about the impetus behind the change. For the time being, I can

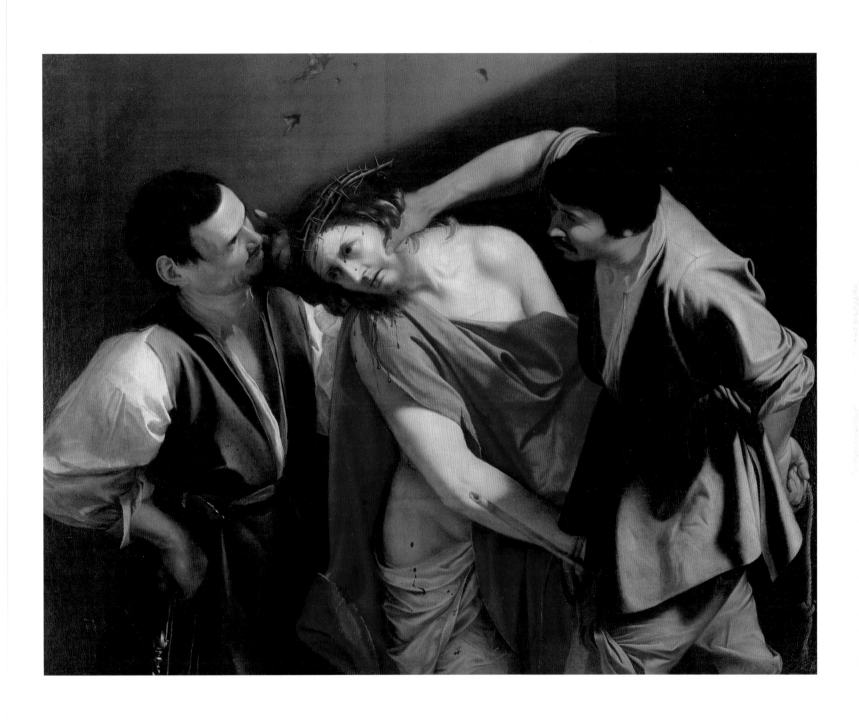

REFERENCES: Constable 1929–30, 756, 758, 761; London 1930, 334 no. 733; London 1931, vol. 1, 159 no. 465; Longhi 1943, 47 n. 38; Milan 1951, 66 no. 114; Millar 1958–60, 231; Nutthall 1965, 302, 304, 308; Millar 1970–72, 266 no. 158; Nicolson 1979, 25, 53; Bissell 1981, 58, 193–94; Nicolson 1990, 66, 116; Finaldi in London–Bilbao–Madrid 1999, 22, 36 n. 50, 99; Wood 2000–2001, 114.

Woman (Metropolitan Museum of Art, New York). This resemblance would be even more compelling if the blue gray background—now scraped down to the preparation—were still intact. Apart from its abraded surface, the panel has been cut down about fourteen centimeters in height and six centimeters in width; it does not show the woman's breasts, as described in the inventory.

Van der Doort notes that the picture was purchased by Charles I. It is thus not a commission but conceivably a painting that Orazio made for himself and kept in his studio: the sort of work he could have referred to in making a large history painting. Indeed, a figure with similar features appears as Pharaoh's daughter in the *Finding of Moses* (cat. 48), suggesting the way in which life and art intersect in Orazio's late career. One of the primary differences between the two versions of the *Finding of Moses*—that exhibited here and the one in the Prado, Madrid—is the way the second one, destined for Philip IV (fig. 87), is further distanced from life and posed models, which we know Orazio continued to use in London.

Vermeer's paintings belong to the Dutch tradition of *tronies*—paintings of heads done not as portraits but as studies of expression, type, physiognomy, or perhaps some exotic characteristic. Such pictures were intended as demonstration pieces. It is interesting to speculate on the possible relationship of Orazio's painting to this tradition. Certainly his picture reminds us how much these kinds of studies owe to the impetus provided by Caravaggio in Rome in the 1590s—for example, his portrait of the courtesan Filide that was owned by Vincenzo Giustiniani (formerly Gemäldegalerie, Berlin; destroyed). The fact that Orazio's painting originally showed the woman with an exposed breast also recalls the Venetian tradition of "portraits" of ideal beauties or courtesans, of which Giorgione's so-called portrait of Laura (Kunsthistorisches Museum, Vienna) is the key work. It is a shame that Longhi did not know the picture when he wrote his groundbreaking article on the Gentileschi in 1916, for he could scarcely have found a more powerful argument for the role he assigned Orazio as the middle term between Caravaggio and Vermeer, and for his notion of light as the keynote of Orazio's work.

1. The terminology is explained in Millar 1958–60, xix.
2. These inventory references are conveniently reprinted in London–Bilbao–Madrid 1999, 99.
3. See Nutthall 1965, 302–9.
4. It is there asserted that the picture belonged to George IV and was displayed at Brighton Pavilion.
5. In Millar 1958–60, 38, 201.

Artemisia Gentileschi

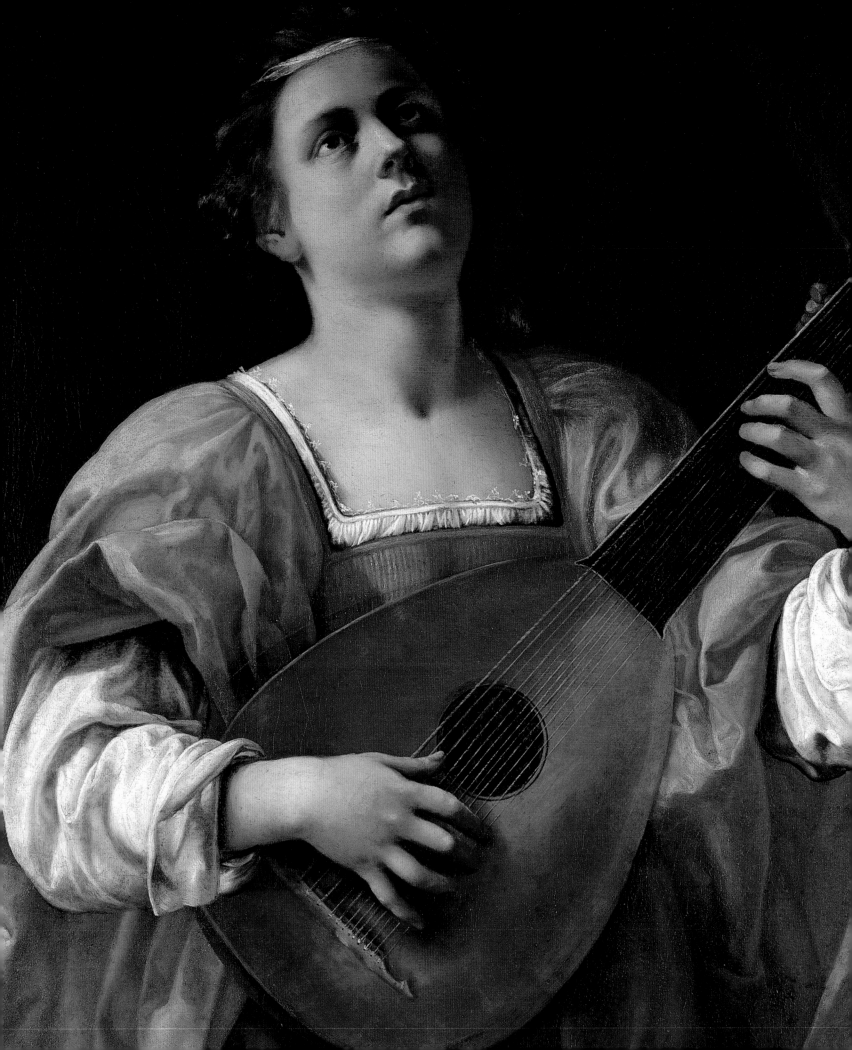

Artemisia and Orazio Gentileschi

JUDITH W. MANN

Orazio and Artemisia Gentileschi, father and daughter, entered the roster of twentieth-century art history together in the seminal 1916 article by the noted Caravaggio scholar Roberto Longhi. It is thus fitting that, eighty-five years later, we re-examine these two exceptional artists side by side, painting by painting. The Gentileschi Longhi wrote about and the Gentileschi we know today only partially overlap. Of the thirty-nine paintings he attributed to Orazio, fewer than half remain in the scholarly arena and only one-third of the works that he gave to Artemisia appear in the latest catalogue raisonné of her paintings, testimony to the maturation of the study of seicento art and to the methodological reorientation of the art-historical endeavor.[1]

After Longhi, critical attention to the Gentileschi came about in the context of exhibitions devoted to Caravaggio and his followers, within the admittedly loose context of Caravaggism. But even when scholarly consideration of Caravaggism was at its height, interest in Artemisia had begun to emerge in a quite different way. In 1947, Longhi's wife, Lucia Lopresti (under the pseudonym Anna Banti), published a novel about Artemisia that anticipated the feminist interest in the artist which blossomed in the 1980s. As Banti sought to understand the historical Artemisia, she also established the biases that continue to inform our ways of thinking about her. Ironically, while Banti struggled to come to terms with the circumscribed parameters of historiography, her focus on the Uffizi *Judith Slaying Holofernes* (which she interpreted as the artist's visual revenge on Agostino Tassi, the painter by whom she was raped in 1611; cat. 62) established its own delimiting framework that plagues us still. Although the novel was not widely read until much later (its translation into English in 1994 attracted a broader American readership), it contained the seeds of the predominating view of the artist. A second key moment in the developing interest in Artemisia came with the 1976 exhibition "Women Artists: 1550–1950," curated by Ann Sutherland Harris and Linda Nochlin, which raised Artemisia's profile by including six of her paintings, a surprisingly large sampling of her works (only Mary Cassatt and Georgia O'Keeffe had a greater number).[2] The seemingly inconsequential illustration of these six paintings (two in color) in the accompanying catalogue led to Artemisia's paintings (particularly the Detroit *Judith and Her Maidservant;* cat. 69) appearing more often in introductory courses on the history of art and surveys on Italian art of the seventeenth century. This burgeoning interest during the next decade was capped by Mary Garrard's insightful and provocative monograph of 1989, in which the author seeks to balance the interest in Artemisia's life with a thoughtful reading of her work. Garrard's book introduces a forceful creative personality that has helped to define Gentileschi's work, and while it argues for the validity of a creative female point of view, it cautions against perceiving the rape as a simple causal factor for interpreting Artemisia's paintings.

Nonetheless, a simple conception of the artist soon prevailed. The Uffizi *Judith* quickly became the exemplar of her entire oeuvre, an emblem of dramatic confrontation and female victory. It appears in more than a dozen survey texts of art history and is usually accompanied by commentary relating the painting to the rape. Artemisia Gentileschi's name now conjures up art that is dramatic, populated with uncompromisingly direct visualizations of forceful women, and integrally related to the events of her life. This characterization describes perhaps less than a quarter of her known paintings, and yet it persists.

Authors have lamented and rejected the now infamous labeling of Artemisia by the eminent historians of Italian Baroque art, Rudolf and Margot Wittkower, in 1963 as "a lascivious and precocious girl."[3] This characterization of Artemisia can be traced back

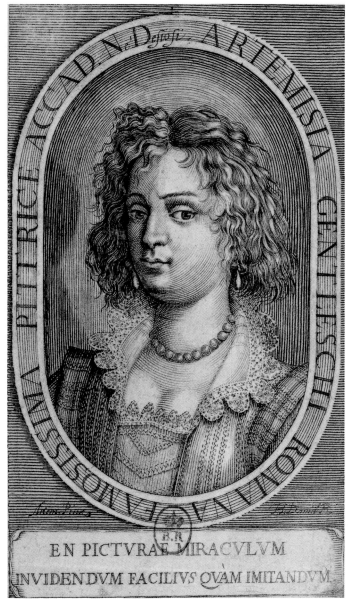

Figure 95. Jérôme David (ca. 1605–after 1670), *Portrait of Artemisia Gentileschi*. Engraving after a painted self-portrait. Bibliothèque Nationale de France, Cabinet des Estampes, Paris

to the discipline of art history, but it is to the prevailing feminist construct that we owe our new stereotype. Without denying that gender can offer valid interpretive strategies for the investigation of Artemisia's art, we may wonder whether the application of gendered readings has created too narrow an expectation. Underpinning Garrard's monograph, and reiterated in a limited way by R. Ward Bissell in his catalogue raisonné, are certain presumptions: that Artemisia's full creative power emerged only in the depiction of strong, assertive women, that she would not engage in conventional religious imagery such as the Madonna and Child or a Virgin who responds with submission to the Annunciation, and that she refused to yield her personal interpretation to suit the tastes of her presumably male clientele. This stereotype has had the doubly restricting effect of causing scholars to question the attribution of pictures that do not conform to the model, and to value less highly those that do not fit the mold. My criticism here refers to what has shaped the popular view, particularly in the United States, of Artemisia's creative personality. A new generation of feminist scholars, particularly Mieke Bal and Griselda Pollock, have not correlated the life with the work, but have posed promising questions for further interpretive exploration.[5]

Current scholarship on Orazio is a bit different. Investigation of his work has included noteworthy contributions by Bissell (his 1981 catalogue raisonné remains the standard reference) as well as by Erich Schleier and Gabriele Finaldi.[6] Yet, in contrast to Artemisia's, Orazio's art remains the domain of the specialist and the connoisseur, and while a few of his paintings have become emblematic of the Caravaggesque tradition (the Hartford *Judith* [cat. 39] is an example), he has not garnered widespread public attention and, unlike Artemisia, he has not become a standard fixture in the college art-history curriculum. So, at century's end, Artemisia's profile, though highly visible, has tended to be based on generalizations, while Orazio's visibility remains undeservedly low and, also, in its own way, stereotyped.

This situation alone demonstrates the timeliness of the present exhibition. Both artists, for very different reasons, require an overview of their respective bodies of work. While a selection of Artemisia's paintings, presented in 1991 at the Casa Buonarroti, focused on the seven-year period she spent in Florence, and while Orazio's late English paintings were featured in an exhibition at the National Gallery, London, in 1999, neither painter has

to posthumous epitaphs that describe her presumed cuckolding of her husband: "To carve two horns upon my husband's head, I put down the brush and took a chisel instead."[4] And it assumes that a woman who had succeeded in a male profession necessarily exploited her gender, if not her sexuality. Nonetheless, the creation of an oversimplified persona seems to have become the defining model for looking at the artist, and we have now exchanged one stereotype for another. Feminist scholarship has made a significant contribution to Gentileschi studies, as well as

received monographic treatment and works spanning the careers of both artists have never been exhibited together.

The timing for Artemisia is fortuitous. The present moment in Artemisia studies, after the 1999 publication of Bissell's monumental catalogue, finds us at a point where the full creative endeavor of the artist can now be explored in depth. While Bissell's omission of the two paintings from the Spada collection (cat. nos. 52, 63) and his unavoidable exclusion of the newly discovered *Self-Portrait as a Lute Player* (cat. 57) deprived us of some key works, his book presents an artist of wide-ranging sensibilities and stylistic variations. Bissell has brought several never-before-published paintings to a broader audience (including the *Aurora*, fig. 96), and his investigations have begun to separate works of the 1630s from those of the 1640s. With the cleaning and restoration of several important paintings within the last few years, we can now bring together a substantial sampling of Artemisia's creative output and present a more balanced and interesting artist, one who clearly followed her own instinct for narrative interpretation, but one who also was keenly attuned to the prospects of patronage that lay before her and the artistic milieus in which she worked.

One by-product of the feminist focus on Artemisia Gentileschi has been the assumption that, were she not female, she would not warrant the kind of scholarly and popular attention that she has received over the last thirty years. The poor condition, inaccessibility, and often murky published photographs of many of her paintings have supported this negative interpretation and precluded a full appreciation of key pictures. The considered study of paintings selected from the entire breadth of the artist's career can now challenge that implication as it questions other misguided assessments.

The timing for examining Orazio's work is also opportune. While there are few of the problems of attribution that plague the study of Artemisia, many issues of dating and chronology—and thus of interpretation—remain unresolved. Only one of the approximately sixty pictures is dated, and although some new supporting documents have come to light since the publication in 1981 of Bissell's catalogue raisonné, many works have been placed at widely divergent moments in his life. That these issues are still pressing was illustrated by the response to the London *Mocking of Christ* (cat. 49), which was presented as a late work in the National Gallery exhibition (as it is here), but about which a number of

viewers expressed the opinion that it should be placed in his early Roman period.[7] Thanks to documentary discoveries, we now know that three altarpieces by Orazio (cat. nos. 7, 9, 11) were painted within a year or so of one another rather than over almost two decades, as Bissell posited. Moreover, what he believed to be the earliest of the three—the *Baptism of Christ* in Santa Maria della Pace (cat. 11)—proves to have been the latest. A comparison of the chronology put forward here with that argued in Bissell's book only emphasizes the need to rethink assumptions about Orazio's development and his contribution to seicento painting. This exhibition, with its remarkable representation of his work, provides an ideal—indeed, a unique—opportunity for just such a reconsideration.

Directly linked to a proper evaluation of Orazio's place in the seventeenth century is an understanding of his patronage. Who were the major collectors of his work, and what part did they play in shaping his art? Both Livia Carloni and Keith Christiansen (see their essays in this publication) attempt to sketch in the network of patrons that sustained him and that led to the magnificent series of altarpieces painted for Ancona and Fabriano in the Marches, works that pose fundamental issues pertaining to the religious thought and culture they seem to exemplify.

Students of the artist have long known the importance of the Genoese patron Giovan Antonio Sauli and his relationship with the artist. Yet none of the paintings that Orazio produced for him during the approximately three years he spent in Genoa were accessible to the public until 1999, when the J. Paul Getty Museum purchased one of the three, the *Lot and His Daughters* (cat. 37). The other two, the *Penitent Magdalene* (cat. 35) and the *Danaë* (cat. 36), are in private collections. For the first time since the eighteenth century, these paintings have been brought together. The means by which Orazio produced variants and replicas of these works for other important clients is also investigated with surprising results.

In much of the literature, Orazio's career after he left Rome in 1621 is seen as a period of decline. If his paintings are evaluated in terms of their adherence to Caravaggism, this judgment is the inevitable result. But here it is argued that in many respects the Genoese paintings mark the high point of his career, that for Orazio Caravaggism was a prelude to the creation of a highly individual poetics, one indebted to Bolognese traditions as well as to Caravaggio. Although the pictures he painted in Paris and

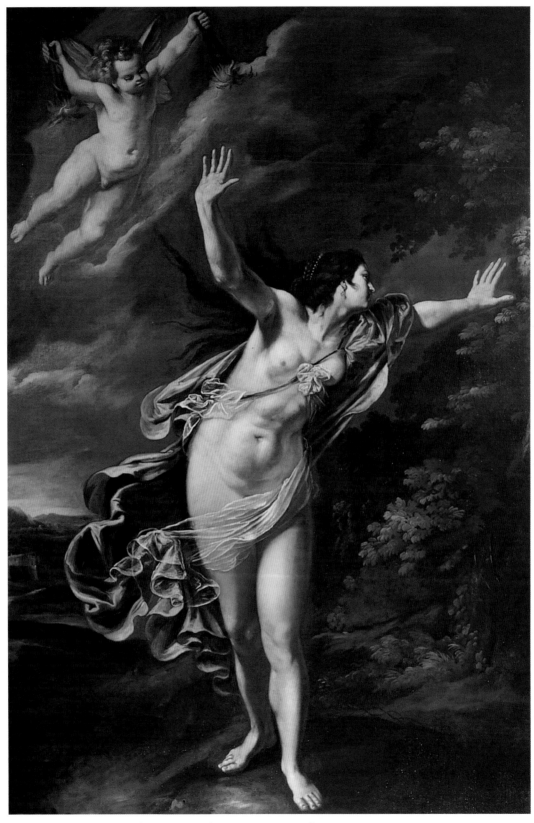

Figure 96. Artemisia Gentileschi, *Aurora*. Oil on canvas. Private collection, Rome

London may not appeal to modern taste, they surely raise interpretive questions as interesting as those raised by his earlier pictures and reveal an artist keenly responsive to the ambient in which he worked.

A single exhibition devoted to both Orazio and Artemisia Gentileschi can accomplish the important task of providing the essential overview of each painter. Given the relatively small size of the known oeuvres of both artists, it is possible, without taxing the patience and stamina of all but the most ardent students of the Baroque, to represent the full scope of each career. But a joint exhibition offers far more opportunities for discovery. Anyone who has delved into recent scholarship on the Gentileschi knows that they are not always perceived as independent artists. Indeed, there remain a few paintings that carry convincing attributions to each—pictures that were probably produced when father and daughter worked together in Rome, from about 1609 (Orazio wrote, in a letter of 1612, that Artemisia had been painting for three years) until 1612 or 1613, at which time Artemisia left Rome following the ordeal of the rape trial.[8]

The key work in this regard is the *Susanna and the Elders* from Pommersfelden (cat. 51). Signed by Artemisia and dated 1610 and presumably the earliest of her paintings, the *Susanna* has engendered much discussion concerning the role of Orazio in his daughter's artistic development. Early confusion over the year of Artemisia's birth (originally thought to be 1597 until her baptismal records of 1593 were published by Bissell in 1968) had caused scholars to question the authenticity of the signature and date, raising doubts that it could actually be by Artemisia's hand.[9] While most scholars now accept Artemisia's participation in the execution of this picture, they have offered a full spectrum of opinion on Orazio's role, ranging from his nearly total responsibility for the work to a belief that it is solely the creation of Artemisia.[10] Included in both "Women Artists" and the Casa Buonarroti exhibition, the picture has never been evaluated alongside important early paintings by Orazio. Certainly, such an evaluation is the necessary first stage in determining whether Orazio assisted Artemisia in this project, and, if so, how.

Evidence indicates that Orazio was an ardent champion of his daughter. The often quoted letter that he wrote to Cristina of Lorraine, grand duchess of Tuscany, in 1612 suggests that he acted almost as her agent. He wrote that Artemisia "has in three years become so skilled that I can venture to say that today she has no peer; indeed, she has produced works which demonstrate a level of understanding that perhaps even the principal masters of the profession have not attained, as I will show Your Very Serene Highness at the proper time and place."[11] Might he not have guided his daughter's execution of the *Susanna*, correcting at times, perhaps even working with her on preparatory drawings? While there is no evidence that such drawings were used, the extraordinary accomplishment of the seated figure of Susanna suggests prolonged study and reworking. The newly discovered oval panel, the *Allegory of Painting* (fig. 97), in which the sophisticated depiction of the hand and face is more advanced than the handling of the costume and drapery, indicates that the very young Artemisia, perhaps under the tutelage of her father, must have devoted considerable effort to the representation of the human figure and the description of anatomical details.

The painting that more or less launched the present exhibition is the small copper *Danaë* (cat. 54) that the Saint Louis Art Museum acquired in 1986 amid a flurry of debate. Attributed to Orazio at the Sotheby's Monaco sale, many scholars at the time were convinced

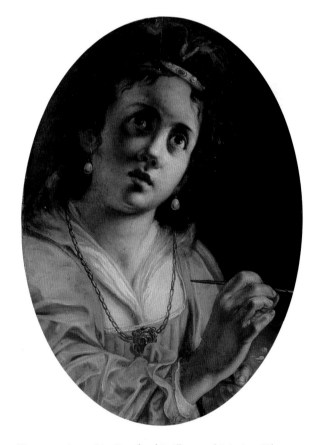

Figure 97. Artemisia Gentileschi, *Allegory of Painting.* Oil on wood. Location unknown

that the painting was by Artemisia. Although exhibited in Saint Louis as by Artemisia, it remains a controversial work, as does the larger, related canvas from the Morandotti collection in Milan, the magnificent *Cleopatra* (cat. nos. 17, 53).[12] Neither picture has been assigned securely to either painter, nor do scholars agree on their dates of execution. The two paintings have not been exhibited together, and perhaps they were never intended as a pair. It is hoped that the opportunity to examine both pictures in the context of this exhibition will help to resolve these questions of attribution. Given the prominent role that the *Cleopatra* has played in Garrard's and Pollock's feminist readings of Artemisia, the clarification of issues relating to connoisseurship remains crucial to an understanding of her career.[13] Should the painting now gain acceptance within Orazio's oeuvre, it will not only reinforce our understanding of his study of the model during the time he was training his daughter, but enable important discussions on the role of gender and its application as a tool for connoisseurship and interpretation.[14]

The correct assignment of the *Danaë* offers as well promising rewards in understanding both artists. If it is a work by Artemisia done as a variant interpretation of Orazio's *Cleopatra,* it would

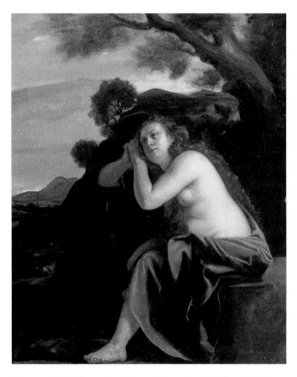

Figure 98. Attributed to Artemisia or Orazio Gentileschi, *Penitent Magdalene.* Oil on copper. Walpole Galleries, London

represent the only known instance in which she appropriated so closely an entire figure from his oeuvre. This kind of examination may open the way to a better understanding of how the Gentileschi workshop functioned in these early years and illuminate the role of patrons in the early careers of the two painters. As a work that dates to around the time of the rape, it forces us to come to terms with an image of overt sexuality produced at the moment Artemisia was going through the duress of the trial. Its presentation of a sexually available heroine not necessarily in control of her fate challenges the tendency to see a strong autobiographical component in Artemisia's paintings, according to which the rape experience is thought to have spurred the artist to represent forceful women who shape their own destiny. A firm attribution to Artemisia may also afford feminist scholars an opportunity to expand on Pollock's acknowledgment of the indirect nature of expression in the artistic production of women. This painting, which embraces rather than rejects sexuality and voyeurism, prompts us to ask why a woman, so soon after her own sexual abuse, should undertake the presentation of a mythological heroine engaged in a sexual act from which she so clearly derives pleasure.[15] Should the *Danaë* prove to be the work of Orazio, as Bissell argues, we must recognize a more varied approach to narrative in his Roman paintings and wonder why he never again experimented as boldly with the expressive potential of a single figure.

Other paintings that have been published under both Orazio's and Artemisia's names include the Oslo *Judith and Her Maidservant* (cat. 13), the Naples *Judith Slaying Holofernes* (cat. 55), and, recently, the Milan *Lucretia* (cat. 67). Although there are fewer differences of opinion about their attribution than is the case with the *Cleopatra* and the *Danaë,* being able to view them in the context of the output of both painters may put lingering doubts to rest.[16] Recently, Gianni Papi has identified the *Lucretia* as a work by Orazio.[17] While this suggestion has not been fully evaluated by scholars, the present exhibition offers the ideal venue for examining this extraordinary image (seen recently in the context of several exhibitions) within the oeuvre of both painters.[18] Of course, not all the pictures that have disputed attributions are represented. A *Penitent Magdalene* on copper, currently on the London art market (fig. 98), has elicited the same dichotomous opinion as the *Cleopatra* and the *Danaë.* In 1998 and 1999, it was included in the exhibition "Copper as Canvas" (Phoenix–Kansas City–

The Hague) ascribed to Orazio, after having been sold at Sotheby's in 1996 as by Artemisia. Bissell, the scholar most comfortably conversant with both artists' work, has reversed his attribution from Artemisia to Orazio.[19] However, the curators of the present exhibition find no compelling argument for assigning it to either painter.

Beyond clarification of attribution, a viewing of the two artists together provides a means for examining the most generally acknowledged aspect of the Gentileschi—their Caravaggism. While some have argued that the designation *Caravaggisti* resists uniformity and cannot be understood as a movement or school per se (indeed, Caravaggio, unlike his great Bolognese contemporary Annibale Carracci, did not take on pupils), it does address key aspects of the style of those painters who worked in Rome in the early seventeenth century or came, through various avenues, into contact with Caravaggio's powerful tenebrist style.[20] The discussion of the Caravaggesque influences on Orazio and Artemisia has informed nearly all interpretations of their art, and their paintings when seen side by side will surely refine our understanding of the ways in which Caravaggio's radical naturalism shaped their early development.

The two artists had very different experiences of Caravaggio. Orazio established contact with him in 1600, shortly after the unveiling of the Lombard master's first public commission, in San Luigi dei Francesi; they were initially on friendly terms and, according to Orazio's testimony in the 1603 libel trial brought by Baglione, even shared studio props.[21] By the time he encountered Caravaggio's paintings, Orazio had been trained and had worked in a late-Mannerist tradition, evident in the *Saint Ursula* he painted at the abbey of Farfa and in the early *Madonna and Child with Saints Sebastian and Francis* (cat. 1), in which we encounter a stiffness and lack of formal cohesion and an ambiguity in the treatment of space. By the end of the first decade of the seventeenth century, he was working directly from the model and embraced a meticulously observed naturalism. By the 1620s, while he never lost the power of tactility or delicately modeled form, his work shows a greater elegance, and there are echoes of a Bolognese classicism in his focus on the artfully posed figure (see the Hartford *Judith* [cat. 39] and the Nantes *Diana* [cat. 47]). Late in his career, this nascent Mannerism sometimes burst forth in his most refined works. In paintings such as the *Finding of Moses* (cat. 48), he adopts a courtly style, attenuating his figures and adjusting their forms as he seeks to transcend strict references to the natural world.

Artemisia's knowledge of Caravaggio was indirect and came in stages. As Patrizia Cavazzini makes clear (see pp. 286–90), her artistic education in early-Baroque Rome was extremely limited. Chaperoned wherever she went, she knew only some of Caravaggio's paintings. While she must have visited prominent churches, such as Santa Maria del Popolo (the Gentileschi's parish), and would certainly have seen the Cerasi chapel with Caravaggio's *Conversion of Saint Paul,* we can't be sure that she knew his Saint Matthew cycle in the Contarelli chapel, and privately owned paintings were probably inaccessible to her. Undoubtedly, she first understood the revolutionary qualities of Caravaggio's vision through her father's work, paintings that Orazio prepared in the studio in the years prior to her own artistic debut in 1610, and perhaps also, to a lesser extent, through selected pictures by the Lombard master himself. In Florence, she must have met the Neapolitan Caravaggesque artist Giovanni Battista Caracciolo (1578–1635; he was there in 1618) and become more profoundly acquainted with Caravaggio's work when she returned to Rome in 1620. As a married woman and an established painter, she had the opportunity to see a fuller range of Caravaggio's canvases. This renewed experience of Caravaggio, however, was inevitably colored by the work of other Caravaggesque painters working in Rome. She obviously learned from Simon Vouet (Garrard has plausibly suggested a friendship between Artemisia and his artist wife, Virginia da Vezzo) and she must have known the paintings of Bartolomeo Manfredi as well.[22] Gerrit van Honthorst has been cited as a source for her imagery and expressive vocabulary, and she may also have known Cecco del Caravaggio and the French Caravaggisti Valentin de Boulogne and Nicolas Tournier.

When she moved to Naples, about 1630, Artemisia came to know yet another group of Caravaggesque painters, as well as Caravaggio's own Neapolitan canvases. She again came into contact with Caracciolo, and seems to have been changed by the art of Jusepe de Ribera. She knew Francesco Guarino, worked with Paolo Finoglia, and collaborated with Massimo Stanzione and, quite possibly, Bernardo Cavallino. As Riccardo Lattuada points out (see pp. 382–86), the old assumption that Artemisia was the main conduit for Caravaggism in Naples cannot be sustained, and in fact the main reason for her relocation to Naples may have been her understanding that there was in that city a taste for Caravaggesque paintings.[23] Be that as it may, during the last two decades of her career, Caravaggism remained one of several sources that she tapped as she moved to a more rhetorical and decorous style. In her late work, unrefined naturalism and observed details of physiognomy and form are less in evidence.

One area in which Artemisia adhered to an accurate transcription of details is in her painstaking depiction of weaponry. Among the seven paintings in the exhibition that include swords or daggers, she has taken great pains to describe weapons accurately and with great precision[24]— the falchion in the Detroit *Judith and Her Maidservant* (cat. 69), for example, or the gauntlet on the table and the scabbard for the sword. This aspect of Artemisia's style, however, relates less to the physicality of objects and the study of light and surface than to an interest in the subjects and the feasibility of the events portrayed.

Herein lies the single most important way in which the sensibilities of Artemisia and Orazio diverge. Although Artemisia does not seek the accuracy of surface and texture that engaged her father, early on she evinced an interest in rendering narrative in a believable manner. Orazio rarely demonstrates such attunement to the dramatic details of his stories. His protagonists often assume masterful poses but rarely poses that further the narrative. In his early work, the *Saint Michael and the Devil* (cat. 14), Michael rests his left knee on a bank of clouds, and Orazio's convincing replication of the soft clouds makes it look as if the knee will be enveloped and thus not provide the stable support the archangel will need to rout his foe. In the later Hartford *Judith,* Orazio achieves an arrestingly beautiful rendition of Judith and her maidservant as they prepare to exit Holofernes' camp, but one that makes little narrative sense. While the two women should be engaged in a common pursuit, to wrap Holofernes' head and depart quickly before their deed is discovered, they seem to be working at cross-purposes. As with many of Orazio's compositions, a moment of potential drama is transformed into an emblematic, formal beauty. The figures appear contrived and arranged, the action arrested. This does not imply a failure in terms of Orazio's skill and the beauty of his paintings, but it does differentiate his approach to representation from that of Artemisia.

Artemisia's renderings of the Judith narrative show her thinking through how these situations could have come about, even at the expense of formal niceties. In the Naples *Judith* (cat. 55), beyond the awkwardly posed arms of the heroine and the problematic scale of Holofernes' hand, is the sense that the women

had a plan. Abra uses her weight to hold the sleeping general down while Judith decapitates him. In the *Jael and Sisera* (cat. 61), Jael kneels down to drive the nail into Sisera's temple, with her dress falling over the sleeping general's hand, in a pose that allows her to carry out her task. Few other representations of Jael position her in such a way that she can actually hammer the peg without losing her balance or missing the mark. The Susanna in the painting from Burghley House (cat. 65) attempts to draw her cast-off linen chemise around her. While the pose itself is based on an ancient type of Venus statuary and is in some ways already a cliché by the seventeenth century, most artists depicted a generic length of sheet or richly colored drape, more for effect than specifically to illustrate Susanna's clothing. For the topmost elder, Artemisia has selected a pose that aptly encapsulates the power of lust and voyeurism, in which he pushes down on his partner as he strains to catch a glimpse of Susanna's body.

Through her pictures of the 1620s and 1630s, Artemisia continued to display these kinds of narrative concerns. Even in the works from the mid-1630s, in which she shows less overt drama or action, she weds her compositions to the details of her stories. The composition of the Columbus *David and Bathsheba* (cat. 80) seems designed to focus on the protagonist's toilette and beauty and the supporting actions of the three maids as they set about their tasks. The grouping of the figures in the *Lot and His Daughters* (cat. 78) is a skilled arrangement in which the sequence of the story is indicated through the poses of the figures and the repetition of certain shared forms. The father will have sexual relations first with one daughter and then the other. The repetition of the attitudes of father and daughter (both in yellow) suggests that such coupling has already occurred, while the daughter with the jug who approaches from the left is about to ply him with wine.

One of the most revealing moments in the parallel stories of Orazio and Artemisia Gentileschi is the early period of the third decade. When Pope Paul V Borghese (r. 1605–21) died and Gregory XV Ludovisi (r. 1621–23) replaced him, Orazio left for Genoa, where he produced some of his most compelling pictures for one of the most important patrons of his career—Giovan Antonio Sauli.[25] The three Sauli paintings—the *Penitent Magdalene,* the *Danaë,* and the *Lot and His Daughters* (cat. nos. 35–37)—while they feature Caravaggesque elements, also mark a turning point in Orazio's stylistic development, a development that was possible only after he had quit Rome once and for all; and it was outside this artistic ambient that his stylistic maturity was realized.

At this same time, Artemisia ended her seven-year sojourn in Florence and returned to Rome, where she had been working since 1620 and where she realized that she could carve out a successful career. Although we are unsure of the exact dates of her departure and relocation, documentary evidence verifies her presence in Rome by 1621, and a letter written in Florence to Grand Duke Cosimo II de' Medici announces her intention of going there as early as February 1620.[26] In 1621, Artemisia sold the contents of her Florence studio to Francesco Maringhi (see appendix 3), perhaps to help finance the move. In 1622, she painted the Burghley House *Susanna and the Elders* (cat. 65), which offers a very different interpretation of the subject from that of her debut composition of 1610 (cat. 51) and seems an obvious nod to the tastes of the newly elected Bolognese pope and his favored nephew, Ludovico, both ardent champions of their compatriots, such as Guido Reni, Guercino, and Annibale Carracci.[27] The present condition of the painting has prompted questions as to whether it is fully autograph. But if indeed the picture is in fact by Artemisia it will underscore the already acknowledged changeability of her work. Having recently left Florence, with her sights set on Rome, Artemisia sized up the way the artistic winds were blowing and showed herself quite capable of providing her would-be patron with a surprising image, one that extends beyond her earlier interpretive expression and stylistic vocabulary. This is the Artemisia who prompted Mina Gregori to write that we must not "undervalue her exceptional (and one could say feminine) receptive capacity and her adaptation to her environment."[28] One may question whether this adaptation is a distinctly female response. Nevertheless, the ascription of this painting to Artemisia means that we can now evaluate still undiscovered or misattributed paintings that may not conform to such a narrow definition of her style.

The careers of the Gentileschi document key aspects of the development and dissemination of the Baroque style. For all practical purposes, both careers began in the ambient of Counter-Reformation Rome, where the foundations of Baroque art were established. Although the manner in which these artists experienced Rome and contemporary Roman art was vastly different, their art was shaped to some degree by Rome and its artistic milieu. Artemisia moved to Florence in 1613 and was ushered into the lively circle of the court of Cosimo II de' Medici. She returned to Rome during the 1620s, the decade that witnessed the emergence of Gianlorenzo Bernini (1598–1680) and the beginning of the papacy of Urban VIII (r. 1623–44), which made Rome an environment in which Baroque art could flourish. Artemisia's peripatetic life—she left Rome in the 1620s, traveled to Venice toward the end of the decade, and settled in Naples—was not uncharacteristic for contemporary artists. The French painter Simon Vouet (1590–1649) went to Venice around the same time, as did the German artist Johann Liss (ca. 1595/1600–1631), who had been in Rome in the first half of the decade but who returned to Venice in the 1620s. Artemisia's arrival in Naples coincided with the period in which the city, already the second largest city in Europe, emerged as an important center for the visual arts.

In the 1620s, Orazio was in Rome, but he completed a number of commissions in the Marches. He then went to Genoa, then Paris, and finally served as court painter to Charles I (r. 1625–49) in London, beginning in 1626. His movement northward parallels, in a somewhat limited way, the development of other centers of Baroque art—Paris in the second half of the century and Versailles in the last three decades. Charles I was arguably the most important collector of his age, and the arrival of paintings at the English court had profound implications for later artists. While the experience of the Gentileschi did not typify that of all seventeenth-century artists, the sort of itinerant careers that both artists led and the specific places they worked cover some of the major geography of the Baroque style.

One aspect of the Gentileschi that still resists full understanding is the relationship between the two painters after Artemisia left Rome and even during the time they spent together in London at the end of the 1630s. Substantial visual evidence suggests some sort of artistic dialogue continued throughout their lives, beyond Orazio's role of mentor. Banti suggests a familial bond between the two painters, and Alexandra Lapierre's recent fictionalized account of the relationship between the two artists emphasizes the strong tie that drew Artemisia to her father. And while her dependence on him has at times been overstated, scholars have found in Artemisia's paintings confirmation of his continuing influence.[29] For example, Gregori, followed by Garrard and Bissell, has noted that Artemisia's Rome *Cleopatra* (cat. 76), a work she probably painted in the 1630s, was dependent on Orazio's *Penitent Magdalene* (cat. 35), although it is also possible

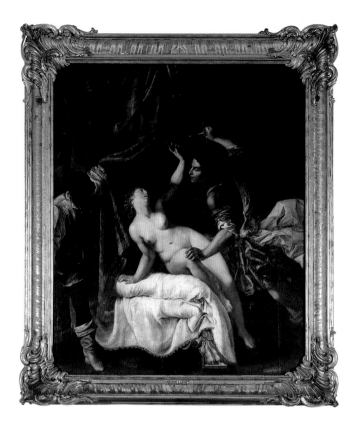

Figure 99. Artemisia Gentileschi, *Rape of Lucretia*. Oil on canvas. Neues Palais, Potsdam

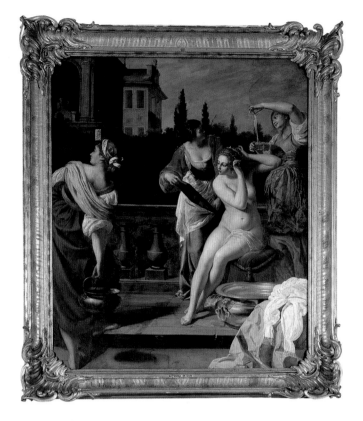

Figure 100. Artemisia Gentileschi, *David and Bathsheba*. Oil on canvas. Neues Palais, Potsdam

that she knew an engraving of a similar figure done by Claude Mellan (1598–1688) which may in turn have been based on Orazio's painting.[30] In Artemisia's late *Rape of Lucretia* (fig. 99), a work obviously based on Titian's prototype (Fitzwilliam Museum, Cambridge), Lucretia's pose is derived from the figure of Saint Francis in Orazio's early altarpiece in San Silvestro in Capite (cat. 25).

Unfortunately, the present exhibition will not be able to throw light on the two years Artemisia spent in London. Other than the magnificent *Self-Portrait as the Allegory of Painting* (cat. 81), we have no certain attributions during this time. This period of her career remains the great uncharted portion of her life. The motivation and circumstances of her trip to London, just prior to Orazio's death in 1639, remain shrouded in mystery. Artemisia does not figure in her father's will, drawn up in the early part of 1639. On the basis of this documentation, Gabriele Finaldi has argued that she must not yet have arrived in London, ruling out her participation in the ceiling paintings for the Queen's House at Greenwich (fig. 85), which had been installed by the middle of

1638.[31] However, her inheritance would probably already have been doled out to her in her dowry, and therefore her omission from the will is not proof that she was not in London. We cannot verify that Artemisia arrived before the canvases were finished in 1638, and the poor state of preservation of these paintings precludes any definitive judgment of her style.[32] Why, then, did Artemisia go to London? Her letters of 1635 indicate that she was an unwilling recipient of Charles's patronage. She was undoubtedly a devout Catholic and the prospect of working for a Protestant king may have elicited from her the same response experienced by Guercino, who described such employment as "dealing with heretics."[33] Familial loyalty was perhaps a factor, and she went to assist her father. Or possibly she was finally ready to quit Naples and was therefore open to other commissions, however disagreeable. In 1636, she wrote to Andrea Cioli, secretary of state to Cosimo II: "I have no further desire to stay in Naples, both because of the fighting and because of the hard life and the high cost of living." Naples suffered an earthquake in 1638–39, and after having already lived through one in 1631, Artemisia was in all likelihood ready to leave; the only situation that presented itself (in spite of concerted effort on her part to go elsewhere) was the Caroline court. Elizabeth Cropper's hypothesis (see p. 270), that Artemisia was employed as an emissary, a suitable successor to her father, may be correct, but this would explain why she was sought by the king, not necessarily why she overcame her initial reluctance to go. The trip was an arduous and dangerous one, requiring at least two to three weeks and entailing considerable discomfort. It could have been made entirely by sea (Livorno to London), entirely by land (through the Mont Cenis Pass and the city of Lyon), or by sea and land in combination, surely a journey not lightly undertaken.

Our assessment of this period and of Artemisia's career and of her attitude toward the work of her father remains of fundamental importance for our understanding of her final Neapolitan period (1640/42–52/53), the more than ten years she spent in Naples after her return from London. We have no evidence that she was in Naples continuously; nor do we know that she traveled. Regrettably, this phase of Artemisia's career cannot be well represented in the exhibition. Few of the late paintings are extant, and the masterworks, the two beautiful paintings in the Neues

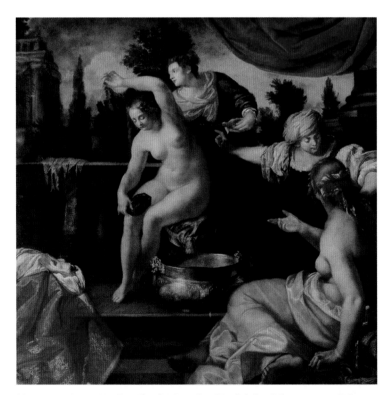

Figure 101. Artemisia Gentileschi, *David and Bathsheba*. Oil on canvas. Private collection, Vienna

Palais in Potsdam (figs. 99, 100), could not be removed from their setting (they are affixed to the wall) at the time of the exhibition. Currently, there are approximately one dozen paintings believed to date from the 1640s. Bissell lists twelve, of which eight seem to me to be reasonable attributions. Of these, three represent Bathsheba. It has been argued that Artemisia's repetition of a single composition testifies to her success in Naples (patrons as a rule requested popular works). But it has also been claimed that she became a far less imaginative and innovative artist while she was there. One is reminded of her letter to Don Antonio Ruffo of November 13, 1649, in which she was obviously responding to her patron's apprehension that she would not provide an original composition: "There was no need for you to urge me to do this, since by the grace of God and the Most Holy Virgin, they [clients] come to a woman with this kind of talent, that is, to vary the subjects in my painting; never has anyone found in my pictures any repetition of invention, not even of one hand."[34] Such an acknowledgment does not necessarily confirm diminished artistic vision, nor does it tell us her pictures were so popular that, incapable of meeting the demands of her clients, she was forced to repeat earlier compositions again and again. We simply do not know.

Yet, this preponderance of late *Bathsheba*s may create a new stereotype of Artemisia during her last decade. Knowing that she repeated the theme of Bathsheba in similar compositions, we expect her to repeat others and are predisposed to reject pictures that do not fit the mold. There may be other, less predictable paintings that have not yet been added to her oeuvre because they deviate from this expectation. One example is the small *Virgin and Child with a Rosary* from the Escorial (cat. 84), which, on first viewing, appears to be almost inconsistent with her production and which, in spite of a signature, still does not have universal acceptance.[35]

On the basis of the opulent appointments and elegant surfaces of the late *Bathsheba*s, some have formed the opinion that Artemisia returned from London reacquainted with the work of her father, having just seen the sumptuous late paintings that he made for the English court. And indeed, her attention to surface and detail, already noticeable in the 1630s, is surely evidence of a renewed interest in his stylistic temperament. Although the Columbus *Bathsheba* (cat. 80) is marked by a tone of poetic reverie, the later reformulations of the story focus on surface richness and material opulence. In this way, the *Bathsheba*s in the Uffizi and in a private collection (fig. 101), for instance, relate closely to Orazio's late *Finding of Moses* in the Prado (fig. 87) or the *Joseph and Potiphar's Wife* in Hampton Court (fig. 88). Certainly, some of this resemblance can be explained simply by Artemisia's voracious receptivity to the work of a range of artists, Orazio among them. The direct influence of one of Orazio's London paintings can be discerned in at least three of her late *Bathshebas*, exemplified by the version in Potsdam. The lovely figure carrying the water bucket at the left is undoubtedly based on a figure in Orazio's *Apollo and the Nine Muses* (fig. 93). By looking at the one picture in the exhibition that definitely dates to the 1640s, the *Susanna and the Elders* from Brno (signed and dated 1649; cat. 83), and seeing it together with Orazio's late canvases, we can begin to test the possible impact that Orazio's late art had on the final phase of Artemisia's career.

However, our assessment of the degree to which Artemisia relied on the work of her father in these late years is skewed by the small number of extant paintings and by the implicit acceptance of the Bathsheba pictures as emblematic of her late style. This paucity of examples is offset by a particularly dense documentation of her life through her letters. Nearly half the surviving correspondence was written between 1649 and 1651, although

it is difficult to know why. Admittedly, our comprehension of Artemisia's entire career is still plagued by conflict and inconsistency. The work often contradicts the evidence of documents and contemporary biographies, and may therefore not be representative. Early biographers tell us that she was known for her portraiture, although no certain examples other than the *Portrait of a Gonfaloniere* (cat. 66) exist. Similarly, the Florentine biographer Filippo Baldinucci, writing in 1681, lauded her talent at painting still lifes of fruit, although there is only one possible candidate.[36] Bissell published 108 lost works, and even if some of them are duplicate references, they outnumber the known works nearly two to one.[37] This is not unusual for artists before the nineteenth century, but, given the changeable nature of Artemisia's style, we are reminded that we have a far from accurate picture. The 1640s are perhaps the most problematic period to decipher. Artemisia Gentileschi is still a work in progress. While we may not yet be in a position to offer a definitive assessment, we can abandon the narrow stereotype of one view or another and accept this extraordinary artist as she presents herself—as incomplete as this picture is—and look forward to more of the unexpected.

1. Longhi (1916) lists forty paintings by Orazio, of which fifteen have general acceptance as autograph works: *Presentation in the Temple,* Rome; *Saint Thaddeus,* Rome; *Baptism of Christ,* Rome; *Saint Francis with an Angel,* Rome (cat. 21); *Saint Francis Receiving the Stigmata,* Rome (cat. 26); frescoes in the Casino of the Muses, Rome; *Madonna and Child,* Rome (cat. 4); *Vision of Saint Cecilia,* Milan (cat. 9); *David Contemplating the Head of Goliath,* Rome (cat. 18); *Annunciation,* Genoa; *Annunciation,* Turin (cat. 43); *Rest on the Flight into Egypt,* Vienna (cat. 45); *Saint Mary Magdalene in Penitence,* Vienna; *The Finding of Moses,* Madrid; *The Finding of Moses,* private collection (cat. 48).

   He lists thirty-one paintings by Artemisia, and of these eleven are currently accepted as authentic works: *Allegory of Inclination,* Florence; *Judith and Her Maidservant,* Florence (cat. 60); *Conversion of the Magdalene,* Florence (cat. 58); *Judith Slaying Holofernes,* Naples (cat. 55); *Annunciation,* Naples (cat. 72); *Judith and Holofernes,* Naples; *Self-Portrait as the Allegory of Painting (La Pittura),* London (cat. 81); *Birth of Saint John the Baptist,* Madrid (cat. 77); *Saints Proculus and Nicea,* Pozzuoli; *Adoration of the Magi,* Pozzuoli; *Saint Januarius in the Amphitheater,* Pozzuoli (cat. 79).

2. The exhibition included seven paintings and prints by Cassatt and seven works by O'Keeffe; Los Angeles 1976–77, 237–43, 300–306.

3. Wittkower and Wittkower 1963, 164.

4. As translated in Barthes et al. 1979, p. 41. The Italian reads: "Ne l'intagliar le corna a mio marito / Lasciai il pennello, e presi lo scalpello" (Battisti 1963). For other poems written about Artemisia after her death, less pointedly sexual in their descriptions but nonetheless focusing on Artemisia's physical beauty, see Bissell 1999, 166–68.

5. See in particular Pollock 1999, 97–167, and Bal 1996, 289–311.

6. Schleier first published the Farnese *Saint Michael* in 1962 and the late *Crowning with Thorns* in 1993, and with Diane De Grazia in 1994 recognized Orazio's shared authorship with Giovanni Lanfranco of the Washington *Saint Cecilia and the Angel.*

   Finaldi's 1999 exhibition "Orazio Gentileschi at the Court of Charles I" (London–Bilbao–Madrid) was the first devoted to Orazio and offered new archival material on his London period. It also presented the first opportunity to see his two versions of the *Finding of Moses* exhibited together.

7. McEwen (1999) noted the close affinity of Orazio's *Mocking of Christ* to his period of closest involvement with Caravaggio, suggesting it appeared to reflect more directly Caravaggio's influence. While no published reviews questioned the dating of this work, many exhibition visitors wondered whether the picture might not have been created earlier in Orazio's career. Schleier (1993) argued for placing the picture in Orazio's Genoese period.

8. See note 10 below.

9. Patrizia Cavazzini has found that Artemisia did not sign her depositions presented in the 1612 trial. In her view, this was because Artemisia did not know how to write, not even in simple block letters. Therefore, this calls into question who actually painted Artemisia's signature on the stone bench in the Pommersfelden painting.

10. Opinions as to the extent of Orazio's participation in the Pommersfelden painting vary widely. Before documentation came to light that established 1593 as the year of Artemisia's birth, the accepted date was 1597. Many scholars had difficulty believing that a thirteen-year-old girl would have had the ability to paint a canvas

with the technical sophistication of the *Susanna and the Elders*. As a result, Longhi (1943), Emiliani (1958b), Moir (1967), and Gregori (1968) attribute the painting entirely to Orazio. Some scholars, believing the date on the painting originally to have been 1616 or 1619, support an attribution to Artemisia: Ortolani (in Naples 1938), Borea (in Florence 1970), Marini (1981), and Rave (in Nürnberg 1989). Harris (in Los Angeles 1976–77), Garrard (1989), Spike (1991b), and Bissell (1999) all support an attribution to Artemisia but acknowledge her father's help in the design and execution of the piece (although Spike and Bissell argue for substantially more assistance from Orazio). Voss (1925), Harris (1989), Lippincott (1990), Papi and Contini (in Florence 1991), and Hersey (1993) all argue for Artemisia as the sole artist.

11. For the full text, see Tanfani-Centofanti 1897, 221–24.

12. For a summary of the opinions on the attributions of both paintings, see Mann 1996, 44 n. 2, 45 n. 5.

13. Garrard (1989, 244–73) devotes an entire essay to the *Cleopatra* as evidence of Artemisia's gendered interpretation of forceful female models, in this case a powerful queen shown just as she gains everlasting life, where the artist has transformed the death-delivering asp into a symbol of "divine immortality." Pollock (1999, 138–53) uses the painting to explore the indirect ways in which traumatic experience (in this case, the death of Artemisia's mother) can inform and inspire works of art.

14. For an overview of recent psychoanalytic and feminist analyses of Artemisia's works, see Spear 2000, 569–71. For the most recent discussion of gender as a tool for connoisseurship, see Garrard 2001, 1–6.

15. Pollock deals with this theme in 1999, chap. 5 (97–127), "The Female Hero."

16. Spike (1991b) raised the interesting possibility that Orazio was the artist of the Naples canvas. This attribution accounts, in his view, for the differences between the dramatic handling of the Capodimonte *Judith* and the more decorative, yet harder, treatment he notes in the Uffizi *Judith*.

17. Papi 2000, 451.

18. Genoa 1999–2000, 330, and Düsseldorf–Darmstadt 1995–96, 300–301 no. 146.

19. Bissell 1999, 338. See also the essay by Roberto Contini, in this publication.

20. Most studies devoted to the influence of Caravaggio acknowledge the wide disparity among those artists seen as followers and the tendency of most artists to adapt only one aspect of his style. Pepper (1987, 3–4) questions the validity of this label.

21. For a transcription in English of Orazio's deposition at the libel suit instigated by Giovanni Baglione in 1603, see Friedlaender 1955, 278–79.

22. Garrard (1989, 70, 504 n. 116) has argued that, given the proximity of the dwellings of Vouet and Artemisia and their shared patrons, it is logical to assume that they would have become friends.

23. See Gregori (in Naples 1984–85, 147), who notes that this view has changed and that Artemisia is instead seen as having learned from her experience of the art and the forces at work in Naples during the 1630s rather than having introduced new stylistic direction.

24. Thanks to Walter J. Karcheski, Senior Curator, Department of Arms and Armor, Higgins Armory Museum, Worcester, Mass., who was kind enough to share his vast knowledge with me; and also to Stuart Pyhrr, Curator in Charge, Department of Arms and Armor, The Metropolitan Museum of Art, who passed along valuable information on Artemisia's weapons via Keith Christiansen.

25. Soprani 1674, 316–17.

26. For the letter, see Crinò 1954, 205–6. For an English translation, see Garrard 1989, 377. The letter itself is dated February 10, 1619, as the calendar in use ended the year in March, just before the feast of the Annunciation (March 25). The modern date is, therefore, given as 1620. The newly discovered inventory for the sale of Artemisia's household and studio furnishings (appendix 3) indicates that she may have stayed in Florence until as late as February 1621 or (more likely, in my view) that she returned to Florence from Rome to settle her personal affairs.

27. On the collection of Cardinal Ludovico Ludovisi, the papal nephew, see Wood 1992, 515–23.

28. Gregori in Naples 1984–85, 150.

29. Lapierre 1998, esp. 13–17, 396–407; 2000, 3–6, 345–47.

30. Gregori in Naples 1984–85, 306; Garrard 1989, 106; Bissell 1999, 230.

31. Finaldi (1999, 32, 37 n. 84) cites a record of payment in the building accounts covering October 1637 to September 1638 for "putting up the Queen's canvases." He argues that this must refer to something more elaborate than the simple hanging of pictures and therefore associates it with the installation of the set of nine canvases for the Queen's House at Greenwich.

32. I wish to thank Patrizia Cavazzini for this information.

33. Malvasia (1678, vol. 2, part 4, 366) lists the reasons that Guercino, having been invited to the English court, chose not to go there, including "non volendo conversar con heretici. . . ."

34. Translated in Garrard 1989, 397.

35. Garrard (2001, 9) asserts that the attribution of the painting to Artemisia represents the perpetuation of "the inflated construct of Artemisia-the-beautiful." This judgment illustrates the difficulty in evaluating paintings that deviate from the established stylistic norms, and, to my mind, the danger of assuming that in all cases a painting by a seventeenth-century artist represents the personal inclination of the painter rather than an attempt to satisfy the tastes and perhaps explicit stipulations of a patron.

36. Bissell (1999, 106–7) has proposed the interesting hypothesis that this reputation for still life reflects a confusion between Artemisia Gentileschi and Giovanna Garzoni (1600–1670), a female still-life painter whose geographic career path paralleled that of Artemisia. The one possible candidate, a picture entitled *Still Life with Pastry Eater* (location unknown), bears an inscription attributing the painting to Artemisia Gentileschi and Giacomo Recco. The assumption has been that Recco (1603–before 1653) painted the still-life elements, given that the only known works by his hand are floral still-life paintings and the only certain attribution is a signed painting of flowers in a vase. If indeed this inscription is correct, it suggests that Artemisia was not a practitioner of still-life pictures, since, had she been known for this genre, it seems highly unlikely she would have relied on a collaborator to paint the foods and dishes.

37. Bissell (ibid., 373 no. L-49) lists lost *Judith Triumphant, with the Head of Holofernes,* recorded in a 1743 inventory among the holdings of the Calabrese nobleman Antonio Maria Lumaga. It seems quite likely that this picture may be the Capodimonte *Judith and Her Maidservant* (one of the three pictures listed in the palace of Ranuccio II Farnese, the sixth duke of Parma, in 1671), which bears an "L" on both the stretcher and the frame and also on the frame "Anticamera." The Lumaga *Judith* was identified as hanging in the Anticamera in the inventory (Getty Provenance Index), and the erroneous title may simply be a common title assigned to images of Judith even though the heroine was not explicitly shown holding the severed head aloft.

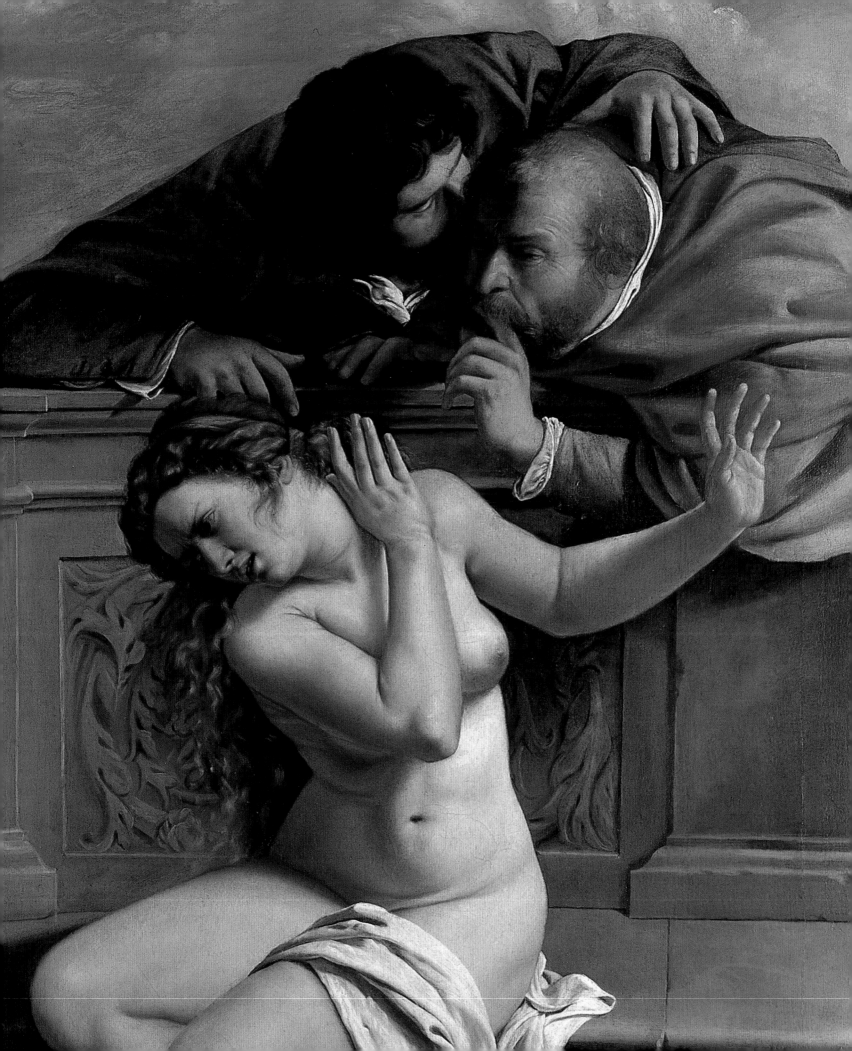

Life on the Edge: Artemisia Gentileschi, Famous Woman Painter

ELIZABETH CROPPER

For anyone who has thought about Artemisia Gentileschi (1593–1652/53) over a period of time, whether after reading Roberto Longhi's landmark essay "Gentileschi padre e figlia" of 1916, R. Ward Bissell's groundbreaking article of 1968, or even Mary Garrard's feminist monograph, published in 1989 (not to mention Bissell's subsequent catalogue raisonné of 1999), it comes as something of a shock to find the painter described as not only famous but even more famous than her father. For example, popular reviews of the small exhibition of Orazio Gentileschi's work at the National Gallery, London, in 1999 claimed that in recent years Orazio has been "condemned to live in the shadow of his daughter," and that in the late twentieth century a quirk of fate rendered Orazio less famous than Artemisia, whose "proto-feminist credentials" were enhanced by the fact that she was raped and by her specialization in subjects portraying victimized and vengeful women.[1]

Certainly, in the United States Artemisia Gentileschi was rediscovered by the first generation of feminist art historians. Her work was displayed to great effect in the exhibition "Women Artists: 1550–1950," organized by Ann Sutherland Harris and Linda Nochlin, which opened at the Los Angeles County Museum of Art in 1976. Harris writes in the catalogue that "Artemisia Gentileschi is the first woman in the history of western art to make a significant and undeniably important contribution to the art of her time," while conceding that "Artemisia was not a feminist by current standards."[2] This epochal exhibition was one of the sources of inspiration for Garrard's long dedication to the study of Artemisia's work, which culminated in the 1989 monograph *Artemisia Gentileschi: The Image of the Female Hero in Italian Baroque Art*. Garrard opens with the charge that "Artemisia has suffered a scholarly neglect that is almost unthinkable for an artist of her caliber," claiming that this neglect began in her own lifetime when she, like other women artists, was treated as an exotic figure in the art world, as a phenomenal woman rather than as an artist whose work mattered.[3] She recognizes the contribution of recent feminist scholarship in bringing Artemisia to public attention, but she regrets the continuing focus on the twin art-historical concerns of what she calls "biographical celebration," on the one hand, and connoisseurship at the expense of analysis of the expressive quality of Artemisia's work, on the other.[4] To occupy the space between biography and connoisseurship, Garrard takes the position that women's art is inescapably different from men's "because the sexes have been socialized to different experiences of the world."[5] As a consequence, she focuses less on the details of Artemisia's biography and more on the visual expression of women's experience, which in several cases leads her to a new (and controversial) conception of connoisseurship based on the gender of the artist.

Artemisia Gentileschi's life and work have since become a magnet for the exercise of every form of new art history. The results, as Richard Spear has recently documented, have been mixed.[6] Frequent connections have been made between Artemisia's rape by her father's colleague Agostino Tassi (1578–1644) in May 1611 and the violence of the subjects of early works, especially the two versions of *Judith Slaying Holofernes* now in Naples and Florence (cat. nos. 55, 62). Some writers consider these canvases straightforward expressions of Artemisia's need for revenge, whereas others have approached the problem psychoanalytically, in terms of the rape as trauma and the paintings as parallel expressions of images of childbirth and castration. Giving greater importance to specifically artistic experiences, Griselda Pollock has interpreted the two paintings as expressions of Artemisia's "self-definition as a painter."[7] The subject had been treated by Caravaggio (1571–1610), her father's great inspiration in the early 1600s (fig. 109), and then by Orazio himself (cat. 13). Pollock offers a reading of Artemisia's representations as signifying the decapitation of her "artistic fathers" in a version of the Oedipal struggle that is all the more violent because waged by a "daughter-painter—a woman in a genealogy of father figures."[8]

Paradoxically, much of this recent interpretation, which has sought to apply methods developing in the wider field of art history to the resolutely exceptional case of Artemisia, has further sensationalized her work. But this is not the same as understanding it. By contrast, the historian Elizabeth Cohen's research into the codes of honor constructed among the ordinary citizens of Rome in the late sixteenth and early seventeenth centuries changes our response to the legal record of Artemisia's rape through explicating its very conventionality.[9] Cohen explores the connections between such crimes as rape, "house-scorning" (or the shaming of a dwelling), and *sfregio* (or the slashing of someone's face) in terms of a complex code of family honor preoccupied by distinctions between "inside" and "outside," and constructed upon the analogy between house and body. Artemisia's enclosure in Orazio's house, described by Patrizia Cavazzini (see pp. 283–95), was an expression of her virginity; the taking of her virginity by Agostino Tassi was not just a violation of Artemisia's body but a penetration of Orazio's honor that brought shame to his whole family.

Today, no scholar would single out Artemisia's sexuality in the way that Longhi did in 1916, commenting that she must have been precocious in "everything, for which see the account of the Tassi trial"; or as Rudolf and Margot Wittkower did in 1963, calling her "a lascivious and precocious girl [who] later had a distinguished and highly honorable career as an artist"; or as even Eleanor Tufts did, in a feminist account written in 1974, claiming that Artemisia had numerous affairs and, despite the violence of her sexual initiation, wrote "superb" love letters.[10] Cohen's warning that Artemisia's reputation "continues to be violated in the present by an overly sexualized interpretation," in which she is both rape survivor and feminist heroine, is nonetheless totally warranted.[11] Cohen wisely declares that she is leaving interpretation of the paintings to the art historians, but her approach to the trial of Agostino Tassi for the deflowering of Artemisia, an approach that historicizes the rape and questions the relative importance of sexuality in the construction of the self in seventeenth-century Rome, has many implications for the analysis of Artemisia's work. Cohen argues that from a legal point of view, the crime of rape in early modern Italy was quite simply not metaphorized as gender oppression, or even necessarily seen by the violated woman as an attack on her self. Personhood, or personal identity, in other words, was more externally than internally directed. Looking at how Artemisia managed her responses within the conventions of the investigation and trial, Cohen identifies the personality of an assertive young woman defending her social honor rather than a victim seeking vengeance for attacks on the integrity of her body.

In Cohen's reconstruction of events, which is based on comparison with other similar cases, the business of the trial had to do with Tassi's failure to marry Artemisia. This would have been the proper conclusion to the familiar scenario of forcible deflowering followed by a promise of marriage, leading to regular sexual relations. Tassi was a liar and a wholly dishonorable man, and Artemisia, betrayed by everyone around her, risked losing far more than her virginity. Writing in 1612 to Cristina of Lorraine, grand duchess of Tuscany, imploring her to intervene in the case against Tassi to make sure that justice was done, Orazio Gentileschi lists his former colleague's dishonorable social characteristics: Agostino has three sisters in Rome who are all prostitutes, his wife is a prostitute, and so is his sister-in-law, with whom he has sexual relations; one brother was hanged, and another exiled for procuring sodomites; Agostino himself has been tried in Genoa, Pisa, Livorno, Naples, and Lucca, and in Rome he has been charged with incest, robbery, and other obscenities, and he has been beaten for theft.[12] In Rome, the only way Artemisia could be made whole was through the public condemnation of this scandalous man, and through providing her with a husband.

After practicing her profession for three years, she was, in her father's justifiable view, without equal, and she now needed the protection of the grand duchess in Florence to fulfill her promise. All of this Orazio accomplished: Tassi was sentenced, Artemisia was married to Pierantonio Stiattesi (born 1584), and after the wedding in 1612 the couple left for Florence. Artemisia's near miss with social ostracism was also a near miss with the destruction of all her hopes as a painter, for without a defined social standing she could not expect commissions for work. As a result of the grand duchess's support, she was to thrive as a female painter at the Medici court, even if simultaneously she suffered all the many familial difficulties of a woman of the artisan class.[13] In 1615, on the other hand, the Roman ambassador advised the grand duke's secretary not to invite Orazio to Florence because he claimed that Orazio was an incompetent figure painter and a thoroughly bad person. Tassi's influence was at work here, and his corrupt ways continued, leading to yet another trial in 1619 for having "amorous relations" with his sister-in-law Costanza.[14]

Not to submit Artemisia Gentileschi to a constant rehearsal of her rape—and to a modern reading of it at that—means not to view her work, especially from the early years, as primarily expressing her conscious or unconscious reaction to that rape. In struggling to find a better way to come to terms with her critical fortune, there is remarkable pressure to begin at the end of her story, for the beginning is just too shocking. It is also too well documented, for, with the exception of a handful of letters, Artemisia's own voice is never again heard so directly, and the "reality effect" of the legal account is overpowering. As a result, it becomes urgent to say that Artemisia Gentileschi had an influential career, which Bissell has now documented, and that she traveled to Venice, Naples, and even London to work for the most eminent patrons.

This need to resist the power of chronological events to condition our understanding of the "real" Artemisia Gentileschi is emblematized by the fact that one of the most important modern treatments of her life is a work of fiction that begins with an ending. Anna Banti's existential *Artemisia* (1947) opens at the end of World War II in 1944. The author looks out from the Boboli Gardens over the city of Florence, devastated by bombs—bombs that have destroyed not only the house she knew Artemisia had lived in, but also her own, and with it the manuscript of her book about the painter. In preparing that book, Banti, in her true, or other, persona as the art historian Lucia Lopresti, had clearly read the same trial documents we have been discussing. Banti / Lopresti was the wife of Roberto Longhi, then Italy's most authoritative art historian, who had written the first modern analysis of Artemisia's work in his expansive and exquisite prose, never, however, concerning himself with biographical details, except to say that Artemisia was "precocious" and that she was "the only woman in Italy who ever understood what painting was, both colors, impasto, and other essentials."[15] Banti's one-hundred-page manuscript, she gives us to understand, had been a history. Its loss turned the author to remembering. In that remembering, she records the voice of Artemisia from the documents concerning the rape, even as the painter herself appears in the novel to approve or correct what is said. This extraordinary

work, prompted by Artemisia's familiar voice coming to comfort the author at the sight of the destruction of so much of Florence's past and present, becomes a dialogue within Banti's conscience over the meaning and character of history and its relationship to fiction. It has often been pointed out that Banti's adoption of the notion of the *verosimile*, or the art of the probable, which permitted the inclusion of the *fatto supposto*, or supposition, as opposed to the literally true, was inspired by the great nineteenth-century novelist Alessandro Manzoni.[16] But though he was committed to telling the story of ordinary lives in his classic novel *I promessi sposi* (first ed. 1827), Manzoni never claimed, as Banti does, that the recounting of such lives—in her case the chronicle of "Agostino acquitted and released . . . ; Orazio Gentileschi returned to intellectual indifference slightly tinged with disgust; Artemisia condemned by her shortlived, scandalous fame to an unruly, besieged solitude"—provided material equal to a second Punic War. "It is not difficult to guess what the African elephants ate in Italy; it is not difficult to imagine how Artemisia passed the evenings in the summer of 1615," she insists provocatively, placing one woman's history on a level with the ancient battles recorded by Livy, and so revered by Italy's discredited fascist regime.[17]

At points Banti is convinced that what she is writing is not only probable but also true, but then, around the middle of the story when Artemisia is in Naples, the authoritative, validating voice of the painter is withdrawn. In her thoughtful study of the novel (1994), JoAnn Cannon argues that at this moment Banti, challenged by Artemisia, sees that she is falling into a patriarchal narrative, criticizing her as a woman who is a bad mother, a painter of doubtful quality, and someone who would rather be a man.[18] But the author's split with her subject, remembered from the earlier text, also comes about, I believe, because Artemisia's historical voice, so vividly present in the trial documents, is no longer to be found. The problem, in other words, is not only one of telling an outstanding woman's story according to the norms and expectations of society (whether hers or ours), but also that Artemisia's history is continually threatened by the overpowering documentary record of the rape, which renders her a victim for posterity.

Banti's novel works on many levels, and these are all relevant to our modern view of Artemisia. A successful writer, who adapted her talents to her life with a very famous man, Banti portrays Artemisia Gentileschi as constantly engaged in the struggle between the role of famous painter, extraordinary *because* female, and the more conventional familial relationships of daughter, wife, and mother. Then there is the closely related question of whether telling the story of Artemisia's life (which Longhi had so resolutely not done) damaged or supported her. As Banti realizes how she has imposed her sense of her own split self on Artemisia the woman and Artemisia the painter, she confesses to having dealt with her "as one woman to another, lacking manly respect."[19] By that manly respect she clearly means Longhi's way of dealing with Artemisia's work to the exclusion of her life, overlooking for the moment his misogynist asides. "Three hundred years of greater experience," she continues, "have not taught me to release my companion from her human errors and reconstruct for her an ideal freedom, the freedom that gave her strength and elation during her hours of work, of which there were many."[20] And yet there is a subtle irony in her comment that she cannot bring Artemisia alive "with these memories of her unhappy motherhood, the usual topic of women's conversation," for in a letter of 1649 Artemisia herself makes excuses to Don Antonio Ruffo for indulging in all this womanly chatter (chiacchiere femenili) about the expense of marrying off her daughter and her dependence on her patron for support.[21] This sort of historical evidence and the use she is making of it produce in the historian-novelist a crisis of conscience. Banti's honesty in confronting this crisis should not go unremarked, especially now that the intertwining of history and fiction is enjoying new popularity. She confesses her failure as follows:

> I now admit that it is not possible to recall to life and understand an action that happened three hundred years ago, far less an emotion, and what at the time was sadness or happiness, sudden remorse and torment, a pact between good and evil. I acknowledge my mistakes; and now that the ruins have been ruins for a year and show no sign of being in any way different from so many other, ancient ones, I limit myself to the short span of my own memory, condemning my presumptuous idea of trying to share the terrors of my own epoch with a woman who has been dead for three centuries. It is raining on the ruins over which I wept, around which sounds had a muffled, frightening quality that the first blow of a shovel dispelled for ever. Artemisia's two graves, the real and the fictitious, are now the same, breathed-in dust.[22]

Banti decides to continue her story, but only as an expiation and as an exercise in perseverance, closing the novel with the aging Artemisia's own realization, as she returns to Italy from London after the death of her father, that her own life might well end without dramatic incident, in her sleep.

The discipline of history itself has been transformed since Banti wrote. Statistical analyses, anthropological studies, and case histories have all advanced claims about the vero, or actuality, of the lives of persons, especially women, previously thought to be without a history, and whose stories are, as a result, now much more interesting than the diet of the elephants in the Punic wars.[23] These techniques have been borrowed by art historians asking new questions about the function, production, and reception of works of art as artifacts. But to determine just how they help us think about Artemisia Gentileschi, female artist, remains problematic. That we can now place Artemisia's rape in the context of the rapes of a Menica, Cecilia, Caterina, or Domenica; or that we can establish that Artemisia, like most young women of her class, probably couldn't read with ease; or—to turn to the familial—that we have recovered the names of her children and their godparents, and even how much she spent on enemas and sweetmeats during her pregnancies, means that we know a great deal more about Artemisia Gentileschi and her world than did Anna Banti, or even Garrard. Yet when we step outside microhistory and comparative historical reconstruction and turn to the particular matter of Artemisia's art we are immediately beset by methodological doubts, as Banti was the first to understand.

The organizers of the first exhibition dedicated to Artemisia Gentileschi, held at the Casa Buonarotti in Florence in 1991, set out to focus on the painter rather than the woman.[24] They did not succeed entirely in making this fresh start (for which they were also criticized), but their point was important. Without questioning the relevance of biography to art history in general, they wanted to call attention to the ways in which sociological and psychoanalytical approaches in particular had become fatally self-validating in Artemisia's case. In what had been, as they put it, a "sacrosanct, and almost ineluctable operation," the dramatic events of Artemisia's life had been turned into a feminist historical model. This operation had, however, just as ineluctably consigned Artemisia's work to second place to her life.[25] Contini and Papi sought to confront the fact that Artemisia had indeed become famous once again in our own times, but, as Banti had feared, and despite Garrard's best efforts, very much at the cost of her professional eclipse. Quite remarkably coming full circle, this position matches early feminist claims that Artemisia was treated only as an exception in her day, and somehow not as a real artist.[26]

Artemisia Gentileschi was, however, indisputably an exception in her day, and her exceptionality had much to do with the very same tension between life and work that continues to mark approaches to her story. In a succinct discussion of the evolving rights and communities available to women in Italy between the sixteenth and seventeenth centuries, Giulia Calvi (1992) emphasizes that neither the convent nor the family—women's two social worlds—were then considered separate or private spheres, as they were to be in the nineteenth century.[27] Rather, they were structures through which women could gain both influence and rights. What was increasingly denied to women was access to the social world of work: "marginal to the inner workings of corporations and confraternities, women were not recognised as having an identity as workers, but only in relation to their family status."[28] This is not to say that women did not work, for they often did. But, Calvi insists, women's work, so amply documented in tax records and censuses, remained "semiclandestine" and informal, both stimulated by and subordinate to family needs.[29] After failing to get Artemisia to join a convent, Orazio succeeded in getting her married, thereby providing her a social environment in which to function. That she had an extraordinary talent and that he passed on to her his skills as a painter made her highly unconventional, however, and immediately raised the issue of how she could continue to work in such a way as to gain public recognition. Work itself was what made her different from other women, and this is probably the single most important fact about her life. She was painting when Tassi seized her, and he shouted as he did so, "Not so much painting, not so much painting," before grabbing the palette and brushes from her hand and throwing them down.[30] It is as if he was as enraged by her working as he was inflamed by carnal lust: stopping her from working was the first step in his attempt to dominate her.[31]

If there were few examples for Artemisia to follow of a woman working at anything at all in a professional manner, for contemporary painters in general the whole question of work had become problematic, as academic discourse, sustained by increasingly aristocratic codes of conduct, emphasized the quality of painting as a liberal and intellectual practice.[32] This redefinition of painting manifested itself in many ways, but placed particular pressure on questions of price. When Artemisia refused to put a price on her mature work, even while complaining about the prices she got, she was participating in the same way as her contemporary Nicolas Poussin (1594–1665) in a highly complex mixed economy that combined feudal honor with market values. Artists of a less stoic outlook than Poussin sought to improve their social status in this hierarchical society through the achievement of knighthood. This meant, as in the case of Velázquez (1599–1660), establishing that one did not live from the fruits of one's labor.[33] For a woman who was not supposed to be engaged in the world of professional work in the first place, nor to be capable of producing more than children, such dissimulating devices presented a double bind. We will never understand Artemisia Gentileschi as a painter if we cannot accept that she was not supposed to be a painter at all, and that her own sense of herself—not to mention others' views of her—as an independent woman, as a marvel, a *stupor mundi*, as worthy of immortal fame and historical celebration, was entirely justified. Whether or not women were taken seriously as artists in the seventeenth century, Artemisia clearly was, and her very exceptionality was a sustaining principle in her career. None of this in any way resembles modern feminist critiques against having to make choices between work and family or of women artists not being taken seriously. None of it justifies Banti's lament that she had not allowed Artemisia the great ideal freedom "that gave her strength and elation during her hours of work," and none of it justifies thinking that Artemisia Gentileschi is "a gift to the twentieth century"[34]—or to the twenty-first.

*　　*　　*

In 1632, Artemisia Gentileschi painted an allegory of History (cat. 75). The muse Clio stands, three-quarter-length, looking upward to her left, her eyes shining and her full mouth slightly open in the hint of a smile, as if in recognition of inspiration or about to speak of a vision. She is identified as Clio by the lush laurel garland—a sign of immortality—on her head, and by the trumpet she balances with her right hand, an emblem of fame. This confident, passionate woman strikes a dominating and heroic pose, her left elbow bent, the back of her left hand resting on her hip. She wears glowing, rust-red sleeves and a low-cut white chemise with an intricate lace border at the neckline, over which is swathed a turquoise drapery of shining silk velvet. The luminous, pear-shaped pearl earring and the large brooches that clasp the drapery at her shoulders, not to mention the gold aglets, or tips on the cords attaching the sleeves, are bold ornaments which add to her majesty rather than serving as mere decoration. Artemisia signed and dated the work on the left page of the book open on the table, with a dedication, so far as can be determined, to François de Rosières (1534–1607), who had been named archdeacon of Toul and counselor to the duke of Lorraine by Cardinal Guise.[35] Garrard has suggested that the work was instead a posthumous tribute to another member of the large Rosières family, Antoine de Rosières II, seigneur d'Euvesin, first maître d'hotel of the duke of Lorraine, who died in Paris in 1631.[36] The garbled letters on the right appear to be Greek and probably refer to Thucydides.

This allegory and its history are both cautionary and exemplary. Given its connection to the Rosières family, the painting was likely made for Charles of Lorraine, fourth duke of Guise (1571–1640), whose family were great patrons of the Rosières.[37] Bissell's proposal that the reference on the book is to the earlier François de Rosières, whom Artemisia could not have known, has to do with the fact that there was good reason to commemorate François in an allegory of history. So great was François Rosières's debt to the house of Guise that he published a history of the family, the *Stemmata Lotharingiae ac Barri ducum* (1580). The genealogy was based on fake and falsified documents, designed to prove that the family was descended directly from Charlemagne. This was highly offensive to King Henry III of France (r. 1574–89), and Rosières only narrowly escaped execution. In 1632, when the picture was painted, Charles of Lorraine had cause to reflect on such turns of fate, for he too had fallen into disfavor with the king of France, Louis XIII (r. 1609–43). As governor of Provence, Charles had incurred the jealousy of Cardinal Richelieu, and went into voluntary exile in 1631. Charles settled in Florence, where Artemisia sent at least one painting to him. From Florence he wrote to a friend in 1631:

> If my oppression is longer than my life, that posterity which preserves dearly the memory of my fathers will judge fairly my own, will praise my constancy and my fidelity, will condemn the authors of my persecution, and will say what is known to good people, and that is that I am guilty of no other crime than the government of Provence.[38]

Artemisia's painting expresses this sense of history looking toward posterity for truth, and for true fame. On the other hand, the reference to Rosières raises the question of what true history is, and puts in doubt the status of documentary facts in the production of a historical work intended to flatter. This bitter yet optimistic invention implies that Rosières's history celebrating the duke's family will contribute to overcoming the calumnies against him. By accepting the allegory from Artemisia, the duke would also have accepted the witty implication of having such a work from the hand of a woman who had also been maligned, but who could now stand, like the figure of Clio, boldly and excitedly looking forward to establishing her fame and immortality.

I have said that the story of Artemisia's *Clio* is cautionary as well as exemplary. The work is cautionary above all because it raises questions about history and truth, implying, if Bissell's argument is correct, that history can be tampered with even if based on documents; and establishing beyond any doubt that in Artemisia's day history was not only about records and texts, but, more important, about posterity and immortal fame. Artemisia constantly identified her own person and skill with such fame, and every image of a forceful woman she painted has to be associated with its author in some sense. In this context the *Clio* is exemplary.[39]

Artemisia Gentileschi was not merely successful. She was famous. The first woman to enter the Accademia del Disegno in Florence, in 1614, Artemisia enjoyed Medici patronage and protection, especially through the grand duchess Cristina, to whom Orazio had recommended her, in 1612, as without equal.[40] She was associated with the Accademia dei Desiosi in Rome in the 1620s, and this reflects her protection by the house of Savoy. Jérôme David's engraved portrait (fig. 95) celebrating her connection with this academy calls her a most famous painter, "a miracle in painting, more easily envied than imitated."[41] Pierre Dumonstier dated his drawing of her hand (fig. 119) in December 1625, calling her the "excellent and knowledgeable Artemisia, Roman gentlewoman," and praising her hands as more beautiful than those of Aurora because they make marvels that ravish the eyes of those who judge best.[42] In Venice in 1627–28, Artemisia was the subject of several literary tributes from academic writers. Antonio Colluraffi's dedicatory inscriptions, published in 1628, address her as "Artemisia Gentilesca Romae concepta fama excepta," and as a greater painter than Apelles, greater than Zeuxis, and rival of the sun.[43] Colluraffi hesitated to attempt to praise the genius of such a "noble and celebrated painter," but did so, and in one of the two rather pedantic madrigals that survive he compares Artemisia to Rome herself: where the latter builds marvels, Artemisia paints *stupori*. In the second he compares her to the ancient painter Parrhasius: where the latter had painted a deceptive curtain over Zeuxis's illusionistic bunch of grapes, Artemisia "Gentil" deceives art itself and conquers nature. While in Venice Artemisia was paid for a *Hercules and Omphale*, commissioned for Philip IV, king of Spain (r. 1621–65), by the conde de Oñate as a companion to the *Discovery of Achilles* by Anthony van Dyck and Peter Paul Rubens for the Salon Nuevo in the Alcázar, Madrid.[44] This was an acknowledgment that she was one of the greatest painters in Europe, and its subject, depicting the demigod subjugated by a woman, deliberately celebrated her conquest of nature.

Artemisia left Venice to flee the plague in 1630. Her decision to go to Naples was motivated by the possibilities for patronage she saw there, given the Spanish viceroy's passion for purchasing paintings. Fernando Enríquez Afán de Ribera, third duke of Alcalá, acquired several paintings by Artemisia during his rule (see cat. 68), and she would receive commissions from Empress María of Austria, sister of Philip IV, and eventually from Philip himself.[45] Whereas in Rome, on her return from Florence, she had cultivated Cassiano dal Pozzo, secretary to Francesco Barberini (cardinal-nephew and a Florentine), and sold pictures to such collectors as the Patrizi, in Naples Artemisia succeeded in manipulating a much grander and more international market. In the 1630s, she was in a position to participate in converting her own reputation as a *stupor mundi* into real fame. Commissions linked her to contemporaries, and provided a showcase for her unique achievement. For example, she contributed, together with Massimo Stanzione and Paolo Finoglia, to the cycle of canvases dedicated to the life of John the Baptist for the hermitage of Saint John at the Buen Retiro in Madrid.[46] Artemisia's canvas (cat. 77) of 1633–35 gives center stage to the four women attending the bathing of the infant Baptist; it is in a mood quite different from that of the *Clio* of the previous year. Artemisia and Stanzione both adopted a humble, natural style for this eremitical commission, drawing out the implications of Caravaggio's Neapolitan works, and her capacity to do this reflects the high level of Artemisia's critical sophistication at the moment of her greatest influence on Neapolitan painting. A commission to a woman to paint an altarpiece was not unheard of—the Bolognese Lavinia Fontana (1552–1614) had painted several.[47] But it was still highly unusual, and in Naples in the mid-1630s Artemisia was commissioned to paint no fewer than three for the cathedral at Pozzuoli (cat. 79) as part of a renovation that also involved Giovanni Lanfranco, Francanzano, Finoglia, and Agostino Beltrano, all called "most famous and skillful" in a 1640 description.[48] In 1636, she received payment for a series of three quite different paintings (all untraced today)—a *Bathsheba*, a *Susanna*, and a *Lucretia*—from Prince Karl von Liechtenstein, an avid collector who obviously associated these alluring female subjects with the famous female painter.[49]

Artemisia was increasingly successful in manipulating her growing fame in this way, painting a limited set of subjects, and sometimes in pairs or larger groups. She continued to sell to local collectors, but her influential studio in Naples was, like Poussin's in Rome, also the center of complex patronage networks conducted either by post or through the agency of her brothers, who were sent throughout Europe in her service. Most illuminating for our understanding of Artemisia's exploitation of these networks and her management of her own fame is her letter of October 9, 1635, to her friend the astronomer and physicist Galileo Galilei (at that point in exile at Arcetri), asking for his help in securing a response from Duke Ferdinand II de' Medici to a painting she had sent him.[50] Describing herself as the duke's vassal and servant, she writes that she has fulfilled her obligation to him by giving him her work: in other words, the painting is in itself a payment from a social inferior, and so no payment is due in reply. What she does anticipate, however, is a favor from the duke as a demonstration of his pleasure, and his failure to respond is humiliating. "I have seen myself honored," she insists, "by all the kings and rulers of Europe to whom I have sent my works, not only with great gifts but also with most favored letters, which I keep with me." Among these Artemisia lists (without exaggeration) the kings of France, Spain, and England, and the duke of Guise, none of whose favors, however, could match that which she expects from her natural prince in Tuscany. By exploiting the conventions of courtly honor in this way, Artemisia could hope to place herself outside the marketplace, enhancing rather than diminishing her independence and dignity. She was also putting together her collection of tokens of respect, which could then be parlayed into yet more.

Artemisia was not afraid to play this game of favors, telling Duke Francesco I d'Este by letter in 1635 that she would rather work for him than for the English crown, and sending gifts of paintings to sway him.[51] She wanted very much to return to Florence in the 1630s, and in July 1635, in another name-dropping letter, she tells Ferdinand II de' Medici that Charles I, king of England (r. 1625–49), knows that her paintings for Philip IV are finished, which means she will have to accept his summons to London.[52] The duchess of Savoy had secured her a safe passage through France, and she would have to make use of it, even though she would rather work for the duke of Modena, Cardinal Antonio Barberini, and, of course, Duke Ferdinand himself.[53] Artemisia understood the value of intermediaries such as Galileo, using Andrea Cioli, secretary to the grand duke, to reach the Medici, and exploiting her friendship with Cassiano dal Pozzo to sell pictures to the papal family. With Cassiano she could be frank, explaining on October 24, 1637, that she is sending paintings for Cardinals Francesco and Antonio Barberini, for Monsignor Filomarino, and for himself, because she needs money to marry off her daughter.[54]

It is worth considering just why Artemisia did not succeed in persuading Ferdinand II to invite her back to Florence under his protection, and why she found herself in England in 1638. Given her obvious reluctance to go, the argument does not ring true that she was driven by filial devotion to help out her aging father as he completed the canvases for the ceiling of the Queen's House at Greenwich. The long-standing invitation from Charles I was obviously related to the presence of Orazio at court, but it was also stimulated by Artemisia's own reputation. Her lost *Tarquin and Lucretia* was almost certainly in the royal collection by 1634, providing the court with an example of the sort of passionate drama about a female protagonist for which she was so famous with other collectors.[55] That she had to make the arduous journey in person and present herself at court was something else, however. Given Francesco Barberini's attempts to live up to his responsibilities as cardinal protector to the Catholic queen Henrietta Maria in the increasingly hostile climate of the Protestant kingdom, it is tempting to see Artemisia as a part of his policy.[56] Artemisia's father had been more than a mere painter on his arrival from Paris in 1626; as the grand duke of Tuscany's ambassador observed, in addition to his art, Orazio "is also engaged in another matter of great importance, as he is often with the Duke of Buckingham and also with the King."[57] After the death of Buckingham, Orazio became the queen's painter rather than the king's. Like Artemisia, he wanted to return to Tuscany, but he was never invited back.[58] As he grew old and feeble, it was perhaps as important for the Barberini to have an emissary

in place, in the person of Gentileschi's daughter, as it was for the queen to get her decorations finished.

Orazio's death in February 1639 did not liberate Artemisia immediately, and in December of that year she wrote to Francesco I d'Este from London seeking his support by sending him a painting and stating quite openly that, despite the honors and favors she had received, she was not content in the service of Charles I. Duke Francesco, she wrote, would inspire her to make yet greater things, although she did not fail to let him know that despite her imperfections she had pleased "all the greatest princes of Europe."[59] Remarkably, we have no secure record of Artemisia between 1639 and 1642, when she was again in Naples, again enjoying great fame, and successfully manipulating it. Three works painted "by a woman called Artemisia" and depicting *Judith Cutting off the Head of Holofernes*, *Lucretia Romana Overcome by Tarquin*, and *Bathsheba Spied on by David*, appear in Giacomo Barri's description of the Palazzo del Giardino in Parma in 1671 (figs. 99, 100).[60] The evidence of the surviving paintings suggests a date in the late 1640s, and the subjects and location reveal that Artemisia was continuing her successful practice of painting images of virtuous and heroic women—often nude or nearly so—in series for patrons elsewhere.

There is no reason to think that Artemisia's fame was in decline before her death in 1652/53. In Naples, her paintings appear in inventories of many noble collections, as well as in those of bankers such as the Genoese Davide Imperiale; in Rome in 1644 her *Sleeping Venus* in the Barberini collection (see cat. 70) was already so prized that it was covered by a green taffeta curtain, just as Caravaggio's *Victorious Cupid* (Staatliche Gemäldegalerie, Berlin) had been in the Palazzo Giustiniani.[61] However, the fortuitous survival of her letters to the famous collector Don Antonio Ruffo in Messina, Sicily, allows us, *pace* Anna Banti, to see the human side of a woman no longer strong or resilient in body.[62] The letters, written between 1649 and 1651, which concern commissions to Artemisia to paint the now predictable favorite subjects with female protagonists—*Galatea* (lost?), the *Bath of Diana*, a *Liberation of Andromeda*, and a *Joseph and Potiphar's Wife* (all three are lost)—are filled with sharp comments on price and value, and Artemisia even states at one point that she needs work desperately because she is bankrupt and has been sick. At the same time, Artemisia never renounces her multiple roles as a faithful vassal serving her lord, as an abject serf needing the protection of his household, and finally as the famous painter whom he must honor. She sends him little painted favors—a *Madonna*, for example, and a *Self-Portrait* (both are lost)—that he is is to hang in his gallery "as all the other Princes do."[63] Least of all does she relinquish her role as *woman* painter, as the following sample of her comments illustrates: "You feel sorry for me because a woman's name raises doubts until her work is seen";[64] "I shall not bore you any longer with this female chatter. The works will speak for themselves";[65] "And I will show Your Most Illustrious Lordship what a woman can do, hoping to give you the greatest pleasure";[66] "You will find the spirit of Caesar in this soul of a woman."[67] Remarkable is her insistence that women have the power to invent and not simply copy, whether nature, the work of others, or even their own. She is deeply upset that Ruffo should have urged her to be sure that a *Galatea* commissioned for his friend should be different from his, for she is fully able to vary her subjects, and no one has ever found the slightest repetition in her work—"not even of a single hand," she exaggerates.[68] Artemisia complains that she has been cheated by people who have taken her drawings in order to have her ideas executed by others, concluding, "If I were a man, I can't imagine it would have turned out like this, for when the invention has been realized and defined with lights and darks, and established by means of planes, the rest is a trifle."[69]

That Artemisia had—and could have—no large fresco commissions did not lessen her fame. As the decades of her life passed, the easel painting became the more prestigious format, collected and hung in galleries large and small. That Artemisia became famous for painting virtuous and heroic women and female nudes might seem at first more compromising for her fame, both during her lifetime and for posterity. It implies that she was prepared to specialize her production for the market, and it suggests, as Harris has put it, that she was prepared to depict "what 20th century feminists have labelled 'woman as sex object'" for a male audience.[70] The first issue is the more quickly disposed of, though it is not uninteresting. The ideal of the universal painter who excelled in everything and in all styles—high, middle, and low—was still current in the 1630s, but it was under considerable pressure in practice. Caravaggio had disdained the tradition of *disegno* and had introduced new subjects for painting, taking his models from the street, preferring the direct imitation of nature to the improvement of nature through the imitation of the great

tradition of art. Given critical authority by his success, a whole generation of artists, especially those Northerners identified as the "gothic plague" by the painter Francesco Albani, ceded the idea of universality to the Italian Old Masters and began to produce scenes of city life, landscapes, and battle pictures for the new market supplying Roman picture galleries. Michelangelo Cerquozzi was known as "Michelangelo delle battaglie" because he painted battles, and Pieter van Laer as "Il Bamboccio," from the clumsy little figures he put in his genre scenes; Claude Lorraine was commissioned by noble and patrician patrons to paint so many landscapes and harbor views, often in pairs, that he had to keep track of them in his *Liber veritatis*; a portrait by Van Dyck was an essential sign of distinction in a noble collection; in Florence, Filippo Napolitano painted detailed still lifes and little landscapes for the grand duke while Artemisia was there, and decades later in Naples the Recco and Ruoppolo families produced lush still lifes of fish, meat, and fruit. Even Poussin, whose inventions belonged to the tradition of universal painting, was known for his easel paintings with small figures that seemed grand, and which had their proper place in galleries, often in pairs or series; he never painted in fresco.[71] By the 1630s and 1640s it would have been unusual, not to say unrealistic, for Artemisia not to have a specialty. In 1651 Andrea Sacchi, a universal painter, lamented that the great tradition of the Carracci was over.[72]

For Artemisia to have made her reputation as a painter of large canvases showing virtuous women and female nudes, sometimes in the same person, is more difficult to explain, and is probably the most controversial issue raised by this exhibition. In relation to the popularity of images of virtuous women in the seventeenth century, Garrard has usefully summarized the literature of feminism and antifeminism in northern Europe, associating this with the rise and fall of Queen Marie de' Medici (1573–1642).[73] She traces the emergence of interest in the *femme forte* to around 1630, and points to the influence of Marie's own patronage and that of her daughter-in-law Anne of Austria in propagating the imagery of such heroic female figures as Minerva, Judith, Jael, and Zenobia. Unfortunately, Garrard dismisses this fascination with the exceptional woman, even in high culture, as just one more manifestation that women could be heroic only when they behaved like men, and that men accepted strong women only in the context of the marvelous and of the world-turned-upside-down—and then only when presented in emblematic or mythological form. Garrard imputes her own rejection of this tradition to Artemisia herself, linking that rejection to her reading of Artemisia's style:

> Unlike the femmes fortes framed by moralizing verses and immobilized by their emblematic format, Artemisia's Judiths are armed with swords that cut, weapons they do not hesitate to use. And unlike the beautiful Susannas, Lucretias, and Cleopatras of men's art, who wriggle seductively even in extremis, Artemisia's nude heroines convincingly experience pain and emotional anguish. In her oeuvre, the stereotypes are inverted: evil women—Cleopatra, Potiphar's Wife—become heroic; saintly characters—the Virgin, Lucretia, Mary Magdalen—exude a meaty vitality.[74]

Garrard's argument is that Artemisia took up the current fascination with images of strong women and, through the lucky accident of her Caravaggesque vocabulary, developed a sort of fusion of real and archetypal female body, reversing traditional expectations of the nude. By providing "a visual model in which mundane women might recognize themselves," Artemisia provided a way through which "all women—beautiful or plain, heroic or ordinary, powerful or powerless—might live vicariously in art."[75] Garrard suspects that this disappointed patrons more accustomed to the "plumply seductive figures" of Titian or Rubens, but that their erotic expectations were satisfied by being displaced onto the idea of the woman painter herself.

Garrard's claims about Artemisia's nudes have not met with general approval.[76] Nonetheless, much of the criticism of her work is marked by similar assumptions that we can read Artemisia's female self and female experience into these pictures, and that we can gain direct access to their eroticism, or lack of it, in relation to either the artist's intention or a work's reception. George Hersey, for example, brings the issue back to Artemisia's rape and the theory that the psychic wound she suffered led her to paint personal protests throughout her life in the form of a public art devoted to meditations on "sex, victimization, and sanguinary death."[77] Agreeing with Garrard that it was the absent artist who titillated rather than the painted body, Hersey suggests that Artemisia succeeded because behind the "gawkiest Susanna and most massive Judith," the collector would always imagine the beautiful artist. Unlike Garrard, he does not regret this, seeing it as part of Artemisia's own successful enterprise. Harris is also interested in how Artemisia Gentileschi marketed herself in her work, but focuses on the Susanna and the Elders of 1610 (cat. 51)

rather than on the bloody Judiths. This was Artemisia's originary statement on the virtuous female nude, painted before her rape, in which the figure is far from "gawky." Harris calls attention to the new popularity of this subject in the early seventeenth century, seeing in Artemisia's deliberate choice of it "an awesome degree of ambition" and in her execution a "brilliant synthesis of the art of Annibale and Caravaggio," which demonstrates her capacity as a painter of human action and her claims to take her place among the painters of her generation.[78] Most significant for Harris is the "striking realism" of the figure of Susanna, and she believes that Artemisia took her proficiency in painting the female nude as a sort of manifesto, suggesting that it was usual for ambitious artists to make such demonstrations at the beginning of their careers.[79] In Artemisia's case, the manifesto was not about victimization or rape but a declaration "that she could paint women better than anyone else then working in Rome."[80] Bissell is largely in agreement with all this, recognizing that Artemisia's themes of violence and eroticism were popular, and proposing that because she was a woman Artemisia would quite naturally have felt a special sympathy with female heroes and a desire to represent them. As time went on she, like other painters, simply became associated with a special repertory that would have been difficult to change.

Harris's idea of the Susanna and the Elders as a kind of manifesto goes very much to the heart of the matter, though the work had to be more than a competitive professional declaration for a young woman to whom such competition was not open. The painting is deeply shocking, perhaps even more so than the fierce drama of the two versions of Judith Slaying Holofernes (cat. nos. 55, 62). Rather than offering a new reading of this work or rehearsing the various feminist and psychoanalytic interpretations already in print, I would hope to help the viewer rediscover its shock value, for this is by no means obvious anymore. So remarkable is this work by the seventeen-year-old Artemisia that attempts have been made in recent years to take it away from her and give it to Orazio, or at least to give credit for its invention to him.[81] Yet Orazio himself was not experienced in painting the nude, and the closest he had come to painting one by 1610 was, probably, the lost Saint Michael the Archangel, exhibited in 1602 at San Giovanni dei Fiorentini, followed by the David Contemplating the Head of Goliath (cat. nos. 18, 19) and the Saint Jerome (lost, and cat. 16), in which male figures are more than decorously draped, with only their limbs and chests bare. Orazio's lack of experience in painting the *female* nude before 1610 is not surprising given the source of his realism in the work of Caravaggio, who, it is often pointed out, for all his attachment to the natural model, never painted one. The Carracci, by contrast—it is also often pointed out—were quite fascinated by female nudes depicted in erotic scenes, but these were usually mythological, and the bodies they introduced reflect little attention to the flesh of the natural model, privileging instead the more ideal forms of ancient sculpture. Yet both the Carracci and Caravaggio were to be implicated in scandals having to do with the depiction of the body.

In the early 1590s, Agostino Carracci (1557–1602) produced a group of prints known as the *Lascivie*, which showed a variety of sexual encounters between men and women in the images of *Susanna and the Elders*, *Lot and His Daughters*, *Andromeda*, *Orpheus and Eurydice*; female nudes in the form of *Galatea*, the *Three Graces*, *Venus Beating Cupid*; and several overtly pornographic images of naked women and satyrs.[82] The *Susanna and the Elders*, in which one of the old men masturbates as the other grabs the frightened woman, is far more sexually explicit than anything in painting around 1600, but it reminds us that erotic readings of these subjects (almost all of them treated later by Artemisia) could never have been far from the surface, regardless of the sex of the painter. Several women in these small, informal works resemble a natural model, even if they are also transformed by art. The prints were wildly successful and made a great deal of money for the artist and the publisher until they were condemned by Pope Clement VIII (r. 1592–1605), much to Agostino's embarrassment and shame.

The suppression of such erotica by the pope, a reprise of Clement VII's (r. 1523–34) condemnation of Marcantonio Raimondi's engravings of *I modi*, was only partly an exercise of predictable moral censorship. On a less obvious level it also manifests awareness on the part of the Church of the potentially dangerous licentiousness of art more generally. The Catholic Reformation encouraged the dramatic expression of religious experience through a greater naturalism in painting and a more direct appeal to the emotions through music and action in drama. This could lead only to an intense concentration on the expressive power of the human body, and with that came the possibility of evoking empathetically passions that were not so easily controlled—those very emotional expressions that have come to define the Baroque style. The Carracci Academy in Bologna, inspired by calls for the reform of religious art, accomplished the reform of art through a return to drawing from nature: out of the natural, through the imitation of art, the Carracci produced painting that was verisimilar, or persuasive, but within the traditions of art and decorum. Caravaggio took a different approach, determined to provide a convincing illusion of the actual through representing the natural without idealizing it. Caravaggio's revolution has been integrated into the history of art, together with its sensationalism, and it is now essential for the understanding of painting in the first years of the seventeenth century to insist once again upon the shocking nature of his practice. As Giovan Pietro Bellori would complain later in the century, Caravaggio led all the young artists in Rome to think that they could simply undress a model, direct a light to the figure, and paint.[83]

Much has been made of the prohibition in the Accademia di San Luca in Rome in the early seventeenth century against the study of the female nude, and later proscriptions in the French Academy against women drawing from the nude have been cited in connection with Artemisia's supposedly limited artistic education.[84] Harris, for example, claims that "the only women that unmarried men could see undressed were prostitutes, when the viewing time was usually brief."[85] By contrast, she complains that Artemisia was denied access to the male body as a young woman, and that she would have had little opportunity to see ancient sculptures. Certainly control over the natural body and its representation was one of the powers that the Accademia di San Luca tried to claim. This academy, founded during the papacy of Clement VIII under the protection of Cardinal Federico Borromeo, was more an instrument for policing the behavior of artists and the moral practice of art than a place for individual education. Such events as the publication of Agostino's *Lascivie*, the appearance of Titian's *Bacchanals* and other secular art in the city, and the parallel difficulty of maintaining a decorum of viewing in new palaces and galleries made for attempts at a policy of repression. Yet informal study of the nude, and even the female nude, was a standard practice in the cinquecento, especially in Venice and in Florence, where it had deep roots in the precepts of Leonardo. What was new about Caravaggio's position, and what made it threatening to the new morality, was not that he produced works of erotic subject matter but that even for religious history paintings he required the constant presence of the model,

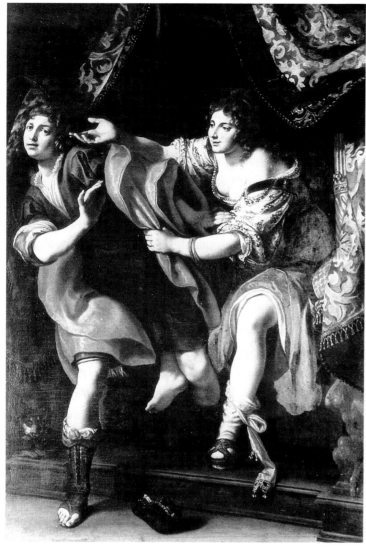

Figure 102. Lodovico Cigoli (1599–1613), *Joseph and Potiphar's Wife.* Oil on canvas. Galleria Borghese, Rome

way as to make her own pact with the viewer. Artemisia the painter seized the moment to make such a contract in the only way that she understood to be open to her from her training with her father, which is to say through her own unique female body, signed and dated. That this self-presentation would inevitably incur shame and charges of licentious display is also already understood in the very subject of *Susanna and the Elders* (which so far as we know was not commissioned), and that immediate threat of shame is an essential part of her self-portrait in this frontispiece to her career.[98]

In the same year that Artemisia signed and dated her *Susanna and the Elders*, Lodovico Cigoli completed a *Joseph and Potiphar's Wife* (fig. 102) for the bishop of Arezzo, which was quickly acquired

by Cardinal Scipione Borghese.[99] An excited, fleshy woman, her fancy embroidered clothes quite disheveled, tries to grab a young man as he flees her richly appointed bed with heavy damask curtains. She succeeds only in grasping his cloak with her left hand, on one finger of which she wears a wedding ring; this cloak is the proof she will use against him when she tells her husband that he has tried to violate her. Cigoli's painting presents an exact role reversal of Artemisia's *Susanna*, and the comparison is instructive. Where Artemisia's picture is a grave masterpiece of concentration, Cigoli's composition is amusing and theatrical, and has been linked appropriately to the popularity of new lyrical styles of musical drama in Florence. In its dramatic hyperbole, the *Joseph and Potiphar's Wife* sets the stage for Artemisia's future works, especially the Naples *Judith Slaying Holofernes* (cat. 55). When she and her new husband arrived in Florence in late 1612 or early 1613, Artemisia found many more examples of this sort of dramatic painting, and also a great taste for it at the Medici court. Cristofano Allori's *Judith with the Head of Holofernes* (Galleria Palatina, Florence; see the version reproduced in fig. 103), for example, famously shows the painter's lover, Mazzafirra, playing the role of Judith, her mother as the old maid, and the features of Allori himself in the head of Holofernes, with Judith decked out in rich silks and satins and furnished with cushions and curtains.[100] Bringing to bear her own special approach of painting from the model, Artemisia quickly adapted this theatrical manner, and out of her experience in Florence she forged the style that made her famous. All the more important, therefore, is the painting of *Inclination* (fig. 110), which Artemisia produced for Michelangelo Buonarroti the Younger in 1615–16. The patron was a close friend, as was Allori, who stood godfather to Artemisia's second son on November 9, 1615. Artemisia was a married woman, twenty-two years old, when she painted this work, and she was fulfilling a prestigious commission for the decoration of the gallery that celebrated the genius of the great Michelangelo Buonarroti. The subject, derived directly from Cesare Ripa's *Iconologia*, was given to her, and it required the appearance of a nude young woman bearing a compass, and with a star above her head.[101] Artemisia, her own body recovering from the birth of her second child, now painted a second version of her Roman nude, one that was no longer threatened by shame.[102] Where Susanna looks away, Inclination looks upward in anticipation, her mouth half open, like a younger version of the Muse of History in the *Clio*.

Opposite: Detail of *Judith and Her Maidservant* (cat. 60)

their limbs and chests bare. Orazio's lack of experience in painting the *female* nude before 1610 is not surprising given the source of his realism in the work of Caravaggio, who, it is often pointed out, for all his attachment to the natural model, never painted one. The Carracci, by contrast—it is also often pointed out—were quite fascinated by female nudes depicted in erotic scenes, but these were usually mythological, and the bodies they introduced reflect little attention to the flesh of the natural model, privileging instead the more ideal forms of ancient sculpture. Yet both the Carracci and Caravaggio were to be implicated in scandals having to do with the depiction of the body.

In the early 1590s, Agostino Carracci (1557–1602) produced a group of prints known as the *Lascivie*, which showed a variety of sexual encounters between men and women in the images of *Susanna and the Elders, Lot and His Daughters, Andromeda, Orpheus and Eurydice*; female nudes in the form of *Galatea*, the *Three Graces, Venus Beating Cupid*; and several overtly pornographic images of naked women and satyrs.[82] The *Susanna and the Elders*, in which one of the old men masturbates as the other grabs the frightened woman, is far more sexually explicit than anything in painting around 1600, but it reminds us that erotic readings of these subjects (almost all of them treated later by Artemisia) could never have been far from the surface, regardless of the sex of the painter. Several women in these small, informal works resemble a natural model, even if they are also transformed by art. The prints were wildly successful and made a great deal of money for the artist and the publisher until they were condemned by Pope Clement VIII (r. 1592–1605), much to Agostino's embarrassment and shame.

The suppression of such erotica by the pope, a reprise of Clement VII's (r. 1523–34) condemnation of Marcantonio Raimondi's engravings of *I modi*, was only partly an exercise of predictable moral censorship. On a less obvious level it also manifests awareness on the part of the Church of the potentially dangerous licentiousness of art more generally. The Catholic Reformation encouraged the dramatic expression of religious experience through a greater naturalism in painting and a more direct appeal to the emotions through music and action in drama. This could lead only to an intense concentration on the expressive power of the human body, and with that came the possibility of evoking empathetically passions that were not so easily controlled—those very emotional expressions that have come to define the Baroque style. The Carracci Academy in Bologna, inspired by calls for the reform of religious art, accomplished the reform of art through a return to drawing from nature: out of the natural, through the imitation of art, the Carracci produced painting that was verisimilar, or persuasive, but within the traditions of art and decorum. Caravaggio took a different approach, determined to provide a convincing illusion of the actual through representing the natural without idealizing it. Caravaggio's revolution has been integrated into the history of art, together with its sensationalism, and it is now essential for the understanding of painting in the first years of the seventeenth century to insist once again upon the shocking nature of his practice. As Giovan Pietro Bellori would complain later in the century, Caravaggio led all the young artists in Rome to think that they could simply undress a model, direct a light to the figure, and paint.[83]

Much has been made of the prohibition in the Accademia di San Luca in Rome in the early seventeenth century against the study of the female nude, and later proscriptions in the French Academy against women drawing from the nude have been cited in connection with Artemisia's supposedly limited artistic education.[84] Harris, for example, claims that "the only women that unmarried men could see undressed were prostitutes, when the viewing time was usually brief."[85] By contrast, she complains that Artemisia was denied access to the male body as a young woman, and that she would have had little opportunity to see ancient sculptures. Certainly control over the natural body and its representation was one of the powers that the Accademia di San Luca tried to claim. This academy, founded during the papacy of Clement VIII under the protection of Cardinal Federico Borromeo, was more an instrument for policing the behavior of artists and the moral practice of art than a place for individual education. Such events as the publication of Agostino's *Lascivie*, the appearance of Titian's *Bacchanals* and other secular art in the city, and the parallel difficulty of maintaining a decorum of viewing in new palaces and galleries made for attempts at a policy of repression. Yet informal study of the nude, and even the female nude, was a standard practice in the cinquecento, especially in Venice and in Florence, where it had deep roots in the precepts of Leonardo. What was new about Caravaggio's position, and what made it threatening to the new morality, was not that he produced works of erotic subject matter but that even for religious history paintings he required the constant presence of the model, posed before him in the studio, without in any way distancing himself from that model through the practice of drawing or the deployment of memory and tradition. The model's subject position could be defined as torture, as it was in ancient criticism, or as sexual exploitation, as in the extraordinary case of Benvenuto Cellini (1500–1571).[86] Caravaggio's practice, which was not at all masked in his work, challenged authority on every level, artistic, religious, and social.

Caravaggio brought scandal upon himself at every turn. The story of his attack in Rome on a young art student who had stopped to buy candles on his way home from a late night session at the Accademia di San Luca is almost too good to be true. But it is telling that he also got into a fight with the notary Mario da Pasqualone, who wanted to marry Lena, the poor young woman who had served as the model for the *Madonna di Loreto* (Sant' Agostino, Rome). Lena had done this with her mother's consent and had been paid for it, but the young man chastised the mother for letting this happen, and so Caravaggio retaliated by attacking him from behind with his sword in the Piazza Navona.[87] There was no suggestion that Caravaggio had misused Lena, but we are again in the world of domestic honor, and of what was allowed to an unmarried young woman's family if it wished to preserve that honor. To insult Caravaggio's shocking *Death of the Virgin* (Musée du Louvre, Paris) critics said that the artist had painted a prostitute who had been his lover.[88] That prostitutes did serve as models (and were not only glimpsed in the dark) is clear from Cardinal Paleotti's warning against just this practice. But whether prostitute or not, a woman, especially an unmarried one, was quickly tainted with scandal if she served as a model, even for a Virgin. And a painting of the Virgin, as much as that of a nude, ran the risk of slipping into lasciviousness if not properly controlled by decorum and the conventions of style.

The matter of the body is central to artistic culture about 1600, and it is especially important to Artemisia's story, for this is where fame and infamy come together in her battle for posterity. The documentation of her rape is rife with bodily reference, going well beyond the account of the event itself to constant implications with the world of work. Tuzia, a woman who was supposed to be chaperoning the motherless Artemisia, mentions an ugly youth named Francesco with long black hair, whom the Gentileschi both used as a model. Marco Antonio Coppino, a Florentine who had lived in Rome for twenty years, and who

mixed ultramarine, claimed that not only was Artemisia a whore but that he had heard in various shops that she "was a beautiful woman, that her father did not want her to marry, made her pose in the nude and liked for people to look at her."[89] When Giovan Pietro Molli of Palermo went to Orazio's house to model, he saw Artemisia there *in the rooms where work was done*.[90] Orazio's barber, Bernardi di Francesco de Francheschi, testified that he had modeled for Orazio over a period of nearly eighteen years, which is to say for almost all of Artemisia's life. A Spaniard, Pietro Hernandes, testified that he had seen Artemisia, his son's godmother, teaching a young man to paint. This was Nicolò Bedino, who testified that he had ground colors for Artemisia to use in her canvases while her father was away working at Monte Cavallo. Margherita, the washerwoman, testified to the presence of four men, each of whom she could name, in Orazio's house, and to the fact that she knew he had used them as models because he had shown her the paintings for which they had posed. Many questions were asked in the inquiry about the layout of the Gentileschi house, which was not large, and where eating and working spaces adjoined. Clearly Artemisia had witnessed her father's experiments in painting from the model, inspired by Caravaggio, and the *Susanna and the Elders* is the evidence that she shared in them. (On this practice, see Christiansen, pp. 9–12.)

We cannot actually prove or disprove the claim that Orazio had Artemisia pose in the nude, though it is thought that Orazio did use her as a model in such works as the *Young Woman Playing a Violin* (cat. 40; but see cat. 39). Nor can we establish beyond doubt that she painted from the various models hired by Orazio to come to the house throughout her early life—in the case of Molli, stripping to his belt to serve as Saint Jerome. But there is ample evidence that by 1612 Artemisia had been painting for several years in a household where models came and went, that she painted while her father was not present, and that she was able to teach youths to paint in her father's absence, and in a way that was based on the study of the model. As in the case of Caravaggio's Lena, for the model to have posed fully dressed would not have been enough to prevent scandal; and, as I have suggested, painting directly from the model at home, as opposed to drawing from the model in the disciplined academy, was in itself still shocking in 1610. In this context, as Keith Christiansen argues here, the attribution of the *Cleopatra* (cat. nos. 17, 53) to Orazio rather than to Artemisia takes on extraordinary power.[91] For even if Harris's view that unmarried men glimpsed female bodies only in brief moments of passion is humorously exaggerated, the difficulty faced by Orazio in obtaining a female model who would pose in the nude should not be underestimated. Working beside him in the studio, Artemisia was an obvious candidate. If indeed the *Cleopatra* and the *Susanna and the Elders* were produced at the same time, in the same house, by father and daughter, with Artemisia serving as model in both cases, then much about these bodily forceful works becomes clearer. Sixteen ten would be the year in which the Gentileschi brand of Caravaggism (practiced by both father and daughter) took its new direction, a direction that Orazio did not pursue after the departure of his daughter for Florence, but which Artemisia would continue to explore in more rhetorical ways. According to this chronology, the new direction in the Gentileschi studio around 1610 involved the bodily presence of Artemisia as both model and painter, and was as shocking as Caravaggio's earlier employment of ordinary, undisguised people as models. That the actors in the studio romance which so fascinated gossips were a widowed father and an unmarried daughter, or a woman painter and young male assistants, could only add to the threat of infamy. The extraordinary *Allegory of Painting* now in Le Mans (cat. 64), whoever painted it, and whether it refers to Artemisia or not, is testimony to a prurient and lascivious fascination with the female body in the context of the studio.[92] It is something like a visual equivalent to the sexually loaded gossip of the rape trial.

We would be wrong to imagine the Gentileschi living in a tidy household such as that portrayed by Federico Zuccari in his frescoes in his own house in Florence, or even in his drawings of the life of his brother Taddeo.[93] In 1603, Baglione's libel suit brought against Orazio, Caravaggio, Onorio Longhi, and Filippo Trisegni for writing slanderous sonnets against him led to Orazio's arrest. Artemisia was ten, with two younger brothers in the house to take care of after her mother's death. She couldn't read the poems and letters taken from Orazio, but the references to bodily functions and the lewd sexual insults included in one of the surviving poems could not have been unfamiliar to her, especially with men like Caravaggio and Tassi around, any more than was the sight of the human body itself, whether in the flesh, in prints such as Agostino Carracci's, or the many reproductive prints after antiquity that were in any artist's studio. It would also be an exaggeration to say that in such an environment anything could happen, but Elizabeth Cohen's argument about the breaching of the household by Tassi, and ideally clear distinctions between inside and outside, needs to be set in the context of the character of Artemisia's life in a space that was both studio and household, a place of work and a place of domesticity.[94] Of course, we must not oversimplify. In 1612, Artemisia was also a godmother who painted natural and sweet scenes of nursing mothers. Her father did so too, even while hanging out with trouble-making friends who enjoyed the risks of literary defamation.

In her father's house, in the midst of all this, Artemisia painted the *Susanna and the Elders*, signing and dating it 1610 (cat. 51). A large painting organized around the figure of a female nude gazed upon by men and painted by a nubile seventeen-year-old female painter could never be *just* a declaration of a skill that would help her compete with other painters who were all men.[95] It was from the very beginning already scandalous, and it is on that knife-edge between the already scandalous and the accomplished and skillful painter that Artemisia's fame balanced throughout her life. Writing of Dürer's *Self-Portrait* of 1500 (Alte Pinakothek, Munich), Joseph Leo Koerner has argued that the meaning of the image derives from "its being *by* someone; that the artist paints, as Dürer himself writes, to 'make himself seen in his works'; and that every signed picture is in some sense a self-portrait."[96] Borrowing a term from Philippe Lejeune, he considers Dürer's portrait a sort of "pact" between painter and viewer, which then becomes valid for the artist's oeuvre as a whole. Like Dürer's *Self-Portrait*, Artemisia's *Susanna and the Elders* is a frontispiece proclaiming the consubstantiality of art and artist, and like the *Self-Portrait* it establishes a pact with the viewer about her work as a whole. That oeuvre will be neither emblematic nor small, but it will be ambitious, dramatic history painting that promises to embody and display the unique physical presence of the woman who made it.[97] Koerner's point is that in Northern art, the reading of an artist's work as the product of a single person begins with the Dürer. Such a reading had much earlier beginnings in Italy, and it permeates all art criticism of the Renaissance. It received a powerful reinvigoration from Caravaggio, whose suppression of tradition and direct way of painting, whether from the model or from the mirror image, were all signatures of his pact with the viewer, making his rare signature all the more shocking. No woman in Italy had achieved that consubstantiality of art and artist, however, and no woman had succeeded in working in such a public

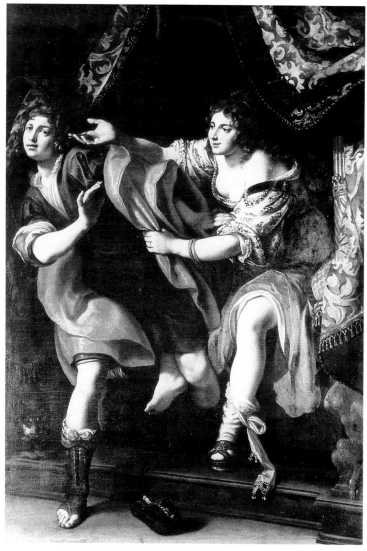

Figure 102. Lodovico Cigoli (1599–1613), *Joseph and Potiphar's Wife*. Oil on canvas. Galleria Borghese, Rome

by Cardinal Scipione Borghese.[99] An excited, fleshy woman, her fancy embroidered clothes quite disheveled, tries to grab a young man as he flees her richly appointed bed with heavy damask curtains. She succeeds only in grasping his cloak with her left hand, on one finger of which she wears a wedding ring; this cloak is the proof she will use against him when she tells her husband that he has tried to violate her. Cigoli's painting presents an exact role reversal of Artemisia's *Susanna*, and the comparison is instructive. Where Artemisia's picture is a grave masterpiece of concentration, Cigoli's composition is amusing and theatrical, and has been linked appropriately to the popularity of new lyrical styles of musical drama in Florence. In its dramatic hyperbole, the *Joseph and Potiphar's Wife* sets the stage for Artemisia's future works, especially the Naples *Judith Slaying Holofernes* (cat. 55). When she and her new husband arrived in Florence in late 1612 or early 1613, Artemisia found many more examples of this sort of dramatic painting, and also a great taste for it at the Medici court. Cristofano Allori's *Judith with the Head of Holofernes* (Galleria Palatina, Florence; see the version reproduced in fig. 103), for example, famously shows the painter's lover, Mazzafirra, playing the role of Judith, her mother as the old maid, and the features of Allori himself in the head of Holofernes, with Judith decked out in rich silks and satins and furnished with cushions and curtains.[100] Bringing to bear her own special approach of painting from the model, Artemisia quickly adapted this theatrical manner, and out of her experience in Florence she forged the style that made her famous. All the more important, therefore, is the painting of *Inclination* (fig. 110), which Artemisia produced for Michelangelo Buonarroti the Younger in 1615–16. The patron was a close friend, as was Allori, who stood godfather to Artemisia's second son on November 9, 1615. Artemisia was a married woman, twenty-two years old, when she painted this work, and she was fulfilling a prestigious commission for the decoration of the gallery that celebrated the genius of the great Michelangelo Buonarroti. The subject, derived directly from Cesare Ripa's *Iconologia*, was given to her, and it required the appearance of a nude young woman bearing a compass, and with a star above her head.[101] Artemisia, her own body recovering from the birth of her second child, now painted a second version of her Roman nude, one that was no longer threatened by shame.[102] Where Susanna looks away, Inclination looks upward in anticipation, her mouth half open, like a younger version of the Muse of History in the *Clio*.

way as to make her own pact with the viewer. Artemisia the painter seized the moment to make such a contract in the only way that she understood to be open to her from her training with her father, which is to say through her own unique female body, signed and dated. That this self-presentation would inevitably incur shame and charges of licentious display is also already understood in the very subject of *Susanna and the Elders* (which so far as we know was not commissioned), and that immediate threat of shame is an essential part of her self-portrait in this frontispiece to her career.[98]

In the same year that Artemisia signed and dated her *Susanna and the Elders*, Lodovico Cigoli completed a *Joseph and Potiphar's Wife* (fig. 102) for the bishop of Arezzo, which was quickly acquired

Opposite: Detail of *Judith and Her Maidservant* (cat. 60)

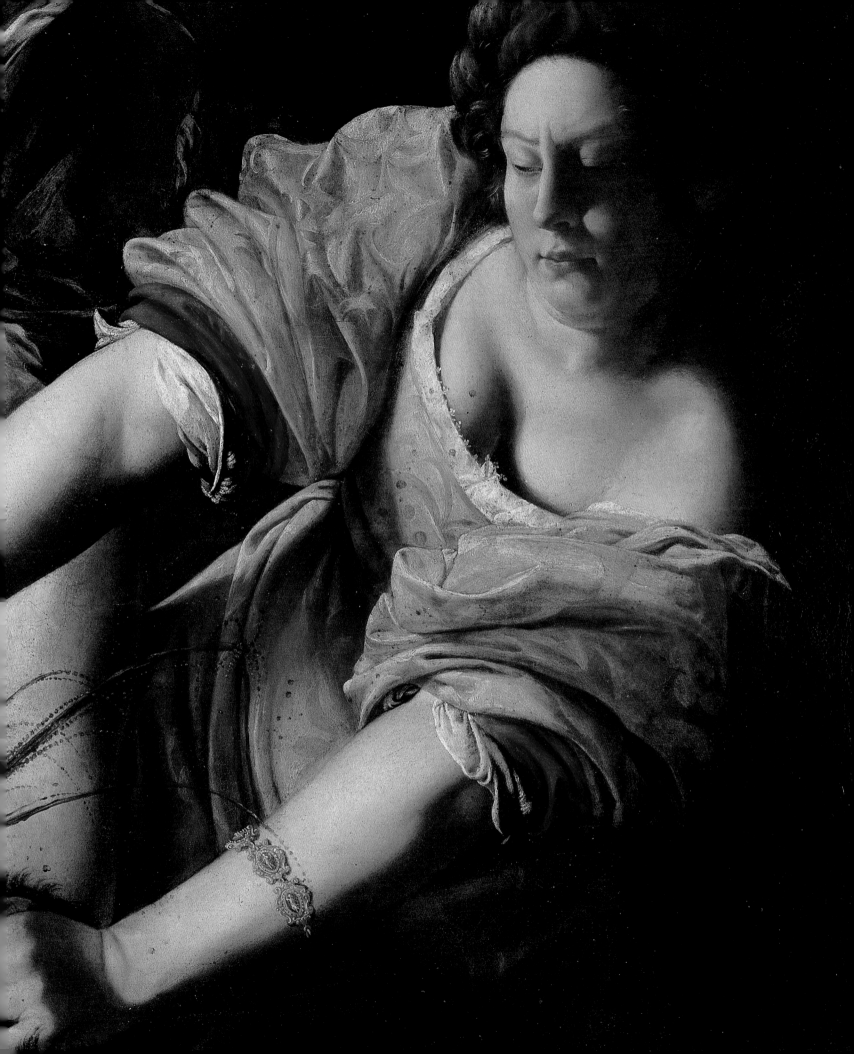

Inclination is Artemisia's second, more optimistic signature painting. The female nude, with her dimpled hand, rosy nipples, and resilient flesh, went well beyond the iconographic requirements of Ripa's nude female, and it was totally unexpected in Florence. So unusual and seductive was it that later in the century, on inheriting the palace, Lionardo Buonarroti had Volterrano cover up the figure with draperies so that his wife and children would not see the nudity. His intention was to do so "without removing any of the beauty of the painting," but of course he destroyed its purpose completely.[103] *Inclination* was a reiteration of *Susanna*, declaring the presence of the artist in her work, whose very subject in this case was the personification of an artist's peculiar inclination toward making art.

The "self-portrait" of Artemisia known as the *Allegory of Painting* (cat. 81) is another such declaration.[104] Much ink has been spilled over its date and the related question of whether or not it is possible that the figure depicted resembles Artemisia. But self-identification with a work has little to do with resemblance. The painting is another signature pact—and it is interesting that Artemisia should have made such a statement when she got to London in 1638, which is when this work almost certainly was painted. As in the case of the figure of Inclination, the attributes of Artemisia's figure of Painting are selected from Ripa, including the female personification, the disordered black hair, the golden chain with a mask hanging from it to stand for imitation, the changing colors of her sleeve, and the brush in one hand. Ripa lists other attributes, but most significant was his suggestion that at the feet of Painting should be some of the tools of the painter, "to show that painting is a noble exercise, and cannot be done without much application of the intellect."[105] The figure of Painting is a passionate young woman, her dark brown eyes looking up to the light, light that emphasizes intellect and body as it falls on her high forehead, and upon her full breast. This shining breast is framed by the lines of the gold chain—that token of esteem usually given by patrons to male painters. The figure holds her brush up to the edge of the actual canvas as if to begin to paint the empty canvas behind her, but she is caught in a moment of meditation or inspiration, as if to show that "painting is a noble exercise, and cannot be done without much application of the intellect." Through this gesture, the entire composition captures the sense of the embodiment of Artemisia's art, her consubstantiality with it, for the moment of inspiration speaks

Artemisia's own name: *Arte-mi-sia*, or "Let art be for me."[106] She signed the work *AGF* (Artemisia Gentileschi fecit).

By this point in her life, Artemisia had learned to objectify her bodily identification with her art, and the threat of scandal was reduced as she aged, even as she would treat her own female models with scorn, complaining about their fees and their chatter. But she never broke her contract as the woman painter, always working, her hair as wild as her imaginings, the embodiment of Painting who was forever young and beautiful. And the threat of scandal, shame, or loss of face was also always there. Garrard sees the constant praise of Artemisia's beauty in poems and letters as "a triple-barrelled weapon": it indicates that she remained on the level of other women in this respect, despite having risen above her sex; it associates her with the potentially corruptive powers of women, which undermined appreciation for her learning and wisdom; and it made it possible to suggest

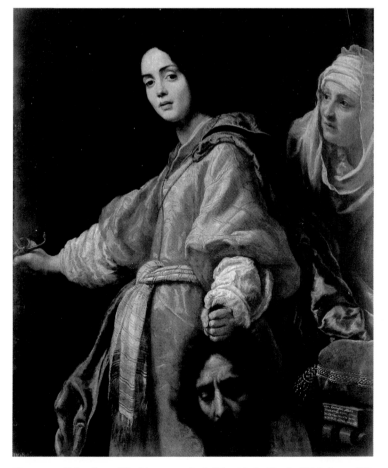

Figure 103. Cristofano Allori (1577–1621), *Judith with the Head of Holofernes*. Oil on canvas. Royal Collection, Hampton Court

that her achievements were a sort of by-product of her looks.[107] Bissell has pointed to various difficulties in Garrard's readings of the texts in praise of Artemisia, but even he, in a feminist gesture, adds that "it was when writers acclaimed Artemisia Gentileschi's physical attributes that they ran a special risk of doing her a disservice by emphasizing that aspect of her person at the expense of her mind (indeed, by implying that she owed her art to her beauty) and by opening the way to those who associated female good looks with lasciviousness and a host of related negative qualities."[108] By singling out Gentileschi as an extraordinary woman, one writer is held guilty of "diminishing women in general."[109] That writer, Gianfrancesco Loredan, addresses Artemisia in a letter declaring himself her vassal, who lacks the words to sing her praises, saying:

I will not say you are a woman in order not to cast doubts on the vitality of your thoughts. I will not say you are a goddess so that you will not doubt the sincerity of my voice. I will not say you are beautiful so as not to associate with you the qualities of every simple woman. I will not say that you make miracles with your brush for me so as not to deprive you of glory. I will not say that you give birth to marvels with your tongue, because only you are worthy of celebrating them. I will just say that the singularity of your virtue requires my mind to invent new words worthy of the greatness of your gifts and expressive of my devotion.[110]

There is every reason to believe that Artemisia would have been delighted by this. Such a tissue of rhetoric protected her, gave her the standing that allowed her to work. She would have been equally, if not more, pleased by the poem dedicated to her by the Neapolitan Giovanni Canale on the occasion of the death of his friend Donati, in which he calls her a "pittrice industre," or hardworking painter, accompanied by Fame.[111] He begs her to take up the depiction of the sorrow he feels, saying, "As famous as you are beautiful, the world praises you, gentle Artemisia." A work by her "saggio pennello," or wise brush, will make his friend immortal,

free from the injuries of time and envy. In another poem dedicated to Artemisia's painting of an Apollo for Girolamo Fontanella, Canale writes of how the "bella Artemisia" has made Apollo fall in love with her. Her hand draws and paints the god, emulating nature and conquering art, so that he seems alive. She seems to have come from heaven, so beautiful is she and so perfect the forms she paints, with the result that Venus must cede to her beauty and Apelles to her painting.

Canale was a notary and not a particularly good poet, working within the tradition of *concettismo* perfected by Giambattista Marino. In praising Artemisia, however, he applies his verses to both her beauty and her work; there can be no sense in which considering her divine is any more demeaning than applying the same term to Michelangelo. Like Loredan's letter, what such poems did was to add more bricks and mortar to the temple of fame that Artemisia had been building for herself since the beginning of her career. The process involved a steady distancing from scandal, but from the very beginning she had understood that to be a woman painter with a body of work, who made a career that lasted her entire life, meant that scandal could never be far away. In Artemisia's case, the only one she knew, this was especially true because of her practice of painting from the model and because of her bodily engagement with the work. She managed to do far more than survive on that knife-edge which divided true fame from infamy until her death, after which she would gradually lose her fame and, more recently, sadly regain her infamy. Artemisia's purpose in living this risky life, and the only thing that made it possible for her to do so, was her work. We should not, in a Longhian way, ignore her life as we look at the work, because the life is in the work. But we should acknowledge, as Banti was compelled to do, that the astonishing output of this woman painter is what counts in the end. Most of all we should not deny her exceptionality, her true independence from her father from the age of nineteen, and the fact that she was indeed a very famous painter during her own lifetime, not just infamous now.

1. See Taylor 1999 and Moore 1999. See also the comments by Richard Feigen in *Tales from the Art Crypt* (2000, 111–13), in which he criticizes the premise of the present exhibition, which is to consider the work of father and daughter together, and insists on Orazio's greater merit. He laments that "[t]he rise of feminism, the scarcity of important women painters, the drama of Artemisia's rape by Orazio's friend Augustino Tassi, and the ensuing trial have recently generated a wave of interest in her work," concluding that "rape and political correctness are irresistible."

2. Los Angeles 1976–77, 118–19.

3. Garrard 1989, 4.

4. Ibid., 5.

5. Ibid.

6. Spear 2000.

7. See Pollock 1990 for an important review of Garrard's book. Garrard 2001, xvii–xxii, replies to her critics, especially Pollock.

8. Pollock 1999, 123. This theory of genealogical struggle lies at the heart of Lapierre's novel (1998, 2000).

9. Cohen 2000, 47–75. See also her earlier, more general study (1991).

10. Longhi 1916, 287; Wittkower and Wittkower 1963, 164; Tufts 1974, 59. I say no scholar, though of course Alexandra Lapierre's novel and Agnès Merlet's popular movie do just that. It seems that the story of the love letters began with Alfred Moir in 1967, for which see Garrard 1989, 533–34 n. 57; see ibid., 206–7, for Artemisia as "the butt of one long historical dirty joke."

11. Cohen 2000, 54.

12. The letter, first published by Leopoldo Tanfani-Centofanti in 1897, is reprinted by Lapierre 2000, 408. The charges all appear to be true.

13. For the hardships of her life in Florence, see Cropper 1992, 203–9; Cropper 1993; and Bissell 1999.

14. Costanza had been married to Filippo Franzini, a pupil of Tassi's, for a year in February 1611, and in May of that year declares that she is fourteen. In 1619 Costanza, Filippo, and Agostino Tassi were living together with two children, for which see Bertolotti 1876.

15. Longhi 1916, 286–87.

16. See, for example, D'Ardia Carraciolo in Banti 1988, 218; and Cannon 1994, esp. 322–25. For a significant discussion of the novel as a whole, see Benedetti 1999, 43–61.

17. Banti 1988, 26–27; and see Cannon 1994, 325–27.

18. Cannon 1994, 330–31.

19. Banti 1988, 111.

20. Ibid.

21. Ibid. For the letter of March 13, 1649, see Garrard 1989, 391–92.

22. Banti 1988, 111–12.

23. Especially the statistical studies of the *Annalistes*, and anthropological studies of law and society by such scholars as Richard Trexler, Elizabeth Cohen, and Thomas Kuehn, as well as case studies of early modern religious belief, witchcraft, sex and gender, by such writers as Carlo Ginzburg, Guido Ruggiero, and Giulia Calvi. Recently, however, historians have voiced increasing concerns about the need to observe distinctions between history, biography, and historical fiction, as new genres gain popularity. Art-historical fiction, whether in print or on film, is now booming.

24. The exhibition was quite modest, but nonetheless aroused comment that Artemisia had beaten her father in the race for a one-man show.

25. Florence 1991, 33. Garrard (2001, 15–17, and 128 nn. 27, 28) rejects this charge, arguing that "[f]or Artemisia Gentileschi, the question is not whether but how feminism enters her work."

26. This is also Bissell's conclusion in his 1999 monograph, though he does not succeed in engaging in the problem. Setting the issue aside does not help, for if the fact of being a woman affected the life experiences of other women

painters such as Lavinia Fontana or Sofonisba Anguissola, this is even more the case for Artemisia, who lived a far more independent life than any of her predecessors.

27. Calvi 1992, vii–xxvii.

28. Ibid., xi.

29. Ibid., xii.

30. Garrard 1989, 415.

31. At the same time, as several scholars have suggested, it is not unreasonable to think that Tassi hoped to use Artemisia's extraordinary ability to work as a guarantee of his own future security.

32. On this issue in general see, most recently, Barzman 2000. See also Lukehart 1993.

33. Brown 1986, 251–52.

34. Garrard (1989, 8), adopting Leo Steinberg's phrase for the late works of Michelangelo.

35. Bissell 1999, 239–41; see also ibid., 385 no. L-95, on the identification of the duke of Guise and inaccuracies in Garrard's account.

36. Garrard 1989, 94–95.

37. Bissell 1999, 240.

38. Ibid., 241.

39. This great work is not among Artemisia's best known because it has been seen by few scholars; it is also an allegory rather than representing a dramatic action. Though female figures in so many earlier works have been identified with Artemisia, only Garrard has suggested that the "absent but ubiquitous artist" is present in the work, but without reading this statuesque allegorical figure as a self-representation, which it surely is.

40. Published by Tanfani-Centofanti 1897, and partially quoted by Bissell 1999, 393.

41. Lapierre (1998, 427) makes the important connection with this academy. See also Garrard 1989, 64. Bissell (1999, 38–39) proposes that the reference is rather to the Venetian academy of the same name. The use of "ne'" in the inscription on the engraving is appropriate for Artemisia's sex, for this is the way to express a woman's connection to her family by marriage.

42. Garrard 1989, 64, 503 n. 103; Bissell 1999, 39.

43. On these verses and their attribution, see Costa 2000.

44. Bissell 1999, 370.

45. Ibid., 56, 387. In Naples it is also possible that Artemisia had a pension from the crown, on the model of that given to Giovanna Garzoni.

46. Ibid., 249–56.

47. Harris in Los Angeles 1976–77, 111–14.

48. Bissell 1999, 256–59.

49. Ibid., 264–66.

50. For the text, see Garrard 1989, 383–84.

51. Ibid., 380–81.

52. Bissell 1999, 164–65.

53. Ibid., 148.

54. Garrard 1989, 387.

55. Bissell 1999, 389–90; see ibid., 150, for the *Fame* and *Susanna and the Elders* also in the royal collection.

56. See most recently Madocks Lister 2000.

57. Cited by Finaldi in London–Bilbao–Madrid 1999, 10.

58. Ibid., 15.

59. Garrard 1989, 388–89.

60. Bissell 1999, 281–86.

61. Ibid., 225–26. See also Harris 1998, 115 n. 37.

62. Garrard (1989, 390–401) publishes the letters in English translation. They were first published by Imparato 1889, 423–25.

63. Garrard 1989, 390.

64. Ibid.

65. Ibid., 392.

66. Ibid., 394.

67. Ibid., 397.

68. Ibid.

69. Ibid., 398.

70. Harris 1998, 113.

71. On this generic division, see Cropper 1998, 210–53, and Cropper 1996a. Bissell (1999, 112–31) also discusses the character of Artemisia's specialization. On the invention of the tableau as such, see Dempsey 2000. Artemisia's *Esther Before Ahasuerus* in The Metropolitan Museum of Art, New York (cat. 71), is probably her most successful tragic history.

72. See Cropper 1984, 106–9.

73. Garrard 1989, 141–71. The concentration on France, unfortunately, means that there is no discussion of the importance for painting of the heroic women of Italian epic, especially in the work of Torquato Tasso.

74. Garrard (1989, 171) also argues that Artemisia aggressively modeled her art on the work of certain male artists—notably Michelangelo and Caravaggio— to produce a sort of "gender-inverted version of androgyny" in her female figures that would not be understood as long as "the unofficial religion of patriarchal misogyny" prevailed. As far as I know, Artemisia produced few Madonnas.

75. Garrard 1989, 179.

76. In her response to her critics, Garrard (2001, 108–13) in part bases her rejection of the reworking of the Burghley House *Susanna and the Elders* on the grounds that Artemisia was not prepared to sell herself by making the work more seductive to the viewer.

77. Hersey 1993, 330.

78. Harris 1998, 113–15.

79. Ibid., 118.

80. Ibid., 119. A word should be said here about Harris's view (ibid., 114 n. 31) that Artemisia could not have used herself as a model. Painters in the sixteenth century indeed depicted themselves from reflections, even in pieces of polished metal.

81. See Bissell 1999, 187–89.

82. De Grazia 1984, 168–76 nos. 176–90.

83. Bellori 1976, 217–18.

84. For an important distinction between life drawing and figure drawing after the model in the academy, see Barzman 2000, 98–101.

85. Harris (1998, 115) also claims that even after the arrival in Rome of Titian's *Bacchanals* in 1598, the depiction of women by men trained in the Carracci tradition remained unreal, and therefore safe.

86. Cropper 1996.

87. For a popular account of the story, see Langdon 1998, 298–99.

88. Ibid., 249–51.

89. Cited by Garrard 1989, 481.

90. Ibid., 482 (my emphasis).

91. Bissell (1999, 306–10) explains his reasons for changing his mind on this, reattributing the work to Orazio and redating it to 1611–12.

92. Ibid., 299–301.

93. See Lukehart 1993, 41–43. Archivio di Stato, Firenze, Med. 6028 contains an interesting reference of July 18, 1614, in a letter to the grand duchess, to the fact that a young Flemish artist wanting to study with Passignano could not live in the artist's house because there were women in the household.

94. For the spaces of Artemisia's life, see Cropper 1992.

95. Nor can it be said that there was nothing else "for her to do all day except to become a painter," for which see Harris 1998, 107.

96. Koerner 1993, xviii.

97. Pollock (1988, 44–46) makes the important point that it was not exclusion from the nude model as such in the academies that denied women power, but their exclusion from the discourse of history painting.

98. Florence 1986–87, 116–17.

99. Ibid.

100. Ibid., 189–91. The picture was begun about 1610–12, but consigned to the Medici only in 1619.

101. Bissell 1999, 205–8.

102. See also Contini (in Florence 1991, 128) for the relationship to the Pommersfelden *Susanna* (cat. 51).

103. According to Baldinucci, as cited by Contini in ibid., 127.

104. Bissell 1999, 272–75.

105. Ripa 1986, vol. 2, 121.

106. Cropper 1992, 215–16.

107. Garrard 1989, 174.

108. Bissell 1999, 40.

109. Ibid., 41.

110. Cited by ibid., 166.

111. Cited by ibid., 166–68.

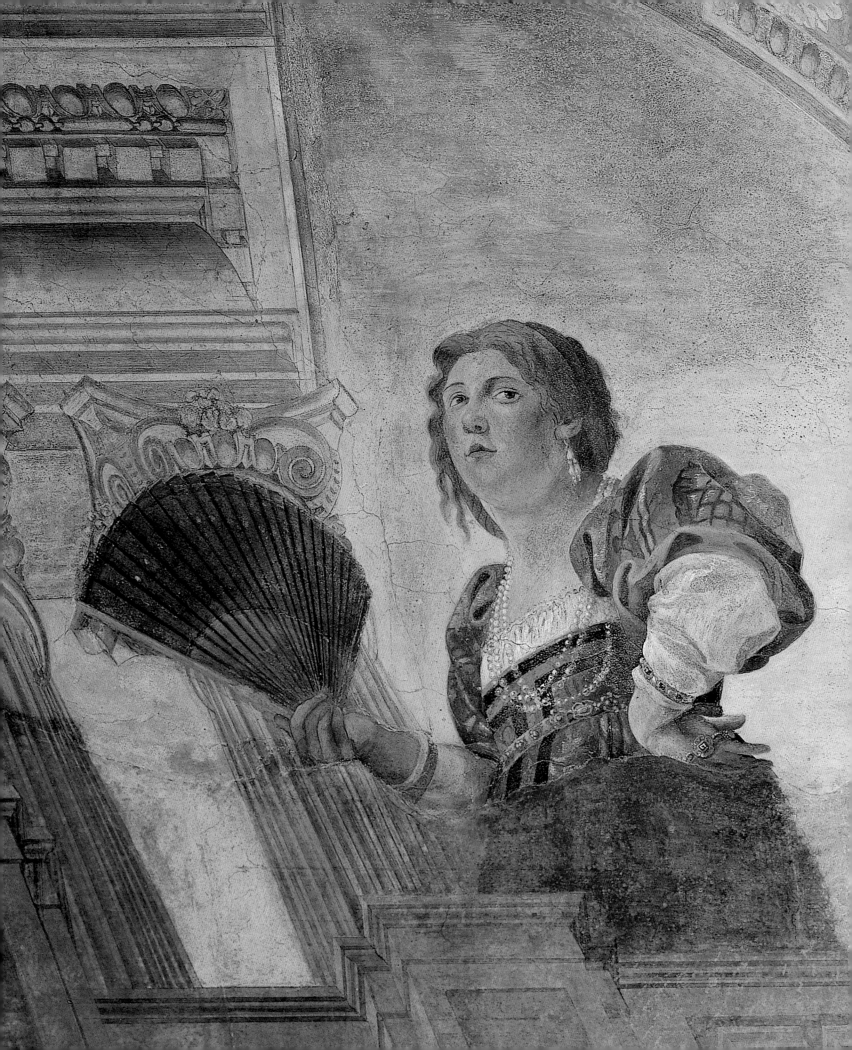

Artemisia in Her Father's House

PATRIZIA CAVAZZINI

An engraving after a lost self-portrait by Artemisia Gentileschi (fig. 95) calls her "famosissima pittrice . . . en picturae miraculum" (celebrated painter . . . a marvel in the art of painting).[1] In an age that was much drawn to what was strange and exotic, Artemisia and her paintings of heroines were probably esteemed as such, as prized curiosities. And as R. Ward Bissell has pointed out in his 1999 publication, her male customers, because they were no doubt titillated by her stories of violence and seduction, continued to commission them from her.[2] But Artemisia did not reach the apex of success during her lifetime. In Rome, in Florence, and in Venice she did not receive a single public commission, even though in Florence she was a favorite at court and gained admittance to the Accademia del Disegno.[3] The Rome of the 1630s, which decreed the triumph of the Baroque, had no room for her, or for any other follower of Caravaggio. Her last twenty years were spent mostly in Naples, a city better attuned to her Caravaggism tempered by Bolognese influences. Here she enjoyed the patronage of the Spanish nobility, including that of Philip IV (r. 1621–65), and even painted altarpieces. But still she was dissatisfied. She did not like the place, repeatedly tried—and failed—to gain steady patronage elsewhere, and often found herself in financial straits.[4]

In the past twenty-five years, captivated by the links that we have seen or imagined between Artemisia's life and work, we have turned her into a marvel of our own time. But for all the feminist studies devoted to her and to her work, not much attention has been paid to what it meant to be a young, unmarried female artist in early-seventeenth-century Rome. It can be argued that in Florence, where she lived from the end of 1612 to 1620, Artemisia became a refined painter, an elegant lady, and perhaps also a sophisticated intellectual. It can at least be proven that there she learned to write.[5] Artemisia's married status, her increasing

success, not to mention her contacts with the Medici court, allowed her a freedom she had not enjoyed before. The situation was certainly different in Rome, before 1612. Almost unconsciously, many art historians have assumed that Artemisia was trained as a history painter and that she was well aware, as a male artist would have been, of everything that was going on in the Roman art world. In her groundbreaking monograph of 1989, Mary Garrard proposes a feminist interpretation of Artemisia's art that assumes her familiarity with a wide range of visual sources and literary texts. But are these assumptions tenable in view of what we know about Orazio and Artemisia around 1610?

Artemisia Gentileschi's social situation was profoundly different, for instance, from that of Lavinia Fontana (1552–1614), the other woman artist of high repute in Rome at that time (fig. 104). Lavinia's father, Prospero (1512–1597), was perhaps the foremost Bolognese painter in the third quarter of the cinquecento. He was a successful, wealthy man, who combined a vast erudition with a wide array of visual sources. When Bishop Paleotti wanted to establish guidelines to help artists follow the dictates of the Council of Trent, he consulted Prospero Fontana. Prospero's patrons included Pope Julius III (r. 1550–55); among his friends were Ulisse Aldrovandi and Achille Bocchi.[6] He had an extensive workshop, called a "studio," where pupils—but almost certainly not his daughter—could study anatomy. For their training, students had at their disposal a collection of antiques (or casts after the antique) and casts of parts of the body, which would have been easily accessible to Lavinia. And although she was a woman, raised in a cultivated, broad cultural context, she became not only a portraitist but also a history painter, practically a unique occurrence in Italian art up to this point.[7] In 1604, Lavinia moved to Rome (where she died in 1614), securing commissions for a number of altarpieces, including one for San Paolo fuori le Mura, which was unfavorably received by the Roman public.[8] In her self-portraits she emphasizes her social station, her intellectual achievements, and her prim virtue.[9]

Compared with Lavinia Fontana's, Artemisia's youth was one of limitations, as clearly emerges from the proceedings of the famous rape—or, more accurately, defloration—trial of 1612. In particular her social station, coupled with her father's notoriously strange temperament, allowed her very limited artistic or intellectual contacts.[10] Artemisia was a motherless child, whose father had long struggled to achieve a minimal recognition in Roman artistic circles.[11] In 1611, although he had lived and worked in Rome for more than thirty years, Orazio was still considered—by a neighbor—a poor man, too poor to keep a servant.[12] His significant commissions were few and far between: in the late 1590s he had painted the apse of San Nicola in Carcere for the cardinal-nephew Pietro Aldobrandini, in 1596 a *Conversion of Saul* in San Paolo fuori le Mura, and after 1607 the *Baptism of Christ* (cat. 11) in the Olgiati chapel in Santa Maria della Pace.[13] Settimio Olgiati seems to have appreciated Orazio and to have been a faithful patron, as was Paolo Savelli, who in the aftermath of the trial assisted Orazio by providing patronage and housing.[14] But the top prizes eluded him; he was never considered for an altarpiece in Saint Peter's and, until 1611, neither Pope Paul V (r. 1605–21) nor his cardinal-nephew, Scipione Borghese, had shown any interest in him. Until the turn of the century, Gentileschi had been one of the many *frescanti* active in the large collaborative enterprises carried out by such painters as Cesare Nebbia (ca. 1536–1614) and Giovanni Guerra (1544–1618). And still in 1610, he was merely transposing in mosaic a drawing by the Cavaliere d'Arpino (1568–1640) on a segment of the dome of Saint Peter's.[15]

At this date, the example of Caravaggio, perhaps coupled with that of Guido Reni (1575–1642), had already profoundly influenced Orazio.[16] From a rather conventional, reformed Mannerist style, he had slowly turned toward observation of nature, especially to painting directly from the model. His works were infused with a lyrical sensibility derived from Caravaggio, but which Caravaggio himself had soon abandoned. If some of his most powerful early canvases, such as the *David* in the Galleria Spada (cat. 18), date approximately from this period, they were probably considered more appropriate for private collections than for public commissions. In particular, Orazio's inability to convincingly handle large multifigure compositions, especially in terms of space, must have limited him.[17]

He had few friends and seems to have been rather distant from many of the most influential and innovative patrons. The Aldobrandini had only a portrait by him, and even Caravaggio's early advocates, such as Cardinal Francesco Maria del Monte, the Mattei, and the Giustiniani, did not consider Orazio a valid alternative.[18] Antiveduto Gramatica (1571–1626), who tempered his Caravaggism with a strong dose of influence from Raphael, seems to have been preferred both by those who esteemed and by those who disdained Caravaggio. His name in fact appears repeatedly both in the Del Monte inventory and in the accounts of Cardinal Alessandro Peretti Montalto.[19]

At least until the time of the trial, in 1612, what we know of Orazio's social life suggests a downward spiral. If in 1594 he was close to the Cavaliere d'Arpino, he soon began to associate with more unsavory characters, such as Caravaggio, Onorio Longhi (1568–1619), and Carlo Saraceni (ca. 1579–1620).[20] Together with Orazio Borgianni, Saraceni and Gentileschi were among the earliest followers of Caravaggio, but the friendship between them did not last long. Already in 1603 there was friction with Caravaggio, and by 1610 Gentileschi's connection with Saraceni—and probably with Borgianni—had been severed.[21]

Orazio had quarreled with Giovanni Baglione (ca. 1566–1643) in 1603. If we can make generalizations from his declarations at this date, many of the arguments were based both on artistic rivalries and on perceived injuries to his honor.[22] Although artistic matters were behind these altercations, the level of discourse was certainly not very profound or elevated. The rhymes composed by Gentileschi, Caravaggio, and Filippo Trisegni begin with "O Giovanni Baglione, great whore," and follow with language so vulgar that they have only rarely been printed. Far from having any intellectual pretense, Orazio declared, "I can write, but I cannot spell properly."[23]

Gentileschi was in touch with Northern painters who lived in his neighborhood, certainly with Wenzel Cobergher (1560?–1632), and perhaps with Adam Elsheimer (1578–1610).[24] With Annibale Carracci (1560–1609) and his followers there seems to have been very little professional contact. The ever-widening circles of the 1612 depositions might mention Passignano (1559–1638) or Cigoli (1559–1613)—at least as friends of friends—but never the Emilian painters.[25]

By 1610, Orazio was left with one close companion, a Cosimo Quorli, understeward to the pope, collector of paintings, and a truly revolting character if ever there was one.[26] In the rape trial, various witnesses attested that he claimed to be Artemisia's father, but evidently he also repeatedly tried to rape her.[27] Perhaps through Quorli, Orazio met Agostino Tassi (1578–1644), who had arrived in Rome in August 1610 with a long criminal record, and became his fast friend.[28]

From Florence, where he stayed only briefly in the early 1590s, Tassi had been banished to Livorno, which was at the time little more than a penal colony. In 1599, in Rome, he assaulted a prostitute who had refused to spend the night with him because of a previous engagement. As punishment for a further crime committed in Tuscany, Tassi spent time on the grand-ducal galleys, but not actually at the oars. When he regained his freedom he married a prostitute, as fulfillment of a vow to redeem one. The woman, called Maria Cannodoli, left him for a rich merchant, ostensibly because Agostino had seduced her sister Costanza. In revenge he tried, probably unsuccessfully, to have her killed.[29]

All of this did not prevent Tassi from being an original and productive painter, much sought after by patrons. Among the members of the Florentine court, Lorenzo Usimbardi, who had been supervisor of construction in Livorno, wrote to Agostino while he was in jail, signing himself, "come fratello" (like a brother).[30] As soon as he arrived in Rome, Tassi went to work in the Palazzo Firenze, under the direction of Cigoli. There he painted a frieze of sea- and landscapes, celebrating the military exploits of Grand Duke Ferdinand I de' Medici.[31] Soon after, he may have been active in the Palazzo Colonna.[32] By February 1611, Tassi was being tried for incest with his sister-in-law, and apparently both Cosimo Quorli and Orazio Gentileschi were instrumental in securing his release.[33]

But one wonders whether Agostino Tassi needed such protection. In March 1611, nine days after his release, he was already receiving 150 scudi from the Camera Apostolica for frescoes in the papal palace on the Quirinal hill, obviously commissioned before the trial.[34] By far the most prominent room he had to paint in the palace was the Sala del Concistoro—also called the Sala Regia—the decorations of which do not survive. Tassi, who was not a figure painter but mainly a painter of illusionistic architecture and landscape, turned to Gentileschi for help. In 1612, the latter complained that he "had" to help Tassi in this task, but actually the opportunity could not have been more timely. Tassi had not only

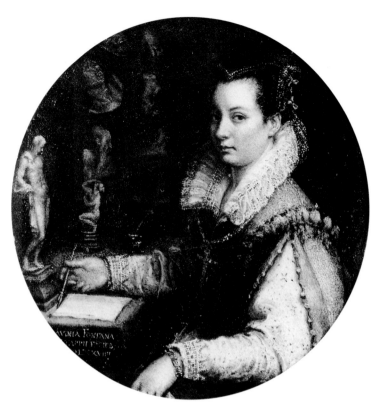

Figure 104. Lavinia Fontana (1552–1614), *Self-Portrait*. Oil on canvas. Galleria degli Uffizi, Florence

finally obtained for him a commission with the papal family, but had provided an ideally suited collaboration.[35] If Gentileschi had trouble arranging figures in space, Tassi was a master of spatial illusionism and supplied a convincing framework into which Orazio could easily insert his personages. And although the latter angrily complained that Tassi was much exalted for this work, he himself received equal praise.[36] The success of this lost fresco—where angels were shown holding a Borghese coat of arms in the center of the ceiling and the Virtues leaned on an illusionistic balustrade—led to further collaborations for the Borghese. The two painters worked together in the Casino delle Muse in Cardinal Scipione's garden palace—from September 1611—and in the so-called apartment of Cardinal Lanfranco still in the Palazzo del Quirinale—from January 1612.

Cardinal Scipione's accounts show that at the Casino delle Muse, the two painters were on equal footing and received equal pay. The situation was different at the Palazzo del Quirinale. Gentileschi must have been paid through Tassi for the Sala del Concistoro and received a single payment for the decoration of Cardinal

Lanfranco's apartment. He may well have obtained more money through Tassi, but this would indicate that Tassi was in charge of the work and that the illusionistic architecture dominated the figures.[37] Perhaps this situation also played a role in Orazio's decision to press charges against Agostino for the defloration of his daughter.

The two close friends were often seen walking together through the streets of Rome, and Agostino often went to Orazio's house.[38] Thus, a fateful chain of events was set in motion; it culminated in March 1612, when Orazio Gentileschi presented a petition to the Tribunale Criminale del Governatore di Roma against Agostino Tassi and Cosimo Quorli. Tassi had forcibly deflowered his daughter, Artemisia, and Quorli had not only abetted him and tried to rape her in turn, but had also extracted from Artemisia a few paintings, including a large *Judith* (fig. 46). Under the pretense of friendship they had inflicted severe damage on Orazio, both on his honor and on his purse.[39]

Although only seventeen, Artemisia was already a painter in fact as well as in reputation. Yet with remarkably few exceptions, nobody knew her personally. Few had ever seen her, not to mention talked to her. Orazio, who had repeatedly tried to convince her to become a nun, kept her almost secluded in their house.[40] He never took her anyplace and hardly ever proposed that she go anywhere. He allowed her to go on a very few excursions organized by others, joining her if he could. Artemisia chafed at these restrictions, which were not, however, unusual for a young woman in the Rome of that time. But she could not bear the thought of becoming a nun, and she was often seen at the window, a major breach of propriety.[41] Many witnesses who tried to steer a middle course between Agostino and Orazio testified to this, while all those who accused Artemisia of being a public prostitute, or in any case of having had lovers, were convinced to do so by Tassi himself. Only Tassi, likely with the intention of discrediting her, claimed to have seen her outside the house.[42] All other witnesses, even those who wished to defame her, said she stayed inside. Thus, the house meant to protect Artemisia became her undoing.[43]

Doubling as a workshop, and without a partition between living and working quarters, the Gentileschi dwelling was much more open to the outside world than was desirable at the time. People of various sorts—fellow artists, patrons, shop boys, models—frequented it. And although Orazio often took care that visitors

did not meet Artemisia, or if they met her, that they did not speak to her, these comings and goings hurt her reputation.[44] At the very least, the judge suspected that they might have caused the rumors about her.[45] At home, Artemisia painted the portrait of a certain Artigenio, again exposing herself to the risk of being criticized for an excessive degree of intimacy.[46] She lied to the judge about the age of her brother Francesco, making him sixteen when he actually would have been no more than thirteen, to give the impression that he was there to protect her.[47] Tassi raped Artemisia in her home, and there they carried on their subsequent relationship. Agostino even claimed that Orazio had given him the task of teaching her perspective.[48] While this may or may not be true, Orazio seems to have granted both Tassi and Quorli, a married man whom he trusted, free access to his daughter, who was sheltered from many other encounters. It is remarkable, for instance, that Carlo Saraceni, a friend of Orazio's from at least 1603 to 1610, had never seen her.[49] Antinoro Bertucci, who owned a pigment store on via del Corso, had seen but not met a girl in Orazio's house and had assumed she was his daughter.[50]

Orazio had clearly used Artemisia as a model, inducing rumors that he had her pose in the nude.[51] Beautiful and provocative, with her unkempt hair and low-cut dresses, she stirred the imagination of many men. In part because she belonged to a different social class, she was far from conforming to the image of the virtuous female artist fashioned by Lavinia Fontana and Sofonisba Anguissola (ca. 1532–1625).[52] After the rape, Tassi's promise of marriage made Artemisia acquiesce "amorevolmente"—her own word—to a relationship.[53] We know little of her feelings, but it would perhaps be well to keep in mind how rarely the word *amore* is used in Italian. True, Agostino was "piccolotto, grassotto, di poca barba" (small, chubby, with a scant beard), but he must have been a charmer and inspired strong loyalties, otherwise it would be hard to explain why so many witnesses lied on his behalf.[54] Even during the trial, Artemisia was seen as behaving affectionately toward him.[55] It was only the discovery that Agostino had lied to her once again—he could not marry her because his wife was still living—that turned Artemisia definitively against him.[56]

The association with Tassi had boosted Orazio's career and his financial situation—he could, for instance, afford a full-time helper only after he started working on the Casino delle Muse (fig. 6)—and a marriage between Agostino and Artemisia would have been the best way of maintaining it.[57] In July 1611, after the rape had already taken place, Orazio moved away from the artists' quarter between the Piazza di Spagna and the Piazza del Popolo, where he had lived all his life, and established himself across the Tiber, near the church of Santo Spirito. Because he was working on the Quirinal hill, such a move would have been rather inconvenient and can be explained only by his wish to be close to Tassi, who lived nearby.[58]

Certainly Orazio did not press suit the moment he knew of the rape. He waited until the works he was carrying out with Agostino were almost finished, and meanwhile tried to see if some other solution could be found.[59] By pressing charges, Orazio probably intended to force the reluctant Agostino into a marriage, or at least into providing a substantial dowry for his daughter. These seem, in fact, to have been the most common legal solutions to a rape. The provision of a dowry would have proven the lack of guilt on the woman's part and made her more attractive in the marriage market, compensating for the loss of virginity.[60]

But according to the famous contemporary lawyer Prospero Farinacci, sentences for rape were somewhat arbitrary. In theory a capital sentence could be pronounced, but in practice this did not happen—unless perhaps the rape involved abduction or arms. A man guilty of rape but unwilling to marry his victim, or to provide a dowry for her, could undergo a punishment, such as fustigation, the galleys, exile, or a fine. Much depended on his and the woman's social condition. For instance, the rape of a maid, even if she was an "honest" woman, was not considered a crime, nor was the rape of a disreputable woman.[61]

In bringing the matter to the court's attention, the Gentileschi underestimated their man and the protections he received. Agostino denied any involvement with Artemisia and produced a number of witnesses declaring she had had several lovers. The crucial one, Nicolò Bedino, who claimed to have lived with Orazio since Lent of 1611, testified that Artemisia went upstairs to her room with various men, "but I do not know what they were doing up there."[62] By proving that Nicolò had been living with him only since the fall of 1611 and had been previously in Tassi's service, Orazio was able to make the court see through Agostino's fabrications. It was, however, a close call for the Gentileschi, implying much legal maneuvering.[63]

Eventually, in November 1612, Tassi was sentenced to five years' exile from Rome under threat of the galleys if he did not leave—but this threat was perhaps more legal wording than a real possibility.[64] The sentence, like many others in seicento Rome, was not implemented. It is not clear how satisfactory this was for the Gentileschi, who gained nothing but the declaration that Artemisia had indeed been raped. Agostino stayed in Rome, even though the nomination of a proxy in January 1613 could be an indication that he was preparing to leave.[65] Not bothering to hide, in March 1613 he initiated a proceeding against Valerio Ursino, a painter who had worked under Passignano.[66] Their friendship had turned sour when Tassi requested payment in exchange for hospitality that Ursino thought had been freely given. In retaliation, Ursino provided one of the key depositions against Agostino and Nicolò.[67] Tassi and Ursino were reconciled on March 20, 1613, but a few days later Agostino assaulted an individual who remains tantalizingly anonymous. Orazio? Ursino? Somebody else entirely? The new crime led to a sentence, on April 9, 1613, of five years' exile from the Papal States.[68] Once again, Agostino did not keep to the terms of the sentence, though for two years he did live elsewhere. From December 1613 to December 1615 he stayed at Bagnaia, not far from Rome, frescoing for Cardinal Montalto, one of the wealthiest and most notable patrons in the city.[69]

The last episode seems to have shaken Orazio, who put himself under the protection of the Savelli and may have left Rome for the Marches in 1613. He can be documented in Rome in 1614 and 1615, exactly when Agostino was in Bagnaia, but not in the years between 1616 and 1620.[70] At least part of this time he must have spent in the Marches (on this subject, see Carloni, pp. 121–24).

In the past, I have misread the document of April 9, 1613, as being a reversal of Tassi's punishment for the rape, causing much confusion in the subsequent literature.[71] But, in fact, the sentence does not seem to have been reversed. However, Nicolò was apparently acquitted, or at least he so declared to a judge in 1619, and Tassi must have spread rumors that he too had been exonerated of any wrongdoing.[72] One of our primary biographical sources, Giulio Mancini, writing about 1620, before the extent of Tassi's criminal career became known, said that Tassi knew how to defend himself and that presumably he was innocent.[73] Giovanni Battista Passeri understood what sort of character Agostino was and condemned him in every instance except the one of the rape. He wrote that Artemisia would have been praiseworthy for her paintings if she had been more virtuous, and that Agostino was acquitted in the trial, even though he may have been guilty.[74]

Tassi's protection possibly came directly from the papal family. In March 1616, soon after his return from Bagnaia, he was again working for Paul V, planning the decoration of the gigantic Pauline chapel in the Palazzo del Quirinale, the equivalent of the Sistine chapel at the Vatican.[75] When the pope decided to have it stuccoed, not frescoed, Tassi was awarded two new tasks, the decoration of the new Sala Regia—now often called the Sala dei Corazzieri—and of the room of Saint Paul. The latter he carried out exclusively with his assistants, the former he shared with Saraceni and Giovanni Lanfranco (1582–1647). The three painters divided into two separate teams—Tassi and his helpers on the long inner wall, Lanfranco, Saraceni, and their collaborators on the other three.[76] There is no question that the Borghese had made their choice; it was Tassi's ability as a quadraturist which was irreplaceable, while Orazio was perhaps not even given a chance to finish his part in the Casino delle Muse.[77] If not as "mediocre" as the Florentine ambassador cruelly labeled him, Gentileschi was one among the many figure painters available in Rome.[78] His lyrical brand of Caravaggism could easily be replaced by Saraceni's, who knew Tassi from at least 1611. (Lanfranco's involvement in the project, and especially his close collaboration with Saraceni, is more difficult to understand. No follower of Caravaggio had worked so closely with a follower of the Carracci, nor had Tassi up to this point shared any project with an Emilian painter.)[79] As a consequence of the trial, Orazio lost the favor of the papal family; never again would he receive a major commission in Rome (but see cat. 25). Artemisia fared somewhat better. On November 29, 1612, the day after Tassi was sentenced to exile, she married Pierantonio Stiattesi (b. 1584), the brother of the man who had helped her father in the legal defense. By December, the newlyweds were preparing to leave Rome for Florence, where a whole new chapter in Artemisia's life was to begin.[80]

What had she painted up to this point? When and how had she been trained? What was the extent of her visual experience? From the trial, we can gather some scant information not so much on her training, but on that of her brother Francesco. In 1610 or early 1611, at the age of thirteen, Francesco was grinding colors, but in late 1611, when he was fourteen, he was learning to draw and was therefore still a beginner.[81] Francesco's companion during his training was the famous Nicolò who would be the main witness against Artemisia. Because Orazio was often out of the house, she helped them.[82] That the traditional method of teaching to draw

first was followed by Orazio and the people around him is confirmed by innumerable testimonies in the trial.[83] Mario Trotta, for example, a day laborer who helped both Tassi and Gentileschi when they frescoed together, declared: "I am a painter—that is, I am a beginner, because I am learning to draw."[84]

If Artemisia had followed the same path as her brother—though it has been argued that women painters were trained at a later age than men—she would have learned to draw around 1607, and started to paint perhaps in 1608.[85] Her father's letter of July 1612, declaring that in three years she had become an extremely accomplished artist, might indicate that she had finished her training by 1609.[86]

Orazio was clearly not a teacher; his household around this time rarely accommodated apprentices, and they never lasted long. He was a loner, carrying out his trade in relative isolation, without an active workshop. When he was frescoing, Orazio hired helpers by the day, and before taking on Nicolò full-time he occasionally borrowed him from Agostino.[87] The contrast between Orazio's various houses and Tassi's could hardly have been more vivid. If both had rather humble abodes, which doubled as workshops, with no clear distinction between working and living spaces, Tassi's lodgings were crowded with a constant flow of apprentices and assistants. Some lived with him, some did not; some paid a fee, some exchanged services for instruction, some received wages.[88] Tassi's own drawings, mainly of landscapes but also after the antique, were their main learning tools.[89] The same was probably true in Orazio's house, where his own drawings and canvases were the key to instruction. Orazio, however, must have been a much less enthusiastic draftsman than Tassi, since there are no definitively autograph drawings by him—and none by Artemisia.

Toward the end of the first decade of the seicento, Orazio seems to have largely abandoned drawing in favor of painting directly from the model, following Caravaggio's example. Largely, though not completely, since he still needed drawings as preparation for frescoes.[90] We also know that he drew, not painted, likenesses of children, probably because they would have become restless if he had made them stand still for too long.[91] But when Gentileschi employed as models Bernardino Franchi, his barber, and Giovan Pietro Molli, a pilgrim who posed as Saint Jerome in the canvas now in Turin (ca. 1610–11; cat. 16), Orazio was painting them directly on the canvas.[92] From their words, it is clear how slow and cumbersome the procedure was. Day after day, Orazio shut himself in a room with them and did not let anyone else in.[93] Did he make an exception for Artemisia? Perhaps. But time and again we have the impression that he did not. On via Margutta, Orazio seems to have painted alone in a room on the main floor, while Artemisia lived, and perhaps worked, upstairs—where Orazio's models never went.[94] On via della Croce, she painted next to her bedroom, possibly an indication that she and her father worked separately.[95] We would imagine that if the disposition of the house permitted, Artemisia's room would have been farther from the space where men came to look at paintings, or partially disrobed to pose.

Because Orazio had so few students, one wonders whether he even owned the teaching tools essential for a figure painter, such as casts of parts of the body and of antique statues. The absence of such implements would help explain Artemisia's rather inept rendering of anatomy, which is evident in her canvases at least until the mid-1610s. It was only in Florence that Artemisia learned to match virtuosity with creativity. The *Saint Cecilia* (cat. 63) and the *Allegory of Inclination* (fig. 110) are highly accomplished works, in which a brilliant rendering of textures is wed to an elegant depiction of the human figure.

Artemisia did learn from Orazio the practice of painting from the model and of posing human figures after famous works of art. In all likelihood Orazio owned a number of prints, which must have been fundamental for broadening her visual experience. From the evidence of the trial, I doubt that Artemisia had in fact seen much art firsthand. As mentioned before, she rarely went out. She went to Mass at her parish church, first Santa Maria del Popolo (she would therefore have been familiar with Caravaggio's canvases in the Cerasi chapel) and then San Lorenzo in Lucina and Santo Spirito in Sassia. She had also gone to Mass at Sant'Onofrio and visited a few of the major Roman basilicas, such as San Giovanni in Laterano, Saint Peter's, and San Paolo fuori le Mura. We hear of a plan to visit Santa Maria Maggiore that fell through.[96] Quorli took her to see the Palazzo del Quirinale, where Agostino Tassi and her father were painting. There, she would have seen Guido Reni's frescoes in the papal chapel. During Carnival, when rules were relaxed even for Artemisia, she spent various evenings at Quorli's house, where plays were staged and where she would have seen his collection of paintings, which included a large *Susanna* in a vertical format like her own.[97]

On these excursions, although she was pursued by both Tassi and Quorli, she took pains to look at works of art, but it is curious that she focused her attention on those which must already have been familiar to her. In San Giovanni, she stopped to look at the Apostles, one of which her father had painted, and in San Paolo she was eager to look at Orazio's altarpiece, the Conversion of Saul.[98] While I certainly do not want to make the claim that this was the extent of Artemisia's visual experience, I want to stress that she had almost no freedom of movement. Churches would have been more accessible to her than private palaces, especially given the few ties Orazio had to many important patrons.[99] The idea of the two of them going to the Palazzo Farnese so that Artemisia could see the Carracci gallery, or even to the Vatican palace to admire the Sistine ceiling is hardly likely; in the year discussed in the trial, that is, between 1611 and 1612, father and daughter never went on such an expedition. It is also hard to believe that Artemisia could have seen works in progress at other painters' houses, given that Orazio never took her to Tassi's or Saraceni's.

What is certainly a historical impossibility is that Artemisia had any role in the Casino delle Muse. Not only would this have been highly inappropriate; it is also clear from the trial that she worked at home. Nicolò ground colors only for Artemisia, since she painted in oil; her father, on the other hand, was painting in fresco.[100] No one, among Tassi's and Gentileschi's various helpers, saw her at the casino, and it is possible that she never went there.[101]

Filippo Baldinucci claimed that in her youth in Rome Artemisia had painted many portraits, and, indeed, at the trial we hear of her painting two.[102] One, of her neighbor's boy, was done for her own pleasure, and one, of a man called Artigenio, was commissioned.[103] When trying to establish Artemisia's oeuvre in these years, we should keep these facts in mind. Because she was the only daughter of a painter who had many sons, there would hardly have been a reason to train her as a history painter, which was at any rate a highly unusual career for a woman.[104] Still lifes, which she apparently painted, images of the Madonna and Child, and little oval panels such as those depicting Poetry and Painting once in the Spada collection (fig. 97), belonged to the realm of a woman painter.[105] Artemisia's illiteracy would also seem to argue against a training as a history painter. In 1612, at seventeen, she declared that she could hardly read and could not write.[106] This must be true because Nicolò, who would have gained by saying the opposite, partially confirmed it.[107] Signing one's name was taught after reading but before writing and, by 1612, Artemisia might not have learned this minimal skill because her deposition is not signed.[108] From the autograph statements appended to each testimony at the trial, it becomes clear how disadvantaged she was in this respect, obviously because of her sex. All the men involved in the trial could write, many in a fluent handwriting and with correct spelling. Such abilities were widespread in seventeenth-century Rome, down to the level of skilled artisans, and certainly including painters and their assistants.[109]

At the beginning, Artemisia may have painted for the market, but her father assisted her career by providing patrons, such as Alessandro Biffi, who owned her first self-portrait as an Allegory of Painting (fig. 97) in addition to her *Madonna and Child* and Orazio's *David,* all of which ended up in the Spada collection (cat. nos. 18, 52).[110] Even at this early stage, Artemisia's work was extraordinarily powerful, as best demonstrated by the Spada *Madonna,* painted in 1609 or shortly thereafter. Gianni Papi aptly underscores the dynamic energy of this composition, perhaps modeled on Sansovino's marble *Madonna* in Sant'Agostino, as well as on her father's painting in Bucharest (cat. 15).[111] Also masterly are the depiction of the emotional relationship between mother and child and the command of space implied by the oblique placement of the chair. Orazio's slightly earlier *Madonna and Child* (cat. 8), obviously known to Artemisia, is more static and less spatially resolved: the pillow, rather than defining the space, seems to stand upright against the canvas.

Works such as the Spada *Madonna,* the unequal length of the Virgin's arms notwithstanding, probably convinced Orazio to make his daughter a history painter. The *Susanna and the Elders* in Pommersfelden (cat. 51) may be the tangible sign of this decision. The anatomical precision, the contrast of textures, the light that strikes Susanna's soft body are so much more accomplished here than in the Naples *Judith Slaying Holofernes* (cat. 55), always considered slightly later, that Orazio must have helped her out, down to the detail of the signature in capital letters, so that she could copy them more easily. Although Susanna's expression, as has often been claimed, may reflect Artemisia's disgust at the passes made at her by various disreputable individuals—though certainly not her revulsion at the rape, since she did not know Tassi in 1610— we also have to come to terms with the fact that neither Orazio

nor Artemisia had any compunction about superimposing her features on a naturalistic and inviting nude body prominently displayed.[112] Was this her own body, admired and copied from a mirror? The notion of Artemisia's owning a large reflecting surface is not implausible, as Ann Sutherland Harris has come to believe, since Cosimo Quorli owned a full-length metal mirror that hung together with his paintings.[113]

Whether Orazio and Artemisia, in addition to the *Susanna,* painted other works together is difficult to say. In the attempt to ascertain whether or not Nicolò did indeed live with Orazio in 1611, many witnesses talk about the household around that time, but in fact nobody saw father and daughter collaborating. Shortly thereafter, Orazio was busy working in fresco for a number of months—perhaps with a gap in the late spring and summer of 1611—with little time for anything else.[114] He would have been more available after the beginning of the trial, in the spring of 1612 and for the remainder of that year. Although it is perhaps hard to imagine father and daughter working side by side at this time, Orazio's letter to Cristina, dowager grand duchess of Tuscany, does betray an affectionate understanding of his daughter's situation more than reproach or anger.[115]

It is unfortunate that we know nothing about the Naples *Judith Slaying Holofernes,* perhaps the first independent history painting by Artemisia. If the picture was indeed started after the rape and painted in Rome, as is generally assumed (but without any proof), then it must have been executed exactly while the trial was going on. Although in Judith's story, the roles of man and woman are almost reversed in respect to Artemisia's own story, still the elements of violence and seduction are fundamental in both, obviously tempting us to read Artemisia's biography into the picture.[116]

But perhaps we should use caution. As Bissell has noted, this kind of canvas was probably commissioned and its subject not chosen by Artemisia.[117] Moreover, we should reconsider the role of Caravaggio's *Judith,* now in the Palazzo Barberini (fig. 109). Even if Artemisia intended her canvas as a personal vendetta against Tassi, the mood with which she infused it is barely distinguishable from that of Caravaggio's picture. The goriness and violence are similar, as is the distaste for the task shown by the two Judiths. In both, a feeling akin to sadness is combined with a finicky fear of dirtying one's clothes.

I think that, at least in part, we should interpret Artemisia's *Judith* as her response to seeing the canvas by Caravaggio for the first time. Because it was in the private collection of a patron not particularly close to her father, it would have been difficult for her to gain access to it, and she can hardly have known it all her life.[118] One wonders if the client who commissioned the painting also told her to take the Caravaggio as a model and arranged for her to see it.

Starting from Caravaggio's almost motionless composition, Artemisia devised a much more forceful and energetic arrangement of figures, one for which no totally convincing precedent can be suggested. In addition, she cast herself as the aggressor, substituting her features for those of Caravaggio's aristocratic heroine. Her Judith is at the same time a more ordinary and a more muscular figure. Again, before we make too much of this, we should remember that Artemisia, in her claustrophobic environment, became obsessed with her own features and repeated them time and again in her paintings, a mirror making up for so many constraints.

It is perhaps true, as it has been argued in the past, that the trial granted Artemisia more freedom—perhaps much more freedom than would have been customary for a young, unmarried woman— since after her loss of virginity became public knowledge, there would not have been much more to protect. For her artistic development it may have been an advantage that Tassi did not marry her. He talked of moving with her to Florence in the service of the court, evidently because he recognized her value as a painter.[119] More learned than her father, more interested in a variety of sources, he could perhaps have broadened the scope of her visual and cultural experience, but at the same time might have absorbed her into his workshop. If she had learned anything from Tassi, she obstinately refused to put it into her pictures. Strong, self-assured, totally in control as she appears during the trial, by marrying a nonentity she ensured her independence as an artist.

I wish to thank Keith Christiansen, Elizabeth and Thomas Cohen, and Alexandra Lapierre, who have most patiently answered my endless queries. A long conversation with Gianni Papi was also extremely helpful. My research on Agostino Tassi was financed by the Getty Grant Foundation.

1. Bissell 1999, 227.
2. For a discussion of the subject matter of Artemisia's pictures, see ibid., 112–31.
3. Spear 2000, 568.
4. See Artemisia's letters in Menzio 1981, 162–73; and translations in Garrard 1989, app. A, esp. nos. 11, 13, 16, 17, 19, 23, 24, 25, 26, 28.
5. See the autograph statement at the end of the inventory found by Francesco Solinas, in the essay by Roberto Contini. See also Bissell 1999, 110, on the issue of Artemisia's literacy. Many of Artemisia's letters survive only in print, and many others are clearly not autograph but written by a secretary, such as those reproduced in Garrard 1989, figs. 328, 329. (Artemisia herself wrote in a letter to Don Antonio Ruffo on June 12, 1649, that she employed secretaries; ibid., app. A, no. 19.) For the approximate date of Artemisia's departure for Florence, see Lapierre 1998, 457.
6. For Prospero Fontana, see Fortunati Pietrantonio 1986, vol. 1, 339–414.
7. For Lavinia Fontana, see Washington 1998 and Murphy 1996. See also King 1999, esp. 51–54, and Glenn 1999, esp. 134.
8. Baglione 1642, 143; Washington 1998, 29.
9. For her self-portraits, see Murphy 1996, 61; Washington 1998, 52, 58; and Glenn 1999, 178–81.
10. For Orazio's strange character, see Baglione 1642, 360: "Se Orazio fusse stato di humore più pratticabile, haverebbe fatto gran profitto nella virtù, ma più nel bestiale che nell'humano egli dava; e di qualsiasi soggetto per eminente che egli fusse conto non faceva; era di sua opinione e con la sua satirica lingua ciasche-

duno offendeva. . . ." Baglione's opinion can hardly be seen simply as a reflection of the 1603 trial, since his biography of Caravaggio is much more charitable. Pietro Guicciardini, the Florentine ambassador in Rome, in 1615 wrote to the Florentine court that Orazio was "uomo sì stratto di vita, di costumi, e d'humor tali che non si può convenir seco, né trattarlo, e con mille maleagevolezze tenerlo intorno" (Crinò and Nicolson 1961, 144). See also Baldinucci's comments on Gentileschi's "stravaganza di umore," 1811–12, vol. 3, 712.
11. See Christiansen, this publication, p. 3, and Contini in Florence 1991, 36–37.
12. Appendix 1, this publication, sect. B, fols. 110, 114, Costanza Ceuli: ". . . so che non ha tenuto mai servitore che veramente il Gentileschi era povero huomo . . . so bene che servitore non ha tenuto che haveva della famiglia assai."
13. Bissell 1981, 134–35, 216; Maniello 1994, 155–60. See Christiansen, this publication, pp. 15–19.
14. Olgiati not only commissioned the altarpiece in Santa Maria della Pace, but was evidently interested in Orazio's work; see appendix 1, sect. A, fols. 432v–433, Bernardino de Franceschi: ". . . mentre ce stetti io all'hora il signor Settimio Olgiati che venne a vedere la loggia . . . in quella casa che habitava detto signor Horatio nella strada di Margutta . . . ho ben visto venire il signor Settimio Olgiati a vedere qualche quadro." For Orazio's relationship with Paolo Savelli, see Pizzorusso 1987, 68–70; Gallo 1998, 334; Testa 1998; and cat. nos. 23, 25.
15. Bissell 1981, 5–6, 147–48.
16. See cat. nos. 9, 16, and the essay by Christiansen, this publication, pp. 5–9.
17. See, for example, the Baptism of Christ (cat. 11) for Santa Maria della Pace.
18. See Frommel 1971 (for Cardinal Del Monte); Rome 1995a (for the Mattei); Cappelletti 1998 (for the Aldobrandini, with previous bibliography); and Rome–Berlin 2001 (for the Giustiniani).
19. In 1611, Gramatica painted a Europa and a Judith for Cardinal Montalto, for which he was paid 50 scudi each. In 1620 and 1621, he painted two more canvases for the cardinal, the first of an unspecified subject, the second of a Madonna.

See Archivio Storico Capitolino (hereafter, ASC), Archivio Cardelli, app. 35 (27 gennaio, 8 agosto 1611, 38, 30 settembre 1621), app. 53 (25 aprile 1620). For Gramatica's presence in Cardinal Del Monte's collection, see Frommel 1971.

20. Bissell 1968, nn. 8, 9; Bissell 1981, 215; Garrard 1989, 14.

21. Appendix 1, sect. A, fol. 412: In August 1612, during the trial, Saraceni declared: "non ho praticato con il detto Horatio che saranno circa due anni." Borgianni seems to have been questioned only once during the trial; see Archivio di Stato di Roma (hereafter, ASR), Miscellanea artistica, b. 2, in Garrard 1989, 475. His deposition is lost, but being presented by Tassi's defense lawyer was certainly in Borgianni's favor, not in Gentileschi's. The cooling of Orazio's friendship with Caravaggio is mentioned in the famous trial of 1603; see Dell'Acqua and Cinotti 1971, 154–57.

22. Dell'Acqua and Cinotti 1971, 156. For the concept of honor in a Roman context, see Cohen 1992a.

23. "Io so scrivere ma non troppo corretto" (Dell'Acqua and Cinotti 1971, 154). See ibid., 155 (for the rather haphazard spelling of Orazio's letter to Baglione), 75 (for Dell'Acqua's comments).

24. Cobergher was godfather to Giulio Gentileschi, baptized on September 16, 1599 (Archivio del Vicariato di Roma [hereafter, AVR], S. Maria del Popolo, Battesimi, 1595–1619, fol. 52v, cited in Hoogewerff 1942, 112). Elsheimer, like Gentileschi, lived on via del Babuino in 1606, 1609, and 1610. According to F. Noack (quoted in Weizsäcker 1952, 160), in 1607 and 1608 Elsheimer lived on via dei Greci, therefore extremely close to Orazio, but his identification of the street might be mistaken.

25. Appendix 1, sect. B, fols. 104v, 106. See note 31 below. For the one reference to Annibale Carracci, see Panofsky 1993, 125.

26. For Quorli, see Lapierre 1998, 429.

27. Menzio 1981, 51, 69.

28. Orazio's isolation and his close ties with Tassi are repeatedly asserted in the trial; see Menzio 1981, 94, Agostino: "Orazio non ha amico nessuno né altro refrigerio che me in questo mondo." See also appendix 1, sect. A, fol. 376, Mario Trotta: "Io non ho mai visto praticare il detto Horatio se non con Agostino Tassi, con il detto Cosmo furiero, con il custode delle fontane di palazzo e con noi altri lavoranti"; and fol. 378r,v, Marcantonio Coppino: "Io non ho mai visto il detto Horatio se non in compagnia di Cosmo Quorlo et di detto Agostino Tassi del resto lo [trovo] quasi sempre solo."

29. For a biography of Tassi during these years, see Cavazzini 1998, 171–74. No proof of Tassi's residence at the Florentine court could be found at the Archivio di Stato in Florence (hereafter, ASF), and I have come to believe that his sojourn in the Tuscan capital was extremely short.

For Tassi and his wife, see ASR, Tribunale Criminale del Governatore, Processi, b. 62, febbraio 1611, fol. 111v, Costanza de Bargellis: ". . . questo Valerio [Ursino] . . . mi ha confessato che detto Agostino gli haveva messo due banditi in casa et che havevano le pistole . . . et che li voleva mandare per fare ammazzare sua moglie et che si troveranno le lettere a quelli che scriveva;" fol. 134, Agostino Tassi: "Mia moglie si chiama Maria e saranno otto anni che la sposai a Livorno, non mi ha mai havuto figli . . . su le galere feci voto di levare una dama di peccato arrivai a Livorno e sposai questa Maria. . . ."

30. ASF, Fondo Mediceo 3506, September 8, 1612; in Weizsäcker 1952, 205.

31. ASF, Fondo Mediceo 1343, August 27, 1610, in Cavazzini 1998, 218; Matteoli 1980, 445; see also appendix 1, sect. B, fol. 104v, Michelangelo Vestri: "Io ho cognosciuto Agostino Tasso pittore sin dal principio che lui tornò a Roma, che mi pare che fosse l'anno 1610 d'estate con occasione che lavorando io nel palazzo dell'ambasciatore di Firenze, ci venne detto signor Agostino a fare certi paesi. . . ."

32. Appendix 1, sect. A, fol. 441, Luca Finocchi: "Io cognosco prima Agostino Tasso che cognoscessi detto Nicolò con occasione che venne ad una commedia che se faceva in casa del contestabile Colonna et con occasione che havendolo io visto praticar lì nel palazzo vedendolo la sera . . . alla comedia gli prestai uno sgabello."

33. Ibid., fol. 427v, Olimpia de Bargellis: ". . . et io una volta querelai [Agostino] in Borgo perché si teneva la cognata e fu assolto per favore che hebbe di Cosimo suddetto che tre-quattro giorni uscì di prigione." This explains why Tassi told Stiattesi that he owed his life to Quorli (Menzio 1981, 69). Orazio, in his letter of July 1612 to Cristina of Lorraine (ASR, Mediceo del Principato, filza 6003; Lapierre 1998, 454), also claimed: "Agostino Tasso . . . in breve tempo mi si dimostrò amico sviscerattissimo et io con reciproca benevolenza, non solo l'amavo, ma con mezzi potentissimi lo liberai della forca. Laonde mostrandomi detto Agostino obbligatissimo fui necessitato aiutarlo nel depingere la Sala Regia fatta da Nostro Signore a Monte Cavallo, della qual pittura, come è notissimo a tutto il mondo, Agostino ne restò assai esaltato."

34. ASR, Camerale I, fabbriche 1537, fol. 155, 19 marzo 1611. For the payments for the decoration of the Palazzo del Quirinale, see Hibbard 1971, 196; Borsi, Briganti, and Del Piazzo 1973, 247; Cavazzini 1998, 219. See also Fumagalli 1992, 226–28.

35. Tassi's primary role is indicated by the payments, from March 19 to September 6, 1611, which never mention Gentileschi's name. See also Gentileschi's letter quoted in note 33 above.

36. See note 33 above. Baglione 1642, 360: "Nella sala grande di Montecavallo verso il giardino, ove tal'hora si suole fare consistoro pubblico, v'ha di suo nel mezo della volta uno sfondato, entrovi un'arme grande del Papa con due angeli che la reggono, e intorno evvi una prospettiva di mano di Agostino Tasso, ove posano diverse figure dal Gentileschi formate con vista di sotto in sù, assai buone, e come giudicarono li professori, sono le migliori che egli facesse, e rappresentano diverse Virtù, le quali al Pontefice Paolo V alludono, con grand'amore, e diligenza a buonissimo fresco condotte." See also Baldinucci 1811–12, vol. 3, 712.

37. For all the payments relating to the frescoes for the pope and for Cardinal Scipione Borghese, see Cavazzini 1998, 218–19, with previous bibliography.

38. See note 28 above and appendix 1, sect. B, fol. 104v.

39. For a brief summary of the trial, see appendix 1, with more documentary material and essential bibliography. It was found by Bertolotti (1876), whose transcriptions are unreliable. Much new material relating to the trial and to the Gentileschi has been found by Alexandra Lapierre, and no full understanding of the events is possible without reading her novel. However, I would caution against quoting directly from her text, and I doubt this was her intention. Her transcriptions from the trial depositions are highly accurate in the appendixes, but her text was meant as fiction, where truth and probability mix. Her appendixes provide invaluable archival citations, and sometimes summaries, to most of her discoveries, not necessarily transcriptions.

40. Menzio 1981, 47, Artemisia Gentileschi: "Tutia disse a mio padre che mi doveva mandare un poco a camminare e che mi noceva il stare sempre in casa"; ibid., 59 (Tuzia Medaglia): ". . . mi disse anco quando ci andai a stare che stessi avvertita e non dir alla sua figliola né parlarli di mariti, ma che li persuadessi a farli monaca et io l'ho fatto più volte, ma lei sempre mi diceva che non occorreva che suo padre perdesse tempo perché ogni volta che li parlava di fari monaca li diventava inimico"; ibid., 61: "il padre haveva gelosia di questa figliola e non voleva che fosse vista." See also Lapierre 1998, 62–63.

41. Appendix 1, sect. A, fol. 366v, Luca Penti: "Detta Artimitia io l'ho vista a una finestra lì alli Greci che c'era l'impanata et anco l'ho vista a San Spirito alla finestra et una volta in casa quando c'entrai con Cosmo furiero e non ho mai parlato"; ibid., 421, Antinoro Bertucci:"Giovanni Battista si lamentava del detto Horatio che l'haveva cacciato di casa perché haveva bravato alla figlia che stava alla finestra." See also ibid., fol. 375, Mario Trotta: ". . . un nipote di Horatio Gentileschi chiamato Giovanni Battista, che è morto all'ospedale di San Giovanni haveva detto che il detto Horatio l'haveva scacciato di casa per una parola . . . che lui haveva detto alla sorella cugina figlia di detto Gentileschi che non stesse alla finestra ch'era vergogna che lui gli l'haveva detto al padre e per questo l'haveva cacciato via." Orazio's eldest brother, Baccio, had a son called Giovanni Battista; see Ciardi, Galassi, and Carofano 1989, 36 n. 4.

In Rome, women belonged inside the house, men outside. Windows and doors were "exciting places, emotionally and sexually charged"; see Cohen 1992, esp. 617, 621. For an example of a woman literally locked inside the house when the husband was out, see Cohen and Cohen 1993, 159–87.

42. Menzio 1981, 98.

43. Cohen 1992, 617, 621.

44. See, for example, Antinoro Bertucci's deposition, note 50 below.

45. If homes were meant to be closed spaces, workshops clearly were not. As often stated in the trial depositions, they were a key point of contact, where painters showed work in progress to patrons and close friends. Orazio, like Tassi and perhaps like many other painters of the time, had no proper space in which to work. He painted in a room next to where the family took their meals, creating an ambiguous situation for Artemisia, who lacked the protection of a mother or of servants. Mario Trotta's statement (appendix 1, sect. A, fol. 376: "Signorsì che in casa di pittori ci praticano gentilhuomini ch'io son stato in casa del Cavalier Giuseppe [d'Arpino] e c'ho visto Monsignor Santoro e altri signori e gentilhuomini e cardinali e mal nome io non ho mai inteso in casa del Cavaliere per la pratica di detti signori") certainly applies to a totally different setup, with a clear distinction between residential spaces and working quarters. Other witnesses were asked what they though of this "andari di gentilhuomini et altri"; see, for example, Coppino's deposition, appendix 1, sect. A, fol. 378v.

46. See Artemisia's answer to Agostino, who is evidently implying she was alone with Artigenio: "Signorsì che fui ricercata a fare un ritratto [di Artigenio] per una donna che diceva essere sua innamorata et lo feci et che volete voi dire per questo et fu Tutia che mi ricercò a fare questo ritratto" (Menzio 1981, 123). The translation of this passage in Garrard (1989, app. B, fol. 128) reverses the meaning of the sentence.

47. Menzio 1981, 124. Francesco Gentileschi was born on May 31, 1597 (AVR, S. Lorenzo in Lucina, Battesimi, fol. 167v; Bissell 1981, 100). Artemisia falsely asserted that Francesco was sixteen when Francesco Scarpellino lived with them, that is, before May 1611; see Menzio 1981, 46.

48. Menzio 1981, 87, 152.

49. Appendix 1, sect. A, fol. 411v, Carlo Saraceni: ". . . so ch'[Horatio] ha una figliola chiamata la signora Artemisia ch'io l'ho sentita nominare ma non la conosco e l'ho sentita nominare con occasione che lei dipingeva. . . ."

50. Ibid., fol. 420, Antinoro Bertucci: "mentre habitava in strada della Croce Horatio . . . mi menò di sopra che mi mostrò certi quadri e viddi lì una giovane ch'io mi imaginai che fosse sua figliola perché havevo inteso dire che haveva una figliola."

51. See cat. 17 and appendix 1, sect. A, fol. 379v.

52. See note 9 above. Both Passeri (1995, 122) and Baldinucci (1811–12, vol. 3, 713) mention Artemisia's beauty.

53. "E con questa buona promessa mi racquetai e con questa promessa mi ha indotto a consentir doppo amorevolmente alle sue voglie" (Menzio 1981, 49). I disagree with Cohen's (2000, 71) interpretation of the word as "willingly."

54. Costanza de Bargellis described the physical appearance of her brother during the trial for incest (ASR, processi, b. 62, 111); Cavazzini 1998, 204; Bertolotti 1876, 199.

55. See appendix 1, sect. A, fol. 383r,v, Fra Pietro Giordano's deposition: ". . . viddi ch'una di quelle donne all'uscir di Cancelleria sin al cancello andava appoggiata al braccio di detto Agostino et al separarsi facero gran segno d'amor et affettione insieme. . . ." See also Porzia Stiattesi's deposition in Menzio 1981, 138.

56. See Lapierre 1998, 169–70, for this interpretation of the development of the trial.

57. See note 12 above and appendix 1, sect. A, fols. 401v–403. Orazio's servant, the Nicolò Bedino discussed below, did household chores in exchange for food, lodging, and instruction in drawing. He did not receive a salary, but, according to Richard Spear, expenses for food were substantial. His position seems to have been common at the time; see Cavazzini 1997, 408–9; and Lukehart 1993, 41, 46–47.

58. On July 16, 1612, Orazio moved to the "portone di Santo Spirito"; Menzio 1981, 57. Tassi had been living at the "salita di Sant'Onfrio" since the late summer of 1610; see, for example, appendix 1, sect. A, fols. 427, 443r,v.

59. Menzio 1981, 124, Artemisia: ". . . non se n'è dato querela prima perché s'era ordinato di fare qualche altra cosa acciò non si divulgasse questo vituperio." The relationship was known to many people, including Artemisia's brothers; ibid., 42.

60. Cohen and Cohen 1993, esp. 173–74; Cohen 2000.

61. Farinacci 1606–49, vol. 4 (1618), Quaestio CXLVII, Stuprum, 519–27, vol. 6, Decisio LXXIV, 579. A man who had violated a woman had to provide a dowry for her even if he married her, but the dowry had to be larger if he did not marry her. A *stuprum* involving abduction was considered a much more serious crime, and for this reason Agostino was also accused of having repeatedly tried to take Artemisia away from Rome, see Menzio 1981, 43. But this accusation was not pursued in the trial.

That a violent *stuprum* could be punished by the gallows is recorded in the *Statuti Almae Urbis Romae* of 1580, where, however, it is also said that charges should be pressed within two months. Elizabeth Cohen has kindly informed me that the punishments established by the *Statuti* were much stricter than the ones applied in practice.

62. Menzio 1981, 154. Nicolò's full name was Nicolò di Bernardino de Felice, but his name is always spelled Bedino—without abbreviations—in this trial. See ASR, Trib. Crim. del Governatore, Processi del secolo XVII, b. 62, i.e., fol. 555, and note 72 below.

63. See appendix 1, sect. C.

64. For the sentence, see ibid.

65. Cardinal Scipione Borghese settled his accounts with Agostino on December 15, 1612. Evidently, more than two weeks after the sentence of exile, Agostino was in Rome. On January 26, 1613, Agostino nominated as his proxy a Giacomo Pavalli from Pisa in the office of a Roman notary; see ASR, 30 Notai Capitolini, uff. 36, vol. 25, fol. 73. I owe this information to Alexandra Lapierre.

66. Appendix 1, sect. B, fol. 106, and sect. C. See Lapierre 1998, 456.

67. Appendix 1, sect. A, fols. 442v–445.

68. For these documents, see appendix 1, sect. C, under March 13, 20, 23, 1613, April 9, 1613.

69. Cavazzini 1993, 318, 325.

70. See note 14 above for Orazio's presence in Rome. Passeri ([1772] 1995, 122, 124) states that after a period of bitter contention, Tassi and Gentileschi became friends again and even painted together at Bagnaia. This was certainly not the case; see Bissell 1981, 199–200, and Cavazzini 1993.

71. See appendix 1, sect. C, under April 9, for the document. My incorrect transcription is in Cavazzini 1997, n. 77, cited in Lapierre 1998, 456. There were not two different pronouncements on April 8 and 9, but only one on the ninth. For various reasons, I suspected that Tassi had been exonerated of the crime. My suspicions seemed to be confirmed by the sentence beginning "in Tassi's favor" and ending with the order to release him from jail, not to accompany him to the border of the Papal States, as in Lapierre 1998, 214. Thus, I misread "iniustum exilium" for "iniucto exilium" and constructed the meaning accordingly. I realize now that these formulas apply to all the sentences of exile, at least to all of those in the Registrazioni d'Atti. A prisoner condemned to exile was evidently released, sometimes under bail, and no provisions seem to have been made to ensure that he actually left the city or the states.

72. ASR, Processi sec. XVII, b. 62, 602, Nicolò di Bernardino de Felice, 19 novembre 1619: ". . . io per la verità m'essaminai a favore del detto Agostino et detto Gentileschi mi fece mettere pregione sotto pretesto che io non havessi detto la verità e saranno da cinque o sei anni in circa e fui assoluto nel tribunale del medesimo che era giudice il signor Girolamo Felice."

73. Mancini (1617–21) 1956–57, 252: "[Agostino] è huomo destro, e nel parlare molto libero e pronto, che per tale prontezza e libertà s'è rotto spesse volte con gli

amici, e per tale rottura ha patito dei travagli; nodimeno con il cervello si è saputo difendere, et si deve credere che vi sia stata accompagnata l'innocenza." Mancini probably knew Tassi well, because he lived nearby the "portone di santo Spirito," in the same neighborhood. See ASR, Stato civile, appendice, Santo Spirito in Sassia, Stati di anime, 1614, unpaged.

74. Passeri (1772) 1995, 122: ". . . Artemisia . . . nella pittura si rese gloriosa, e sarebbe stata degna d'ogni stima se fusse stata di qualità più onesta e onorata . . . Agostino . . . fu da Orazio querelato, ch'egli l'havesse stuprata, e successe veramente il caso; ma che fusse stato Agostino non se ne ha certezza . . . uscì dalla prigione innocente, se pure era tale. . . ."

75. ASR, Camerale I, fabbriche 1544, in Borsi, Briganti, and Del Piazzo 1973, 251–54, and Cavazzini 1998, 220. For the chapel, see Fumagalli 1992, 240–42, and Laureati and Trezzani 1993, 58–75.

76. Cavazzini 1997, 419; Laureati and Trezzani 1993, 76–135.

77. The Casino delle Muse was not quite finished when Tassi was imprisoned in early March 1612, even though work on the apartment of Cardinal Lanfranco had already started by that January. See note 37 above. Both painters were paid by Scipione Borghese on April 20—Tassi was in jail at that point—and the account was settled in December 1612 only with Tassi. Gentileschi seems to have worked on the casino after the beginning of the trial. A painter called Pietro Hernandez saw him there after Nicolò had left his service, and therefore after Tassi's arrest; see appendix 1, sect. A, fols. 418v, 413. However, Gentileschi may have been prevented from completing the figures on the lower register, between the arches, which do not seem to be by him, especially those on the outside wall; see Bissell 1981, 157.

78. Crinò and Nicolson 1961, 144–45.

79. See ASR, Tribunale Criminale del Governatore, Registrazioni d'Atti, 165, fol. 208v, 10 gennaio 1612, "Pro fisco contra Carolum Saracium venetum pictorem degentes in via [tinda] versus Populum et Augustinum Tassum pictorem in iudicium coram Ill.mus et excell. Anselmo Ciolo locumtenens meque et Portio Camerarius subst. locumtenens [fasto] reportavit moniturium de non descendendo de domo. . . ."

Lanfranco had already worked for the Borghese, but in a relatively minor capacity; see Fumagalli 1990.

80. AVR, Santo Spirito in Sassia, matrimoni, fol. 17; Bissell 1981, 103. For the date of the couple's departure for Florence, see Lapierre 1998, 457.

81. Appendix 1, sect. A, fol. 395v, Molli: ". . . io ci viddi in casa [in via Margutta] oltre detto Signor Horatio una sua figlia grande e tre figli maschi che uno dei quali che era il più grande macinava li colori e anco un nipote del Signor Horatio che andava apprendere. . . ." As discussed in the appendix, it is not precisely clear at what time Molli posed on via Margutta. Appendix 1, sect. A, fol. 403, Caterina Zuccarini: ". . . prima che detto Nicolò s'accomodasse con detto signor Horatio [this must have happened around November 1611] io ce l'ho visto venire in casa non so che volte che sarà doi o tre volte in circa che veniva a imparare di disegnare e disegnavano insieme lui e Francesco figliolo di detto signor Horatio che imparavano da loro. . . ."

82. Appendix 1, sect. A, fol. 403, Pietro Hernandez: ". . . et [Nicolò] imparava di disegnare et anco l'ho visto dipingere che la signora Artemisia gli insegnava." See note 81 above.

83. For artists' training, see, for example, Goldstein 1996, 10–14; Lukehart 1993, 41–43.

84. Appendix 1, sect. A, fol. 374v: ". . . l'essercitio mio è di pittore, cioè principiante, che vado disegnando."

85. Glenn 1999, 123.

86. See note 33 above for the letter.

87. Appendix 1, sect. B, fols. 112v–113.

88. For Tassi's workshop, see Cavazzini 1997.

89. An album of drawings sold by Sotheby's in 1964 seems to have included not only autograph drawings by Tassi, but also copies of them by his students; see Cavazzini 2000.

90. Appendix 1, sect. A, fol. 407.

91. Ibid., sect. B, fol. 114v.

92. For Orazio's practice of making drawn studies from the model, see Christiansen, pp. 9–12, in this publication.

93. Appendix 1, sect. A, fols. 395, 431v; see also fol. 424v, Margherita milanese lavandaia: ". . . poche volte io l'ho visto dipingere et in casa sua ho visto praticare li supradetti che lui li ritraheva in camera che non si poteva vedere, ma mi mostrava bene li quadri che lui faceva a similitudine di costoro."

94. Various depositions give this impression; see, for example, ibid., fol. 424, where Margherita the washerwoman from Milan lists Orazio's models and repeatedly says that Orazio, not Orazio and Artemisia, painted them. Both Molli and Bernardino de Franceschi claim that Orazio, not father and daughter, employed them; for a description of the house, see also fols. 395, 396v, 397, 399. In particular, see Franchi's deposition, fol. 410v: ". . . di sopra so che ci sono dui stanze dove ci stava la zitella che di sopra io non ci andai mai. . . ." Nicolò (in Menzio 1981, 150–51): ". . . son stato in detta casa del signor Horatio in strada Margutta . . . di sopra ci stanno doi stanze che in una ci dipingeva nell'altra si faceva la cucina . . . e la signora Artemitia dormiva in una camera in alto a capo le scale."

95. Menzio 1981, 48.

96. Ibid., 61, 68.

97. Ibid., 70. ASR, 30 Notai Capitolini, uff. 34, 11 maggio 1612, cc. 446–56, "S. Cecilia in ginocchio sopra un cuscino rosso, palmi 10 di altezza, S. Susanna con doi vecchi con la cornice tutta indorata con la medesima altezza. . . ." The inventory of Quorli's possessions has been found by Lapierre (1998, app. 3).

98. Menzio 1981, 61, 112.

99. For a contrary opinion, see Harris 1998, 110.

100. Appendix 1, sect. A, fols. 407v–408.

101. Ibid., sect. B, fols. 107v–108: "Io come ho detto ho visto dipingere il sig. Horatio Gentileschi nella sala al Monte Cavallo dove ci dipingevo io ancho . . . Ho visto anco di poi dipingere la loggia del Card. Borghese dove ho lavorato ancora io . . . Io so che il sig. Horatio Gentileschi ha figli maschi e femmine che l'ho sentito dire et conosco un figlio maschio che si chiama Francesco che l'ho visto venire su nel [lavoro] a Montecavallo." See also ibid., sect. A, fols. 375v–376v, Mario Trotta's deposition: "Io conosco Horatio Gentileschi et Agostino Tasso perché ho lavorato a giornate con loro a Montecavallo . . . Signor no che io non conosco Artimitia figliola di Horatio et io non so di che fama e conditione si sia" (also in Lapierre 1998, app. 5). Menzio 1981, 109, Antonio Mazzantino: ". . . io incollavo al giardino del signor Cardinale Borghese dove dipingevano . . . Io lo so [che Orazio ha tre figli maschi e una femmina] perché li ragazzi li ho visti, e della femmina l'ho inteso dire dal Gentileschi che l'haveva."

102. Baldinucci 1811–12, vol. 3, 713. See also De Dominici 1840–46, vol. 3, 82; Costa 2000, 36.

103. Artemisia Gentileschi: "Et il medesimo giorno, che era tempo piovoso, stando io pingendo un ritratto di un putto di Tutia per mio gusto"; Menzio 1981, 48. See note 46 above.

Glenn (1999, 122) argues that women needed a man to mediate between them and their clients, while here we seem to witness a chain of mediation by women: Artigenio's lover talks to Tuzia and Tuzia to Artemisia. However, Artigenio may have discussed the matter directly with Orazio. Tuzia brought him to see Orazio, who was painting, and the two talked together; see Menzio 1981, 123.

104. Glenn (1999, 123–30) convincingly argues that women were trained as history painters only for lack of a better alternative, that is, if they had no brothers.

105. For Artemisia as a painter of still lifes, see Baldinucci 1811–12, vol. 3, 714, and Costa 2000. For the paintings by Orazio and Artemisia in the Galleria Spada, see ASR, 30 Notai Capitolini, uff. 28, 1637, 969, in Cannatà and Vicini 1992, 103. The inventory mentions "due ovati piccoli con due teste rappresentanti Pittura e Poesia una che ha la cornice rifatta." One of these is probably the *Self-Portrait as*

Painting, once in a private collection in Brazil, rejected by Bissell 1999, 327; see also Spear 2000, 574, and Papi 1994, 198–99.

106. Menzio 1981, 124: "Io non so scrivere e poco leggere."

107. Ibid., 151: "Io ho visto leggere detta signora Artimitia litere stampate et anco scritte a mano ma lei non sa scrivere." Appendix 1, sect. A, fol. 392.

108. Chartier 1989, 112.

109. Harris's claim (1998, 120) that artists became more learned in the second half of the seicento is unwarranted. Depositions in trials and receipts of payment are reliable documents by which to test the writing skills of painters and assistants, much better than letters, which are often dictated. The formula "Io . . . ho deposto quanto di sopra mano propria" indicates autograph statements by people who could both sign—and therefore read—and write. (Receipts of payment usually include similar statements, "Io . . . ho ricevuto quanto di sopra mano propria.") See appendixes A and B for various examples. Previous transcriptions of the 1612 trial do not include these formulas, which are present throughout. Spelling and handwriting give an indication of the literacy of the author. It was not unheard-of for young women to read and write; see Ottavia, daughter of a merchant, in Cohen and Cohen 1993, 113–14. For literacy in Rome, see Grendler 1989, esp. 78–80, and Petrucci 1982, esp. 12–17. For the education of artists in Bologna, see Dempsey 1980.

110. See note 105 above.

111. Papi in Florence 1991, 114.

112. An engraving and a medal identify Artemisia's features for us; Bissell 1999, figs. 97, 100. It has often been suggested, but not unanimously accepted, that the woman with a fan painted by Orazio in the Casino delle Muse (see frontispiece, p. 282) may be a portrait of Artemisia. I believe the identification to be correct, and I see a similar face, with slight variations, repeated endlessly in Orazio's and Artemisia's works, certainly in the *Susanna*. For another example of Artemisia's features on a nude body, see fig. 110. A self-portrait of her Florentine years, published by Papi (2000), may show her countenance after numerous pregnancies.

113. "Uno specchio grande di valore di scudi tre in circa quale è di acciaro con cornice e due colonnette." See note 97 above for Quorli's inventory. Full-length glass mirrors were indeed invented later, as Harris states (1998, 114).

114. See note 37 above for payments from the Borghese, which establish the timing of Orazio's work for them.

115. See note 33 above.

116. Pollock 1999, 116–19.

117. Bissell 1999, 117, 122. For a contrary opinion, see, for example, Harris 1998, 113.

118. Among the vast literature on the painting, see Spezzaferro 1975 and Vodret in Rome 1999, 24–26. No early engraving after the painting is known.

119. See Orazio's letter cited in note 33 above.

51.

Susanna and the Elders

Oil on canvas, 66⅞ × 46⅞ in. (170 × 119 cm)

Signed (on wall behind figure): ARTIMITIA/ GENTILESCHI F/1610

Collection Graf von Schönborn, Pommersfelden (inv. 191)

1610

New York, Saint Louis

Figure 105. Michelangelo (1475–1564), *Expulsion of Adam and Eve from the Garden of Eden*. Fresco. Sistine chapel, Vatican City

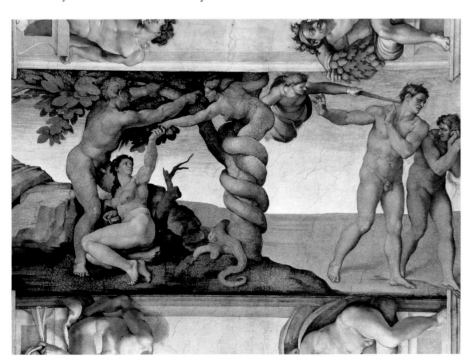

The story of Susanna in the Apocrypha tells of a beautiful matron who is seen and desired by two elders who frequently spy on her house. One day Susanna decides to bathe in her garden and sends her servants for oil and balsam. When the servants leave, the elders approach Susanna, demanding sexual favors and threatening to declare they had seen her with a young lover if she refuses them. Susanna does reject them, and true to their promise, they falsely accuse her. Eventually, a young man named Daniel questions the elders separately, and when details of their stories do not agree, he knows they have lied and condemns them to death. Susanna, in refusing to yield to the elders' demands, came to exemplify virtue, chastity, and marital fidelity, although sixteenth- and seventeenth-century artists often depict her as an alluring temptress—or at least a willing victim—prominently posed for the viewer's admiration, notably in Paolo Veronese's painting in Dresden and in the Cavaliere d'Arpino's on copper, dated about 1607, now in the Pinacoteca, Siena.

The Pommersfelden *Susanna* reveals a painter acutely attuned to narrative nuance. While the Susanna story is most often represented as a lateral composition, Artemisia's version is arranged vertically, allowing the elders graphically to press the heroine to comply with their demands. By spreading the two elders across the top of the fountain wall and depicting them as dark elements literally on top of the pale, nearly nude Susanna, the artist enables the viewer to empathize with the terrible plight of the defenseless woman. Treated as a unified pair, in collusion, the elders maintain power over their victim; Susanna triumphs only after they are interrogated separately. The solid stone wall behind the heroine enhances our understanding of her entrapment. Annibale Carracci's 1590 engraving of the subject, a likely source for the picture, uses an open balustrade, a motif copied by most other artists. But Artemisia grasped the implications of such a seemingly small detail. The extreme simplicity of the setting must also be seen as Artemisia's invention. Gone are the details of fountain and foliage that appear in nearly every other *Susanna*, and their absence contributes to the stark power of the image.

No other artist had interpreted the psychological dimension of the biblical story in such an effective format, and this aspect alone indicates that Orazio did not design the composition or develop the interpretation. Orazio rarely focused on the logical denouement of his narratives, and he often ignored essential details of a story altogether. The Dublin *David Slaying Goliath*, for example (cat. 12), presents the protagonist trying to wield (with one hand!) an oversized sword in a position that will in fact not allow him to decapitate the giant. His David is not tall enough to maneuver such a large weapon, nor are his feet firmly planted on the ground to offer the solid footing required to land the blow.

Garrard (1982, 1989) has argued eloquently that the picture reflects a specifically female point of view, which had autobiographical meaning for Artemisia, noting that she was raped in 1611 by Agostino Tassi and may already have received sexual overtures from

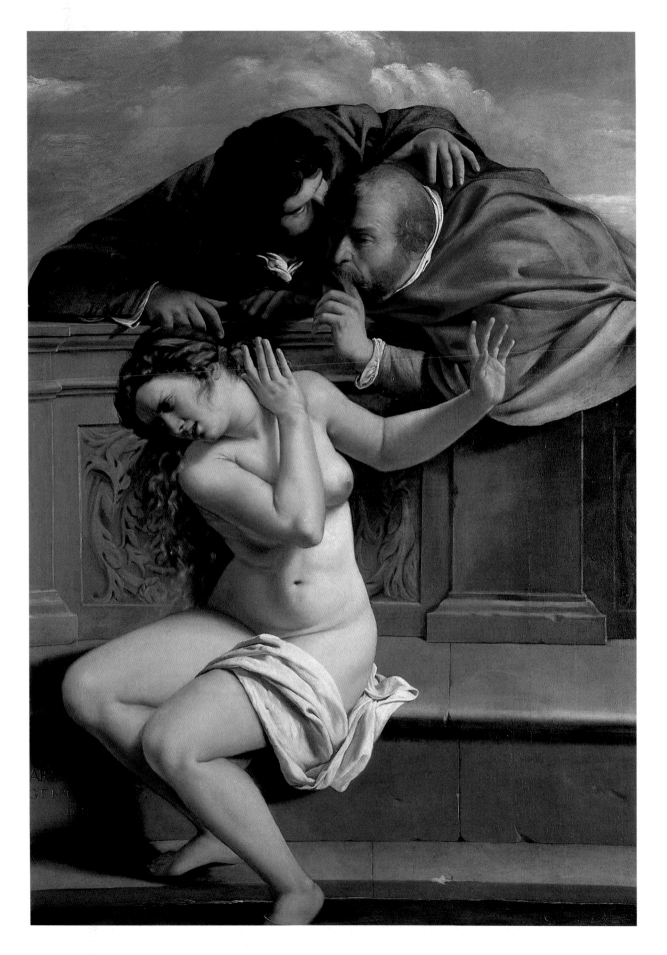

PROVENANCE: Benedetto Luti, Rome (until 1715?); family of Dr. Karl Graf von Schönborn, Schloss Weissenstein, Pommersfelden (from the early 18th century).

REFERENCES: Heller 1845, 23; Longhi 1916, 475–92; Boll 1928, 235–36; Schönborn Collection catalogue 1935, 22; Longhi 1943, 47 n. 38; Emiliani 1958b, 42; Bissell 1966, vol. 2, 262; Bissell 1968, 153, 157; Gregori 1968, 415; Borea in Florence 1970, 71, 414–21; Harris in Los Angeles 1976–77, 119–20; Greer 1979, 191; Bissell 1981, 64, 92 n. 5; Garrard 1982, 146–71; Slap 1985, 339–41; Hagen 1988, 78–79; Garrard 1989, 15–18, 182–209, 528–34 nn. 1–63; Rave in Nürnberg 1989, 373–75; Berti, Contini, and Papi in Florence 1991, 21, 34, 58, 109–33 no. 7; Spike 1991b, 732–33; Stolzenwald 1991, 18–19, 69–72; Bionda 1992, 21–22; Cropper 1992, 195, 202; Merkel 1992, 350, 352; Harris 1998, 115–17; Bissell 1999, 187–89 no. 2.

him that paralleled Susanna's story. Papi (Florence 1991) has supported this interpretation by identifying the two elders as Orazio Gentileschi and Agostino Tassi. However, it is difficult for us to re-create the specific experience of Artemisia as of 1610, and male artists also presented sensitive portrayals of Susanna's anguish, including Ludovico Carracci in 1598 and Gerrit van Honthorst in 1655.[1]

This superb painting must serve as the touchstone for understanding Artemisia's early development, her artistic relationship with her father, and her evolving artistic personality. Nevertheless, we must acknowledge that, notwithstanding its signature and the date of 1610, it has been challenged on both its attribution and its date of execution. These last two issues are closely intertwined and must be discussed together.

The painting is first mentioned in a 1715 letter from the Florentine artist Benedetto Luti to his patron Hofrat Bauer von Heppenstein. Working in Rome at the time, Luti offered to send a picture (the *Susanna*) by Orazio Gentileschi from his own collection.[2] The first published acknowledgment of Artemisia's authorship came in 1845, in Joseph Heller's guidebook to the Pommersfelden collection. Heller may, in fact, have been the first to correctly read the signature, which, as Boll posited in 1928, was made legible when the picture was cleaned by a Nuremberg restorer in 1839. However, the proficiency in the modeling of the body of Susanna and its unclear date led some scholars (Longhi 1943, Emiliani) to question whether Artemisia, who was only seventeen at the time, was actually the author. The problem was exacerbated by the incorrect identification of her birth date as 1597. This error was corrected by Bissell (1968), who discovered and published her birth records. Nevertheless, scholars continued to question the date, suspecting it should read 1619 rather than 1610. Hagen and Berti have suggested that the picture was made in Florence and backdated to 1610, the Roman period, while Rave believes that the last digit is either a 6 or a 9, placing the picture in Artemisia's Florentine period. In 1977, during the touring exhibition "Women Artists: 1550–1950," the picture was analyzed in the lab of the Brooklyn Museum of Art by Susanne P. Sack, then Chief Conservator. Her analysis, with ultraviolet-light photography, indicates

that the signature and date are original to the picture and were neither altered nor overpainted. These results, published by Garrard (1982), have been accepted by most scholars.

While, for some, the naturalism of the unidealized body of Susanna remains the most important argument for seeing the painting as exclusively by Artemisia, the issue of her sole authorship is still questioned, and several scholars (Greer, Garrard 1989, Contini, Stolzenwald) have found strong evidence for Orazio's guidance. Indeed, it makes sense that Orazio would have assisted Artemisia in this endeavor. His much quoted letter of 1612, written to the dowager grand duchess of Tuscany, Cristina of Lorraine, claiming that Artemisia had "no peer," shows Orazio to be an ardent advocate of his daughter's art.[3] The conception of the picture, a female nude seated in an expressive contrapposto attitude, seems designed to reveal the virtuosity of its maker, as Harris also points out. Might not Orazio have worked with his daughter to design such a vehicle for the display of her talents, a painting to which she must have devoted herself for some time in his workshop, given that she was only seventeen?

Orazio surely assisted his daughter in her choice of models. Garrard (1982, 1989) argues that Artemisia's source for the pose of Susanna was a figure on a Roman sarcophagus illustrating the story of Orestes and that this same sarcophagus inspired her father in his conception of the *David*, a painting that Artemisia must have observed as her father painted it. More likely, the model was Michelangelo's figure of Adam being expelled from Paradise, from the Sistine ceiling (fig. 105). There, the gesture is used to fend off the threat of the avenging angel, a function analogous to Susanna's rejection of the elders' demands. As in Michelangelo's figure, Susanna's left hand is shown with an open gesture, the thumb extended, and with the back of the hand to the viewer—rather than the palm, as in the sarcophagus. Artemisia may never have seen the Sistine chapel itself, but it is likely that she knew the imagery through a print made after the ceiling paintings. Testimony at the 1612 rape trial paints a picture of Artemisia's leading a sheltered life in those early Roman years. An outing in 1611 to see the frescoes that Orazio was completing for Scipione

Borghese is described as an unusual event and suggests that such excursions for the young painter were not routine. Artemisia's models must therefore have been drawn from a restricted repertoire.

Other models available to Artemisia may have been her father's pictures, her own or her father's drawings (it is unfathomable to imagine that Orazio, trained in the 1580s as a Mannerist painter, did not base his practice on the execution of preparatory drawings, in spite of the absence of any such drawings today), and various prints. The general configuration (Susanna seated in the foreground with the elders behind) may indeed have been originally inspired by Annibale Carracci's engraving. And Artemisia undoubtedly knew an important representation of Susanna in Rome, Baldassarre

Croce's fresco in Santa Susanna—a church she could well have visited—whose seated, gesturing heroine is echoed in Artemisia's composition. The quieting gesture of the gray-haired elder so closely echoes Domenichino's 1603 *Susanna and the Elders* (Doria Pamphili, Rome) that Artemisia must have known it or the lost original by Annibale Carracci that inspired it.[4]

1. For Carracci's painting, see Bologna–Fort Worth 1993, 116–18. For the Van Honthorst, see Judson and Ekkart 1999, no. 18, pl. 6.
2. Rave in Nürnberg 1989, 373–75.
3. The original letter is stored in Florence, Archivo di Stato, *Mediceo*, fil. 2 LVI segn. di N moderno 6003, 1612, and is published in Tanfani-Centofanti 1897, 221–24.
4. For the picture, see Rome 1996–97, 380–81 no. 6.

52.

Madonna and Child

Oil on canvas, 45⅞ × 34 in.
(116.5 × 86.5 cm)

Galleria Spada, Rome (inv. 166)

1610–11

This engaging rendition of the Virgin breast-feeding her child can be traced back to its first owner, Alessandro Biffi, in the early seventeenth century. It entered the Spada collection through the owner's indebtedness. Biffi rented living quarters near the Veralli family. When he fell behind in his rent, he entered into an agreement with the administrator, Virgilio Vespignani, allowing him to discharge his obligation by consigning to the family some of his property. Biffi owned several works of art, and these were bequeathed to the Veralli heirs in an inventory signed by Biffi on December 22, 1637. Marchese Maria Veralli married Orazio Spada in 1636, and the painting may have entered the Spada collection sometime after 1643, when Giulia, Maria Veralli's only (unmarried) sister, died. Among these works was the present painting, described as "A Madonna by Artemisia with the child in her arms."

These inventory notices were published only in 1992. Prior to that date, the painting had a varied attribution history. An 1862 inventory lists it as by Bernardo Strozzi, while in 1925 the painting was given a tentative attribution to Francesco Cozza (both in Cannatà and Vicini). Porcella gave the picture to Artemisia, while Zeri attributed it to Giovanni Francesco Guerrieri, to whom it was, until recently, ascribed by the Galleria Spada. Emiliani, following Longhi, assigned the picture to a Baglionesque artist. Alfred Moir questioned its attribution to Angelo Caroselli. However, since the publication in 1968 of Bissell's important chronology of the artist, most writers (Borea, Gregori, Garrard, Papi in Florence 1991, 1994) have acknowledged the attribution to Artemisia. Surprisingly, in his new catalogue raisonné, Bissell rejects Artemisia's authorship, evidently unaware of the early provenance and the 1637 inventory. He

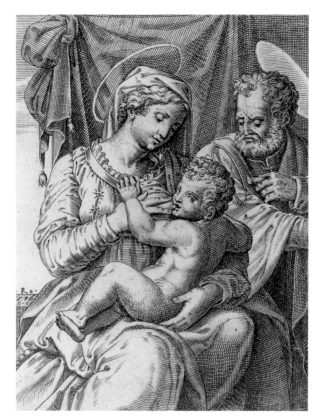

Figure 106. Agostino Carracci (1557–1602), *The Holy Family.* Engraving. Graphische Sammlung Albertina, Vienna

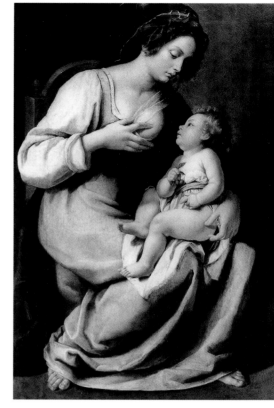

Figure 107. Attributed to Giovanni Francesco Guerrieri (1589–1655/59), *Madonna and Child.* Oil on canvas. Palazzo Pitti, Galleria Palatina, Florence

PROVENANCE: Alessandro Biffi, Rome (until 1637; 1637 list of paintings, as by Artemisia); Veralli collection, Rome (1637–43/86); Spada collection, Rome (after 1643/86); Galleria Spada, Rome.

REFERENCES: Porcella 1931, 7, 215; Lavagnino 1933, 9, 12; Longhi 1943, 41 n. 28; Zeri 1954, 88–89 no. 298; Francini Ciaranfi 1955, 63; Emiliani 1958b, 19–20, 50; Moir 1967, vol. 1, 55–56, vol. 2, 64; Paolucci 1967, 78; Bissell 1968, 155; Borea in Florence 1970, 74 no. 46, 125; Nicolson 1970, 641; Volpe 1970, 116–17; Sricchia Santoro 1974, 44; Neppi 1975, 144; Bissell 1981, 92 n. 4, 147; Menzio 1981, 40, 48, 64; Gregori in Naples 1984–85, vol. 1, 147; Emiliani in San Severino Marche–Bologna 1988, 15, 33–35, 68–69 no. 3; Garrard 1989, 23–35, 411, 415, 423 and n. 57, 492–93 nn. 19–20; Berti, Contini, and Papi in Florence 1991, 19, 24, 114–15 no. 8, 150–51; Stolzenwald 1991, 18, 25 fig. 9; Bionda 1992, 26; Cannatà and Vicini 1992, 188, 192, 195; Vicini 1992, 44; Sotheby's, London, sale cat., May 20, 1993, under lot 55; Szigethi in Milan 1993, 93; Papi 1994, 198–99; Vicini 1998; Vicini 1999; Bissell 1999, 327 no. X-19; Papi 2000, 450; Vicini 2000, 7–12.

finds the composition lacking in originality and has revived Emiliani's attribution to an artist in the circle of Baglione. Nevertheless, the style of and approach to the subject fit well within Artemisia's early Roman oeuvre.

In several respects the painting recalls the Pommersfelden *Susanna and the Elders* (cat. 51). The physiognomy of the Virgin closely resembles the features of the Susanna, and the choice of similar coloration for the drapery of the Madonna and for the elder on the right reinforces the placement of the *Madonna and Child* around the same date as the *Susanna.* A comparison with the Pommersfelden picture is telling and reveals the artist working simultaneously in two different styles. Where Artemisia's sophisticated treatment of the human figure in the Pommersfelden painting suggests careful working and reworking of a posed female model through drawings, perhaps under the guidance of her father, the Madonna in the Spada painting is not nearly as accomplished. The Virgin's

right arm is awkwardly proportioned and its placement not thought through, while the left arm, of which only the hand is shown, appears to be longer than its mate. The graceful, elongated fingers of the right hand are not repeated in the fleshier proportions of the left. Pentimenti along the Madonna's right elbow indicate that Artemisia reworked the contours of the arm, never reaching a fully satisfactory solution.

The painting may have been made in response to Orazio's 1609 *Madonna and Child* (cat. 15), an intimate portrayal of mother and infant as the baby suckles at the mother's breast. The picture is filled with examples of minutely observed details—the flexed feet and wrinkled left hand of the child, the mother's braided hair and carefully observed facial features, a rendering which suggests that Orazio painted directly from the model. Nevertheless, the sitter is obviously posed, and the image ends up being somewhat contrived.

Artemisia's version, on the other hand, though not based on the observation of two individuals, portrays

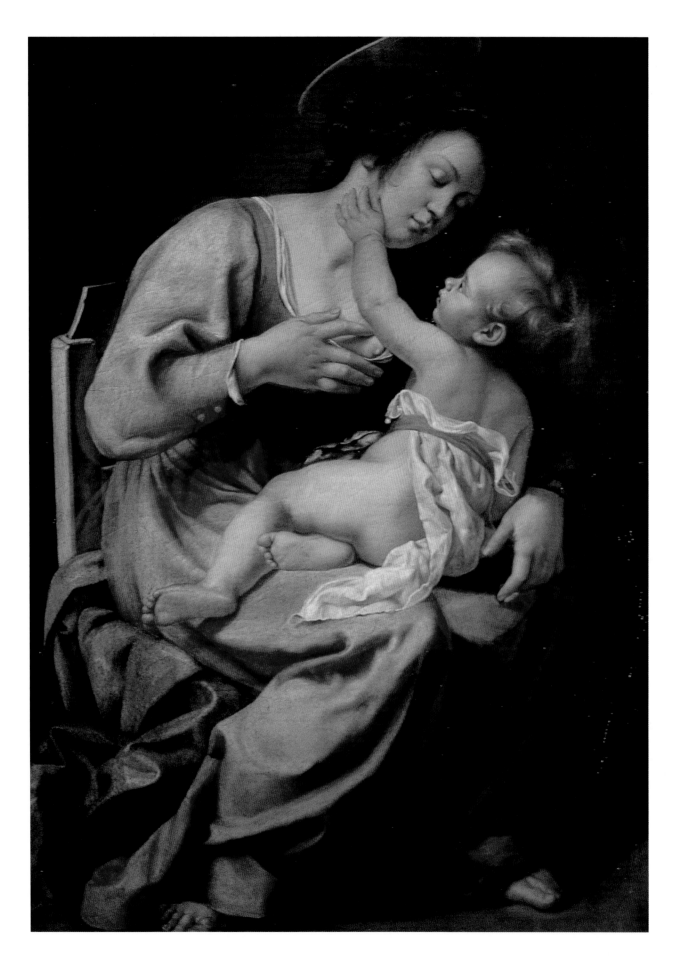

an intimate interaction between mother and child. Artemisia has chosen a less static moment, in which the child reaches up to caress his mother's cheek, holding his head in a corresponding angle to that of his mother, while she in turn bows her head in sympathetic response. The Virgin is based on a type, and her physiognomy, similar to that of the Susanna in the Pommersfelden painting, shows that Artemisia used this general image on at least two occasions. The Virgin's left hand may derive from that of her father's painting. Artemisia's arrangement integrates elegance of pose with an affective use of gesture—traits that reappear in the artist's mature production but that here strike a distinctly juvenile and unresolved note.

Bissell (1999) correctly observes that while Artemisia's *Madonna* clearly derives from the painting by Orazio—specifically the left hand of the Virgin— another source for the composition is undoubtedly an engraving of the *Holy Family,* either the original, from the workshop of Marcantonio Raimondi, or, less likely, a copy by Agostino Carracci (fig. 106). Although Vicini has most recently related the pose to Titian's *Madonna and Child with Saints Maurice and Jerome* (Louvre, Paris), it makes much better sense to see the artist working from the Carracci print, which would have been easily available to her and which exhibits much closer parallels to key elements of the composition. Undoubtedly,

Artemisia may initially have been inspired by the pose of the Virgin and the reclining position of the Christ child and his grasping gesture, but the painting has the sense of a child responding to his mother. The treatment of the baby, in particular his enlarged forehead, long golden curls, and tousled hair, suggests the artist had experience working with a real child. A number of writers have associated this picture with a passage in the summation of the testimony for Agostino Tassi's rape trial, in which Artemisia is described as "painting, accompanied by Tuzia with her son seated on her lap."[1] Tuzia was the Gentileschi's tenant, who often served as Artemisia's chaperone.

A second version of this composition, in the Galleria Palatina, Florence, has been closely linked to the present picture (fig. 107) and has been attributed to Artemisia by a number of writers (Menzio, Gregori, Contini, Stolzenwald, Bissell 1999). Its more studied positioning of the child and correction of the awkward right elbow and left hand indicate it was made at a later date. And while the two paintings must be related, the Madonna and the child in the Palatina *Madonna* lack the physiognomies characteristic of Artemisia's other figures and cannot be considered autograph.

1. "... dipingeva et con lei assisteva Tutia con il figlio suo fra le gambe a seder ..." See Menzio 1981, 40.

53.

Cleopatra

Oil on canvas, 46½ × 71¼ in. (118 × 181 cm)

Amedeo Morandotti, Milan

ca. 1611–12

PROVENANCE: See cat. 17.

REFERENCES: See cat. 17.

Painted when Orazio and Artemisia worked together in Rome in the early 1610s, the Morandotti *Cleopatra* falls within a period when their styles were very similar, and it has been attributed to both artists (see cat. 17). Conceptions of the building up of form as well as the depiction of similar physiognomies and drapery textures seem characteristic of the work of both father and daughter during this period; the case for Artemisia's authorship of this remarkable painting must therefore focus on its interpretive tone.

After the death of her lover, Mark Antony, the Egyptian queen Cleopatra takes her own life to avoid the indignity of being paraded in a triumphal procession by Octavian, the future Roman emperor Augustus. Sources vary as to how this deed was actually accomplished. The most popular account tells of an asp, concealed in a basket of figs, whose poison Cleopatra administers to herself after sending a request to Octavian that she be buried alongside Mark Antony. Octavian, upon receiving Cleopatra's letter, sends

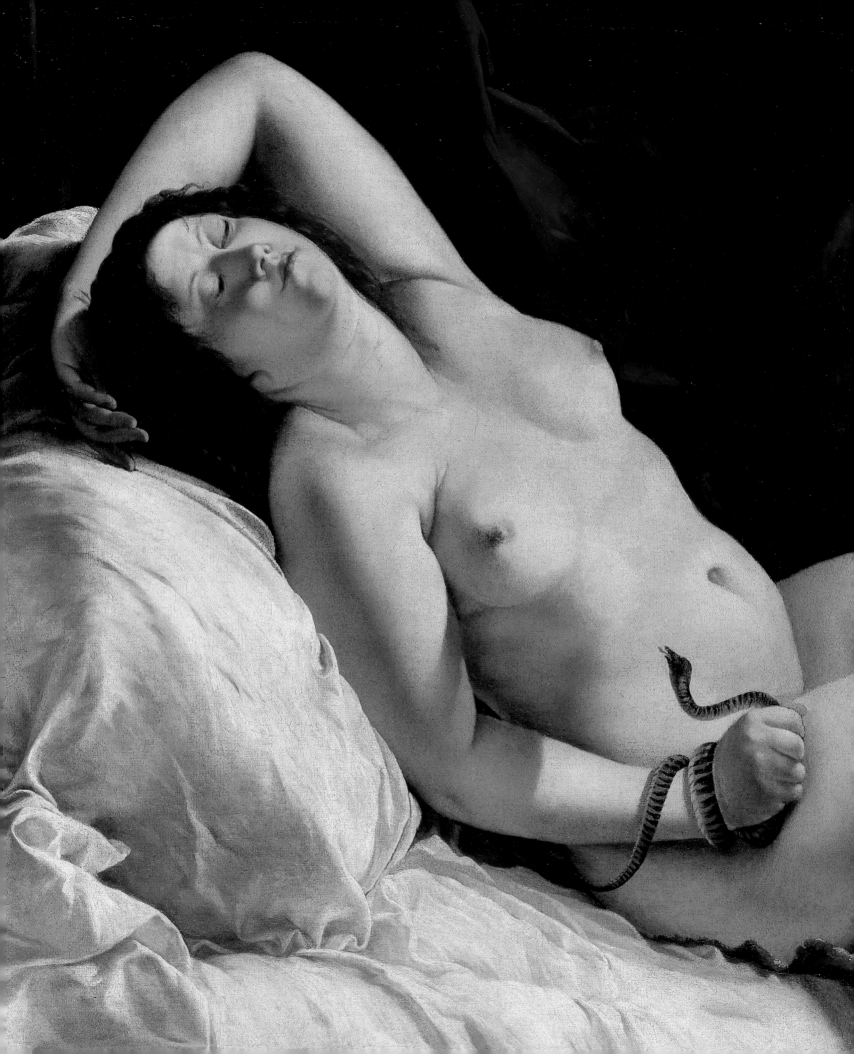

soldiers to find her, and when they arrive and enter her chamber, they discover the dead bodies of Cleopatra and her maid Iras. A second maid, Charmion, is found replacing the crown upon her mistress's head. Charmion, too, succumbs soon after. The most thorough account of the death of Cleopatra is told by the Greek historian and biographer Plutarch, and it is his version that probably informed most artists who represented this infamous event.

The painter of this picture, in my view Artemisia Gentileschi, has focused on the moment when the solitary Cleopatra (as described by Plutarch) prepares to administer the asp's venom. Traditionally, artists portrayed the act itself or its immediate aftermath, when, as the poison begins to take effect, the heroine writhes in agony. These pictures derive their erotic power from the juxtaposition of the asp (with its obvious phallic symbolism) and the bare and vulnerable breasts of the expiring queen. Here, Cleopatra pauses before she positions the serpent, arresting the action and deviating from tradition, an approach to narrative that we find in both the *Jael and Sisera* (cat. 61) and the later *Lucretia* (cat. 67).

Artemisia's penchant for displaying her talent at the handling of the nude figure (already demonstrated in her debut composition of the *Susanna* in 1610; cat. 51) and her predisposition for original narrative interpretation suggest she, and not Orazio, is the author of this painting. The powerful gesture (no other Cleopatra grasps the snake so forcefully), coupled with the glaring nakedness of the body, in this bold rendition of the last moments of the Egyptian queen's life, is unmatched. The coiling snake may have been suggested by Agostino Veneziano's 1515 engraving in which a standing Cleopatra brings the serpent, wrapped around her wrist, to her breast, but here the artist has infused the gesture with new dramatic intensity, silhouetting the flicking tongue against the pale abdominal flesh.

The parting of the background drapery on the far right also exemplifies the kind of attention to narrative detail that specifically characterizes Artemisia's work of the first several decades of her career. While initially it reads as simply the source for the light that floods over Cleopatra's body, other interior images painted by both Gentileschi do not always include an identifiable source. Rather, the curtain aperture reminds us that although Cleopatra was alone at the moment of her suicide, her lifeless body was discovered, first by her own two maids who also killed themselves, and then by Octavian's soldiers, who discovered all three. The maids figure prominently in Artemisia's later *Cleopatra* (cat. 76) from the 1630s.

Unlike Artemisia, Orazio did not typically invent new interpretive moments; rarely does he stray far from the established norms for representing specific narratives. Nevertheless, he did at times introduce original elements into his compositions that enhanced the setting or the tone of the story, such as the endearing donkey peering over the masonry wall in the Birmingham *Rest on the Flight into Egypt* (cat. 34). Although he painted moving and affecting images of individuals in contemplation (the Fabriano *Magdalene* [cat. 24] and his Spada *David* [cat. 18] come to mind), the novel aspect of the present painting, in which Cleopatra's gesture underscores her will to carry through her suicide, does not comply with Orazio's way of thinking. Rather, it recalls other paintings in Artemisia's oeuvre. The *Cleopatra*, which as Bissell (1981) has pointed out shares the physiognomy of the Uffizi *Judith* (cat. 62), also brings to mind the tormented isolation of the Seville *Magdalene* (cat. 68) and the Milan *Lucretia* (cat. 67).

Garrard (1989) has identified the particularized anatomy of the figure as a mark of Artemisia's being a female painter. Christiansen (see pp. 11, 98) argues that such realism testifies to Orazio's use of the living model during the three-year period between 1609 and 1612. Orazio's other nudes, the two versions of the *Danaë* from the 1620s (cat. nos. 36, 41), certainly do not exhibit such brutal naturalism and show a far different anatomical form. But in the work of Artemisia, with the exception of the Burghley House *Susanna* ([cat. 65], where, I believe, she intentionally selected another figural type), the rounded stomach, swelling conical breasts, and ample hips reappear—as, for example in the later Bathshebas—over and over again. This is the same body type that we find in the earlier *Susanna*, and although some have argued that the *Susanna* was designed by Orazio, he did not reuse the figure type, while Artemisia did.

While not necessarily advancing an Artemisia attribution for the picture, Pollock has used the painting to analyze its possible indicators of female authorship. She finds it yields contradictory meanings, since its individualized body rejects the conventional generic nude and represents a real woman, while at the same time the pose can be interpreted as connoting eroticism and as intending to suit the tastes of male clients. She has related the portrayal of an expiring woman in this painting as well as in the later *Cleopatra* (cat. 76) to the artist's own experience of the death of her mother in 1605, making the works indirect expressions of the painter's personal trauma.

While Christiansen identifies the model for Cleopatra's head as the woman with a fan from the Casino delle Muse (traditionally understood as an image of Artemisia; frontispiece, p. 282), to my eye the head of the lute player in the casino ceiling (fig. 6) remains the more probable source.[1] Not only do they share the same angular orientation, but Cleopatra's nose and mouth appear to be duplicated from the fresco. Whether Cleopatra may represent Artemisia herself remains a tricky subject. Given that Orazio's primary motive for bringing suit against Artemisia's rapist was the honor of his family, it seems highly unlikely that in the middle of the trial proceedings he would have created a large-scale picture (undoubtedly intended for a patron) of his naked daughter. Nearly everyone who has written about the picture has noted its erotic expression, and it seems problematic that Orazio would willingly have subjected himself to the kind of tongue wagging and street gossip that such an obvious personal reference would have engendered.

1. Garrard (1989, 19–20) maintains that the figure with the fan is an image of Artemisia. Bissell (1981, 202) notes the similarity of the physiognomy of the lute player to that of Cleopatra.

54.

Danaë

Oil on copper, 16 × 20 ⅝ in. (40.5 × 52.5 cm)

The Saint Louis Art Museum (inv. 93:1986)

ca. 1612

First appearing in the 1986 Sotheby's Monaco sale, this small painting on copper has generated active discussion among Gentileschi scholars, who have disputed its authorship as well as its dating. Freedberg, Schleier, and Bissell have argued that Orazio painted the picture, although Schleier has more recently questioned this view.[1] Matthiesen first published the picture as a work by Artemisia, and that attribution is accepted by Nicolson and by Papi and Contini. Garrard has suggested that a third artist, perhaps one of Artemisia's daughters, made this reduced version, clearly intended as a copy of the nude figure from the Morandotti *Cleopatra* (cat. nos. 17, 53).[2]

Bissell has most recently and most extensively argued for an attribution to Orazio, based on the high quality of the handling and the assumption that both this painting and the *Cleopatra* were executed by the same hand. His argument for Orazio's authorship of the *Cleopatra* is based on several points, including the correspondence of the head to a figure in the Casino delle Muse frescoes, the similarity of the linens to those in Orazio's Pommersfelden *Madonna and Child* (Schloss Weissenstein), and a reference in a 1615 letter indicating that Orazio had a *Cleopatra* in his studio that he intended to send to Florence. To these Bissell has added further points specifically germane to the *Danaë*. He has related the headdress of the maidservant to Orazio's ex-Colnaghi *Judith* (fig. 46) and notes similarities in the lost profile of the maid with the same motif in the Oslo *Judith* (cat. 13). He further argues that Orazio specialized in working on copper.

None of these assertions, however, offers a definitive argument for an attribution to Orazio; the *Danaë* can be related to Artemisia as well. The face of the protagonist in Artemisia's Uffizi *Judith Slaying Holofernes* (cat. 62) bears a close resemblance to a figure in

PROVENANCE: Private collection (sale, Sotheby's, Monaco, February 22, 1986, lot 243, as by Orazio); Kate Ganz Ltd., London (1986); The Saint Louis Art Museum.

REFERENCES: Settis 1985, 219; London 1986, 52; Nicolson 1990, vol. 1, 110; Contini and Papi in Florence 1991, 48, 51 fig. 34, 61; Mann 1996, 39–45; Mann 1997, 6–9; Zarucchi 1998–99, 13–16; Bissell 1999, 310–13 no. x-7, 377–78.

Figure 108. Titian (ca. 1485/90–1576), *Danaë*. Oil on canvas. Museo del Prado, Madrid

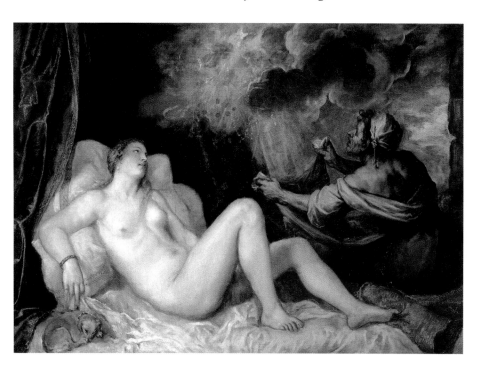

Orazio's Casino delle Muse frescoes (as Bissell himself has noted), and it would not be uncharacteristic to see Artemisia using that same source in this earlier picture. Orazio's reputed proficiency on copper in his Roman works (five by his hand are known, of which four are included in the present exhibition; cat. nos. 10, 19, 27, 38) does not preclude Artemisia's having worked on this support, as painting on copper was widely practiced by Italian painters of the early seventeenth century. We know that Artemisia made at least two, and perhaps three, other copper pictures—the late *Virgin and Child with a Rosary* (cat. 84), a lost *Saint Apollonia,* and a lost *Sleeping Putto.*[3] And the inventory of her household effects, drawn up in Florence in 1621, lists three works on copper (see appendix 3).

The narrative sensitivity displayed in the interpretation of the mythological story certainly conforms more to Artemisia's approach than to that of her father. The story, treated as a bold assertion of sexual union and sensual eroticism, derives from the earliest complete version told by the Greek author Apollodorus (2nd century B.C.). King Acrisius of Argos had a daughter named Danaë. It was prophesied that Danaë would bear offspring who would kill the king, and Acrisius locked his daughter in a brazen chamber. But the amorous Zeus was able to penetrate Danaë's protective fortress by transforming himself into a shower of

gold, and gaining entry he impregnated her. Danaë's son, Perseus, the offspring of this union, would later fulfill the prophecy by murdering the king.

The painting depicts the sexually aroused Danaë, who clutches some coins in her right fist (a brilliant adaptation of the *Cleopatra*) while others accumulate on the tender flesh between her thighs, an entirely original conceptualization of the myth. The coins had by the sixteenth century replaced the golden shower as the visual reference to Zeus, tangible indicators of the god's forceful entry into her chamber and into her body.[4] Danaë's fist, the coins pushed between the clenched fingers, also becomes a metaphor for sexual embrace, suggestive of the fact that the god was not initially invited by the young and vulnerable Danaë.[5] This is one of the few images where Danaë is shown actually experiencing the consummation. More typically, she is portrayed either as a sexually aggressive temptress or as a chaste innocent unaware of her impending fate.

The artist who made this painting was surely familiar with sixteenth-century variations on the Danaë story and has expanded on these earlier prototypes.[6] The placement and pose of the maid were undoubtedly inspired by Titian's masterly rendition (or some version of it) in the Prado (fig. 108). Titian's maid has assumed the characteristic gesture of Danaë (found already in early antiquity) in which she holds up one end of the drapery to cover her lap.[7] In Titian's painting, Danaë still fingers the sheet, whereas Artemisia's Danaë has abandoned any reference to this tradition.

Tactile sensation has assumed primacy in this painting. The artist has used the suggestive device of metal coins resting on bare flesh, and while Tintoretto had also portrayed Danaë with coins lying on her thighs (Musée des Beaux-Arts, Lyons), no other artist had positioned them for such obvious erotic meaning. The play between clothed and nude, seen in Titian's image, has been further developed by contrasting the maid's head scarf and covered shoulders with the stark nakedness of Danaë, whose longer hair caresses the upper part of her right arm to maximize the sensual force of the picture.

The Saint Louis *Danaë* displays the subtle variations in skin tone and the tightly composed format that are

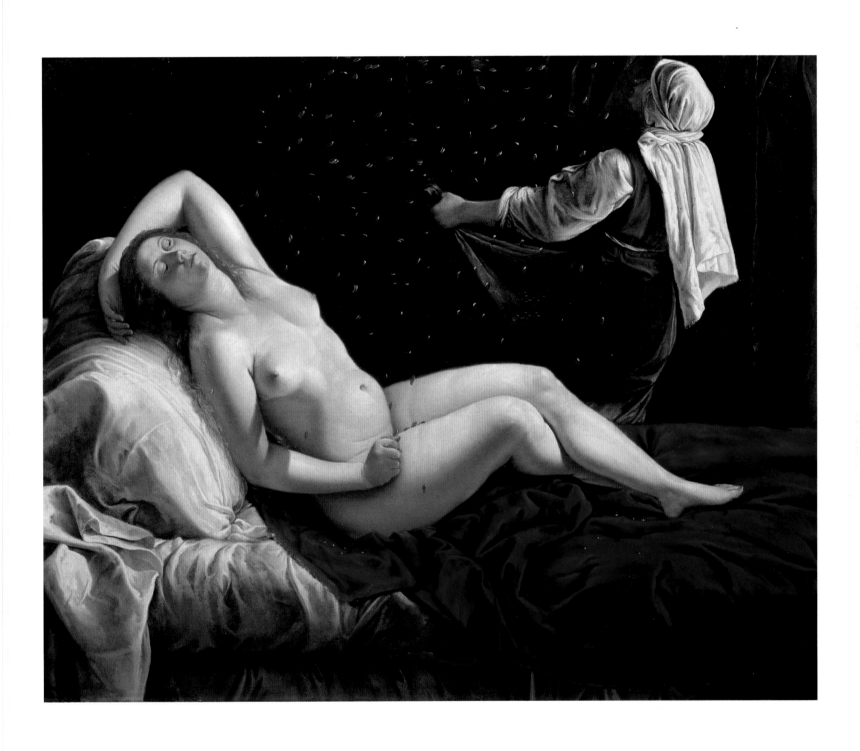

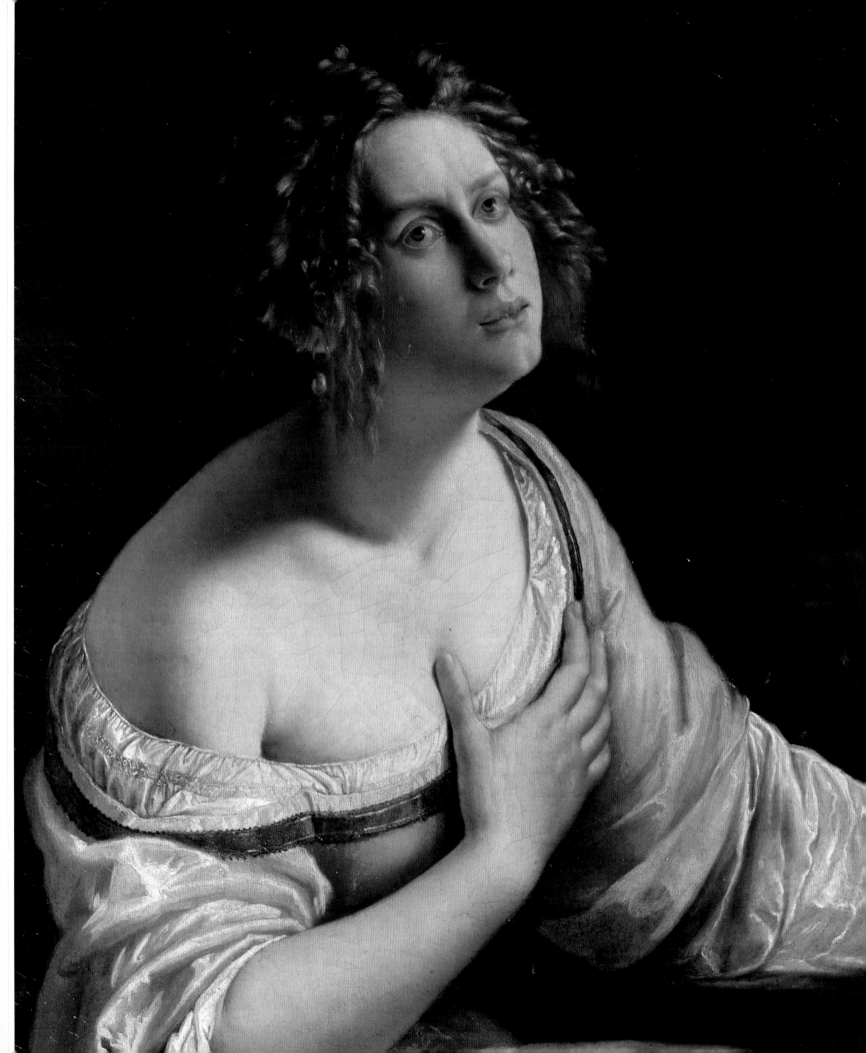

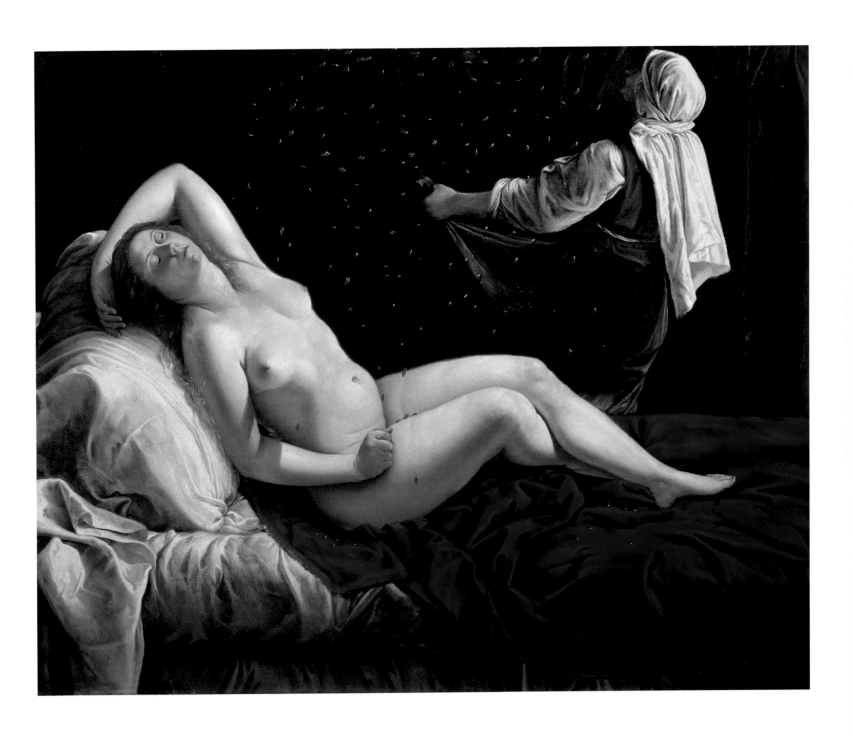

characteristic of Artemisia's Roman work and cannot sustain a placement in the early 1620s, a dating that originally developed from a belief (now discredited) that Artemisia must have visited Genoa with her father at that time. Most important, the picture was done in the period during which Artemisia painted in the workshop of her father, employing the techniques that he had taught her, which are evident in the handling of pigment and glazes in the skin tones. The Caravaggesque shading in the body and the treatment of the velvet and linen bedclothes also derive directly from the work of Orazio. The somewhat looser handling of the bed linens when compared with those of the *Cleopatra* results from the polished surface of the copper support rather than an obviously different hand. This is the period in Artemisia's career when technically her work is as close as it will ever be to the work of her father.

1. Sidney Freedberg, conversation with James Burke, Director, The Saint Louis Art Museum, June 19, 1986; Erich Schleier, letter, February 16, 1988, document file, The Saint Louis Art Museum; Bissell 1999, 310–13.

2. Conversation with author, April 1990, The Saint Louis Art Museum. For further reading on this hypothesis, see Garrard 1989, 539 n. 85.

3. Bissell 1999, nos. L-68, L-11.

4. On the developing iconographies for this myth in the sixteenth and seventeenth centuries, see Kahr 1978, 43–55.

5. I wish to thank Leo Steinberg, who on a visit to the Saint Louis Art Museum in March 1999 shared his astute reading of visual forms that enabled the true nature of this gesture to be understood.

6. See Santore 1991, 412–27.

7. The maid herself becomes a fixture of this imagery in the sixteenth century, derived perhaps from a late-fifteenth-century Danaë drama that featured a servant named Syro who was entrusted with the task of guarding the chaste princess. Ancient sources describe Danaë as having her lap covered; an early visual means for representing this element becomes the drape held in her hand. See Settis 1985, 225–29.

55.

Judith Slaying Holofernes

Oil on canvas, 62½ × 49⅜ in. (158.8 × 125.5 cm)

Museo di Capodimonte, Naples (inv. Q378)

1612–13

J udith, one of the "worthy women" whose story is told in the Old Testament Apocrypha, plots to kill the Assyrian general Holofernes as he lays siege to her town. Having donned her finest attire, she is permitted entry to the military encampment. Holofernes, smitten by her beauty, invites her to dine with him. Initially Judith refuses, but finally she accepts the offer. Holofernes becomes inebriated at dinner, and after he falls into a drunken slumber, Judith seizes his sword and cuts off his head. With the assistance of her maidservant Abra, she wraps the head, conceals it in the basket she had used for her food, and escapes the camp. The embodiment of such virtues as chastity and fortitude, Judith was often identified with the Virgin Mary and during the Counter-Reformation came to symbolize the Church's triumph over heresy. Some sixteenth-century artists, rather than focusing on her virtues, depicted the widowed heroine as a temptress who seduced Holofernes with her charms and lured him to his death. While most artists favored the scene of Judith and Abra fleeing after the assassination, Caravaggio's more dramatic depiction of the moment of the general's decapitation (fig. 109) was crucial to Artemisia's conception of the theme.

The Capodimonte painting and a related version in the Uffizi (cat. 62) have come to be associated with the presumed independent and fiery personality of the young Artemisia. This picture, which has been cut down, offers the more restrained interpretation of the story and was long assumed to be the second version. However, Garrard in her 1989 monograph places it early in Artemisia's career, dating it to 1612–13. Her conclusions are based in part on X radiography, which indicates numerous pentimenti (most notably in the arms and position of Holofernes and in the placement of Abra's arms), and in part on its dependence

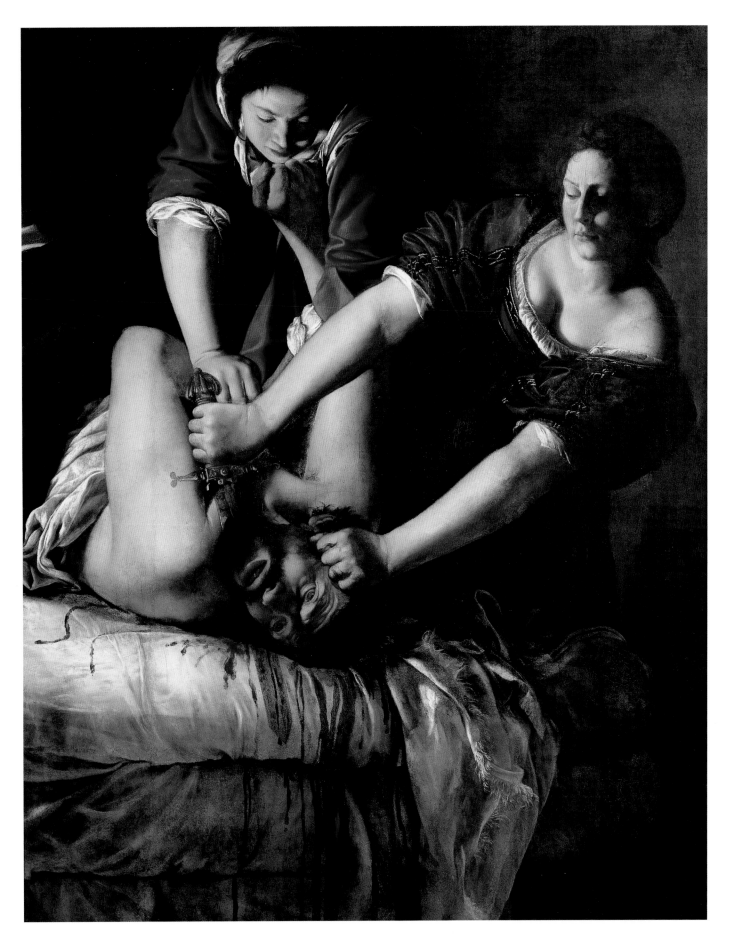

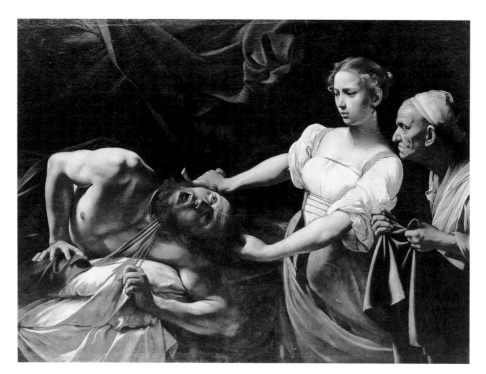

Figure 109. Michelangelo Merisi da Caravaggio (1571–1610), *Judith Beheading Holofernes.* Oil on canvas. Galleria Nazionale d'Arte Antica, Rome

on prototypes by other artists working in Rome. While earlier scholars, on the basis of the Capodimonte provenance, have dated the picture to the 1630s, Artemisia's first Neapolitan period, more recent literature has followed an earlier dating.[1] The modeling and skin tones resemble those of the Pommersfelden *Susanna* (cat. 51), and the bold Caravaggesque presentation and the awkward treatment of space and anatomy further support an early Roman dating.

Garrard also associates the violence against a sexual aggressor with Artemisia's presumed rejection of traditional patriarchal interpretations (that is, Judith as temptress), inspired in part by the artist's response to her own rape in 1611 by Agostino Tassi. This interpretation has found wide currency in the literature, where the image is linked inextricably to the events of Artemisia's personal life. Other writers have focused on reconstructing Artemisia's psychological response to the trauma of the rape without, however, linking her experience directly to her paintings. More recent scholarship has attempted to enlarge the discussion by exploring the notions of the self in the seventeenth century, when rape was more bound up with family honor than with a sense of personal violation.[2] Furthermore, a definitive reading of the image as a

revelation of personal struggle is complicated by the unknown circumstances of patronage for the picture. Pollock maintains that while Artemisia's response to her own rape may have informed the way in which she composed the picture, reactions to trauma are often sublimated and rarely emerge consciously: indeed, she cautions against an autobiographical reading of Artemisia's imagery in general. Recognizing that the painting cannot be read literally but represents a complex interaction of woman artist and historical context, she notes that the picture can be analyzed as an assertion of agency, "an active woman who can make art."[3] Most recently, visual rather than psychological motives have been emphasized, to the point of dismissing the rape almost entirely, with Adam Elsheimer's version and Orazio's Hartford *Judith* (cat. 39) cited as the primary formal sources for the picture.[4]

As Garrard, followed by Papi and Bissell, has claimed, the painting is inconceivable without the experience of the earlier treatment of the theme by Caravaggio, who also rejected the more popular moments in the narrative, the escape of Judith and Abra and the triumphant elevation of Holofernes' severed head. Artemisia's Judith repeats—even

PROVENANCE: Saveria de Simone, Naples (until 1827); Museo di Capodimonte, Naples.

RELATED PICTURES: Galleria dell'Arcivescovado, Milan, on touchstone 32 × 22 cm; Pinacoteca Nazionale, Bologna, 161 × 138 cm; location unknown, documented in a photograph in the Istituto Centrale per il Catalogo e la Documentazione, Rome, no. E44973.

REFERENCES: Sandrart (1675) 1925, 290; Valentiner 1935, 101–4; Molajoli 1955, 51; Longhi 1961, 149–50, 259, 281; Moir 1967, fig. 160; Bissell 1968, 157–58; Borea in Florence 1970, 77; Greer 1979, 194; Bissell 1981, 149–50; Pointon 1981, 343 n. 2; Whitfield in London 1982, 168; Gregori in Naples 1984–85, 147; Pérez Sánchez in Madrid 1985, 164–65 no. 56; Cohen and Cohen 1989, 66–67; Garrard 1989, 32–34, 131–35, 306–13; Papi in Florence 1991, 116, 119–20, 182, pl. 9a,b; Stolzenwald 1991, 24, 33, 89, pl. 54; Bionda 1992, 22–24; Cohen 1992, 617; Hersey 1993, 327–28; Baumgärtel in Düsseldorf–Darmstadt 1995–96, 244–47; Daprà in Chambéry 1995, 90–91; Levenson in Atlanta 1996, 126; Bissell 1999, 191–98 no. 4; Pollock 1999, 117–24; Brown in London–Rome 2001, 296 no. 110; Christiansen 2001, 384.

exaggerates—the stiff-arm pose and the spatial relationship of killer and victim from Caravaggio's picture. Garrard, followed by Bissell, correctly argues that Artemisia probably also mined Peter Paul Rubens's painting the *Great Judith* (now lost) or the Cornelius Galle engraving after it for the lurid details of violence and that the reclining figure of Holofernes was inspired by Orazio's prone Goliath in the Dublin *David* (cat. 12). Brown and Christiansen have recently noted the formal debt to Elsheimer's small copper, clearly a reference point for Artemisia's work.

What has not been adequately discussed is the nature of Artemisia's borrowing from her sources. In adapting the pose of Holofernes from Rubens's *Judith* and in taking as her point of departure Caravaggio's representation, Artemisia builds on both in her effort to create a bloodbath, violence as a real occurrence. Rubens's Judith is no match for her formidably muscular victim. And Caravaggio's Judith, who approaches her victim gingerly and receives no help from her geriatric assistant, challenges credibility as an assassin. Artemisia's painting, by contrast, is a visualization of how such a grisly deed could actually be accomplished. As Garrard briefly acknowledges, what is most important about Artemisia's interpretation is that Abra is not only a loyal follower but a participant in the decapitation, what Baumgärtel (in Düsseldorf–Darmstadt 1995–96) calls "an active partner." Artemisia had already seen her father paint two versions of *Judith and Her Maidservant* (cat. 13 and fig. 46), allowing her ample time to reflect on the details of this biblical story and its presentation. Her impulse toward naturalism is not, however, like Orazio's, limited to recording the specifics of surface and the physicality of form; rather, she has amplified his vision by presenting the story in strongly expressive terms.

The painting has suffered from abrasion and harsh cleaning, and the dark tones have deteriorated in the shadow areas. That it has been cut down on the left (by how much cannot be determined) has also compromised our full understanding of the artist's narrative intent. Discussion has been complicated by the existence of a copy, presumably made before the picture was cut down. Bissell (1999) summarizes the issues involved in determining the original appearance of the painting, drawing the conclusion that a precise reconstruction of the picture may continue to elude us. While Garrard argues that the original, complete, picture more closely approximated the Uffizi version, Papi's assertion (in Florence 1991) that the two pictures offer divergent sensibilities and that the Capodimonte painting never included as much of Holofernes merits consideration. In this first attempt to present the story of Judith, Artemisia creates a composition (an inverted triangle) that underlines the struggle of the three protagonists and offers the immediacy of an observed event. In so doing, she avoids the more balanced, less contentious, arrangement that she embraces in the later picture, in which the sword defines the midpoint of the composition.

1. Among those who have argued for a later dating are Longhi, Borea, Whitfield, and Pérez Sánchez. More recent assignments of an earlier dating include Papi, Stolzenwald, Bionda, and Bissell.

2. Cohen 1992, 617.

3. Pollock 1999, 123.

4. Brown, who characterizes arguments that seek to tie this picture to Artemisia's rape as explaining the painting as "a personal reaction to her 'date-rape' trial of 1612," grossly distorts the nature of the rape. Not only is the term inappropriate for the seventeenth century, but its colloquial usage denies the seriousness of the charges brought against Tassi.

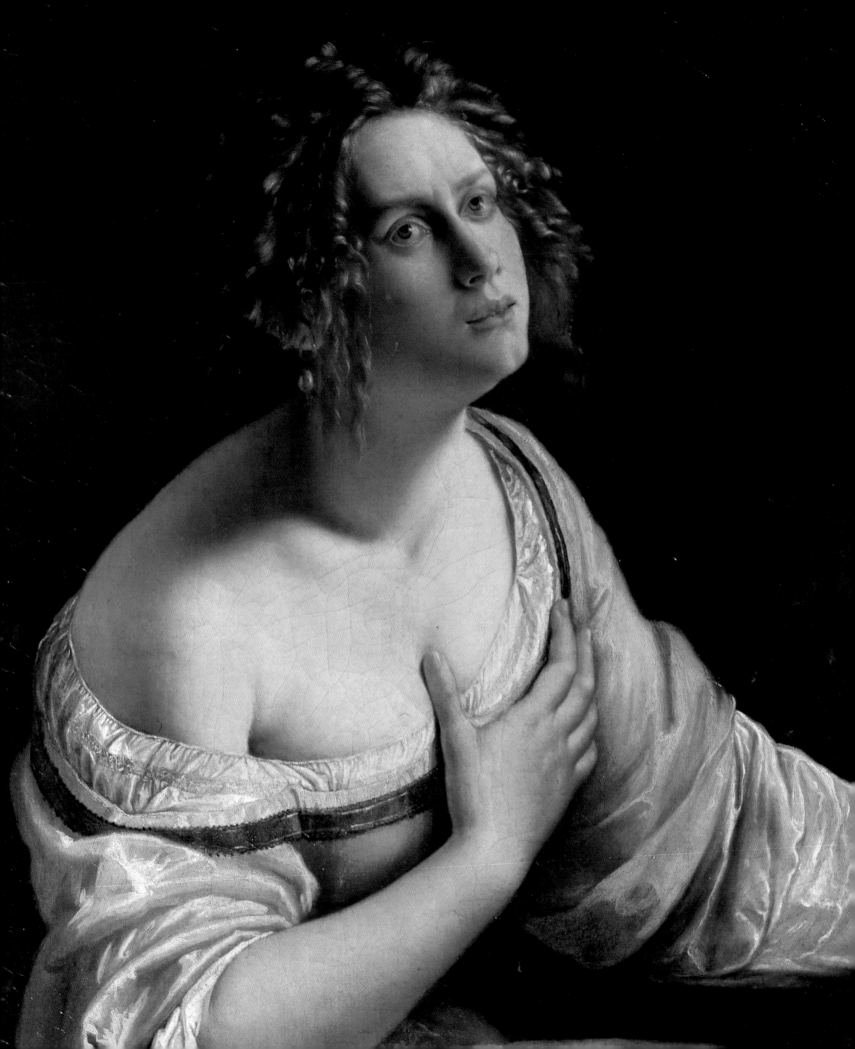

Artemisia Gentileschi's Florentine Inspiration

ROBERTO CONTINI

T en years after the first monographic exhibition devoted to Artemisia Gentileschi, it is still, I fear, almost futile to wonder about the influence Florence had on her art, for there are so many concrete indications that it had none. Unanticipated documentary discoveries relating to the chronology of Orazio's work and radical revisions in the assessment of Artemisia's Neapolitan production—both beyond the scope of this essay—remind us of the fragile basis of our knowledge of this remarkable painter, an artist endowed with a greater ability than her father to constantly transform her art in a naturalistic vein.[1]

We can be reasonably certain that Artemisia had shown considerable promise even before she arrived in Florence, as demonstrated, for example, in the Pommersfelden *Susanna and the Elders* (cat. 51). Nevertheless, it is easy to play the devil's advocate and consider the signature and very early date of 1610 that appear on the painting to be fraudulent, or at least later additions, done either for commercial or for propagandistic reasons. There is the *Saint Cecilia* (cat. 63) and the *Madonna and Child* (cat. 52), both often considered autograph works done before 1612. And, above all, the *Judith Slaying Holofernes* (cat. 55), which may be unfinished and is now generally acknowledged to be one of Artemisia's earliest representations of this violent and bloody subject (and thus a product of her Roman years). When we think of the accomplishment of this last-mentioned work, we must ask ourselves what additional sustenance Artemisia could have found in Florence in the second decade of the seventeenth century. Florence was not exactly provincial, though the city's best artists had moved to Rome. However, it was still dominated by a generation of painters who were older than the almost twenty-year-old Artemisia, if only by a few years.

Florence had become a small center of "magnificent" painting following the example of Cigoli (1559–1613), who from 1604 increasingly worked in Rome, and the more austere Domenico Cresti, known as Passignano (1559–1638). If Artemisia arrived in Florence a decade too early to fully appreciate the talents of her local contemporaries, or slightly younger artists, so much the better. Otherwise, we would likely have witnessed an inexorable (though probably fascinating) tempering of her Caravaggesque inclinations and virile compositions in favor of a mawkish adherence to the Florentine current of decorative painting, which was dominated by Venetian-inspired color and a shamelessly epicurean vaunting of its own graphic style. In short, she would have become the most sumptuous of propagandists. Instead, nothing of what was happening there—whether on the scaffolding erected by Cardinal Carlo de' Medici in the casino on via Larga or in the work commissioned by Maria Maddalena of Austria for her residence at Poggio Imperiale—pertains to Artemisia's figural style. Slowly, however, and for decades after she lived along the Arno, an awareness of her presence took root in the grand-ducal city.

What did Florence mean for Artemisia as a context in which to affirm herself as an autonomous artist—beyond her father's supervision, though not necessarily out of his reach (was anybody in the Tuscan capital even acquainted with his art prior to 1615?)? An answer is perhaps to be found in the guise of her release from the shackles of illiteracy—in every sense of the term (for at the time of the rape trial, Artemisia claimed she could not write and could barely read).

It would seem that in Florence, Artemisia reached a turning point, in terms not of style but of a sense of color. Her indulgence in painting rich and brilliantly colored costumes, for example, must have been influenced by her stay in a place particularly prone to superficial extravagence. Yet, in the *Saint Catherine of Alexandria* (cat. 59), rediscovered by Luciano Berti, and the

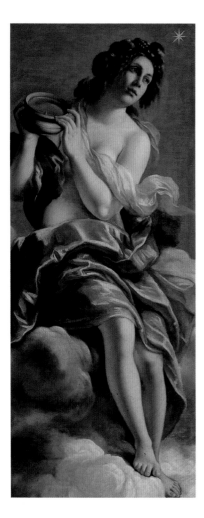

Figure 110. Artemisia Gentileschi, *Allegory of Inclination*. Oil on canvas. Casa Buonarroti, Florence

painter's work without being particularly concerned about his or her training, and this, it seems to me, was the case with Buonarroti, who played something of a Pygmalion to the young artist.

As part of its dowry, Florence also brought Artemisia to the attention of, and indeed nurtured her friendship with, Galileo, who had visited Rome in 1611. It is not implausible that Cigoli—a close friend of Galileo's—was the connection between the scientist and the young artist, possibly also her father. And yet, based on the later, ample correspondence between Artemisia and the Palermo nobleman Don Antonio Ruffo and the sparse exchange of letters between the artist and that most cultivated and learned patron Cassiano dal Pozzo, there is no indication that she was ever expected to speak of herself as other than an artist—indeed, one ever better remunerated for her work. Nor did the correspondent, eminent or not, need to be anything other than an admirer of her work.

Who can say what illuminated Artemisia's relationship with Galileo, to whom she claimed in 1635 to be "infinitely obliged"? Perhaps theirs was something more than mere camaraderie, a kinship between the painter's strong artistic soul and the scientist's attraction to grandness of expression rather than to the mumblings of which he, a strong proponent of the poetry of Ludovico Ariosto (1474–1595), accused Torquato Tasso (1544–1595) of being guilty. That Artemisia should seem to some modern critics a woman of letters is somewhat mystifying. It is true that she was a lively correspondent during the years she spent in Naples (which is more than one can claim for the difficult years in Rome). It is also true that she denounced her illiteracy in the famous note in the Buonarroti archives in which she and her husband seem to compete with each other about who had more causes for complaint. Hers is a fine vernacular prose, more pleasing than the affected and cumbersome style of the tiresomely anecdotal Filippo Baldinucci, the biographer of Florentine artists. Although it is unlikely that Artemisia was, in any sense, a "Professore del Disegno" (professor of composition), her association with Buonarroti had the effect of redeeming her from the suspicion that she could not write and had only a very limited ability to read. I cannot deny that I would be gratified to be proved wrong on many of these points, for the image of an Artemisia who was literate, intellectually engaged, a fixture of the drawing room—perhaps even a delight to those in her company—would greatly increase the complexity of her personality.

Pitti *Conversion of the Magdalene* (cat. 58), I see no diminution in aggressiveness or in the brazen declaration of her personality, which indeed the artist rarely abandoned. It is this powerful mode of expression that constitutes the strength of her work and for which she received the numerous commissions from her broad-minded admirer Cosimo II de' Medici.

It does not seem to me that Artemisia's membership in the official art establishment, the Accademia del Disegno—an institution that regularly listed her on its roster from 1616 until 1620 (she is mentioned earlier, in 1614, but only because of unresolved debts)—necessarily means that she had obtained a privileged position, except in an arid, bureaucratic sense (she was the first female member). Nor can I believe that her friendship with Michelangelo Buonarroti the Younger (1568–1646), a truly erudite man and present in Rome in 1610, indicates that she had been launched in society. Did she have a temperament that could be educated? Certainly her father did not. One can be enamored of a

Artemisia was, in any case, surely in contact with the Tuscan community before leaving Rome at the end of the first decade of the seventeenth century and the beginning of the second. It seems indisputable that she knew Cigoli in Rome, the city in which he then lived and would stay until he died. Some of Passignano's more experimental works, such as the sinister *Burial of Saint Sebastian* (Capodimonte, Naples), painted, perhaps, for Cardinal Pompeo Arrigoni, may also have been of interest to her. Artemisia arrived in Florence just at the time of Bernardino Poccetti's (1548–1612) death. Little known outside his native city, Poccetti was a great master in the tradition of Andrea del Sarto (1486–1530). He may have been only a name that Artemisia heard from her father, but the monumentality of his compositions and his nostalgic deviation from the expressive norms of his day likely exercised some small influence on her.

Although Artemisia had no lasting interest in the neo-Mannerists in Florence in the 1620s, their coloristic pyrotechnics seem to have influenced the high-pitched range of hues in her Florentine work. We need only think of such examples as the *Saint Catherine of Alexandria* (cat. 59), the *Conversion of the Magdalene* (cat. 58), or the *Jael and Sisera*, of 1620 (cat. 61). These coloristic qualities, familar to the young artist from her father's work (and especially evident in the Naples *Judith*; cat. 55), may have been reinforced by the work of artists associated with Cigoli, such as Giovanni Bilivert (1585–1644) and, later, the less talented Sigismondo Coccopani (1583–1643).

The gallery in the Casa Buonarroti (fig. 110), where Artemisia worked alongside Bilivert, Coccopani, and Matteo Rosselli (1578–1650), provided an occasion for young artists such as Giovan Battista Ghidoni—who was by no means a minor figure—to learn from her. It is possible that Bilivert's sumptuous *Tobias and the Angel* of 1612 (Palazzo Pitti, Florence) influenced Artemisia's color choices, though she may also have known, in Rome, his now largely unappreciated *Saint Calixtus Thrown into the Well*, painted in 1610 for the church of San Callisto in Trastevere, Rome. Cristofano Allori (1577–1621) was certainly the more talented painter, both in terms of his color choices and in the overall quality of his work, and his pictures would have been more congenial to Artemisia. She would have been drawn to the *Judith* in the Uffizi (now somewhat deteriorated) and to the noble expressiveness of his paintings, which display his own brand of naturalism. And she would have been interested in his drawings.[2]

As her career evolved, Artemisia would also make use of what she had observed in Tuscany, both in her compositions and in the mannered—or Mannerist—aspect of some of her figures. The *Esther Before Ahasuerus* (cat. 71), for example, has a suggestive relationship with works by the Sienese painter Rutilio Manetti (1571–1639)—although one does not know in which direction the influence ran. The *Esther* also has something in common with the *Theseus and Ariadne* (private collection), by the Florentine Bartolomeo Salvestrini (doc. 1600–1633), though he was still quite young when Artemisia was in Florence.

It is almost an assumption today that Tuscan painters were indebted to Artemisia, with the almost inevitable result that studies refer to now-lost "prototypes." And when all is said and done, little that is Florentine appears to have made much of an impression on Artemisia's stylistic development, at least from what we can glean from her extant work. That Artemisia proudly followed her own path seems unquestionable. Thus, the considerable influence she exercised on Florentine painting took some time to emerge. Works whose manner seems most to resemble Artemisia's appear many years after the eight that she spent in the city. Numerous cases could be added to those already cited in the literature,[3] but I believe that even as late as the early 1640s, Artemisia's *terribilismo* could not have been better interpreted than it is by Ottavio Vannini (1585–1644) in the monochromatic ovals (greenish with gold outlines) that he painted to simulate cameos on faux marble within festoons, in the window embrasures of a ground-floor room of the Palazzo Pitti (today the Museo degli Argenti; fig. 111). The oval on the right side of the second window is a particularly good example. The Medusa-like treatment of the woman's hair presupposes a knowledge of Artemisia's more Baglionesque works, perhaps even her *Self-Portrait* as it appears in the famous print by Jérôme David (fig. 95).[4]

Concealed among these later Baglionesque painters—a sort of Berensonian "Amico di Artemisia"—is Anastasio Fontebuoni (ca. 1580–1626), one of the most talented Florentines to go to Rome. In 1599, we find him staying with Agostino Ciampelli. Fontebuoni was open to Caravaggesque naturalism as practiced by Gentileschi and by Giovanni Baglione, Tommaso Salini, and Giovanni Francesco Guerrieri. It seems most likely that when Fontebuoni returned to Florence, before the end of July 1620 (thus crossing paths with the departing Artemisia), part of the commission to decorate the vault in the Ajax courtyard, on the ground

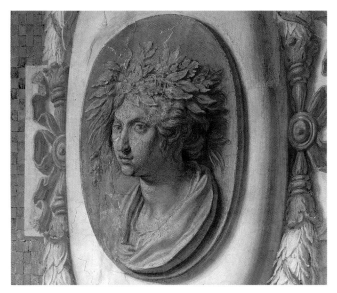

Figure 111. Ottavio Vannini (1585–1644), *Allegorical Figure*. Fresco. Palazzo Pitti, Museo degli Argenti, Salone di Giovanni da San Giovanni, Florence

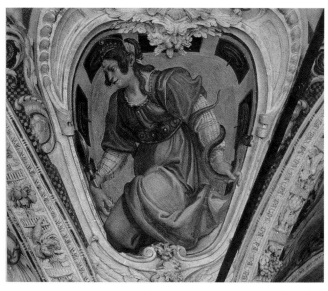

Figure 112. Anastasio Fontebuoni (ca. 1580–1626), *Allegorical Figure of Prudence*. Fresco. Palazzo Pitti, Loggetta del Cortiletto, Florence

floor of the Palazzo Pitti, awaited him (fig. 112 offers a small example of that decoration).[5]

This interest in Artemisia after her departure might explain the presence in Florence not only of pictures she had executed for the Medici—which, as a matter of course, were accessible—but also of unfinished or undelivered paintings that had perhaps remained in the artist's studio. Knowledge of such pictures would justify and even help to resolve the debates surrounding the attribution of some single-figure compositions currently ascribed to her Florentine contemporaries. The argument can be constructed, at least in part, from an inventory of the goods that she left in Florence and that were sold, in February 1621, to Francesco Maria Maringhi for 175 ducats.

Maringhi was most likely a close acquaintance, if not a friend, of Artemisia's, and he appears in other Florentine documents that pertain to her. More interesting here than her relationship with Maringhi, however, are several entries in the 1621 inventory. This recent discovery in the Frescobaldi family archives (see appendix 3) was made by Francesco Solinas, who, with exceptional generosity made it available for publication. In truth, not all that much can be inferred from the inventory (does the sale of her household effects imply that Artemisia returned to Florence?).[6] Yet it is suggestive. For example, from a number of surviving paintings, one might suspect that some Florentine forgeries were

based on prototypes that she had made—sweetened versions of works that were too potent for local tastes. One might also imagine Artemisia's half-disguised grimace when confronted with certain pictures marked by a pronounced Florentine style. (I am thinking here of that masterpiece of Florentine seicento painting, the *Apollo and Marsyas* in the Palazzo Pitti, the composition of which can be understood only in a Florentine context, although the details have a robust Roman flavor that does not quite overcome the neo-Mannerist poetry of Bilivert or of the less talented Salvestrini.) With the inventory in hand, we are in a position to suggest that some of these works were indeed unfinished autograph canvases, put into circulation and completed by Artemisia's Florentine colleagues—though not until the 1620s. These were the painters of the great Medici decorations—but we should not expect any particular compatibility between the style of these artists and the vigorous naturalism of Artemisia.

Among the pictures listed in the inventory—untraced or possibly just misidentified—are a "large canvas, half painted" and a "picture of a Magdalene, just begun, two *braccia* high." The latter is especially interesting if it can be identified with the Pitti *Conversion of the Magdalene* (cat. 58), even though the Pitti picture's height is greater than the two *braccia* listed in the inventory (146.5 × 108 cm as opposed to a height of only 120 cm). Nevertheless, the inventory should be taken into account, especially by those who see stylistic inconsistencies in the painting, which is Artemisia's most Florentine work in terms of color. It has been thought the picture was enlarged on the left side with a strip of canvas that includes the signature on the back of the red velvet chair and along the bottom (an arc including the terminating folds of the yellow-gold drapery, the saint's left foot, and an ointment jar, which would have been an indispensable iconographic attribute in an early design for the composition).[7] These additions have been ascribed to a second hand. Yet such speculation must be treated with the utmost prudence. It is one thing to take note of these unpublished documents and quite another to approach them with the caution required for a live grenade.

In addition to these two unfinished paintings, the inventory lists six more pictures; a seventh work, referred to simply as a "Crucifix," is probably a three-dimensional devotional object of very little value. Thus, the search is on for a "picture of a clothed Magdalene, two *braccia* high," a "Madonna" of the same size, a "portrait of a woman in a walnut frame," and "3 small paintings on copper." The latter would represent novel additions to our knowledge of the painter's work.

The inventory indicates that Artemisia did not lack for commissions in Florence. Also listed are four walnut palettes, four "legij da dipingere"—that is, easels—and fifteen canvases for paintings, both large and small. If the Florentine art market was indeed consumed by a passion for Artemisia's violent images (Orazio's work was not, it should be noted, part of the Medici's ambitions as collectors),[8] there was probably a market for substitutes, which brought pressure to bear on local artists to make pictures "in the manner of" the painter. At the same time, there is a continuing obligation to look for Artemisia's work among small pictures, even those painted on copperplates. No Florentine examples of paintings on copper survive, unless one dares ascribe to her the splendid *Penitent Magdalene* in London (fig. 98). Although it was auctioned in 1996 as "attributed to Artemisia Gentileschi," Bissell suggested, after it was cleaned, that it might be by Orazio.[9]

Maringhi also interceded on Artemisia's behalf after she failed to deliver a *Hercules* commissioned by Grand Duke Cosimo II de' Medici. Having told the duke that she was going to Rome for a few months, she promised, on February 10, 1620, to send the finished painting in, at the most, a couple of months (she had received an advance of fifty scudi). Just five days later, the likelihood that this commitment would not be met seemed quite clear.

Artemisia had failed to pay for an ounce and a half of ultramarine blue that she had already received, as a result of which her household goods were sequestered. Maringhi then stepped in and guaranteed that she would finish the picture within six months, offering personally to pay her debt if the work were not delivered. Maringhi, who continued as Artemisia's agent in Florence, is mentioned again some fifteen years later in a feverish letter addressed by the artist to Galileo. In the letter, sent from Naples on October 9, 1635, Artemisia expressed her concern that she had received no notice of receipt (and thus no expression of appreciation) from Grand Duke Ferdinando II de' Medici for two large pictures. She thus implied to her illustrious correspondent the disparity between the treatment she received from the Florentine court and her reception by her patrons elsewhere in Europe. If the grand duke would deign to reply to her, Artemisia told Galileo, the correspondence could be forwarded to Maringhi.[10]

One can speculate endlessly on the relationship between Maringhi and Gentileschi, and on the identification of the generically described paintings in the correspondence. However, a picture that should not be overlooked (at least as a possible prototype) is, unfortunately, not a *Hercules* but a *Samson Victorious* (fig. 113). This work, which was ceded by the Medici collection to the Palazzo Mansi in Lucca in the second half of the nineteenth century, has not yet received the attention it merits. Attributed to Domenichino (1581–1641),[11] it is instead the product of the "gentileschiana methodus," although perhaps softened in ways that are unlike Artemisia's approach. Nonetheless, the painting is rooted in a manner whose tempered naturalism and volumetric compactness seem alien to the school from which Domenichino—a pupil of Annibale Carracci (1560–1609)—came, yet not distant from the manner of the Gentileschi (both father and daughter).

I would like, finally, to discuss a painting that may have nothing to do with Artemisia's activity in Florence. I know this picture, the *Portrait of a Nun* (fig. 114), only from photographs, but it seems to me important since, if it is by Artemisia, it would represent both an addition to her oeuvre and a possible document of her trip to Venice in the late 1620s. The hypothesis that it was painted for a Venetian patron hangs by a slender thread: its appearance in the Italico Brass collection in Venice in the nineteenth century. Despite the risks of judging from a photograph the saturnine appearance of the nun, and despite the picture's evidently rather compromised state, one can dismiss outright the

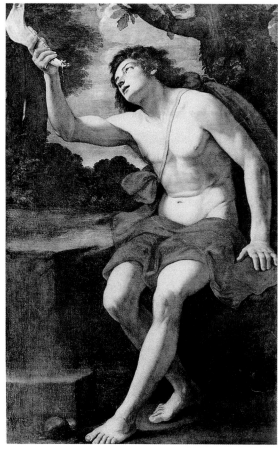

Figure 113. Seventeenth-century Tuscan painter, *Samson Victorious*. Oil on canvas. Museo Nazionale di Palazzo Mansi, Lucca

but few cards to play in establishing a chronology for Artemisia during the years 1622–30, but there is in the painting evidence of a renewed familiarity with the Roman scene. Yet this is, perhaps, only a captious argument, since the most relevant point of reference seems to me to be the masterfully rendered angel in the *Resurrection* (Art Institute of Chicago), by the Lombard artist Francesco Buoneri (Cecco di Caravaggio; fl. 1610–20). That painting was executed (as we now know thanks to Gianni Papi's addendum to Corti's important documentary discovery)[12] for the Guicciardini chapel in Santa Felicità in Florence. Unfortunately, like Caravaggio—his compatriot and mentor—Buoneri suffered the shame of having his work refused. Nonetheless, one cannot help but think that Artemisia saw it.

Could the *Portrait of a Nun* conceivably be a canvas by Artemisia, painted in Florence or shortly after she left? Surely a work of this power serves as a provocative reminder of the limits of our current knowledge.

current attribution to Bernardo Strozzi (1581–1644). The surface of this psychologically penetrating, bust-length image appears to be dry and controlled—in short, naturalistic—and could not be further from the frothy impasto that characterizes the work of the Genovese painter.

I believe instead that the nun, fixedly gazing out of the picture with a feverish lack of indulgence either for the viewer or, in truth, for herself, has a well-known antecedent. It is to be found on the ceiling of the Casino delle Muse (fig. 6) as well as, in certain respects, in the *Susanna and the Elders* (cat. 51), whose Florentine descendants include the Baglionesque *Conversion of the Magdalene* (cat. 58), the *Self-Portrait as a Female Martyr* (cat. 56), and the *Saint Catherine of Alexandria* (cat. 59). There is a contradiction here, for although Artemisia is recorded in Venice between 1627 and 1628, the style of this intriguing portrait—assuming it is by her—is not that of the artist during this time. We have, it is true,

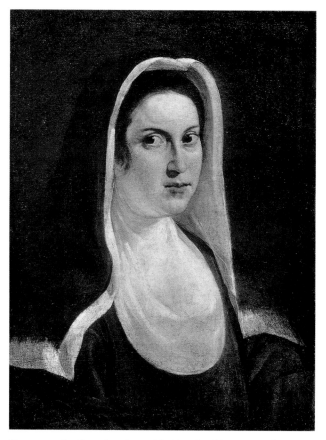

Figure 114. Attributed to Artemisia Gentileschi, *Portrait of a Nun*. Oil on canvas. Formerly private collection, Venice

1. Causa 1993, passim.

2. It is also important to note that Allori could be counted as one of Artemisia's true friends in Florence and not just a professional acquaintance. He was godfather to Artemisia's son, who was named for him and baptized on November 9, 1616. See Cropper 1993, 760 n. 6.

3. Contini in Florence 1991, 181–96.

4. The inscription on the tablet below the allegorical image reads, "ROS MARGARITAS GIGNIT, / PRINCIPIS GRATIAS CANDIDA IN PECTORE / VIRTUTUM PARENS."

5. Contini in Fossombrone 1997, 10–11, 16 n. 19.

6. Critics (Spike 1991b, 732–34) have taken aim particularly at the small *Female Martyr* (32 × 24.5 cm) in the Zeri collection (see cat. 56) and the *Saint Cecilia* (92 × 72 cm) in a private collection in Trent. Neither subject is mentioned in the Frescobaldi inventory. The *Saint Cecilia* seems to me at the very least Gentileschiesque and may even derive from a prototype by Artemisia. It would, however, require someone well trained in divination to discover its author (the picture is in less than ideal condition). Any reservations about the lovely painting in the Zeri collection seem to me gratuitous; there really is no alternative to an attribution to Artemisia. The only Florentine artist perhaps capable of rendering its powerful sweetness (if one will excuse the oxymoron) is Fontebuoni, in whose work there is always a trace of the academic (derived from Campelli). Nor should we take as an excuse the obvious disparity with the painting exhibited here (cat. 56). If the latter, like the Pitti *Magdalene*, reveals a dominant, stereotypical Baglionesque style, the Zeri picture reflects a later moment, with the *Allegory of Inclination* (fig. 110)

the middle term. Certainly, when I see the *Aurora* (fig. 96) peddled as a work by Artemisia and the attribution of the *Mary Magdalene* at West Wycombe Park changed to "circle of Angelo Caroselli" (Bissell 1991, 220–22 no. 15, 340–41 no. x-35, figs. 87, 90, 232), even though there should be no doubt of Artemisia's authorship, I see also that the often seductive exercise of attribution should sometimes be autocratically self-censured.

7. Spike 1991b, 732–34.

8. Decisive here is the opinion of Orazio's abilities submitted to Cosimo II de' Medici by the Florentine ambassador to Rome, Pietro Guicciardini, on March 27, 1615; see Crinò and Nicholson 1961, 144–45. Guicciardini considered Cristofano Allori and Jacopo Ligozzi to be more talented than Orazio. Beyond the clear misrepresentations of the relative merits of these Florentine artists at the expense of Orazio (whose work can, however, bring to mind that of artists such as Ligozzi), his verdict does call attention to possible disagreements among the most avant-garde figures in Tuscany (the proto-Caravaggisti). This is especially important to bear in mind when evaluating the relationship of the later work of a sober Florentine naturalist such as Giovanni Martinelli to that of Artemisia.

9. Bissell 1999, 338 no. x-32, figs. 240, 241.

10. Biblioteca Nazionale Centrale, Florence, mss. Gal. P.I.T. XIII, ff. 269–70; Galilei 1929–39, vol. 16, 318–19, and, more recently, translated into English in Garrard 1989, 383–84.

11. Borella and Giusti Maccari 1993, 268 (where the picture is also attributed to Domenichino).

12. Corti 1989, 131, payment number 49; Papi in Florence 1991, 39–50; Papi 1992a, 7–26.

56.

Self-Portrait as a Female Martyr (Female Martyr)

Oil on panel, 12½ × 9¾ in. (31.75 × 24.76 cm)

Inscribed (on the reverse): Di mano di Artemisia figlia di A.rili.Lomi/Pisano Nipote di Orazio F[G?] . . . . E . . . /

Private collection

ca. 1615

New York, Saint Louis

PROVENANCE: Ignazio Hugford (until 1779?); Wollaston family? (19th century); by descent to Martha Beavan, née Wollaston, of Leintwardine, Herefordshire; Newhouse Galleries; private collection (1995?).

REFERENCES: Fleming 1955, 106–10, 197–200, 203–6; Del Bravo 1967, 82 n. 11; Sotheby's, London, December 9, 1987, lot 13; Bissell in New York 1989, no. 3; Contini in Florence 1991, 140–43, fig. 84; Spike 1991b, 734; Bissell 1999, 204–5 no. 7; Papi 2000, 452.

This picture is one of two works by Artemisia Gentileschi painted on panel. A bill sent to Artemisia dated February 12, 1615, lists materials and household furnishings that had been supplied to the artist by a joiner, and includes "a small wood panel for painting on," although as Bissell (1999) has correctly pointed out, the word *tavoletta* can mean both "panel" and "table."[1] The term is used in both ways in the February 1615 account. The 1621 inventory of Artemisia's Florence studio (see appendix 3) lists four "tavolozze" (which has been translated as "palettes," but which may also be interpreted as "panels") and three "tavolini" (translated as "small wooden tables," though it could be understood to mean "panels" as well).

While the palm frond identifies the subject as a martyr, most scholars (Contini, Bissell 1999, Papi) have accepted it as a self-portrait of the artist, noting the characteristic bow lips, slight dip in the nose, and full face evident in the engraved portrait of Artemisia by Jérôme David (fig. 95) of about 1628. Contini has likened the face to that of a figure in Orazio's ceiling at the Casino delle Muse (fig. 6), Rome, one of several understood to record the features of the adolescent Artemisia. The painting has convincingly been placed in the artist's Florentine period and can easily be compared with two key pictures of that time, the Pitti *Magdalene* (cat. 58) and the *Allegory of Inclination* (Casa Buonarroti, Florence; fig. 110), both of which share the same facial type, dimpled hands, and wavy, disheveled hair. It also warrants comparison with the Uffizi *Saint Catherine* (cat. 59). The accomplished handling of paint in the rose drapery and lapis blue turban is not unlike the flourish of paint more robustly displayed in the Pitti *Magdalene*. A Medici inventory dated March 17, 1625, lists a *Saint Apollonia* by Artemisia, a copper oval

of relatively small size, attesting to her having produced small-format images of at least one saint while she was in Florence.[2]

Bissell (1999) associates the picture with the "Testa di Santa" lent by the Italian-born Englishman Ignazio Hugford to an exhibition at the Santissima Annunziata, Florence, in 1767. An inscription on the back of the panel, "By the hand of Artemisia daughter of A[u]r[e]li[o] Lomi/ Pisan, niece of Orazio," which confuses Orazio Gentileschi with his brother, Aurelio (such errors are common in early notations), specifies Lomi's Pisan origins, a fact that would have been noteworthy for Hugford, who was himself born in Pisa.

Counter-Reformation zeal to reaffirm the original teachings of the Church engendered a particular interest in the lives of the early Christian martyrs. Cesare Baronio, the Church historian and follower of Saint Philip Neri, completed important revisions to the *Martyrologium romanum* in 1586, and representations of saints who were put to death when they refused to forsake their Christian ideals were popular as devotional images among early-seventeenth-century patrons; this small panel may have served such a purpose. However, the absence of an identifying attribute is unusual, and the depiction of the sitter with a turban wrapped loosely around her head conforms more to the standard artist portrait than to images of martyred saints. The painting appears to have been used as the model for a similar canvas in the Zeri collection, included by Contini in the 1991 Florence exhibition as an autograph work, though in my view by another hand.

1. The date in the account is recorded as 1614. As the new year in Florence did not begin until March, it is actually 1615, however.
2. Cited by Gregori 1968, 419 n. 18.

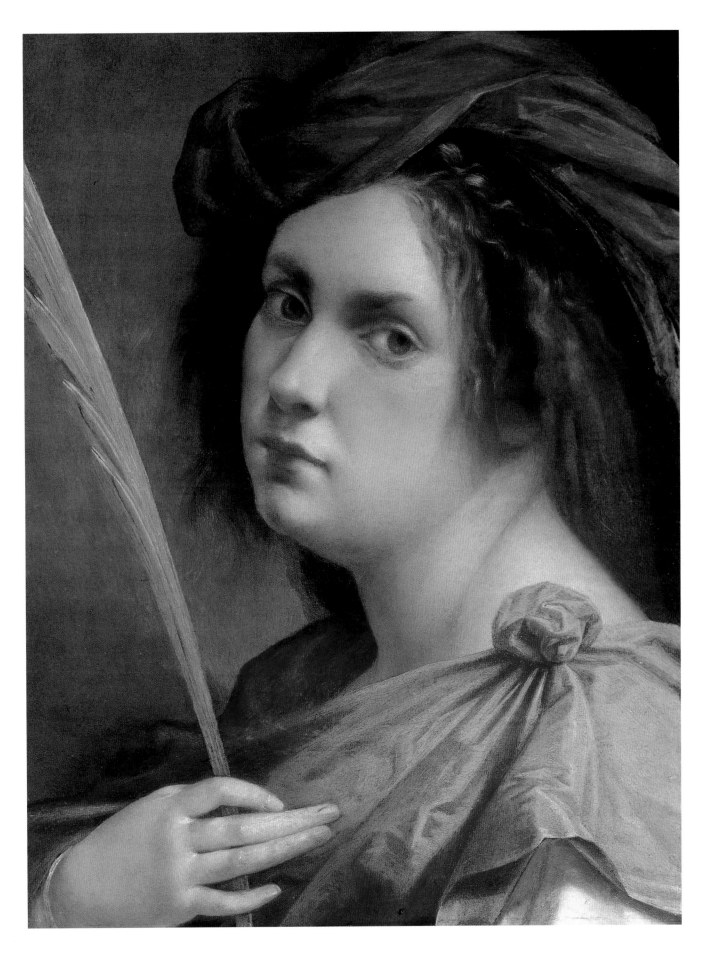

57·
Self-Portrait as a Lute Player

Oil on canvas, 30½ × 28¼ in. (77.5 × 71.8 cm)

Curtis Galleries, Minneapolis

ca. 1615–17

A 1638 inventory of the Villa Medici at Artimino records "Un Quadro in tela alto b. 1½ largo b. 1¼ con adornam.to nero filettato d'oro entrovi dipinto il ritratto della' artimisia di sua mano che suona il liuto" (A picture on canvas 1½ *braccia* high and 1¼ *braccia* wide in a black frame bordered in gold, the portrait of Artemisia playing a lute painted by her own hand), a description that most certainly refers to the present painting, as Papi has recently pointed out (a Florentine *braccia* equals 58.4 cm). A comparison with the Jérôme David engraving of Artemisia's face (ca. 1628; fig. 95) confirms this as a likeness of the painter, notable in such details as the full chin, the configuration of the nose, and the pursed, bow lips. Unknown until it appeared at the Sotheby's London sale of July 1998, the painting has now been accepted by most scholars, and its Medici provenance establishes it as an important reference point for Artemisia's career in Florence; it was perhaps even a commission from Grand Duke Cosimo II de' Medici himself.

There has been a tendency among writers to assume that Artemisia used her own countenance as her model in nearly all the works that include young women, and it is important to weed out the true self-portraits in order to come to grips with her oeuvre and its meaning. All her Judiths at one time or another have been considered self-representations, as have the Pitti *Conversion of the Magdalene* (cat. 58), the *Allegory of Inclination* (fig. 110), the Milan *Lucretia* (cat. 67), and the Pommersfelden *Susanna* (cat. 51). These interpretations in part relate to the tendency to read the narratives in autobiographical terms as well (see, for example, cat. nos. 51, 55). However, while there is clearly an Artemisia "type" in the early paintings, she employs a range of physical features, and not all of them appear to be drawn from the same model. Furthermore, we know that Artemisia had people model for her. In her trial testimony, she describes how she was sketching her neighbor Tuzia's little boy when Agostino entered her room prior to the rape itself,

establishing this practice as early as 1611. And later in her life, in a letter written on June 12, 1649, to her Sicilian patron Don Antonio Ruffo, she lamented the difficulties of completing a commission for a figure painting given the problem of finding suitable models: "Because out of the fifty women who undress themselves, there is scarcely one good one."[1]

Stylistic affinities with other pictures from Artemisia's Tuscan period confirm the placement of the *Self-Portrait as a Lute Player* within her Florentine sojourn. There are similarities with the *Allegory of Inclination*, the one documented picture of the period (we know that the patron, Michelangelo Buonarroti the Younger, made the final payment in 1616): in the type of the eye, the handling of the hair, and the configuration of the hands. Furthermore, the lighting along her left forearm and hand seems analogous to the more filtered, enveloping light of the Buonarroti picture. The facial type links it as well to the *Self-Portrait as a*

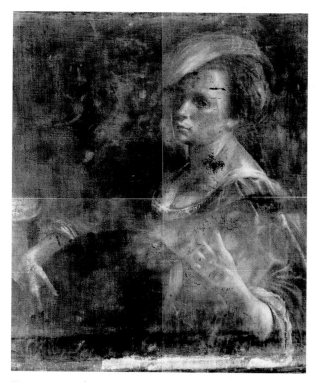

Figure 115. X radiograph of cat. 57

PROVENANCE: Possibly Medici collection, Villa Medici, Artimino (inv. 1638); sold, Sotheby's, London, July 9, 1998, lot 68; Curtis Galleries, Minneapolis.

REFERENCES: Garrard 1982, 163; Garrard 1989, 204, 393; Florence 1991, 34; Papi 2000, 452.

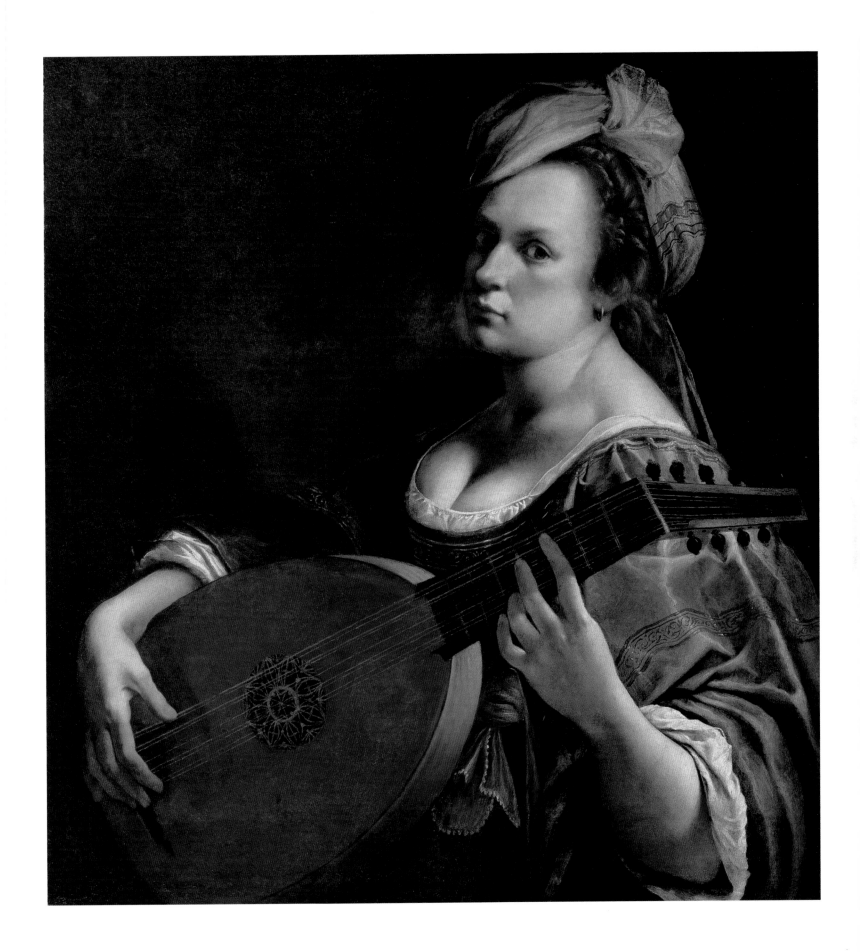

for a female nude. One must wonder whether the Pitti *Magdalene* as well, with its virtuoso technique and flashy signature, was intended as a demonstration piece.

1. Jacobus de Voragine 1993, vol. 1, 375. Other sources regarding the iconography of the Magdalene include Janssen 1974, 516–41;

Moltmann-Wendel 1982, 61–90; Ingenhoff-Danhaüser 1984; and Florence 1986.

2. Hart 1995, 75–76.

3. Paleotti 1582, cited in Barocchi 1960–62, vol. 2, 267.

4. Aikema 1994, 58.

5. On the use of Lomi in and out of Florence, see the Burghley House *Susanna and the Elders* (cat. 65).

6. I wish to thank Patrizia Cavazzini for providing this information.

59.

Saint Catherine of Alexandria

Oil on canvas, 30⅜ × 24¾ in. (77 × 63 cm)

On the reverse of the original canvas, before relining: 123, 39, 4344, 1725, 4778

Galleria degli Uffizi, Florence (inv. 8032)

ca. 1618–19

Rome, Saint Louis

PROVENANCE: Galleria dell'Accademia, Florence (1890 inv., as by follower of Artemisia); Soprintendenza alle Gallerie, Florence (until 1970); Galleria degli Uffizi, Florence.

REFERENCES: Solerti 1905, 92; Sricchia 1963, 251; Gregori 1968, 416; Borea in Florence 1970, 72–73; Nicolson 1970, 641; Volpe 1970, 116; Schleier 1971, 89; Bagnoli in Siena 1978, 103–4; Gregori in Naples 1984–85, vol. 1, 147; Valli in Bologna–Los Angeles–Fort Worth 1988, 186; Garrard 1989, 48, 499–500 n. 72; Contini in Florence 1991, 147–49 no. 18; Hersey 1993, 329; Bissell 1999, 203–4 no. 6; Schleier 2000, 168.

First cited as by an unknown follower of Artemisia Gentileschi in an 1890 inventory of the Galleria dell'Accademia in Florence, this painting was initially attributed to the artist in 1966 by Berti when it was restored, and confirmed by Borea in 1970 when it appeared in Florence in the exhibition "Caravaggio e Caravaggeschi nelle Gallerie di Firenze." Although Bissell did not include it in his 1968 chronology of Artemisia's paintings, he lists it as autograph in his catalogue raisonné of 1999, a view shared by all major scholars on the artist.

Saint Catherine, the daughter of King Costus of Alexandria, was a fourth-century convert to Christianity. Catherine pleaded with the pagan emperor Maxentius (r. 306–12) to spare the lives of the persecuted Christians. So Maxentius selected a group of fifty learned thinkers to debate with Catherine the tenets of Christianity. Catherine's oratorial skills intimidated the philosophers and enraged Maxentius, who ordered that she be starved and then placed between two sets of revolving wheels studded with spikes and nails. An angel stayed her torture by breaking the wheels, but, incensed, Maxentius had her beheaded.

Saint Catherine's attributes are a wheel, shown here on the left, a book, which testifies to her erudition, and a sword. She is often portrayed, as she is here, wearing a crown and holding a martyr's palm. Her royal lineage led to her being portrayed in sumptuous costume, as in Caravaggio's *Saint Catherine* (Thyssen-Bornemisza Collection, Madrid), and

Artemisia has given her a lavishly jeweled crown and a gown embroidered with bands of gold. While Hersey has suggested that Catherine's assertive resistance to authority made her an ideal subject for Artemisia's repertoire, this representation of the saint adheres to a more contemplative model and in that way can be associated most closely with Guido Reni's image of the saint (Prado, Madrid) painted in Rome about 1606. The upturned gaze, palm frond, and sumptuous attire may relate to that often copied model or, as Valli has suggested in the case of Reni's saint, to Agostino Carracci's 1581 engraving. As she rests her left hand on the instrument of her most heinous torture, she casts her eyes heavenward, assuming an expression recommended in Giovanni Paolo Lomazzo's 1584 treatise on painting as a means to represent contemplation.[1]

In spite of its relationship to Roman prototypes, the picture must be placed in Artemisia's Florentine period, when the facial type, wispy halo of hair, and dimpled knuckles are particular features of Artemisia's style, established in the *Allegory of Inclination* (fig. 110) painted for Michelangelo Buonarroti the Younger in 1616. The heavily jewel-encrusted crown, the elaborately embroidered edging bands within her red garment, and the finely wrought veil across her chest fit the Florentine taste for opulent fabric and refined coloration. The 1998 discovery of the *Self-Portrait as a Lute Player* (cat. 57) has established a group of Florentine pictures that share similar formal and stylistic qualities and appear to derive from a common

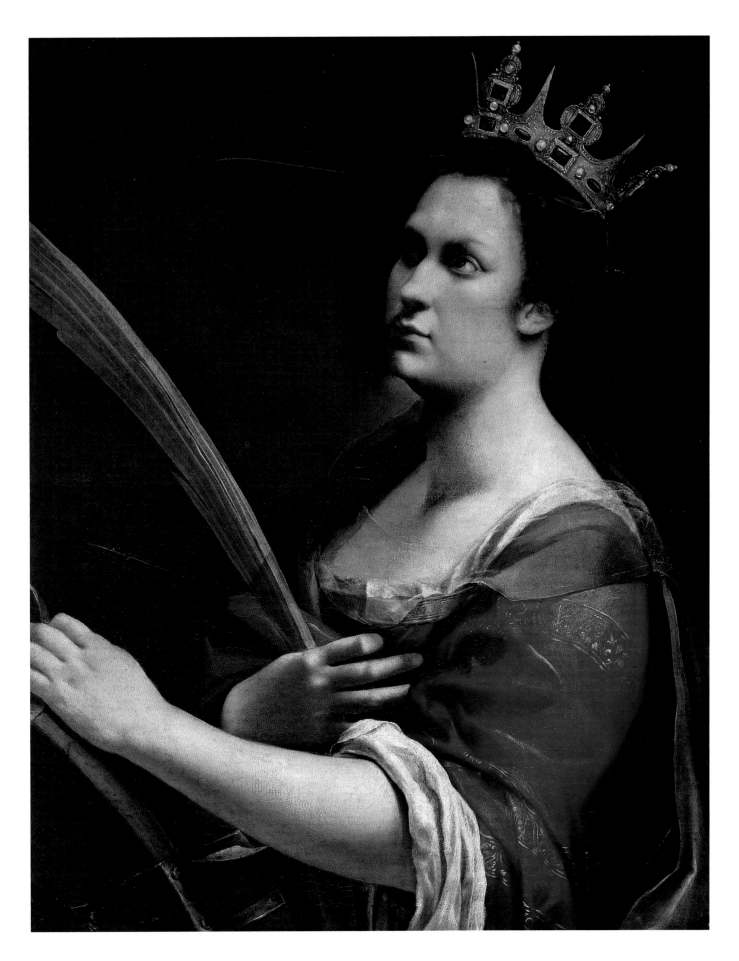

model. And while the *Saint Catherine* has generally been recognized as from Artemisia's Florentine period, opinions differ as to the precise sequencing of the works Artemisia created in that city. Bissell assigns a date of 1614–15, placing it slightly before the *Self-Portrait as a Female Martyr* (cat. 56) and the Pitti *Judith and Her Maidservant* (cat. 60), while Contini places it after the *Allegory of Inclination,* of 1616. Undoubtedly, the painting relates to the *Female Martyr,* but it is logical to suppose that it expands on the smaller depiction of the unidentified martyr rather than serving as a preliminary phase of that composition. The contemplative tone of the picture places it closer to the *Jael and Sisera* (cat. 61) than to the more active and exuberant *Conversion of the Magdalene* (cat. 58).

The dating of the picture has been complicated by a reference Artemisia made to a *Saint Catherine* in a letter she wrote in 1635 to Andrea Cioli, Cosimo's secretary of state, in which she refers to a painting of the saint that she had made "a while ago." Now it is generally assumed that the reference is not to the present picture, and attempts have been made to relate it to two other images that have been variously attributed to Artemisia, a painting on slate in the Uffizi[2] and a three-quarter view of a standing Saint Catherine in the

El Paso Museum of Art.[3] I do not believe either of these paintings is autograph, however, and it is likely that the 1635 reference is to a still-unknown or lost work.

The selection of Saint Catherine as the subject for this painting has been associated with the Florentine court of Grand Duke Cosimo II de' Medici. After Artemisia moved to Florence in late 1613 or early 1614, she certainly associated with members of Cosimo's court. Indeed, she may even have been present at a court ball in 1618, when a contemporary document describes "a lady Artemitia" who danced at one of the lavish court spectacles. Catherine de' Medici was Cosimo's sister. She lived in Florence until her marriage in 1617 to the duke of Mantua, and several writers have posited that the association of Catherine and her patron saint, Catherine of Alexandria, may explain the popularity of the image. Although nothing is currently known about the circumstances surrounding Artemisia's *Saint Catherine,* it is not unlikely that it was painted in reference to the Medici Catherine.

1. Lomazzo 1584, vol. 2, 150, as cited by Valli in Bologna–Los Angeles–Fort Worth 1988, 186.
2. Sricchia 1963; Borea in Florence 1970.
3. Gregori 1968; Gregori in Naples 1984–85; Schleier 2000.

60.

Judith and Her Maidservant

Oil on canvas, 44⅞ × 36¾ in. (114 × 93.5 cm)

Galleria Palatina, Palazzo Pitti, Florence (inv. 398)

ca. 1618–19

New York

In a dramatically darkened setting, presumed to be the interior of Holofernes' tent, Judith and her maidservant Abra pause, perhaps in response to something they have heard. Having devised a plan to free her city of Bethulia, the recently widowed Judith had cast aside her widow's attire, donned her most elegant clothing, and gained entry to the enemy's camp by promising to help their leader, Holofernes. Accompanied by Abra, she is permitted to see the general, who is attracted by her beauty. On the

fourth day, Holofernes invites Judith to dine with him. He drinks heavily and falls asleep. Judith seizes the opportunity and, using Holofernes' scimitar, cuts off his head. Abra places it in their bag, and the two women leave the camp. Judith takes the general's head and displays it to the Israelite army, galvanizing the troops and ensuring victory.

Clearly a masterwork within Artemisia's oeuvre, this *Judith and Her Maidservant* is best understood as the culmination of a series of Judith paintings by both

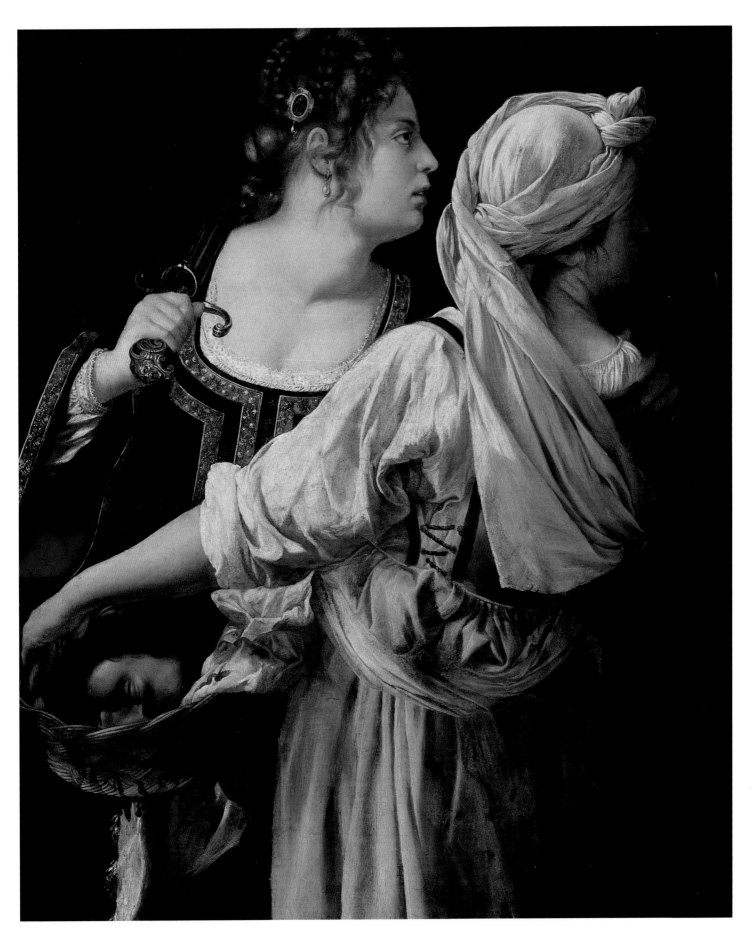

PROVENANCE: Medici collection (1637 inv.); Palazzo Pitti, Florence (by 1638).

RELATED PICTURES: Smaller replica, formerly in Galleria Corsini, Florence (present location unknown; attributed to Artemisia by Longhi 1916, 29); copy in storage in the Galleria di Palazzo Rosso, Genoa; replica in the Quirós Collection, Madrid; closely related version that belonged to the dealer De Boer, Amsterdam; *Judith with Her Maidservant*, signed, in a private collection, Milan, exhibited by Relarte as by Artemisia in 1964; *Judith with Servant*, in the Puerto Seguro (Aveyro) Collection, Málaga (cited by Pérez Sánchez 1965, 500); a *Giuditta eretta chre impugna la spada*, once belonging to Barone Staffa at Montegiorgio (cited by Ortolani 1938, 45–46); replica in Galerie Charpentier, Paris (cited by Richardson 1952–53, 83 n. 2); three additional copies are listed by De Witt 1939, 51.

REFERENCES: Longhi 1916, 293–94, fig. 30; Valentiner 1935, 101–4; Gregori 1962, 38, 39; Bissell 1968, 155 n. 22, 159 n. 51; Borea in Florence 1970, 44, 75–76; Greer 1979, 189–91, 194; Whitfield in London 1982, 168; Hagen 1988, 80; Garrard 1989, 8–9, 39–41, 200, 305, 313, 314, 318, 319, 497 n. 55; Florence 1991, 120, 122, 124, pl. 10a,b; Stolzenwald 1991, 22 fig. 13, 23, 24, 36, 86, pl. 24; Bionda 1992, 22; Hersey 1993, 327, 333 n. 50; Lapierre 1998, 144, 146–47, 157, 445–48; Bissell 1999, 198–203 no. 5.

father and daughter. Artemisia had illustrated the biblical story of Judith once before, in her riveting visualization of assassination, the Naples *Judith Slaying Holofernes* (cat. 55), which she probably completed before she came to Florence. That work, inspired by Caravaggio's *Judith* (fig. 109), focused on the moment of death, Holofernes' bloody struggle as Judith pulls the sword through his neck. This second Judith follows a more long-standing tradition for depiction of the Judith narrative, showing the moments after the killing, when mistress and servant flee the Assyrian camp. Memorable works by Andrea Mantegna and Sandro Botticelli record the flight of the two women as they hurry from the military encampment with their grisly prize.[1] Artemisia has chosen the beginning of their escape, with Judith shouldering her sword and Abra holding the trophy head in a basket.

Most scholars have acknowledged that the Pitti *Judith* is related in some way to the *Judith* in Oslo (cat. 13), accepted by many scholars as the work of Orazio.[2] While Greer sees it as an improvement on the Oslo composition, Garrard has argued that the Oslo painting must derive from the Pitti version, an unlikely scenario. With the emergence of another early *Judith and Her Maidservant* by Orazio, the ex-Colnaghi picture (fig. 46), a reasonable relationship can be posited among these three early representations of the story, as Gregori also has noted. The Pitti *Judith* is the logical third version. The ex-Colnaghi *Judith*, most likely a picture of the first half of the first decade, was a painting that Artemisia undoubtedly knew quite well. Although it was probably completed before Artemisia herself began to paint, the supposition that it was the famous *Judith* "of large size" cited in the 1612 testimony given in Agostino Tassi's rape trial[3] indicates that the picture remained in Orazio's studio for the rest of the decade. Because Artemisia herself painted an important representation of the Judith narrative in the early 1610s, she must have noted the picture and thought about its version of the story as she painted her own. The ex-Colnaghi picture records a similar moment of arrested action, when Judith and Abra respond to some nocturnal disturbance. Judith's awkward grasp of the sword in front of Holofernes' head and Abra's nearly untenable position as she holds the basket but bends

backward as she strains to listen demonstrate Orazio's typical narrative style where details of feasibility have not been worked out.

The Oslo painting represents a thoughtful improvement on the depiction of this particular moment. Judith's grasp of Abra's shoulder allows the repetition of their profiles, a far more effective dramatic representation, and the gesture of the mistress toward her servant unites the two protagonists in common purpose. The Oslo picture was executed by Orazio during the time when Artemisia herself was beginning to paint, and it represents the one instance in Orazio's oeuvre in which he shows the same kind of attention to narrative detail that characterizes Artemisia's early paintings. We don't know whether Artemisia had any input into the conception of the painting, but clearly she remembered the picture when she created her own version.

Artemisia has built upon the Oslo picture and refined the composition. By moving the two figures closer together (now Judith rests her left hand on Abra's right shoulder) and by framing the picture more closely, she has made an image in which the two women are united. The majestic diagonal sweep of the composition confers greater monumentality and hence greater theatrical force. The sensitive adjustment in the interpretation of the story, complete with the screaming face on the pommel of the sword, again reveals an artist sensitive to narrative detail. Garrard's suggestion that the women's poses recall those of Christ and Saint Peter in Caravaggio's *Calling of Saint Matthew* (Contarelli chapel, San Luigi dei Francesi, Rome) may indeed be correct. However, rather than confirming a Roman origin or a dating early in Artemisia's Florentine period, it merely indicates that she filed away examples of successful dramatic interpretation for later use, especially since the relationship to Caravaggio's picture is of a general nature rather than an example of borrowing a specific motif.

Listed and published for the first time in a Medici inventory of 1637, the Pitti *Judith* is securely accepted within the oeuvre of Artemisia Gentileschi by all major scholars. What has remained unresolved is the dating of the picture and the city of origin. Several scholars have argued that it must have been made in

Rome, shortly before Artemisia left for Florence in late 1613 or early 1614.[4] Evidence garnered in support of this dating includes references to works the artist would have known in Rome. The pose of the maid has been related to that of the seated swordsman in Caravaggio's *Calling of Saint Matthew* and to a fresco decoration in the private burial chapel for Paul V in Santa Maria Maggiore, by the Florentine painter Cigoli.[5] Contini, who does not place the picture definitively in either Rome or Florence, also notes a dependence in the Pitti painting on the works of the Roman painter Giovanni Baglione. Bissell (1999) posits that the relationship of the painting to the two earlier works by Orazio is ample evidence for placing it in Artemisia's early Roman period. A second group of writers places it early within the period Artemisia spent in Florence, finding that the more sumptuously conceived costume reveals the impact of courtly taste and opulent appointments.[6] The looser handling of paint is more typical of her Florentine pictures than of her early Roman work.

The painting may date to an even later within Artemisia's Tuscan career. The quietly dramatic tone of the picture and its close-up view of the protagonists relate to her work at the end of the second decade. The picture can be associated with the *Saint Catherine* of 1618–19 (cat. 59), in which the subject shares the same heavy-lidded physiognomy of Judith,

and to the Budapest *Jael and Sisera* of 1620 (cat. 61). The use of the expressive face on the sword pommel, described by Garrard as a Gorgon but more likely a reference to Holofernes, as an interpretive element can be related to the Budapest picture, in which the face on the sword pommel slumbers, perhaps a surrogate for the sleeping general.

The picture has suffered considerably over the years; numerous areas of loss and retouching are visible. Garrard, followed by Bissell (1999), notes that the painting has been cut down, most likely on the top and left side, as evidenced in an engraving of 1837 and several extant copies.

1. There is a large and growing body of literature on Judith in art. Garrard (1989, 278–305) offers a good introduction to the subject, with good bibliographic citations. See also Anderson 1997; and Düsseldorf–Darmstadt 1995–96, 238–79.

2. Garrard 1989; Bissell 1999.

3. Whitfield and Banks (in New York 1984) and Pepper (1984a) have argued that the inscriptions on the back of the canvas relate to the trial, and Lapierre (1998, 447–48) believes that the inscription "Piz" may well be a reference to trial notary Tranquillo Pizzuti, whose name is abbreviated in the records as "Pizz°."

4. Whitfield in London 1982; Hagen 1988; Papi in Florence 1991; Hersey 1993; Bissell 1999.

5. Contini (in Florence 1991, 120) likens Abra's pose to that of an apostle in Cigoli's fresco decoration of the private burial chapel for Pope Paul V in Santa Maria Maggiore.

6. Garrard 1989; followed by Stolzenwald 1991 and Bionda 1992.

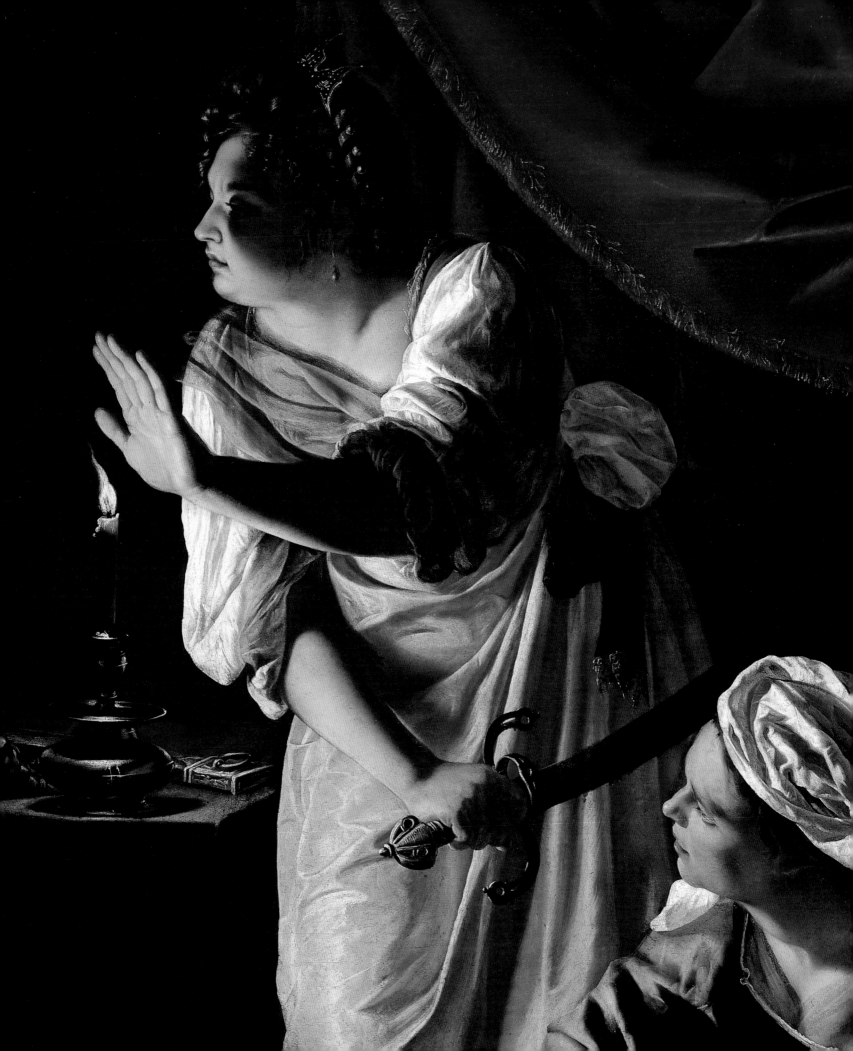

"I have made up my mind to take a short trip to Rome"

RICHARD E. SPEAR

Evidently frustrated with her life in Florence, where for eight years she had to juggle her duties as professional artist, wife, and mother, cope with debts run up by her husband, and bear the strains of four pregnancies (still, only one of the four children survived), Artemisia wrote to Cosimo II de' Medici in February 1620, telling him about her travel plans: "I have made up my mind to take a short trip to Rome," she said, because she hoped to recover there from "my many past illnesses [indispositioni]" and "not few troubles at home and with family." She told the grand duke that she expected to spend "a few months with my people [i miei]" in Rome, undoubtedly meaning her father and brothers.[1]

This brief essay addresses the social and artistic context—chiefly politics and patronage, which so often were intertwined—of Artemisia's Roman activity.[2] The few months that Artemisia envisioned in Rome actually became at least six years. It is not recorded when she left Florence, or if she ever returned, but by March 1621, she was in the papal capital, accompanied by her husband. His name disappears from the records in 1623. In 1627–28 she was in Venice, where possibly she stayed longer, for no documents pin down her whereabouts at the end of the decade. It nonetheless is likely that she returned to Rome at least briefly before settling in Naples by 1630.[3]

During Artemisia's absence, the papal capital inevitably had changed. The population had crept up to about 110,000, three times its size after the disastrous Sack of 1527. It was half again the size of Florence, but still smaller than Venice and only half as big as Naples, Italy's largest city and one of the great metropolises of Europe. A new pope, Gregory XV Ludovisi (r. 1621–23), who was Bolognese in origin, had been elected that February. Giovanni Baglione's eyewitness account of the main Roman projects undertaken by his predecessor, Paul V Borghese (r. 1605–21),[4] includes the Pauline chapel in Santa Maria Maggiore, which had been lavishly decorated on the eve of Artemisia's departure in late 1612 or early 1613; the Borghese's own palaces and villa; major additions to the Palazzo del Quirinale, the Vatican palace, and Saint Peter's; a host of restoration projects; and new granaries, which must have interested the Roman public more than all the pope's art projects combined, since the supply and price of grain, and weight of a loaf, were constant and contentious issues in heavily taxed, debt-ridden Rome.

Upon her return to Rome, Artemisia also would have seen some large churches under construction, most prominently Sant'Andrea della Valle for the Theatine order, and San Carlo ai Catinari for the Barnabites. Together with numerous smaller projects, they promised lucrative commissions for the favored artists, though private sponsorship, not that of the religious orders, typically would determine who got work. Artemisia was not to be among the lucky ones.

The church of Santa Maria della Vittoria was under way, too, for the Discalced (Barefoot) Carmelites. The vittoria of its name refers to the Battle of the White Mountain (1620), near Prague, where, in an early phase of the wars known collectively as the Thirty Years' War (1618–48), the Catholics won a decisive victory over the Protestants, thanks, it was thought, to a miraculous image of the Madonna that was carried into battle and then brought to Rome. It was welcomed in 1622 by Gregory XV and installed in Santa Maria della Vittoria.[5]

The image displaced a painting by Gerrit van Honthorst, the Caravaggesque Dutch master of nocturnes who in 1620 had returned to his native Utrecht, but not before making a strong impression on Roman art, as Simon Vouet's recently completed paintings in San Francesco a Ripa (1618–20) and his decoration of the Alaleoni chapel in San Lorenzo in Lucina (1623–24; fig. 117) both attest. As discussed below, Artemisia's own *Judith and Her Maidservant* in Detroit (cat. 69) brilliantly builds on this Caravaggesque tradition.[6]

In 1622, Gregory XV canonized Saint Teresa of Ávila, the founder of the Discalced Carmelites (Bernini's famous chapel in Santa Maria della Vittoria showing an angel piercing the saint's heart was built a generation later). The founder of the Oratorians, Saint Philip Neri, was also canonized in 1622, as were the first Jesuits, Saint Ignatius of Loyola and Francis Xavier. And in the same year, Gregory XV established the Sacra Congregatio de Propaganda Fide, in an effort to spread the Catholic faith.

Clearly, this was a vital time socially and politically. As the fabric of Rome and the city's response to Protestant threats expanded, the pan-European war was bringing about a basic realignment of church and state, which resulted in the emergence of our modern, secularized nations. The war was in essence a political struggle for European hegemony between Spain and the Austrian Hapsburgs on one side and France on the other, but complex issues of faith, trade, and trust drew virtually every European power into the bloody conflict.

While a few of the theaters of war were in northern Italy, most were well beyond the Alps. Nevertheless, it is hard to imagine that anyone in Rome could have been unaware that a great conflict was tearing Latin Christianity apart, especially because, like President Bill Clinton with the Palestinian leader Yasir Arafat, the Vatican tried, with scant success, to appear neutral and broker

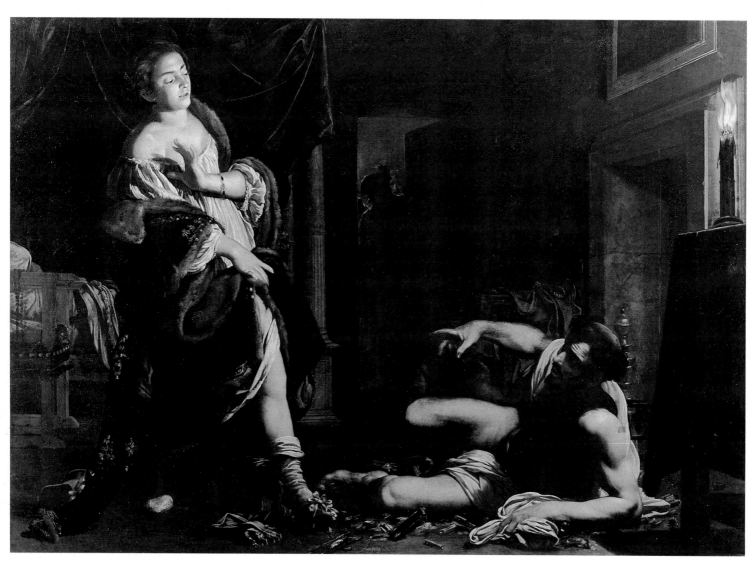

Figure 117. Simon Vouet (1590–1649), *Temptation of Saint Francis*. Oil on canvas. San Lorenzo in Lucina, Rome

peace between two stubborn sides. Not surprisingly, by the end of the war the Roman Church had lost its historical authority in European politics.

How much Artemisia personally cared about these affairs is impossible to know. On the basis of her patronage and travel, it would seem that she, like many artists of the time, was far more concerned with where the money flowed (as one Renaissance writer bluntly put it) than with political or religious allegiances.[7] Venice, for instance, despite being Catholic, earlier in the century had created a major crisis between church and state by refusing to recognize Rome's authority, and then during the Thirty Years' War for economic self-interest allied itself with anti-Hapsburg and anti-Catholic factions. Worse, from the Vatican's perspective, in an early phase of the War of Mantuan Succession (a complicated struggle about religion and control of Alpine passes that broke out in 1628, just when Artemisia was in Venice), France, with Savoy and Venice as allies, had attacked papal troops in the Valtelline.

Officially, the Vatican was neutral on the Spanish-French struggle, but under Gregory XV and Urban VIII (r. 1623–44) its leanings were strongly pro-French. This did not discourage Artemisia or others from working for the Spanish king, Philip IV (r. 1621–65), and his ambassadors and viceroys. In 1621, both Orazio and Simon Vouet (1590–1649) sought fortune by moving to a Spanish client-state, mercantile Genoa, as had Agostino Tassi a decade before them. Orazio was even willing to settle in Protestant England (1626) when it was at war with Spain, and he remained there after England engaged France in war as well (1627). In doing so, Orazio accepted a position rejected by Guercino, who took the unusually principled stance that he "didn't want to live with heretics."[8]

Jacques Thuillier's conclusion—"we must admit that if the Thirty Years' War left little mark on the arts [Callot is an obvious exception], it is because artistic creation is most often detached from everyday life"—undoubtedly is too sweeping, unless everyday life is narrowly defined as professional politics, and one disregards how politics can determine opportunities and affect taste.[9] In Artemisia's case, there is a pattern of support from Spanish patrons that provocatively, if elusively, corresponds with her relative neglect in Rome.

Orazio's departure for Genoa in 1621 coincided with Artemisia's return. If their paths crossed is unknown. Had Artemisia decided to stay in Rome to fill a gap left by her father? Presumably she went around the city to see what was new, not just to study what she did and didn't like but also to catch up on what her potential competitors were doing. Most of the leading painters of her youth were long dead, including Federico Zuccari and Annibale Carracci (both in 1609), Caravaggio, Adam Elsheimer, and Francesco Vanni (all in 1610), Barocci (1612), and Cigoli (1613). A group of less-celebrated Mannerists, who played a major role in decorating Rome's sixteenth-century churches, all died in 1614–15: Cesare Nebbia, Giovanni de' Vecchi, and Cherubino Alberti, as well as Lavinia Fontana, the other important woman painter active in Rome. Bartolomeo Manfredi, who more than any other artist was responsible for the survival and transformation of Caravaggio's innovations, died in 1622, about a year after Artemisia arrived, so she could well have met him and been encouraged by his success.

From the old guard, four prominent painters remained, of whom two, like Artemisia's family, were Tuscan: Domenico Passignano (1559–1638), whom she would have known from Florence, and Agostino Ciampelli (1565–1630), whose support from the Florentine Sacchetti family she should have envied. Cristoforo Roncalli, called Pomarancio (ca. 1553–1626), was still alive, as was the indefatigable Cavaliere d'Arpino (1568–1640).

Although Caravaggio and Annibale Carracci were dead, their followers were flourishing. Foreign artists in particular poured into Rome and embraced Caravaggio's, or more often Bartolomeo Manfredi's, manner. The Dutchman Hendrick ter Brugghen, the Frenchman Guy François, and perhaps the Fleming Gerard Seghers arrived before Artemisia first left, but by the time Vouet took up residence in 1613 and Dirck van Baburen by 1615, she was in Florence. Van Honthorst reached Rome by 1616, more likely earlier; Nicolas Tournier before 1619, Valentin de Boulogne before 1620, and Nicolas Regnier by 1621, among others. The mysterious Frenchman Trophime Bigot, who perhaps is the Candlelight Master, probably arrived in Rome when Artemisia did.

Jusepe de Ribera had been in Rome during 1613–16, just when Cecco del Caravaggio (Francesco Buoneri) collaborated with Tassi at Cardinal Montalto's villa in Bagnaia. The list of Caravaggio's other main Italian followers active in Rome while Artemisia was in Florence—Orazio Borgianni, Carlo Saraceni, Spadarino, Angelo Caroselli, Giovanni Baglione, Antiveduto Gramatica, Bartolomeo Cavarozzi—makes evident that Caravaggism had a strong, if fragile, presence in Rome when Artemisia returned, fragile because

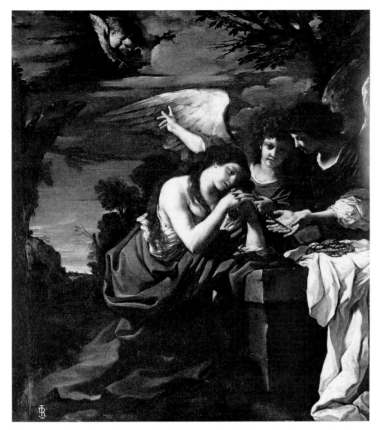

Figure 118. Guercino (1591–1666), *Saint Mary Magdalene with Two Angels.* Oil on canvas. Pinacoteca Vaticana, Vatican City

its tenebrism was entirely unsuited to fresco work and its naturalism increasingly seen as being more suited to easel than to altarpiece painting.

Inasmuch as Artemisia had no opportunities to paint frescoes or altarpieces in Rome, Caravaggism remained compatible with her assignments. None of them, however, included the Caravaggesque street themes that were so popular at the time— fortune-tellers, cardsharps, musicians, gypsies, drinkers, and soldiers—possibly because they were understood as being unsuited to a woman, but more likely because by then Artemisia was known as a painter of stories with powerful female protagonists.

Conversely, frescoes and altarpieces were the bread and butter of the Carracci's followers and the real measure of artistic success, but alongside them was a burgeoning market for genre subjects, portraiture, landscapes, and still lifes (female artists traditionally specialized in the last). A group of Northerners in Rome called the Bamboccianti, who were known for their genre scenes of street life, organized themselves into a society in 1623 and became quite successful. Artemisia, however, chose to compete at the loftiest level as a history painter, that is, as a painter of elevated religious, historical, and mythological scenes meant to instruct, although she also had a reputation as a portraitist and perhaps did some still lifes.

One of the most celebrated history paintings of the time, Guido Reni's *Aurora* (Casino dell'Aurora, Palazzo Pallavicini-Rospigliosi, Rome), had been commissioned by Scipione Borghese and completed in 1614, but Reni, like his compatriot Francesco Albani, had gone back to Bologna before Artemisia was in Rome again. Three of Domenichino's greatest works, the *Last Communion of Saint Jerome* (1614; Musei Vaticani), his fresco cycle of Saint Cecilia in San Luigi dei Francesi (1612–15), and the *Hunt of Diana* (1616–17; Galleria Borghese, Rome), also were painted while Artemisia was in Florence. Meanwhile, Lanfranco completed his first public Roman commission, the Buongiovanni chapel in Sant'Agostino (1616), and he decorated the Sala Regia in the Palazzo del Quirinale (1616–17), in collaboration with Tassi, Saraceni, Turchi, and Spadarino. Then he was awarded the commission to fresco the vault of the Benediction loggia of Saint Peter's (1620), although the job fell through when Paul V died the following year. Unlike Reni and Albani, however, Domenichino and Lanfranco chose to stay in Rome during the 1620s. It was their work that defined the highest artistic achievement and presented a daunting challenge.

Another Emilian painter, Guercino (1591–1666), arrived in Rome just when Artemisia did because the election of a Bolognese pope promised him patronage. His star rose quickly, thanks to former connections with the Ludovisi family, which gave him major commissions in Rome, including the Benediction loggia of Saint Peter's (again nothing came of it); a ceiling painting of *Aurora*, set illusionistically in fictive architecture by Tassi in their villa's casino; and the enormous *Burial and Reception into Heaven of Saint Petronilla* for Saint Peter's (Pinacoteca Capitolina, Rome), which was finished just before Guercino left Rome, in 1623.

If Artemisia's *Judith and Her Maidservant* (cat. 69) challenges Van Honthorst and Vouet on their own terms, then her *Susanna and the Elders,* dated 1622 (cat. 65), demonstrates that she could paint in an Emilian way as well, for she must have recognized that the Carracci's followers had the upper hand in Rome. Its design is Carraccesque while its coloration, lighting, expressive gestures, and background evoke Guercino's work in particular, for example, his *Saint Mary Magdalene with Two Angels* (fig. 118), painted in 1622 for Santa Maria Maddalena delle Convertite al Corso. Emulation of Guercino's manner was a clever strategy at a time when the Bolognese Ludovisi were ascendant, all the more so if the picture was painted for them (see cat. 65 regarding this likelihood).[10]

Artemisia's strikingly veristic *Portrait of a Gonfaloniere* (cat. 66) can also be dated to 1622, which means it was done just when Van Dyck was in Rome and painting portraits of the shah of Persia's emissary to Gregory XV, Sir Robert Shirley, and Lady Shirley in a more astonishingly free, neo-Venetian manner. Sixteen twenty-two was a productive year in Rome altogether, despite the "mortalità grande" (big loss of life) that the diarist Giacinto Gigli observed sweeping the city.[11] Domenichino had begun designing the most important commission in Rome, frescoes for the crossing and apse of Sant'Andrea della Valle, a project he shared with Lanfranco. Concurrently, with Guercino, Paul Bril, and Giovanni Battista Viola, he was painting another ceiling in the casino of the Ludovisi's villa, and a second in the Palazzo Costaguti (at the time the Palazzo Patrizi), with Tassi as collaborator. Another ceiling in the Palazzo Costaguti was decorated by Guercino and Tassi. Tassi had further work in the Palazzo Lancellotti, both on his own and together with Guercino. One wonders what Artemisia thought of her rapist-lover's conspicuous success.

In 1622, Andrea Sacchi painted his earliest surviving work, the *Vision of Saint Isidore* (Sant'Isidoro, Rome). Vouet signed and dated his *Circumcision* for Sant'Angelo a Segno in Naples. The gallery of the Palazzo Mattei had been begun, with frescoes by Pietro Paolo Bonzi and a rising talent from Tuscany, Pietro da Cortona. Its walls soon would display oils by Cortona, along with others by Serodine, Gramatica, Riminaldi, Turchi, and Valentin. Gianlorenzo Bernini (1598–1680) was carving two of his youthful masterpieces that year, *Pluto and Persephone* and *Apollo and Daphne*, and was ready to start his *David* (all Galleria Borghese, Rome). Lanfranco was busily at work with his powerful decoration of the Sacchetti chapel in San Giovanni dei Fiorentini.

Marcello and Giulio Sacchetti were Florentines, but they never supported Artemisia, despite the fact that Baroque patronage so often was determined by regional loyalties and friendships. Poussin, for instance, shortly after arriving in Rome in 1624, was introduced to Marcello Sacchetti by the poet Giambattista Marino, whom he knew from Paris. Sacchetti, in turn, became

Poussin's link to Barberini patronage. Pietro da Cortona benefited from the same Sacchetti-Barberini link. It is surprising, therefore, that during the 1620s, when Tuscan patrons were so prominent in Rome (not by coincidence, the Barberini were Florentines), Artemisia fared so poorly with them.

Like the Sacchetti, Cardinal del Monte, another Tuscan, apparently bought nothing from her. A *Donna con un'amore* is the only painting by her that appears in the numerous Barberini inventories (see cat. 70), together with a lost "libro con molta diversità de fiori et erbe" (book with many different flowers and plants)—the kind of work one would have expected from a woman artist, such as Giovanna Garzoni—cited in 1649 as a Barberini commission.[12] In the 1630s, Artemisia sent paintings to Francesco and Antonio Barberini from Naples, hoping in vain to win their patronage. Even her later correspondent Cassiano dal Pozzo, who was nominally Tuscan, evidently owned only a *Self-Portrait* (see cat. 81).

This same pattern of scattered support persists with the other main Roman collectors of the 1620s. As far as one knows, the Ludovisi, who amassed a large collection of ancient sculptures and many paintings, owned only a *Susanna* by Artemisia, very likely the Guercinesque picture at Burghley House dated 1622 (cat. 65). At the time of his death in 1624, the Roman-born papal treasurer Costanzo Patrizi, whose family was Sienese, owned a lost *Cupid and Psyche*. Vincenzo and Benedetto Giustiniani's important collection included only a lost *David with the Head of Goliath*, probably from the 1630s. The Mattei family acquired nothing from her hand, nor did Enzo or Guido Bentivoglio or Paolo Giordano Orsini, despite the implications of Pierre Dumonstier le Neveu's unusual, encomiastic drawing of "la digne main de l'excellente et sçavante Artemise" (the worthy hand of the excellent and skillful Artemisia), dated, in Rome, 1625 (fig. 119).

It was probably during the Jubilee Year of 1625, which witnessed more than fifty thousand Masses celebrated in Saint Peter's (Bernini's *Baldacchino* for the crossing in the church had been started the previous year), or in early 1626, when the new Saint Peter's finally was consecrated, that the Spanish ambassador to the Vatican, the duke of Alcalá, acquired Artemisia's *Penitent Magdalene* (cat. 68), along with two (now lost) pictures of *Christ Blessing the Children* and *David with a Harp* (for a candidate for the former, see fig. 132). Later, as viceroy in Naples, Alcalá bought three more of her works.

Artemisia must have valued his support, given that she was entirely ignored as commissions for altarpieces in Saint Peter's were being awarded, some even to old-fashioned painters of the *maniera* like Gaspare Celio and others to die-hard Caravaggisti, such as Valentin.[13] Artemisia's absence from that list of who's who in Roman painting is conspicuous, probably the result of her lacking sufficient support from any of the prominent patrons, since it mattered as much in the art world then as it does now whom you knew. Domenico Passignano uniquely was given three commissions in Saint Peter's; he also was the best paid. He was Tuscan and, of course, male.

Artemisia enjoyed further support from Spain—why is unknown. In 1625, after France had attacked papal forces in the Valtelline (this was the year the siege of Breda ended, which Velázquez commemorated a decade later), Cardinal Francesco Barberini was sent to Paris by his uncle Urban VIII to negotiate peace between Spain and France, but he failed to make headway with a more clever cardinal-politician, Richelieu. The next year he was sent to Spain, with Cassiano dal Pozzo in his retinue. That great antiquarian and partisan of Poussin kept a diary of this second, equally unsuccessful diplomatic mission. For this time, Philip IV's chief minister, the count of Olivares, candidly revealed that Spain already had negotiated with France without any need of papal input. In his diary, Cassiano notes seeing in a private collection in Madrid a (lost) *Mystic Marriage of Saint Catherine* by Artemisia.

Two years later, when the conde de Oñate, on behalf of Philip IV, awarded the king's first Italian commissions, Artemisia (then in Venice) was among the artists chosen. She was asked to paint a very large *Hercules and Omphale*, for which she received the equivalent of 147 Roman scudi, a reasonable but not generous sum, at least not compared with the one thousand scudi that Domenichino was paid at the same time for two pictures for Philip IV. Of course, Domenichino was much more famous than Artemisia. By contrast, Poussin, who had recently settled in Rome, was paid only sixty scudi for his *Death of Germanicus* (Minneapolis Institute of Arts) commissioned by Francesco Barberini right after he returned from Spain, far less than the two hundred to four hundred scudi Manfredi commanded for his easel paintings toward the end of his career.

Our principal contemporary source, Giulio Mancini, estimated that a good painter could earn three to six scudi a day, so by that measure 147 represented about a month's to six weeks' labor. Guercino, who was more in demand than Artemisia, on average made about fifteen hundred scudi a year; Domenichino earned two thousand a year while in Naples during the 1630s. Canons of Saint Peter's were paid about eight hundred scudi annually, which was roughly the going minimum rate for a new altarpiece in their basilica.

Scipione Borghese's income of 140,000 scudi in 1612, like Francesco Barberini's of eighty thousand to one hundred thousand scudi in 1630, dwarfs such earnings, yet on a comparative basis artists were well off, their constant complaints notwithstanding. For instance, a field hand or tailor was paid only about one-fifth of a scudo a day, half the cost of a pair of shoes, and a skilled construction worker just fifty to sixty scudi a year. Cardinal Francesco Barberini's majordomo received just six scudi a month, while musicians working for the family were paid anywhere between three and fifteen scudi a month. Therefore, had a

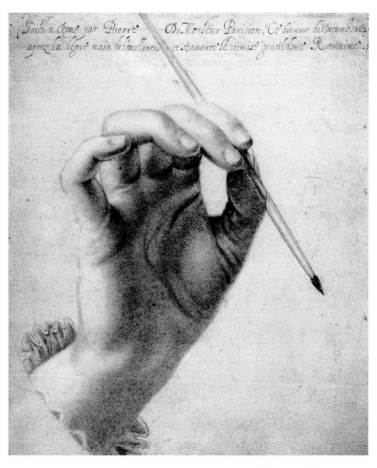

Figure 119. Pierre Dumonstier le Neveu (1585–1656), *Right Hand of Artemisia Gentileschi Holding a Brush*. Pen and ink on paper. The British Museum, London

musician wanted to buy even a copy of a painting by Caravaggio, it would have taken a good month's salary, for Mancini reveals that such copies at the time cost fifteen scudi apiece, more than Caravaggio was paid for some of his youthful originals.[14]

The smaller of Domenichino's two pictures for Philip IV, a *Sacrifice of Isaac*, is still in Madrid in the Museo del Prado, but his large *Solomon and the Queen of Sheba*, like Artemisia's *Hercules and Omphale*, is lost. Both were part of a group of similar-size canvases for the Salón Nuevo, or Hall of Mirrors, of the Alcázar in Madrid, whose iconographic unity was stories of women. In addition to Artemisia's and Domenichino's pictures, Reni was asked to paint an *Abduction of Helen*. The catalyst for the series was *Achilles Discovered among the Daughters of Lycomedes* by Rubens and Van Dyck in the royal collection, which, like Artemisia's work, showed a man in a woman's role. Orazio's dazzling painting of the daughter of Pharaoh finding Moses, now in the Prado (fig. 87), was sent to Madrid in 1633. Ribera contributed *Jael and Sisera* and *Samson and Delilah*. By 1686, four Tintorettos also were hanging in the room: *Judith and Holofernes*, the *Abduction of Helen* (Reni's picture of that subject never reached Spain), *Pyramus and Thisbe*, and *Venus and Adonis*.[15] Perhaps Cassiano dal Pozzo helped Artemisia get a commission for the Salón Nuevo, or maybe Alcalá put in a good word. In either case, the depiction of a powerful, possibly nude woman fit Artemisia's reputation and probably contributed to her being selected.

A variety of circumstances account for Artemisia's limited success in Rome, but it is difficult to recover their relative significance. That she was a woman working in a man's world doubtlessly impeded her chances for winning church commissions, particularly because, unlike Lavinia Fontana earlier, who painted traditional altarpieces, she had established a reputation for specializing in female nudes, whether by choice or market necessity. The absence of any paintings by her of Christ, for instance, is quite remarkable for the time, and probably indicative that patrons thought of Artemisia as suited only to certain subjects. The two exceptions that depicted Christ—*Christ Blessing the Children* and *Christ and the Samaritana*—were stories about children and about a woman (both are lost).

It is possible that had Gregory XV lived longer and the Ludovisi remained the papal family, Artemisia would have developed the Bolognese manner she explored in her *Susanna*, dated 1622, and thus moved further away from the chiaroscuro-based work that by the mid-1620s in Rome, unlike in Naples and Florence, was becoming old-fashioned. Her harshly tenebristic *Lucretia* (Etro collection, Milan, cat. 67), if painted as late as the 1620s, would have looked especially *retardataire*, which is why Ward Bissell's counterproposal of an earlier date, when Artemisia was working in a more starkly realistic style, is attractive. The Barberini, it is true, supported Valentin's earthy Caravaggism throughout the decade, but how much they tilted toward his art because of their French leanings is hard to say. Poussin had their backing as well. And another Frenchman, Vouet, was enormously successful in Barberini Rome, winning major commissions, including an altarpiece for Saint Peter's, and being elected to the presidency of the Roman academy, in 1624.

Artemisia may have thought that the Barberini would like her work, for if stylistically she identified with anyone other than Orazio, it would have been with Vouet.[16] He, too, had been drawn to the naturalism, dramatic lighting, compositions, and subjects of Caravaggism, and, like Artemisia, tempered its realism not only with demonstrative expressions of the passions derived from Bolognese art but with the decorative effects of elaborately tailored, colorful costumes. Artemisia's *Penitent Magdalene* in Seville, like her more openly Caravaggesque *Judith and Her Maidservant* (cat. nos. 68, 69), parallels Vouet's complex style, which had assimilated a variety of up-to-date traits, including the painterly qualities of Borgianni's work, the boldness of Lanfranco's compositions, and the elegance of Reni's art. By the time Vouet left Rome in 1627, however, practically all signs of Caravaggism in his paintings had disappeared and were replaced by a lighter, clearer palette, more idealized figures, more graceful, curvilinear designs, and a tendency toward Venetian colorism in fabrics.

At that date, Artemisia probably felt that she was stuck at the margins of the Roman art world. She would have sensed that while the Barberini were supporting the new "Baroque" style of Bernini and Cortona as well as the "classicism" of Poussin and Sacchi, her work did not fit in either of those (oversimplified) categories. Moreover, absolutely nothing by her was on public display in Rome, which is why her local influence, unlike that in Florence and Naples, was negligible, probably limited to those who shared her penchant for embellishing dramatically lighted, quasi-Caravaggesque types in fancy dress—not only Vouet, but an older Roman artist, Antiveduto Gramatica. While Vouet's

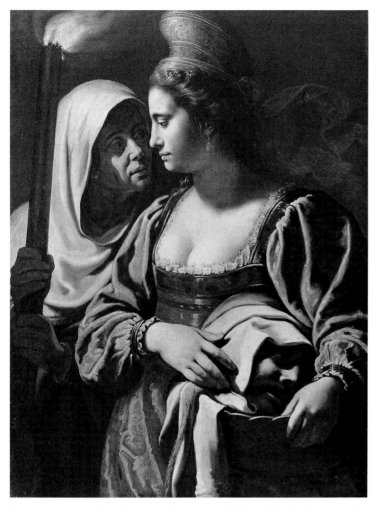

Figure 120. Antiveduto Gramatica (1571–1626), *Judith and Her Maidservant with the Head of Holofernes.* Oil on canvas. Nationalmuseum, Stockholm

Peter's, but because he had shipped his huge *Trinity* to Rome the year before, his contemporary, lighter, more elegant style already was known and admired. In 1627, too, Tassi's former student Claude Lorrain (1600–1682) settled in Rome, one year after its leading landscape painter, Paul Bril, had died. Another "foreign" artist was there in 1627, the Neapolitan Massimo Stanzione (1585?–1656). In view of Artemisia's decision to settle in Naples shortly thereafter, it might be noted that Ribera visited Rome again in 1626, in order to be knighted. Stanzione already had worked in Rome in 1617–18, and is documented there in 1621 as well, when he was knighted by Gregory XV. One wonders if and to what extent Artemisia may have had contact with Stanzione at this time, given that, perhaps of all artists, his fusion of Bolognese and Caravaggesque elements most closely parallels her own later path in Naples.

Apart from issues of taste and patronage, Artemisia's work of the 1620s is arguably her most impressive (I leave aside the much-damaged *Jael and Sisera* of 1620 in Budapest; cat. 61), for on one end stands the bold *Judith Slaying Holofernes* (cat. 62), commissioned in Florence probably by Cosimo II, followed by the *Portrait of a Gonfaloniere* (cat. 66), *Susanna and the Elders* (cat. 65), the *Penitent Magdalene* (cat. 68), and *Judith and Her Maidservant* (cat. 69), and, on the other end, *Esther Before Ahasuerus* (cat. 71), one of Artemisia's most ambitious and brilliant achievements. Like *Susanna and the Elders*, it demonstrates her gift for quickly adjusting to local taste, in this case a Venetian, more specifically Veronesan, manner, though it is possible, too, that the "neo-Venetian" strain in Vouet's, Poussin's, and Cortona's art already had pushed her in this direction. Unfortunately, nothing is known about the commission or critical response to *Esther Before Ahasuerus*, nor do we know for certain who wrote three verses published in Venice in 1627 dedicated to three of Artemisia's (lost) paintings, an *Amoretto*, a *Lucretia*, and a *Susanna* (though Bissell plausibly argues that Gianfranco Loredan may have been their author).[17]

Artemisia in any case decided in 1629–30 to move again. Considering her success with Spanish patrons, she made a wise choice. Naples was under Spanish control and rich in opportunities for artists, as Domenichino and Lanfranco recognized by moving there in 1631 and 1634, respectively. As fate would have it, although Artemisia managed to avoid the terrible plague of 1630 that ravaged northern Italy (Venice lost a third of its population), and then she survived the huge eruption of Mount Vesuvius in

public commissions undoubtedly were influential, it is hard to pin down all the interactions between these three artists because so many of their works are undated, including Gramatica's *Judith and Her Maidservant with the Head of Holofernes* (fig. 120), which used to be attributed to Artemisia herself and probably preceded her picture in Detroit (cat. 69). Gramatica's Judith represents the kind of elegantly clothed, full-bodied, calm figures that Vouet and Artemisia also preferred to the boisterous, brash, sinister types who populate Valentin's world and that of most of Manfredi's followers.

In 1627, Artemisia decided to try her luck in Venice—the same year, by coincidence or not, that Vouet left Rome for Paris by way of Venice. For a painter to pull up stakes for fame and money was not unusual. Reni, for example, despite his success in Bologna, was persuaded to return to Rome that year to work in Saint

1631, she still had her former Roman rivals to contend with. Nonetheless, she made an impressive start. In 1630, she signed and dated the first altarpiece of her career (cat. 72). Three years later she was engaged in a prestigious commission for the Buen Retiro in Madrid (cat. 77). And by mid-decade she had secured the job to paint three big canvases for a major church, the cathedral of Pozzuoli (cat. 79), an opportunity that had eluded her in Florence, Venice, and Rome.

1. See Crinò 1954 for the full text of the letter.
2. Magnuson (1982–86) provides a rich overview of Roman art, politics, and patronage during the seventeenth century. For further information on individual patrons, see the pioneering study by Haskell (1963) and the entries in the *Dizionario biografico degli Italiani* and Grove's *Dictionary of Art*, all with additional bibliography.
3. Bissell (1999, 37) assumes that Artemisia visited Florence again in the later 1620s. Costa (2000) speculates that she may have remained in Venice as late as 1630.
4. Baglione 1642, 94–97.
5. On the Battle of the White Mountain and Santa Maria della Vittoria, see Bätschmann 1998.
6. For discussion of all the paintings by Artemisia, see the fundamental studies by Garrard (1989) and Bissell (1999), the latter also with a detailed catalogue of the preserved and lost works alike.
7. Francesco Sansovino, as cited in Spear 1997, 210.
8. Malvasia 1841, vol. 2, 261.
9. Thuillier 1998, 23; see also the many other essays on the Thirty Years' War and the arts in Münster–Osnabrück 1998–99.
10. Garrard (2001, 101–5) speculates that Guercino himself may have been the "second hand" that she believes reworked Artemisia's *Susanna and the Elders*, though elsewhere she excludes him (ibid., 111).
11. Gigli 1958, 69.
12. See Costa 2000 on the book of still-life drawings.
13. Rice 1997 provides an excellent history of the commissions in Saint Peter's.
14. These matters of money are discussed in Spear 1994 and Spear 1997, 223, with further references; on the cost of copies after Caravaggio, see Maccherini 1997. An overview of Rome's economy in the seventeenth century is given by Petrocchi 1970.
15. See Gerard 1982 and Orso 1986 on the decoration of the Salón Nuevo.
16. See cat. 61 for the suggestion that Artemisia's *Jael and Sisera* was painted in response to a picture by Vouet. In my view, both an engraving of the subject by Philips Galle and especially a lost painting of about 1620 by Guercino (Garrard 2001, 66, fig. 37) are closer models; moreover, I do not believe that the alleged prototype is by Vouet. Stylistically, Artemisia's *Jael and Sisera*, whether painted in Florence or Rome, does not emulate Guercino's manner.
17. Bissell 1999, 355–56.

61.

Jael and Sisera

Oil on canvas, 33⅞ × 49¼ in.
(86 × 125 cm)

Signed (on column at center):
ARTEMITIA.LOMI / FACI-
BAT / M.D.CXX; marks (on
back of frame): KK [branded] /
1115.

Szépmüvészeti Múzeum,
Budapest (inv. 75.11)

1620

PROVENANCE: Transferred
from the imperial collection in
Vienna to the royal palace at
Pressburg (1781); royal palace,
Buda (from 1784 until July 1856?);
Enterprise des Magasins de
Commission, Budapest (sale 38,
1974, lot 85); Szépmüvészeti
Múzeum, Budapest.

REFERENCES: Salerno 1960,
95, 682; Garas 1969, 91, 97–98,
102 n. 29, 116, 193; Szigethi 1979,
35 n. 4, 38–44; Lattuada in
Naples 1984–85, 40–42; Papi in
Florence 1991, 143–47 no. 17;
Stolzenwald 1991, 33, pl. 23;
Szigethi in Milan 1993, 90, 92–93;
Baumgärtel in Düsseldorf–
Darmstadt 1995–96, 232–33
no. 101; Bissell 1999, 211–13
no. 11; Pollock 1999, 161;
Garrard 2001, 64.

The story of Jael and Sisera, from the Old Testament Book of Judges (4:11–22; 5:24–31), concerns a time when Israel, having done evil in the eyes of the Lord, is given, in retribution, to the Canaanites. Sisera, the commander of the Canaanite army, has abandoned his chariot in the midst of battle. While his entire force is slaughtered, he flees on foot to the tent of Jael, the wife of Heber the Kenite, who was at peace with the Canaanites. Jael gives him refreshment, and when he falls asleep, she goes to him and drives a nail from the tent through his temple. The Israelites then defeat the Canaanite army. In the following chapter, Jael is feted and extolled: "Blessed above women shall Jael [be]. . . . With the hammer she smote Sisera, she smote off his head, when she had pierced and stricken through his temples. At her feet . . . he fell down dead. . . . So let all thine enemies perish, O Lord: but let them that love him be as the sun when he goeth forth in his might."

Jael was often represented in cycles of the lives of biblical heroines. Artists most often depicted the moment when she raised her mallet to strike the murderous blow. Sometimes Sisera is shown sleeping peacefully, while at other times he wakens and writhes in pain. In some representations, Jael exhibits the slain Sisera to attentive observers. A third variation, an extrapolation of the text, includes a standing Jael raising her hammer in triumph over her victim's recumbent body. In Artemisia's painting, Jael kneels beside the sleeping general. As she places the nail against his temple, she raises the hammer in her right hand. Her forearm, highlighted against the darkened interior, provides the only real drama within the painting. True to the biblical text, the general lies between her feet, unaware of his impending doom. His abandoned sword rests beside him, its hilt carved in the form of a sleeping lion in obvious reference to his own imminent fate.[1]

Bissell describes the manner in which Jael holds the mallet as awkward and nonfunctional, while Szigethi finds the lack of dramatic action and quiet tone of the picture "feminine." And indeed the overall tenor of the painting is restrained and contemplative. Artemisia has abandoned a dramatic interpretation and strives, instead, for greater elegance and refinement, eschewing the eyewitness drama of the Naples *Judith Slaying Holofernes* (cat. 55). At the same time, details such as the sword hilt and the position of the general's body in relation to Jael show the artist's attentiveness to the specifics of her narrative. Jael's grip on the mallet suggests a symbolic raising of the weapon; she will need to adjust her hold in order to deliver the deathblow. Pollock has noted the same sort of rhetorical gesture in Artemisia's *Lucretia* (cat. 67) where the dagger is oddly positioned, not aimed as it would be by someone about to stab her own body. Artemisia's prominent signature indicates that she considered her efforts worthy of recognition.

This picture was painted either just before Artemisia left Florence to return to Rome in 1620 or just after

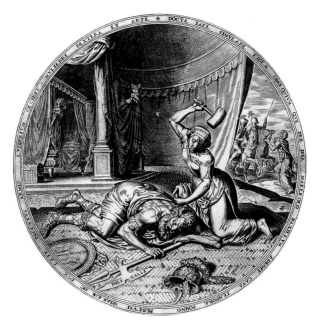

Figure 121. Philip Galle (1537–1612), *Jael and Sisera* (from the series *Women's Tricks in the Old Testament*). Engraving. Rijksmuseum, Amsterdam

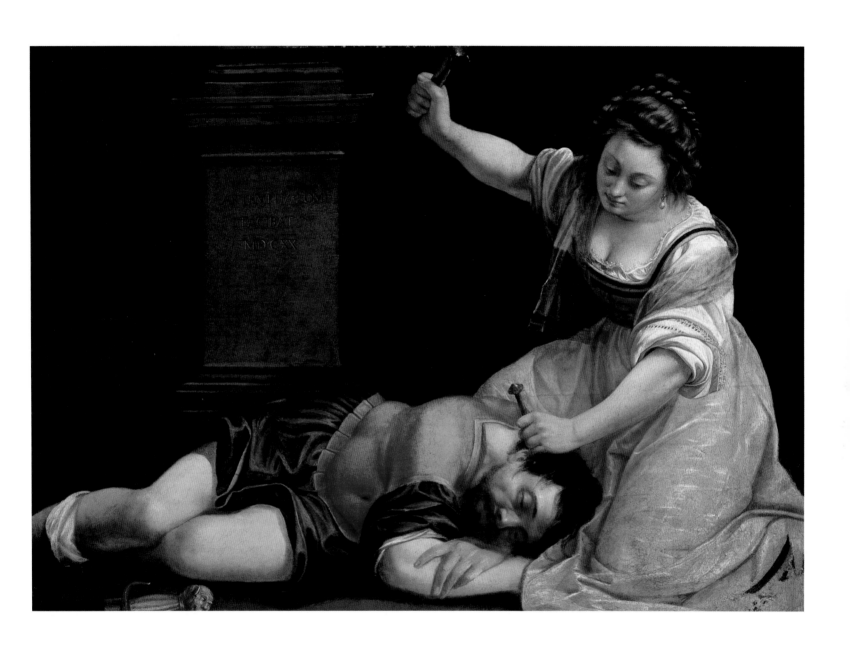

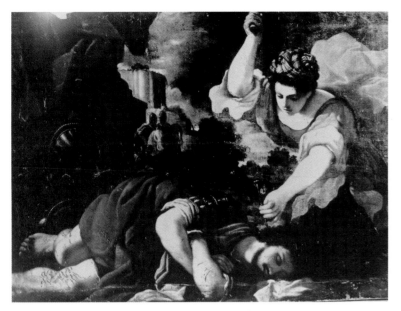

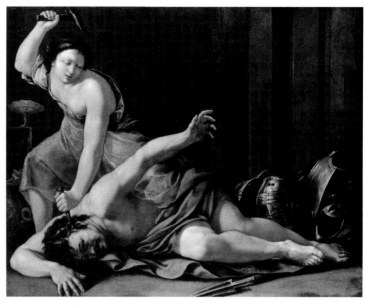

Figure 122. Copy after Guercino (1591–1666), *Jael and Sisera*. Oil on canvas. Location unknown

Figure 123. Attributed to Simon Vouet (1590–1649), *Jael and Sisera*. Oil on canvas. Whitfield Fine Art, Ltd., London

she resettled there. Scholars have linked its style to both phases of her career. Papi sees the less brutal depiction as more Florentine and places it in the context of the work of artists such as Santi di Tito or Jacopo da Empoli. Without ruling out a Roman origin, he notes that the form of the signature, in which Artemisia's paternal surname, Lomi, appears, may indicate a Florentine patron, as that is the manner in which she signed her Tuscan paintings. Bissell also points out that the general style and treatment of Jael's costume relate to Artemisia's Tuscan work, and several scholars have compared the picture with the Florentine painter Cigoli's interpretation of the subject (private collection, Florence).[2] The arrangement of the two protagonists may have been suggested by Philip Galle's 1610 engraving from a series entitled *Women's Tricks in the Old Testament* (fig. 121), as Bissell has noted.

Garrard identifies a clear similarity between Artemisia's *Jael and Sisera* and a lost canvas painted by Guercino, probably in 1619–20 (fig. 122), most likely for Cardinal Giacomo Serra, papal legate to Ferrara. How Artemisia knew this picture is not possible at present to determine. Certainly the poses are nearly identical, although Artemisia has replaced the ambitious

landscape background with a darkened and monumental interior. This element may have been inspired by a *Jael and Sisera* (London art market; fig. 123) which has been attributed to Simon Vouet and which certainly seems to have been painted in Rome during the second decade of the century. The palettes are similar, and the evocative use of dark, empty space, where the figures occupy only a portion of the pictorial field, may also derive from this Roman version and suggests that Artemisia conceived this composition in Rome rather than in Florence. Moreover, Artemisia's interpretation typifies her Roman paintings of the 1620s, as she responds anew to Caravaggism, either through her reacquaintance with the pictures themselves or through the work of Caravaggio's followers, who were translating his style into a more international idiom.

It is uncertain when Artemisia could have seen the London *Jael and Sisera*. The newly discovered inventory of Artemisia's household effects in Florence, sold to Francesco Maringhi in 1621 (see appendix 3) may indicate that she was still in Florence as late as February 1621. However, since she wrote, on February 10, 1620, to Grand Duke Cosimo II, telling him of her impending "short trip to Rome," she may have been living in Rome in 1620, returning to the Tuscan city in 1621 in order to raise money and settle affairs before moving again to Rome, where she resided for the next seven years.

The provenance for the painting has been thoroughly discussed in the literature, and most authors accept this work as having come from the imperial collections in Vienna, based on the KK (Königlich Kaiserhaus) burned into the frame, which dates from the eighteenth century.[3] Szigethi and Garas link the picture to an inventory compiled in 1781, when the collection was moved from Vienna to Pressburg and in turn transferred to Buda in 1784. The collection was dispersed in the nineteenth century.

The ruinous condition of the painting's surface limits a full appreciation of the work. The surface has been badly rubbed and substantial losses appear, most evident along the far left and right edges. Jael's drapery has been reworked and Sisera's costume has been partly repainted. Surprisingly, as Bissell has noted, the base of the background pillar, where the artist's signature appears, is still intact.

1. It would appear that Artemisia attempted some sense of an actual weapon here. The pommel of the sword, depicting a grotesque head, resembles drawings for weaponry by Filippo Orso of Mantua, dating to the mid-sixteenth century. I wish to thank Walter J. Karcheski Jr., Senior Curator, Arms and Armor, Higgins Armory Museum, Worcester, Massachusetts.
2. Affinities with Cigoli's work can be found in the angle of Jael's face, the general positioning of her upper body, and the conception of her left arm. Bissell also notes that Sisera's position derives from a drawing made by Cigoli in preparation for his finished painting.
3. See Bissell 1999, 212, for an overview of the information relevant to the painting's history.

62.
Judith Slaying Holofernes

Oil on canvas, 39 3/8 × 64 in. (100 × 162.5 cm)

Signed (at bottom right, on sword blade): EGO ARTEMITIA / LOMI FEC.

Galleria degli Uffizi, Florence (inv. 1567)

ca. 1620

Rome, New York

If the name Artemisia Gentileschi has come to be associated with any single image, it is this one of Judith slaying Holofernes. Its frequent inclusion in survey texts of the history of art has made it a famous and easily recognized picture that has profoundly shaped the understanding and expectation of Artemisia's art. A grandly conceived image of violent struggle, it was undoubtedly made as a variant of the Naples *Judith Slaying Holofernes* (cat. 55). Given the Florentine provenance, the signature that includes the paternal surname "Lomi" (a form of signature Artemisia used mostly in Florence), and Artemisia's mention in a letter written in 1635 to Galileo of a *Judith* painted for Grand Duke Cosimo II de' Medici, it was almost certainly commissioned by the grand duke in Florence. Most recent discussions of the painting have argued that it was painted in Rome after Artemisia returned from Florence in 1620 and then was sent back to Florence.

The painting's emblematic status within Artemisia's oeuvre has prompted a wide range of scholarly interpretation. Its most exceptional feature, the spurting, seeping blood, makes it among the most violent of all the representations of the biblical story. In light of Artemisia's own sexual history, writers have often associated the image with her personal experience.[1] Psychoanalytic and feminist studies have explored various associations for such violence, including references to childbirth and castration.[2] Pollock has offered a particularly rich feminist analysis of both this picture and its Naples prototype (cat. 55), arguing that the painting should perhaps be read less in terms of its overt references to Artemisia's experience than as an encoding of the artist's sublimated responses to events of her life and the historical context in which she worked. The painting certainly exemplifies Artemisia's penchant for representing strong heroines. But it also documents Artemisia's response to

PROVENANCE: Probably Cosimo II de' Medici, Florence (from about 1620); Palazzo Pitti, Florence (by 1638?–1774); Galleria degli Uffizi, Florence (from 1774).

RELATED PICTURES: Reduced copy in the collection of Luiz de Rocka Machado a Funchal, Madeira (notation on a photograph in the Musée du Louvre, division of documentation, cited in Papi in Florence 1991, 153).

REFERENCES: Baldinucci 1767–74, vol. 12 (1772), 11; Lastri 1791–95, vol. 2, pl. 84; Longhi 1916, 194–95; Voss 1925, 463, pl. 119; Milan 1951, 62 no. 101; Zürich 1958, 12 no. 20; Longhi 1961, 258, 281; Bissell 1968, 156; Borea in Florence 1970, 76–78; Greer 1979, 189, 191; Nicolson 1979, 50; Gorsen 1980, 76; Hofrichter 1980, 9–15; Parker and Pollock 1981, 21; Pointon 1981, 350–59; Slap 1985, 337–38; Garrard 1989, 38–39, 51–53, 326, 337–38; Nicolson 1990, vol. 1, 111; Papi in Florence 1991, 49–50 no. 19, 150–53; Cropper 1992, 204, 209; Wachenfeld and Barthes 1992, 30–31, 33–34; Bal 1996, 297–300; Topper and Gillis 1996, 10–13; Anderson 1997, 60–66; Bissell 1999, 43–44, 104–5, 213–16 no. 12; Pollock 1999, 115–24; Spear 2000, 569–71.

the presumed tastes of her patron, to which the adjustments made from the earlier Naples version in composition, size, and coloration all testify.

Compared with the Naples *Judith*, the Uffizi painting presents a more refined image of the protagonist. She wears an elegant gold damask dress that contrasts strongly with the arc of blood spurting from Holofernes' neck. Her hair is more tightly curled compared with the disheveled wispiness of the Naples heroine. The biblical account says specifically that Judith "dressed her hair" and that she wore necklaces, bracelets, rings, and earrings. The bracelet on Judith's right arm may have been inspired by the text and was most certainly encouraged by the Florentine taste for stylish attire. It is decorated with cameos or enamels depicting figures, interpreted by Garrard as images of Diana (Artemis in Greek) and hence referring to the artist's own name to suggest an autobiographical association. By contrast, Bissell views the bracelet medallions as showing Mars, the valiant god of war, intended as an ironic contrast with the vanquished Holofernes and a Bacchante intended to be juxtaposed with the forceful victor Judith. Color combinations have been refined, notably in the counterpoint of Abra's predominantly blue garment with the golden color of Judith's dress. Red, used to accent Judith's and Abra's sleeves, repeats the rich red of Holofernes' velvet drape and his spurting blood.

More significantly, the entire composition of the Uffizi picture is more studied and contrived than the Naples version, an effect that may derive in part from the discrepancy in size. The Naples picture has been cut down along the left side, making it smaller than the Uffizi version, although it has been suggested that the two were originally close in size. Papi and Bissell have argued, correctly in my view, that the two versions represent two different compositions, a suggestion that makes sense given the more symmetrical arrangement of the Uffizi picture. Pentimenti evident in the right leg of Holofernes suggests that the artist worked to achieve greater symmetry, an effect reinforced through the central axis of the nearly vertical sword blade and the central—also vertical—placement of Abra. The parallel arms of Judith, the analogous angle of the legs of Holofernes, and the placement of

Abra form a triangular composition, with the head of Holofernes at the center. Such a self-consciously manipulated composition differs considerably from the Naples version, where the more skewed arrangement underscores the sense of an observed event. Artemisia signed her work prominently on the blade of the sword, and she clearly intended the picture as a demonstration of artistic prowess. In this sense, the gushing arc of blood, which many scholars have associated with her reacquaintance in Rome with the realist work of Caravaggio, seems an ostentatious display, assuring that this second version would surpass its earlier model in every way, including horror.

The argument that the picture was made (or at least finished) in Rome (about 1621) rather than in Florence has been based on the presumed availability in Rome of the earlier painting. However, we have no evidence for the early ownership of the Naples work, which Artemisia may have taken to Florence with her. Cosimo could have seen it there and requested a copy or a variant version. The placing of the picture as a Roman work finds support in Papi's observation of a stylistic similarity to the Milan *Cleopatra* ([cat. 53], which he attributes to Artemisia) and to the Milan *Lucretia* ([cat. 67], which he dates earlier than 1620), both of which he conjectures were still in Rome.

Borea first associated the painting with a 1637 (1638 New Style) inventory of the works of art in the Palazzo Pitti; the same picture is mentioned again in a Pitti inventory of 1663.[3] Papi questions whether this citation in fact refers to the painting, since there is no attribution in the inventory while our painting is signed. And Bissell notes a discrepancy between the measurements of the canvas cited in the inventory and those of the present, Uffizi version. The earliest certain reference to the picture is a 1774 notice of the transfer to the Uffizi of a *Judith* ascribed to Caravaggio, in which the biographer Filippo Baldinucci notes that he had seen the work and praises it, saying it caused "not a little terror." In 1791, an engraved copy of the painting was included in a history of Tuscan painting by Marco Lastri. The author remarks that the painting had been relegated to a remote corner of the gallery, since the grand duchess did not wish to be subjected to such horror.

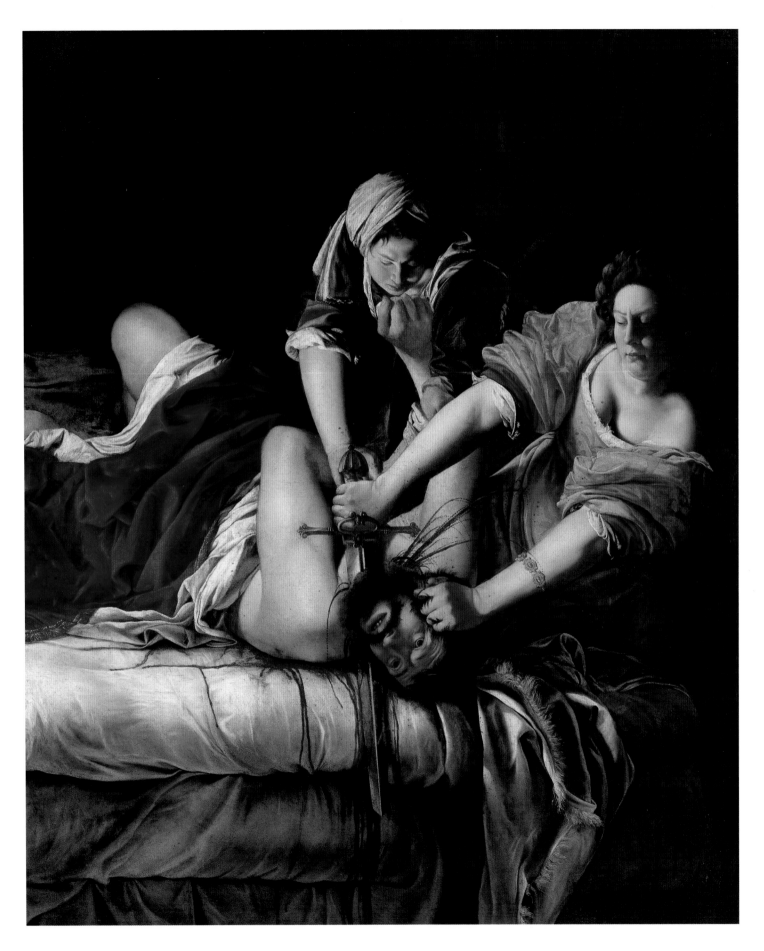

The picture has suffered considerable damage, most recently in the 1993 bombing of the Uffizi, when it sustained as many as seven discrete losses. Even before this latest damage, there were considerable losses and repaintings throughout. The most severe losses have been noted in Holofernes' head, and there has been damage to Abra's face around her left eye. The background curtain is barely discernible as a result of sinking.

1. Bissell (1968) has noted that it is difficult not to see Holofernes as a stand-in for Agostino Tassi. Garrard (1989, 278), while noting the importance the theme seems to have had for Artemisia, acknowledges in discussing the Uffizi painting, "It is impossible to ignore the echo of personal experience in this *Judith* . . . ;

indeed, the very imagery of the bloody bedroom scene invokes Artemisia's own description of Tassi's bedroom assault upon her, with its tangle of knees, thighs, blood, and knives." Whitfield (in London 1982, 168) has noted in general that Artemisia's own life caused her to select themes of women "whose lives were threatened by men." Daprà (in Chambéry 1995, 90) notes that the artist's taste for the decapitation theme must be put in relation to her life. Most recently, Levenson (1996, 126) has noted, after summarizing Artemisia's rape and trial, that "Artemisia's choice of themes for the Naples picture, as well as the extreme violence of the depiction, have not unreasonably been connected with the trauma of those events." Anderson has noted that the paintings of the Judith story reflect the trauma of Artemisia's rape experience.

2. See Pointon (1981, 343–67), who argues the picture can be read as a scene of childbirth; and Slap (1985, 335–42), who on the basis of dubious formal similarities in the objects portrayed has suggested castrated male genitalia.

3. The beginning of the year in Florence coincided with the feast of the Annunciation, on March 25.

63.

Saint Cecilia

Oil on canvas, 42½ × 30⅞ in. (108 × 78.5 cm)

Galleria Spada, Rome (inv. 149)

ca. 1620

New York, Saint Louis

Like the Spada *Madonna and Child* (cat. 52), this painting was once owned by Alessandro Biffi and came to the Spada collection through an agreement to offset debts. It is listed in an inventory that Biffi signed in 1637, where it is described as "una Santa Cecilia . . . sona un leuto" (a Saint Cecilia . . . playing a lute) by the hand of Artemisia.[1] In spite of its early documentation, the attributional history of the painting is long and varied, including eighteenth-century assignments to the school of Titian and to Caravaggio. While Venturi sustained the attribution to Caravaggio, Voss assigned the picture in 1911 to Artemisia, although he identified the subject as a generic female lute player rather than the Roman saint. A cleaning in 1988 rendered the background organ more visible, making it identifiable as an image of Saint Cecilia. Most writers have accepted an attribution to Artemisia, including Gregori, Garrard, Papi, and Vicini, although Bissell (1999) places the picture generally within a Roman workshop of the first decade of the seventeenth century.

Saint Cecilia, an early Christian martyr, enjoyed considerable popularity during the Counter-Reformation, with a particularly fervent following in Rome. Her body, still intact after over twelve centuries, had been discovered on October 20, 1599, when her church was rebuilt and her tomb was opened. Cecilia, born to a Roman patrician family, is fervent in her devotion to God and remains a virgin, although she has been given in marriage. Her husband, Valerian, together with his brother, is converted by Cecilia to Christianity. Cecilia's refusal to follow the practice of pagan sacrifice angers the Roman prefect, and he orders that she be suffocated. This attempt to end her life fails, and he has her beheaded. The executioner delivers three blows to her neck, but she lingers for several days. A celebrated sculpture by Stefano Maderno made in 1600 (church of Santa Cecilia, Rome) represents the saint in the fallen position in which she dies.

Saint Cecilia is often portrayed with musical instruments. In Jacobus de Voragine's *Golden Legend*, she is described as arriving at her wedding to the sounds of

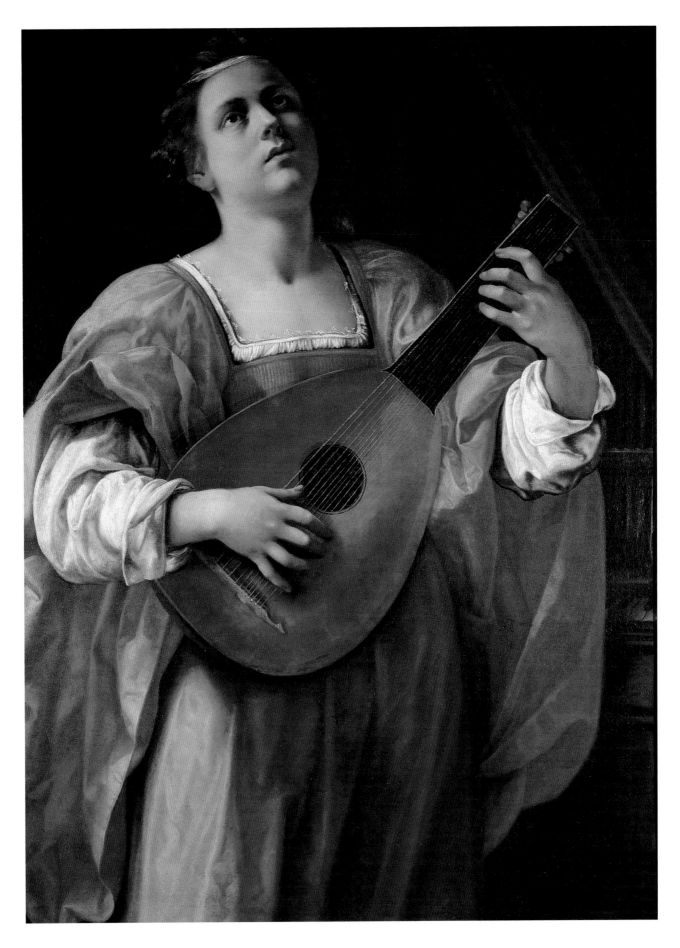

PROVENANCE: Alessandro Biffi, Rome (until 1637); Veralli collection, Rome (1637–1643/86); Spada collection, Rome (from 1643/86).

REFERENCES: Venturi 1910, 268; Voss 1911, 124; Voss 1925, 463; Porcella 1931, 222; Lavagnino 1933, 9; Marangoni 1945, 55; Zeri 1954, 85–86, no. 293; Longhi 1961, vol. 1, 502; Moir 1967, vol. 1, 55–56; Bissell 1968, 167; Nicolson 1979, 51; Gregori in Naples 1984–85, vol. 1, 147; Garrard 1989, 26–28; Nicolson 1990, vol. 1, 111; Papi in Florence 1991, 132–35 no. 13; Vicini 1992, 44; Szigethi in Milan 1993, 93; Papi 1994, 198–99; Bissell 1999, 333–34 no. x-28; Papi 2000, 451; Vicini 2000, 20–22; Brown in London–Rome 2001, 99.

music, although "she sang in her heart to the Lord alone."[2] By the fourteenth century, she is shown with instruments, and in the fifteenth century the organ becomes her most common attribute.[3] Nevertheless, she continued to be depicted playing a variety of instruments. Guido Reni's *Saint Cecilia* (The Norton Simon Museum, Pasadena) plays a violin; Peter Paul Rubens shows her playing the virginals (Gemäldegalerie, Staatliche Museen, Berlin), and Pierre Mignard paints her strumming a harp (Louvre, Paris).

Artemisia's saint stands in a murky interior, her attribute, the organ, barely visible behind her while she plays a lute. Her deep yellow garment recalls the costume of Orazio's Washington *Lute Player* (cat. 22), although the elegiac mood of that painting is absent here. Brown has also noted the direct influence of that picture. Giovanni Paolo Lomazzo's treatise on painting and Cesare Ripa's iconographic handbook advocated that yellow garments be worn in painted representations of Saint Cecilia, coloration that symbolized the desire for God. Artemisia's saint is shown in the pose recommended by Ripa, with the face turned upward and the eyes gazing toward heaven. While Artemisia may not herself have consulted these sources (in her 1612 trial testimony she stated that she could neither read nor write), the characteristics she uses were part of the general iconography of Saint Cecilia in the seventeenth century. Artemisia's saint, standing close to the picture plane and nearly filling the allotted space, is one of the most monumental representations of this figure from the seventeenth century.

Theories on dating range from Artemisia's Roman period to the end of her years in Florence. A number of scholars (Porcella, Lavagnino, Zeri, and Garrard) have associated this image with the frescoed musicians made in 1611 by Orazio for Scipione Borghese's Casino delle Muse (fig. 6). While Zeri dates the picture to as late as 1620, Papi, followed by Vicini, finds the association with the earlier works from Artemisia's Florentine period more viable. In particular, he links the treatment of her dress to the drapery of the Pitti *Judith and Her Maidservant* (cat. 60), the palette to that of the Pitti *Magdalene* (cat. 58), and the coiffure to those found in other Florentine works, such as the *Allegory of Inclination* (fig. 110) and the *Saint Catherine of Alexandria* (cat. 59). Papi notes a correspondence to the work of Cristofano Allori, and he places the work in the early years of Artemisia's Florentine career. Vicini emphasizes the Venetian character of the picture.

Zeri's dating to the end of the Florentine period may warrant reexamination. Not only is the painting in tone and in color associated with the *Jael and Sisera* (cat. 61), but its more contemplative mood also conforms to the *Saint Catherine*. The importance of Saint Cecilia in Rome during the early seventeenth century may lend further weight to a Roman origin. The similarity of the pose of Cecilia and that of musicians in Orazio's Casino delle Muse frescoes may reflect Artemisia's reacquaintance with those paintings upon her return to Rome from Florence in 1620. The general demeanor of the saint recalls Caravaggio's *Boy with a Basket of Fruit* (Galleria Borghese, Rome), which was owned by Scipione Borghese in the early 1620s.

1. See Vicini 2000.

2. Jacobus de Voragine 1993, 318.

3. There are various theories as to how music in general and the organ in particular came to be identified with Saint Cecilia, ranging from the association with virginity and virtue to the use of the word "organum," meaning "instrument," for the more specific "organ." See, for example, Stefaniak 1991, 345–71, and Connoly 1983, 121–39.

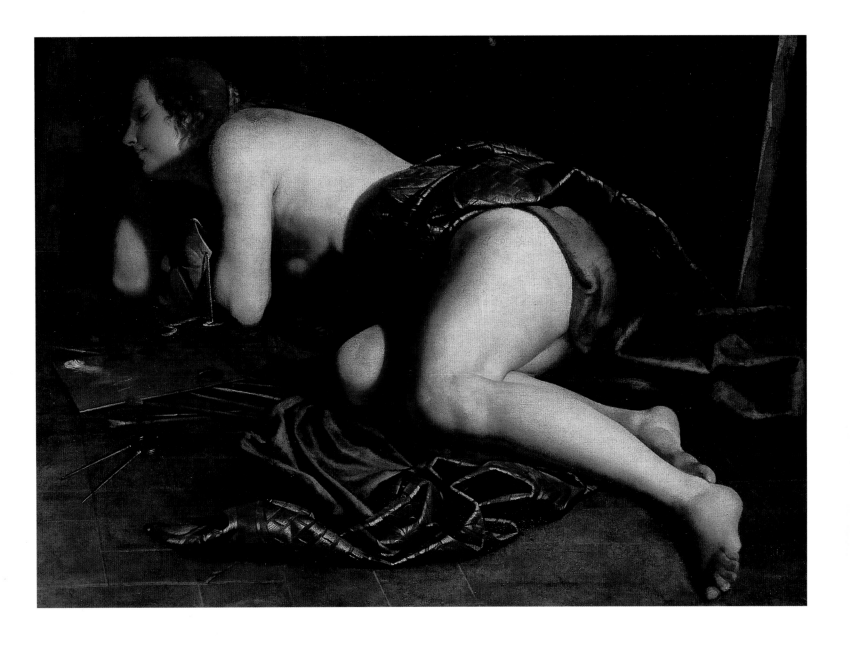

64.
Allegory of Painting

Oil on canvas, 37 ⅝ × 52 ⅜ in.
(95.5 × 133 cm)

Musée de Tessé, Le Mans
(inv. 10.69)

1620s

During the past decade, a number of new paintings have been ascribed to the hand of Artemisia Gentileschi. While a few that have received general acceptance are works in this exhibition (*Self-Portrait as a Lute Player; Self-Portrait as a Female Martyr; Penitent Magdalene;* cat. nos. 57, 56, 73), the curators wanted to avoid including too many pictures for which the attribution is tenuous. However, this painting from the Musée de Tessé, Le Mans, is perhaps the most provocative to receive this attribution. First published by Arnauld Brejon de Lavergnée as autograph in 1988, the attribution is sustained by Chaserant. The picture takes up a theme, the Allegory of Painting, that Artemisia herself addresses in two other works, and

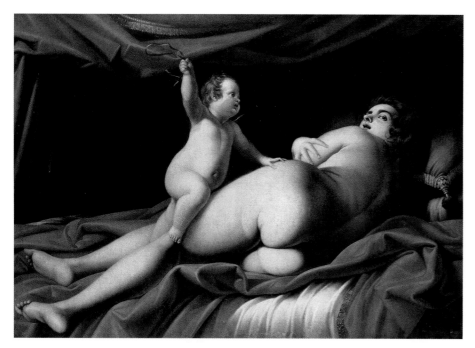

Figure 124. Giovanni Baglione (ca. 1566–1643), *Cupid and Venus*. Oil on canvas. Private collection

proportions, that had dominated Italian painting of the sixteenth century.

Bissell has focused on the erotic quality of this painting, drawing comparisons with two works by the Roman painter and nemesis of Orazio, Giovanni Baglione. The figure's position, the placement of the drapery (which draws attention to the genital area), and the known animosity between Orazio and Baglione warrant, Bissell argues, an attribution to Baglione. Baglione had been the victim of vulgar and derisive poems circulated in Rome by Caravaggio and Orazio, among others, in the first years of the century. Baglione sued for libel, and a trial ensued in 1603. According to Bissell, Baglione, who never completely reconciled with Orazio, made with this painting another crude barb, this one visual and designed to refer to Orazio's daughter, who would have been immediately recognizable in the picture. The painting can certainly be related in terms of composition and type to a work by Baglione (fig. 124) in which Venus reclines, with her back to the viewer, while Cupid chastises her. In a companion painting (Museo Provinciale, Valencia), Cupid restrains a libidinous satyr who approaches a provocatively displayed Venus. However, the softness of the modeling and the suppression of outline in the Le Mans painting distinguish it from the two paintings by Baglione. Although several scholars have placed the picture in Rome in the second or third decade of the seventeenth century, it has not been definitively assigned to any one hand.

The painting is undoubtedly an allegory but may present a meaning far more subtle than the one Bissell proposes. The quality of the work suggests that it was perhaps painted for purposes other than crude revenge by Baglione. The limited color scheme also indicates that it could have been made in accordance with a patron's very specific directives.

The conception of the picture seems designed to demonstrate the abilities of the artist, since the foreshortening of the figure, who is positioned diagonal to the picture plane, is a difficult pictorial exercise. It certainly has been handled with more refinement than is evident in Baglione's two overtly erotic canvases. Furthermore, this reinterpretation of the Allegory of Painting and the daring composition relate to other

PROVENANCE: Le Popelinière family; Musée de Tessé, Le Mans (from 1836).

REFERENCES: Lecoq in Dijon 1982–83, 40–41; Brejon de Lavergnée and Volle 1988, 161; Laboratoire de Recherche des Musées de France, conservation report, 1994; Chaserant in Chambéry 1995, 92–93; Bissell 1999, 299–301 no. X-1.

its overt Caravaggesque manner and the particular female physique relate to a number of works within the oeuvre.

In a dimly lighted room with a tiled or brick floor, a young woman lies sleeping, her head resting against the legs of an easel. A mahlstick, a canelike rod used to steady an artist's hand, has been propped through the legs of the easel. Next to the woman's left hand lie a palette, several brushes, and a drawing compass; a grimacing mask leans against her left forearm. A canvas can be discerned at the right side of the picture. Clearly the figure is based on the iconographic illustration of "Painting: La Pittura" in Cesare Ripa's artists' reference, the *Iconologia*. The mask, brushes, and palette are all standard attributes of painting, as is the shot fabric that she wears. Here, the description may refer to the rich damask drapery that lies across her body, painted in varying shades of dark blue and a rich maroon woven with golden threads. Lecoq has argued that the overt Caravaggesque style combined with the mask's expression—denoting falsehood—may have been intended as a kind of manifesto of the naturalistic manner of Caravaggio as opposed to the false style of Mannerism, exemplified by contrived compositions, unresolved spatial formulas, and exaggerated

works by Artemisia: the dramatic pose of Susanna in the Pommersfelden painting (cat. 51) and the London *Self-Portrait as the Allegory of Painting* (cat. 81).

Given its format and its dependence on the prototypes of Baglione, the picture (if autograph) should be placed among Artemisia's works of the 1620s. Chaserant, however, based on the play of light and shadow that he traces to the influence of Caravaggio, assigns it to her Neapolitan period (presumably before 1638).

The painting has pinpoint losses throughout, with larger losses on the left cheek and within the flesh areas along the hip at the drapery line. X radiographs reveal another, inverted image, beneath the left arm, apparently depicting a bishop wearing a miter.[1]

1. I wish to thank Genevieve Aitken, Documentation peinture, Ministère du Culture, Direction des Musées de France, for providing the composite X radiations of the painting.

65.

Susanna and the Elders

Oil on canvas, 63 ⅝ × 48 ⅜ in. (161.5 × 123 cm)

Signed (lower center): ARTEMITIA GENTILESCHI LOMI/ FACIEBAT. A D. M DC XXII

Collection of the Marquess of Exeter, Burghley House, Stamford, Lincolnshire

1622

New York, Saint Louis

First listed as by Artemisia by the ninth earl of Exeter in an eighteenth-century inventory of his collection, this beautiful painting was attributed the following century to Caravaggio. Restored to Artemisia by Gregori in 1968, it has also been given to an anonymous seventeenth-century artist (Bissell 1999). Its style has confounded many viewers, for its lushly sensuous Susanna, who looks devoutly heavenward to beseech God's help in her predicament, does not conform to the type of dramatic, aggressive heroine that has become associated with the artist. There is, however, strong evidence that links the picture to her work.

Most obvious is the signature, near Susanna's right knee, which reads ARTEMITIA GENTILESCHI LOMI / FACIEBAT. A D. M DC XXII. Although visible today, it had become obscured through accumulations of dirt and varnish and was revealed only when the canvas was cleaned prior to the 1995 exhibition of works from Burghley House. Bissell (1999) and Garrard (2001) have been reluctant to accept the signature because of its unique format—which combines Orazio's maternal and paternal surnames—and repainting around the letters. However, there is really no consistency in Artemisia's signatures; of the seventeen signed works believed to be autograph, there are fourteen different variations. The use of "Lomi" has been associated exclusively with the Florentine period.

But if the *Jael and Sisera* (signed ARTEMITIA.LOMI / FACIBAT / M.D.CXX; cat. 61) was indeed made in Rome, the circumstances for her usage of the name are not so easily understood. In fact, Artemisia is still recorded as "Lomi" by a Roman notary on November 17, 1621.[1] A technical analysis made at the Indianapolis Museum of Art in 1995 indicates that the signature is consistent with the rest of the painting and appears to have been inscribed by the same artist.[2]

There are also stylistic details that support an attribution to Artemisia. The worn stone bench, the physiognomies of the two elders, and the handling of the white linen chemise all relate to her 1610 rendition of the subject now in Pommersfelden (cat. 51). The substantial proportions of the thigh and leg, as well as the handling of the fleshy joint, recall both that painting and the Milan *Lucretia* (cat. 67). Nevertheless, such elements as Susanna's face, the more traditional rather than boldly innovative iconography, and the reworking of the canvas evident in the pentimenti have caused a number of scholars to hesitate over its attribution.[3] The configuration of the fountain is completely altered (there is also evidence of a fountain much farther back from picture plane), a branch above Susanna's head has been painted out, and a head directly above that of Susanna and turned to the viewer's right can be discerned even in photographs.

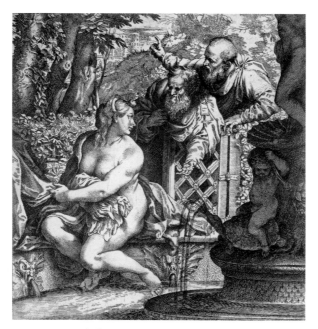

Figure 125. Annibale Carracci (1560–1609), *Susanna and the Elders*. Etching. National Gallery of Art, Washington D.C.

PROVENANCE: Possibly Cardinal Ludovico Ludovisi, Rome (by 1623–before 1633); the ninth earl of Exeter, Brownlow Cecil (before 1793); collection of the marquess of Exeter, Burghley House, Stamford, Lincolnshire.

RELATED PICTURE: Castle Museum and Art Gallery, Nottingham (copy of nearly identical size).

REFERENCES: Waagen 1854, 405; Bissell 1968, 167; Gregori 1968, 414–19; Nicolson 1974, 418 fig. 87; Harris in Los Angeles 1976–77, 121 n. 18; Garrard 1989, 202–4; Contini in Florence 1991, 113; Wood 1992, 515–23; Hersey 1993, 327; Brigstocke in Pittsburgh 1995, 80–81 no. 20; Harris 1998, 117–18; Bissell 1999, 348–53 no. x-42; Brigstocke 2001, 276; Garrard 2001, 77–113.

These changes, however, may simply argue that Artemisia had a hard time bringing the composition to realization or that she made corrections based on the directives of a patron; they do not necessarily provide evidence of another hand. In fact, the ghost head above Susanna recalls the general form of the elder on the left in the Pommersfelden picture. Finding the grouping of the three figures in the earlier painting crowded, Artemisia may have placed the second elder's head above that of the other in order to underscore their licentious curiosity. This adjustment, in turn, may have required an alteration in the form of the fountain; the putto (who originally stood on the top) has been replaced by a broad basin, an enlargement that provided needed compositional balance.

Garrard (2001) has most recently argued that an initial composition was begun and finished by Artemisia but that the painting was significantly altered by a second, later hand, who added the present form of the signature, revised the expression of Susanna, and eliminated the original fountain. A key element of her argument holds that Susanna's demeanor, of the compliant seductress who casts her eyes invitingly back toward the elders, exemplifies an interpretive mode that she finds inconsistent with the work of Artemisia at this point in her life. Susanna, however, gazes toward

heaven rather than toward the elders, in a pose drawn directly from the description in the Apocrypha, which appears in many seventeenth-century representations of the story: When Susanna is confronted by the two men, "Through her tears she looked up toward Heaven, for her heart trusted in the Lord." By the seventeenth century, there was a fairly well-established tradition that conflates the two narrative moments—the elders' lusting and their approach to Susanna—into a single scene, as Artemisia has done.

An important feature of this painting is its obvious dependence on the print *Susanna and the Elders* by Annibale Carracci, made between 1590 and 1595 (fig. 125), and its reliance on a work from the Carracci circle, a *Susanna and the Elders* (The John and Mable Ringling Museum of Art, Sarasota; it bears the signature "Agostino Carracci" but is also attributed to Sisto Badalocchio) painted in Rome about 1600. The landscape background has also been associated with Guercino's paintings of the late teens and twenties (Brigstocke). In other words, the picture, which seems intended to emulate a Bolognese style, was perhaps designed to appeal more to Bolognese taste. This makes sense when we consider the inscribed date of 1622, the second year of the very brief papacy of Gregory XV (r. 1621–23). While Gregory himself patronized artists to a limited degree, his favored nephew, Cardinal Ludovico Ludovisi, was a major player in Roman art of the 1620s, a formidable collector who acquired three hundred paintings in a frenzy of buying between 1621 and 1623.[4]

In fact, the Burghley House *Susanna* may be the one listed in the 1623 inventory of the Ludovisi collection, which includes a painting described as "a Susanna with the Elders . . . by the hand of artimitia."[5] This reference has previously been associated with the Pommersfelden *Susanna*, since it roughly matches the inventory dimensions and because the owners of the painting, the Schönborn, originally bought the picture in 1715 in Florence from the Florentine artist Benedetto Luti. Because Luti spent time in Rome, it made sense to suppose that Luti had somehow acquired the picture from the Ludovisi collection when he was in Rome and took it back to Florence before selling it. But it is far more logical to assume that the Burghley

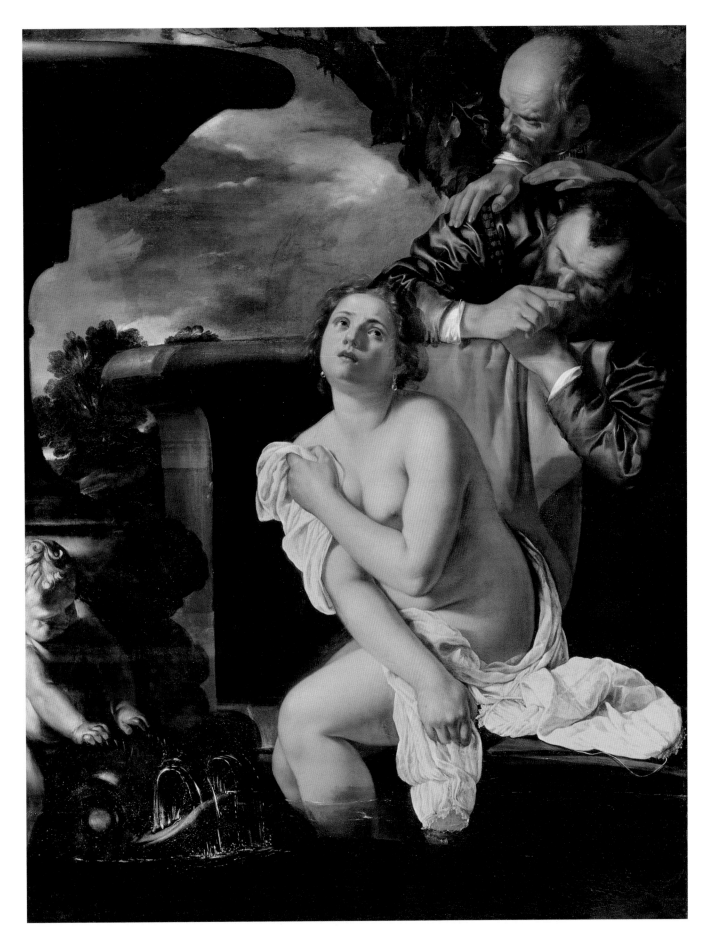

House painting is the one in question, since it would have appealed to the Ludovisi, noted for patronizing compatriot Bolognese artists. The Burghley House canvas and the painting in Pommersfelden are very close in size, so the former picture fits the inventory description just as well as the latter. It does not appear in the more detailed 1633 Ludovisi inventory, so we can assume that the picture had been sold by that date.[6]

At this point, we have no further information as to the painting's whereabouts between its inventory listing in 1623 and its probable purchase in the eighteenth century by the ninth earl of Exeter, Brownlow Cecil (1725–1793). It is described in a list made in his handwriting as "Susannah and ye Elders by Arta: Gentileschi from ye Barbarini Pallace at Rome." Nevertheless, we must note that inventory listings made over a century after a picture was painted are often inaccurate, and the earl's citation does not argue definitively for an assignment to Artemisia, especially given that many of his attributions are, in fact, inaccurate.[7] Bissell (1999) questions the Barberini provenance, and indeed the painting does not appear in any of the Barberini inventories.

Should this painting prove to be the picture listed in the Ludovisi inventory, the ramifications for understanding Artemisia's oeuvre are immense. Certain pictures have already suggested an artist capable and willing to amend her style as conditions warranted; the Bologna *Portrait of a Gonfaloniere* (cat. 66) and the *Virgin*

and Child with a Rosary in the Escorial (cat. 84) are both stylistic anomalies, yet both are signed and the *Virgin and Child* is documented in a letter of 1651. Garrard's earlier assertion that the "nature of expression is sharply out of character for the artist" may be precisely the point—that this artist was capable of adapting her style and expressive mode to accommodate the expectations or stipulated wishes of her patrons.

1. I wish to thank Patrizia Cavazzini, who unearthed this information and was so generous as to share it with me. This document, without a notation of its designation of Artemisia, is referred to in Bissell 1999, 144.

2. Ibid., 349.

3. Bissell (1968, 167) considered the painting as possibly by Artemisia, although in his 1999 catalogue raisonné he rejects this attribution. Harris (in Los Angeles 1976–77, 121) also considered it a possible attribution, which she later accepts definitively (1998, 117–18). Contini (in Florence 1991, 113) is skeptical and suggests a follower of Simon Vouet. Garrard (1982; 1989, 202–4) initially rejected the attribution, although in her most recent essay (2001), she argues that the painting was originally by Artemisia but substantially altered by a later artist.

4. See Wood 1992.

5. Wood (ibid., 522) lists the inventory, where item 284, among a group located in a "Sala di Sopra," is described as "Un a Susanna Con li vecchi alta p. i 8 Cornice nere proliferate e rabeseate d'oro di m.o di artimitia. . . ."

6. Garrard (2001, 96–97) also suggests that the painting may indeed be the work listed in the Ludovisi inventory.

7. Bissell (1999, 351) notes that one-fifth of the pictures included in the 1995 Burghley House exhibition had their original Cecil attributions changed.

66.

Portrait of a Gonfaloniere

Oil on canvas, 81⅞ × 50⅜ in. (208 × 128 cm)

Signed (on back of canvas, visible before relining): ARTEMISIA. GENTILSCA. FA-/CIEBAT ROMAE 1622.

Collezione Comunali d'Arte, Palazzo d'Accursio, Bologna (inv. 6)

1622

Titian is credited with developing the tradition of standing male portraiture that became the definitive means for recording the likeness and power of wealthy patrons and influential rulers in the sixteenth century. Standing, and in elegant finery or full military regalia and accompanied by physical attributes of prosperity and influence, these figures command respect and exude authority. Artemisia here shows herself an accomplished practitioner of this form of celebratory painting. In an interior of minimal

description stands a man in full armor, adorned with a sash worn diagonally across his chest. He rests his fingertips on the velvet-covered table to the left, upon which sits an elaborately plumed helmet (a cavalry type known as a close helmet). At the right hangs a banner (a *gonfalone*), the source of the portrait's title, as it suggests that this individual carried such a banner in processions or military engagements.

Artemisia's gift for describing the quality of disparate surfaces is abundantly evident in this

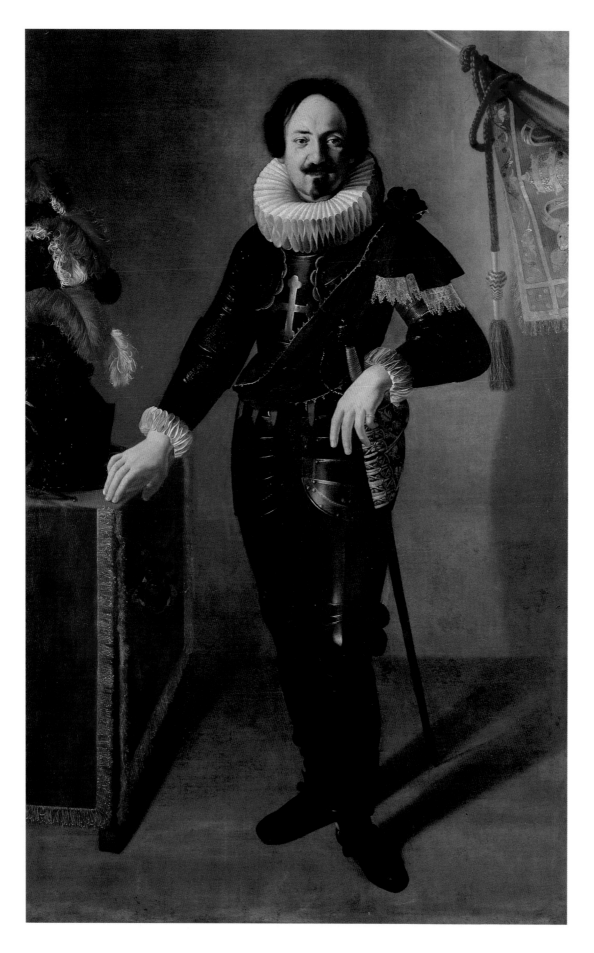

PROVENANCE: Agostino Pepoli, Bologna; Pinacoteca, Bologna (from 1920?); Palazzo d'Accursio, Bologna (from 1934).

REFERENCES: Baldinucci 1767–74, vol. 12 (1772), 9; De Dominici (1742–43) 1979, 45; Malaguzzi Valeri 1926, 30, 33; Zucchini 1938, 22, 24; Bissell 1968, 157; Harris in Los Angeles 1976–77, 121–22; Gregori in Naples 1984–85, 147; Garrard 1989, 59–62; Papi in Florence 1991, 157–60 no. 21; Bissell 1999, 44–45, 216–19 no. 13.

fine portrait. The steely hardness of the armor, the golden lace edging of the green silk sash, the feathery softness of the helmet plumes, the soft velvet coverlet on the table, and the starched stiffness of the ruff have all been captured with tactile exactitude heralded as the mark of a Caravaggesque painter. Harris suggests that this picture, while possibly an accurate likeness, does not demonstrate the kind of virtuosic gift that Titian often brought to this type of composition, in which dazzling brushwork and coloristic boldness lend majesty to his portraits. Nevertheless, it would appear that Artemisia gives a true likeness of the anonymous gonfaloniere, expressed through his balletic pose and the tentative yet energetic touch of his fingers on the edge of the table; more magisterial flourishes may have been inappropriate. We might note that the sword he carries is a civilian form known as a rapier and was employed by the artist more for visual impact than for military accuracy.[1]

The cross on the man's chest and the green sash and papal banner (its small size may indicate that it is a cavalry guidon) all suggest that he is a knight of the Order of Saints Maurice and Lazarus. Papi is surely correct in noting the similarities between this painting and the *Portrait of Asdrubale Mattei* (Musée Condé, Chantilly), which has been attributed to Caravaggio himself. And Gregori (in Naples 1984–85) describes the painting as one of "gli esempi più sensazionali della ritrattistica caravaggesca" (the most sensational examples of Caravaggesque portraiture).

Inscribed on the back with Artemisia's name accompanied by "ROMAE 1622," this portrait has been accepted as autograph from the early years of her second period in Rome. In a census document taken during Lent of 1622, Artemisia is listed as living on via del Corso together with her husband, Pierantonio Stiattesi, her daughter Palmira, and her brothers Giulio and Francesco.[2] The only point of controversy surrounding the picture is the identity of the model. The coat of arms on the table cover was revealed in the cleaning of 1964. Prior to restoration, it comprised fifteen squares arranged in a checkerboard pattern. The restored emblem, a

chevron of two silver bands flanking a black band, has not been identified. Garrard's assertion that it was a generic template designed to be covered by a replacement coat of arms is untenable, as Bissell (1999) has recently argued. Further complicating attempts to identify the insignia is the fact that it is aligned not with the right side of the table, which is foreshortened to suggest spatial recession, but rather with the picture plane. This would suggest that it may not, in fact, be original to the painting. It does not, however, rule out the possibility that it relates to the subject.

This picture offers the sole testimony to Artemisia's celebrated gifts as a portrait painter (not counting the possible self-portraits), an important component of her artistic career according to the various seventeenth-century accounts. One, written by the Florentine Filippo Baldinucci and published between 1681 and 1728, states that "she dedicated herself first to making portraits, of which she made very many in Rome." Another, by the Neapolitan Bernardo de Dominici, offers the most eloquent praise of her portraiture when he writes that her acclaim was based on "portraits of important personages that she had so excellently painted." Scholars have struggled with the discrepancy between these accounts and the available evidence. Garrard suggests that these writers were merely repeating an assumption about women painters, who, not admitted to the academies or allowed access to representing the male nude, necessary for making narrative images, were forced to specialize in portrait painting. As Bissell (1999) correctly points out, however, a reference to a portrait by Artemisia in the 1612 rape trial testimony supports Artemisia's early accomplishment in the genre. An engraving of about 1628 by Jérôme David of another knight of the Order of Saints Maurice and Lazarus, inscribed as having been copied from a "Portrait of Antoine de Ville by Artemisia Gentileschi," lends further support to Artemisia's activity as a portraitist. However, were the *Portrait of a Gonfaloniere* not inscribed on the back (the inscription is now obliterated as a result of relining), its attribution to Artemisia Gentileschi may not have gained the general acceptance it now has. For this reason and because of its extraordinary quality, we may assume that other portraits by her hand await identification and correct attribution.

1. I wish to thank Walter J. Karcheski Jr., Senior Curator, Arms and Armor, Higgins Armory Museum, Worcester, Mass., for his enormous help in identifying the armorial elements of this portrait.

2. The document, listed in Bissell's chronology (1999, 144), was originally published in Bousquet 1978, 106.

67.

Lucretia

Oil on canvas, 39 ⅜ × 30 ⅜ in. (100 × 77 cm)

Gerolamo Etro, Milan

ca. 1623–25

The story of Lucretia, the virtuous wife of Tarquinius Collatinus, who takes her own life after having been sexually assaulted by one of her husband's kinsmen, Sextus Tarquinius, was originally told in the Roman history of Livy.[1] While off at battle, Tarquinius Collatinus regales his men with claims of the loyalty of his wife, Lucretia, and challenges them to return home immediately to see whether their own spouses live up to her exemplary model. The soldiers accept this challenge and steal back to their homes to spy on their wives. While they find Lucretia innocently spinning wool, they discover the other wives engaged in various forms of idle revelry. Sextus Tarquinius is smitten with Lucretia's beauty and later returns to her house. To test her virtue, he attempts to rape her. In order to force her compliance, he threatens to kill Lucretia and, worse, to malign her character saying he will kill a slave and place his nude body beside Lucretia's, claiming they were lovers. Lucretia, loath to bring dishonor upon herself by the appearance of infidelity, succumbs to Sextus so that he will not spread this story. The next morning, after confessing to her husband and her father (and receiving their pardon), she stabs herself with a knife.

Although Livy's account makes clear that Lucretia is not alone when she commits suicide, she is, conventionally, depicted as a solitary figure, usually nude or at least with chest bared, posed provocatively as she wields the knife against her pale skin. Occasionally, she is represented as having already pierced her flesh with the blade. Sometimes, she wears elaborate jewelry

and rich costume and, in a few instances, even lavish furs. This may echo the sentiments expressed by the sixteenth-century English reformer William Tyndale, who wrote that Lucretia, by taking her life, sought to preserve her own honor and thus fell prey to vanity. Typical of these images is the portrayal of Lucretia as a submissive female; this together with her nudity and the presence of weapons—with phallic connotations—heightened their erotic charge.

Selecting the close-up view and truncated figure she had used for the *Saint Cecilia* (cat. 63), Artemisia, in her presentation of Lucretia, invigorates the composition. In a pose that may have been inspired by her father's image of the reflective *David Contemplating the Head of Goliath* (cat. 18) and drawing upon an early-seventeenth-century *Susanna* attributed to Agostino Carracci (The John and Mable Ringling Museum of Art, Sarasota), Artemisia has conveyed the drama of the heroine's decision rather than the pathos of her death. While other artists had focused on the action of the story, Artemisia stills the action. Garrard has noted that the blade is shown pointing heavenward, and Pollock has commented that the weapon is not grasped so that it can be used.[2] The artist, therefore, shows us a new dramatic moment, as Lucretia pauses between life and death, symbolized by the nurturing breast in her right hand and the death-dealing blade in her left.

Save for Papi's recent suggestion that the painting should be included in Orazio's oeuvre, scholars have universally attributed the painting to Artemisia. There

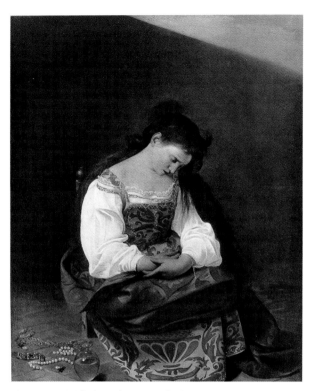

Figure 126. Michelangelo Merisi da Caravaggio (1571–1610), *Penitent Magdalene.* Oil on canvas. Galleria Doria Pamphili, Rome

PROVENANCE: Pietro Maria I Gentile, Palazzo Gentile, Genoa (until 1640/41); Gentile collection, Genoa (1640/41–1811/18); Palazzo Durazzo-Adorno (now Cattaneo-Adorno), Genoa (perhaps by 1818 and certainly by 1846–1980s); Piero Pagano (until 2001); Gerolamo Etro, Milan (2001).

REFERENCES: Ratti 1780, 119–20, 122; Tyndale 1848; Morassi 1947, 102 no. 138; Bissell 1968, 42–43, 56–57; Gregori in Naples 1984–85, vol. 1, 147; Garrard 1989, 55, 216–39; Contini in Florence 1991, 109, 160–62 no. 22; Cropper 1992, 209; Pesenti in Genoa 1992, 192; Volland in Düsseldorf–Darmstadt 1995–96, 300–301; Lapierre 1998, 462, 471–72; Pollock 1999, 158–64; Bissell 1999, 36–37, 189–91 no. 3; Boccardo 2000, 205; Papi 2000, 451–52.

is less consensus about its date. The picture has traditionally been placed in the early 1620s, argued initially by Bissell (1968), who posited a Genoese trip that Artemisia made with her father when Giovan Antonio Sauli invited Orazio to the Ligurian city in 1621. The proposed trip by Artemisia to Genoa was based primarily on the presence of a *Lucretia* in Genoa as early as 1780, when Carlo Giuseppe Ratti noted it in the palace of Pietro Gentile. Although Ratti attributed the painting to Orazio, most scholars assumed it to be this *Lucretia* by Artemisia, as indeed it probably is. Some writers challenged the idea of a trip to Genoa, and Bissell (1999) has now abandoned the argument, noting that documentary evidence for Artemisia's continued presence in Rome between 1621 and 1626, including recent discoveries by Lapierre, makes a Genoese trip improbable.[3] Boccardo's conjecture that Gentile may have purchased the painting from the duke of Alcalá, who would presumably have bought the work in Rome or Naples, must be treated with caution, since no such work occurs in the inventories of his collection.

While Garrard's dating of about 1621 (Garrard 1989) is based on the painting's similarity to the work of the teens, most notably the Pitti *Magdalene* (cat. 58), other writers have associated it with Orazio's paintings from the first two decades of the century. Gregori notes the influence of Guido Reni on Artemisia's oeuvre and also suggests the influence of Cecco del Caravaggio, while Pesenti emphasizes the importance of Artemisia's renewed acquaintance with the work of Caravaggio. This last point is an important one, for certainly Artemisia's experience of the Roman art world was substantially different when she returned to Rome in 1620 (as a married woman and an accomplished artist) than it had been in her earlier years in Rome, when she had limited access to collections and churches. The heightened chiaroscuro and harder contours notable in the *Lucretia* can be likened to the Seville *Penitent Magdalene* (cat. 68), a painting undoubtedly based on Caravaggio's *Penitent Magdalene* in the Doria Pamphili (fig. 126). The interpretive tone is similar as well to the *Jael and Sisera* (cat. 61), and Cropper has also associated that painting, made in 1620, with the *Lucretia*. The rendering of the impressive thigh and knee comes close to the treatment of the leg in the Burghley House *Susanna* (cat. 65), a controversial picture, but, should it prove to be an autograph work, the 1622 date and signature will undoubtedly help in establishing the dating for such paintings as the *Lucretia*. A reference to a *Lucretia* that Artemisia presumably either brought to Venice in 1627 or painted while she was there indicates that she treated the subject during the 1620s.[4] Bissell (1999) has courageously offered the earliest date (followed by Spear and Christiansen, in the present volume) by placing the painting in 1611–12, noting stylistic similarities to pictures by Orazio dating to the first decade, as well as the strong Caravaggesque quality of its conception and execution.

The *Lucretia* may have been produced in Rome at the same time as a *Lucretia* painted by Simon Vouet in 1624–25 (fig. 127). Like Artemisia's image, Vouet's shows a solitary figure, in her draped bedchamber, holding her dagger aloft and casting her eyes heavenward. The picture was engraved in 1627 by Claude Mellan with an added Latin inscription that expounds

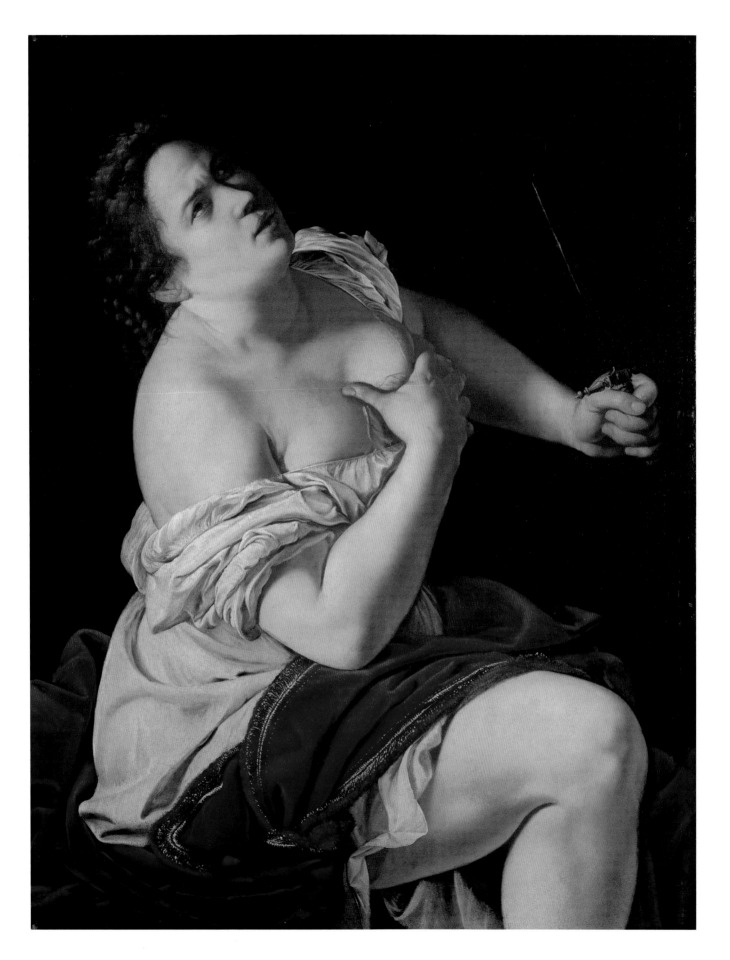

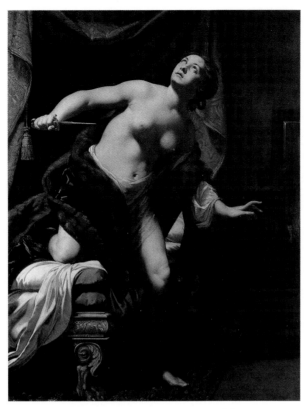

Figure 127. Simon Vouet (1590–1649), *Lucretia*. Oil on canvas. Národni Galeri, Prague

upon the heroine's motivation. In translation, it reads, "Did he violently cling to me with a shameful embrace? Were these breasts touched by a strange hand? For shame, O evil act. You rend with your right hand your side, profaned not with impunity avenging your chastity. So had she spoken, and with chaste sword she pierced her groin, confessing herself guilty, though not having committed a crime. By her proud wound, she thus heals the wounds of love and wipes clean the impure stains with the stream of her own blood."[5] While the Vouet picture represents a radically different Lucretia, a nobly posed beauty exemplifying an ideal, the inscribed lines may reveal a more general contemporary understanding of Lucretia's story and in that way may also apply to Artemisia's dramatic rendering. Given the vehemence with which Lucretia distorts the contour of her left breast by the pressure of her fingers and grasps her body in anger at the violence

so recently perpetrated against her, we might also associate this verse with Artemisia's heroine.

Further preventing our understanding of this important picture is its change in format. When it was exhibited in Florence in 1991, there were strips on all four sides, judged to be eighteenth-century additions. These were removed in 1995. Bissell (1999) argues that although the strips were painted over, they may reflect Artemisia's original conception, and he believes that the present configuration does not reflect the original format. But the power of the composition in its reduced form—minus the rather awkward lower portion of the right leg—is considerably strengthened, suggesting that it is, in fact, the smaller format which reveals the artist's true intentions. Cusping along the top and bottom edges confirms the reduced size as the original format.

1. The most popular source was Livy, *Ab Urbe Condita*, 1:57—note also the story occurs in Ovid's *Fasti* and Dio Cassius's *Roman History*. See Garrard (1989, chap. 4), who gives a good introduction to the depiction of Lucretia in the context of the representation of female suicide as well as the historical development in both visual and literary interpretations of the story.

2. Pollock (1999, 163) comes to a different conclusion, however, about the oddity of Lucretia's grasp and suggests that the heroine holds the knife as if to wound another (Sextus/Tassi?) rather than herself.

3. See Archivio di Stato (hereafter ASR), Rome, *30 Notai Capitolini*, Officio 19, vol. 121 (1621), fols. 385r,v, 396r; ASR, *Tribunale Criminale del Governatore*, processo no. 181 (1622), fols. 52–55; ASR, *30 Notai Capitolini*, Officio 19, vol. 136 (1625), fol. 735; ASR, *Tribunale Civile del Governatore, Sentenze*, busta 309 (1621–32); ASR, *30 Notai Capitolini*, Officio 19, vol. 138 (1625), fol. 523; as cited in Lapierre 1998, 462, 471–72.

4. A pamphlet dated 1627 lists three paintings by Artemisia that were in Venice: a "Small Love [Amoretto]," a *Lucretia*, and a *Susanna and the Elders*. See Toesca 1971, 90–91.

5. *Hoc latus indigno cinxit violentia nexu?*
Haec sunt externa pectora tacta manu?
Proh pudor, o facinus. Tu non impune prophanum,
Vlta pudicitium, dextera scinde latus.
Dixerat, et casto traiecit viscera ferro,
Se, non admisso crimine, fassa, ream.
Vlunere magn.mo. Sic vulnera sanat amoris.
Tergit et impuras sanguinis amne notas.
Sim. Voüet paris. Pinx. Cl. Mellan Gall'.
Sculp. Romae
Superiorum pmissu.

68.

Penitent Magdalene

Oil on canvas, 48 × 38¼ in.
(122 × 97 cm)

Seville Cathedral

1625–26

PROVENANCE: Fernando Enríquez Afán de Ribera, third duke of Alcalá, Rome and Casa de Pilatos, Seville (by 1626–37; inv. 1632/36, as by Artemisia Gentileschi); Seville Cathedral (by the late 17th century?).

REFERENCES: Valdivieso 1978, 131 no. 511; Brown and Kagan 1987, 239–40; Bissell 1999, 222–25 no. 16; Garrard 2001, 14–75.

While modern scholars have seen Mary Magdalene as a privileged follower of Christ, the first witness to his resurrection and apostle to the apostles, the seventeenth century understood her as the prototype of the reformed sinner, a prostitute who sets aside a life of sin and vanity and embraces one of penitence.[1] In a departure from conventional paintings, which show the Magdalene at the moment of her conversion, Artemisia presents her disheveled, seated in a chair, her head resting on the back of her hand (her eyes, slightly open, suggest a wakeful state). This genrelike approach—so different from the emotionally charged picture Artemisia had painted in Florence (cat. 58)—recalls that of Caravaggio in his early *Penitent Magdalene* (Doria Pamphili, Rome; fig. 126). Artemisia's original conception included a more provocative penitent. The linen chemise revealed her bare shoulder and the swelling flesh of the upper part of her left breast. The sheer scarf that surrounds her neck has been amplified by a later hand; the clumsy brushwork and heavy fabric do not match the quality of the rest of the painting.[2]

Bellori described Caravaggio's picture as showing a woman drying her hair and suggested the artist had transformed it into a depiction of the Magdalene by adding jewelry and an ointment jar on the floor beside her.[3] Similarly, Artemisia's Magdalene caresses her hair and, in the syntax of seventeenth-century imagery, identifies the object of her meditation. The emphasis on hair, coupled with her visible tear, is appropriate to this saint, who washed Christ's feet with her tears and dried them with her hair as her initial act of penance and who later, in the wilderness of Sainte-Baume, where she lived for thirty years, let her hair grow long in order to cover her nudity. Artemisia had already—in the *Danaë* (cat. 54)—used the tactile sensation of long, luxuriant hair to refer to sensuality.

No other artist—not even Caravaggio—had gone so far in envisaging guilt and penitence. There is in this picture a quality of self-projection that takes precedence over pictorial tradition, although the extreme tilt of the head recalls the posture of lamentation associated with mourning figures at the Crucifixion and Entombment, embodying the enormity of the saint's penitential grief. It also suggests a woman completely unresponsive to physical comfort and can be read as the aftermath to the kind of violent soul-searching so vividly expressed in the sermon given by Francesco Panigarola (see cat. 58). By combining such a reference to mourning with the pose of the head resting on a hand that is associated with contemplation (the Magdalenes of Georges de La Tour come to mind), the artist adds another layer of meaning.

In her rich and thoughtful essay, Garrard maintains that the Seville Magdalene represents the saint as a visionary, making reference to Artemisia herself and to Artemisia's own identification with the intellectual and prophetic aspects of creativity. The artist, Garrard argues, has fused the masculine role of melancholic seer with that of the Magdalene as female contemplative and, in doing so, legitimizes the feminine representation of inspiration. While gendered readings of Artemisia's imagery need not necessarily be discounted, there is little evidence to support such intellectual responses to the subjects of her work. The pose and attributes can be readily explained simply within the contemporary understanding of the Magdalene, to which Artemisia has given a compelling realization.

An inventory of the duke of Alcalá's collection, drawn up between 1632 and 1636, includes a description that must refer to the present painting: "A Magdalene seated in a chair sleeping on her arm by artemissa Gentileça pintora romana."[4] The duke went to Rome in July 1625 to serve as ambassador to the Holy See. He stayed there until February 1626, and two seventeenth-century sources indicate that he was one of Artemisia's patrons.[5] When he returned to Seville after serving as viceroy in Naples from 1629 until 1631, he transferred his collection from Naples; each item was marked

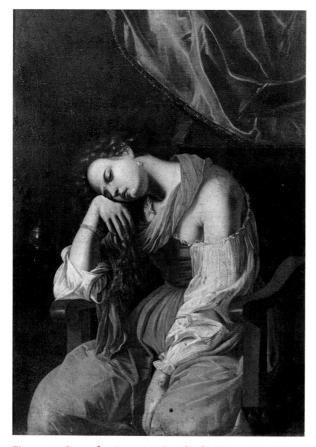

Figure 128. Copy after Artemisia Gentileschi, *Penitent Magdalene*. Oil on canvas. Private collection

which displays neither the subtlety nor the sensitivity of the Seville canvas. Bissell, joined by Garrard, accepts both versions as autograph and links the Seville painting to the one executed for the duke.

The *Penitent Magdalene* is dated by Garrard to the early 1620s and by Bissell to the mid-1620s. On balance, Bissell's date seems more viable and has the advantage of coinciding with the duke's residence in Rome. This later date also fits well in the context of Artemisia's other work of this period, in which she is rediscovering the art of Caravaggio. Her *Portrait of a Gonfaloniere* (cat. 66), for example, registers a response to Caravaggesque portraiture, as does her second and more forcefully violent version of the *Judith Slaying Holofernes* (cat. 62), which developed out of a reacquaintance with Caravaggio's *Judith* (Galleria Nazionale, Palazzo Barberini, Rome; fig. 109). The Seville *Magdalene* must be more or less contemporary with the Detroit *Judith and Her Maidservant* (cat. 69) and, like that work, shows Artemisia's interest in the example of such Caravaggisti as Gerrit van Honthorst and Simon Vouet.

with the number of the crate in which it was shipped, and the number was recorded in the inventory. Brown and Kagan have deduced that because the Seville painting bears no crate number, it must not have been shipped from Naples, but was instead purchased during the duke's tenure in Rome.

A second version of the painting was exhibited at the Richard L. Feigen Gallery, New York, in 1998.[6] It is nearly identical save for the absence of the added drapery and the greater height of the copy and what appears in the Seville version to be a pillow behind the Magdalene. The close replication of compositions was not Artemisia's usual practice. Furthermore, the Feigen picture has all the hallmarks of a copy: hard contours, a lack of delicacy in the modeling, and an inept rendering of the Magdalene's left hand and head,

1. On Mary Magdalene and her depiction in art, see Florence 1986. On the historical development of interest in Mary Magdalene, with a summary of some of the newer feminist scholarship as to the identity of the Magdalene, see Haskins 1993, esp. chaps. 1–3; and Moltmann-Wendel 1982, 61–90.
2. It is possible that the family of the patron (the duke of Alcalá) presented this picture to the cathedral in Seville in the late seventeenth century and that its placement in this religious setting required a more modest presentation.
3. Bellori 1672, as cited in Garrard 2001, 43, 137 n. 49.
4. "Una Mag. na sentada en una silla durmiendo sobre el braço de artemissa Gentileça romana." See Brown and Kagan 1987, 239–40.
5. The art historian Francisco Pacheco reiterates in his famous *Arte de la pintura*, published posthumously in 1649, that the duke of Alcalá had purchased paintings from the artist; Pacheco 1956, vol. 1, 148. Lazaro Diaz del Valle, in 1656, described Artemisia as "Pintora de Roma; desta mujer trajo el Duque de Alcalá a España algunas famosas pinturas / Roman painter [From this woman the duke of Alcalá brought to Spain several famous paintings]"; see Sánchez Cantón 1933, 361.
6. Timed to coincide with the New York premiere in 1998 of Agnès Merlet's film *Artemisia*, a brochure was produced for the exhibition at the Feigen gallery in which the twelve works that appeared in the exhibition were listed.

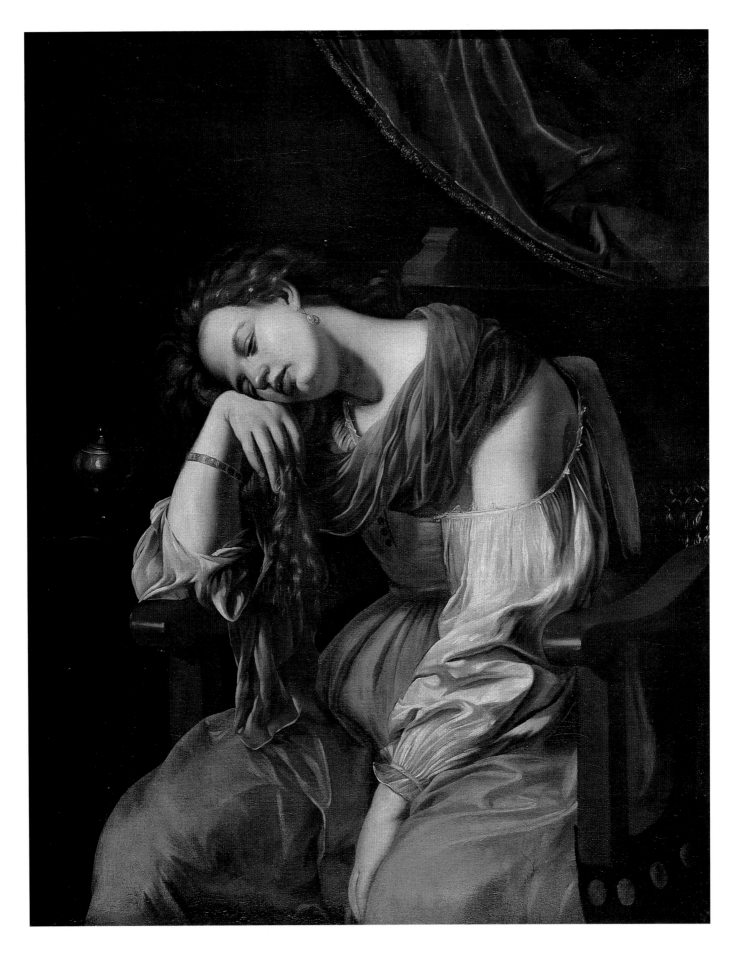

69.

Judith and Her Maidservant

Oil on canvas, 72 × 56 in.
(182.8 × 142.2 cm)

The Detroit Institute of Arts,
Gift of Mr. Leslie H. Green
(inv. 52.253)

ca. 1625–27

New York, Saint Louis

PROVENANCE: "Prince
Brancaccio," Rome; Alessandro
Morandotti and Adolph Loewi;
Leslie H. Green (until 1952);
Detroit Institute of Arts.

RELATED PICTURE: *Judith and
Her Maidservant*, Museo di
Capodimonte, Naples.

REFERENCES: Richardson
1952–53, 81–83; Moir in Detroit
1965, 29–30 no. 8; Bissell 1968,
157–58; Spear in Cleveland 1971,
96–97 no. 28; Harris in Los
Angeles 1976–77, 122 no. 13;
Garrard 1989, 67–72; 328–35;
Papi and Contini in Florence
1991, 53–54, 141; Bissell 1999,
219–20 no. 14.

By the light of a single candle, Judith and her maidservant, Abra, prepare to depart the military encampment of Holofernes and his Assyrian army. Artemisia has depicted the moments immediately following the general's murder, when Abra wraps his head to carry it away and before Judith has sheathed her sword. Both women pause momentarily, responding to some unseen disturbance.

The painting is generally recognized as Artemisia's finest work. A number of scholars are in agreement as to its date, placing it in the middle of the 1620s, when the artist was living in Rome (Spear, Papi, Garrard, Harris, and Bissell 1999). Garrard relates the use of dramatic chiaroscuro, most evident in the shadow cast across the heroine's face, to Simon Vouet's *Temptation of Saint Francis* in San Lorenzo in Lucina (fig. 117), painted in the 1620s, and the lighting, more generally, to the work of Gerrit van Honthorst. Dissenting views are those of Contini, who dates the picture to the first years of the decade, and Moir, who places it in the late teens. Bissell argues for a Neapolitan provenance, suggesting that Artemisia must have taken the painting with her when she moved to Naples, in 1629 or 1630. There, she reused Abra's pose in a kneeling figure found in several Neapolitan paintings; it served, for example, as the model for the maid in her late *Judith and Her Maidservant*, now in the Museo di Capodimonte, Naples, probably painted for the duke of Parma in the 1640s, although some have argued that the Capodimonte picture is a copy of a lost work.

The Detroit canvas represents Artemisia's most complex rendering of the Judith narrative. Garrard analyzes the picture in terms of its multivalent feminist imagery, arguing that this forceful presentation of Judith disguised as a warrior (she appears in heavy, more military shoes rather than, as traditionally, barefoot or wearing sandals) represents an inversion of the antique goddess of beauty, transforming sensuality into power. Many writers have noted its expressive potency and almost textbook illustration of

Baroque drama. Certainly, Artemisia has gone beyond the Pitti *Judith* (cat. 60), in which the two women, turning in profile to the right, also pause at the same moment. The composition is certainly more interesting in the present version. The impressively described elements of the scene—Holofernes' head, the sword and scabbard, the candle, the gauntlet—recall Baldinucci's assertion that Artemisia developed a reputation for still life.[1] And indeed, the sword and gauntlet were most certainly painted from life. Artemisia has accurately depicted a falchion in Judith's hand, a dress weapon worn with armor, favored by artists who sought visual means to create an exotic Eastern tone in their representation of biblical events.[2]

The inclusion of the gauntlet, unusual in Judith paintings, warrants special comment. Because Holofernes was a military leader, the representation of armorial elements, however anachronistic, is appropriate. The general's decapitation occurred in his tent,

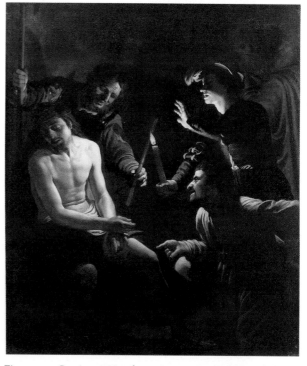

Figure 129. Gerrit van Honthorst (1592–1656), *Mocking of Christ*. Oil on canvas. Brentwood Holdings Assets Ltd., Spier Collection

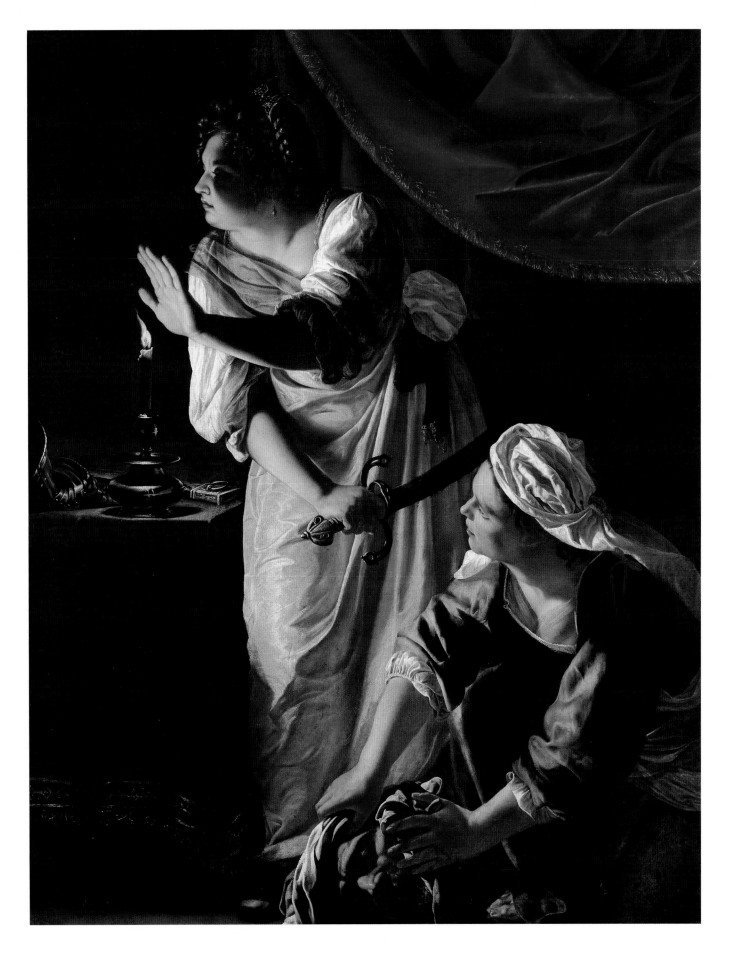

and presumably he would have cast aside his armor and shield as he prepared for his meeting with Judith. Antonio Tempesta, for example, etched the subject in 1613 and included the discarded breastplate, shield, and helmet hanging at the back of the tent.[3] Artemisia, however, has represented only the gauntlet, a choice that must not have been arbitrary. A medieval reference to the challenge of battle, the cast-off glove becomes emblematic of Judith's successful challenge to the Assyrian general. Positioned close to the heroine's raised hand, the gauntlet encourages the viewer to consider the defeat of the seasoned military hero by the hand of the young widow. In an image primarily of female camaraderie, Artemisia introduces a novel reminder of the decapitation itself, by means of a symbolic reference to Judith's challenge to the authority of Holofernes.

Artemisia drew upon several sources for the composition. Garrard and Bissell (1999) have traced the nocturnal setting to Adam Elsheimer's small copper *Judith* (Wellington Museum, Apsley House, London), in which a candle also illuminates a darkened interior. Artemisia may also have emulated the paintings of Gerrit van Honthorst, a Northern painter from the city of Utrecht, who, while in Rome between 1613 and 1620, developed a specialty in the representation of candles and their attendant luminous effects. Artemisia appears to have drawn from his work, as both Bissell (1999) and Garrard have noted.[4] And Spear correctly points out that Artemisia creates a far greater drama than had the Utrecht painter. Van Honthorst's *Mocking of Christ* (fig. 129), which may have been available to Artemisia in Rome during this period, bears a strong formal likeness to the Detroit painting.[5] The two works share a basic compositional structure, an interior illumination, and an obscuring shadow across the face of the protagonist.

The unresolved spatial inconsistency of the interior suggests that Artemisia had not yet completely worked out the formal relationships. The placement of the candle, on top of the table, precludes its being the source of light on Judith's palm. While Garrard argues that the light comes not from the candle but from the opening of the tent, the illumination on the kneeling Abra does not conform to the more generalized glow issuing forth from the left. This would suggest that the candle was added later, after the composition had been designed, perhaps to create a more showy effect—a nod to contemporary currents popular in Rome introduced in hopes of pleasing a patron.

1. "Ebbe costei un altro bel talento, che fu di ritrarne al naturale maravifliosamente ogni sorte di frutti . . ."; Baldinucci 1811–12, vol. 10, 254.
2. Thanks to Stuart Pyhrr, Curator, Department of Arms and Armor, The Metropolitan Museum of Art, and Walter J. Karcheski Jr., Senior Curator, Arms and Armor, Higgins Armory Museum, Worcester, Massachusetts, for providing me with information regarding the history of the arms in this piece.
3. For the Tempesta engraving, see Bissell 1999, fig. 76.
4. Leonard Slatkes, writing in the entry on Van Honthorst's Los Angeles *Mocking of Christ* (London–Rome 2001, 319), has associated Artemisia's painting with Van Honthorst's work.
5. This painting, a recent addition to the Van Honthorst oeuvre, does not have an early provenance, but Richard Judson (in Judson and Ekkart 1999, 32) considers it possible that the picture could have been in Rome at the time.

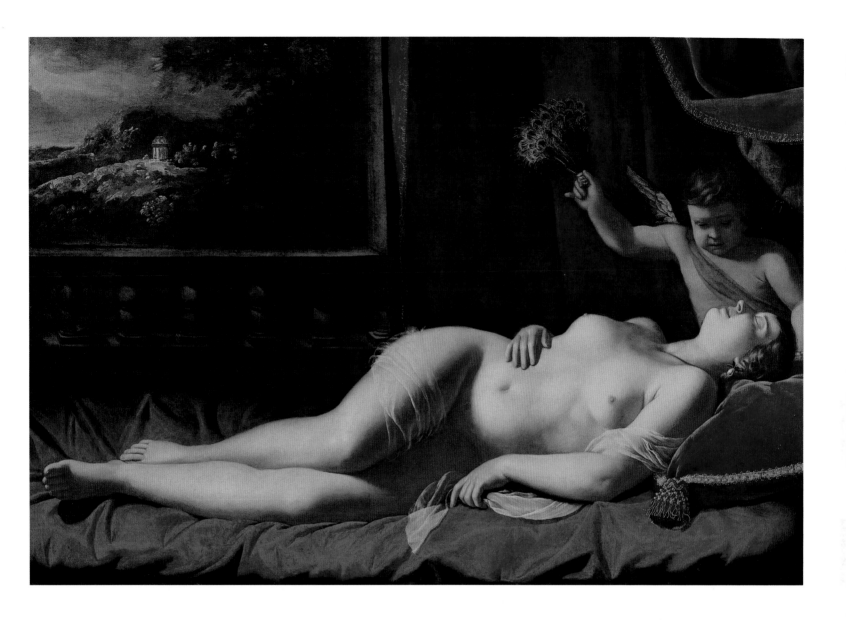

70.

Sleeping Venus

Oil on canvas, 37 × 56¾ in.
(94 × 144 cm)

The Barbara Piasecka
Johnson Foundation,
Princeton, New Jersey

1625–30

New York, Saint Louis

Artemisia's recognized mastery of the female nude is evident in this fascinating painting, which must have been made during the artist's second Roman stay. Venus, sound asleep and almost completely nude save for a diaphanous scarf around her upper arm and thigh, as a passive participant in the viewer's visual enjoyment enhances the erotic charge of the picture. Cupid stands behind his mother's couch and raises a peacock feather to fan her.[1] Garrard and Matthiesen initially dated the painting to the mid-1630s. Its reference to Titian's Venus paintings, the *Venus with a Lute Player*, in the Prado, for example, led Grabski to suggest in 1985 that it was painted after the artist went to Venice, in 1627–28. However, as Matthiesen and Bissell (1999) have recently pointed out, such imagery would already have been available to Artemisia in

Florence, since one such painting, the *Venus and Cupid with a Partridge* (Uffizi, Florence), was owned by Cosimo de' Medici as early as 1618. Furthermore, Bissell notes that the closest parallels to the picture were not Venetian but Roman, and relates the painting to Annibale Carracci's *Danaë* (formerly Bridgewater collection) and his highly sexual print, *Sleeping Venus with a Satyr and Cupid*, made in 1592.[2]

Garrard, on the other hand, identifies the more likely source for Venus's pose—Caravaggio's *Sleeping Cupid* (Galleria Palatina, Florence), whose early presence in Florence can be demonstrated, since it served as a model for Giovanni da San Giovanni in 1620 for his facade fresco for the Palazzo dell'Antella in Piazza Santa Croce.[3] While the references to the Titian prototypes are generic at best (sharing elements such as the reclining Venus, attendant figure, balustrade, and open window onto a landscape vista), the similarity in pose between Artemisia's goddess and Caravaggio's young Cupid suggests that the model was either close at hand or clear in her memory when she painted her Venus. But the painting does not fit comfortably into her Florentine style, and we do not know of a return visit to Florence after she sold the contents of her studio in 1621.[4] It is reasonable to assume that she began preliminary plans for the picture soon after returning to Rome, raising the possibility that she made drawings to record the distinctive pose of Caravaggio's *Cupid*. This heavy reliance on Caravaggio characterizes other pictures of Artemisia's second Roman period, most notably the Seville *Penitent Magdalene* (cat. 68), the *Portrait of a Gonfaloniere* (cat. 66), and the *Lucretia* (cat. 67). The gold-fringed velvet curtain at the upper right appears in the Seville *Magdalene* and the Detroit *Judith and Her Maidservant* (cat. 69), while a similar veil swirls about the standing Aurora (fig. 96).

The rich and generously painted cobalt cover of the couch (it is painted in two layers of lapis lazuli) suggests that the picture was intended for an important patron, as it is unlikely that the artist would otherwise have applied such expensive materials so liberally.[5] We must ask whether it is the one that Artemisia sent (via her brother Francesco) from Naples to Cardinal Antonio Barberini in Rome—mentioned in a letter that she wrote in 1635 to Cassiano dal Pozzo in Rome[6]—

which may also be the picture inventoried nine years later in the Barberini collection as "a woman with a cupid."[7]

If so, then the *Sleeping Venus* stayed in Artemisia's workshop for some time before she actually sent it off. Given its highly accomplished handling of the body and its use of expensive materials, it seems just the sort of painting that Artemisia might have presented to a potential patron in hopes of securing a position. Bissell has suggested that the *Venus Embracing Cupid* (cat. 82) should be identified with the Barberini gift, but this would seem an impossible scenario if that picture proves to have been painted in the 1640s.

Matthiesen notes that the recent cleaning reveals that the window and landscape were painted separately and by a different hand, something Bissell has already suggested. Although no extensive outdoor scenes by Artemisia exist, there are partial landscapes in some works of the 1620s that may be autograph, notably the *Aurora* (fig. 96) and the Burghley House *Susanna* (cat. 65). However, if the *Sleeping Venus* was in fact intended as a showpiece, Artemisia may have focused her efforts on the figures and sought assistance for the outdoor vista from an artist with greater experience in painting landscape. Matthiesen posits that it may be the work of a Northern painter.

The subject follows a tradition that goes back to ancient representations of sleeping nymphs and goddesses, the most famous of them undoubtedly the Hellenistic sculpture of the sleeping Ariadne (Museo Vaticano, Rome; fig. 141).[8] Giorgione's *Sleeping Venus*, of 1508–10 (Gemäldegalerie, Dresden), represents one of the most arresting of these images, in which the slumbering goddess reclines in a pastoral setting. Artemisia surely knew this tradition through prints as well as paintings. Annibale Carracci portrayed the sleeping Venus, arm raised over her head, lying in a landscape and surrounded by cavorting putti (Musée Condé, Chantilly). His painting was famous in the early seventeenth century and was enthusiastically described first by Agucchi and later by Bellori in his life of Annibale.[9] Obviously derived from the antique *Ariadne*, it may well have been known to Artemisia, although she has given the subject a slightly different interpretation. As Cupid fans his mother on her right

PROVENANCE: Private collection, Rome; private collection, London; The Barbara Piasecka Johnson Foundation, Princeton, New Jersey (1980s?).

REFERENCES: Bellori 1672, 89–92; Marini 1981a, 370; Grabski 1985, 56–63; Bober and Rubinstein 1986, 113–14, fig. 79; Matthiesen in London 1986, 52; Garrard 1989, 105–6, 274–76; Kultermann 1990, 137–40; Contini in Florence 1991, 85 n. 40; Bissell 1999, 225–26 no. 18; Matthiesen 2001, 264–69.

side, the viewer gazes upon her from her left. The circular temple outside the window recalls similar structures dedicated to the pagan goddess Vesta, which Artemisia may have known in Rome, and may be intended to allude to pagan veneration, suggesting that the viewer participates in surreptitious worship of the goddess of beauty.[10]

The representation of a slumbering female raises questions about reading Artemisia's imagery in terms of forceful heroines with whom Artemisia could identify. While she has minimized some of the patently sexual references used by other artists, she has presented a vulnerable female, unaware of the viewer's gaze, who becomes the inadvertent object of male desire, evidence of Artemisia's willingness to respond to the requests of male patrons.

1. Matthiesen has described Cupid as trying to waken his mother. However, while artists often depicted a mischievous Cupid who willingly teased his mother, there is none of that playfulness in the present picture.

2. Both are illustrated in Bissell 1999, figs. 105, 106.

3. Friedlaender 1955, 212.

4. See appendix 3 for the contents of that sale. Rather than assuming that she did not move to Rome until she is recorded there in March 1621, I find it perfectly plausible that Artemisia moved to Rome in 1620, returning to Florence briefly the following year to conclude the sale, and then returning to Rome,

5. I wish to thank David Chesterman, a private restorer in London, who so graciously allowed me to see the picture while it was in his lab and generously shared his information with me.

6. See Garrard 1989, 380–81.

7. Lavin 1975, 165.

8. See Bober and Rubinstein, 113–14, fig. 79.

9. See Posner 1971, vol. 2, 59–60 no. 134. Agucchi's description was recorded by Malvasia (1678, vol. 1, 503). For Bellori's description, see Bellori 1672, 89–92.

10. Matthiesen describes this as a Temple of Venus, but circular temples were generally not dedicated to the goddess of beauty, and the two that Artemisia may have known in Rome were believed in the early seventeenth century to have been dedicated to Vesta. Recent scholarship has identified the one near the Tiber as originally dedicated to Hercules.

71.

Esther Before Ahasuerus

Oil on canvas, 81⅞ × 107½ in. (208 × 273 cm)

The Metropolitan Museum of Art, New York. Gift of Elinor Dorrance Ingersoll, 1969 (inv. 69.281)

ca. 1628–35

Esther's appearance before the throne of her husband, King Ahasuerus, is a central scene in a complicated story of love, death, virtue, palace intrigue, power, and social status. Ahasuerus was a proud and powerful ruler. His queen, Vashti, refused his summons to appear before his guests at a feast, and she was disavowed. The king replaced her with Esther, a renowned beauty, not knowing she was a Jewess. Some time later, hearing that Ahasuerus had signed an edict that all Jews be slaughtered, Esther agreed to intervene, though aware that to appear unbidden before her husband would result in death. Before her audience, Esther ordered that all Jews fast for three days. Weakened from her fast, she appeared before the king and fainted. Ahasuerus, however, did not punish Esther but showed favor toward her, touching her with his scepter to indicate her special status.

The details of Artemisia's imagery derive from Greek additions made to the original Hebrew narrative, popularly used in the seventeenth century, after the Council of Trent gave them canonical status in 1546:[1]

On the third day, when she had finished praying, she took off her supplicant's mourning attire and dressed herself in her full splendor. Radiant as she then appeared, she invoked God who watches over all people and saves them. With her, she took her two ladies-in-waiting. With a delicate air she leaned on one, while the other accompanied her carrying her train. Rosy with the full flush of her beauty, her face radiated joy and love: but her heart shrank with fear. Having passed through door after door, she found herself in the presence of the king. He was sitting on his royal throne, dressed in all his robes of state, glittering with gold and precious stones—a

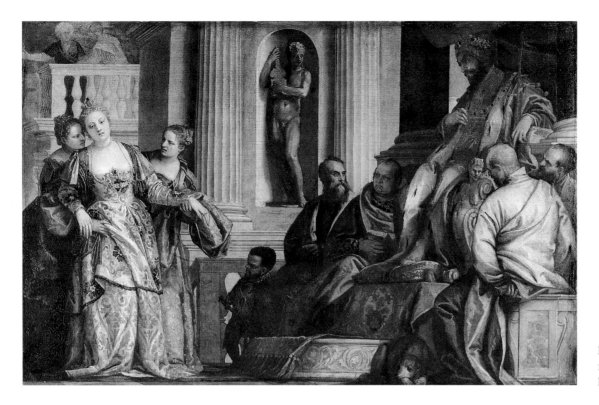

Figure 130. Workshop of Veronese (1528–1588), *Esther and Ahasuerus.* Oil on canvas. Musée du Louvre, Paris

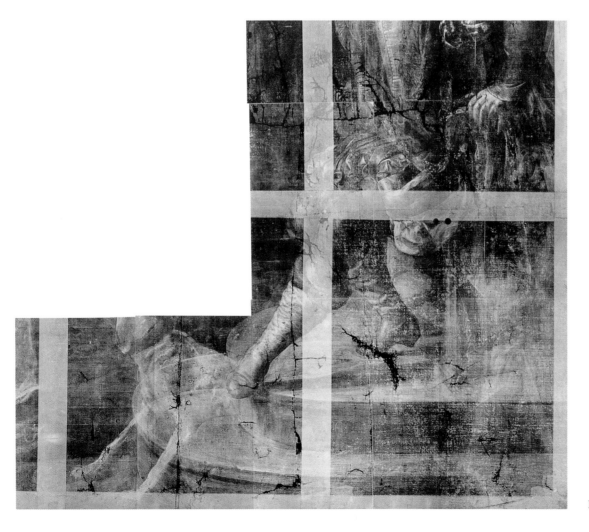

Figure 131. X radiograph of cat. 69

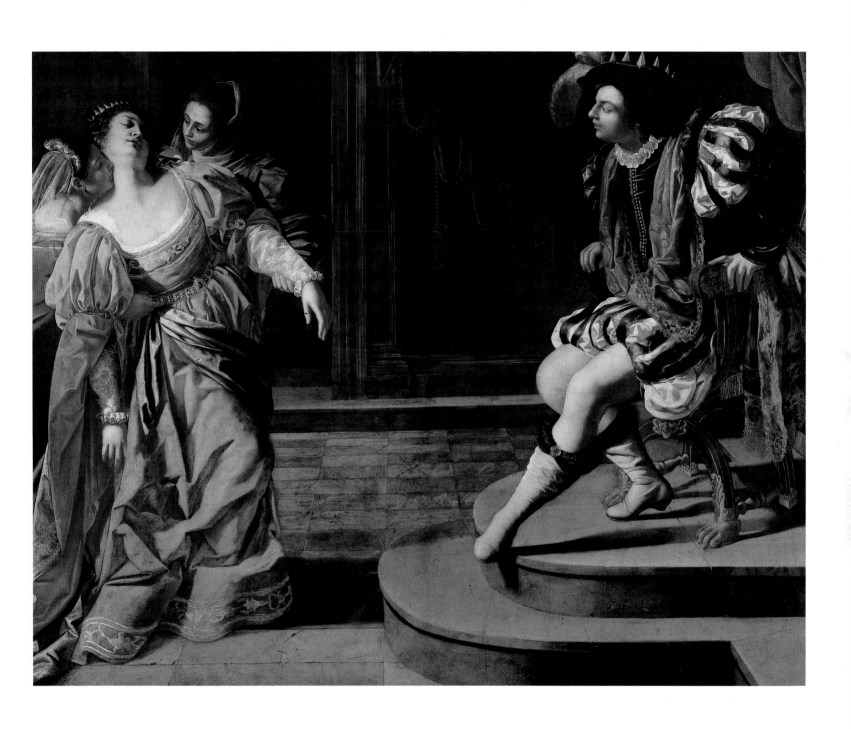

formidable sight. He looked up, afire with majesty and, blazing with anger, saw her. The queen sank to the floor. As she fainted, the color drained from her face and her head fell against the lady-in-waiting beside her. But God changed the king's heart, inducing a milder spirit. He sprang from his throne in alarm and took her in his arms until she recovered, comforting her with soothing words. "What is the matter Esther?" he said. "I am your brother. Take heart, you are not going to die; our order applies only to ordinary people. Come to me." And raising his golden sceptre he laid it on Esther's neck, embraced her and said, "Speak to me."

Artemisia has followed her text closely: the king prepares to "spring" forward from his throne as he sees his queen swoon; Esther's pale skin shows that the color has indeed ebbed from her face; and as she faints, her head falls against her lady-in-waiting. Esther's attire evokes the "full splendor" described in the text, with its extravagantly embroidered bodice and hem, splendid damask sleeves, bejeweled belt, and elaborately ornamented sleeve caps. And Ahasuerus presents a "formidable sight" in his velvet doublet, lace ruff, richly ribboned sleeves and breeches, and white kid boots trimmed in dyed fur and capped with ruby brooches, a costume unique within the repertoire of Ahasuerus depictions.

Many of these details were integral to an earlier version of Esther from the workshop of the Venetian painter Paolo Veronese (fig. 130), as Garrard, followed by Bissell, has noted. Artemisia must have known this image when she made her own painting, as the two share a number of details. Pentimenti (confirmed by X ray; fig. 131) throughout Artemisia's picture indicate that other elements from the Veronese painting were once part of the composition, including a servant at the base of the stairs and a seated dog. The curving steps that support Ahasuerus's throne may also derive from the Veronese painting, although they also occur in a number of other Venetian examples of the story.

Esther was typically portrayed either kneeling or assuming the posture of supplicant. In the Veronese version, she stands, although she is about to faint and is held up only with the support of her maids. This pose evidently appealed to Artemisia. Garrard has

argued that the pose and the masculine head, derived from Michelangelo's Haman in the Sistine chapel, present Esther as a stronger heroine, not subservient to the king.[2] But since Esther has clearly fainted and will soon fall, it was surely some other objective that was served by selecting the Veronese model. Furthermore, Artemisia did not base her Ahasuerus on the Venetian prototype but created an absolutely original king, something of a dandy with a youthful swagger. The artist designed a composition in which each protagonist echoes the movement of the other, to create a balletic quality shared by no other representations of this narrative. Given that Artemisia's interpretation relies on a careful reading of the text, she may well have understood the nature of the complete biblical book where status constantly changes; the mighty fall and the weak are elevated. In designing the figures of Esther and Ahasuerus, the artist selected poses that suggest imminent change—Esther will fall and Ahasuerus will rise.

The extraordinary number of changes and corrections throughout the picture suggest that Artemisia had difficulty in satisfactorily resolving the composition, as is evident in the X ray. At one time, a dog sat at the foot of the throne. The steps were changed from their original location and reconfigured. A page or servant stood in the space between Esther and Ahasuerus; the pose of the servant was adjusted at least once. And visible pentimenti reveal that the king's legs were repositioned. While a number of writers (Kaufmann, Greer, Garrard, Contini, Spike, Bionda, and Bissell) have noted its expressive power and the pregnant void in the center, the painting lacks real compositional rigor; the beauty of its parts overwhelms the whole.

Artemisia could have seen the Veronese painting during her Venetian sojourn since, on the authority of Carlo Ridolfi, we know that the picture was in the Bonaldi collection until it was bought in 1662 by the Parisian banker Everard Jabach, who, in the same year, ceded the picture to Louis XIV.[3] Indeed, Artemisia came close to copying portions of the Venetian work. Artemisia's Esther borrows the general design of Veronese's costume, the close proximity of the heads of Esther and one of her maids, and the configuration

PROVENANCE: Grafen Harrach, Vienna (by 1856–after 1926); Alessandro Morandotti, Rome (by 1956); Acquavella Galleries, New York (1959–60); Elinor Dorrance Ingersoll, New York (1960–69); The Metropolitan Museum of Art, New York (gift of Elinor Dorrance Ingersoll, 1969).

REFERENCES: Voss 1925, 105–8; Salerno in Rome 1956–57, 131; Bissell 1968, 163; Kaufmann 1970, 165–69; Greer 1979, 197–98; Garrard 1989, 72–79; Contini in Florence 1991, 165–69 no. 24; Spike 1991b, 734; Bionda 1992, 28; Bissell 1999, 75–76, 241–44 no. 28.

and position of Esther's left hand. In fact, the left hand so faithfully reproduces the prototype (which has been edited and strengthened by eliminating the drapery) that we cannot doubt the source. Artemisia most certainly began work on the *Esther* in Venice in 1628, when the Veronese picture was available to her or at least the impression of it was still fresh in her mind. It would also seem reasonable to assume that she took the canvas with her when she left Venice, that she still had it (indeed, was still working on it) when she moved to Naples around 1630, and that she continued to rework it there in the ensuing years. The numerous pentimenti and the incompatibility of the various compositional stages support this conclusion.

In nearly every other representation of the story, Ahasuerus is shown sitting on an elevated throne and holding a scepter. Artemisia's rejection of this most common format may indicate that she chose not to allude to the popular understanding of Esther as an Old Testament prefiguration of the Virgin Mary, in that the king's touching Esther with his scepter was identified with Mary's special designation as the immaculate mother of Christ.[4] In fact, Artemisia's interpretation of Ahasuerus, normally represented as either an Oriental potentate or a forbidding warrior king, stands as an entirely original creation and warrants further investigation.

Most scholars have placed the *Esther Before Ahasuerus* in Artemisia's first Neapolitan period. The Harrach provenance has been interpreted as an indication of a Neapolitan origin, first presented by Voss and subsequently accepted by Salerno, Kaufmann, and Contini, all of whom assume that the picture was purchased in Naples by Aloys Thomas von Harrach, who served as viceroy to the city from 1728 until 1733. Bissell (1999)

has pointed out that the painting could have come into the Harrach collection via Spain instead. Garrard assigns the painting to Artemisia's Roman period of the early 1620s, based on what she sees as the overtly Caravaggesque garb of King Ahasuerus, on her assumption that Artemisia saw the Veronese-school *Esther* during a Venetian trip in the early 1620s, and on her reading of the strong heroine, whom she argues is more typical of the 1620s than the 1640s. Bissell (1968) originally assigned the picture to the late 1630s but revised the date to the early 1630s in his catalogue raisonné of 1999, asserting that Artemisia's use of the Veronese painting meant that she had to have completed it after 1627–28 (when she is documented as having been in Venice) based on its similarities to other pictures of the early 1630s. Contini also finds stylistic analogies to Artemisia's paintings of the 1630s and posits a renewed acquaintance with Florentine sources, most probably the work of Rutilio Manetti, which may have occurred during a trip to Pisa to raise money for her daughter's wedding, an opinion also endorsed by Bissell. The strong associations between this picture and Artemisia's *Saints Proculus and Nicea* (Capodimonte, Naples; fig. 143), painted for Pozzuoli cathedral in the mid-1630s, as well as the energy and originality of the iconography, suggest that it was reworked during the early part of the 1630s.

1. On the history of the Greek text, see Levenson 1997, 27–34.
2. Lippincott (1990, 447) also has noted the obvious influence of Michelangelo's figure on Artemisia's rendering of Esther.
3. See Pignatti 1976, 200 no. A237.
4. On Esther as typological parallel to the Virgin, see Perlove 1989, 133–47.

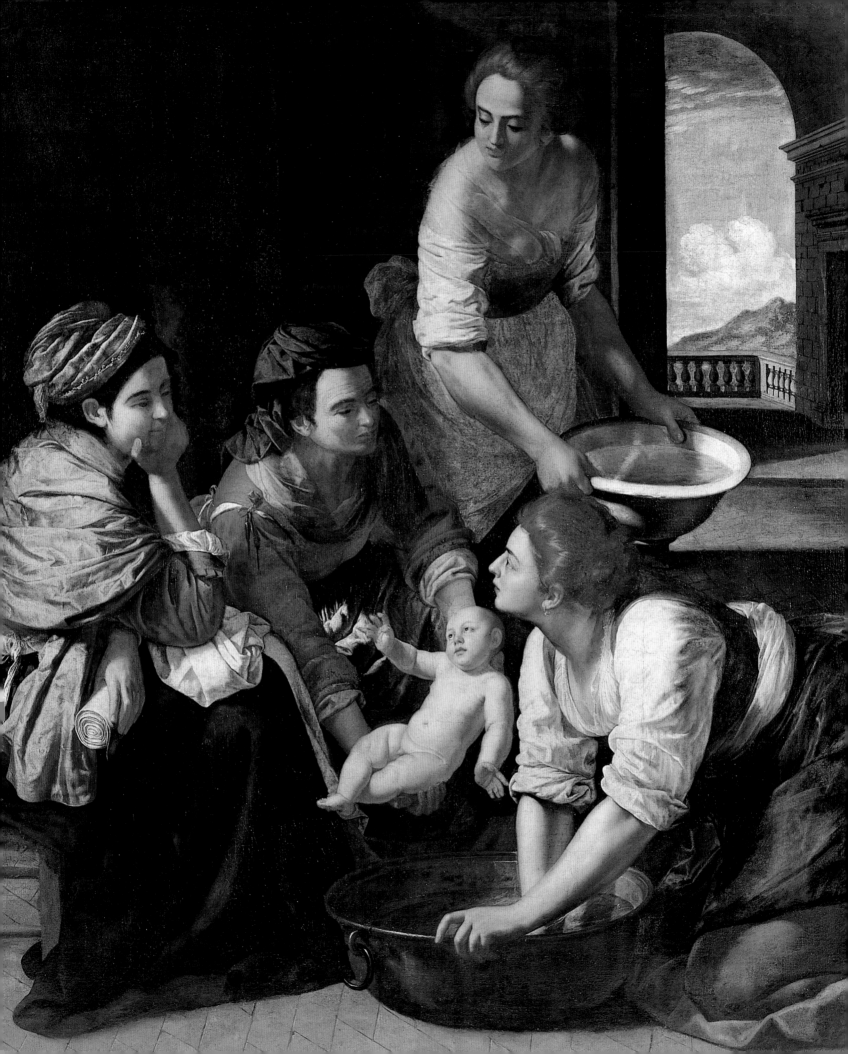

Artemisia and Naples, Naples and Artemisia

RICCARDO LATTUADA

Naples in Artemisia Gentileschi's day was one of the great as well as most turbulent cities of the world and, with Paris, one of the two largest metropolitan centers in Europe. It was also a place of political ferment and natural disasters. In 1631, Mount Vesuvius erupted, and the lava flow devastated the towns on its slopes. Naples was only just spared, and an outpouring of popular devotion followed in its wake. In 1647, a popular insurrection, directed first at the powerful Neapolitan nobility and then at the authority of Spain itself (Naples had been under Spanish rule since 1504), engulfed Naples and then all of southern Italy.[1] The insurrection took its name from a fishmonger, Masaniello, who was chosen to lead the protest, and it would be commemorated by a medal with his profile on one side and on the reverse that of Oliver Cromwell (ca. 1599–1658), the notorious English rebel and regicide. Eight years later, an outbreak of the plague carried off approximately two-thirds of the city's nearly half-million inhabitants.

Despite the image that these and other disasters have created of Naples in the seventeenth century as a kind of urban inferno, the city was complex and richly faceted. Naples retained its vitality during each of these dramatic events and throughout the seicento.[2] It is interesting that they are barely mentioned in Artemisia's correspondence, even though she was in Naples both when Vesuvius erupted in 1631 and during the insurrection of 1647.

To imagine the artist in the midst of a turbulent, anarchical, and tragic world would not be historically accurate.[3] Artemisia's patrons, Neapolitans among them, had the means to enjoy a life of pleasure and to indulge in complicated social rituals, and they were, for the most part, sheltered from any turmoil by the considerable class differences typical of Italian society at that time.[4] The cultural life of Naples, the political and administrative capital of all southern Italy, with the exception of Sicily, was rich, and the

city filled with sophisticated people whose outlook was not only Neapolitan but European. The poet Giambattista Marino (1569–1625) and the natural philosophers Giordano Bruno (1548–1600) and Tommaso Campanella (1568–1639) lived and studied in Naples at the end of the sixteenth and the beginning of the seventeenth century. From the middle of the fifteenth century, the city had been controlled by the principal families of the Kingdom of Naples (known simply as il Regno); the Carafa, Sanseverino, Caracciolo, d'Avalos, Pignatelli, and Orsini families held thirty percent of the kingdom's territory by feudal right. If we include such families as the Di Capua, Gonzaga, Spinelli, De Lannoy, Sforza, Acquaviva, Piccolomini, Colonna, Fernández de Córdoba, and Farnese in this group, we find that sixty percent of southern Italy was subject to feudal governance.[5]

The wealth amassed in the provinces of southern Italy flowed into Naples, and the great families became ever more entrenched in the construction and perpetual renovation of their palaces, in an effort to make them ever larger and more lavish as their households expanded.[6] As the capital city, Naples also offered enormous possibilities for doing business with the Spanish administrative machine. Indeed, at the time of the Masaniello revolt, Naples accounted for a full third of the revenue deposited in the treasury of the Spanish crown, a situation that changed little in the second half of the seventeenth century.

In addition to the great feudal families, the important religious orders—the older ones like the Carthusians, the Franciscans, and the Dominicans, as well as the newer ones, such as the Jesuits, Theatines, and Oratorians—established impressive houses and monasteries that were firmly rooted in the urban fabric of the ancient Greco-Roman city. As late as 1872, Gennaro Aspreno Galante listed 343 sacred buildings in the historical center of Naples, nearly all of which were constructed between the thirteenth and

Opposite: Detail of the *Birth of Saint John the Baptist* (cat. 77)

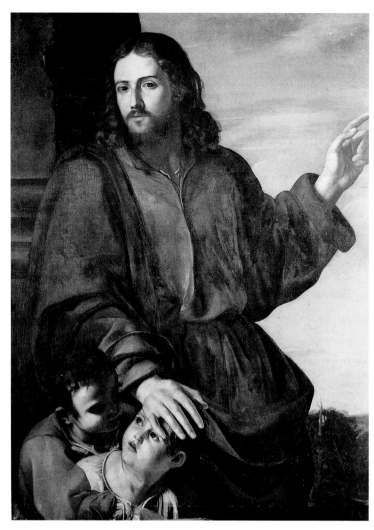

Figure 132. Attributed to Artemisia Gentileschi, *Christ Blessing the Children*. Oil on canvas. Formerly The Metropolitan Museum of Art, New York

the eighteenth century.[7] The most active period in the history of ecclesiastical construction was from the end of the fifteenth through the seventeenth century. Naples thus had one of the richest art markets in Italy. The enormous number of projects, both secular and religious, carried out by Cosimo Fanzago (1591–1678), the most important architect in the city, involved the employment of hundreds of architects, contractors, and marble workers.[8] Bartolomeo and Francesco Antonio Picchiatti, Dionisio Lazzari, Giuliano Finelli, and the young Ercole Ferrata all produced the best of their work during these years.

In the area of painting, too, the number of commissions grew continuously, natural disasters, rebellions, and epidemics notwithstanding. In the first half of the seicento, Annibale Carracci, Caravaggio, Guido Reni, Simon Vouet, Diego Velázquez, Pietro da Cortona, Domenichino, Giovanni Lanfranco, Charles Mellin,

Nicolas Poussin, and Giovanni Benedetto Castiglione either passed through, sent paintings to, or, in the majority of cases, worked in Naples. The city also enjoyed the advantage of being the Italian metropolis closest to Rome,[9] which was the natural destination for the training of a young Neapolitan artist and often offered him the opportunity of work. Massimo Stanzione (1585?–?1656), for example, presumably matured as an artist in Rome and then traveled continuously between the papal city and Naples from 1617 to about 1630. Indeed, it was from Rome, in 1630, that a Carthusian priest, Carlo Filippo de Ferrariis, recommended Stanzione to one of his Neapolitan brothers as the artist best qualified for the commission to paint the first frescoes at the Certosa di San Martino.[10]

The Spanish presence in Naples was essential to the development of the local school of painting. The first round of commissions for paintings to decorate Philip IV's (r. 1621–65) Buen Retiro palace in Madrid, for example, was awarded to artists working in Rome by agents of Gaspar de Guzmán y Pimentel, count-duke of Olivares. The second and much larger group of commissions was entrusted to Olivares's brother-in-law, the Spanish viceroy Manuel de Zúñiga y Fonseca, count of Monterrey, and assigned in Naples between 1631 and 1637. In addition to Jusepe de Ribera, Stanzione, Aniello Falcone, Domenico Gargiulo, Andrea di Lione, Cesare Fracanzano, Viviano Codazzi, and Scipione Compagni all worked at the Buen Retiro, as did Giovanni Lanfranco (1582–1647) and Domenichino (1581–1641), each of whom was in the process of transferring his professional activity to Naples.[11] As never before, Naples and Rome served as the two culturally interdependent poles of the artistic world, guided by such men as the viceroys Fernando Enríquez, Afán de Ribera, third duke of Alcalá, and the count of Monterrey. Artemisia, who was evidently aware of this great project, knew that moving to Naples could provide important opportunities for her career. It is likely that Artemisia's fame reached Naples on the basis of work, now lost, made for Neapolitan or Spanish patrons and perhaps traded for Neapolitan products. This was the case, for example, with a painting that showed Christ blessing the children—"un lienço de un Salvador con la mano derecha sobre unos muchachos"—which was acquired by the duke of Alcalá when he was the Spanish ambassador to the Holy See in Rome (1625–26).[12] The painting was perhaps taken from Rome to Naples when the duke was viceroy (1629–32),[13] and there copies were made.[14] It seems to me that this work can be identified with a painting in the collection of The Metropolitan Museum of Art from 1927 until 1979 (fig. 132). In a letter of 1936 in the Museum's files, Hermann Voss attributed it to Pacecco de Rosa (1607–1656), and this is the attribution recorded on the photograph of the painting in the Fondazione Roberto Longhi in Florence, which is where I first saw it. More recently, Bologna attributed it to Carlo Rosa (1613–1678).[15] But in an unpublished catalogue entry Federico Zeri notes that "[t]he strong reminiscences of Massimo Stanzione's types are modified by a closer approach to Guido Reni's [1575–1642] classical forms; the group of two children seems somewhat related to Artemisia Gentileschi."[16] It is my hope that this work, with its obvious connection to Artemisia, will sooner or later be available again for close study.

The admiration Artemisia may have garnered in Rome, before she went to Naples, has been much discussed; it is likely that she was given privileged access to the court of the duke of Alcalá through Cassiano dal Pozzo (1588–1657).[17] Artemisia's ability to find support throughout her career perhaps explains the confidence with which she worked from the moment of her arrival in Naples.

Artemisia's first work in Naples, the *Annunciation* (cat. 72), signed and dated 1630, reflects the painter's awareness of an artistic center similar to but at the same time profoundly different from Rome. The picture, recently restored and in less than perfect state, is an example of the changeable nature of Artemisia's style. It indicates an interest in the work of Simon Vouet (1590–1649)—the *Scenes from the Life of Saint Francis* at San Lorenzo in Lucina, Rome (fig. 117), for example, or the *Circumcision* in Sant'Angelo a Segno, Naples—and the contrasts of light and shadow are more dramatic here than they were in her earlier Roman works.[18] The composition, however, is a reworking of Scipione Pulzone's (1544–1598) *Annunciation,* originally in San Domenico at Gaeta and then transferred, in 1821, to Capodimonte. It would not have been at all unlikely that a traveler from Rome to Naples, such as Artemisia, would have made a stop in Gaeta. The *Annunciation* is one of the most famous of those works whose artless style, in accordance with the tenets of the Council of Trent (1545–63), Zeri memorably characterized as "senza tempo."[19] It is not the only example of Pulzone's work to have influenced Artemisia. The composition of the *Madonna and Child* (cat. 52) is another instance, since in many ways it depends on Pulzone's *Holy Family* in the Galleria Borghese, Rome.[20] Artemisia does away with much of the background in her 1630 *Annunciation*, contracting the space around the

figures, so that they project a greater sense of immediacy; it is a clear demonstration that she wanted her work to be in harmony with the formal aspects of the late-Caravaggesque style prevalent in the city. It would seem that Artemisia, who found herself in a cultural milieu similar to that of Rome but with its own idiosyncracies, used her personal archive of sources of what Vasari referred to as the "maniera moderna" to make her mark on the Neapolitan scene. With the *Annunciation*, she adapted to local taste a work that, to judge from its size and formal elements, was intended for a public space. It is curious that Giovanni Battista Caracciolo (1578–1635) would have used a similar source for his 1631 fresco of the *Annunciation* in the chapel of the Annunciation in San Martino, Naples.[21] Caracciolo's frescoes in this chapel have been described as exhibiting an impulse toward simplicity.

In 1630, the entire art world in Naples was undergoing profound changes. Diego Velázquez (1599–1660), painter to Philip IV of Spain, had arrived in the city that year in the retinue of the Spanish infanta, and he most likely visited Jusepe de Ribera's (1591–1652) studio.[22] In turn, Ribera revised the violent, Caravaggesque style of his youthful works, adopting ever lighter and more brilliant colors. This transformation is evident in his *Democritus*, signed and dated 1630, as well as in the pendant canvases of *Saint Roch* and *Saint James Major*, both signed and dated 1631 (all three are in the Prado, Madrid).[23] In Ribera's *Jacob and His Flocks*, signed and dated 1632 (El Escorial), the animals, the rocks, and Jacob's robes are all illuminated by a diffuse, transparent light, although the forms and shadows remain sharply defined.[24] The same can be said of his *Trinitas Terrestris* (Capodimonte, Naples), in which the Venetian-based coloration—now highly developed—poses a difficult problem related to the influence of the work produced by Anthony van Dyck (1599–1641) during his stay in Italy.[25] In this case, Pietro Novelli (called Il Monrealese; 1603–1647), may have played a significant role. Novelli was in Naples shortly after 1630, having come from Palermo, where he saw the great works Van Dyck had made there. At the same time, Novelli also absorbed the styles of Ribera and Stanzione in Naples.[26]

Stanzione raises the same issues, as his style is often—and incorrectly—contrasted with that of Ribera. In the Raleigh *Assumption of the Virgin* (North Carolina Museum of Art), dated to the late 1620s or early 1630s,[27] Stanzione turns to the altarpieces of Annibale Carracci (1560–1609) for his composition, but the brilliant colors he uses are closer to Vouet's last Italian works. There are, furthermore, motifs that can still be traced to the French Caravaggisti, such as the so-called Master of the Judgment of Solomon. The detail of the pair of figures in the right background is drawn from Caravaggio's *Martyrdom of Saint Matthew* (fig. 4). But in 1630, Stanzione updated his Caravaggesque style, in keeping with the current of the Roman Baroque.[28] Stanzione had many of the same objectives as Artemisia, a commonality that led to productive exchanges and even the sharing of important commissions. Yet in this relationship, Artemisia certainly took more from Stanzione than she was able to offer him.

The first important commission that they carried out together is the five canvases with scenes from the Life of Saint John the Baptist intended for the hermitage of San Juan, and built by the count-duke of Olivares in 1634 in the park of the Buen Retiro in Madrid.[29] The paintings were executed in about 1633–34.[30] The five scenes include Artemisia's *Birth of Saint John the Baptist* (cat. 77) and Stanzione's *Annunciation to Zaccharias, Saint John the Baptist Taking Leave of His Parents* (fig. 133), *Saint John the Baptist Preaching,* and the *Beheading of Saint John the Baptist.* A sixth scene in the series—Paolo Finoglia's *Saint John the Baptist in Prison*—is now lost.[31] Artemisia's work seems to be the first real fruit of Cassiano dal Pozzo's connections at the court of the Spanish viceroy in Naples; the count of Monterrey oversaw the commissions for these works. The proportional division of the commission (four paintings to Stanzione and only one each to Artemisia and Finoglia) gives an indication of the respective status each artist had in the eyes of the patron.

Stanzione's canvases for the series are among his finest;[32] the variety of the compositions is enhanced by a striking diversification of stylistic choices. In the *Annunciation to Zaccharias,* for example, the monumental figures are grouped in a classical composition, and the figure seen from the back reveals a study of ancient sculpture, as does the altar. It is not surprising, then, that Francesco Guarino (1611–1654) recycled this composition with little alteration in his work of the same subject for the transept ceiling in the Collegiata at Solofra (1637).[33] The *Saint John the Baptist Taking Leave of His Parents* is perhaps the most original work in the cycle. Here, Stanzione transfers the formal world of the Roman Caravaggisti to a plein-air setting. Again, the composition is marked by a strong sense of harmony among the figures, yet the rustic character of the clothing has none of the harshness seen in the manner of the early Ribera or the Master of the

Annunciation to the Shepherds (fl. ca. 1620–40?). The emotional tenor is one of rural simplicity.

In the *Saint John the Baptist Preaching,* Stanzione grafts the figures and colors of French Caravaggism onto his recollections of both Annibale Carracci and, especially, Domenichino. For example, the seated woman holding a child in the lower right corner is a reworking of a similar figure in Domenichino's Polet chapel frescoes in San Luigi dei Francesi, Rome (1612–15), as is a figure in the *Presentation of the Virgin at the Temple,* in the Santuario della Madonna della Misericordia, Savona (ca. 1623–27).[34] The seated woman also recalls—in this case, with only minor variations on the part of Stanzione—the figure in the lower right corner of Vouet's *Saint Francis Taking the Habit,* in San Lorenzo in Lucina, Rome (1624).[35] A Caravaggesque topos, it also reminds us of the figure in the lower right in Caravaggio's *Martyrdom of Saint Matthew,* in San Luigi dei Francesi. The rustic setting of the *Saint John* appears to follow the biblical sources, and it is likely that the picture was intended to share in the veneration for the pastoral that led Philip IV to build hermitages throughout the park of the Buen Retiro palace.[36]

The *Beheading of Saint John the Baptist* also reflects Stanzione's acquaintance with the work of the French and Northern Caravaggisti in Rome, in particular, that of Dutch painter Gerrit van Honthorst (1592–1656). Stanzione's studied eclecticism, which takes him well beyond the source of his traditional sobriquet, the "Neapolitan Guido" (Reni), seems frankly more advanced than what Artemisia achieves in her *Birth of Saint John.* In Stanzione's canvas, the wealth of stylistic references is not an end in itself but also a means of expressing emotion; indeed, his style presents an alternative in Neapolitan painting to that represented in the work of Ribera. Artemisia's composition is more stilted, and the sense that the artist was uncomfortable representing a religious subject was evident even to a supporter of her work as enthusiastic as Roberto Longhi.[37] The horizontal format of the painting also seems to have given Artemisia problems: the figures, seen in a large space, are detached from one another, both compositionally and emotionally. It is certainly possible that the speed with which the commission was executed—"at a breakneck pace," as R. Ward Bissell has noted[38]—had an impact on the end result, as perhaps did the fact that Artemisia had to adapt not only to the general scheme of the cycle but to the instructions given to her by Stanzione.

The other major commission was for a cycle of paintings to decorate the choir of the cathedral at Pozzuoli (see cat. 79). A

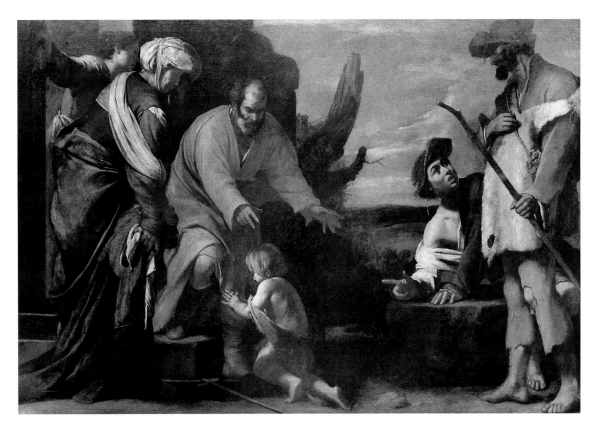

Figure 133. Massimo Stanzione (1585?–?1656), *Saint John the Baptist Taking Leave of His Parents.* Oil on canvas. Museo Nacional del Prado, Madrid

veritable army of Neapolitan and Roman artists worked on the cathedral from 1635 to about 1638.[39] The genesis of the cycle is usually explained by the renewed devotion to Saint Januarius (San Gennaro; ca. 272–ca. 305) engendered by the eruption of Vesuvius in 1631. The patronage might be more fully explained by a careful look at the relationship between the bishop of Pozzuoli, Martino de Leòn y Cárdenas, and the count of Monterrey, who, as a key player in the Neapolitan art scene, may have had substantial input into the directives given by the church administration.[40]

Pozzuoli, which had been an important city in the Phlegraean Fields since Roman times, was situated in front of the Castello di Baia, a defensive outpost in Campania. The fact that the city was significant in the strategic defense of the Kingdom of Naples meant that it had a strong Spanish presence beyond that of its bishop. The seventeenth-century revival of the cult of Saint Januarius, which culminated in the completion of the spectacular chapel housing the saint's relics in the Neapolitan cathedral, also led to a renewed interest in the various places the saint spent the last days before his martyrdom.

The paintings for the choir of the cathedral of Pozzuoli, painted by Stanzione, Lanfranco, Agostino Beltrano (1607–

1656), Finoglia, and Cesare (ca. 1605–1651) and perhaps Francesco (1612–?1656) Fracanzano, as well as Artemisia, represent an essential anthology for the understanding of the artistic trends in Naples at the end of the 1630s. The deplorable state of these pictures (among the devastations to which they have been subject over the years, the last was a fire in 1964) is evident also in Artemisia's *Saint Januarius in the Amphitheater* (cat. 79), the *Adoration of the Magi* (fig. 142),[41] and the *Saints Proculus and Nicea* (fig. 143). (As is often the case with works from the disaster-prone area around Naples, the three canvases are today housed in the Capodimonte.) The paintings exemplify Artemisia's integration into the Neapolitan scene and, as has been noted, exhibit no connection with her Florentine and Roman works.[42] They are characterized by a certain conventionality and, for precisely this reason, their style is difficult to define. "Dignified, even solemn, and approached with a seriousness of purpose, they are nonetheless without much expressive passion."[43]

At Pozzuoli, Artemisia again appears to have turned to Stanzione for more than just advice. Her Saints Proculus and Nicea, as they stand in a Tuscan portico, are both splendid figures. A Corinthian loggia in the background suggests a vaguely antique setting that alludes to the historical period in which the two saints were martyred. The monumental figures are as solemn as two polychromed statues, and they attest to Artemisia's confidence in handling the human figure. Many scholars have suggested that another artist was responsible for the architecture—Giovanni Bottari, Mina Gregori, David Ryley Marshall proposing Viviano Codazzi (ca. 1604–1670) and Bissell suggesting Domenico Gargiulo (1609–?1675).[44]

It has also been consistently suggested in the literature that the *Adoration of the Magi* is a collaboration between Artemisia and Stanzione. When the work is seen in the brightly lit galleries of the Capodimonte, this argument seems somewhat implausible. In composition, the painting recalls Caracciolo's *Adoration of the Magi* in the chapter house of the Certosa di San Martino, Naples, while the figures of the Madonna and child and the kneeling magus bring to mind Vouet's painting the *Virgin Appearing to Saint Bruno*, executed at about the same time and for the same place.[45] Artemisia's picture is also close to Stanzione's *Adoration of the Magi*, painted in the second half of the 1620s (private collection, Philadelphia),[46] but it exhibits the same insecurity on the part of the painter that we have encountered in the *Birth of the Virgin*. Stanzione's unmistakable style is difficult to discern in Artemisia's treatment of the figures; here, she seems instead to be looking to those Neapolitan painters who were building on the decorative aspects of Stanzione's poetic style—Agostino Beltrano, for example, who was also active at the cathedral in Pozzuoli and whose *Lot and His Daughters* (fig. 134) reveals his inclination toward the ornamental.

The *Saint Januarius in the Amphitheater* (cat. 79), in Pozzuoli, is a work of linguistic richness.[47] It is almost universally agreed that Gargiulo executed the background, which shows the amphitheater of Pozzuoli, with its emphatic diagonal perspective. There is as well a strong link to the work of Paolo Finoglia (ca. 1590–1645). Associated with Artemisia for the Buen Retiro commission, Finoglia also worked at the cathedral at Pozzuoli, where he executed the *Saint Peter Consecrating Sant'Aspreno*.[48] Finoglia and Artemisia had much in common, sharing a love for fabrics rendered in a brilliant, changeable light and for figures with a monumental presence. In the mid-1630s, Finoglia's style was less developed than that of such Neapolitan masters as Ribera, Stanzione, and Cavallino, but his skill in describing textiles in minute detail has led to some confusion of his work with Artemisia's, as in the case

of the *Joseph and Potiphar's Wife* (fig. 135).[49] The composition of this sumptuous painting is still tied to late-sixteenth-century formulas, not entirely absent from the work of Ribera of about 1630–35; it provided ideas that proved to be important for Artemisia as well.

The commissions for the Buen Retiro and the cathedral at Pozzuoli thrust Artemisia into the very center of professional life in Naples—a world well known for its hostility to foreigners (the case of Domenichino is notorious). Neither Artemisia nor Lanfranco, however, seems to have had any problems in this regard. This would indicate that entry into the art scene also depended on social skills, which both Artemisia and Lanfranco possessed, and that the art market in Naples between 1630 and 1650 was expanding as never before. Thus the prospects for finding work were excellent— despite Artemisia's continual complaints to the contrary.

The collaboration between Artemisia and Neapolitan masters such as Stanzione, Gargiulo, and Cavallino, as well as the Bergamasque-Roman-Neapolitan Viviano Codazzi, creates considerable confusion having to do with the division of labor, attribution, and shared interests. Each of these local painters had a well-established professional and business identity long before Artemisia arrived in Naples. Bernardo Cavallino (1616–ca. 1656), for instance, whose early works date to about 1635, was already an important figure in Stanzione's circle when Artemisia received her first Neapolitan commissions. One example of Cavallino's independence can be found in his *Meeting at the Golden Gate* (Szépmüvészeti Múzeum, Budapest).[50] This work, the subject of which is taken from Jacobus de Voragine's *Golden Legend*, combines Ribera's manner with that of Stanzione in the sensitive evocation of feeling. Thus, in my opinion, we succumb to the myth of Artemisia if we consider that the artists with whom she worked in Naples were her followers. In fact, as our knowledge of Neapolitan painting in the first half of the seventeenth century expands, it becomes increasingly difficult to ascribe to Artemisia a central role in the collaborative efforts in which she participated.[51]

The dynamic of these collaborations is exemplified in the powerful *Susanna and the Elders* that was sold at Sotheby's in London in 1995 (fig. 144).[52] A collaboration between Artemisia, Cavallino, Gargiulo, and Codazzi, this work is perhaps one of the finest accomplishments of Neapolitan painting in the first half of the seventeenth century. It is also almost certainly the picture Bernardo de Dominici saw in 1742 in the Neapolitan collection

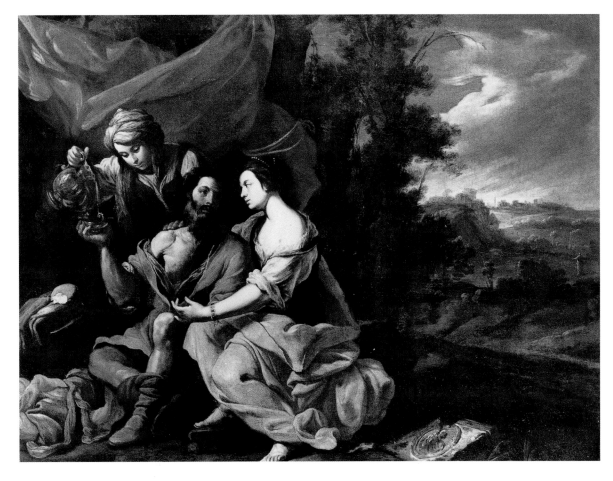

Figure 134. Agostino Beltrano (1607–1656), *Lot and His Daughters*. Oil on canvas. Molinari Pradelli collection, Marano di Castenaso

of Luigi Romeo, baron of San Luigi, where it was hanging with a *David and Bathsheba* attributed to Artemisia alone, now in Columbus, Ohio (cat. 80).[53] The number of artists to whom various parts of these two paintings have been attributed is indicative of the exceptional degree of interaction between Artemisia and her Neapolitan colleagues. Current opinion holds that in the ex-Sotheby's picture, Gargiulo executed the landscape and architectural passages (after a design by Codazzi),[54] while Artemisia painted the figure of Susanna—but not the elders (who are, in fact, not very aged), which were painted by Cavallino.[55] In the Columbus *Bathsheba*, the architecture is attributed to Codazzi, and the young woman who offers the necklace of pearls to Cavallino. Bissell has asserted that in both paintings, Artemisia had "full responsibility for the compositions and overall expressive thrusts."[56] It is understandable that Roberto Contini should have remained uncertain about the attribution of the *Susanna*, which he termed a "noterole, ma difficile."[57] The figural composition, the color scheme, the drapery, and the beautiful transparency of the shadows seem, on balance, the work of Cavallino. Given what we know

about Artemisia, it is difficult to see her hand in the subtle passages of light and shadow on Susanna's face and torso, the golden reflections of her hair, the tapering hands, the soft drapery—more flowing than anything we see in her Neapolitan work—or in the emotional tenor of the figures. Indeed, the two male figures can easily be compared with those in the Cavallino *Apostles* (Spafford Establishment, London) and, in particular, a *Saint Paul* and a *Praying Saint* (present location unknown).[58] The manner of painting in these works is not the same as what we find in the Columbus *Bathsheba*. There, the maidservant holding the pearls is not executed with the same fluency, and the drapery of the other figures has the more solid, stiff quality that is typical of Artemisia. In my opinion, the best stylistic comparison with the *Bathsheba* is the *Lot and His Daughters* in Toledo (cat. 78).[59] In sum, we have three works that, in their composition and homogeneity of color, are typical of the Neapolitan art scene at this time.

Discussion of the Columbus *Bathsheba* and the ex-Sotheby's *Susanna* could be extended to include the magnificent *Galatea*, now in the National Gallery of Art, Washington.[60] Yet for the

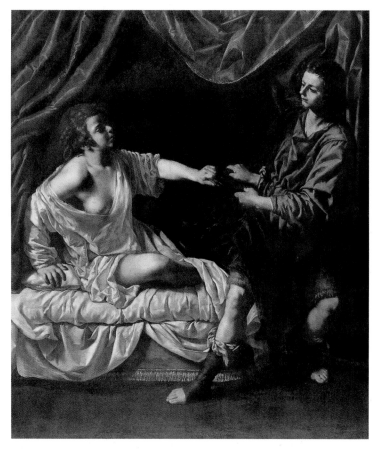

Figure 135. Paolo Domenico Finoglia (ca. 1590–1645), *Joseph and Potiphar's Wife.* Oil on canvas. The Fogg Museum of Art, Cambridge, Mass., Kress Collection

sake of brevity, I will speak more generally on the nature of these collaborations. Do they derive from Artemisia's inability to handle specific parts of the paintings, such as architectural backdrops or landscapes? Or did collaborations simply offer the possibility of a faster execution? It is hard to say. Artemisia was certainly capable of painting all the figures in the *Susanna* herself, and she had and would again paint ambitious backgrounds. Such collaborations were already far from unusual in Rome—Andrea Sacchi and Jan Miel, Codazzi and Michelangelo Cerquozzi, as well as the many collaborations between figure painters and specialists in still life, landscapes, and architecture come to mind—and they took root quickly in Naples. A sort of pictorial *certamen*, in which each artist offered elements, figures, and motifs typical of his or her own style, animates these splendid collaborations, which are not just instances of commercial partnerships but truly interactive productions. The source of this practice was in Rome, but the results in Naples were long-lasting, culminating in 1684 in the collaboration of Luca Giordano, Paolo de Matteis, Giuseppe

Recco, Giovanni Battista Ruoppolo, and Francesco della Quosta on fourteen canvases for the feast of Corpus Domini, organized at the royal palace in Naples by Gaspar de Haro y Guzman, seventh marquis of Carpio.[61]

The *Corisca and the Satyr* (cat. 74), a work of the mid-1630s, presents yet another example of Artemisia's full participation in the Neapolitan art world.[62] It is not surprising that in 1990 the picture was sold at Christie's in Rome with an attribution to Stanzione and that only the discovery of Artemisia's signature, uncovered during the cleaning of the canvas, allows us to restore it definitively to her oeuvre. Here, too, we see an intelligent reading of the dominant style in Neapolitan painting around 1630–35. The mise-en-scène, with a glimpse of landscape in the background, recalls Stanzione's *Orpheus Beaten by the Bacchantes* (Banca Manusardi & C., Milan) and reminds us again of the close ties between these two artists.[63] The playfulness and irony of the scene, which depicts one of the most comic moments in Giovanni Battista Guarini's pastoral drama *Il pastor fido* (act 2, scene 6),[64] is narrated in muted tones. Artemisia seems to have fully understood Guarini's text, which is permeated with a classicism quite distinct from the moralism of the Counter-Reformation. Corisca is an embodiment of the elusive, seductive power of women, the source of frustration for her suitors. But she too knows the suffering of love, the love she bears for Mirtillo. The stunned satyr falls back, Corisca's hairpiece in his hand, his dejected pose contrasting with the buoyant flight of the girl who tricked him.

The painting was guided by an informed patron, one who was well aware of the implications of the subject. It is one of Artemisia's finest Neapolitan works, and there is much appeal in the fact that she was asked to represent one of the key moments in the drama. As described by Fassò:

> The male characters are certainly rather pallid, especially Mirtillo and Silvio. But not the female characters, Amarilli, Dorinda, and Corisca. The first two are delineated [by Guarini] with a delicacy and sureness of touch born of an understanding of the nature of women. The third [Corisca] is incised as if with a burin. An experienced and cunning seductress, Corisca openly proclaims her sensuality, which is fueled by true passion. If, however, she is [betrayed and] disillusioned, she takes revenge with calumny and deceit. Yet she can redeem herself when faced with the happiness of her loved one. I would say that Corisca is the most felicitous character in this tragicomedy

and that, in her psychological complexity, she foreshadows modern drama. The scene in which she mocks the brutal satyr has rightly been defined as the most perfect in the play. But one might add that every time Corisca is onstage, the dramatic poet does his best work.[65]

During the same years that Artemisia executed her commissions for the Buen Retiro and the cathedral in Pozzuoli, she also became known for the kind of paintings that were more characteristic of her work. Her heroines are dramatis personae, and they convey the ambiguous and fascinating interplay between Artemisia's work and her complicated private life;[66] here, too, the history of Neapolitan painting offers precedents and parallels.

While Ribera's work centered on the representation of saints and hermits—examples of what Raffaello Causa in his survey of Neapolitan seicento painting of 1972 called "heroic old age" ("senescenza eroica")—Stanzione was the first Neapolitan painter to make a series of images of female martyrs. These were especially influenced by the work of Vouet, who was an important model both for Stanzione and for Stanzione's pupils Francesco Guarino and Bernardo Cavallino, who also excelled in paintings of this subject. In his mature works, Stanzione developed his own personal style, combining Vouet's manner with that of Reni, sometimes Sassoferrato (1609–1685), and, occasionally, even Artemisia. The women Artemisia painted presented new problems for Neapolitan painters. The sweet and seductive figures painted by Stanzione, the young Guarino, and Cavallino were replaced in about 1640 by figures that are more courtly and solemn in their bearing and express as well a certain imperiousness.

Stanzione approaches Artemisia's manner in his splendid *Death of Cleopatra* (Pushkin Museum of Fine Arts, Moscow), a painting datable to about 1640.[67] As Sebastian Schütze and Thomas Willette have noted, "the hardness of the modeling and the frigid emotions expressed by the figures recall the style of Domenichino more than that of Reni."[68] The magisterial figure of the queen, however, is closer still to the protagonist in Artemisia's *Bathsheba* in Columbus or the later version of the same subject in the Neue Palais, Potsdam.[69] Indeed, the isolated nude figure, surrounded by rich materials of red, yellow, white, and a touch of ultramarine, seems an obvious homage to Artemisia. It is also symptomatic of Stanzione's acquaintance with Artemisia's style that this painting seems to be unique in his oeuvre. The tone set by Cleopatra's expression of exhaustion and despair in Stanzione's painting is

very different from that in Artemisia's, but the general composition of the two works is similar.

This kind of mutual borrowing can be found in two additional images of female figures, inspired by the stoic models that enjoyed such success in seventeenth-century Naples. These are Guarino's *Saint Cecilia*, dated about 1643,[70] and his *Saint Christina* (versions in the Musée de Picardie, Amiens, and in Pesaro; fig. 136), both dated about 1645.[71] In the *Saint Cecilia*, Guarino makes an elaborate study of the saint's white, blue, and yellow drapery— a veritable homage to Artemisia's masterly rendering of color. Elsewhere, I have argued that the *Saint Christina* reveals a close link to Finoglia in the frontality of the figure and in the protagonist's arrogant expression, as well as in the execution of the rich and satiny material, with its artfully arranged folds. The relationship of these paintings—Guarino's *Saint Christina* (especially the Pesaro version) and *Saint Cecilia*, and Stanzione's *Cleopatra*—to

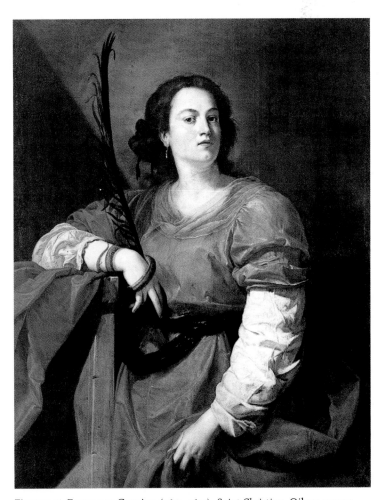

Figure 136. Francesco Guarino (1611–1654), *Saint Christina*. Oil on canvas. Collezioni Comunali d'Arte, Museo Civico, Pesaro

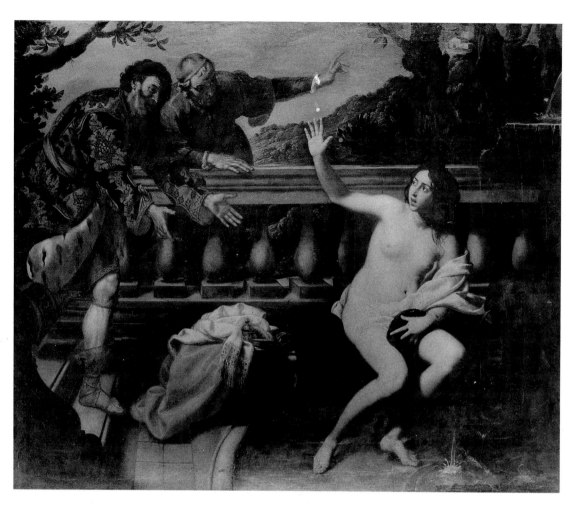

Figure 137. Pacecco de Rosa (1607–1656), *Susanna and the Elders*. Oil on canvas. Museo e Gallerie Nazionali di Capodimonte, Naples

the work of Artemisia derives from a general recollection of her work rather than from an imitation of her style. Yet neither Stanzione nor Guarino was unaffected by her manner, as reflected in the fact that the impact of Vouet, which is visible in such paintings as Guarino's *Saint Agatha* (Museo di San Martino, Naples)[72] and Stanzione's *Cleopatra* (Palazzo Durazzo Pallavicini, Genoa), diminishes in about 1640–45.[73]

The mature works of Pacecco de Rosa (1607–1656), a painter of very different abilities, show a perhaps not coincidental similarity with Artemisia's most successful works.[74] His *Susanna and the Elders* (fig. 137), one of his most accomplished paintings, illustrates aspects typical of his style—vivid colors, a subtle rendering of shadows, and careful attention to decorative detail (note the damask material worn by the elder on the left). A nude figure was required by the subject matter, but Pacecco also uses it to convey the protagonist's heroic behavior. Pacecco is always successful at concealing the eclecticism of his manner behind a recognizable

style, but here the strong influence of Artemisia—who produced so many pictures on this theme—is easily discernible. It is also perhaps not by chance that the series of mythological paintings Pacecco made for the d'Avalos family beginning in the 1640s prominently features the female nude: *Mars and Venus*, *Venus Discovered by a Satyr*, *Diana at her Bath*, the *Judgment of Paris*, and even *Dido Abandoned* create a gallery of goddesses and heroines that makes Artemisia's specialty in this kind of image less atypical.[75] It would be worth exploring the fact that Pacecco, Stanzione, Cavallino, and even Andrea Vaccaro (1604–1670) all painted similar subjects during the years Artemisia was in Naples and that their work constitutes a counterpart to hers.

The work of Onofrio Palumbo (fl. mid-17th century), the only Neapolitan artist whom Bernardo de Dominici identified as a pupil of Artemisia's, poses a more complicated problem.[76] The contours of Palumbo's career have taken shape only over the last fifty years. Ferdinando Bologna, in an exhibition held in

Salerno in 1955, was the first to identify the *Annunciation* and the *Nativity* at Santa Maria delle Salute, Naples, as Palumbo's work, and documents later established that payments were made in 1641.[77] Raffaello Causa has made important contributions to our knowledge of the artist's oeuvre in his discussion of the lovely *Saint Januarius Interceding on Behalf of Naples during the Plague of 1656* (Trinità dei Pellegrini, Naples), which has a view of the city attributed to Didier Barra (ca. 1590–after ca. 1652).[78] Bologna returned to his study of Palumbo in 1991, having made occasional contributions (unpublished) about the artist.[79] Here, he gives some paintings traditionally attributed to Artemisia to Onofrio, and assigns new works to him as well. And Bissell, in his 1999 monograph, comments on Bologna's thesis. A fair number of the works that Bologna noted or discussed were then published again by Stefano Causa, who was the first to attempt to make a systematic study of the artist.[80]

A nonspecialist reading this material on Palumbo will be confused, at the very least, by the complexity and fluidity of the attributions. Stefano Causa, for example, attributes the *Galatea* in Washington to Cavallino and Palumbo (it is generally attributed to Cavallino and by Bissell to Cavallino and Artemisia), and he gives the *Lot and His Daughters* in Toledo (cat. 78) and the *Cleopatra* in a private collection (cat. 76) to Palumbo alone. Bologna and Stefano Causa give a *Samson and Delilah* in the collection of the Banco di Napoli to Palumbo, while Bissell, who does not discuss Causa's attribution, calls it a copy after a work by Artemisia. These differences in perception, which are far too complicated to explore fully in this essay, do not derive simply from different schools of thought or subjective opinions (which are often a factor in the history of art). The history of Neapolitan painting in the first half of the seventeenth century is still in a fluid state, a situation that pertains especially to the relationship between the work of individual painters—the subject of important ongoing research—and the available documentation. We can therefore look forward to this type of discussion for some time to come.

An apt candidate for the subject of such discussion is the *Saint Catherine of Alexandria* (fig. 138), which Stefano Causa attributes to Palumbo.[81] This is a notable painting that demonstrates the artist's debt to Artemisia. The saint's proud posture, her inspired expression, the rich treatment of the drapery—which resembles Finoglia's—are an intelligent rereading of Artemisia's images, although within the context of the Neapolitan art scene.

At this time, too, it is not possible to go beyond merely suggesting that there is an analogy between the biography of Artemisia and that of Annella de Rosa (b. 1602), Pacecco de Rosa's niece. Considered one of Stanzione's most brilliant pupils, Annella was murdered by her husband, Agostino Beltrano, who was also a painter.[82] Her story is noteworthy in that it gives voice, in a Neapolitan context, to the predicament of the female artist who is as talented as her male counterparts but whose career as a painter is stifled by their envy.[83] It is also notable that, according to De Dominici (our principal seventeenth-century source for Neapolitan painting), there were in Naples other women who followed Annella's example and, "motivated by a virtuous envy, took up painting."[84] Interestingly, there have been no studies of the similarities between Annella's and Artemisia's situations, which is all

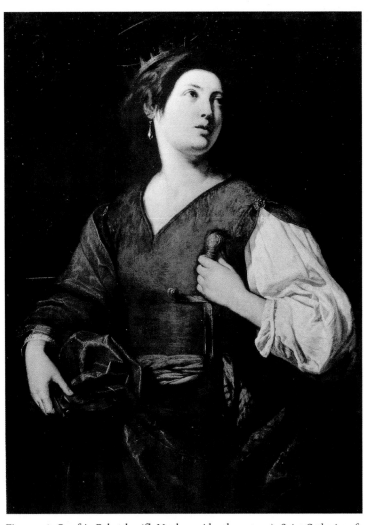

Figure 138. Onofrio Palumbo (fl. Naples, mid-17th century), *Saint Catherine of Alexandria*. Oil on canvas. Location unknown

the more curious in that the two painters lived and worked in the same city and at the same time. Clearly this subject, which would also have to include painters such as Elisabetta Sirani (1638–1665), requires a broad reevaluation. Heretofore, primarily the province of feminist literature, it is now open to approaches that are more specifically art-historical.[85]

The intensity with which Artemisia Gentileschi measured herself against her male colleagues in Naples is a most pertinent subject. And the relationship she established with the world of Neapolitan painting is so important because it challenges the notion that she worked in a kind of enforced seclusion, spending all her time serving only foreign patrons and ignoring the work of the other painters in the city. To the contrary. She was, in fact, highly sensitive to the dynamics of exchange, influence, and style. This would suggest that she had a major role in the development of Neapolitan art, and it makes her an important player in the genius loci. As so many scholars have said, to ask the most important questions, we must turn to the work, for it is only through the paintings, taken one by one, that we can find the answers to her legendary life and career.

1. Villari 1976.

2. Galasso 1982.

3. See Prohaska 1995, 13–19, for some interesting observations that also raise objections it is not possible to discuss here.

4. Sella 2000, 200–210, and passim.

5. "Dislocazione territoriale e dimensione del possesso feudale nel Regno di Napoli a metà Cinquecento," in Visceglia 1992, 64–65.

6. Labrot 1979 and Labrot 1993.

7. Spinosa in Galante (1872) 1985, xi.

8. Cantone 1984.

9. Lattuada 1988, 17–43.

10. Novelli 1974a; Schütze and Willette 1992, 41–57.

11. Brown and Elliott 1980, 123–40, and passim; the first list of Neapolitan works destined for the Buen Retiro was compiled by Pérez Sánchez 1965.

12. See Brown and Kagan 1987, 239–40 item 7: "que es copia del original de artemisia que esta entre los que su Ex.a trujo de Ytalia para la cartuxa." Brown and Kagan note that the original, acquired by the duke during his stay in Rome, was given to the Cartuja de Santa María de las Cuevas.

13. Coniglio 1967, 219–32.

14. Bissell 1999, 359 no. L-14.

15. Bologna 1958, 33 n. 12.

16. I am grateful to Keith Christiansen for the information he so graciously provided about this painting, and for having shared with me his idea of its probable connection with the picture already in the collection of the duke of Alcalá. The painting was sold at auction at Sotheby's, New York, on May 30, 1979, lot 143.

17. Contini in Florence 1991, 65–66; Bissell 1999, 56–61.

18. Contini in Florence 1991, 66.

19. Zeri 1957, 73; Cassanova in Gaeta 1976, 96–97 no. 39; Leone de Castris 1991, 300 colorpl. 52.

20. Bissell 1999, 184–87, figs. 1–6.

21. Causa 2000, 203–4 no. A112f, 314, fig. 320.

22. See Lattuada 2000, 62 n. 11, for a critical history of the problem of Velázquez's visit to Naples.

23. Pérez Sánchez in Naples 1991–92, 170–71 no. 1.32, 177–79 nos. 1.37, 1.38.

24. Ibid., 189–90 no. 1.45.

25. Prohaska 1994–95.

26. Paolini in Palermo 1990, 60–64.

27. Schütze and Willette 1992, 195–96 no. A23.

28. Leone de Castris 1992, 545–68; for a more complete discussion, see Schütze and Willette 1992, 69–78.

29. Brown and Elliott 1980, 76–77, fig. 42.

30. Bissell 1999, 249–53.

31. For the history of this cycle, see ibid., 249–56.

32. Schütze and Willette 1992, 200–202 no. A30.

33. Lattuada 2000, 52, 125–27 no. A8.

34. Spear in Rome 1996–97, 460–61 n. 44; Lavalle and Di Matteo in ibid., 237–52.

35. Thuillier in Rome 1991, 94, 143–48 nn. 12, 13, colorpls. 12, 13.

36. Brown and Elliott 1980, 77.

37. Longhi 1916, 263.

38. Bissell 1999, 253.

39. Ibid., 256–57.

40. D'Ambrosio 1973.

41. Bissell 1999, 257.

42. Contini in Florence 1991, 68.

43. Bissell 1999, 81.

44. For the critical history of this problem, see ibid., 258.

45. Ibid., 81, 259 no. 33a.

46. Schütze and Willette 1992, 21, colorpl. 3, 193 no. A13.

47. Bissell 1999, 258–59; Barbone Pugliese in Conversano 2000, 141, colorpl. 52, 173.

48. Bissell 1999, 256–57; Barbone Pugliese in Conversano 2000, 114, colorpl. 34, 162. These two authors disagree on the dating of this work; Bissell puts it at about 1635 and Barbone Pugliese to the second half of the 1630s.

49. See Simonetti in Conversano 2000, 104, colorpl. 21, 153–54, for the critical history of this work.

50. Tzeutschler Lurie in Cleveland–Fort Worth–Naples 1984–85, 50–53 no. 1 (American ed.), 85–87 no. A.1 (Italian ed.).

51. Bissell 1999, 82–87.

52. Sotheby's, London, December 6, 1995, lot 53; see Bissell 1999, 266–67 no. 38, for the critical history of this painting.

53. Bissell 1999, 263–66 no. 37. The date of 1742 is deduced by Bissell from De Dominici 1742–44, vol. 3, 199, in his life of Domenico Gargiulo.

54. Bissell 1999, 267 no. 38.

55. Ibid., 85; Ryley Marshall 1993, 153–55 nos. vc-55, vc-56; Sestieri (in Sestieri and Daprà 1994, 91–92 nos. 21, 22) attributes these two works to a collaboration among Gargiulo, Codazzi, and Artemisia.

56. Bissell 1999, 84.

57. Contini in Florence 1991, 113.

58. Percy in Cleveland–Forth Worth–Naples 1984–85, 110–13 nos. 30, 31 (American ed.), 120–22 nos. A.21, A.22a–d (Italian ed.).

59. See Bissell 1999, 267–69 no. 39, for a critical history of the painting, which he attributes to Artemisia with the likely collaboration of Cavallino.

60. See ibid., 287–92 no. 49, for a critical history of the painting, which Bissell attributes to a collaboration between Artemisia and Cavallino.

61. Lattuada in Naples 1997–98, 150–69.

62. Bissell 1999, 245–47 no. 30.

63. Schütze and Willette 1992, 38, colorpl. X, 199 no. A28, 295, fig. 141.

64. Fassò 1956, 169–75, verses 840–1005.

65. "Pallidi sono certamente i personaggi maschili, in ispecie Mirtillo e Silvio, ma non le figure femminili, Amarilli, Dorinda, Corisca: delineate, le due prime, con la finezza e la sicurezza di tocco che nasce dalla conoscenza dell'animo muliebre, incisa, la terza, con uno scaltro bulino che ne ha fatto una vera creazione. Corisca, la lusingatrice cinica ed esperta, che proclama senza veli il suo sensuale ardore, e pur sa elevarlo al grado di passione, e che poi, delusa, riesce sì a vendicarsi con la calunnia e con l'inganno, ma anche sa redimersi da ultimo davanti alla felicità che l'amato raggiunge. Corisca, dico, è la figura più felice della tragicommedia, e prelude, con la sua complessità psicologica, al dramma moderno. La scena in cui beffa il Satiro brutale è stata definita, a ragione, la più perfetta del dramma; ma si può aggiungere che tutte le volte che Corsica è in scena il poeta drammatico fa le sue prove migliori." Ibid., xiv.

66. Garrard 1989.

67. Vsevolozhskaia and Linnik 1975, colorpl. 72; Vsevolozhskaia and Kostenevich 1984, 250 n. 143; Schütze and Willette 1992, 213 no. A55, 323, fig. 194.

68. Schütze and Willette 1992, 213.

69. Bissell 1999, 284–85 no. 48a.

70. Lattuada 2000, 202–3 no. E26, colorpl. E26.

71. Ibid., 232–33 nos. E52, E53, colorpl. E53.

72. Ibid., 179–81, colorpl. E9.

73. Schütze and Willette 1992, 213 no. A56.1, 322, fig.192; Lattuada 2000, 281–83 no. G69.

74. See Lattuada 1991, for a preliminary catalogue of Pacecco de Rosa's work.

75. Leone de Castris in Naples 1994–95, 96–101 nn. 47–49, 104–7 nn. 51–52.

76. De Dominici 1742–44, vol. 2, 241.

77. Bologna in Salerno 1954–55, 64 n. 2; see Lattuada 2000, 272–73, for a summary of the bibliography for these two works.

78. Causa 1972, 956 n. 81.

79. Bologna in Naples 1991, 162–64 no. 142, fig. 147, 145–48, figs. 150–57.

80. Causa 1993.

81. Lattuada 2000, 271–72 no. G42, with earlier bibliography.

82. De Dominici 1742–44, vol. 3, 96–100. The doubts about the circumstances of the artist's death are conspicuous.

83. Novelli 1989.

84. De Dominici 1742–44, vol. 3, 97.

85. Salvatori 1999, an essay which is also useful for its numerous references to Artemisia Gentileschi.

72.

Annunciation

Oil on canvas, 101 1/8 × 70 1/2 in.
(257 × 179 cm)

Signed (at lower right):
Aertemitia Gentilischa F:1630

Museo di Capodimonte, Naples
(inv. Q375)

1630

PROVENANCE: Francesco
Saverio di Rovette, Naples
(until 1815); Museo di
Capodimonte, Naples.

REFERENCES: Bissell 1968, 158–
59 n. 50; Greer 1979, 199, 200;
Gregori in Naples 1984–85, 147–
50; Stoughton 1985, 193–94;
Garrard 1989, 91, 92, fig. 92;
Contini in Florence 1991, 65;
Düsseldorf–Darmstadt 1995–
96, 162–63; Bissell 1999, 56–57,
233–34 no. 24.

Signed and dated 1630, this picture must serve as the standard for understanding Artemisia's early Neapolitan career. We don't know when the artist first arrived in Naples. On August 24, 1630, she posted a letter from Naples to Cassiano dal Pozzo in Rome. She may have been invited to Naples by Fernando Enríquez Afán de Ribera, third duke of Alcalá, as Garrard has posited, or gone there with expectations of further patronage from the duke, as Bissell (1999) has suggested. Given Alcalá's earlier interest in her work (he purchased three pictures from her in Rome, a *Penitent Magdalene* [cat. 68], *Christ Blessing the Children* [private collection, Rome; fig. 132]), and a *David with a Harp* [untraced]), it is highly plausible that he played a role in her decision to relocate to Naples.[1] In a second letter to Dal Pozzo dated a week later, Artemisia notes that she hopes to come to Rome soon to serve him but that she is currently working on some pictures for "the Empress."[2] Bissell (1999) conjectures that the artist must have arrived in Naples considerably earlier than August 1630 if she was already contemplating her departure. Indeed, her studio must have been set up, and we know that by August she was producing paintings for patrons. Her arrival can therefore be placed sometime in 1629 or early 1630, and the *Annunciation* may be among her earliest productions.

In a darkened interior, the angel Gabriel arrives amid a flourish of sumptuous gold and rose drapery and announces to the Virgin Mary that she will bear the son of God. Gabriel's words (as recounted in Luke 1:35), "[T]he power of the Highest shall overshadow thee," are made manifest in the image that Artemisia has created, as the splendor of the heavenly apparition overwhelms the humble clothing, paler tonality, and downcast gaze of the Virgin. Gabriel's left arm, dramatically thrust toward the descending dove, reinforces the angelic message, and a lily, symbol of the Virgin's purity, is emblematic of her celibacy and the exceptional nature of her pregnancy. Mary greets Gabriel with her left hand extended while she holds her right hand to her breast, in an expression of submission and maternity; Artemisia had used the same gesture in the Pitti *Conversion of the Magdalene* (cat. 58), and a somewhat more emphatic version adds dramatic tension to the Milan *Lucretia* (cat. 67).

The composition may have been inspired by an altarpiece completed in 1584 by Federico Barocci for the Della Rovere chapel in the basilica of Loreto. A kneeling Gabriel who looks up toward the kneeling Virgin is not a format typical of representations of the Annunciation, and this one may have been based on Barocci's design, which he repeated in an etching (fig. 139). The similar color scheme suggests that Artemisia may have known the altarpiece itself; it is

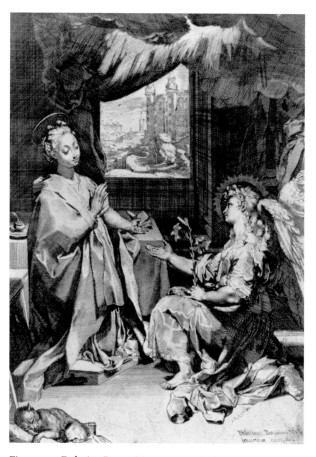

Figure 139. Federico Barocci (ca. 1535–1612), *Annunciation*. Etching. Saint Louis Art Museum

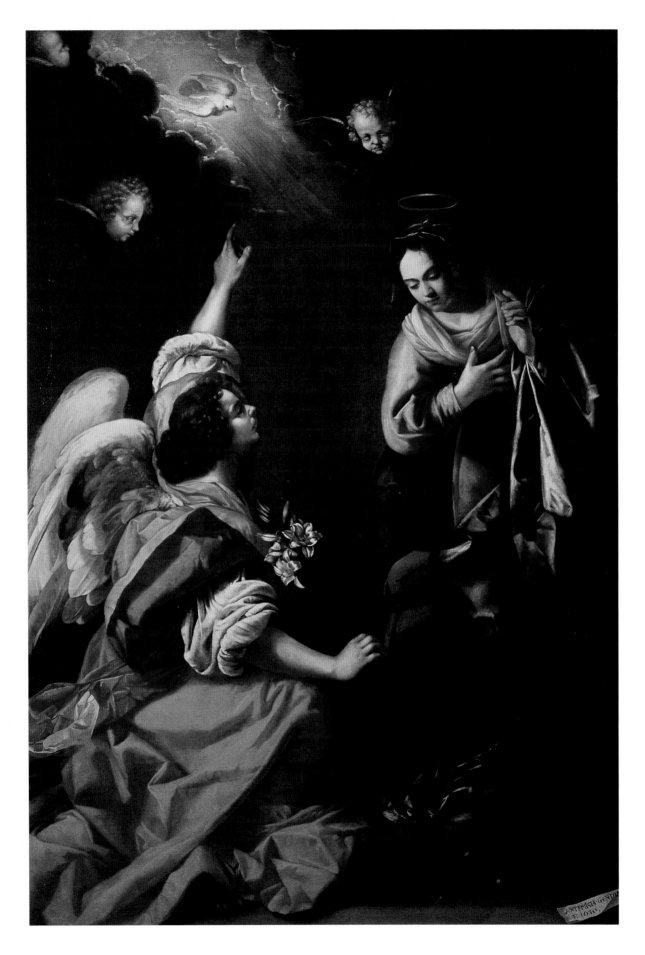

possible that she visited Loreto (a popular pilgrimage site) during her Venetian trip in 1627–28.

The painting's traditional iconography, and its sensitive and quiet tone, has made it less popular than her other work among art historians, but as it may have been commissioned for a Neapolitan church, these aspects would have been appropriate to the setting. Bissell (1968) first posited that it was a church altarpiece, although his suggestion that it was the unidentified painting by Artemisia mentioned in an order for removal from San Giorgio de' Genovesi in 1811 is not tenable, as he himself has acknowledged, since the altarpiece for that church, by Domenico Fiasella, is in situ, as it has been since it was installed.

Its newly cleaned state may help to revise our understanding of Artemisia's Neapolitan career. She uses, to some degree, a more Caravaggesque presentation, evident in the intense light and shadow and the convincing representation of the Virgin's gesturing left hand. A number of scholars have noted (Whitfield, Gregori, Bissell 1999) that it may have been a climate more receptive to Caravaggism that led Artemisia to relocate to Naples, although her art of the 1620s is not necessarily marked by a total embrace of Caravaggio's style. Contini describes the painting as exemplifying a new style, and in many ways it does augur some characteristics of the artist's manner of the next decade; its looser, sometimes cursory handling of paint reappears in other works of the 1630s, most notably the *Clio* (cat. 75). Artemisia is already demonstrating the interest in lavish coloration and decorative drapery treatment that has been associated with the second period of her Neapolitan career. Bissell (1999) posits that this decorative richness may derive from a renewed acquaintance with Florentine art during the late 1620s, although some elements of the florid drapery style may have been influenced by her Roman experience; Gabriel's rich costume calls to mind some of the last works created by Simon Vouet before he departed Rome to return to Paris, as Gregori has noted. The handling of the angel's drapery also recalls a painting that Artemisia may have known while she still lived in Rome; in 1627, prior to leaving for Venice, Vouet painted *Time Vanquished by Hope, Love, and Beauty* (Prado, Madrid), in which animated garments cling to the bodies of the female protagonists and the figure of Venus is encircled by a band of drapery painted in the same color scheme as Gabriel's sash. And Gabriel's open left hand may have been inspired by the airborne angel in Caravaggio's *Seven Acts of Mercy* (Pio Monte della Misericordia, Naples), an altarpiece that had profound impact on Neapolitan artists of the early seventeenth century. During the decade of the 1630s, Artemisia seems to combine this interest in rich color and bold decorative effects with an often intense naturalism and the use of dramatically selective lighting to meet the demands, in at least this case, of imagery especially suitable for religious devotion.

1. The *Christ Blessing the Children* was in the collection of The Metropolitan Museum of Art until 1979, when it was sold at Sotheby's, New York, to a collector in Italy; see Lattuada, pp. 380–81.

2. The letter, translated into English, is reprinted in Garrard 1989, 377–78.

73.

Penitent Magdalene

Oil on canvas, 25¾ × 19¾ in.
(65.7 × 50.8 cm)

Private collection

ca. 1630–32

PROVENANCE: Sale, Los Angeles (mid-1970s); private collection.

REFERENCES: Bissell 1999, 208–9 no. 9; Mormando 1999, 119–20; Papi 2000, 450–52.

One of the newest additions to the oeuvre of Artemisia Gentileschi, this picture was first identified by Burton Fredericksen in the 1980s. It was published by Bissell in his recent catalogue raisonné, but has not as yet had the scholarly vetting that many other attributions have received. Papi has also expressed support for the picture. Several stylistic features argue persuasively for attribution to Artemisia, including the physiognomy (particularly the mouth and nose), hand gesture, and somewhat muted palette of ochre and pale rose. Especially when viewed together with the Naples *Annunciation* (cat. 72), this picture must be accepted as having been produced by the same hand.

Like the scenes from the life of Mary Magdalene—at the Crucifixion, at Christ's tomb after the Resurrection, the drying of Christ's feet with her hair—single images of the saint were also widely produced in seventeenth-century Italy. Guido Reni, or his studio, may have executed as many as fifteen such pictures, while there are over twenty attributed to Guercino. Most of these pictures show a half-length figure of the Magdalene, with her hand held against her chest and either gazing heavenward or with her eyes downcast, and surrounded by objects of meditation—a book, a human skull, a crucifix (the *Golden Legend* tells us that her meditational focus was Christ's Passion). These images were, for the devout, simple aids to contemplation, a function reflected in a popular devotional treatise published in 1611 by the Capuchin preacher Michelangelo da Venezia: "Who will ever be able to express fully the happiness of that soul who, imitating the glorious Magdalene, gives himself to the meditative life and with a burning spirit, through the practice of elevated contemplation, desires and procures for himself union with the sweet and beloved Jesus?"[1]

Whereas Artemisia's first representation of the Magdalene focuses on the saint's vigorous renunciation of sin and turn to contemplation (cat. 58), this later image focuses on the final, meditational period of her life, when she lived as a hermit in a grotto near Sainte-Baume, in France. Alone in a dark setting, she places her right hand on her breast and her left on the skull lying before her, gestures that refer to the dual stages of her life, her early devotion to sensual pleasures and her later renunciation of worldly vanity.

The similarity in the gesture of her right hand and that of the Virgin in the Naples *Annunciation* may not be simply stylistic but may indicate an intended association of the Magdalene with her namesake, the Virgin Mary, based on a perception of her as the "other" Mary, whose sin, though forgiven, made her a more appropriate model for those in search of redemption.[2]

Bissell has suggested placing the *Penitent Magdalene* in Artemisia's Florentine period, comparing the head of the Magdalene with Judith in the Naples *Judith Slaying Holofernes* (cat. 55) and the "rosy complexion, small bow mouth, and dimpled chin" with those of figures in other paintings, including the *Self-Portrait as a Female Martyr* (cat. 56), the Pitti *Conversion of the Magdalene* (cat. 58), and the *Allegory of Inclination* (fig. 110). However, the Naples Judith has more highly defined cheekbones, smaller eyes, and a sharper nose, while the general configuration and physiogomy, pose, and expressive nature of the Magdalene are more in accordance with Artemisia's Neapolitan paintings. The similarity of Mary Magdalene to the Virgin Annunciate in the Naples painting, dated 1630, offers strong support for a dating of about 1630–32, and, when examined in the context of Artemisia's other images of the Penitent Magdalene (cat. nos. 58, 68), demonstrates the more pious, conservative turn that can be observed in her work after she relocated to Naples around 1630. Papi has also endorsed placing the picture among the Neapolitan works.

Artemisia may have been familiar with a version of a nearly identical composition by the Florentine painter Lodovico Cardi (Il Cigoli), who completed a painting of the Penitent Magdalene in Rome about 1610 (fig. 140). The two pictures share not only composition

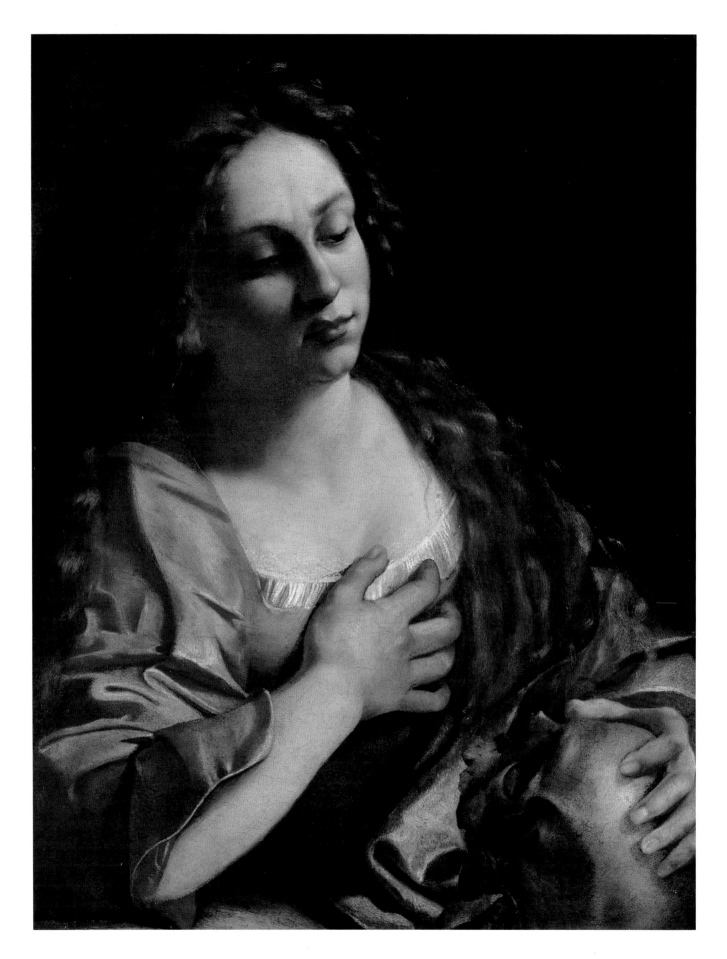

but also the Magdalene's hair treatment, her focus on a skull in the lower right, and her contemplative demeanor. Cigoli's painting, however, displays a more sumptuous detailing of the dress and chemise, and Mary appears made up—both features one expects from a Florentine painter in the early years of the seicento. Cigoli's painting, though similar in external form, demonstrates how far removed Artemisia's *Magdalene* is from the sensibility of early-seventeenth-century Florentine painting.

1. Mormando 1999.
2. The contemporary theologian Francis of Sales notes this association between the Magdalene and the Virgin Mary when he says that they were both vehicles for prayer in his sermon for the Feast of Saint Mary Magdalene, delivered on July 22, 1621. He discusses the two Marys in these terms, writing, "It is these two grand queens, your mistresses and protectresses, which you should know [,] the sacred Virgin Mary your Mother, and Mary Magdalene, who are both named Mary"; in Sales 1892, 96.

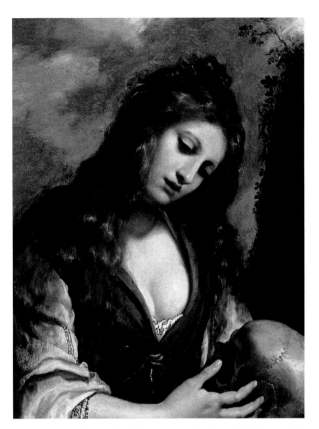

Figure 140. Lodovico Cigoli (1599–1613), *Penitent Magdalene.* Oil on canvas. Cassa di Risparmio di San Miniato

74.

Corisca and the Satyr

Oil on canvas, 61 × 82 ⅝ in. (155 × 210 cm)

Signed (on a tree at right): ARTIMISIA / GENTILES / CHI.

Private collection

1630–35

A recent addition to Artemisia's oeuvre, this painting was unknown until 1989, when Novelli published it as an Annella de Rosa of the 1630s. The painting appeared at auction the following year and entered a private collection, where it remains today. Identified by Garrard as "the kind of narrative that seems to have appealed to Artemisia," this picture does indeed portray a heroine who outwits her male tormentor. The subject is based on a popular play originally published in the late sixteenth century, Giovanni Battista Guarini's *Il pastor fido*, a work that,

as Garrard notes, was usually read rather than performed. The particular scene that Artemisia has depicted is from act 2, scene 6, in which a lustful satyr pursues the nymph Corisca and finally catches her, holding fast to her hair. A struggle ensues, and Corisca emerges the victor, as she is wearing a hairpiece that eventually ends up in the hand of the satyr, allowing her to escape.

Using standard visual language to represent triumph, Artemisia portrays a running Corisca, a majestic figure whose richly colored golden gown and rose-colored

PROVENANCE: Private collection, Naples (1989; sale, Christie's, Rome, March 8, 1990, lot 129, as by Massimo Stanzione); private collection.

REFERENCES: Longhi 1916, 308; Novelli 1989, 149, 151–52; Rocco in Naples 1991–92, 326 no. 2.97; Garrard 1993, 34–38; Bissell 1999, 245–47 no. 30.

cape offer some of the most beautiful passages of drapery that the artist ever painted. She towers above the kneeling and defeated satyr, rubbing her head where the hairpiece has been dislodged. The composition is a masterly achievement, aligned along an extended diagonal arc from the satyr's left arm, through his torso, head, and right arm, and beyond Corisca's billowing cape (see also Lattuada pp. 386–87).

Garrard argues that the subject represents Artemisia's gendered interpretation of the story, seeing in Corisca not the more prevalent example of a wily and deceiving female (in the play she is lustful and immoral) but rather the "bold woman who wrought havoc in Arcadia and got away with it." She suggests that Artemisia perceives Corisca's situation as parallel to her own sexual history. Bissell questions this identification by the artist with the nymph, noting that the viewer would undoubtedly have been aware of the negative connotations of the heroine and not found in her a positive model of resistance to male oppression. Indeed, it remains difficult to judge Artemisia's intent in the *Corisca* until the circumstances of patronage are known. Bissell is certainly correct in his assertion that it must have been made on commission, especially given how seldom the story seems to have inspired visual representation; extant paintings are overwhelmingly Northern; few Italian examples exist. Artemisia seems to have stayed very close to the details of the story, dressing Corisca in the gown and open-toed buskins that the satyr had earlier stolen for her. Scholars are still not certain of Artemisia's education and the extent of her knowledge of contemporary literature. It would thus seem far more likely that a patron requested the subject rather than Artemisia's having selected it on her own.

The painting has been generally dated to the 1630s, with Rocco placing it in the first two years of the decade, while Bissell dates it to about 1633–35. Garrard

assigns it to the second Neapolitan period, during the early 1640s. A date in the early 1630s seems warranted. Both Bissell and Rocco note the similarities between Corisca's gown and the sumptuous drapery and palette of the angel Gabriel in the 1630 *Annunciation* (cat. 72). A similar association can also be made to the clothing in the *Esther Before Ahasuerus* (cat. 71). Bissell points to the Riberesque character of the satyr, likening it to the satyr in the Prado *Ixion*, and reiterates the relationship of Stanzione in the figure of Corisca. Rocco was the first to note an echo of Simon Vouet in the naturalistic yet simplified rendering of Corisca's head. Certainly Artemisia maintained a close relationship with Vouet during the 1620s in Rome, and similarities can be detected in a number of their works. Vouet's 1633 etching the *Holy Family with a Bird*, made in Paris, features a woman with a profile not unlike that of Corisca.[1] Corisca's pose can also be compared with that of Guido Reni's Dejanira in his *Nessus and Dejanira* (Louvre, Paris), painted around 1621 in Bologna for the duke of Mantua. It seems hard to believe that Artemisia was not familiar with this figure in some form—although we do not know that she saw it in either Mantua or Bologna, and the painting was not engraved until the 1660s—but the advancing pose of the nymph, with her left foot forward as she turns back to look over her shoulder, echoes the pose of Dejanira in Reni's work.[2] Other scholars have also noted Reni's apparent influence on Artemisia, beginning with Roberto Longhi's pioneering article of 1916.[3]

1. For the etching, see Crelly 1962, 231 no. 161, fig. 50.
2. Artemisia's *Aurora* (fig. 96), dating probably to the 1620s (Bissell 1999, no. 15), demonstrates the same free and expressive approach, where a female figure is posed so that it charges the surrounding space—another instance in which Artemisia took Reni's work as her model.
3. Longhi 1916, 308.

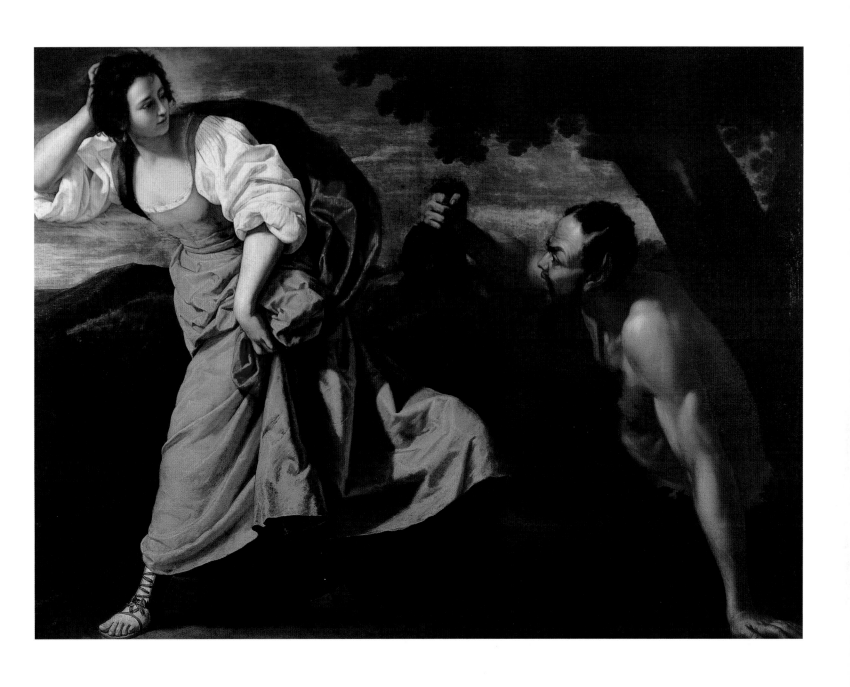

75.
Clio, Muse of History

Oil on canvas, 50 × 38⅜ in.
(127 × 97.5 cm)

Signed (in book): [1]632 /
ARTEMISIA / [F]aciebat / All
[?] illstr mo isg [nre] tr [in
monogram] osier [s?]

Private collection

1632

PROVENANCE: Oswald T.
Falk, Oxford; C. R. Churchill,
Colemore, Alton, Hampshire;
London and New York art mar-
kets (since 1943); Arcade
Gallery, London (1955);
Sotheby's, London, February
26, 1958, lot 55; Wildenstein
(1958); private collection (1997).

REFERENCES: Fröhlich-Bume
1940, 169; Harris in Los Angeles
1976–77, 122; Gregori in Naples
1984–85, 147; Garrard 1989, 92–
96, 384, 514 n. 191, figs. 84, 85;
Florence 1991, 66, 84 nn. 14, 15,
165 n. 24, 67, fig. 50; Rowlands
in New York 1995–96, no. 2;
Bissell 1999, 239–41 no. 27, 367
under no. L-30.

Signed and prominently dated, this painting was unquestionably made during the early years of the artist's first stay in Naples. A statuesque woman dressed in a bluish green mantle with richly textured rust-colored sleeves worn over a lace-edged linen chemise stands with her left hand on her hip and her right hand resting on a trumpet. She wears a crown of laurel leaves, and to her right lies an open book with a legible inscription. Garrard, Bissell, and Rowlands have reconstructed the inscription as "1632 Artemisia faciebat all'Illustre M., smemorato Rosiers / 1632" (1632 Artemisia made this for the Illustrious M., in memory of Rosiers /1632). These scholars have related it to the fourth duke of Guise, Charles of Lorraine (1571–1640), who ruled Lorraine in the sixteenth and seventeenth centuries and employed as maître d'hôtel a nobleman named Antoine de Rosières, who died in 1631. We know that Artemisia worked for the duke of Guise, since she wrote in a letter on October 9, 1635, to the astronomer Galileo Galilei that the duke had paid her 200 *piastre* for a painting.[1] The Rosières of the inscription, however, is more likely to have been François de Rosières (1534–1607), who had been under the protection of the cardinal of Guise and had written a history of the duchy that traced its origins to the time of Charlemagne. Based on spurious sources, the work so offended Henry III that he imprisoned Rosières in the Bastille; he was released—in 1583— only on the intervention of the duke of Guise. It is likely, as Bissell suggests, that in commemoration of the twenty-fifth anniversary of Rosières's death in 1607, the duke commissioned a work in his honor.

How the duke came to commission the painting from Artemisia is unknown, although the fact that she mentions payment for the work in her letter to Galileo may be a clue. We do know that the duke requested and received permission to leave France in 1631. Guise had supported Marie de' Medici in her dispute with her son Louis XIII, and in so doing had roused the ire of the powerful Cardinal Richelieu. By applying for permission and undertaking a pilgrimage to Loreto, an important religious site, the duke in essence escaped to Italy. He later moved to Tuscany to take up permanent residence. In Tuscany, he may have met Galileo, who, in turn, referred him to the services of his friend Artemisia Gentileschi.

Previously known under the title *Fame,* this painting may have been altered by the artist to represent Clio. Cesare Ripa's 1625 edition of the *Iconologia* describes Clio, the Muse of History, as carrying a book and a trumpet and wearing a laurel crown, all elements of this portrayal. The attributes of Fame also include a trumpet, but the figure usually has wings, holds an olive branch, and wears a gold chain with a heart pendant. Recent cleaning has revealed the presence of wings in an earlier version (visible in the darkened areas at the shoulders), and it appears that the figure's left hand may once have held an olive branch.

The prominent signature may be Artemisia's own gloss on the notion of celebrity. The chief attribute of Fame is the book into which the names of noted individuals are recorded. Clio is usually depicted carrying a closed book, but Artemisia may have included an open book in her original rendition, one that she later retained when she changed the iconography. Artemisia has not only inscribed the name of Rosières, to whom the painting is dedicated and the patron's honoree; she has also signed the picture herself, thereby entering her own name into the book of Fame. The placement of the book, open for both Clio and the viewer to read, establishes a more interactive relationship between the viewer and the subject, whose statuesque pose and distant gaze do not otherwise invite the viewer's approach. In a similar reading, Garrard notes that the three-way relationship between Clio, Rosières, and the artist is, in effect, a commentary on the Renaissance notion of the pivotal role of the artist in the establishment of fame, while Hersey maintains that the picture serves as evidence that Artemisia was concerned about her own fame.

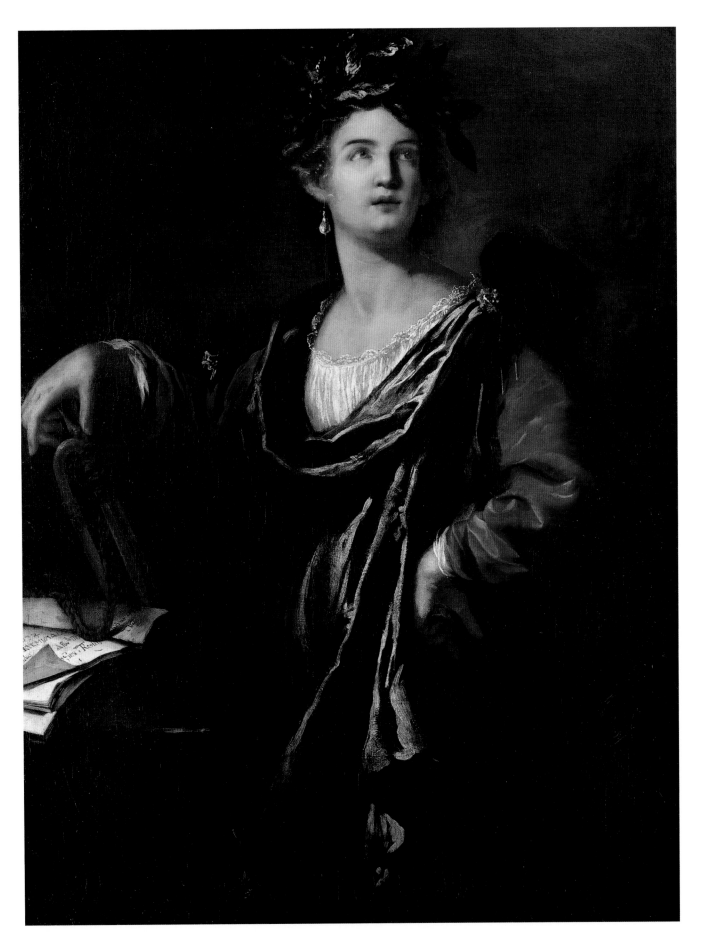

The relationship of this picture to a citation in a seventeenth-century inventory of the English royal collection has yet to be sorted out. Abraham van der Doort, the keeper of pictures and antiquities to Charles I, recorded a similar painting by Artemisia, "Done by Artemesio Gentellesco Item a woemans picture in some bluish draperie . . . with a trumpett in her left hand Signifying ffame with her other hand having a penn to write being uppon a Straining frame painted uppon Cloath. Hight 3 f 3–Breadth 2 f 5." Inventory descriptions are notoriously inaccurate, but the absence of a pen in the present painting and the discrepancy in size between the two pictures have led scholars to discount the inventoried painting as being the same as the *Clio*. Garrard and Fröhlich-Bume have suggested that the inventory entry describes a reduced copy.

The dark tonality of the picture, in which velvety rust complements a cooler dark green, lends a somber air to the statuesque figure. Harris comments on the "bravura" handling of paint, most clearly evident in the freedom and surety with which the edges of the green drapery and folds along the shoulder have been defined. The tighter, more meticulous technique of many of Artemisia's paintings executed in the 1620s (the *Portrait of a Gonfaloniere* [cat. 66] or the Seville *Penitent Magdalene* [cat. 68], for example) has yielded to a looser, and perhaps more showy, application of paint.

The picture sustained some damage when it was first transferred to an oak panel in the eighteenth century. It was returned to a canvas support prior to the 1976 "Women Artists" exhibition and now displays surface cracking. It is trimmed along the left side.

1. The original letter can be found in the Biblioteca Nazionale, Florence, Mss. Gal., P.I.T. XIII, car. 269–70. It is published in English translation in Garrard 1989, 383–84.

76.

Cleopatra

Oil on canvas, 46⅛ × 69⅛ in. (117 × 175.5 cm)

Private collection, Rome

ca. 1633–35

PROVENANCE: Matthiesen Fine Art Ltd., London (1982–1988?); private collection, Rome.

REFERENCES: Gregori in Naples 1984–85, 306; Grabski 1985, 56–63; Matthiesen in London 1986, 49–52; Garrard 1989, 105–6, 274–76; Contini in Florence 1991, 70, 73; Bissell 1999, 50, 53, 230–31 no. 22.

In this, perhaps Artemisia's second representation of Cleopatra, the artist is unusually faithful to Plutarch's story. Plutarch recounts the arrival of Octavian's soldiers to find Cleopatra's body. Artemisia has selected the moment just preceding, when the maidservants Charmion and Iras have discovered the deceased queen and have not yet replaced the crown on her head. No evidence of the asp's bite is found on her body. The reclining figure of Cleopatra is tilted forward toward the picture plane and presented invitingly to the viewer. In the background, Iras and Charmion enter the closed chamber. The first maidservant registers no response; the second wipes tears from her eyes. But otherwise, neither shows any visible shock or horror. The jeweled crown and tasseled

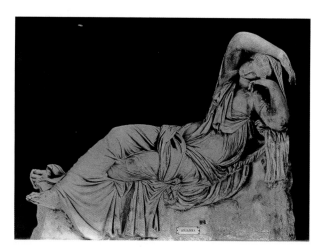

Figure 141. Roman, third century A.D., *Sleeping Ariadne*. Marble. Museo Vaticano

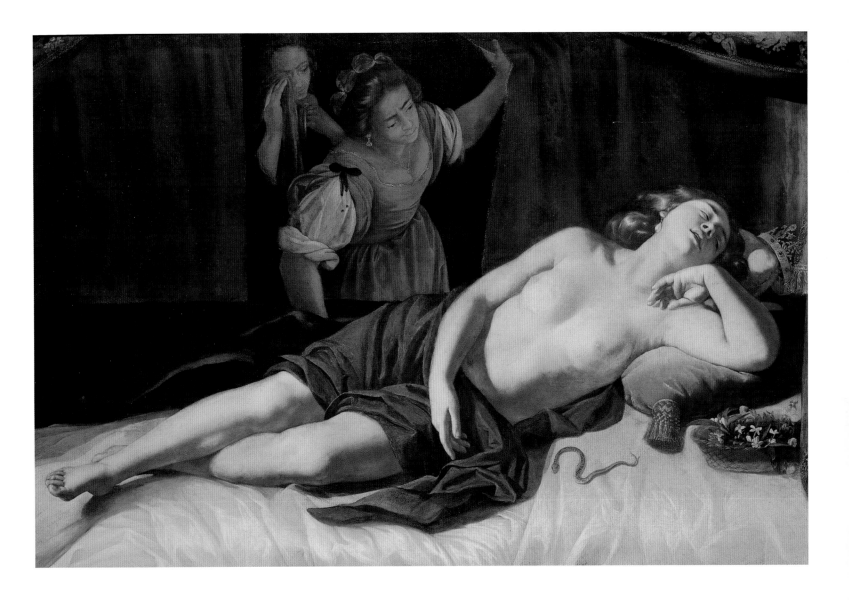

velvet pillow suggest regal adornment, and the fig basket of Plutarch's story has been changed to one of flowers.

Rarely, however, did artists follow the details of the story so closely, and the discovery of Cleopatra (either by Octavian's soldiers or by her own attendants) is seldom isolated for representation. The French artist Jacques Blanchard, whose 1630 painting (Musée des Beaux-Arts, Rheims) portrays Cleopatra discovered by the soldiers, is among the very few. Most painters present Cleopatra as a tormented sexual temptress, placing the serpent (sometimes two) on her bared breast; she is not usually attired in royal garb, and few artists follow Plutarch's description of the snake as biting her arm.

There is general consensus that the original idea for the composition derived either from Orazio's *Penitent Magdalene* (cat. 35), made in Genoa in the early 1620s, or from Claude Mellan's 1629 engraving (which may in turn have been based on Orazio's painting), with which it has a closer formal affinity.[1] Particularly noteworthy is Artemisia's use of the stiffened, slightly unnatural pose to convey the early stages of rigor mortis that have set in, suggesting that Cleopatra's death was indeed a solitary event and that only later was she discovered by her faithful maids. The fallen crown reminds us that Charmion, when discovered later by the Roman soldiers, was in the act of replacing it upon Cleopatra's head. It is very likely that Artemisia intended to refer to the most famous antique image of Cleopatra then in Rome, a sculpted reclining figure now known as the *Sleeping Ariadne* (fig. 141) but believed, in the seventeenth century, to represent the Egyptian queen.

Having been initially attributed to Massimo Stanzione, the *Cleopatra* was first published as by Artemisia by Gregori, and accepted at that time by Schleier, Spinosa, Matthiesen, and Bologna; this attribution has since gained wide acceptance. The painting has been dated by many scholars to Artemisia's first Neapolitan period, the most notable exception being Bissell, who dates it to the 1620s, having found its eroticism more acceptable in the ambience of Rome and Venice than Naples and noting the Titianesque brushwork in the bedclothes. Grabski notes the picture's general Neapolitan character, citing its affinities with Ribera's *Drunken Silenus* (Capodimonte, Naples), as well as its logical placement within the Neapolitan naturalistic tradition, first established by Caravaggio and then carried on in the work of Caracciolo. Furthermore, correspondences exist between this picture and other works that date to Artemisia's first Neapolitan period. Cleopatra's pose, for example, has been compared with that of the foreshortened head in Artemisia's *Esther Before Ahasuerus* (Contini, Gregori, Garrard; cat. 71), as well as to the physiognomy of Saint Nicea in one of the paintings for Pozzuoli cathedral (fig. 143). The conception and execution of Iras and Charmion have been likened to those of the kneeling maid in the Columbus *David and Bathsheba* (cat. 80) and the servant with rolled-up sleeves in the Prado *Birth of Saint John the Baptist* (Garrard; cat. 77). The similarity in expressive tone between the *Cleopatra* and Ribera's 1637 *Pietà* (Certosa di San Martino, Naples) reinforces the argument that it was made in Naples rather than Rome.

Artemisia places the two maids directly at the center of the composition, and contrasts the rich blue of Cleopatra's drapery against the muted ochre coloration of Charmion's dress. This combination of colors also marks the Columbus *David and Bathsheba* and the Toledo *Lot and His Daughters* (cat. 78), and the carefully balanced composition fits in well with other paintings of the middle years of the 1630s. While many works from the 1620s are now lost, surviving examples testify to an artist who is still drawn to Baroque drama and compositional majesty (both absent here), evident in the Seville *Penitent Magdalene* (cat. 68) as well as in the Detroit *Judith and Her Maidservant* (cat. 69).

Garrard suggests that by replacing the basket of figs with a basket of flowers, Artemisia introduces the idea of rebirth, recalling Cleopatra's association with the Egyptian earth goddess, Isis. While Artemisia seems to have been well aware of a broad range of visual traditions that she continually introduces into her works—she may even have read some of the literary texts herself—we have little evidence to suggest that she was acquainted with the broader associations and metaphoric allusions of her protagonists.

The canvas is in generally good condition. The blue in the heroine's drapery has had some chemical interaction, and darkening in the shadows has eliminated the original sense of background space. There has been some loss in the glazing of Cleopatra's skin.

1. Bissell (1999, 230) argues that the pose is based primarily on Mellan's print, which is in turn based on a lost Roman work by Orazio. Matthiesen mentions only Artemisia's use of her father's image. Scholars who maintain that Artemisia used both the print and her father's painting include Contini and Gregori.

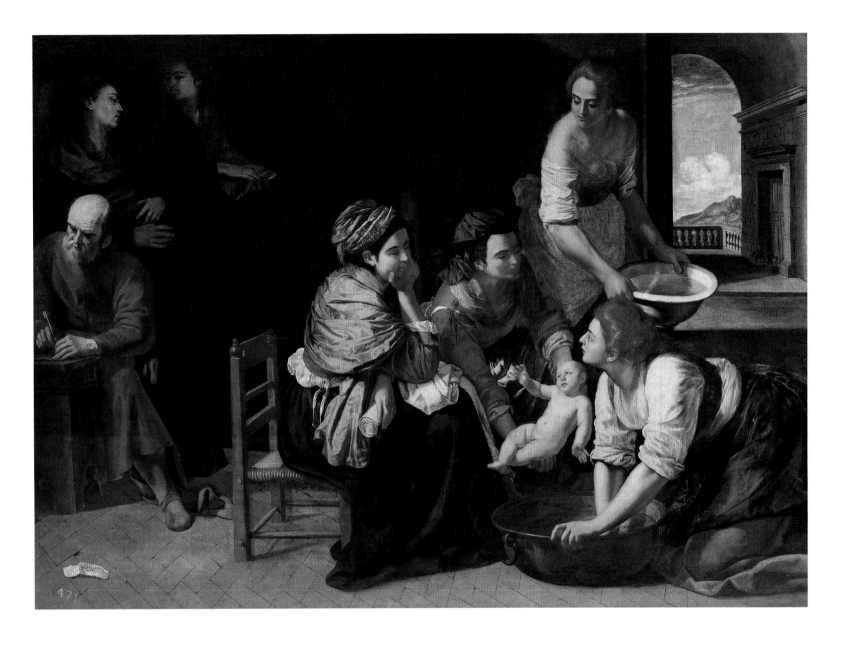

77.

Birth of Saint John the Baptist

Oil on canvas, 72½ × 101⅝ in.
(184 × 258 cm)

Signed (on piece of paper at lower
left): ARTEMITIA / GINTILES

Museo Nacional del Prado,
Madrid (inv. P149)

ca. 1633–35

Rome, New York

The story of John the Baptist is told in Luke 1:5–80. The priest Zacharias and his wife, Elizabeth, are old and childless. While Zacharias is performing his service in the temple, the angel Gabriel appears and tells him that his wife will bear him a son. Incredulous, Zacharias asks Gabriel how he could know such a thing and the angel, angered that Zacharias does not believe him, strikes him dumb. When the child is born, the neighbors and midwives announce that he will

be called Zacharias, after his father. But Elizabeth protests, and names him John. Because no one in the family bore that name, the midwives appeal to the mute Zacharias, who motions for a writing tablet to be brought to him; upon the tablet, he inscribes the words "His name is John."

Artemisia has followed a formula in use at least since the eleventh century for the representation of this scene from the life of Saint John.[1] On the left, the elderly

Elizabeth reclines on her bed, attended by a servant, while in front of her Zacharias writes the words of the naming. The central focus, however, is the group of midwives who tend to the bathing and swaddling of the infant. This emphasis on the bath and its implication of ritual is not unlike that found in most images of the birth of the Virgin Mary, a subject with a similar representational tradition. It is appropriate for an event with a popular feast day and undoubtedly alludes to the role of Saint John in the baptizing of Christ.

The painting is one of a series of six pictures. The Neapolitan painter Massimo Stanzione made four of them, the *Annunciation to Zacharias, Saint John Taking Leave of His Parents* (fig. 133), *Saint John Preaching*, and the *Beheading of Saint John* (all Prado, Madrid), while another Neapolitan artist, Paolo Finoglia, painted the sixth scene, now missing, *Saint John in Prison*. It remains uncertain if the event of primary importance in John's life, the Baptism, was included in the cycle. If so, as Bissell (1999) and Vannugli argue, it was probably an earlier painting integrated into the group.

Ever since Roberto Longhi wrote of the painting's effective re-creation of a domestic interior, in his pivotal article of 1916, it has generally been acknowledged to be an important example of Artemisia's Caravaggesque, tenebrist leanings. The figures appear to emerge out of darkened shadows, although the poor state of preservation perhaps intensifies this sense of chiaroscuro. Details of the floor tiles, the simple furniture, and the fabric textures add to the sense of observed individuals performing everyday tasks. Andrea Sacchi, who depicted the same scene in the early 1640s for the baptistry of the church of San Giovanni in Laterano in Rome, represented Zacharias with a heavenward gaze, confronted by gesturing onlookers who respond to the divine intervention. No such acknowledgment of the miraculous appearance of Gabriel can be found in Artemisia's picture.

Garrard notes evidence of her reliance on the prototypes of Simon Vouet, whose *Circumcision of Christ* (Capodimonte, Naples) arrived in Naples in the 1620s, and Artemisia undoubtedly knew Vouet's heavily Caravaggesque *Birth of the Virgin* in the Roman church of San Francesco a Ripa. Vouet's realism and dramatic illumination combined with a carefully

balanced composition and classical figural style come close to Artemisia's *Saint John*, since her naturalist conception has been tempered by a beautifully composed and balanced figural grouping and some of her most accomplished figures, such as the kneeling maid at the right. The beautifully realized tactility of the midwife's shawl combines a naturalist tendency in the rendition of texture and surface with a growing interest in the representation of opulent fabrics and richly appointed interiors.

Pérez Sánchez notes that Artemisia's naturalism is tempered with the influence of classicism, a phenomenon that emerges in much Neapolitan painting of the 1630s, while Vannugli describes the picture as a transitional work, between the Caravaggism and drama of Artemisia's paintings of the 1620s and her more elegant later works, which responded to Bolognese classicism. It has been noted, by Garrard and Bissell (1999), that Artemisia attempted to conform stylistically to the work of Stanzione, and indeed the physiognomies of the pensive maid and the attendant holding the baby are comparable. The biographer Bernardo de Dominici, writing in the eighteenth century, describes a close relationship between the two painters, and mentions that Artemisia was mentor to the older Stanzione. While De Dominici's assertion may not be altogether accurate (see Lattuada, p. 384), Garrard's observation that the two artists "appear to have met each other halfway in the interest of creating a harmonious ensemble" must certainly be correct.[2]

Artemisia's *Saint John* is first mentioned as in the palace of the Buen Retiro in Madrid in the 1650s together with Stanzione's pictures, and is believed to have been commissioned by the king of Spain, Philip IV, for a chapel dedicated to Saint John, though nothing certain is known of such a commission.[3] Artemisia, in a letter written in Naples in July 1635 to Grand Duke Ferdinand II de' Medici, tells her patron that she had to finish "some works" for "His Catholic Majesty" (meaning Philip IV).[4] No other pictures currently known by Artemisia could have been done for him, and most writers concur that the Madrid *Saint John* must be among the pictures to which she refers. We know that the paintings were commissioned in Naples, for in the same letter she says that the

PROVENANCE: Buen Retiro, Ermita de San Juan, Madrid; Palacio del Buen Retiro, Madrid (by the 17th century); Palacio Real Nuevo; Capilla de la Calle del Tesoro, Madrid (by 1772); Museo Nacional del Prado, Madrid (by 1820).

REFERENCES: Longhi 1916, 301; Pérez Sánchez 1965, 394, 452–54, 499; Bissell 1968, 161; Pérez Sánchez in Madrid 1970, 272–73 no. 83, 530–37 nos. 175–78; Brown and Elliott 1980, 67–68, 73 fig. 39, 79, fig. 42, 77, 78, fig. 46, 80–82, 89, 92, 123, 125, 217, 244, 251, 254, 263 n. 52, 264 n. 87, 266 n. 27; Gregori in Naples 1984–85, 304 no. 2.113; von Barghahn 1986, 29, 34, 152, 302, 306–8, 391–99, 447 n. 234, 533 n. 423; Garrard 1989, 97–99, 511 n. 163; Contini in Florence 1991, 67–70, 178; Vannugli 1991, 25–33; Vannugli 1994, 59–73; Bissell 1999, 249–56 no. 32.

viceroy had ordered the pictures on the king's behalf. Several scholars (Brown and Elliott, Gregori, Garrard) have identified this agent as Manuel de Guzmán, count of Monterrey and viceroy to Naples between May 14, 1631, and November 12, 1637.

The date of the commission is still not confirmed, although it has been placed between 1633 and 1635. Bissell (1999) posits that the paintings must have been under way before the artist made her claim of patronage in 1635. And a copy after Stanzione's *Annunciation to Zacharias*, by Francesco Guarino for the church of San Michele at Solofra, was painted in 1637. Paolo Finoglia must have already received his commission, which he presumably completed by 1635, when he departed Naples for Puglia, where he is documented in January 1635 and where he apparently stayed, precluding his having made his painting any later than that date. Garrard, followed by Contini, argues that the paintings must have been finished by 1633 and that they were part of a shipment sent by Monterrey from Naples to Spain in that year. (Monterrey also brought a second shipment with him when he returned in 1638, too late a date for the paintings to have arrived, given that Guarino had access to them in 1637.) Several writers have suggested that the Neapolitan architectural painter Viviano Codazzi must have inspired the open archway in the background of Artemisia's painting. Because he did not arrive in Naples until at least 1633 and is first documented as in the city in January 1634,

if Artemisia did respond to Codazzi's work, she could not have completed the painting before 1634.

Bissell (1999) has suggested that the painting may have been completed by the middle of 1634. He has identified the space in which the cycle was installed as the chapel of the Hermitage of San Juan at the Buen Retiro, begun in the spring of 1633. He submits that the pictures were ordered then and shipped in November, although he acknowledges that it would have been difficult for them all to have been painted so quickly. Evidence that they were completed by 1634 is provided by a couple of factors. Artemisia's letter of July 1635 uses the imperfect tense in mentioning works she had done for the king, suggesting that a period of time had elapsed since she had painted them. Second, other pictures commissioned from Artemisia were finished by January 1635, and Bissell has assumed that the *Saint John* must have been finished well before these paintings were begun. This would mean that it was completed sometime in the earlier part of 1634.

1. For these early traditions, see Réau 1955–58, vol. 1, 443–47.
2. "Vita del Cavalier Massimo Stanzione," in De Dominici (1742–44) 1979, 45, describes how Stanzione went each day to watch Artemisia paint and how he attempted to imitate the "freshness of her beautiful color."
3. For hypothetical reconstructions of how the paintings were originally installed, see Vannugli 1994, 65–69; and Bissell 1999, 251–54. The present discussion of this commission is based largely on these works.
4. For the letter, see Fuda 1989, 170–71.

78.

Lot and His Daughters

Oil on canvas, 90¾ × 72 in.
(230.5 × 183 cm)

The Toledo Museum of Art,
Clarence Brown Fund
(inv. 1983.107)

1635–38

New York, Saint Louis

PROVENANCE: Luigi Romeo,
baron of San Luigi, Naples?;
private collection, Switzerland;
New York art market (1983);
The Toledo Museum of Art.

REFERENCES: De Dominici
(1742–44) 1979, 414–15; Percy in
Cleveland–Fort Worth–Naples
1984–85, 16–17; Spinosa and
Kopelman in Cleveland–Fort
Worth–Naples 1984–85, 107–9
no. 29; Grabski 1985, 23–40;
Stoughton 1985, 194; Garrard
1989, 123, 214–17; Novelli 1989,
152–53; Bologna in Naples 1991–
92, 162; Contini in Florence 1991,
76, 79, 87 n. 86; Stolzenwald
1991, 94, fig. 58; Sestieri in
Sestieri and Daprà 1994, 88;
Bissell 1999, 267–69 no. 39.

The story of Lot and his daughters is told in
Genesis (19:31–36). Following God's destruction
of Sodom and Gomorrah, Lot and his two daughters
flee, seeking refuge first in the town of Zoar and then
in a cave. The daughters, realizing they will have no
opportunity to marry and thus to ensure that their
father will have male descendants, decide that their
only hope is to ply their father with wine and seduce
him. The first night, the older daughter makes her
father drunk and lies with him; the younger daughter
does the same on the second night. Both daughters
become impregnated and give birth to sons.

Visual representations of this story proliferated in
the sixteenth and seventeenth centuries. The subject
offered an opportunity to portray erotic scenes of sensuous carousing, and Lot and his daughters were
often shown in various stages of undress. The Dutch
painter Hendrick Goltzius depicted all three figures
completely nude, and his conception of the scene was
hardly unusual. Seductive poses, strategic caresses,
and suggestive gestures all served to carry the narrative message of the impending incestuous acts.

Artemisia's painting, by contrast, is an exemplar of
restraint and illustrates how compositional grouping
can convey narrative meaning. While Spinosa identifies
the moment depicted as that when the daughters convince their father to drink wine, it is in fact after the act
has been committed, as suggested by his embracing of
his daughter, his less than upright stance, and the glass
in his hand. Garrard has noted in the figure of Lot "a
lack of full expressive definition," which may actually,
with his drowsy gaze, be intended to represent a besot-
ted state. The relationship between Lot and the daughter in yellow is subtly implied through the formal
rhyming of their left legs. The second daughter, who
approaches from the left with a wine jug and places
her hand lightly on her father's shoulder, indicates
that she, too, will soon begin a similar liaison. The
artist, presumably Artemisia Gentileschi, has developed a repertoire of visual devices for suggesting

the similarities of the situation while indicating that
there remain differences in the specific stages of the
incestuous relationships.

The authorship of this picture has been the subject
of much animated debate, triggered in part by the
appearance of the painting in an exhibition devoted
to the work of Bernardo Cavallino, held in 1984–85
and organized by Ann T. Lurie and Ann Percy, where
it was ascribed to Cavallino. In the catalogue, Spinosa
notes that, interestingly, neither Lurie nor Percy
endorses the Cavallino attribution. The work has
been variously given to Antonio de Bellis or Francesco
Guarino (Causa), Agostino Beltrano (Grabski),
Annella de Rosa (Novelli), and Artemisia Gentileschi
(Stoughton, Garrard). Spinosa raises the possibility of
joint authorship, while Bissell assigns the major portion to Artemisia and identifies Cavallino's hand in the
upper part of the figure of Lot. Bissell further suggests
that Domenico Gargiulo painted the landscape. The
Toledo Museum of Art has recently changed the attribution from Cavallino to Artemisia. (On the issue of
collaboration, see Lattuada, pp. 384–86.)

Close affinities between this picture and the
Columbus *David and Bathsheba* (cat. 80) support this
attribution. The two paintings share color harmonies,
and the diaphanous drapery of Lot's daughter on
the right is echoed in the garment worn by one of
Bathsheba's maids. Additionally, the physiognomy of
the kneeling servant in the Columbus painting closely
resembles that of the left-hand daughter in the present
work. Beyond the similarities to the *Bathsheba,* the
painting can be related to other works by Artemisia
from her first Neapolitan period, 1630 to 1638. The
model for the right-hand daughter may also have
been the model for the kneeling servant on the right
in the Madrid *Birth of Saint John the Baptist* (cat. 77).
And the accomplished handling of the texture of the
soft fabric of Lot's mauve shirt is analogous to the same
effect in the dalmatic of Saint Proculus in the *Saint
Januarius in the Amphitheater* (cat. 79).

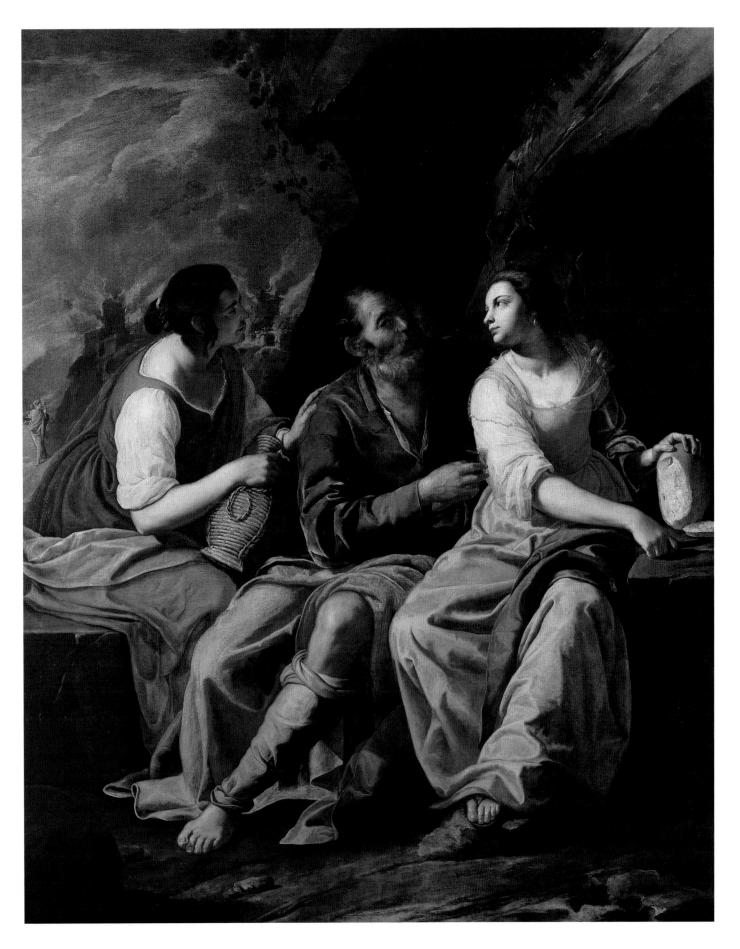

These visual associations have some textual support in an eighteenth-century biography of Neapolitan painters written after 1740. Bernardo de Dominici mentions in his biography of Gargiulo a *Lot and His Daughters* by Artemisia Gentileschi that is discussed together with the *Bathsheba*. While it is not possible to relate this reference definitively to the present picture, the combination of strong affinities to Artemisia's work with this contemporary reference to the painting constitutes persuasive evidence in support of her authorship. To this should be added the anomalous situation that the painting poses within the oeuvre of Cavallino. Grand compositions of relatively large-scale figures are not common in Cavallino's work. While Cavallino may have been influenced by Artemisia's figures, these still find little echo in Cavallino's accepted paintings. Furthermore, and most to the point, the depiction of Lot and the two daughters lacks the dramatic liveliness normally so characteristic of Cavallino, what Stoughton describes as "nervous dynamism."[1] There are two additional versions of the Lot story that

Cavallino painted, which represent radically divergent interpretations. While the Toledo painting exhibits elegant economy in its masterly rendering of a reserved composition, demonstrating the balance and return to classical ideals that is evidenced in Neapolitan painting from the 1630s, the *Lots* that we know Cavallino to have painted (for example, Louvre, Paris) are marked by bawdy carousing and playful eroticism; they are, as Bissell has noted, "ribald and low-life."

The painting is in good condition. The thinly applied pigment, in conjunction with a large proportion of medium to pigment, has resulted in the pink robe on Lot's knee and the lining of the left-hand daughter's skirt having become transparent glazes.

1. Grabski (1985, 25–26) develops this point thoroughly and demonstrates through diagrams that the kind of static composition found in the Toledo *Lot* is not characteristic of Cavallino. Percy also contends that the expressive sense of this *Lot,* its "unenergetic poses and composition," is quite different from the "dynamic, tightly knit organization" found in Cavallino's *Lot* in the Louvre.

79.

Saint Januarius in the Amphitheater

Oil on canvas, 118⅛ × 78¾ in. (300 × 200 cm)

Signed (lower right): Artemi . . . Gentilesc. / F

Museo di Capodimonte, Naples (on deposit from the cathedral at Pozzuoli)

1636–37

PROVENANCE: Cathedral at Pozzuoli (until 1964); Certosa di San Martino, Naples; Museo di Capodimonte, Naples (on deposit from the cathedral at Pozzuoli).

REFERENCES: Longhi (1916) 1961, 264, 277 n. 66; Brunetti 1956, 60, 63 n. 28; Bologna 1958, 127; Scavizzi 1963, 37 n. 26; Moir 1967, vol. 1, 100 n. 105, vol. 2, 74; Bissell 1968, 159–60; Whitfield in London 1982, 148, 166; Gregori in Naples 1984–85, 148, 150; Garrard 1989, 99–104, fig. 100; Stolzenwald 1991, 37, 40, pl. 29; Sestieri and Daprà 1994, 91–92; Bissell 1999, 256–59 no. 33b.

Saint Januarius in the Amphitheater is one of three paintings that Artemisia executed for the cathedral at Pozzuoli, a coastal town approximately seven miles west of Naples, along the bay. By 1631, when Martín de Leòn y Cárdenas was elected bishop of Pozzuoli, the cathedral had fallen into disrepair. Leòn y Cárdenas set out to refurbish the church, signing a contract in 1632. He also undertook the construction of a high altar, which was completed by 1636. Commissions were probably under way before the completion of the building, since one of the artists who contributed to the project, Paolo Finoglia, is documented as having left for Puglia in 1635, and scholars believe he remained there until his death in 1645. As noted in the bishop's report, the *Relatio ad limina* of 1640, eleven of the paintings that formed the decorative program for the choir, including the three canvases by Artemisia, were completed and installed by that date. These paintings, not mentioned in the *Relatio ad limina* of 1635, present scenes from the lives of Christ and the Virgin Mary as well as from the lives of saints who had some particular connection to

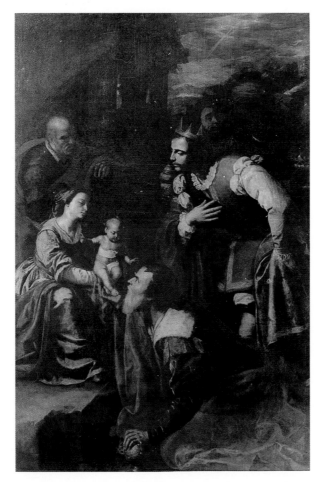

Figure 142. Artemisia Gentileschi, *Adoration of the Magi*. Oil on canvas. Museo Nazionale di San Martino, Naples

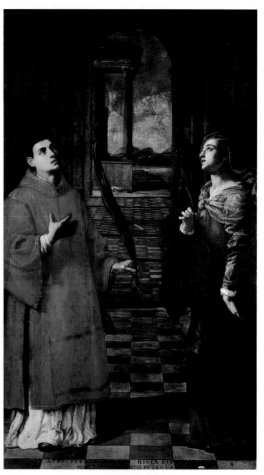

Figure 143. Artemisia Gentileschi. *Saints Proculus and Nicea*. Oil on canvas. Museo e Gallerie Nazionali di Capodimonte, Naples

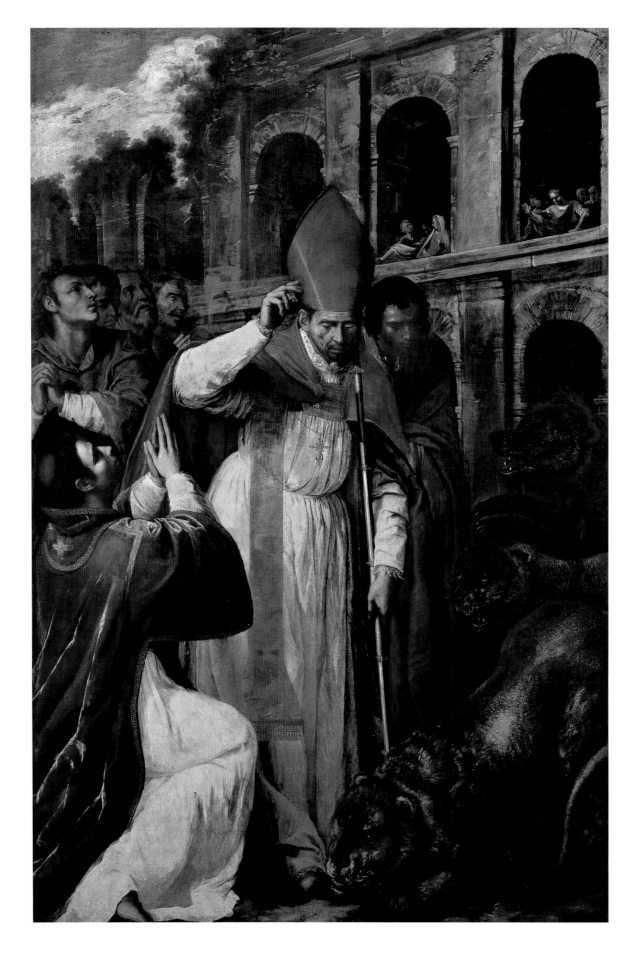

the history of Pozzuoli. In addition to this image of Saint Januarius, Artemisia made a *Saints Proculus and Nicea* (fig. 143) and an *Adoration of the Magi* (fig. 142).

Januarius, the patron saint of Naples, was bishop of Benevento. In the year 305, he returned to his hometown, where with other Christians he was the victim of persecution imposed by the emperor Diocletian. He was accompanied by his deacon, Festus, and five other followers, Proculus, Socius, Desiderius, Eutyches, and Acutius. Timotheus, the ruler of Campania, where Pozzuoli is located, condemned the seven men to death, first by casting them into a fiery furnace and then by throwing them to the lions and bears in the amphitheater. Januarius tamed the animals, which, rather than attacking the Christians, licked their feet and left them unharmed. Timotheus, in a rage, had the men beheaded. Januarius's body was taken to Naples in the fifth century, and although the relics were moved elsewhere in the course of the following centuries, they were ultimately returned to Naples and interred in the cathedral. A vial of the saint's blood, also kept in the cathedral, has since 1389 miraculously liquified on the saint's feast day.

Artemisia has represented Januarius in the Roman amphitheater for which the city of Pozzuoli had become famous. The saint raises his right arm in benediction, making the sign of the cross over the two lions and bear in the lower right, while Proculus, the deacon of Pozzuoli, raises his hands to pray for divine intervention. Most scholars have noted the traditional and conservative composition that Artemisia has chosen. No evidence of the drama of the Detroit *Judith* (cat. 69) or the flair of her assured treatment of Gabriel in the 1630 *Annunciation* (cat. 72) appears here. Rather, she has placed Januarius at the center of the painting and dressed him in a simple cope over a beautifully rendered white linen alb. The iconography for images of Januarius was well established by this time; he is almost always shown wearing the golden bishop's miter seen here, and usually his cope is elaborately embroidered or fashioned from rich damask. Artemisia has opened the cope to focus on the simpler white linen, and selected a pose reminiscent of fifteenth-century images of the Madonna della Misericordia, in which the Virgin, invoked as protectress, raises her arms and spreads her cape to safeguard her followers. This analogy is reinforced by the manner in which the saint's followers surround him as they look to him to perform the miracle.

While Whitfield has suggested that this more balanced and conservative composition may have been Artemisia's response to Bolognese classicism (Domenichino and Guido Reni had worked in the cathedral of Naples, and Lanfranco was involved in the Pozzuoli commission), Garrard argues that Artemisia proves herself a steadfast adherent of Caravaggesque naturalism through her attention to an accurately rendered setting and the individualized treatment of the animals. Bissell (1999) has rightly pointed out that although we can no longer reconstruct the placement of the pictures in the cathedral, Artemisia was obviously responding to the requirements of the location in which her painting would be seen. We do know that the *Saint Januarius* was the middle painting along the left-hand wall of the choir, and the orientation of Januarius, who faces east, was designed to accommodate the picture to its site.

The painting has been carefully realized and, rather than a sense of Baroque drama, offers a comforting image of blessing by the local patron saint. The figures on the left look up in prayer, while Saint Januarius looks down to the animals at his feet. The austere format of Artemisia's other choir picture, the *Saints Proculus and Nicea* (fig. 143), suggests that Artemisia has chosen to provide devotional pictures for liturgical use. She does not, therefore, attempt to capture the horror of Januarius's confrontation with ferocious beasts. Artemisia's paintings of the 1630s demonstrate an impulse to use balanced, static compositions rather than the more explosive, active images of her earlier career.

Evidence provided by the bishop's report of 1640 gives a terminus ad quem for the completion of the picture. The commission probably was given to Artemisia in either 1634 or 1636, and most scholars have assigned to the three paintings a date of 1635–37, since she may have left Naples as early as 1638 to relocate in London. Gregori finds evidence in this painting of Artemisia's adaptation to the artistic environment of early seicento Naples, and has noted similarities to the paintings of Aniello Falcone, Agostino Beltrano, and Artemisia's collaborator on the John the Baptist cycle, Massimo Stanzione.

The *Saint Januarius* appears to include the work of a second hand, detected in the handling of the amphitheater wall; opinions differ as to the painter's identity. Bologna and Garrard see the hand of Viviano Codazzi in the architecture, while Brunetti, Sestieri and Daprà, and Bissell have identified the collaborator as Domenico Gargiulo. We know through a contemporary biography that both painters worked with Artemisia in her later *David and Bathsheba* in Columbus (cat. 80).[1] The stylistic disparity in the background is not as obvious as in the Columbus picture, however, and Garrard's idea that Artemisia "gave the composition its final painterly unity" seems correct.

Pozzuoli cathedral was engulfed by fire in May of 1964, and many of its appointments were lost. The choir and high altar survived the blaze, as did the chapel of the Holy Sacrament. After the fire, the surviving paintings, the *Saint Januarius* among them, were moved to Naples and stored in the Certosa di San Martino before being transferred to the Capodimonte over the last several years. The painting was cleaned after the fire, at which time the signature was revealed, having been covered by a later, spurious signature. The picture has suffered through the centuries, with particular damage in the saint's left cheek and chin and some damage and repair in the cope and at the upper left.

1. Bernardo de Dominici ([1742–44], 1979, 414) described the *David and Bathsheba* in Columbus as including architecture painted by Viviano Codazzi and trees and background elements by Domenico Gargiulo.

80.

David and Bathsheba

Oil on canvas, 104 ½ × 82 ½ in. (265.4 × 209.5 cm)

Columbus Museum of Art (inv. 1967.006)

ca. 1636–38

While Artemisia is known for having made at least five versions of the story of Judith, she painted the biblical story of David and Bathsheba (2 Sam. 11, 12) perhaps as many as seven times. King David, unable to sleep, is strolling on the roof of his palace when he observes Bathsheba, the wife of the Hittite soldier Uriah (who is away at war), bathing in her garden. Attracted by her beauty, David dispatches messengers to summon her to his palace. When Bathsheba meets with him, he seduces her, after which she conceives. Hoping that the child would appear to be her husband's, David makes repeated but unsuccessful attempts to send Uriah home to his wife. Finally, the king orders him into battle, specifying to his commander that he be "set . . . in the forefront of the hottest battle . . . that he may be smitten, and die." Uriah is slain, and after Bathsheba's period of mourning, David takes her for his wife.

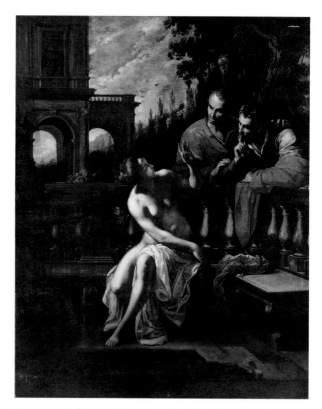

Figure 144. Follower of Bernardo Cavallino (bapt. 1616–?1656), *Susanna and the Elders.* Oil on canvas. Private collection

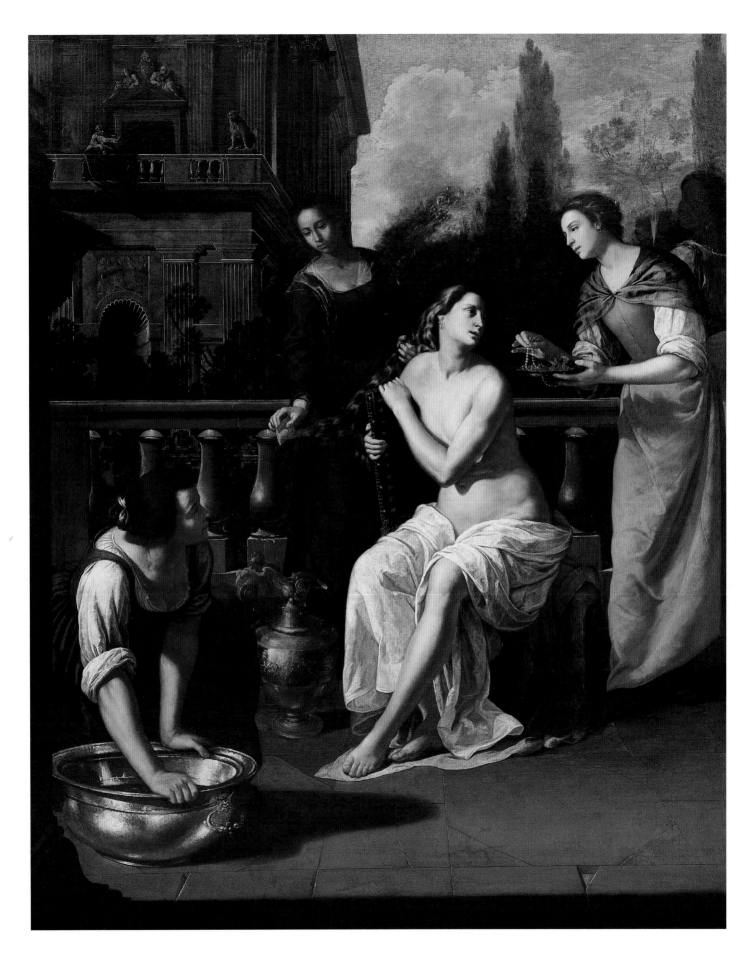

Gentileschi follows the popular preference, traditional since as early as the thirteenth century, for depicting David's first sight of Bathsheba at her bath. At the extreme upper left, David, resting his arm on the railing of his balcony, gestures toward his future wife. She, in turn, appears oblivious of his gaze as she turns toward her maidservant, who offers to her mistress a tray of jewelry. Bathsheba's expression, one of thoughtful reverie, imbues the painting with a sense of wistful contemplation.

The picture demonstrates the sophisticated construction of one of Artemisia's most accomplished works. The entire composition is defined by a strong central vertical formed by the side of David's palace and a comparable horizontal division provided by the balustrade. The figures introduce two sweeping diagonals. One, beginning with King David's gesture at the upper left, continues through the maid who combs Bathsheba's hair, through the angle of the chair, and is reinforced by the turn of Bathsheba's head. A second diagonal leads from the kneeling maidservant on the left, through Bathsheba's torso, and toward the attendant at the right. The composition, marked by elegant color harmonies of blue and gold and the sumptuous surfaces of the washbasin and water jug, becomes a carefully studied masterpiece of grace and rigor. Although Artemisia has certainly not avoided the theme of the bath and the pampered elegance of a wealthy woman, she has played down the sensual qualities of the heroine while still offering the viewer a commanding figure of the female nude. But she has not included a standard feature of Bathsheba iconography, a mirror, which is present in the five versions of the story, painted during the 1640s, one of which may not be autograph. The absence of the mirror allows the picture to focus more on Bathsheba's expression of thoughtfulness and less on her vanity or her role as an object displayed for the viewer's delectation.

The picture is first mentioned in 1742, by Bernardo de Dominici in his biography of Domenico Gargiulo, as being in the Neapolitan house of Luigi Romeo, baron of San Luigi. De Dominici describes it as primarily the work of Artemisia Gentileschi, with architecture painted by Viviano Codazzi and with trees and background by Gargiulo. Most writers have assumed that David's palace was painted by Codazzi, whose designs often include the multilayered application of architectural detail. Marshall has suggested that the foreground pavement and large balustrade may also have been painted by Codazzi. However, these elements appear in as many as six other paintings by Artemisia, and these offer no evidence of collaboration. The group attribution to Gentileschi, Codazzi, and Gargiulo of the Columbus Bathsheba has been accepted by most scholars, and it fits comfortably in a period when Artemisia was engaged in collaborative projects, including the three canvases for Pozzuoli cathedral (cat. 79) and the joint commission with Massimo Stanzione for Philip IV (cat. 77).

While De Dominici's reference confirms the work as a Neapolitan picture, opinions have been divided as to whether it was made shortly before Artemisia went to London, in 1638–39 (Bissell, Contini, Sestieri), or whether she completed the work immediately upon her return to Naples, in the early 1640s (Schleier, Garrard, Stolzenwald). Complicating the matter is a record of a final payment to Artemisia on May 5, 1636, of 250 ducats of a contracted 600 for three paintings, a Bathsheba, a Susanna, and a Lucretia, for Prince Karl Eusebius von Liechtenstein.[1] Although the measurements given for the height of the Liechtenstein Bathsheba are larger than the Columbus picture, there remains the possibility that the latter was indeed a commission for the prince. However, as Bissell has noted, it seems unlikely that Artemisia would not have delivered a paid commission for such an important patron. Given the wide disparity between Artemisia's known oeuvre and the many documents and references to now lost or unknown paintings, it is more than likely that the Liechtenstein pictures were part of a different group, which are now lost. The date of the Liechtenstein payment indicates that in the 1630s Artemisia was working on groups of pictures for individual patrons, as Bissell has also suggested.

Dating the painting to the mid-1630s places it within a context of works with similar formal concerns and establishes this period as a high point in Artemisia's compositional refinement, echoed in the subtle balance of the Cleopatra (cat. 76) and the Birth of Saint

PROVENANCE: Luigi Romeo, baron of San Luigi, Naples (by 1742); Antiquario Tarchini, Rome; Carlo Sestieri, Rome (1960?); P. and D. Colnaghi, London (1962); Columbus Museum of Art (from 1967).

RELATED PICTURES: Neues Palais, Potsdam (autograph); formerly Ramunni collection, currently in private collection, Naples; ex-Leipzig (appears to be autograph); Palazzo Pitti, Florence (autograph); Gosford House, Scotland (destroyed); Haas collection, Vienna, horizontal format (very damaged condition; appears to be autograph; fig. 101).

REFERENCES: De Dominici (1742–44) 1979, 414; Richardson in Phillips 1976, 173–75; Schleier in London 1982, 47; Garrard 1989, 121–22; Contini in Florence 1991, 178–79; Stolzenwald 1991, 95; Marshall 1993, vol. 2, 153–55 no. vc55; Sestieri in Sestieri and Daprà 1994, 90–91 no. 22; Sotheby's, London, sale cat., December 6, 1995, lot 53; Bissell 1999, 82–86, 263–66 no. 37.

John the Baptist (cat. 77). Bissell compares the kneeling maidservant in the *Bathsheba* with the maid in the *Saint John*, and the maid holding the jewelry bears a strong resemblance to the seated Virgin in the Naples *Adoration* (fig. 142). As Bissell also notes, the *Bathsheba* does not share the more opulent appointments and overt emphasis on material richness that characterize the few paintings dating to the last decade of the painter's life, after she returned from London.

Bissell suggests that the picture may reflect the work of the young Bernardo Cavallino. Partly on the stylistic evidence of a *Susanna and the Elders* (fig. 144) that appeared on the London art market in 1995 (argued to be the painting pendant to the present canvas; see Lattuada, pp. 384–85), he posits the participation of Cavallino in both pictures. However, on the basis of photographs (I have not examined the *Susanna* first-hand), the attribution to Gentileschi seems problematic, although the figures of the elders appear to fit easily into the oeuvre of Cavallino (London 1995). Without a secure attribution of the *Susanna* to Artemisia, it is difficult to conjecture that Cavallino's participation in that painting suggests he worked with her on the *Bathsheba*. That need not rule out the possibility that the London picture records a now lost pendant to the Columbus canvas.

The painting has suffered a great deal and has undergone two substantial courses of restoration, the first in 1979 at the Intermuseum Conservation Association Laboratory at Oberlin, and the second in 1996 by Mark Tucker, of the Philadelphia Museum of Art. The painting has three major tears that have been repaired, and the background landscape has suffered abrasion. Some of the colors have been absorbed, and areas of reworking in Bathsheba's chest, right knee, and left wrist have rendered those areas much flatter than they must originally have appeared.

1. "A Lorenzo Cambi e Simone Verzone D. 250. E per loro ad Artemisia Gentileschi, dite se li paghino a compimento di D. 300 che li altri D. 50 l'ha recevuti contanti, dite in conto di D. 600 che l'ho dato d'ordine dall'eccellentissimo principe Carlo de Lochtenten si li pagano per valore di tre quadri consistenti in una Betsabea, una Susanna et una Lucretia, ognuno del quale d'altezza d'undici palmi e mezzo da dare e consignare di tutto punto. E per lei all'Alfiere Costantino del Cunto per altritanti"; Nappi 1983, 76.

81.

Self-Portrait as the Allegory of Painting (La Pittura)

Oil on canvas, 38⅞ × 29⅝ in. (98.6 × 75.2 cm)

Signed (on right corner of tabletop): A.G. F.

Her Majesty Queen Elizabeth II

1638–39

Saint Louis

An inventory of the "Pictures Statues Plate and Effects of King Charles I," drawn up between the king's execution in 1649 and the sale of his effects in October 1651, lists four pictures by Artemisia, including "A Pintura A painteinge" (An allegory of Painting in the act of painting) and "Arthemesia gentelisco. done by her selfe." Beginning with Michael Levey, whose 1964 catalogue of the later Italian paintings in the royal collections includes the picture, scholars have understood these citations as referring to a single work. However, as Bissell has now clarified, the two are given different valuations in the 1649 inventory and therefore the references must identify two separate items.

Certainly, this splendid picture must be associated with the inventoried "Pintura A painteinge," as it conforms convincingly to key elements of Cesare Ripa's description of *Painting (La Pittura)*: "A beautiful woman, with full black hair, disheveled, and twisted in various ways, with arched eyebrows that show imaginative thought, the mouth covered with a cloth tied behind her ears, with a chain of gold at her throat from which hangs a mask, and has written in front 'imitation.' She holds in her hand a brush, and in the other the palette, with clothes of evanescently colored drapery. . . ."[1] This painting is generally believed to be the work of Artemisia Gentileschi, and her initials, A.G.F. (the *F* most likely refers to some variation of the Latin verb *fecere*, meaning "to make"), appear at the corner of the foreground tabletop.

Because the picture has gained wide acceptance as a self-portrait (if not the self-portrait in the inventory), we must consider the possibility that the artist intended it to be self-referential. When compared with other sixteenth- and seventeenth-century self-portraits, it poses interesting problems. Artists' self-portraits as independent works developed in the fifteenth century and, as Woods-Marsden has argued, became vehicles for the affirmation of the artist's elevated status in society.[2] These portraits usually include the artist standing at an easel or seated at a desk, brandishing brushes or a palette, and sometimes holding a drawing (*disegno*), a reference to artistic inspiration, thereby emphasizing the intellectual rigor of the profession. A portrait in the Palazzo Barberini demonstrates the artist self-portrait at its most straightforward: a female artist stands at her easel, her palette in the left hand and a paintbrush in the right. She gazes toward the viewer as she applies finishing touches to the portrait of a man. Interestingly, a number of writers have attributed this picture to Artemisia, though it has most recently been given to the workshop of Simon Vouet.[3]

Not all subjects of self-portraits address the viewer directly, in spite of the required use of a mirror in their production. Titian employed this pose with particularly fine results in his impressive *Self-Portrait* from the 1550s in Berlin (fig. 145), which shows him staring off to the viewer's right, effectively denying his use of a mirror in the painting's execution. The early Baroque saw the creation of one of the most eloquent and novel self-portraits by any artist, a painting by Annibale Carracci (Hermitage, Saint Petersburg), in which his own painted self-portrait stands alone on an easel in a simple interior space.

There were noteworthy precedents for self-fashioning by female artists. Sofonisba Anguissola (ca. 1532–1625) and Lavinia Fontana (1552–1614) made impressive self-portraits: Anguissola's *Self-Portrait at the Easel* (Muzeum Zamek, Lancut), for example,

and Fontana's *Self-Portrait in the Studiolo* (Uffizi, Florence). In both cases, they emphasize their noble status through refined costume and references to appropriate talents. Both women include within their repertoire self-portraits before a keyboard, in demonstration of their musical abilities, and both also portray books, attesting to their intellectual achievements. Fontana, who held a doctorate from the University of Bologna, depicts herself at a desk in her study, pen poised over paper, surrounded by sculpture.

The London *Allegory of Painting* does not fit easily into any of the established self-portrait types. The sitter does not address the viewer directly, and while such a pose is not mandatory, it is understandable why the compiler of the 1649 inventory may not have recognized the image as a portrait. Bissell, Haskell, and Gregori have questioned its representation of a self-image of the artist on the basis of likeness, not finding the facial features similar to those in the engraving by Jérôme David of Artemisia made around 1628 (fig. 95) or to the anonymous portrait medal of approximately the same date (Staatliche Museen, Berlin). Nevertheless, the wide forehead, full cheeks, ample chin, and bow lips do, in fact, resemble the artist's face. And although her hair was auburn rather than black, it is possible that she adjusted the color in the painting to conform to Ripa's formula, as many scholars have suggested. Garrard argues eloquently and, in my view, correctly that Artemisia painted *La Pittura* as an image of herself to comment on her unique role as a woman painter, conflating two images that male artists would have to make separately. While Garrard goes on to discuss Artemisia's image as an assertion of the artist's role as intellectual and the elevated status of the profession, we can perhaps view the painting—in which virtuoso execution and the cleverness of the concept are paramount—as simply expanding the repertoire of self-imaging in much the same way that Annibale Carracci accomplished in his easel portrait.

It seems hard to imagine that Artemisia, in making an image of Painting, did not reflect on the special significance this allegory held for her as a woman artist. As Garrard has pointed out, there was precedent for the combination of the image of a female artist and the representation of the act of painting.

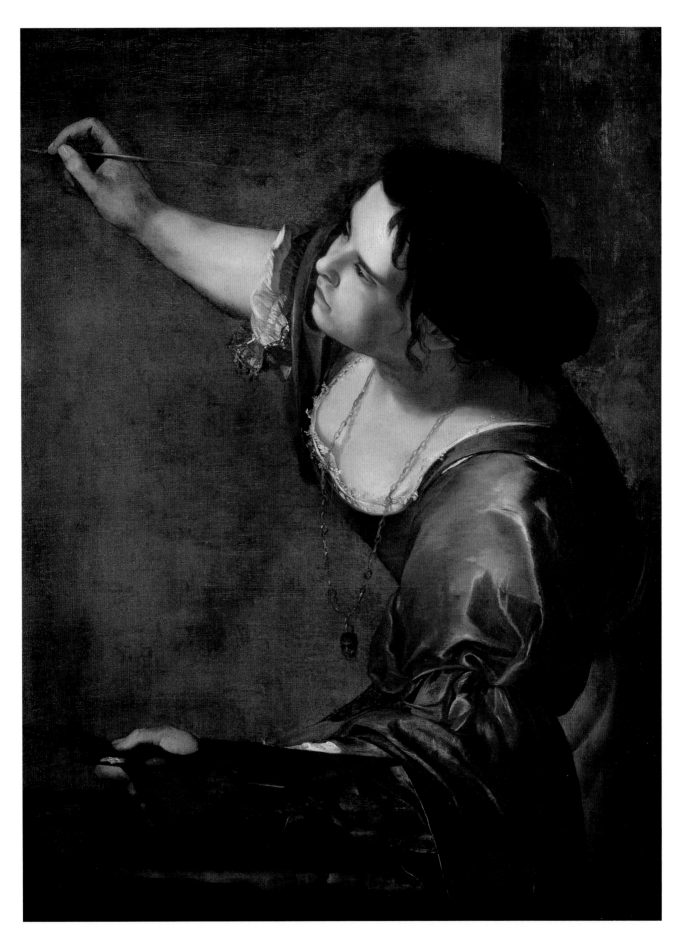

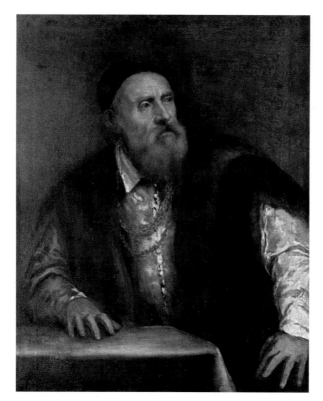

Figure 145. Titian (ca. 1485/90–1576), *Self-Portrait*. Oil on canvas. Gemäldegalerie, Staatliche Museen zu Berlin

PROVENANCE: Charles I (1639–49); recovered for the crown at Hampton Court (1651); Kensington Palace (since 1974); Hampton Court.

REFERENCES: Levey 1964, 91 no. 499; Spear in Cleveland 1971, 98–99 no. 29; Millar in London 1972–73; 65 no. 90; Garrard 1980, 97–112; Whitfield in London 1982, 167–68 no. 59; Gregori in Naples 1984–85, vol. 1, 150; Garrard 1989, 85–88, 337–70; Haskell 1989, 37; Contini in Florence 1991, 74–75, 172–75; Levey 1991, 91 no. 499; Cropper 1992, 215; Bissell 1999, 175, 272–75 no. 42.

Fontana was honored in a celebratory 1611 medal on which her profile portrait on the front is paired with a representation of Painting on the reverse (fig. 146). In similar fashion, Bissell suggests that the present image of *La Pittura* was intended to be paired with the lost "Arthemesia gentilisco. done by her selfe," although until that picture is identified, the proposal is difficult to verify. Especially at the court of Charles I, where Artemisia undoubtedly observed the elevated position of such flamboyant figures as Anthony van Dyck, she may have pondered her status within her profession and her anomalous role as a woman painter. Surely, she knew Van Dyck's famous *Self-Portrait with a Sunflower* of 1633 (Collection the Duke of Westminster), which shows the sitter wearing a prominent chain and holding a sunflower; these have been interpreted as emblems of the artist's devotion to his patron.[4] Artemisia's portrayal of herself as Painting, with an unusually small mask and more prominent chain, may also have been intended to represent the artist as serving her current (or future?) patron. Especially

if one of her first pictures is the small oval *Allegory of Painting* (fig. 97), in which, by necessity, she relied on her own likeness in a far more traditional rendering, it is likely that for this later representation she once again used her own image, but in a highly original fashion.

As Garrard points out, Artemisia addresses these issues in her comments to Don Antonio Ruffo in Sicily. In a letter dated August 7, 1649, she notes, "And I will show Your Most Illustrious Lordship what a woman can do," and on November 13, "You will find the spirit of Caesar in this soul of a woman." The representation, by its sheer difficulty of execution (a self-portrait from the side required a two-mirror setup), made its own eloquent case for her abilities as an artist. This is the same spirit that infused the Pommersfelden *Susanna* (cat. 51); the Pitti *Magdalene* (cat. 58) played a similar role as a demonstration piece for her considerable talents at coloring and compositional dynamism.

Gentileschi made several self-portraits (which we know from references in her letters), and scholars have assumed that they adhere to the model of the Barberini painting. However, because they are mentioned only cryptically in her correspondence, it is difficult to determine whether they were easily recognizable as self-portraits. In letters to the Roman collector Cassiano dal Pozzo, she discusses two of them. In 1630 she notes, "I have painted my portrait with the utmost care," and later, in 1637, she tells him she is sending "my portrait, which you once requested."[5] (Scholars have speculated that the portrait referred to in 1630 can be associated with the Barberini painting, while the second, 1637 reference may indicate the London *Allegory*.) The artist's letters to Don Antonio Ruffo, of January and June 1649, mention "my portrait," and the January letter goes on to refer to a painting "which you may keep in your gallery, as all the other princes do," suggesting that her patron placed stipulations on format, size, and so forth. However, we have no other description to help us determine how that painting must have looked. The *Self-Portrait as a Lute Player* (cat. 57) may well have been executed for a patron who requested a self-portrait, and we know that Artemisia presented herself as an Amazon in another Medici picture.[6] Only David's engraving (inscribed as recording a self-portrait) provides evidence

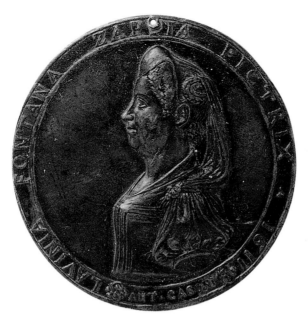

Figure 146. Felice Antonio Casoni (1559–1634), *Portrait Medal of Lavinia Fontana*. Bronze. Biblioteca e Musei Comunali, Imola

dating that is supported stylistically by the painting itself. The physiognomy, particularly the treatment of the forehead, eyes, and mouth, corresponds more to the pictures of the mid-1630s than to those dated to the early part of the decade. Similarities can also be found with the *Birth of Saint John the Baptist* (cat. 77), of about 1633–35, including the features of the midwives and the sophisticated coloration. Bissell rests his dating on the correspondence of this picture to the references in the queen's inventory and the stylistic relationship to the ceiling paintings done for the royal residence at Whitehall in 1637–38. Finaldi's suggestion that Artemisia may not have been involved in this project, as well as the paintings' state of almost total ruin, makes it difficult to base the dating of *La Pittura* on this evidence.

of how Artemisia may have fashioned her own image. Therefore, while it is clear that she produced several self-likenesses, few of them have been identified, and they seem to cover a variety of types. Indeed, we may not yet know what constitutes a proper Artemisia Gentileschi self-portrait, which suggests that the London *Allegory* could be more representative of her self-imaging than we have previously realized.

Some writers have dated *La Pittura* to 1630, based largely on the assumption that the picture is a self-portrait and that the age of the sitter would correspond with a woman in her mid-thirties, Artemisia's age in 1630.[7] These writers have also argued that it is the picture referred to in the 1630 letter to Cassiano dal Pozzo, and that Artemisia held on to the painting and brought it with her to London. That scenario, however, appears unlikely, since she obviously valued her relationship with Cassiano—particularly in light of her often expressed wish to return to Rome, her city of birth—and her hopes of continued rapport would have mandated providing him the promised picture.

Contini, Bissell, and Cropper have all dated this work to 1638–40, when the artist was in London, a

1. Ripa (1618) 1986, 357: "Donna bella, con capelli negri, & grossi, sparsi, & ritorti in diverse maniere, con le ciglia inarcate, che mostrino pensieri fantastichi, si cuopre la bocca con una fascia legata dietro à gli orecchi, con una catena d'oro al collo, dalla quale penda una maschera, & abbia scritto nella fronte, *imitatio*. Terrà in una mano il pennello, & nell'altra la tavola, con la veste di drappo cangiante, . . ."

2. See Woods-Marsden 1998, esp. 1–9, 71–77.

3. It was most recently included in an exhibition devoted to Cassiano dal Pozzo, in which it was attributed to a follower of Simon Vouet, based on its listing in several inventories, most notably an inventory of 1740 that describes the painting in detail and assigns it to Vouet (Volpe in Rome 2000, 49). The condition of the picture is very poor, making a definitive attribution difficult, although I am inclined to agree with the Vouet atelier attribution.

4. On the significance of symbolism in Van Dyck's picture, see Edgerton (in Antwerp–London 1999, 244), who suggests that Van Dyck's chain may be intended as a reference to *La Pittura*.

5. English translations of the letters are published in Garrard 1989, 378, 387. For Italian transcriptions of the letters (both are now lost), see Bottari and Ticozzi 1822–25, vol. 1, 352–53, nos. 139, 141.

6. There are, in addition to these references to self-portraits, other mentions of portraits of the artist, but which may or may not have been self-portraits. The collection of the duke of Alcalá, for example, included two portraits of Artemisia described merely as "un retrato di Artemissa gentilesca."

7. Levey 1962, 79–80; Spear in Cleveland 1971, 98–99; Millar in London 1972–73, 65; Garrard 1989, 85–86. Levey (1991, 91) changed the date to coincide with Artemisia's visit to England, identifying the painting with the self-portrait mentioned in her correspondence of 1637.

82.

Venus Embracing Cupid

Oil on canvas, 47 ⅝ × 63 in.
(121 × 160 cm)

Private collection

1640s

Hermann Voss published a short article on this splendid painting in 1961 after it had been shown in exhibitions in Zürich (1958) and Bordeaux (1959) bearing an attribution to Artemisia Gentileschi. Voss supported the attribution and argued that it fit most securely with her paintings from the 1640s. Schleier and Marini also assigned the picture to Artemisia, and Bissell (1999), most recently, has included it among her autograph works. Garrard maintains that the picture was "wrongly ascribed to Artemisia," while Contini finds that it more closely matches the style of Francesco Guerrieri. The painting bears provocative affinities with Artemisia's work, and should it prove to be a product of her brush (I have not examined it firsthand), it most probably belongs to the last decade of her life.

This presentation of a languorously reclining Venus attended by her young son includes many luxurious appointments and comes closest to the sensibility of Artemisia's late paintings, most notably the two she painted for the duke of Parma, the *David and Bathsheba* and the *Rape of Lucretia* (Neues Palais, Potsdam; fig. 99). The three paintings share specific details, such as the triangular lace edging of Lucretia's sheet and Venus's cover and the elaborately adorned coiffures, as well as more general features of rich surface texture and an emphasis on opulence. The *Venus* also corresponds to other late paintings. Its intense color recalls the hues of the *Virgin and Child with a Rosary* (cat. 84), in which deep red and blue dominate. The ribbon that binds Venus's hair as well as the tight curls that frame her face can also be found in the reclining figure in the right foreground of the Vienna *Bathsheba* (private collection; fig. 101).

Other qualities suggest Artemisia's authorship in general, even if they do not argue specifically for a dating to the final decade. Venus's body type certainly belongs among Artemisia's nudes. The conical breasts, swelling stomach, flared hips, and high navel relate closely to the physical forms of the Columbus *David and Bathsheba* (cat. 80), the *Aurora* (private collection,

PROVENANCE: Segesser de Brunegg family (with F. von Segesser, Lucerne, by 1958); private collection (by 1963).

REFERENCES: Zürich 1958, 12, no. 22; Bordeaux 1959, 36–37 no. 69; Voss 1960–61, 79–82; Bissell 1968, 167; Schleier 1971, 89; Lavin 1975, 165; Marini 1981a, 370; Garrard 1989, 105–6, 274–76; Contini in Florence 1991, 85 n. 40; Bissell 1999, 247–49 no. 31.

Rome; fig. 96), and the Saint Louis *Danaë* (cat. 54). Bissell finds the physiognomy to be comparable to that in the Columbus painting, and indeed the same woman may have posed as Artemisia's model in both cases.

Bissell has posited that the painting may have been the one owned by the English diplomat and collector Matthew Prior (1664–1721), described as a "Venus and Cupid Kissing. Big as the life," which was attributed to either Orazio or Artemisia. He also identifies it as the painting listed in the Barberini inventories of 1644, where it is cited as a "woman with a cupid."[1] Although it seems unlikely that the picture would have been described in such vague terms, the compiler of the inventory may have intentionally ignored the obvious sexuality of the image, as Bissell also suggests.

Those scholars who have attributed the *Venus* to Artemisia, with the exception of Voss, have placed it in the early 1630s. Bissell links it to a reference in a letter of 1635 that Artemisia wrote to Cassiano dal Pozzo in Rome.[2] In the letter, she mentions a painting that she had sent to Cardinal Antonio Barberini, also in Rome, having given it to her brother Francesco, who took it from Naples.

Troubling to Bissell and perhaps among the reasons that Garrard has eliminated the *Venus* from Artemisia's oeuvre is its overt, if not gratuitous, eroticism. The subject recalls Bronzino's famous *Allegory with Venus and Cupid* (National Gallery, London), to which it may allude in the nearly touching profiles and proximity of lips. Images of Venus as lover, goddess, sex queen, and Olympian ideal were popular among sixteenth- and seventeenth-century patrons. Less subtle references to physical gratification were made in paintings such as Baglione's *Cupid and Venus* (private collection, Rome; fig. 124). The Cavaliere d'Arpino had painted the goddess literally romping in bed with her son, her legs spread provocatively while she fondles Cupid's buttocks (Fabio Failla collection, Rome).

Artemisia's *Venus* certainly demonstrates far greater restraint. Its elegant presentation of female beauty

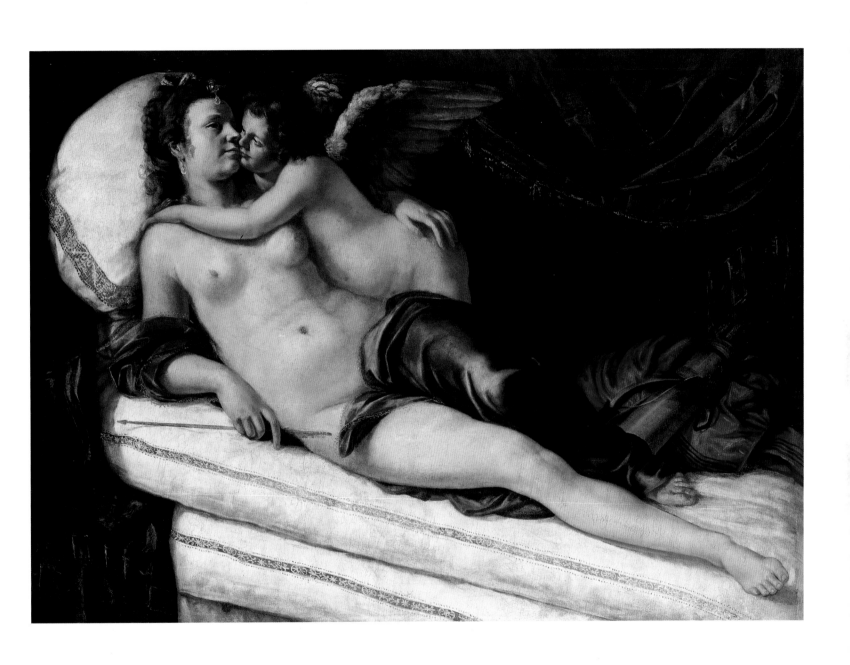

dominates the canvas. However, by including such details as Cupid's pressing up against his mother, her hand resting gently on his rump, and the subtly evocative elongated leg, the artist has underscored the eroticism inherent in the image; it is unlikely that the picture was conceived as an allegory.[3]

Should this picture prove to be by Artemisia, it presents persuasive evidence of her mastery of the female body. Rejecting the less subtle passion of its prototypes, the artist offers one of the most stunning representations of female nudity of the seventeenth century. The handsome profile, the gracefully curving torso, and glorious outstretched leg present a body both exquisitely beautiful and erotically charged. The leg recalls the provocative display of the vase-bearing angel in Parmigianino's *Madonna of the Long Neck* (Uffizi, Florence), and indeed a Florentine elegance and almost Mannerist sensuality pervade the work. Contini and Bissell posit that Artemisia may have

returned to Florence at some time during her career. The most logical placement for such a visit would be during her trip to England in 1637–38. Indeed, it is unthinkable that after her repeated efforts to secure Florentine patronage in the early 1630s, she did not visit the Tuscan capital, most likely before she finally relocated to London. The sensibility of this picture certainly suggests some contact with Florentine artists—Cesare Dandini, perhaps, or Rutillio Manetti—and reminds us yet again how little we really understand of the final decade of Artemisia Gentileschi's life.

1. The inventory lists a "donna con un'amore." Lavin 1975, 165.
2. I find it far more likely that the *Sleeping Venus* (cat. 70) was the picture Artemisia sent to Cardinal Barberini.
3. Venus's seizing of Cupid's weapons was traditionally intended as a reference to the power of beauty to overwhelm, or disarm, love. But the disarming of Cupid usually alludes to the suppression rather than arousal of desire; the decidedly sensual cast of this painting negates such allegorical symbolism.

83.

Susanna and the Elders

Oil on canvas, 80¾ × 66⅛ in. (205 × 168 cm)

Signed (at right, on socle of balustrade): ARTEMITIA / GENTILESCHI. F. / MDCIL

Moravská Galerie, Brno (inv. M246)

1649

Given the meager evidence from Artemisia's last Neapolitan period (after her return from London in the early 1640s until her death in the early 1650s), this signed and dated painting of 1649 must serve as an important guide to understanding the direction of her art in this final phase. Artemisia here repeats some of the formal elements of her earliest representation of the story of Susanna (cat. 51), but has chosen a far more traditional interpretation. While Susanna resists the elders' sexual demands, the heroine now looks heavenward, seeming to implore divine assistance. In fact, her pose refers to a later moment in the story, when, confronted by the elders, Susanna "looked up toward Heaven, for her heart trusted in the Lord," a passage that seems to have inspired many representations. Ludovico Carracci, Guercino, and Peter Paul Rubens, among many others, followed this convention.

The tightly framed composition and stark setting that distinguished the 1610 version have been abandoned for a grander stage, complete with sculpted fountain and lush flowers, visible through the balusters—what Garrard has termed the "Garden of Love"—which emphasizes the associations of Susanna with overt sexuality. The striking compression of space that created the dramatic tension in the earlier work has given way to a more rigid compositional structure, achieved through the spacing of the elders farther to the right offset by the diagonal of Susanna's pose and the presence of the substantial washbasin beside her. Her gesture is more rhetorical than dramatic, and the vocabulary now integrates late-seventeenth-century notions of *bellezza* with the powerful naturalism of the Pommersfelden painting.

The seated heroine is still a commanding presentation of the female nude, although greater attention

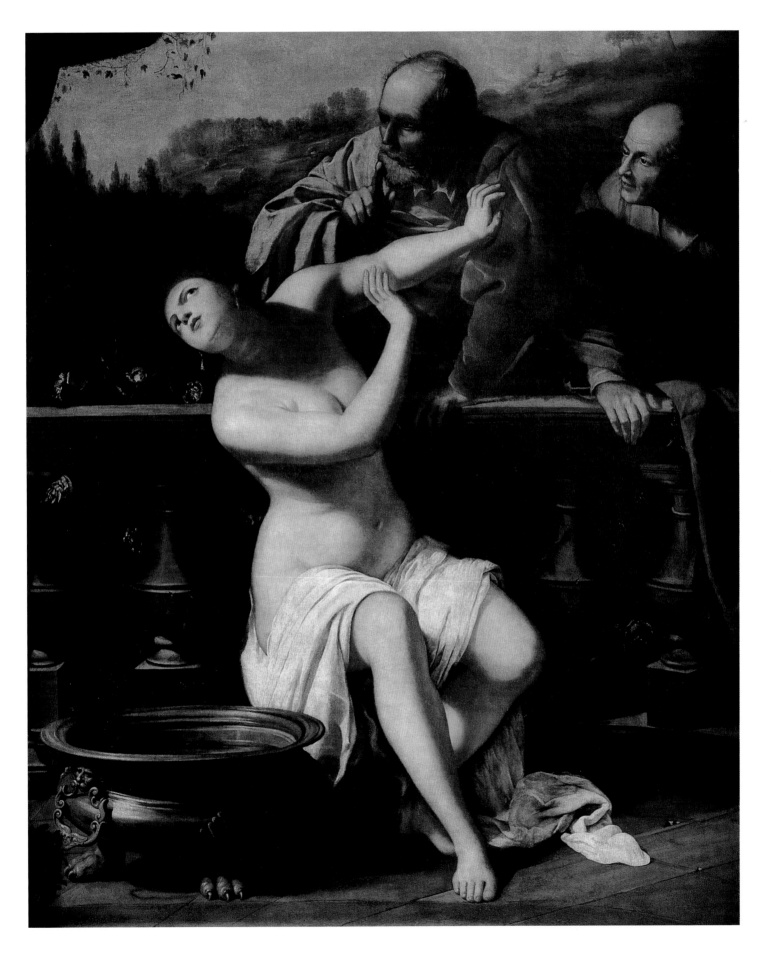

has been given to the drapery of the elders (the lovely blue of the right elder's sleeve seen against the railing must once have been a beautiful passage but is now somewhat damaged) and the accomplished rendering of the polished pewter basin with grotesque handles and robust claw feet. Susanna's pose has become a stock type within Artemisia's oeuvre, for we see comparably seated figures in the Columbus *David and Bathsheba* (cat. 80) and the Toledo *Lot and His Daughters* (cat. 78). The washbasin also occurs in at least two other paintings, and may have been inspired by Simon Vouet's *Circumcision of Christ* (Capodimonte, Naples), which was in Naples in the 1620s, as both Garrard (1989) and Bissell (1999) have noted. Contini comments on similarities to such artists as Francesco Guarino in the foreshortened presentation of Susanna's face, and finds the picture comfortably placed within the Neapolitan ambience of Bernardo Cavallino.

In spite of several disastrous events of the 1630s and 1640s—the volcanic eruption and earthquake of the 1630s and the popular revolt led by the fisherman Masaniello in 1647—the demand for pictures in Naples apparently did not wane. Artemisia's repetition of forms, as well as her five versions of Bathsheba from the 1640s, may testify to the high number of commissions the artist received during this late period of her career. In spite of the celebrated claim in her November 13, 1649, letter to Don Antonio Ruffo in Naples that "never has anyone found in my pictures any repetition of invention, not even of one hand," it is quite clear that Artemisia did repeat herself; her assertion may have been made in response to criticism of this practice or to a request for assurance

that a forthcoming commission would indeed be a new composition.

Rarely seen by scholars, this painting has generated only limited discussion. Bissell (1999) accepts it within Artemisia's oeuvre, noting that layers of old varnish still covered the signature in the 1950s, precluding alteration prior to its initial restoration. Garrard (1989) originally questioned the attribution, but has recently (2001) accepted it in her oeuvre. Garrard (1989) and Hersey have suggested that this picture may have been the one cited by Alessandro da Morrona as in the collection of Averardo de' Medici late in the eighteenth century. Bissell has noted that the Medici picture, signed and dated 1652, was of horizontal format and described as showing Susanna with covered breasts, and must therefore be understood as a different work.

The landscape, a rarity among Artemisia's autograph paintings, has been attributed by Daniel to the hand of Domenico Gargiulo, a known collaborator with the artist in the Columbus *David and Bathsheba*. Bissell suggests that the landscape appears to be Artemisia imitating the work of Gargiulo, and certainly the touch does not demonstrate the light, feathery quality that distinguishes the latter's style.

The condition of the painting and its probable reduced size make definitive judgments difficult as to Artemisia's late style. The composition seems to have been cut down, at least on the left and top edges, and it is likely that it may have been cut on all sides, as Bissell (1999) has posited. Losses and cracks have occurred throughout the surface, with heaviest damage in Susanna's left arm and right leg, the head of the left elder, and the shadowed areas immediately surrounding Susanna's lower torso.

PROVENANCE: Heinrich Gomperz, Brno (until 1894); the city of Brno (by the Gomperz testament of 1892); Moravská Galerie, Brno.

RELATED PICTURE: Bassano del Grappo, Museo Biblioteca Archivio, variant, studio version of reduced size.

REFERENCES: Böhmová-Hájková 1956, 307–8; Bissell 1968, 164–65; Garrard 1989, 99, 130–31, 134–35, 189, 518 n. 234; Contini in Florence 1991, 76–78; Hersey 1993, 330–31 n. 3; Daniel in Prague 1995, 56–58 no. A11; Bissell 1999, 72, 292–93 no. 50; Garrard 2001, 81, 92–93.

84.

Virgin and Child with a Rosary

Oil on copper, 22⅞ × 19¾ in. (58 × 50 cm), affixed to a panel measuring 28⅜ × 20½ in. (72 × 52 cm)

Signed (across front edge of table): Artemitia Gentileschi

El Escorial, Casita del Principe (inv. 10014628)

1651

Saint Louis

This small gem of a picture is first mentioned in a 1749 inventory of the furnishings in La Granja, the eighteenth-century royal palace built by Philip V of Spain. It is not known exactly when it was transferred to the Escorial—but it is cited there in a catalogue of 1857. In a letter dated August 13, 1650, to the collector Don Antonio Ruffo in Sicily, Artemisia refers to "this little Madonna [Madonina in piccolo]," and later, on January 1, 1651, she writes, "Your little copper is nearly half finished." Bissell has concluded that this "copper" is indeed the painting referred to in Artemisia's letter, while Pérez Sánchez and Nicolson date the picture to much earlier in her career, between 1614 and 1620.

Devotion to the rosary, a string of beads used as an aid to meditative prayer (each bead refers to one of the Mysteries in the life of Christ or the Virgin), experienced renewed vigor in the later sixteenth century. Particularly after the naval victory over the Turks at Lepanto in 1571, attributed to rosary prayer, the practice became more widespread, prompting Gregory XIII to institute the Feast of the Rosary in 1573. The practice offered a personal means of prayer, and this small painting, with its reference to the rosary, was unquestionably intended for private devotion. The rosary was often represented by a rose crown and sometimes by angels placing a rose garland on the head of the Virgin. Here, the allusion is made by the roses in the infant's right hand and the spray of roses resting on the table.

The painting was largely ignored until Pérez Sánchez included it in his 1973 exhibition, "Caravaggio y el naturalismo español." In spite of the signature, the picture is not universally accepted as autograph, given its unique format and style. The simple, vivid palette of rich green, bright red, and blue appears in no other picture by Gentileschi. Contini understandably describes its style as incongruous, and Borea suggests an attribution to Caroselli, positing that the signature was added to increase the painting's value.

Garrard challenges the attribution to Artemisia on the ground that its more delicate and clearly feminine representation of the Virgin is symptomatic of a tendency to associate a feminine style with a female artist. She suggests the possibility that the painting is "a weak replica of a lost original by Artemisia."

There are, however, some similarities between this small copper and paintings from the last decades of the artist's career. The transparent veil of the Madonna recalls a scarf worn by a maidservant in a *Bathsheba* of the 1630s (private collection, Halle, Germany); the same veil also appears on one of the maidservants in the Columbus *David and Bathsheba* (cat. 80) and on Saint Nicea in Artemisia's painting for Pozzuoli cathedral (fig. 143). The daughter on the right in the Toledo *Lot* (cat. 78) wears a similar delicately sheer covering.

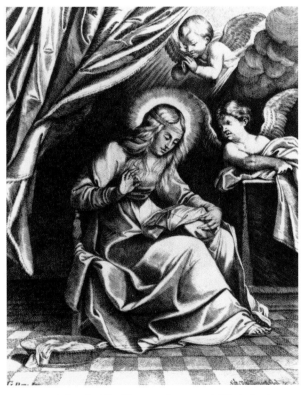

Figure 147. Sébastien Vouillement (b. ca. 1610), *Virgin Sewing*. Engraving after Guido Reni (1575–1642). Bibliothèque Nationale de France, Paris

PROVENANCE: Collection of
Isabella Farnese, La Granja
(by 1749); sacristy, El Escorial
(by 1857); Casita del Principe,
El Escorial.

REFERENCES: Pérez Sánchez
1965, 500; Pérez Sánchez in
Seville 1973, no. 22; Borea 1974,
46–47; Nicolson 1974, 611;
Garrard 1989, 399–400; Contini
in Florence 1991, 84 n. 23, 86
n. 78; Bissell 1999, 99, 293–95
no. 51; Garrard 2001, 9, 127–28,
n. 20.

Bissell notes that the identical pose of the Virgin's
right hand and arm occurs in several other late paintings, including the *Bathsheba* in the Neues Palais,
Potsdam (fig. 100), and a *Bathsheba* of reduced format
in Vienna (fig. 101).

The *Virgin and Child with a Rosary* is similar to small
devotional pictures of the Virgin sewing; the hand
gesture of the Virgin holding the rosary can be traced
to representations of the Virgin sewing from the school
of Guido Reni. Artemisia herself may even have known
the example that Reni painted in 1609 for Paul V in
the private papal chapel in the Quirinal palace, or a
small, earlier version on copper that Reni painted for
the Borghese in 1606.[1] Although the latter is now lost,
there still exist painted and printed variants, such as the
engraving by Sébastien Vouillement, which eliminates
one of the angels and the crown of roses from Reni's
original (fig. 147). It seems evident that Artemisia knew
the original painting, as she employs not only the
same hand gesture but the same palette (Reni's
Madonna wears a red dress and sews on a brilliant blue
cushion in her lap). The Reni work, which should accurately be titled *Virgin and Child with a Rosary*, would
have been a logical source for Artemisia, since the
imagery of the Virgin sewing was often combined
with allusions to the rosary, usually the presentation
of a rose crown.

Artemisia had replicated Bolognese models earlier
in her career, most notably in the Burghley House
Susanna and the Elders (cat. 65). Scholars have also found
other stylistic evidence of Reni's influence in additional
examples of Artemisia's work.[2] Interestingly, his *Virgin
Sewing* was given by Scipione Borghese to Cardinal
Ludovisi, a gift recorded on September 8, 1622. If
Artemisia's Burghley House *Susanna* was a Ludovisi
commission, painted in 1622, then she may have known
the Reni picture early in her career and drawn on it as
the inspiration for her late copper. Whether this was
a specific request from Ruffo or whether the artist
thought such a style would appeal to his taste, we
cannot determine.

We can only speculate as to why Artemisia turned
to such a model late in her career. The exactness with
which she reproduces Reni's hand gesture suggests
that either she had recently renewed her acquaintance
with the picture (or some version of it) or that she
had made drawings of it when she had seen it earlier.
This latter point is still a very little understood aspect
of Artemisia's working procedure. There is evidence,
however—including her own letters—that she did
employ drawings. On November 13, 1649, she wrote
to Don Antonio Ruffo in Sicily: "As for my doing a
drawing and sending it, I have made a solemn vow
never to send my drawings, because people have
cheated me. In particular, just today I found myself
[in the situation] that, having done a drawing of souls
in purgatory for the bishop of Saint Gata, in order to
spend less, he commissioned another painter to do
the picture using my work. I can't imagine it would
have turned out this way if I were a man, because
when the concept has been realized and defined with
lights and darks, and established by means of planes,
the rest is a trifle."[3] No drawings by Artemisia's hand
are known today.

The current size of the painting reflects an augmentation at the top and on both sides. A clumsy addition
to the green curtain in the upper part of the painting
mars its original beauty (it is reproduced here without the additions). Bissell, noting that an inventory
number and the Farnese fleur-de-lis overlap the
joint, has suggested that the enlargement occurred
in the eighteenth century, a judgment confirmed
by Juan Martinez, a conservator at the Palacio
Real, Madrid.[4]

1. On the Reni paintings, see Pepper 1984b, 294.
2. For a discussion of Reni's influence on Artemisia, see Longhi
    1916, 308; Gregori (in Naples 1984–85) notes that the Morandotti
    Cleopatra (cat. nos. 17, 53) which she attributes to Artemisia,
    shows evidence of the artist's having followed "Renian" models.
3. For the translation of the letter, see Garrard 1989, 397–98.
4. Letter to the author, June 21, 1995.

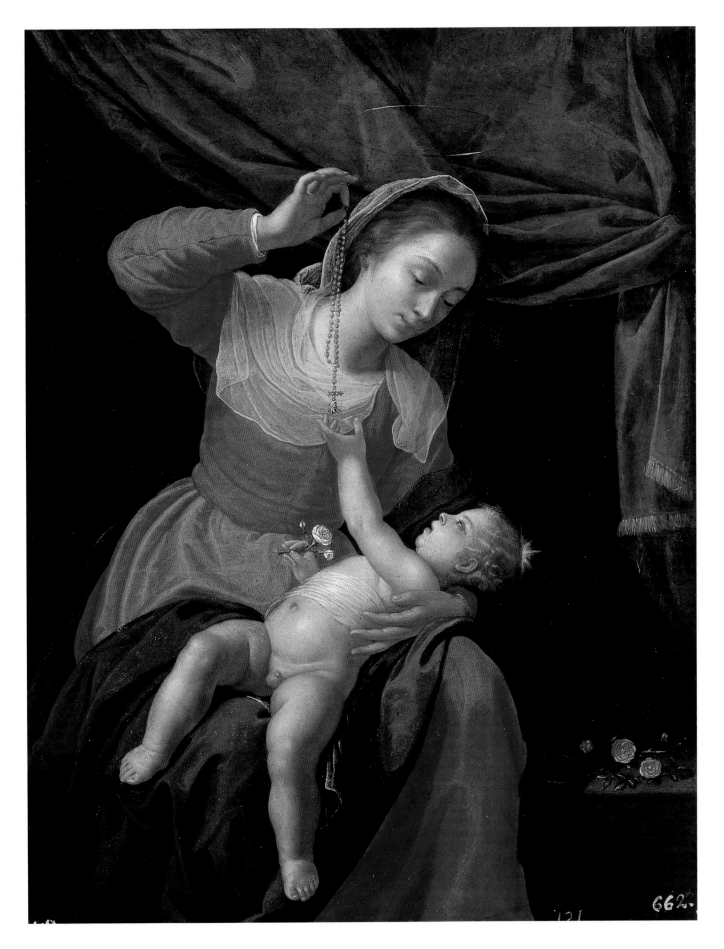

85.

ADDENDUM: ORAZIO GENTILESCHI

Conversion of the Magdalene

Oil on canvas, 52⅜ × 61 in.
(133 × 155 cm)

Alte Pinakothek, Munich
(inv. 12726)

ca. 1613–15

New York

PROVENANCE: Possibly Conte
Francesco Maria Carpegna,
Rome (until 1749); Freiherrn
von Wendlant, Berlin (by 1911,
when lent to the Kaiser Friedrich
Museum, Berlin); his heirs
(until ca. 1930); private collec-
tion, Germany; Julius Böhler,
Munich (1954); Georg and Otto
Schäfer, Schweinfurt (1954–57);
Alte Pinakothek, Munich.

REFERENCES: Longhi (1916)
1961, 264–65; Voss 1920b, 409;
Gamba 1922–23, 256; Voss 1925,
462; Redig de Campos 1939,
322; Longhi 1943, 47 n. 38; Moir
1967, vol. 1, 75 n. 22, vol. 2, 77;
Cummings 1974, 578; Nicolson
1979, 53; Bissell 1981, 172–73
no. 44; Pepper 1984a, 316;
Gregori in New York–Naples
1985, 251; Brown in Washington–
Cincinnati 1988–89, 57–59 no. 7;
Garrard 1989, 46, 499 n. 69;
Nicolson 1990, 115; Contini in
Florence 1991, 103–5 no. 5;
Spike 1991b, 732; Heiden 1998,
398–400.

This picture, Orazio's most compelling translation of a dialogue between two people into
gesture and expression (the *affetti*), made its debut in
Longhi's seminal article of 1916 as by either Artemisia
or Orazio. Despite this initial hesitation, there is now
consensus that the picture is indeed by Orazio. But at
what date? Longhi, Gamba, and Contini all date it to
after Rome; Bissell suggests about 1620. Like Moir
and Brown, I believe that the style points to an earlier
moment. The figures possess a plebeian sort of
beauty derived directly from the models who posed,
and the wonderfully subtle light is used to confer on
them a quality of physical density. They seem almost
to have descended from Orazio's concert on the vault
of the Casino delle Muse (fig. 6), discarding their
musical instruments to act out a religious pantomime.
Surprisingly, no one has suggested that Artemisia
posed for the figure of the Magdalene. The picture
seems to me to serve as a middle term between the
lyrical poetry of the *Lute Player* (cat. 22) and the
frozen drama of the Braunschweig *Crowning with
Thorns* (cat. 23).

Longhi, ever ready to emphasize the secular slant
of the Gentileschis' work, christened the picture "two
women at their toilette" Gamba suggested it might
show Leah and Rachel or Modesty and Vanity. Yet, as
Voss (1925) was quick to point out, "the pronounced
dramatic character of the representation leaves no
doubt that a fixed incident was intended": the story of
Martha reproving her sister Mary (usually identified as
Mary Magdalene) for her vanity.

The story is based very loosely on an incident told
in Luke 10:41–42, in which Christ rebukes Martha for
complaining that her sister did nothing to help her
with the chores. This episode has been elaborated
into the moment of the Magdalene's conversion from
her life of sin.

The subject achieved popularity only in the seventeenth century. However, as Cummings has shown,

it had a literary tradition going back at least to the
fourteenth century and was treated by Bernardino
Luini in a painting that, in the early seventeenth
century, was ascribed to Leonardo da Vinci and
belonged to Cardinal Francesco Maria del Monte
(Fine Arts Museum, San Diego). The moment Orazio
illustrates—when, to appropriate the words from a
hymn composed by Cardinal Robert Bellarmine
around 1597–99, the light of God's glance "Fills the
Magdalene with holy love / And melts the ice within
her soul"—is typically Counter-Reformation in its
emphasis on spiritual conversion. Seventeenth-century
writers focused on key episodes in the spiritual life
of the Magdalene for meditation and, hence, pictorial
(and musical) treatment: the Magdalene at the tomb
of Christ; her conversion while meditating in her
chamber; or, as here, her dialogue with her sister.
There is Riccardo Riccardi's *Conversione di Santa Maria
Maddalena*, of 1609, the *Pentimento di Santa Maria Maddalena* by Francucci, of 1615, and the *Maddalena lasciva e
penitente* by Gian Battista Andreini, of 1617, set to
music by Monteverdi. Garrard points out that in July
1622, a dialogue between Mary Magdalene and
Martha was performed at the Medicean court contrasting the contemplative versus the active life,
and it is just such a dialogue that Orazio has portrayed in his painting.

Orazio's model was unquestionably the influential
painting by Caravaggio that belonged to the Genoese
banker Ottavio Costa (Detroit Institute of Art; see
both Cummings and Gregori). In Orazio's picture, the
story has been rendered at its most basic. The hardworking Martha, on the left, dark-haired and modestly
garbed, her hands arranged in discourse, leans forward in intimate conversation with her idle sister, who
is seated in a somewhat wanton pose, her auburn hair
falling luxuriously over her shoulder, the ivory skin of
her bosom displayed to view, her arms resting listlessly
on the black frame of a rectangular mirror. The last

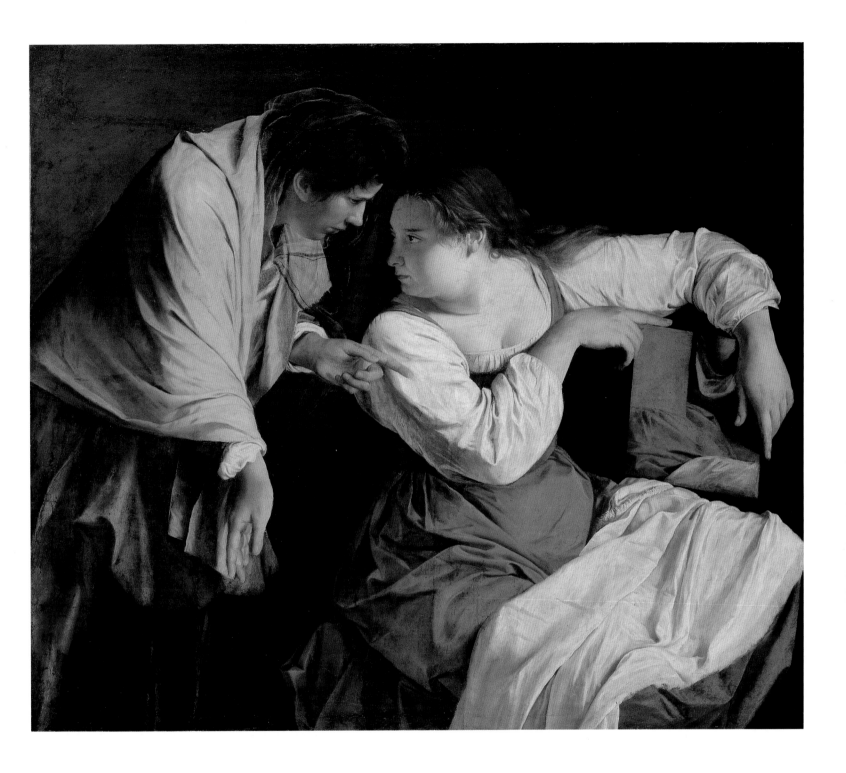

is a tour de force of artistic invention that suggests a simile of Caravaggesque painting as the mirror of nature. As had Caravaggio, Orazio uses light to suggest the enlightened path of Martha and Mary's conversion from her sinful life to one of pentitence, as she turns her head from the mirror to her sister.

Bissell has noted that in 1716 a picture of two women by Orazio was owned by Count Carpegna. The dimensions he quotes, seven by nine *braccia*, included the frame. The picture measured seven by five *braccia* (156 × 112 cm) and could be the Munich painting (see De Marchi 1987, 330).

Appendix 1. Documents Relating to the Trial of Agostino Tassi

PATRIZIA CAVAZZINI

The never-ending fascination of historians and art historians with the trial of Agostino Tassi for the defloration of Artemisia Gentileschi has yet to produce a complete transcription of the documentary material. Approximately half of the depositions in the Archivo di Stato di Roma (hereafter, ASR), Tribunale Criminale del Governatore, Processi del secolo XVII, vol. 104 (hereafter, Processi 104), were accurately transcribed by Eva Menzio (1981) in what is now an extremely rare publication. Mary Garrard, in her book on Artemisia (1989), includes an English translation, not always reliable, of this evidence, and adds a few more pages from ASR, Tribunale Criminale del Governatore, Miscellanea Artistica, b. 108 (hereafter, Miscellanea 108). For the sake of convenience, I am providing the briefest of summaries of what has already been transcribed, while inviting the reader to consult the two publications mentioned above. Also fundamental to an understanding of the trial are Elizabeth Cohen's writings (1991, 1992a, 1992b, 2000), for her unerring sense of the judicial proceedings and social customs of the time, and Alexandra Lapierre's novel (1998), based on an astonishing amount of new archival research on the Gentileschi and their circle of friends.

With the help of the notary Giovanni Battista Stiattesi, Orazio Gentileschi in early 1612 presented a petition to Paul V against his close friend and fellow painter Agostino Tassi. Gentileschi accused Tassi of having deflowered his daughter, Artemisia, and having then carried on a sexual liaison with her for many months. Tassi had had two accomplices. One was Tuzia, a neighbor who had moved into Orazio's house to serve as a chaperon for Artemisia and to protect her virginity but who had instead betrayed her. The other was Cosimo Quorli, a cousin of Stiattesi's, a close friend of Orazio's, and a papal official, who had extracted from Artemisia a few paintings belonging to her father, including a *Judith* of "rather large size" (probably fig. 46).

In all likelihood instructed by the same Stiattesi who had helped Orazio with his brief, Artemisia was well prepared for her deposition. With reserve and dignity, she told the judge how Agostino had taken her by force, at the beginning of May 1611, in her house on via della Croce. Confronted by her desperation, Tassi had promised to marry her, and she had then acquiesced to a relationship, always trusting that a marriage would follow. Artemisia was strengthened in this belief when Tassi took care to thwart any other marriage arrangements for her. She had heard that his wife, Maria Cannodoli, was alive, though he had always denied this. She believed it was Cosimo Quorli's fault that Agostino had not married her; the painter had apparently been disgusted by Quorli's failed attempt to rape her. Later during the trial Artemisia learned—or was lead to believe—that Tassi's wife was indeed still alive, and thus there was no hope of a marriage.

Stiattesi, once a friend to both Agostino and Quorli, testified that Tassi had confessed the defloration to him. Apparently, Quorli had encouraged the painter by leading him to believe that Artemisia had already lost her virginity. Moreover, Quorli's disapproval prevented the marriage, because Agostino, who owed him his life, did not want to act against his wishes. (As will become clear from these transcriptions, Quorli, who died shortly after the beginning of the trial, had arranged for Agostino's release from prison when, in 1611, the latter had been tried for incest with his sister-in-law.) According to Stiattesi, Quorli's spiteful behavior toward Artemisia was dictated by his failure to rape her himself. He had, in fact, repeatedly assaulted her, although he also claimed to be her father.

Everybody in the Gentileschi's small circle of friends—with the exception, for a while, of Orazio himself—knew about Artemisia's relationship with Tassi, and various people testified to this end. Agostino resolutely denied any wrongdoing, at the same time taking care to tarnish Artemisia's reputation. The judge mistrusted his version of events, but in a dramatic confrontation with Artemisia, the painter stood by his story. So did Artemisia—even under torture. Having lost her virginity and thus her honor, she was not necessarily regarded as a reliable witness. But her withstanding of torture—the tightening of strings around her fingers, which was considered to be a relatively minor form—confirmed the veracity of her accusations (Cohen 2000).

At this point Agostino produced a new witness, Nicolò di Bernardino de Felice, an apprentice known as Nicolò Bedino. Nicolò testified on June 8, 1612, accusing Artemisia of all sorts of improper behavior. Not only had she exchanged love letters with various men, but she had also had a number of lovers. According to his depositions, Nicolò knew this because he had worked for Orazio and had lived in his house on via Margutta since Lent of 1611, before the rape and at the time of Tassi and Gentileschi's collaboration on the Sala Regia in the Palazzo del Quirinale (their frescoes have been destroyed). Nicolò denied ever having been in Tassi's service, thus giving the impression that he had no reason to lie in his favor.

For unknown reasons, both Menzio and Garrard stop their transcriptions of the trial at this point. Garrard provides a brief summary of the remaining depositions. Agostino produced five more witnesses, in addition to Nicolò, to further damage Artemisia's reputation and to cast doubt on the motives of those who had accused him. It was suggested in the depositions that Orazio had fabricated the entire story to avoid repayment of a debt, that Stiattesi was acting to avenge an insult, and that Tuzia was angry at Agostino because they had had a violent quarrel.

Then, presumably in July 1612, Orazio brought new charges of slander and perjury against Tassi and four of the witnesses who had testified in his favor—Nicolò Bedino, Giuliano Formicino, Luca Penti, and Marcantonio Coppino. Only Tassi and Bedino were actually prosecuted. The rest of the trial focused on trying to establish Bedino's credibility, which largely depended on the question of who had employed him during Lent of 1611. If Bedino was in fact a reliable witness, then Agostino had commited no crime, for the rape of a dishonorable woman would not be prosecuted.

From the new round of questioning, it becomes clear that until the fall of 1611, Nicolò was in Agostino's service and only at this date did he move in with Orazio in the house near the city gate of Santo Spirito. During this time, Orazio must have been in particular need of an assistant since he was making frescoes in Cardinal Borghese's Casino delle Muse (fig. 6), where his role was larger than it had been in the Sala Regia. Nicolò had worked for Orazio before and had been in his house on via della Croce, though only on an occasional basis, when Agostino felt he could spare him. Nicolò also went back to work for Agostino a few days after the latter's incarceration. His loyalty lay with Agostino, and he was indeed a false witness, as Orazio had claimed. But as Nicolò was willing to confirm his version of the story even under torture and had in any case helped Orazio now and then from Lent of 1611, it must have been difficult for the judge to see through his tangle of prevarications. To complicate matters, some of the witnesses in Orazio's favor lied or were confused about dates, weakening his argument that Nicolò was living with Agostino at the crucial time. Tassi was eventually sentenced to five years' exile from Rome, though he did not bother to leave the city until a new sentence of exile, for a different crime, was pronounced against him.

The material in this appendix is divided into three sections:

A. Taken from the main volume of the trial, ASR, Tribunale Criminale del Governatore, Processi 104. From the 170 pages of depositions following Bedino's, I have extracted fragments relating to artistic education in general, to Orazio's workshop practice, to his circle of friends and patrons, and to his house. While I have not transcribed all or even most of what is there, I have tried to convey the gist of what happened during the trial. Among my omissions are all the questions posed by the judge (they are stated in Latin and can be easily deduced from the answers). The page numbers given are those of the bound volume, not the modern pagination in pencil. The same material has been summarized by Garrard, but her focus is very different from mine. Some depositions can be found verbatim in Lapierre—I have indicated when this is the case—and short fragments are also in Bissell's notes.

B. Consisting of two more depositions in Nicolò Bedino's favor, from a different volume, Testimoni 201. To my knowledge, no one has seen or cited these before. They should be inserted toward the end of the interrogations, in Processi 104, according to their date—that is, just before Nicolò final questioning. I have abbreviated these as well, but less substantially than the depositions from section A, which tend to be more repetitive.

C. Involving legal steps taken by the court, by Orazio Gentileschi, and by Tassi, which can be found in Registrazioni d'atti, vols. 166, 167. (The series should be called "Manuali d'atti," but this citation often causes confusion in the retrieval of the proper volume and so is best avoided.) Lapierre has used this material in the past, without a transcription.

I am much indebted to Simona Feci, to Augusto Pompeo, and, in particular, to Michele Di Sivo for having helped me with the transcriptions—especially, but not only, of the material in section C, which I could not have approached without them. Even with their assistance, many words in the Registrazioni d'atti remained indecipherable. I trust, however, that the sense is correct. A few pages of the main volume, Processi 104, have been substantially damaged by the acid ink used at the time of the trial and thus are impossible to transcribe in their entirety.

Parentheses indicate my interpolations; brackets indicate that I have doubts regarding the transcription; ellipses within brackets indicate a word that I was not able to transcribe. I have added a minimum of punctuation and avoided the abbreviations in the Italian text.

It is conceivable that further evidence from the trial will turn up. The file discovered by Garrard in Miscellanea 108 suggests that at least seven depositions, including that of the painter Orazio Borgianni, have been lost. These testimonies must all have been in Tassi's defense, since they were presented by one of his lawyers.

The following is a list, in order of their appearance before the court, of witnesses in the sections of the trial that are transcribed below:

Witnesses for the defense of Agostino Tassi in the rape trial:
Giuliano Formicino, a youth of independent means who had met Tassi in prison at Corte Savella, where his brother was also a prisoner
Luca Penti, a tailor
Fausta Ciacconi, a washerwoman employed by Agostino
Mario Trotta, an apprentice painter
Marcantonio Coppino, a mixer of ultramarine.

Witness for the prosecution in the rape trial:
Fra Pietro di Giordano, a prisoner in Corte Savella.

Witnesses for the prosecution in the perjury trial:
Giovanni Pietro Molli, a pilgrim used as a model by Orazio Gentileschi and other painters
Margherita from Milan, a washerwoman who had worked for Orazio for twenty years
Bernardino Franchi, Orazio's barber of twenty years
Pietro Hernandez, Orazio's neighbor at Santo Spirito
Caterina Zuccarini, Orazio's maid at Santo Spirito
Carlo Saraceni, a painter from Venice
Olimpia de Bargellis, Agostino's half sister
Marta de Rubertis, Agostino's neighbor at Sant'Onofrio
Antinoro Bertucci, the owner of a pigment store on via del Corso
Valerio Ursino, a painter from Florence.

Witnesses for the defense in the perjury trial:
Luca Finocchi, an innkeeper and Tassi's friend since 1610
Michelangelo Vestri, a painter (section B)
Costanza Ceuli, Orazio's neighbor on via della Croce. Her husband had been Orazio's tailor for many years (section B)
Nicolò Bedino, who was also repeatedly questioned in this section of the trial.

SECTION A

ASR, Tribunale Criminale del Governatore, Processi, secolo XVII, busta 104

Giuliano Formicino romano 18 anni
(363v) July 9, 1612 Giuliano Formicino claims he heard Stiattesi declare that he had instigated Agostino's imprisonment as revenge for the latter's maligning him as a cuckold and sodomite. He had also heard that if Agostino lent Stiattesi fifteen scudi, the latter would make Artemisia confess that she had lost her virginity not to Tassi but to Pasquino from Florence—now conveniently dead. In order to help Tassi, Formicino wants to prove that Stiattesi's deposition against the painter was dictated by spite. See Menzio 66–74, 128 for Stiattesi's accusations.

(364)—Io habito in Piazza Mattei e non ho nessun essercitio che vivo del mio.
—Io mi son venuto ad esaminare perché me l'ha detto il sollecitatore di Agostino Tassi pittore che non so il suo cognome che stava a [. . .] dirmelo hier sera in Corte Savella dove io stavo a servir il signor Fabio mio fratello carcerato . . .
(365v)—Io ho inteso raggionare con detto Agostino una volta doppo pranzo un'huomo alto che pranzò con esso e con mio fratello, chiamato per quanto dicevano lo Stiattese, quale ragionava e diceva che se Agostino gli voleva imprestare 15 scudi che gli avrebbe restituiti in qualche suo bisogno perché si haveva gran necessità, e ch'avria fatto disdire quella zitella che si pretendeva che lui havesse sverginata e fattoli dire colui che l'haveva sverginata, cioè un tale Pasquino fiorentino, che diceva che gli l'haveva detto detta zitella da quattro anni fa l'haveva sverginata detto Pasquino, e disse anco ch'haveva fatto mettere priggione detto Agostino perché gli haveva detto quelle parole, cioé becco fottuto e che li voleva dare e che lui non bastava l'animo di vendicarsi altrimenti.
(366v) Io Giuliano formicino romano ho deposto come di sopra

Luca fu Aloisio Penti romano anni 25 circa
(367) June 15, 1612 The tailor Luca Penti, who knows both Tassi and Gentileschi, states that—as was common in every painter's house—people of all sorts frequented Orazio's residence. He has seen Artemisia at a window but has never talked to her. She had had sexual relationships with both Quorli and Pasquino. Stiattesi had declared that Artemisia was a whore, and Cosimo had told him that Tassi was in love with her. More of Penti's deposition can be found in Lapierre, app. 4.

—Io habito in Campo Martio e l'arte mia è di sartore.
—Io conosco Agostino Tassi . . . [da] circa tre anni con occasione che era amico

di Cosimo furiere et l'ho servito di vestiti et Horatio lo conosco da due anni con occasione che praticavo di là su dal Babuino dove habitava lui et anco per via di detto Cosmo . . .

(368)—Io ho visto conversare detto signor Horatio da che l'ho conosciuto con diverse persone quando con gentilhuomini e gente di prezzo e quando con gente bassa, ch'io non so chi siano.

—Io credo ch'in una casa dove ci sia da vedere delle figure et historie ci sogli praticare ogni sorta di gente e gentilhuomini e di altra qualità e non so che ci vadano per far male e bene o si da questo andare ci possa nascere sospetto alcuno.

(369)—Io ho visto Artemisia non so che volte da che stava alli Greci e così la conosco.

—Detta Artimitia io l'ho vista a una finestra lì alli Greci che c'era l'impanata et anco l'ho vista a San Spirito alla finestra et una volta in casa quando c'entrai con Cosmo furiero e non c'ho mai parlato.

(369v)—Io non so quanto tempo sia che detta Artemisia sia stata sverginata né da chi, ma è un pezzo che ci praticava un mio amico chiamato Pasquino da Fiorenza ch'era guardiano di Ripagrande.

(370v)—Sì che può essere che detto Pasquino si vantasse di conoscere carnalmente detta Artemisia e che poi non fosse vero . . .

(370v)—E' un pezzo che sono tre o quattro anni che Cosimo mi cominciò a dire che lui aveva avuto che fare con detta Artemisia . . .

— . . . in compagnia di Cosmo, Agostino et uno che si chiama il Stiattesi che sta in casa di detto Horatio . . . si venne a raggionare di detta Artimitia et il Stiattesi disse che era una poltrona e una puttana.

371—Io ho inteso dire da Cosmo suddetto che Agostino era innamorato di detta Artimitia . . .

(372) io luca pentis ho deposto quanto di sopra

Fausta fu Domenico Ciaccone alias Palumbara
(372v) June 18, 1612 Fausta Ciacconi, a washerwoman, testifies about Tassi's quarrel with Tuzia, the woman who was supposed to protect Artemisia but had instead helped Agostino. Fausta intends to show that Tuzia's deposition against Tassi cannot be trusted since she had reasons for enmity toward the painter. (See Lapierre, app. 6.)

—Io habito alla Longara e son lavandara.

(373v)—Questa donna che io ho detto che contrastò con detto Agostino in casa sua si chiama Tutia et habita in casa del signor Horatio Gentileschi . . . Agostino gli disse poltrona se tu vieni più qua ti voglio buttare per queste scale.

Mario fu Filippo Trotta, circa 21 anni
(374v) June 23, 1612 Mario Trotta, an apprentice "learning to draw," declares that Orazio had evicted from his house his nephew Giovanni Battista, now dead, who had told him that Artemisia spent time at the window. During the winter, Trotta worked with both Orazio and Agostino in the Palazzo del Quirinale for three giulii a day. According to Trotta, Orazio is a loner, whose only friends are Agostino, Quorli, and the keeper of the Vatican fountain. Orazio employs day laborers. Trotta does not know Artemisia. He has heard she was a virtuous woman but has also heard that she was seen by Carlo Saraceni standing "very brazenly" at the window. He does not think that the comings and goings in Orazio's house would cause rumors. (See Lapierre, app. 5.) Mario Trotta was not included by Orazio in the list of false witnesses.

—Io habito in una camera a locanda a Montecitorio et l'essercitio mio è di pittore, cioè principiante, che vado disegnando.

(375) . . . un nipote di Horatio Gentileschi chiamato Giovanni Battista, che è morto all'ospedale di San Giovanni haveva detto che il detto Horatio l'haveva scacciato di casa per una parola . . . che lui haveva detto alla sorella cugina figlia di detto Gentileschi che non stesse alla finestra ch'era vergogna che lui gli l'haveva detto al padre e per questo l'haveva cacciato via.

(375v)—Io sono a Roma dalla canonizzazione di San Carlo [November 1, 1610] in qua . . . io stetti un mese in casa di monsignor Santoro e poi lui mi accomodò con Antinoro Bertucci . . . con il quale stetti tre mesi . . . sono stato anco sei mesi con il Cavalier d'Arpino e dopo tornai in casa di monsignore dove sono stato sino alli 15 di maggio prossimo passato et hadesso habito a camera locanda a Monte Citorio appresso a Monsignore.

—Io conosco Horatio Gentileschi et Agostino Tasso perché ho lavorato a giornate con loro a Monte Cavallo quest'inverno e mi davano tre giulii il giorno . . . l'un e l'altro mi han dato da lavorare . . .

(376)—Io non ho mai visto praticare il detto Horatio se non con Agostino Tassi, con il detto Cosmo furiero, con il custode delle fontane di palazzo e con noi altri lavoranti che ci dava da lavorare.

—Io non ho habitato nè praticato in casa dal detto Horatio, nè son stato mai a casa sua . . .

—Signorsì che in casa di pittori ci praticano gentilhuomini, ch'io son stato in casa del Cavalier Giuseppe [d'Arpino] e c'ho visto Monsignor Santoro e altri signori e gentilhuomini e cardinali e mal nome io non ho mai inteso in casa del Cavaliere per la pratica di detti signori.

—Signorno che io non conosco Artemisia figliola di Horatio et io non so di che fama e conditione si sia. Io (376v) la lasso nel grado e honore suo.

—Io ho inteso sempre dire da diversi pittori, che uno è Carlo Venentiano e delli altri non mi ricordo delli nomi, che la figliola di Horatio è virtuosa e buona zitella . . . quando stavo in casa di Antinoro Bertucci che vendeva li colori e lì ci praticavano delli pittori . . . e raggionavano qualche volta della figlia di detto Horatio et dicevano che era virtuosa e buona zitella come di sopra e la tenevano tutti per zitella se non che il signor Carlo disse l'aveva vista alla finestra molto sfacciatamente . . .

(377) Mario Trotta

Marcantonio Coppino fiorentino di anni 34
June 23, 1612 Marcantonio Coppino, who prepares ultramarine, claims that in Antinoro Bertucci's pigment store, at a time when Carlo Saraceni was also present, he had heard that Artemisia was a whore. When a neighbor reported this to Orazio, the latter had told him to mind his own business. According to Coppino, Orazio is almost always alone; his only friends are Tassi and Quorli. He does not want Artemisia to marry, has her pose in the nude, and likes people to come and see her. Orazio, who has brought charges against Agostino to avoid repayment of a debt of 200 scudi, has repented this action, but it is too late to do anything about it. Orazio wants Agostino to marry Artemisia and go to the devil. (See Lapierre, app. 7.) The painter from Modena mentioned here must be the Girolamo modenese, said by Bedino to be one of Artemisia's lovers. (See Menzio 153.)

—L'essercitio mio è di fare il colore azzurro oltremarino e habito alli Cesarini.

(377v) . . . in particolare una volta l'intesi dire nel corso in bottega di Antinoro Bertucci e che c'era presente Carlo Venetiano pittore e un gentilhuomo sbarbato chiamato Giovanni Battista per quanto credo e un prete che sta lì in casa e altre genti che non so il nome e un modenese pittore del quale non so il nome e si discorreva di questa figliola del Gentileschi come se fosse stata madonna pubblica del bordello e quel modenese disse che (Orazio) era stato avvertito da un suo compare falegname che si stava (378) accanto alli Greci e che lui gli haveva risposto bada a casa tua per favore.

—Io non ho mai visto il detto Horatio se non (378v) in compagnia di Cosmo Quorlo e di detto Agostino Tassi del resto lo [trovo] quasi sempre solo.

—Io in casa di pittori c'ho visto delle volte di gentilhuomini e di prelati e altre genti di buona conditione e fama che per questo andari di gentilhuomini e altri in casa loro ci possi nascere mala fama contra detto pittori o suspitione io non lo so.

(379v)—Io ho sentito dire quella volta nella bottega di detto Antinoro . . . che detta figliola del Gentileschi non fosse zitella, et l'ho sentito dire anco in bottega di uno scultore in Piazza di Sciarra da certi pittori che non so chi siano, dove c'era tra li altri un certo Mario che non so il cognome ma è pittore ed è giovane sbarbato, et il padrone di detta bottega si chiama Angelo . . . diversi dissero molte cose della figlia del Gentileschi, cioè che era una bella giovane e che il padre l'haveva trovata da maritare e non l'haveva voluta maritare e che quando faceva qualche ritratto nudo la faceva spogliar nuda e la ritraheva e che gli piaceva che c'andassero le genti a vederla e dicevano che non era zitella e che faceva servitio a qualcheduno e questo disse haverlo sentito dire anco detto Angelo scultore e così anco disse detto Mario . . . (380) et anco ho inteso dire da Giovanni Battista nipote di detto Horatio ch'hora è morto che disse di haverlo fatto avvertire il padre di detta giovane e che per questo c'era discordia tra loro e l'haveva mandato via e mi disse anco ch'uno zio che stava a Pisa voleva maritare del suo detta figliola del Gentileschi e che lui non ce la voleva mandare, ma chi l'habbia sverginata io non l'ho inteso dire.

(380v) quando Agostino fu fatto prigione io intesi dire da diversi che il detto Horatio l'haveva fatto (381) mettere prigione per non darli 200 scudi che gli haveva da dare e per fargli pigliar per moglie la figliola . . . et io dissi [ad Orazio] ch'haveva fatto male a scoprirsi di questa cosa e lui mi rispose è fatto mò pagherei la man dritta di non haverlo fatto e ne son pentito e poi che ci sono voglio vedere di fargliela pigliare per moglie e poi vada al diavolo.

Io Marco Coppino per la verità ho deposto quanto di sopra

Fra Pietro di Giordano
(381v) June 29, 1612 Friar Pietro di Giordano claims that Tassi and Quorli had instigated Stiattesi's imprisonment, and that they had previously arranged for Stiattesi to live at Orazio's house in order for Agostino to better carry out his affair with Artemisia. Tassi had confessed to the friar his obligation to marry Artemisia because he had deflowered her. However, he was worried that his wife was still alive, even though he had received letters to the contrary. The friar had seen the lovers in Corte Savella behaving affectionately with each other. He had also seen Nicolò Bedino bringing food to Tassi in prison and knew that the latter had arranged for witnesses to declare that Artemisia was a prostitute. (See Lapierre, app. 17.)

The deposition of the friar, so damning for Tassi, also touches on the key point of Tassi's wife. Was she indeed still alive? If this was the case, obviously he could not marry Artemisia. In both the trial of 1611—in which Agostino was accused of incest with his sister-in-law Costanza—and the trial of 1612, we hear that Agostino had actively tried to dispose of her by sending assassins to Livorno).

(381v)—Essendo io questa settimana santa andato carcerato in Corte Savella ci trovai il signor Giovanni Battista Stiattesi il quale mi dette comodità di dormire vicino il suo letto . . . mi disse che era stato un suo cugino chiamato Cosmo a requisitione di Agustino Tasso, il quale havendo sverginato una zitella e lui cercando di farla prendere per moglie, per dispetto l'havevano fatto prendere prigione. Per poter haver maggior (382) comodità detto Agostino lo fece andare ad habitare nella propria casa di quella zitella che non volendo detto Stiattesi tener mano a simil'amori né fare tradimento al padre di detta giovane si corrocciorono e per questo l'havevano fatto metter priggione . . . (382v) detto Agostino confessò . . . come lui doveva prenderla per moglie e che saria stata sua senz'altro giacché l'haveva havuta zitella ma che un sol dubbio li rimaneva ch'era questo che lui sospettava che la moglie fusse viva se bene gli era stato scritto che era morta . . . (383)—. . . viddi doi donne in Corte Savella con il Stiattesi e li figli, dopoi ch'havevano parlato in Cancelleria un pezzo con detto Agostino et il Stiattesi, viddi ch'una di quelle donne all'uscir di Cancelleria sin al cancello (383v) andava appoggiata al braccio di detto Agostino et al separarsi fecero gran segno d'amor et affettione insieme e dimandando io la matina a detto Agostino chi era quella donna che andava appoggiata al suo braccio come di sopra lui mi disse che era la sua cara Artemisia e moglie e così li domandai che havevano ragionato; lui mi disse che havevano concluso il parentado e che lui gli haveva dato le fede di sposarla e mi disse che restava in obbligo infinito al Stiattesi che gli haveva fatto uno dei più grandi servitii che si potessero fare al mondo.
(384)— . . . Nicolò . . . l'ho veduto venir altre volte a veder detto Agostino et a portarli robba da mangiare . . .

—. . . Agostino mi disse che voleva far dire a detti testimoni che Artemisia era stata una puttana pubblica . . .
Io fra Pietro Giordano ho deposto quanto di sopra

(384v) July 5, 1612 Agostino is again interrogated and urged to confess, but he continues to deny everything of which he is accused, even when he is confronted by the friar.

(391) Undated. Orazio brings new charges against Agostino—for slander and for subornation of witnesses—and against four of the six witnesses testifying for Agostino: namely Luca Penti, Marcantonio Coppino, Giuliano Formicino, and Nicolò Bedino. He points out contradictions in their depositions. Bedino, for example, has declared that Artemisia wrote love letters, but she cannot write. He cannot properly describe the house on via Margutta (actually, Nicolò's description of the house [Menzio, 150–51] matches those by Molli and Franchi below). Orazio also lies about Artemisia's age. See Garrard 481–82, for a summary, with some inaccuracies, of Orazio's new charges.

(391) . . . havendo io una figlia chiamata Artimitia zitella d'età d'anni 15 in circa detto Agostino hebbe ardire di Maggio dell'anno prossimo passato d'entrar in casa mia in strada della Croce et con lusinghe e promesse di sposarla voleva conoscerla carnalmente et non volendo lei consentire gli fece violenza addosso . . .
(393) Però vedendosi dalle cose sopradette che detto Agostino ha prodotto articoli falsi e calunniosi et infamatorii et indotti e fatti anco essaminare testimoni falsi dò querela tanto contro detto Agostino quanto anco li sodetti 4 testimoni subornati e falsi et domando che siano castigati conforme il giusto . . .

Giovanni Pietro fu Angelo Molli di Palermo
July 27, 1612 Giovanni Pietro Molli, a pilgrim from Palermo, declares that during Lent of 1611, Orazio used him as a model for a *Saint Jerome* (cat. 16) and other paintings. He went often to Orazio's house and received payment and meals. In the house he saw Orazio's grown daughter and three sons, one of whom ground colors, as well as Orazio's nephew. They had neither a servant nor a shopboy, and he has never seen Nicolò Bedino. During the time Molli was employed as a model, Orazio moved. Thus, he has been in two of Orazio's houses, one "alli Greci" (near the Greek church on via Paolina [present-day via del Babuino]) and one "sopra il Babuino" (that is, on via Margutta). He briefly describes the house "alli Greci" and, in more detail, the one on via Margutta, where the main floor had two rooms: a dining room and a studio where Orazio painted. He has not been in the other rooms. Molli may have been confused about dates, or was perhaps lying, in order to help Orazio prove that Nicolò was not living with him during Lent of 1611. In his second deposition Molli stated he had returned to Rome from Naples on the Tuesday before Easter 1611, after an absence of seven months. Thus, he could not have been in Orazio's house "ai Greci" during Lent of 1611, since Orazio was living on via Margutta by, at the latest, February 16 of that year (Bissell 1981, 102). In her second deposition, of September 14, the washerwoman, Margherita, claimed that Gentileschi lived on via Margutta about two years ago. The barber, Bernardino Franchi, who was admittedly very vague about dates, estimated that Orazio lived on via Margutta six months or a year. Since we know that Orazio moved out of this house on via Margutta by April 10, 1611, he had probably arrived there at some point in 1610 (Menzio, 57). According to Franchi's second deposition, Molli had posed for Orazio during Lent of 1610 at via Margutta, certainly the wrong time for the pilgrim to have helped Orazio prove Nicolò's perjury. The judge must have suspected that something was wrong with Molli's deposition because he continued to question him. Molli eventually refused to answer, saying he was about to faint.

(395; the page is badly damaged)—In quanto Vossignoria mi domanda io gli posso dire per la verità che quest'anno passato nel tempo di quadragesima cioè questa quadragesima prossima passata ha fatto l'anno il signor Horatio Gentileschi pittore si serviva . . . per ritrare una testa simile . . . , alcuni quadri che lui faceva, et . . . un San Girolamo intiero; mi fece spogliare dalla cintura in su per fare un San Girolamo simile a me et per questo effetto mi tenne in casa tutta la quadragesima perché tre et quattro giorni della settimana sempre mai mi bisognava andare a casa sua et in qualche giornata che ci andavo ci stavo dalla mattina a la sera e magnavo e bevevo in casa sua e mi pagava le mie giornate ma a dormire ritornavo a casa mia et mentre il signor Horatio si servì di me per fare (395v) questi ritratti che ho detto lui habitava alli Greci e poi si partì et andò a stare sopra il Babuino in una casa dove . . . io continuai ad andare per l'effetto che io ho detto e mentre praticai in casa in detta quadragesima et anco alcuni giorni dopo Pasqua, che continuò il signor Horatio di servirsi di me che non haveva ancora finito li lavori che voleva fare, io ci viddi in casa oltre detto Signor Horatio una sua figlia grande e tre figli maschi che uno dei quali che era il più grande macinava li colori e anco un nipote del Signor Horatio che andava apprendere . . . [magnavamo] tutti insieme la sera io ritornavo a magnare . . . et in quel tempo perché io praticavo in casa per questo effetto, così alli Greci dove stava prima come anco in quell'altra casa di sopra al Babuino dove andò poi a stare non ci vidi mai nessun altro a tavola sua eccetto questi che ho detto.

—Mentre io praticavo in casa di detto signor Horatio non viddi che havesse garzone o servitore o serva che se l'havesse havuto (396) ci andai tante volte che li avrei veduti. Veddi bene praticarci una donna che era lavandara di casa la quale veneva molte volte a pigliare li panni e drappi.

—Il nipote del detto signor Horatio era quello che spendeva et anco [serviva] alla cucina.

—Mentre io andai in casa di detto Signor Horatio non ci praticò nessuno in casa che servisse a detto Signor Horatio nell'essercitio della pittura che se ci fusse venuto io l'havrei veduto in tanti giorni che io ci andai in casa. Io non conosco né so chi sia questo Nicolò che Vossignoria mi domanda . . .

(396v)—Io ho detto che mentre il signor Horatio si cominciò a servirsi di me lui habitava alli Greci in una casa poco lontano dalla chiesa la quale è una bella casa et ha una stanza a mano destra che s'entrava dalla porta dove lavorava detto signor Horatio, come se sia fatta dalla banda sinistra io non lo so perché non ci andai mai, et mi portavano da magnare in quella camera che in quelli principi finché non presero pratica della persona mia non mi sbrigava a magnare con loro. Partendo dalli Greci detto signor Horatio andò poi ad habitare (397) sopra il Babuino in una casa la quale nell'entrare oltre la porta c'è nell'andito c'è anco il cancello et dopo si trova una stanza a mano manca e poi si salisce su ad alto per una scala di due pezzi e a capo le scale a mano manca sono due stanze una avanti l'altra che nella prima si magnava e nell'altra lavorava e in questa ci sono due finestre che risponde nella strada et dall'altra banda c'è un poco di scoperto col pozzo e la cocinetta e di qui ci sono delle stanze ancora ma io non ci andai et sopra la cocina c'è un giardino con certi arbori che mi dicevano essere del padrone della casa.

Margherita fu Agostino milanese lavandaia
July 20, 1612 Margherita, a washerwoman, has worked for Orazio for eighteen or twenty years. She used to do the laundry and occasionally helped Artemisia with household chores. She has been employed in all of Gentileschi's homes but has met Nicolò Bedino only since Orazio moved near Santo Spirito. If the boy had lived in the other houses, she would, in all likelihood, have seen him.

—Di quanto Vossignoria mi domanda posso dire per verità che saranno fino a 18 o 20 anni che servo per lavandara il signor Horatio Gentileschi (397v) da quando lo cominciai a servire stava nella strada diritta di Ripetta et poi andò a stare nella piazza della Trinità et dopo partito dalla piazza della Trinità andò a stare alli Greci e partito dalli Greci andò a stare alla strada di Margutta sopra il Babuino . . . et alle volte anco mi mandava a chiamare la zitella che gli aiutassi a fare qualche cosa . . . et quanto a questo Nicolò che Vossignoria mi domanda vi dico che ho conosciuto un giovane sbarbato che si chiama Nicolò in casa del signor Horatio Gentileschi da che lui venne a stare alla casa di San Spirito che sarà un anno in circa che faceva in casa molti servitii e imparava anco la pittura, quale Nicolò mentre detto signor Horatio habitava in questi altri luoghi . . .

(398) io non l'ho mai visto in casa d'esso Horatio.

—Ogni cosa può essere ma saria gran cosa che non l'havessi mai visto (Nicolò) in queste altre case se ci fusse stato . . . .

Bernardino fu Francesco Franchi barbiere
(398v) July 31, 1612 Bernardino Franchi has been Orazio's barber for eighteen or twenty years and has often been to his house in different capacities, as a barber, to let blood from family members, and to pose as a model. He has never been to the house at Santo Spirito. During all these years in Orazio's various residences he has seen only Francesco Scarpellino, Giovanni Battista the nephew, Pasquino from Florence, a washerwoman called Margherita, her husband, and a few people who came to see the paintings. He also remembers having seen a young apprentice in the house on via del Babuino. The house on via Margutta had a laundry room on the ground floor, two rooms on the main floor, and two upstairs rooms where Artemisia lived and where he has never been. In this deposition, he gives answers regarding the time of Orazio's move to via Margutta that contradict those in his second interrogation.

(399) . . . saranno da 18 o 20 anni in circa ch'io conosco Horatio Gentileschi et da detto tempo in qua l'ho servito nell'essercitio della barberia che ho praticato in casa sua liberamente . . . se bene adesso è andato a stare a San Spirito dove io non sono mai stato . . . che alle volte ci sono stato una volta la settimana e qualche volta sono stato dieci o dodeci giorni e delle volte ci sono stato quattro et cinque volte il giorno perché lui più volte si è servito di me per modello; ho cavato sangue a lui alla figliola, alla moglie et alli figli, et ho fatto la barba a lui et mentre che in questo tempo ho praticato in casa del detto Horatio ho visto praticare in casa un certo Francesco Scarpellino, un certo Giovanni (399v) Battista nipote di esso Gentileschi et Pasquino fiorentino, un'altra donna lavandara chiamata Margherita et il marito di essa Margherita . . . forsi alle volte ho visto qualcun che veniva per vedere quadri che non so chi siano quali parlavano con lui e se ne andavano via.

—Io non conosco questo Nicolò che Vossignoria mi nomina.

(400)— . . . mi sovviene che habitando esso alli Greci ci veddi più volte in casa un ragazzo sbarbato che all'hora poteva havere da 13 o 14 anni in circa il quale imparava di disegnare et credo che questo ragazzo fosse stato accomodato col signor Horatio dal Cavalier Gioseppe d'Arpino . . . quando designava lo vedevo star basso con la testa ma del nome non me ricordo.

(400v)—Io non ho visto questo ragazzo se non mentre il signor Horatio habitava alli Greci l'ho visto; nelle altre case dove andò ad abitare dipoi io non ce l'ho visto.

(401)— . . . potria essere che il giovine sia stato anco in altri luoghi, in questo io non li posso rispondere con sodisfatione della coscienza mia.

—A me pare che il signor Horatio partisse dalla strada dei Greci et andasse a strada Margutta questo Carnevale ha fatto un (hole in the page) . . .

—Non ci stette molto il signor Horatio nella strada di Margutta ma credo [passasse] sei mesi o simil cosa e come ho detto io ci sono stato in questa casa dove lui habitava la quale all'entrare dalla prima porta c'è un poco di annito e poi si trova un cancello, entrati nel cancello (401v) si trova una porta a mano manca dove si fa il bucato e poi si va su per una scala che torcia e a capo la scala si trovano dui stanze a mano manca che una va nell'altra e l'ultima guarda le finestre nella strada a man dritta. In faccia c'è un cortiletto e se ben mi ricordo credo ci sia due vasche; di sopra so che ci sono dui stanze dove ci stava la zitella che di sopra io non ci andai mai e altre stanze non so che ci fusse.

(The deposition was signed and sworn, but the page has been torn by the ink.)

Pietro Hernandez Spagnolo
(401v) August 4, 1612 Pietro Hernandez is one of Orazio's neighbors at Santo Spirito. He states that Artemisia is his son's godmother and that Nicolò Bedino began living in Orazio's house in November or December 1612. He knows this from a neighbor, Caterina, who was employed as a housemaid

by the Gentileschi but who worked there less frequently after Nicolò arrived. The boy, who was learning to draw, also painted and was taught by Artemisia.

Hernandez was also a painter; see ASR, Stato Civile, app., Stati di anime di Santo Spirito in Sassia, 1614, 1615, where he is called *pittore*. He was a neighbor of Olimpia de Bargellis, Agostino's half sister, who was also a witness for the prosecution.

(The page is damaged.)

— . . . io conosco il detto Horatio Gentileschi da ottobre passato in qua con occasione che essendomi nato un figlio maschio feci comare (402) la signora Artemitia figliola di detto signor Horatio et mentre io il detto mese di ottobre cominciai a praticare in casa sua non ci viddi mai un certo giovane sbarbato che si chiama Nicolò il quale s'accomodò pur con il detto Horatio circa un mese o due di poi e questo lo so perché una donna mia vicina che si chiama Caterina la quale era solita andare in casa sua, ch'aiutava alla cocina et altri servitii di casa mi disse un giorno che detto Horatio haveva preso un ragazzo . . . e che perciò non c'andava più così spesso in casa . . . et (questo ragazzo) imparava di disegnare et anco l'ho visto dipingere che la signora Artemisia gli insegnava.
Io Pietro Hernandez o deposto come di sopra

Caterina Zuccarini
(402v) August (the page is damaged). Caterina Zuccarini says that Artemisia used to employ her as a maid in the house at Santo Spirito, but since Nicolò Bedino has come to live with the Gentileschi she does not go there as often. Previously, Nicolò had come to the house now and then for instruction in drawing, and he would draw with Orazio's son Francesco. They learned by themselves—or perhaps "from them" (da loro) meaning Orazio and Artemisia—but this is less likely. Nicolò used to live with Agostino Tassi.

— . . . l'anno passato nel mese di luglio o di agosto venne ad habitare in faccia a casa mia il detto Horatio Gentileschi pittore con la sua famiglia nel mese di luglio e con questa (403) occasione io cominciai a bazzicar a casa sua intorno a mezzo agosto che la sua figliola chiamata la signora Artimitia mi chiamò un giorno e mi disse s'io li volevo aiutar a far li servitii di casa cioè rifar li letti e quel che bisognava e così io gli risposi di sì e cominciai a praticar in casa sua non avendo loro nessuno che li facesse li servitii e così io seguitai di andare in casa sua ogni due o tre giorni sino a novembre che qualche volta anco mi facevano anco restar a magnar lì in casa e di novembre poi detto signor Horatio pigliò un servitore che era un giovanotto piccoletto sbarbato chiamato Nicolò e doppo che Nicolò venne in casa io non ce andai più così spesso . . . prima che detto Nicolò s'accomodasse con detto signor Horatio io ce l'ho visto venire in casa non so che volte che sarà doi o tre volte in circa che veniva a imparare di disegnare e disegnavano insieme lui e Francesco figliolo di detto signor Horatio che imparavano da loro, e questo Nicolò prima di venire a stare con detto signor Horatio stava (403v) con un pittore chiamato Agostino Tasso ch'abitava al monte di Sant'Honofrio . . .

Nicolò Bedino
(405) August 8, 1612 Nicolò Bedino testifies that he went to live with Orazio during Lent of 1611. According to Nicolò, while he was working in the Palazzo del Quirinale together with other painters, Orazio asked him to live at his house on via Margutta. Nicolò received instruction in drawing, plus food and lodging. In exchange, he cleaned the house, ground colors, made the beds, and sometimes went grocery shopping. At via Margutta, Orazio did not usually paint; at night and on feast days, however, he would make drawings for the frescoes in the Quirinale. Nicolò ground oil colors for Artemisia, who painted on canvas, but not for Orazio, who painted in fresco. He did not sleep in this house, but in the houses on via della Croce and at Santo Spirito —where Orazio is still living—in Orazio's room.

In fact, Nicolò was not employed on a regular basis by Orazio when the latter lived on via Margutta during Lent of 1611, but by Agostino. However, because

the two painters worked together and were close friends, Nicolò may have been to the house on via Margutta occasionally, as he later was in the house on via della Croce.

—Io andai a stare a casa del detto Horatio questa Quaresima ha fatto l'anno. (405v)—Fu a Montecavallo che il detto signor Horatio mi incitò ad andar a stare in casa sua che mi haverebbe imparato a disegnare.
(406)—Non si parlò né di tempo né di altro solamente che s'io havessi voluto andar a star in casa sua m'havrei imparato a disegnare et havrei bevuto e mangiato a casa sua e così ci andai.
—Io portai al detto Agostino (al Palazzo del Quirinale) per parte della cognata una camicia che fu un sabato sera et un'altra volta li portai pure una camicia et un'altra volta certi quattrini prima che m'accomodassi con detto Horatio . . .
(406v) Detto signor Horatio stava a Monte Cavallo a dipingere con altri pittori la sala fabricata nuovamente da nostro signore e la sera andava a dormire a casa sua con la sua famiglia e il giorno dopo stava a mangiare e a bevere lasù a Monte Cavallo.
(407)—Il nipote di detto signor Horatio si partì di casa sua quatro o cinque giorni ch'io andai a star con lui non so dove andasse. Io scopavo la casa e macinavo li colori e facevo li letti et alle volte andavo a comperare da mangiare.
(407v) Mentre stette in strada Margutta il detto Horatio non fece pitture, né opere alcune, solamente che la sera e le feste faceva delli disegni per servirsi a Monte Cavallo.
—Li colori ch'io macinavo in casa mentre stessimo a strada Margutta erano macinati a oglio e se ne serviva la figliola per pingere su le tele e non servivano altrimenti al padre perché (408) a Montecavallo le pitture sono a guazzo.
(408v)—Nel partir della via della Croce detto Signor Horatio andò a stare a San Spirito, dove è stato [per tempo] (409) e sta ancora . . .
(409v)—Io andai a dormir a casa di mio zio mentre il detto Horatio stette a strada Margutta e quando andò nella via della Croce cominciai a dormir in casa nella detta casa di via della Croce e sempre vi ho dormito di poi . . .
—Io dormivo su una cassa a canto al letto del detto Horatio il quale dormiva in una delle camere che ho detto.
—A San Spirito io dormivo in certe tavole in quella medesima camera dove dormiva il detto Horatio e dormivo da me solo.
(410)—Il nipote del signor Horatio si chiamava Giovanni Battista et era un giovane sbarbato poco più grande di me ed era tutto pieno di rogna.

Carlo Saraceni pittore veneziano
(411v) August 17, 1612 Saraceni declares he has known Gentileschi since he came to Rome eight or ten years ago. He does not know Artemisia, but he has heard that she paints. He has not heard anything about her or talked about her in Antinoro Bertucci's pigment store. Saraceni believes that Artemisia and Orazio are honorable people and that she is a virgin. He has not seen Orazio for two years, however, and during this time he has never heard Artemisia mentioned.

—Io conosco il detto Horatio Gentileschi da che son venuto a Roma, che saranno otto o dieci anni con occasione che è della stessa professione che son io e so ch'ha una figliola chiamata la signora Artemisia ch'io l'ho sentita nominare ma non la conosco e l'ho sentita nominare con occasione che lei dipingeva e conosco anco Antinoro Bertucci che vende li colori passato San Ambrosio al Corso con occasione che io qualche volta sono andato alla sua bottega a comperar [. . .], e so che lui in bottega sua ha tenuto un giovane chiamato Mario che non li so il cognome né donde sia che credo macini li colori quale io ho visto (412) in bottega sua . . . ma io non mi ricordo il tempo precisamente.
—Potria essere ch'io conoscessi questo Marco Antonio Coppino . . .
—Io non mi ricordo di havere raggionato né sentito raggionar alcuno nella bottega di Antinoro Bertucci né io ho raggionato che mi ricordi della signora Artemisia né in male né in bene.
—E quando io ne ho sentito raggionare in qualche luogo mentre detto Horatio habitava alli Greci che io conversavo con lui sempre lo conobbi per persona

molto honorata e per tale era tenuta si lui come la detta signora Artemisia sua figliola che sempre di quel tempo intesi dire che era zitella, ma dipoi ch'io non ho praticato con il detto Horatio che saranno circa due anni io non mi ricordo haverne raggionato, né sentito raggionare né in male, né in bene.
—Io Carlo saraceni

Olimpia moglie di Salvatore de Bargellis
(412) August 24, 1612 Olimpia de Bargellis, Agostino's half sister, testifies that in the fall of 1610 she had been instrumental in arranging for Nicolò Bedino to live with Agostino. He stayed with Tassi a year and then went to live with Gentileschi, where he was during Lent of 1612. Soon after, when Agostino was in prison, Nicolò returned to his service. Olimpia cooked for her brother, and Nicolò brought him food in prison.

(412v)—Saranno doi anni finiti adesso . . . ch'essendo io un giorno andata a casa di Agostino Tasso mio fratello che abitava al monte di San Honofrio non havendo detto Agostino in casa alcuno che li facesse servitii, se ben in casa sua habitava anco una donna chiamata Marta moglie di un Paolo che era una volta cavalleggero, io parlai una volta con una donna chiamata Vincenza serva di Giulio de Felice che abitava poco lontano di lì e le dissi che . . . vedesse di trovarli un ragazzo che fosse andato a comperar della roba fuori e a farli qualche servitio che li bisognava in casa e lei mi rispose che c'era un nipote di messer Giulio che lei gli avria fatto havere se gl'imparava di dipingere e così si accordarono che detto Agostino mio fratello gli promise di impararli e lo pigliò in casa (413) e ci stette non so che mesi che credo arrivasse all'anno, o poco più o poco meno, e stava in casa continuamente e lì mangiava, beveva e dormiva . . . e detto ragazzo doppo che si partì da detto Agostino andò a stare con il detto Horatio Gentileschi ch'io non so dire se c'andasse subito ma so che questa quadragesima ci stava e si partì da lui e tornò a stare con detto Agostino ch'era prigione a Corte Savella et io gli facevo da mangiare e detto ragazzo gli lo portava a Corte Savella . . .

Marta de Rubertis
August 24, 1612 Marta de Rubertis, who used to live in the same house as Agostino, confirms that Nicolò Bedino had been in his service.

(414)— . . . mentre io habitavo al Monte di Sant'Honofrio nella medesima casa dove stavo io di sopra c'habitava Agostino Tasso pittore con la cognata chiamata Costanza alias la frittelletta et il cognato chiamato Filippo, ch'havevano doi stantie, cioé una sala et una camera, che gli l'appigionava uno zoppo che era calzettaro e quando io partii da detta casa al monte di Sant'Honofrio Agostino habitava in una casa incontro a me, che c'era andato a stare un pezzo innanzi partitosi dalla casa sopra me.
—. . . detto Nicolò mentre che Agostino habitava sopra a me venne a stare con detto Agostino . . . e ci stette non so che mesi . . . (414v) che detto Agostino l'imparava a dipingere e lui lo serviva e faceva li servitii che li bisognavano e detto Nicolò veniva alle volte in casa mia per il fuoco o per l'acqua che le portava per servitio di detto Agostino . . .
—. . . e loro havevano una porta separata che potevano entrare senza passar per casa mia . . . che c'erano li muri in mezzo . . . (415) et Agostino e gli altri che stavano di sopra per andare alle sue stanze bisognava che passassero dalle stanze di detto zoppo che si chiamamava Pietro Paolo Turci.

Nicolò Bedino
August 26, 1612 Nicolò Bedino repeats his version of the events given on August 8, adding that he had helped Agostino for only four or five days before moving in with Orazio. He also accuses Olimpia and Marta of bearing false witness.

(415v)— . . . in casa di Agostino ci cominciai a praticare cinque o sei giorni prima ch'andassi a stare con il detto Horatio e li feci alcuni servitietti.
(416) Olimpia dice il falso e Marta non la conosco.

Pietro Hernandez
(417v) September 12, 1612 Pietro Hernandez does not know when Orazio started to paint the loggia (that is, the Casino delle Muse) on the Quirinale belonging to Cardinal Borghese (this must have happened during the fall of 1611) but knows that Nicolò Bedino served him as shopboy there. He does not know whether Orazio had any other helper; there might have been a boy called Ippolito. He has been to the Borghese casino only once to see Orazio paint, and this was after Nicolò had left Orazio.

(418) . . . il signor Horatio ha habitato da che io lo conosco al portone di San Spirito dove al presente habita.
—Io non so di che tempo detto signor Horatio habbia cominciato a servire l'illustrissimo signor cardinale Borghese in pingere la loggia a Montecavallo; ho ben inteso dire dalla detta Artimitia da poi ch'io la conosco che lui dipingeva a Montecavallo e quando dipingeva a Monte Cavallo con lui ci stava Nicolò che venne a stare con lui mentre ha habitato a San Spirito e non so se havesse altro garzone che detto Nicolò, ma con lui ci praticava qualche volta un ragazzo chiamato Hippolito.
(418v)—Io non son stato a Monte Cavallo a veder dipingere il detto Horatio se non una volta e quella non mi ci fermai e perciò io non posso dire chi ci dipingesse con esso e chi lo servisse di altri essercitii e quella volta che io ci stetti Nicolò s'era partito dal signor Horatio.
(419) . . . Nicolò . . . può havere da 15 a 16 anni poco più o poco meno et è un tozzotto sbarbato e grassotto e vestito di corame.
(419v)—Io ho detto nel mio esamine che conobbi il detto Horatio il mese di ottobre prossimo passato con occasione che la signora Artemisia fu comare di un putto che mi nacque il giorno di San Francesco e che, cominciando io a praticar in casa sua, una donna chiamata Caterina li faceva li servitii di casa e che da doi mesi in circa dopoi c'andò a stare detto Nicolò qual'io viddi in casa . . .
Io Pietro hendes (sic) confermo quanto di sopra

Antinoro di Alessandro Bertucci, bolognese
(420) September 12, 1612 Antinoro Bertucci, who owns the pigment store on via del Corso, has known Orazio for six or seven years. Once, when he was walking on via della Croce, Orazio called him into his house to show him some paintings. Inside, Bertucci saw a young woman whom he assumed was Artemisia. He has heard no rumors about her, but Orazio's nephew Giovanni Battista had told him that Orazio had ousted him from the house because he had scolded Artemisia for staying at the window.

— . . . io conosco il signor Horatio Gentileschi da sei o sette anni . . . e so che lui ha una figliola ch'io non so come si chiama, ma la viddi una volta mentre habitava in strada della Croce che passando di là il signor Horatio stava sulla porta e mi chiamò e mi menò di sopra che mi mostrò certi quadri e viddi lì una giovane (420v) ch'io mi imaginai che fosse sua figliola perché havevo inteso dire che haveva una figliola.
—Mentre che detto Mario Trotta stette con me né inanzi io non ho mai inteso raggionare nella mia bottega di detto signor Horatio nè della detto figliola né in male né in bene . . . se non che un nipote suo che si chiama Giovanni Battista che praticava con detto Mario si lamentava del signor Horatio che l'haveva cacciato di casa perché haveva bravato alla figlia che stava alla finestra.

Pietro fu Angeli Molli di 73 anni
(421) September 12, 1612 Molli says that he arrived in Rome the Tuesday before Easter 1612 (that is, March 19) from Naples, where he had been for seven months. Previously, he had lived in Rome for a year and a half, and other painters had used him as a model. He posed for Orazio at both via del Babuino and via Margutta, but he does not remember the details and refers to his previous deposition of July 27.

(421)—Io fui invitato ad essaminarmi dal detto Horatio Gentileschi che mi disse come io ero stato tante volte in casa sua mentre lui mi ritraheva in un quadro su chi havevo visto praticar in casa sua che volessi essaminarmi per la verità e così venni ad essaminarmi e dissi quel che sapevo . . .

(421v)—Io venni a Roma il martedì santo prossimo passato che venni da Napoli e sempre son stato ad habitar in Campo di Fiore, eccetto un mese e mezzo che stetti sotto San Pietro in Borgo et a Napoli ci stetti sette mesi che m'ero partito da Roma dove ero stato in Borgo un anno e mezzo che molti pittori si servivano di me per ritrarmi et non so chi siano le parti che litigano . . . ma quando mi ritraheva lui habitava acanto a una chiesa di Greci e poi andò in un'altra casa di sopra a quella in un'altra strada che non mi ricordo adesso come si chiami ma nel mio essame l'ho detto.

— . . . non mi ricordo (422) di che tempo fosse ma io vi andai parecchie volte in dette case perché il signor Horatio mi ritraheva e faceva un quadro di San Geronimo . . . e non mi ricordo adesso come era fatta detta casa . . .

Margherita moglie di Girolamo milanese, lavandaia
(423) September 14, 1612 The washerwoman, Margherita, describes the house on via Margutta and says that in the house, where Orazio's nephew Giovanni Battista also lived, she had seen Francesco Scarpellino, Pasquino Fiorentino, and Pietro Molli the pilgrim, all of whom posed for Gentileschi. Orazio lived there approximately two years ago. She does not know when he began painting for Cardinal Borghese, and she has seen him painting only rarely. When Orazio was painting from the model, he did not let anyone in the room, although he would later show her the canvases.

(423v)— . . . mentre lui habitava in strada Margutta saranno hora vicino o intorno a doi anni, e questa casa che ha la porta nella strada grande e quando s'entra c'è un andito, e ci sta una stanza a man manca dove si faceva la bugata e si salivano su le scale e poi si trovava una sala et una camera et anco una cocina piccolina et un cortile e di sopra ci sta [medesimamente] camera e sala e ci sono le finestre che rispondono nella strada pubblica e c'habitava il detto Horatio, Artimitia sua figliola e tre (424) suoi fratelli et un nipote di detto Horatio chiamato Giovanni Battista.

—In casa del signor Horatio mentre habitava a strada Margutta io c'ho visto praticare Bernardino stuffarolo che il signor Horatio se ne serviva per ritrarlo et anco un Francesco scarpellino et anco un fiorentino chiamato Pasquino che è morto e una volta ci vidi quel vecchio che s'esaminava poco fa che è pilligrino, che il detto Horatio li ritraheva nelli quadri e non c'ho visto altro pellegrino che questo . . .

—Io come ho detto non so dire in che (424v) tempo il detto Horatio cominciasse a servire il signor cardinale Borghese in pingere a Montecavallo e poche volte io l'ho visto dipingere et in casa sua ho visto praticare li supradetti che lui li ritraheva in camera che non si poteva vedere, ma mi mostrava bene li quadri che lui faceva a similitudine di costoro.

(426) September 16, 1612 Pietro Molli is again questioned, but he refers to his previous interrogations and says he is about to faint.

—Io vi ho detto e vi dico che non mi ricordo più come era fatta quella (casa di via Margutta) . . .

—Fatemi confessare e comunicare perché io sento che vengo meno e non posso star più qua.

Olimpia de Bargellis
(426) September 17, 1612 Olimpia de Bargellis describes how her brother Agostino pressed charges against her, under the pretense that she had tried to have him killed by the hand of Giovanni Angelo Rinaldi, one of his friends. He had done this because her husband owed him money. She stayed in prison for a day, after which Quorli helped her out. She, in turn, pressed charges against Agostino for committing incest with Costanza, his wife's sister. Agostino was in prison only a few days before he was acquitted as a result of Quorli's intervention. Until their

argument over the money, Olimpia and her brother had been friends, and in April, or perhaps November, 1611 they made up. During Carnival of 1612, Agostino fell ill. During Lent of 1611, Nicolò Bedino was living with Agostino, certainly not with Orazio, and she would see them walking together toward the Palazzo del Quirinale when she lived near ponte Sant'Angelo. (See Lapierre, chap. 21 and app. 6.) Olimpia at this date was living in Tassi's neighborhood, where she had moved from her previous house at the "immagine di Ponte." Thus, it is likely that they had indeed stopped quarreling for a while. (See ASR, Stato Civile, appendice, Santo Spirito in Sassia, Stati di anime 1614–18.)

(426v)—Io fui querelata una volta nel tribunale del Vicario che era giudice il [Confidato] che fu Agostino Tasso mio fratello che mi querelò per malevolenza di certi denari ch'haveva d'havere da mio marito ch'io l'havessi voluto far ammazzare da Giovanni Angelo Rinaldi suo amico e stetti priggione un giorno e doppo un anno (sic) fui liberata perché Cosimo furiero mi faceva [. . .] ch'ora è amico di detto Agostino et altre volte non sono stato mai in giustitia né processata per causa alcuna. (la prima volta fu Stiattesi che la fece testimoniare)

(427)— . . . Agostino mio fratello venne a Roma nel Corpus Domini prossimo passato ha fatto doi anni e ce stette in casa mia tre mesi e poi andò ad abitare con la cognata che era venuta di fuori poco inanzi a lui al monte di Sant' Honofrio che tutti partirono di casa mia e doppo si partì di lì et andò ad abitare alla Lungara dove habitava quando fu preso et Horatio Gentileschi che litiga con lui io non so dove habbi habitato si non da Carnevale in qua che habitava al portone di San Spirito che mi ci menò detto Agostino una volta che tornavamo da casa di Cosimo furiero, dove eravamo stati a una commedia.

(427v)—Io conosco Agostino perché mi è fratello carnale da canto di madre . . .

—Io so che detto Agostino è stato prigione a Livorno che me lo disse la moglie però non so per che causa et io una volta lo querelai in Borgo perché si teneva la cognata e fu assoluto per favore che hebbe di Cosimo suddetto che tre-quattro giorni uscì di prigione . . .

—Signorsì che quando Agostino andò a stare al Monte di Sant' Honofrio che partì da casa mia io ci praticai et andai in casa sua spesse volte per tutto il mese di novembre sin che ci rompessimo per conto (428) delli detti denari che dopo ci [. . .] criminalmente che poi da Santa Caterina in qua facemmo pace e c'ho praticato anco da poi che lui s'amalò questo carnevale.

(429)— . . . Nicolò andò a star in casa di mio fratello e ci stette un anno in circa e ci andò a stare nel mese di agosto di modo che della quadragesima dell'anno seguente lui stava con detto Agostino mio fratello e certo non poteva stare con Horatio di detta quadragesima e di quel tempo Agostino dipingeva a Monte Cavallo e si menava con esso questo Nicolò ch'io li vedevo passare assieme quando stavo all'Imagine di Ponte.

Bernardino fu Francesco de Franchi stuffarolo
(430) September 27, 1612 Bernardino, the barber, again testifies that he often went to Orazio's house on via Margutta, both as a barber and to pose as a model. Francesco Scarpellino was there, and he too was employed as a model. He went only once to the Borghese casino—to clean Orazio's teeth—and while he was there Settimio Olgiati came to see the casino. He does not know who was Orazio's assistant for this project. At the house on via Margutta, he saw Settimio Olgiati and some Theatine fathers, who had come to see paintings. For more than a month, he saw an old pilgrim there who looked like a Saint Paul and who posed for a full-length *Saint Jerome*. Sometimes he was asked to undress. Orazio used him for other paintings as well, especially studies of heads. Whenever Bernardino went to Orazio's house, he saw him painting, especially during Lent of 1610 (sic), when he saw Orazio painting the pilgrim. He has also seen Orazio working on small paintings on alabaster. The barber's statement that Molli had frequented the house on via Margutta during Lent of 1610 partially invalidates the pilgrim's deposition, since he had talked about Lent of 1611. (See fol. 395 above.)

(431)— . . . non sono ancora tre anni che (Orazio) se partì da quella casa (agli Greci) et andò ad abitare nella strada di Margutta a man dritta passate tre o quattro case nel [partir] dal Babuino et andare per detta strada, che il batocchio della porta è una campanella de ferro o metallo grande e grossa a foggia di maschera, et in questa casa ci stette un anno in circa che no sò manco se il finì l'anno o forse più. So bene che l'altra quadragesima che questa prossima passata ha fatto l'anno se mal non me recordo perché io non ho a memoria bene il tempo so bene che un anno o poco più o poco manco c'è stato in detta casa della strada de Marguta e partendo da questa andò a stare alla strada della Croce in una casa sopra un sartore in faccia ad un saponaro che in questa della strada della Croce io credo che ce habbia habitato da sei mesi in circa da dove partito se ne andò a stare a San Spirito per quello che me ha detto lui che io non la so la casa e ne meno ce so stato mai e lì [dice] che sta adesso . . .

(431v)—Io in casa de Horatio Gentileschi mentre che lui è stato ed ha habitato in quella casa che ve ho detto di sopra dentro strada di Margutta ci sono stato più volte che a mio giuditio e per quello che posso ricordare sarà da sessanta volte in circa in diverse volte che ogni settimana ce andavo due o tre volte e qualche settimana ce stavo in quella casa due o tre dì alla volta et quando ce sono andato ce sono andato a far la barba al detto signor Horatio a tosare agli figlioli a cavare sangue alla figliola e perché si cercava di me per modello cioè per ritrarre . . . (432) . . . Horatio in quella casa (di via Margutta) c'haveva Francesco (432v) scarpellino che pure se ne serviva per modello depingeva [. . .], ogni volta che ce andavo ce il trovavo; ci stava Giovanni Battista suo nepote, Francesco detto Ceccho suo figliolo, Giulio suo figliolo, Marcellino pure suo figliolo, Artimitia sua figliola, la balia lavandara che non me recordo il nome che questa balia ce veniva di continuo ma non ce habitava.

—Io non me ricordo in che tempo Horatio Gentileschi cominciasse a depingere la loggia del Cardinal Borghese ne quanto tempo ce sia stato a depingerla e non so chi fosse garzone di Horatio all'hora e chi ci sia stato assieme nel dipingere detta loggia a Monte Cavallo nel giardino del signor cardinal Borghese; ne meno so se detto Horatio ce tenesse uno o più al suo servitio in detta loggia perché io in tutto il tempo ce fui solo una volta che detto Horatio me ce fece andare solo una volta a nettargli li denti; mentre ce stetti io all'hora il signor Settimio Olgiati che venne a vedere la loggia di modo che se ce tenesse o havesse potuto tenere gente io non lo so perché non ce praticavo e poteva tenere o non tenere gente che io nol potevo sapere perché non praticavo . . . (433) questa loggia a Monte Cavallo. In quella casa che habitava detto signor Horatio nella strada di Margutta [come] ho detto di sopra non ho visto stare altre persone che quelle che ve ho nominate; ho ben visto venire il signor Settimio Olgiati a vedere qualche quadro, i Teatini che pure venivano a vedere quadri come ho visto per più di un mese di continuo tante volte quante ce andavo la settimana in casa un vecchio vestito da pellegrino che è un huomo più presto grande che altrimenti, vestito da pellegrino come ho detto, huomo di bello aspetto d'una faccia che pare un San Paolo testa calva tutto canuto con una bella barba [tonda] grande cioè tanto nelle guancie quanto nella barba istessa e questo pellegrino detto Horatio il teneva che il . . . retraheva per un San Girolamo in un quadro che il ritraheva tutto e molte volte il faceva spogliare et se ne serviva anco per fare altre cose e delle teste e a questo fine ce veniva (433v) il suddetto pellegrino e altri che questo pellegrino io non ce ho visti in casa suddetta che habitava il detto Horatio.

—Ogni volta che io sono andato nella casa del detto . . . sempre l'ho trovato che pingeva et in particolare di quadrigesima dell'anno 1610 io ho trovato in casa più volte detto signor Horatio che depingeva et io non me raccordo che habbia più certa memoria che de quel San Gerolamo che ritraheva detto pellegrino e l'ho visto anco che faceva certi quadretti di alabastro e quant'altro . . .

—Io Bernardino o deposto (in capital letters).

Marta de Rubertis

September 27, 1612 Agostino's neighbor Marta de Rubertis confirms that Agostino had instructed Nicolò Bedino and that they had lived together, but she cannot remember whether this happened in 1611 or in 1610.

(435)—Io no so altro che quanto ve ho detto di sopra e detto Nicolò io non l'ho conosciuto se non mentre stava alla salita di San Nofrio nel tempo che ho detto e non so se fu del 1610 o 1611 che di questo ve ne potete rendere il conto e che Agostino [. . .] lavorato da prima a Monte Cavallo nelle loggie de detto Cardinale . . .

Luca fu Carlo Finocchi da Palliano, locandario

(436) September 30, 1612, in Nicolò Bedino's defense. The innkeeper Luca Finocchi met Orazio's nephew Giovanni Battista during Carnival of 1611, at a play staged in the Palazzo Colonna in Piazza Santi Apostoli. Together with Giovanni Battista, he saw Nicolò at Orazio's house during Lent of 1611. He has also seen him helping Orazio with the shopping. He does not know Artemisia, but he knows Orazio, who has asked him to testify that Agostino confessed to the rape. Agostino was often in the Palazzo Colonna, where they met at a play. Orazio is about fifty, with a black beard that is turning white, and is of medium height; he dresses in black.

—Io sono venuto qui pregato dal signor Agostino Tassi che mi ha detto se me raccordavo quando, in casa del contestabile Colonna, Giovanni Battista . . . (436v) ha menato me a spasso a casa del Gentileschi se non ho visto mai che questo Giovanni Battista chiamasse Nicolò et che me venissi ad affermare per la verità e qui me ce ha menato il signor Pompeo procuratore del Signor Augustino Tassi acciò mi esamini per la verità . . .

(436v)—Io ho fatto una fede per la verità al detto Augustino la quale contiene che io conosco Giovanni Battista nipote del Gentileschi che lo conosco che essendo io in una commedia del contestabile a Carnevale del 1611 e venendo lì detto Giovanni Battista con alcune altre persone per la folla io gli imprestai uno sgabello . . . et altro non contiene la fede che me recordi. Mi ricordo bene che contiene ancora che Giovanni Battista ne menò quattro o cinque (437) volte con occasione che ero andato in quella casa con Giovanni Battista che Giovanni Battista et io andavamo assieme a spasso che lui veniva a trovarmi a Santi Apostoli in casa del Contestabile [. . .] altre volte a casa del Gentileschi e che chiamava Nicolò anche veniva a basso. (Giovanni Battista) era giovane sbarbato e gli diceva se il zio era in casa e quello giovanetto rispondeva quando sì e quando no . . . contiene ancora che l'ho visto questo Nicolò in pescaria alla rotonda mettergli (ad Orazio) il pesce nella sporta e il Gentileschi il pagava . . . et de questa fede me ne ha richiesto Agostino in Corte Savella dove io stavo prigione . . .

(437v)— . . . quando io feci la fede Agostino me domandò ancora se havessi visto la figliola del Gentileschi io gli risposi di no che non l'havevo vista né la conoscevo.

(438)—Io conosco Horatio Gentileschi pittore e lo conosco da quadragesima quando andai con Giovanni Battista et l'ho visto una volta o due a casa sua et l'ho visto anco in piazza di [Montegiordano] . . . mi disse che io mi volessi essaminare a favore suo che havessi inteso dire ad Agostino che havesse sverginato la figliola . . . et io gli risposi che Agostino non haveva detta mai tal cosa . . .

(438v) Io ho visto Nicolò in casa de Horatio nel modo che ho detto di sopra in una casa alla strada Margutta di quadragesima del 1611 e ce l'ho visto quattro o cinque volte con occasione che ero andato in quella casa con Giovanni Battista che Giovanni Battista et io andavamo assieme a spasso (439) che lui veniva a trovarmi ai Santi Apostoli in casa del Contestabile . . .

Luca fu Carlo Finocchi

(439) October 2, 1612 (Finocchi's deposition continues)

(441)—Io cognoscevo prima Agostino Tasso che cognoscessi detto Nicolò con occasione che venne ad una commedia che se faceva in casa del contestabile Colonna et con occasione che havendolo io visto praticar lì nel palazzo vedendolo la sera come ho detto alla comedia gli imprestai uno sgabello.

(442)— . . . Horatio è un huomo di 50 anni di barba negra che ora comincia ad imbiancarsi un poco, di giusta statura [asciutto] vestito di negro . . .

(442v) Io luca finocchi da paliano ho deposto quanto di sopra per la verità

Valerio figlio di Francisco Ursino fiorentino pittore abitante a Roma

October 5, 1612 The painter Valerio Ursino has known Agostino for more than two years, since the latter came to Rome. They were introduced by the Florentine painter Antonio Cinatti. At the time, Agostino was looking for paintings of sibyls to send to Livorno. Ursino obtained them from a painter called Grassino (perhaps Marzio Ganassini), and thus they became friends. He then moved in with Agostino, who later demanded to be paid for his hospitality. Agostino first lived on the right side of the road in via di Sant'Onofrio, then he moved to the left side, where Ursino and Nicolò Bedino also went to live. Ursino left at Easter of 1611, but Nicolò, who had come in the summer of 1610, continued to work for Agostino. Nicolò has confessed that Agostino persuaded him to lie. While in prison, Agostino asked Ursino to testify that Orazio owed him 200 scudi. Ursino first agreed but then changed his mind, since he learned that Agostino had also asked Marcantonio Coppino to perjure himself. (See Lapierre, chap. 21.)

—Io vi posso dire per la verità che conosco Agostino di Domenico Tassi ch'egli è pittore e lo conosco da due anni e più (443v) et dal principio che detto Agostino venne a Roma e suddetto Agostino havendo di bisogno e cercando [dodeci] sibille per mandarle a Livorno a un gentilhuomo suo amico, Antonio Cinatti fiorentino pittore mio amico il menò in casa dove habitavo io alla guglia di san Macuto et in quella casa trattò meco esso Agostino per le mie sibille che detto Cinatti gli haveva detto che io l'avrei fatto trovare siccome feci, che gli li feci dare dal Grassino pittore che stava al Corso et con questa occasione io e Agostino Tasso pigliassimo amicitia et [conoscenza] insieme et havemo praticato sempre per alcuni mesi . . . che ce separassimo poi perché essendo stato in casa sua a magnare et dormire sotto amicitia poi mi mosse una lite che voleva che gli pagassi gli alimenti et perciò ce separassimo et lasciassimo la conoscenza et amicitia et mentre siamo stati [stretti] nella conoscenza et amicitia nel modo che ora ho raccontato detto Agostino stava alla salita di San Nofrio, che prima stava in una casa a man dritta vicino al notaio accanto (443v) quella di Martino Cappelletti, che lì ce habitò da due o tre mesi, e poi si partì in tempo de [meloni] et andò a stare in una strada a man manca la suddetta strada più di un anno et io in quel tempo che ho havuta pratica seco et è stato in quella casa a man dritta et in questa a man manca che in questa finì la conversazione nostra . . . ne l'una e ne l'altra casa io ho praticato da un anno in circa ma otto mesi di continuo son stato a magnare bevere et dormire con Agostino in quella casa a man manca vicino a San Nofrio . . . et in questo tempo che ci sono stato io c'è stato anco sempre un giovanotto di diciotto anni in circa che si chiama Nicolò quale è nepote de uno che gli si dice Brugiavigne et imparava di disegnare e serviva detto Agostino, la cognata, cognato et altri in casa. Il detto Agostino il teneva come servitore, se bene veramente il ragazzo stava lì per imparare perché aveva (444) le spese et il dormire, faceva tutti i servizi in casa et io, quando lasciai l'amicitia di detto Agostino, ce lasciai anco detto Nicolò che pure stava con Agostino che l'amicitia nostra per causa di quella lite finì l'anno passato che saranno più di 14 mesi e quando Agustino andò a stare in quella casa a mano manca anche io cominciai a stare fermo con Agostino a magnare e bevere e dormire . . . Nicolò . . . per alcuni giorni . . . se ne tornò a dormire a casa che stava vicino . . . pui ce se accomodò come ho raccontato di sopra . . . alla sera ce restava a dormire nella stanza da basso che serviva per cocina et ce venne a stare d'estate dell'anno già passato et io me partii dopo Pasqua dell'anno prossimo passato et detto Nicolò ce lo lasciai lì et ho visto (444v) che continuato il servitio.

(445)—Agostino ha fatto dire queste cose al ragazzo, che stava a strada Margutta e agli Greci . . . Agostino mi rispose io gli ho detto che dica la verità et non le bugie et intanto fu chiamato Agostino da un gentilhuomo et io (parlando) con detto Nicolò gli chiesi perché l'hai detto et Nicolò mi rispose Agostino mi ha fatto dire che io son stato con Horatio Gentileschi alla strada Margutta et agli Greci . . . (Agostino inoltre domandava) che io volessi esaminarmi contro Horatio Gentileschi che gli era restato debitore de 200 scudi che io gli promisi all'hora ma poi non ho voluto fare questo esamine falso perché non è vero . . . et tanto più che essendomi incontrato con Marco Antonio Coppino lui mi ha raccontato che Agostino l'haveva richiesto di simile testimonianza et che per non farla non c'era voluto più andare che questo è quanto io vi posso dire per la verità.

Nicolò Bedino

(445v) October 29, 1612 Under torture, Bedino confirms his version of what happened.

— . . . Io son stato in casa di Horatio et ho veduto che Artemitia sua figliola mentre stava in strada Margutta fece questi atti disonesti . . .

SECTION B

ASR, Tribunale Criminale del Governatore, serie Testimoni, vol. 201
The following two depositions, although they come from a different series—witnesses for the defense—are part of the trial and should be inserted before Bedino's last deposition. Stiattesi, on Gentileschi's behalf, asked for their transcription. (See section C below.)

Michelangelo figlio di Silvestro Vestri da Montelupo pittore

(103) October 12, 1612 Michelangelo Vestri from Montelupo, a painter, confirms his written statement that during Lent of 1611, when he was working on the illusionistic architecture of the vault in the Sala Regia in the Palazzo del Quirinale, he saw Nicolò Bedino carrying cartoons for Orazio. Orazio himself told him that he employed Nicolò, and he has also seen the boy in the Gentileschi house on via Margutta. Vestri met Tassi during the summer of 1610, in the Palazzo Firenze, where they both worked. He has often seen Orazio and Agostino walking together on the streets of Rome. He knows that Nicolò helped Agostino "on the Quirinale"—which probably still means the Sala Regia, although this partially contradicts his former claim that Nicolò was Orazio's assistant there—but he does not know whether Nicolò has ever been Agostino's servant or shop-boy or whether he has ever slept at Agostino's house. Vestri met Valerio Ursino in Passignano's workshop and knows that he quarreled with Agostino. Vestri has painted both in the Sala Regia and in the Casino delle Muse. Of all Orazio's children, he has met only Francesco, at the Palazzo del Quirinale. The "Giovanni sollecitatore" is probably the lawyer Giovanni Salvarani of section C below. Tassi also employed the lawyer Pompeo Trococia or Tracagna. (See Cavazzini 2000 and Lapierre, app. 6.)

—Io son comparso qua per esaminarmi e sono stato menato qua da un Giovanni sollecitatore di un Agostino Tasso, et sono stato menato qua (103v) sotto pretesto che dovevo dire la verità quando mi esaminavo et fui cominciato ad essere menato qua da San Michele prossimo passato in qua et io non so sopra che materia mi habbia da esaminare ma mi ho da esaminare ad istanza di Agostino Tasso pittore.

—Signorsì che io ho fatto una fede sottoscritta di mia mano et la fede ch'ho fatta contiene che lavorando io a Montecavallo con il detto Agostino Tasso nella Sala Regia a quella prospettiva ho visto venire in detto luogo il signor Horatio Gentileschi pittore a far le figure da Quaresima passata ha fatto l'anno da che ho visto più volte venire appresso a lui a portar li cartoni un certo ragazzo che si chiama Nicolò e lì su nel lavoro ho visto che più volte ha comandato al detto ragazzo et vedendo io che detto Horatio comandava tanto alla libera al detto ragazzo gli dimandai con chi stava et detto Horatio rispose sta con me [perché].

— . . . perché andando io una volta a spasso per strada Margutta e vedendo uscire detto ragazzo d'una casa [sita] lì in detta strada e dimandando io una matina che ero andato con il detto Augustino Tasso (104), et fu la domenica dell'oliva di quella Quaresima, su chi habitava in quella casa dove lui haveva chiamato il detto Horatio Gentileschi mi disse che ci habitava il detto Horatio et questa fede io feci in Torre di Nona dove io fui mandato a chiamare più volte dal detto Agostino Tasso ed ad instanza sua e da lui pregato io feci la detta fede per la verità et facendo la detta fede io pensava che fosse a favore del detto Horatio.

—Io di questa lite o causa che è tra Agostino Tassi et Horatio Gentileschi non ho parlato mai con altri che con il detto Agostino, et li ragionamenti sono stati che detto Agostino si doleva e lamentava meco dicendo ch'era assassinato in questa causa et anco fu ragionato della detta fede che lui desiderava da me per la verità ma con Filippo cognato di detto Agostino e con Nicolò io non ci ho mai parlato di questa causa.

postea-Con Filippo incontrandomi con lui me ricordo haverci parlato, dimandandolo della causa di Agostino, alcuna volta mi rispondeva che andava bene at altra volta che andava in longo et io ho parlato anco con altre persone della fede ch'io havevo fatto per servitio di detto Agostino per la verità.

(104v)—Agostino per quanto io ho inteso dire da lui e da altri è prigione per causa della figliola del detto Horatio, ma Nicolò non so per che causa et lo [sentii] dire ch'Agostino era prigione per questa causa dal principio che fu carcerato et lo sentii dire da Filippo sua cognato che lavorava con me.

—Io ho cognosciuto Agostino Tasso pittore sin dal principio che lui tornò a Roma, che mi pare che fosse l'anno 1610 d'estate, con occasione che, lavorando io nel palazzo dell'ambasciatore di Firenze, ci venne detto signor Agostino a fare certi paesi et non ho havuto mai che trattare con detto signor Agostino se non questo ho lavorato con lui, et questo Nicolò Bedino lo cognobbi dall'anno 1611 di Quaresima et non ho havuto altro mai che trattar con lui di negotio nissuno et lo cognobbi nella Sala Regia di Montecavallo.

—Signorsì ch'io cognosco il detto Horatio Gentileschi pittore et lo cominciai a conoscere di vista se ben prima lo conoscevo per fama della sua virtù, dopo che cognobbi Agostino Tasso, che li vedevo spesso assieme (105) andar per Roma et li salutavo, l'ho poi conosciuto et visto a Montecavallo quando veniva a far le figure dove lavoravo ancora io et non ho hauto mai che trattar con lui et io non ho né da dare né da havere cosa alcuna da detto signore Horatio Gentileschi.

—La professione mia è di pittore et al [momento] mi esercito a lavorare nella fabrica del Signor Francesco Colonna a Piazza di Sciarra et quando io vado a giornata mi guadagno cinque giulii il giorno et io adesso habito in Piazza di Sciarra solo. Io non ho havuto cosa nessuna per venirmi ad esaminare in questa causa sono stato ben ridutto ad esaminarmi altre volte ma in cause civili

—Io non so dove al presente habiti il detto Horatio Gentileschi, questo carnavale habitava al Monte di Santo Spirito, ma io adesso non so se ci sta più overo se si è partito et prima che andasse ad habitare al monte di Santo Spirito, dove habitava io, ho visto che habitava in strada Margutta et che poi è stato una volta nella strada della Croce, ma io non so in che luogho (105v) perché io non sono stato mai in casa sua.

—Io non so che detto Nicolò sia stato mai per servitore o garzone di detto Agostino, so bene che lavorando io a Monte Cavallo detto Nicolò serviva lì nel lavoro di detto Agostino ma [se] poi ci andasse a dormire et mangiare io non lo so ch'io lavoravo a giornata et la sera quando era hora me ne andavo a dormire et anco ce lo lasciavo a rassettare et la mattina quando ce ritornavo ce lo ritrovavo.

. . .

—Signorsì che io cognosco Valerio Orsino pittore fiorentino che lui venne a Roma che puol essere 6 o 7 (106) anni in circa et lo cominciai a cognoscer perché praticando lui con il Passignani pittore dove praticavo ancora io con certi altri giovani et come tutti di una professione cominciassimo a praticar assieme et io non sono creditore né pretendo di essere debitore di detto Valerio che io gli fossi stato debitore mi haverebbe fatto pagare per via di giustizia havendo noi litigato assieme, et in quanto a me io tengo il detto Valerio per huomo dabene et honorato.

—Io so che Agostino Tasso et Valerio Orsino pittori hanno litigato assieme del dare e del havere che l'uno e l'altro di loro pretendono essere creditori che non fa l'anno hanno havuto tra loro questa lite et lo so perché l'uno e l'altro di loro me l'hanno detto, et io veddi il sopradetto Valerio tre o quattro giorni sono che passava così per strada, et non ho parlato mai più con lui doppo che cominciassimo a litigare et l'ultima volta che mi ricordo parlai con il detto Valerio fu nell'hosteria dell'Aquila in piazza di Sciarra dove venne a cena con certi huomini che lui teneva et non discorsero di altro senò del lavoro che lui haveva di una carrozza del signor [Marangolanti].

(106v)— . . . mi comunicai nella chiesa di San Marcello all'hora mia parrochia . . .

—Io cognosco Antinoro Bertucci, il signor Carlo Venitiani et Mario Trotta pittori ma il signor Carlo Venitiano non lo cognosco se no per vista et in quanto a me io li tengo tutti per huomini da bene.

. . .

(107) Sunday, October 14, 1612 Michelangelo Vestri's interrogation continues

—Io non so il stato suo [di Nicolò] et non so che se sia stato per servitore con nessuno sebene che è stato con li pittori a imparare ne so se ha havuto salario sì o no.

—Io non so che arte si faccia detto Nicolò ma l'ho visto servire al lavoro mentre si dipingeva la sala di Monte Cavallo et non so se sia stato per garzone sì o no, ma l'ho visto servire al lavoro come ho detto di sopra et non l'ho visto praticare mai in casa di Agostino perché io non ci son stato mai.

—Io come ho detto ho visto questo Nicolò servire nel lavoro di Monte Cavallo che haveva preso Agostino Tasso et l'ho visto anco alcune volte andar anco appresso a lui.

—Io so che detto signor Agostino ha dipinto la sala grande di Monte Cavallo assieme con altri pittori et lo so perché ci son stato a pingere ancora io et so come ho detto di sopra che per servitio del lavoro ci stava il sopradetto Nicolò che andava (107v) a fare li servitii che bisognava.

—Signorsì che io conosco il signor Horatio Gentileschi pittore che lo conosco con occasione che detto signor Horatio venne a lavorare di figure nella detta sala di Monte Cavallo di quaresima farà l'anno come ho detto di sopra e non ho mai havuto che trattare con lui.

. . .

—Io non so se il signor Horatio Gentileschi da che io lo conosco ha tenuto servitori e quanti et non so altro se non quanto ho detto di sopra che ragionando io lì sul lavoro su con chi stava detto Nicolò lui rispose sta con me.

—Io come ho detto ho visto dipingere il signor Horatio Gentileschi nella sala al Monte Cavallo (108) dove ci dipingevo io ancho et altri e non so che abbia tenuto altri se no quanto ho detto di sopra. Ho visto anco di poi dipingere la loggia del Cardinal Borghese dove ho lavorato ancora io et ci venivano a servire lì dui ragazzotti questo Nicolò et un Napolitano.

—Io so che il signor Horatio Gentileschi ha figli maschi e femmine che l'ho sentito dire et conosco un figlio maschio che si chiama Francesco che l'ho visto venire su nel [lavoro] a Monte Cavallo.

—Io posso dire per la verità come ho detto anco di sopra che ho visto questo Nicolò servire nel lavoro della sala di Montecavallo et il signor Horatio ho visto che gli commandava et la mattina ho visto che veniva il detto signor Horatio quando veniva su nel lavoro ci menava appresso il detto Nicolò con li cartoni come anco più apieno ho detto nelli interrogatori alli quali mi riferisco.

. . .

(108v) Io Michelagnolo o deposto per la verità quanto di sopra

Costanza moglie di Onofrio Ceuli

(110v) October 21, 1612 Costanza, the wife of Onofrio Ceuli, used to be Orazio's neighbor on via della Croce, but she had known him earlier, because her husband was his tailor. She testifies that Orazio never had a live-in servant, as he could not afford one. However, now and then, from her window she saw Nicolò Bedino working in the Gentileschi house, often grinding pigments. Artemisia told her that Nicolò lived with Agostino, but that occasionally he helped them as well. Costanza has been in their houses—both on via della Croce and on via del Babuino—because Orazio made drawings of her children. She has never seen Orazio paint, only draw.

. . .

(111)—Io non ho fatto fede alcuna ma mio marito ha fatto fede come non c'è stata alcuna persona con il Gentileschi che è un pezzo che io conosco la quale fede e la fece fare il Gentileschi una sera ma se ce fussi stata io non ce l'avria lasciata fare . . . et lui gliela fece fare con dare ad intendere che questo servitore gli domandava scudi trenta per causa di mercede et mio marito due giorni dopo mi domandò dicendomi chi diavolo è questo ragazzo che domanda il salario a costui. Io non me recordo non so chi sia e so che non ha tenuto mai servitore che veramente il Gentileschi era povero huomo e come stimo io che [. . .] alla giornata che quando haveva quatrini spendeva alla grande e quando non ne haveva faceva niente . . . (111v) . . . non so quello gli potesse giovare questa fede che gli fece mio marito.

—Io con Agostino non ho parlato nemeno con Nicolò, ho bene parlato con Filippo che così me pare che si chiama (il) cognato di detto Agostino che è venuto qui due o tre volte acciò mi essamini che altro non me ha detto et io sopra il grembo che sto per partorire ho detto la verità et circa la fede io ho detto quanto che ne sapevo et io non ho parlato con nessuno.

—Io ho inteso che detto Agostino et Nicolò che stanno prigione qui in Roma ma non so in qual carcere che l'ho inteso per il vicinato.

—Io conosco detto Agostino da un anno in qua et da tanto tempo ancora conosco detto Nicolò et non gli sò cognome ma è un ragazzo di sedici o diciotto anni con occasione che detti Agostino et Nicolò praticavano in casa de Horatio Gentileschi che habitava in questa strada et sopra questa casa dove sto io et io al signor Agostino poi gli ho parlato mai ma a Nicolò può essere che gli habbia parlato una volta o due che non me reccordo che cosa gli habbia detto et questo ragazzo se gli ho parlato gli avrò parlato dal cortile di casa che risponde in quello della casa dove stava il Gentileschi . . .

—Io conosco Horatio Gentileschi da quatrodeci anni in qua che mio marito serveva lui di vestiti et la moglie che gli faceva le vesti che quando il cominciai a conoscere habitava nella piazza della Trinità a casa de Pietro Pauluzzi et poi andò a stare agli Greci, di là alla strada di Maruta et poi qui sopra me. Con esso non ho havuto altro che trattare se non che mio marito il serviva et da lui non ho da havere nè gli ho da dare.

—Io [. . .] in bottega con mio marito et guadagnamo da sei a otto giulii il giorno et quando più et quando manco (112v) et sono tredici anni che io sto in questa casa con mio marito.

—Io non so dove habita adesso detto signor Horatio ma quando se partì di qui . . . disse che andava a stare a San Spirito che manco il sò et in casa de detto Horatio mentre habitava in questa casa sopra me ci [stetti] tre volte in casa sua che me ce faceva menare il mio parto per ritrarlo.

—Io so che mentre stava qui il Gentileschi ce praticava in casa con il medesimo ragazzo . . . la figliuola del Gentileschi lo chiamava Nicolò e questo Nicolò rispondeva lui, ma se gli fosse servitore o garzone io non lo so, ma un giorno dimandai ad Artimitia figliuola del Gentileschi chi era quel ragazzo che haveva gli era rispose che non gli era cosa alcuna ma che gli faceva qualche servitio et che stava col detto Agostino che è quel gentilhuomo (113) che sta prigione adesso et questo fu un giorno nel cortile di casa mia che sarà da un anno in circa e poco prima che se partissero da questa casa, ma quanto tempo sarà stato detto Nicolò con Agostino non vorrei dire come io non lo so nè altro ne so che quanto me disse quella figliola del Gentileschi ma quel Nicolò come ho detto praticava in casa del Gentileschi e faceva gli servitii.

—Io ho visto detto Nicolò in casa del Gentileschi mentre ha habitato con la famiglia in questa casa sopra me et ce l'ho visto tre o quattro volte con occasione che me afaciavo quando [cavavo] l'acqua che l'ho visto due volte macinare il colore nel cortile di casa . . . et una volta quando il Gentileschi sgombrò dalla strada Maruta che gli veddi portare certi quadri et una tinozza da fare la [bocata] et sempre l'ho visto solo.

Io mi sono confesata e comunicata quest'anno più volte . . .

. . .

(114)—Io ho visto detto Nicolò col detto Agostino due o tre volte veniva a chiamare il detto Horatio, che detto Horatio con il detto Agostino s'erano come fratelli, et detto Nicolò come ho detto mentre il detto Horatio è stato in questa casa è venuto due o tre volte con detto Agostino che altre volte non ce l'ho visto et quelle volte perché bussarono alla porta e domandarono del signor Horatio che non so altro.

—Io ho inteso dagli figlioli del Gentileschi che Agostino dipingeva la sala di Monte Cavallo assieme con loro padre et me lo dissero quando vennero stare in questa casa in quel principio ma se Agostino tenesse servitore alcuno io non lo so.

. . .

—Io ho detto un'altra volta che ce sono stata in casa del detto Horatio mentre stava qui tre o quattro volte et una volta (114v) [. . .] agli Greci che ce menai gli putti a retrahere.

—In casa del detto Horatio non ci ho visto altri che quel Nicolò come vi ho detto di sopra et . . . se stesse per servitore non lo so, so bene che servitore non ha tenuto che haveva della famiglia assai et agli Greci si faceva servire da Giovanni Battista suo nipote che è morto.

—Io non ho visto il detto Horatio dipingere in luogo alcuno. Io lo ho visto quando designava i putti miei dove et come ho detto et quando ancora et io non ci ho visto mai servitore come ho detto di sopra.

—Il signor Horatio ha quatro figli tre maschi et una femina che si chiama Artimitia che credo habbia adesso da venti anni in circa e dei maschi uno si chiama Francesco che haveva quatrodeci anni, l'altro Giulio di 12 anni in circa, l'altro Marco che può havere da 9 anni . . .

SECTION C

ASR, Tribunale Criminale del Governatore, Registrazioni d'atti, vol. 166

(9v) October 23, 1612 The notary Giovanni Battista Stiattesi, on behalf of Orazio Gentileschi, pays a small tax to receive a copy of the two depositions in section B, both of which are in Nicolò Bedino's defense. Lapierre has argued persuasively that it was Stiattesi who guided Gentileschi through the trial, as this payment surely verifies. (See Lapierre, chap. 21.)

Pro d. Horatio gentilescho contra Nicolaum Bidinum in off. mei Jo bapt. Stiattesi petiit copiam depositionis Michelis Angelis pictoris et Costantiae uxoris Honofrii Ceuli sutoris [. . .] beneventius pro presente d. Nicolai pro qua habenda pro Arra dedit julios tres officium
Io (Giovanni Battista) Stiattesi detti la sopradetta Arra et in fede

(26v–27) October 30, 1612 The day after Nicolò's Bedino's final interrogation— where, under torture, Nicolò repeated that he had been in Orazio's house on via Margutta and had seen Artemisia's lascivious conduct— Orazio reaffirms to the court that he has heard that Nicolò is a false witness. Seven other witnesses have demonstrated that Nicolò was never in Orazio's house, either in 1609 or in 1610, in fact, not until the summer of 1611; nor was he in the houses on via Margutta and via della Croce—but this is not precisely what the witnesses said —and asks that Nicolò not be released from prison.
Pro fisco et adherentes contra Nicolaum Bidinum
In off. mei D. Horatius Gentileschus et interrogato sibi de iure competenti et dixit ad eius aures devenisse dictum Nicolaum fuisse testium super falsa depositiones sine preiuditio confessatos et convictos [. . .] et qua d. Nicolaus est [. . .] falsam depositionem convictus per septem testis qui concludenter deposuerunt et in repetitionionis [dixerunt] Nicolaum nunquam fuisse de anno 1609 et 1610 cum dimidio anni 1611 in domo viae Marguttae nec Crucis et propae protestationis non deveniri ad aliquam ipsius excarcerationem nisi prius data sibi [. . .] ad Nicolaus sit comitus [. . .] Hieronimum Felicium locumtenens

(57) November 10, 1612 Orazio Gentileschi appeals a decree in favor of Tassi and Bedino, which is evidently lost.
Appellatio
Pro D. Horatio Gentilesco contram Augustinum Tassum et Nicolaum Bidinum ex iuramento coram Hieronimo Felicio locumtenens neque [. . .] et a decreti facti ad favorem d. Augustini et Nicolai aliisque appellavit ut in cedula decretis cui dominus dedit refutationis in forma camerae.

(101) November 27, 1612 Agostino Tassi is sentenced to exile from Rome for five years under threat of the galleys for the defloration of Artemisia Gentileschi, for the subornation of witnesses, and for defamatory statements against Orazio Gentileschi. He is released on bail from the prison in Corte Savella, promising to carry out his sentence and not to offend Orazio, under threat of a fine of two hundred scudi. The sentence is pronounced in front of Calisto Paravicino and the prison guards. This document that pronounces the sentence against

Agostino is not the original, which is lost, but a record of it for the benefit of the court. Indeed, the phrase "pro Agostino Tasso," that is, in his favor, is rather baffling. But for some reason all sentences of exile are listed in these volumes as "pro." Lapierre's translation of the sentence, in her chapter 22, is slightly fictionalized. Clearly, it was Orazio's honor that was at stake much more than Artemisia's.

Exil.
Pro Augustino Tasso pictore sabellis carcerato pro pretenso stupro praetensaque subornatione testium de articulis infamatoriis contra Horatium Gentileschum productis et aliis de quibus in processu contra eum fabricato Ill. et ecc. d: Hieron. Felicius sostitutus locumtenens iniucto eius exilio ab urbem sub pena triremium per quinquennium ac data cautionem de servandum dictum exilium ac de non offendendum dictum Horatium sub poena scutorum ducentorum eum relaxari mandavit. Deinde fuit per me intimatum exilium presentibus Calisto Paravicino et carceris custodibus

(103v) November 28, 1612 The sentence is here repeated, with one modification. Not being able to find bail, Agostino is released under the guarantee of a Captain Pietro Paolo Arcamanni. See Lapierre, app. 3, for a Francesco Arcamanni, close friend of Quorli's.
Pro Augustino Tasso pictore sabellis carcerato pro praetenso stupro et praetensa subornatione testium ac productione articulis infamatoriis [. . .] contra d. Horatium Gentileschum et aliis de quibus in processu [. . .] Ill. et ecc. Hier. Felicius habito verbo cum Illm. ut asseruit decretum hinc ex quo ante extensionem decreti et postea fecit de reperienda fideiussionem et non potuit [. . .] fide Cap. Petri Pauli Arcamanni de servando exilio et de non offendendum dictum Horatium ac iniucto exilio ut in alio eundem relaxari mandavit
Deinde fuit per me intimatum exilium presentibus carceris custodibus

ASR, Tribunale Criminale del Governatore, Registrazioni d'atti, vol. 167. The following documents are unrelated to the trial of 1612. See Lapierre, app. 21; her slightly different interpretation results in part from my misreading of the act of April 9. This is not a reversal of the original sentence, as I had believed, but a new sentence of exile for a different crime.

(165v) March 13, 1613 The quarrels between Valerio Ursino and Tassi continue in 1613. Apparently Ursino, who lived in the house of Antonio Maria Bertucci, was about to be released from prison, because there seemed to be no reason to keep him there. At this point, Agostino Tassi appeared in the office of the notary Stefano Faina and asked that more witnesses be interrogated in a new lawsuit that he had filed against Ursino for insulting him. By means of this new filing, Tassi wanted to expose the crimes perpetrated against him by his adversary. Ursino is here called a color grinder. Antonio Maria Bertucci, cousin of Antinoro, used to own the pigment store on via del Corso. (This information is in Processi 104, fol. 420.)

Pro d. Augustino Tasso contra d. Valerium Ursinum macinatorem colorum degentem in domo Antonii Mariae Bertuzzi in Platea Nicosia fiscum adherentem ac instigationem Antonius Cur.li [. . .] in dicta domo eius [. . .] at eius [. . .] excarcerari Infra pt. instantiam [. . .] D. quibuscumque non obstari ad

[. . .] presens e compari in off.o meis [. . .] non posse excarcerari [. . .] ex carceribus secretis ad effectum examinari posse alios testes repertos super nova querela porrecta insultus cum [. . .] de quo in processo et sus locus et tempus petiit sibi accomodari de toto processu ad effectum dimostrandi manifesta delicta per adversarium perpetrata D. insta (instanza) reponit in iudicium coram Ill.m et ecc. D. Anselmo Ciolo locumtenens neque D. Stephanus Faina tamquo uno de populo petiit sibi accomodari de eo processum ad effectum demostrandum manifesta delicta perpetrata D. insta ut coram ill. Anselmo Ciolo locumtenens meque Stephanus Faina . . .

(183) March 20, 1613 This act records the reconciliation between Tassi, a prisoner in Tor di Nona, and Valerio Ursino, a painter from Florence living on via dei Condotti. They promise to forget all wrongs and insults and to be reconciled now and in the future; as a gesture of peace, they embrace and kiss.
Pace
Pro Augustino Tasso Nonae Carcerato contra quosquumquem In meis presentia Augustinus Tassus q. Domenici de Tassis romanus pictor ex una et Valerii q. Francisci Ursini flo. pictor incola urbis in via Conductorum nuncupata [. . .] nunc pacem fecerunt inter se et unum alteri et alter alteri promiserunt [. . .] reconciliationem ac pp. [pacem] duraturam [. . .] et singulis injuris cum armis quibuscunque [. . .] usquem in presentem diem et in signum pacis amplexi fuerunt hosculo interveniente quam pacem promiserunt . . . , et qu sit mihi put et contra nos facere per se ipsam alium [. . .] In ampl. forma camera apostolica

(192) March 23, 1613 Giovanni Salvarani, the lawyer defending Tassi, asks that no sentence be pronounced on his client, who is in prison, until he receives a copy of the evidence (on payment of a small tax). If this and the following act have anything to do with the litigations between Tassi and Ursino, their "long-lasting reconciliation," mentioned in the previous act, was short-lived indeed. The following document may, however, be part of a yet another judicial proceeding. It was not unusual for Tassi to be involved in more than one trial at a time.
Arra
Pro Domino Augustino Tasso carcerato contra fiscum et adherentes, in officio D. Ioannes Salvaranus defensor, Dominum Joannis Salvarani defensor et procurator quaesivit non deveniri ab aliquam sententiam preiudicialem nisi prius habuit copiam indiciorum pro qua habenda pro Arra dedit iulios tres offerendi pro ut

(222v) April 9, 1613 In consequence of a fight—probably with arms—Agostino Tassi, who is in prison, is exiled from the Papal States for five years. The phrase "eundem relaxari mandavit" (I ordered him set free) states, in effect, that after being sentenced to banishment, a prisoner is actually released, at times under bail. We do not know how common it was to ignore such a sentence, as Agostino did in 1612. This time he seems to have left the city, but not the Papal States, for two or two and a half years.
Exil.
Pro Augustino Tasso pictore hodie carcerato pro rixa cum [. . .] de mandato contra fiscum Illustrissimus iniucto eidem exilium toto statu ecclesiastico per quinquennium eundem relaxari mandavit
Deinde fuit per me eidem intimatum exil. presentibus Iulio Martellio et carcerorum custodibus

Appendix 2. Orazio Gentileschi in Rome: Two New Documents

LIVIA CARLONI

March 22, 1601

Orazio Gentileschi petitions to execute cartoons for the mosaics in the cupola of Saint Peter's in order that he may demonstrate his abilities. He was, in fact, among the painters working under the Cavaliere d'Arpino who were paid for cartoons both for the drum of the dome (the account for these was closed on April 15, 1609) and for the cupola, for the latter of which he designed an angel and the Virgin (payments in 1609 and 1610, respectively: see Bissell 1981, 148).

22 marzo (1601)

Beatiss.^{mo} P[ad]re

Oratio Gentileschi Pittore, et humil.^{sso} oratore della S[anti]tà V[ost]ra ha infinito desiderio di poter fare li desegni de Cartoni del restante della Cupola di S.to Pietro per poter cognioscere in concorso di altri valent'huomini se egli è buono da qualche cosa; n'ha supplicato li Si[gno]ri deputati della fabbrica et l'han'dato buona intenzione, però supplica con ogni humiltà V[ostra] B[eatitudi]ne degnarsi farlo gratificare di detta opera, quale farà con ogni diligenza et riceverà a molta gratia da V[ostra] B[eatitudi]ne per la cui felicità pregarà sempre Dio benedetto. Quas Deus

(sul retro): Alla S[anti]tà di N[ostro] S[igno]re

al card.^e di Cosenza [Pallotta]

Per Oratio Gentileschi Pittore

Die 22 mensis martij 1601 in Congregatione

All. Ill. card. del Monte

All. Ill.e Rev. card. del Monte

(Archivio Reverenda Fabbrica S. Pietro, Arm. I, B. 19 N. 42, f. 185)

July 24, 1619

Orazio Gentileschi writes a supplication to decorate the Benediction loggia at Saint Peter's. Having heard of the *fabbrica*'s intention to decorate the Benediction loggia at Saint Peter's, he puts himself forward as a candidate, promising to do his best. The commission was awarded to Giovanni Lanfranco, who in 1616–17 had frescoed the Sala Regia of the Palazzo del Quirinale together with Carlo Saraceni and Agostino Tassi. With the death of Pope Paul V on January 28, 1621, the commission collapsed.

Ill[ustrissi]mi et R[everendissi]mi S[igno]ri

Horatio Gentileschi Pittore humil[is]s[i]mo serv[ito] delle S[ignorie] V[ostre] Ill[ustrissi]me havendo inteso che si doverà dipinger in S. Pietro la loggia delle benedittioni, supplica le S[ignorie] V[ostre] Ill[ustrissi]me à servirsi dell'opera sua promettendo che s'impiegarà con ogni diligenza et lo ricevera per grazia delle S[ignorie] V[ostre] Ill[ustrissi]me. Quas Deus

(sul retro): All: Ill[ustrissi]mi et Rev[erendi]ssimi domini S[igno]ri Cardinali della S. Congregaz[ione] della Rev. Fab.

Per Horatio Gentileschi pittore

die 24 Julij 1619 in Congreg[azione] guando sene trattara

(Archivio Reverenda Fabbrica S. Pietro, Arm. I, B. 14 N. 76)

Appendix 3. Artemisia Gentileschi in Florence: Inventory of Household Goods and Working Materials

FRANCESCO SOLINAS AND ROBERTO CONTINI

On February 10, 1620, Artemisia Gentileschi, then residing in Florence, wrote to Grand Duke Cosimo II de' Medici that she intended to make a trip to Rome. She had begun a painting of Hercules for the grand duke and promised to finish it for him within two months. For this picture, one and a half *oncie* of ultramarine had been advanced to her, and when payment was not received, the ducal *guardarobba* sequestered some of her possessions. These were released on February 15, 1620, when Francesco Maria Maringhi stood as guarantor for the payment. It is unclear whether the picture was ever painted, but by the following year Artemisia had decided to move permanently to Rome and sold her household goods to Maringhi. Maringhi's relationship with Artemisia is not altogether clear; Bissell (1999, 161) has suggested that they may have been lovers. They certainly remained in touch, since in 1635 she wrote to Galileo Galilei indicating that his reply should be addressed to the care of Maringhi.

The inventory provides an indication of the projects Artemisia was involved in at the time of her move to Rome as well a glimpse of her lifestyle in Florence. This previously unpublished inventory was discovered by Francesco Solinas in the private archives of the Frescobaldi family. He has generously permitted its publication here.

Frescobaldi Archive, Florence
1623 [modern calendar: 1624] 10. February

Inventory of furniture and [other objects] sold by Artemisia [cancelled: Margherita] Lomi to Francesco Maringhi for the price of 165 ducats.

X February '620 [1621]. In Florence.

This certifies that Signora Artemisia Lomi sells to Signor Francesco Maria Maringhi the items listed below for the price of 165 ducats, which the above-named Lady will receive in ready money, and she gives this to Signor Francesco as a receipt. They agree that this is valid as a public document, and they have asked me, Francesco Conti, to prepare the present list. The items are as follows:

2. large solid walnut chests
3. other Venetian walnut-veneered chests
1. large walnut cupboard with shelves
12. walnut stools with backs
1. small walnut socle [or plinth]
4. chairs with seats of various colored damasks and their covers
1. wooden chest
4. wool mattresses
4. rough linen mattresses
4. straw mattresses
3. bedsteads, one with walnut columns
76. golden and green leather hangings, Spanish size
18. gold and red columns with their frieze

1. red *ormesia* [?] and taffeta blanket
1. turquoise cloth blanket, trimmed with green taffeta
1. other turquoise blanket, trimmed with rose-colored cloth
3. blankets quilted with cotton wool
1. turquoise and white cotton wool canopy, made in the Turkish manner
2. feather cushions
1. quilted blanket of 30, stuffed with down
1. kneading trough

1623 10. Febb.o [1624 stile comune]

Inventario di Mobili et venduti da Artemisia [canc. Marg/gherita] Lomi a Francesco Maringhi per prezzo di d[ucati] 165.

Adi X febr[ai]o 620 [1621]. In Firenze

Si dichiara per la pre[sen]te qualmente la S[igno]ra Artemi=/sia Lomi vende al S[igno]r Fr[ances]co Maria Maringhi / li robbi qui Sotto notati per il prezzo di ducati / 165, quali d[ett]a S[igno]ra riceve di contanti, e con la p[rese]nte / ne fa quietanza al sud[dett]o S[igno]r Frances]co, restando di accor=/do che questa p[rese]nte sia, e vagli come pub[bli]ca iscrittura, / ed han pregato me Fr[ances]co Conti, che glie ne stenda / la p[rese]nte scrittura. Le robbe sono l'infra[scri]tte /

2. Casse grandi tutte noce
3. altre casse impiallacciate di noce viniziane
1. Credenza di noce grande co' suoi gradini
12. Scabbelli di noce con le spalliere
1. zoccoletto di noce
4. sedie di damasco d'appoggio di colore mischio con fodere
1. cassa d'albero
4. matarazzi di lana
4. matarazzi di capeccio
4. sacconi
3. littiere una con le colone di noce
76. pelli di oro, e verdi misura di Spagna
18. collonne d'oro, e rosse, e suo friscio //

1. coltre di ormesia rosso, e taffetano
1. coltre di tela turchesca bendata di taffetá verde
1. coltre pur turchesca bendata di tela incarnatina
3. coltroni di bambace
1. padiglione di bambace turchino, e bianco fatto alla turchesca
2. piumacci di piuma
1. coltrice di 30 tutto di piuma
1. madia

1. kneading board	1. Asse da pane
1. wooden bed warmer	1. Prete di legno
1. small wooden table	1. tavolino d'Albero
2. other small wooden tables	2. altri tavolini d'albero
1. wooden cabinet with drawers	1. Armarino d'albero coi suoi cassetti
1. big pot	1. caldina grande
1. cauldron	1. paiolo
2. warming pans	2. scaldaletti
1. large pan for starching	1. teglia da dare l'amido
1. vessel for cold water with brass dishes	1. rinfrescatoio con piatti d'ottone
1. small brass bucket with handle	1. secchino fornito d'ottone, e suo manico
1. bucket	1. secchio
1. brass fountain	1. fontana d'ottone
1. copper pan	1. caldano di rame
1. chain for the fireplace	1. catena del foco
2. iron fire shovels	2. palete di ferro
3. tripods	3. trepiedi //
1. big tripod for the cauldron	1. trepiede grande per la caldaia
3. round tin plates	3. tondi di stagno
5. Pistoiese stools	5. seggiole alla Pistolese
4. wooden stools	4. scabelli d'albero
4. easels	4. leggij da dipingere
1. large canvas, half painted	1. tela grande mezza dipinta
1. picture of a clothed Magdalene, 2 *braccia* high	1. quadro alto 2 braccia di una Maddalena abbilata
1. picture of a Madonna, 2 *braccia* high	1. quadro alto 2 braccia di una Madonna
1. portrait of a woman in a walnut frame	1. Ritratto di dona incorniciato di noce
4. walnut palettes for colors	4. tavolozze di noce da dipingere
2. brass candlesticks	2. candelieri d'ottone
3. iron oil lamps	3. lucerne di ferro
1. pair of fire tongs	1. paio di molle per il foco
1. brass snuffer	1. smoccolatore di ottone
3. boards to be put crosswise on the easels	3. assi per metter a traverso a legij
15. stretchers for paintings, including large and small ones	15. telaj da quadri tra grandi, e piccoli
1. picture of a Magdalene, just begun, 2 *braccia* high	1. quadro d'una Maddalena cominciato alto 2. braccia
1. lamp holder with an iron candlestick	1. Lucerniere con il candeliere di ferro
3. small paintings on copper	3. rametti dipinti
1. crucifix	1. Crocifisso
4. small feather pillows [cancelled: viciria]	4. guancialetti di piuma [canc. viciria]
1. mortar with pestle	1. mortaio col pestello
1. large vessel and clay strainer	1. concone, e colatoio di terra
140. gold and red common leather hangings and 13. turquoise and gold cotton ones, decorated on the top and the bottom	140. pelli d'oro, e rosse ord[ina]rie e di cotone 13. turchine, e d'oro, con suo friscio sotto, e sopra
24. majolica dishes, including large and small ones, with other clay utensils for the kitchen	24. piatti di maiolica tra grandi, e piccoli, con altre mas / serizie di cucina di terra

The above-named Signor Francesco Maria Maringhi declares that he has received the items listed above and the above-named Signora Artemisia [declares] that she has received the aforementioned 165 ducats; in witness thereof they undersign [the document] in their own hand, together with their attestation.	Quali robbe il S[igno]r Fr[ances]co Maria Maringhi sud[det]o / confessa havere ricevuto, e la S[igno]ra Artemisia / sud[dett]a ricevuti li sud[dett]i ducati 165 ed in fede / del vero si sottoscriveranno di lor propria / mano con gli infra[scri]tti testimonij
I, Francesco Conti, am the author of this document.	Io. Fr[ances]co Conti ho scritto la presente
I, Artemisia Lomi, confirm the above.	Io Artemisia lomi affermo quanto di sopra
I, Francesco Maria Maringhi, confirm the above.	Io Fran[ces]co M[ari]a Maringhi affermo q[uant]o di sopra.

Appendix 4. Orazio Gentileschi at the Court of Charles I: Six Documents

GABRIELE FINALDI AND JEREMY WOOD

Transcriptions of six documents from Orazio Gentileschi's years in England are included here. There are three letters from Gentileschi to the secretary of state, Lord Dorchester, dating to 1629 and 1630; a report of payments received by Gentileschi and his two sons; a postscript from a letter by Balthazar Gerbier of 1633 that mentions the artist; and Gentileschi's nuncupative will of 1639. The original punctuation and spelling have been retained, but contracted words have been given in full.

I.

Letter from Orazio Gentileschi, in his own hand, to the secretary of state, Dudley Carleton, Lord Dorchester, undated but written in March 1629.

Orazio Gentileschi offers a lengthy and defensive account of the activities of his sons Francesco and Giulio during their recent trip to Italy, where they had been sent to acquire a picture collection in Genoa for Charles I. He explains that Nicholas Lanier, the English musician and art dealer who was then resident in Italy working for the king, had vetoed the purchase, and Gentileschi's sons had been authorized by the English ambassador in Venice to use the money intended for the acquisition to pay for the travel and living expenses of their extended stay.

London, PRO (Public Records Office), SP16/139, no. 88, fols. 168r–169r

Listed in *Calendar of State Papers, Domestic* 1859, 510, no. 88; published in English in Sainsbury 1859b, 311–13.

Ill[ustrissi]mo et Ecc[ellentissi]mo Sig[no]r et p[ad]ron Mio Col[endissi]mo

Acciò V[ost]ra Ecc[ellen]za resti informata delle spese fatte da Francesco, et Giulio miei figlioli, nell'occasione del viaggio fatto da loro in Italia, per ordine di S[ua] M[aes]tà, è necessario con questa sappia, come dal S[igno]r Tomas Cari il di 20 d'Agosto l'anno 1627, furno inviati per commando di S[ua] M[aes]tà à Genova, per far compra d'uno studio di quadri del S[igno]r Filippo San Micheli, con l'intervento del Sig[no]r Nicolas Lanier, quale di già si trovava à Venetia, et per il loro viaggio sino in d[ett]o luogo, gli fù dato per le mani del S[igno]r Cari Lire cento cinquanta, con parola di d[ett]o S[igno]re haverebboro trovato il S[igno]r Lanier à Genova, essendo che per lettere gli haveva inviato tal'ordine, con dover somministrargli danari per la loro stanza, et per il loro ritorno, accompagnandoli con proprie lettere in suo favore; ma quando furno à Milano, intesero che il S[igno]r Lanier si trovava à Venetia, et che era fra poco tempo di partenza per Inghilterra. (Tear in paper, one word missing) uno di loro determinò andare à Genova, et l'altro à Venetia à trovarlo (tear) così fecero, et quando quello arrivò à Venetia, gli fù detto da D(tear) in casa del quale abitava d[ett]o S[igno]r Nicolò, che erano già quattro giorni (tear) per Genova; per il che Giulio immediatamente, risolse in posta andare (tear) per ritrovarsi con il fratello à stabilire con il S[igno]r Nicolas in compagnia del fratello quel tanto, per il quale erano stati mandati in Italia; ma quando Giulio fù arrivato, et abboccatosi con il fratello Francesco, gli dimandò se haveva parlato con il S[igno]r Lanier, et egli gli disse che non l'haveva veduto, per essersi fermato

solo un giorno in Genova, il che fece maravigliare il proprio mercante, al quale erano dirette le lettere di Cambio; si che Giulio di nuovo senza intervallo di tempo, giudicò bene ritornar'à Venetia, per saper chiaramente l'intentione di d[ett]o S[igno]r Nicolas; dove arrivato, et abboccatosi seco, et trovato non voler acconsentire alla compra di quello studio, gli disse che li provedessi de denari perche disegnavano ritornarsene, al che rispose che voleva prima parlar con il S[igno]r Ambasciatore di S[ua] M[aes]tà, et che la mattina seguente serebbe [*sic*] venuto à trovarlo, come fece in compagnia del Nipote del S[igno]re Amb[asciato]re; et per risposta gli disse che al d[ett]o S[igno]r Amb[asciato]re pareva bene che loro dovessero fermarsi in Italia, (tear in paper; fol. 225v:) al che Giulio disse voler obbedire, ma che se si fermavano sino à quel tempo, che sarebbe sopragiunto l'impeto dell'inverno, essendo all'hora il mese di Novembre; che perciò sarebbero stati forzati prolungar il loro ritorno sino à Primavera, et che non havevano commodi di danaro per trattenersi tanto tempo, al che rispose il S[igno]r Lanier, che dovessero valersi delli cinquecento scudi datigli dal S[igno]r Tomas Cari, per comprar pitture, et che ciò era servitio del Rè, et che lui haverebbe fatto scusa con d[ett]o S[igno]r Cari, et avvisatolo esser stato suo ordine, come fece, et doppo questo Giulio gli disse haver fatto dui viaggi in poste à Venetia, per li quali non haveva hauto denaro alcuno, et che haveva speso quanti denari haveva del suo, che però gli facesse gratia provedergliene tanti almeno per il ritorno, et perciò detto S[igno]r Nicolas gli fece dare da Daniel Niis trenta doppie di Spagna, et egli riceutole ritornossene à Genova, dove riscosse unitamente con il fratello li sudd[ett]i cinque cento scudi dal S[igno]r Federico Saminiati, et fermatosi Francesco costà, et Giulio andato à Pisa a passar l'inverno, con alcuni suoi parenti, in capo a cinque ò sei mesi io gli scrissi à tutti dui li miei figli per ordine del S[igno]r Tomas Cari, che dovessero ritornarsene in Inghilterra, chè così era l'intentione di S[ua] M[aes]tà, quale voleva riconoscerli delle loro fatiche, et che il Sig[no]r Nicolas Lanier teneva ordine provederli della medesima somma di danaro, che gli fù dato quando furno inviati in Italia, et loro subito riceuto la mia lettera, scrissero all S[igno]r Nicolò à Venetia, che gli mandasse li denari per il loro ritorno, et doppo haver aspettato la risposta un mese, e mezzo, Francesco si risolse andare à Venetia per il denaro, et in quello instante venne a Genova al S[igno]r Saminiati l'ordine di pagarli cento cinquanta doppie, mà Francesco arrivato à Venetia, et trovato il S[igno]r Lanier gli disse, volessi dargli à lui il denaro; mà il S[igno]r Nicolò gli dette la poliza di cambio in confermatione di quella di prima, pagabile à Giulio, et Francesco unitamente, delle sudd[ett]e doppie cento cinquanta, et poi gli dette per ritornarsene à Genova, et per altri suoi bisogni altre doppie cinquanta sette, che fanno in tutto la valuta delle Lire cento cinquanta sterline riceute da loro (fol. 226r:) per la gita à Genova, et ciò è il denaro ri (tear) per tutto, con la dichiaratione della cagione delli loro viaggi fatti à Venetia, che quando vogli V[os]tra Ecc[ellen]za retifichino il tutto alla sua presenza con il S[igno]r Nicolò Lanier, resterà servita, non havendo io messo nella presente informatione cosa nessuna, che loro prima non l'habbino data in simil forma à S[ua] M[aes]tà et all S[igno]r Tomas Cari, per scarico d'ogni oppositione gli fussi fatta, et quì con reverente affetto gli bacio humilmente le mani.

Di V[ostra] S[ignoria] Ill[ustrissi]ma et Ecc[elentissi]ma
Ser[vito]re Humiliss[i]mo et Obidientiss[i]mo
Oratio Gentileschi

2.

An account of payments received by Orazio Gentileschi and his sons between 1627 and 1629 (addressed to the secretary of state, Lord Dorchester).

The list covers payments received by Gentileschi from the king and from George Villiers, first duke of Buckingham, for living expenses, for the purchase of canvases and pigments, and for payment of male and female models. The list also includes monies received by his sons Francesco and Giulio for their trip to Italy. The document, in Orazio's hand, probably accompanied the letter the artist sent to Lord Dorchester in March 1629 (item 1 in this appendix).

London, PRO, SP85, bundle 6, fol. 333r,v. At the end of the document is an annotation stating that in 1953 it was removed from SP84/104.

Published in Finaldi 1999, 33.

Conti delli denari ricevuti da Oratio Gentileschi, tanto per le sue provisioni, quanto per le spese fatte per colori, tele, accurro Oltramarino, et modelli, per ordine di S[ua] M[aes]tà

In primis lire cinquecento per le mani del s[igno]r Porter, date à Oratio Gentileschi per la provisione d'un anno, assegnateli da sua M[aes]tà si per bocca del s[igno]r Duca per ciascun'anno per il suo vitto, et mantenimento della sua casa _____ 500

Item altre lire cento cinquanta sterline date da S[ua] M[aes]tà per comprar colori, azzurro, tele per dipignere, et Modelli _____ 150

Conto delle spese fatte in Colori

In primis per azzurro oltramarino scudi _____ 225
Per altri colori grossi delli quali ce n'è ancora bona parte __ 45
Per tele impremite scudi _____ 30
Per modelli tanto di femine quanto di huomini, non ce n'è conto preciso, non havendo mai messo in lista il denaro pagato per tal servitio

_____

Conto delli denari ricevuti dalli figlioli d'Oratio Gentileschi per il viaggio fatto da loro in Italia in servitio di S[ua] M[aes]tà, et fermatisi sette mesi

In primis lire cento cinquanta sterline pagate dal segretario del s[igno]r Tomas Cari alli d[ett]i Francesco, et Giulio per andare a Genova, per uno studio di quadri del S[igno]r Filippo San Micheli, conforme appare nell'informatione data a V[ost]ra Ecc[ellen]za _____ 150

Item trenta doppie date dal S[ignor] Nicolas Lanier à Giulio, per il suo ritorno à Genova havendo fatto dui viaggi in poste à Venetia, come appare nella d[ett]a informatione _____ doppie 30

Item riscossi da Francesco, et Giulio, con ordine del S[igno]r Nicolas Lanier in Genova, cinquecento scudi di quella moneta, per la loro stanza in Italia _____ 500

Item doppie cento cinquanta date à Francesco in lettera di Cambio, et altre cinquata sette in contanti, per il loro viaggio in Inghilterra come appare nella d[ett]a informatione dovendo ricever tutta d[ett]a somma, in conformità delle cento cinquanta lire pagategli per la lor gita
Doppie _____ 207

3.

Letter from Orazio Gentileschi, in his own hand, to the secretary of state, Lord Dorchester (by whom endorsed on April 24, 1629).

The painter gives an account of the money he has received from the duke of Buckingham, who had recently died, and from the king. He requests that the money owed him by the king be paid immediately, since he is in financial difficulty.

London, PRO, SP16/141, no. 35, fol. 46r,v

Listed in *Calendar of State Papers, Domestic* 1859, 527, no. 35; published in English in Sainsbury 1859a, 313–14.

Ill[ustrissi]mo et Ecc[ellentissi]mo S[igno]r et p[ad]ron Mio Col[endissi]mo

Poiche Vo[st]ra Ecc[ellen]za mi commanda, per parte di S[ua] M[aest]à ch'io dia conto di quello, mi fu donato dall'Ecc[ellentissi]mo Sig[no]r Duca Bocchingam, gloriosa memoria, alche non pensavo mai di venire, come cosa separata dalle mie pretentioni, et dall'interessi di S[ua] M[aest]à havendolo da sua Ecc[ellen]za riceuto in dono, con sua parola, non per cosa nessuna ch' havessi fatta in questo Regno; mà per essermi appreso à questo servitio, et lasciato quello di Francia a sua devotione, et venutomene à mie spese in Inghilterra, differentemente à quando sono stato chiamato dalla Repub[b]lica di Genova, dal Gran Duca di Toscana, del Ser[enissi]mo di Savoia, et ultimamente dalla Regina Madre di Francia, dalli quali Prencipi hò riceuto buona somma di denaro per il mio viaggio; et ancora per haver perso molto tempo per attendere il commodo di quella casa, fatta da sua Ecc[ellen]za fabricare per mio servitio, et hora per mancamento della sua persona ne devo uscire: gli dirò quello, che hò riceuto da S[ua] Ecc[ellen]za in Inghilterra; che mentre servivo altro Prencipe fuori di questo Regno, credo V[ost]ra Ecc[ellen]za non voglia riceverne conto alcuno, tanto più che il tutto mi hà dato per li quadri inviatigli di Parigi, et per ricompensa dell'opere mie, che ne l'uno ne l'altro m'assicuro non potrà fare pregiuditio alcuno alle mie pretentioni, et al credito che hò con S[ua] M[aes]tà per la servitù fattagli, sapendo non esser l'intention sua satisfarmi del denaro donatomi dal S[ignor] Duca, ma benignamente riconoscermi, conforme me n'hà dato intentione, et come è accostumata di fare si gran M[aes]tà benche sin'hora non habbia riceuto da quella, solo che la prov[v]isione d'un anno, et le cento cinquanta Lire per l'azzurro, Modelli, et altri colori, come di già n'hò informato V[ost]ra Ecc[ellen]za, quale pol ben sapere dalla bocca di S[ua] M[aes]tà se hà ordinato mi sia dato altro denaro, ò vero si trova alcun pagatore del Rè, che m'habbia dato cos'alcuna, che cosX resterà chiara V[ost]ra Ecc[ellen]za del mio credito, et del mio debito; mà per venire à quello di che son ricercato, gli dirò come non ho riceuto altro solo che il denaro di quella gratia che donò S[ua] M[aes]tà al S[igno]r Duca con le sudd[ett]e parole di S[ua] Ecc[ellen]za havendo d[ett]o S[igno]re prima fattone rice[v]uta di sua mano à quel Visconte, al quale ordinb S[ua] M[aes]tà che dovessi pagare il denaro al S[igno]r Duca, et non ad altri, et egli per sua benignità, et per li suddetti particolari me ne fece dono; la qual gratia importb in tutto lire mille, et cinque cento, mà di quelli me ne toccorno solo mille, et trecento, havendone date doicento ad alcuni interessati in quel negotio, essendo quelli che la proposero, et che la trattorno con queste conditioni, et delli lire mille et trecento, parte ne hò spese in mio figliolo, stato qualche tempo al servitio di S[ua] Ecc[ellen]za et il resto nel mantenimento della mia casa, qual figliolo, non hà riceuto cos'alcuna à quella servitù (fol. 46v:) com' hanno fatto gl'altri, delche non ne haverei parlato mai, come delli suddetti particolari, se non fossi stato forzato dar questi conti; si cura che se non era il commodo di questo denaro, mi bisognava esser molto più sollecito per non dir importuno, in risquoter quello, che mi è stato assegnato per il mio vitto. Hora credo non haver altri conti da dare à V[ost]ra Ecc[ellen]za, et questi sò li conoscerà di nessun momento per quello che mi si deve; rest'hora la preghi vogli farmi gratia terminar il tutto, acciò possa far riscossione delle mie provisioni, essendo del tutto scarso di denaro, anzi di più indebitato, per haver mandato li miei figlioli in Italia, sicondo l'intention di Sua M[aes]tà come pol sapere da un Mercante che mi ha accommodato del denaro per tal servitio che di ciò ne resterò obligatiss[i]mo alla cortesia di V[ost]ra Ecc[ellen]za alla quale humilmente bacio le mani

Di V[ostra] S[ignoria] Ill[ustrissi]ma et Ecc[ellentissi]ma

Ser[vito]re Humiliss[i]mo
Oratio Gentileschi

4.
Letter from Orazio Gentileschi, in his own hand, to the secretary of state, Lord Dorchester, October 13, 1630.

Gentileschi asks for money that is owed him to be paid by the lord treasurer as soon as possible, so that he can clear his debts. He asks also for passports for two men returning to Paris who had been with him at Windsor and were concerned that they might be inconvenienced by customs officials when they departed.

London, PRO, SP16/174, no. 33, fol. 45r,v

Listed in *Calendar of State Papers, Domestic* 1860, 359, no. 33. Unpublished.

Eccelent[i]ssimo Sig[no]r e P[ad]ron mio Col[endissi]mo

Pensavo di poter venire costà per sollecitare la rescussione delli denari promessimi dall'Eccelentiss[i]mo Sig[no]r Tesauriere che già sono passati gli otto giorni ne quali havava promessomi sodisfarmi; ma sono stato sopresso da una furia si grande di cattarro che perciß sono stato forzato inviare à Vostra Eccelenza questo huomo à posta e con la presente infastidirla e sono in stato tale che se lei vi fussi presente haveria compassione di me non sendomi mai trovato in peggiore stato, nel quale al presente sono con debiti, che giornalm[en]te mi danno travaglio non essendo io a questo accostumato. Per tanto supplico l'eccelenza vostra à fare qualche cosa p[er] me app[ress]o il sig[no]r Tesauriere à fine che io possa sodisfare i miei debiti e vivere con qualche sorte di quiete del che gli sentirß infinite obligat[io]ni. Quelli ss[ignor]i che à Vinsor in mia compagnia vennero sono di partenza p[er] Parigi et hanno comperato qualche poche cose p[er] loro uso, e p[er]chè non hanno la lingua temono d'essere alle Dogane trattenuti; percio loro, et io insieme la supplichiamo d'un passaporto, à fine che con quello li sia permesso fare il loro viaggio liberam[en]te non have[n]do intentione di defraudare in alcun modo le dette Dogane. Replico che non ho migliore speranza interno alli miei interessi di quella che s'e degnata porgermi la supplico à favorirmi col sudetto passaporto di due linee in risposta con che à vostra Eccelenza inchinandomi prego dal sig[no]re Idio contento di Londra li 13 8bre 1630
di vostra Eccel[en]za ser[vito]re Humiliss[im]o e Devotiss[im]o

Horatio Gentileschi

(45v)
Londra 12 8b[re] 1630
Il Sig[no]r Gentileschi all'Ill[ustrissi]mo & Eccelentiss[im]o Sig[no]r Viconte di Dorcestra

5.
Postscript in a letter from Sir Balthazar Gerbier, in Brussels, to King Charles I, October 14, 1633.

Gerbier informs the king that Queen Maria de' Medici, the exiled mother of Louis XIII of France, and Archduchess Isabella, infanta of Spain, had admired a work by Gentileschi in Brussels.

London, PRO, SP105/10, fol. 260

Gentilesco hath prayed me to [*sic*] in a letter to witnesse to Your Majesty the Queen Mother and the Infanta have admired here his worke; being the truth I cannot refuse him to sett it downe in this postscript, for which I humbly crave pardon.

6.
Orazio Gentileschi's will

Gentileschi did not make a formal will, but before he died he orally declared before witnesses his intentions for the disposal of his estate (nuncupative will). It was to be divided between his three sons, the largest portion to Giulio, his second son, and the smallest to Marco, his youngest. He appointed Francesco, his eldest son, his executor.

London, PRO, Prob 11/180, fol. 473r

Published in Finaldi 1999, 33.

In the margin: T[estamentum] nuncupatinu[m] Horatio Gentileschi: def[unct]i

Memorandum that upon the one and twentieth day of January anno Domini iuxta (?)[?]; one thousand six hundred thirty eight or thereabout Horatio Gentileschi late of the p[ar]ishe of Saint Martin in the fields in the Countie of Midd[lesex] gent[leman] beinge sicke in bodie of the last sicknes whereof he died but of p[er]fecte mynd and memorie with an intention to declare his last will and testam[en]t nuncupative did utter and declare as followeth: I will that after my debts are paied my sonne Julio shall have a little more of my estate then my sonne Francisco because he hath a greate charge of children and is not soe well able to gett his livinge as my sonne Francisco is, and that my sonne Francisco shall have a little lesse then my sonne Julio, and that my sonne Marco shall have leaste of all because he hath beene an undutifull child to me and hath putt me to great charges, and I will that my sonne Francisco shall have all my wearinge apparell and ready monyes to defray the charges of my buriall. And I will that my Servant Francis Tarilli shall have tenn poundes which I owe him for worke and all my household goodes and alsoe that my said three sonnes shall give him (meaninge the said Francis Tarilli []) five poundes apeece, in all fiefteene poundes for his paines taken in attendinge me in my sicknes and he made his sonne Francis Gentileschi sole executor, which wordes or the like in effecte were soe spoken and declared by the said Horatio Gentileschi as aforesaid in the presence and hearinge of Joannes Dumoriceaux (?) # # Joannes Copatus (?) fui presens Francis Tarilli.

The will was proved on July 2, 1639, by Francesco Gentileschi.

Bibliography

COMPILED BY JEAN WAGNER

Abrate, Alessandro, ed.
1989   *Il castello di Carrù da luogo fortificato a dimora a sede di banca.* Carrù, 1989.

Abromson, Morton C.
1981   *Painting in Rome during the Papacy of Clement VIII (1592–1605): A Documented Study.* New York, 1981. Originally the author's dissertation, 1976.

Acanfora, Elisa
2000   "Cigoli, Galileo e le prime riflessioni sulla cupola barocca." *Paragone* 51, no. 31 (2000), 29–52.

Acidini Luchinat, Cristina
1998–99   *Taddeo e Federico Zuccari: Fratelli pittori delcinquecento.* 2 vols. Milan, 1998–99.

Adriani, Gert
1940   *Anton van Dyck: Italienisches Skizzenbuch.* Vienna, 1940.

Aikema, Bernard
1994   "Titian's Mary Magdalen in the Palazzo Pitti: An Ambiguous Painting and Its Critics." *Journal of the Warburg and Courtauld Institutes* 57 (1994), 48–59.

Albani, Alessandro
1980   *Il Cardinale Alessandro Albani e la sua villa: Documenti.* Quaderni sul Neoclassicismo, 5. Rome, 1980.

Albertini, C.
n.d.   "Storia di Ancona. Vol. LXI, 1540–1610." Ms. 263, Biblioteca Civica Benincasa, Ancona.

Alessandrini, Ada, et al.
1986   *Francesco Stelluti, linceo da Fabriano: Studi e ricerche.* Fabriano, 1986.

Alexander, Michael van Cleave
1975   *Charles I's Lord Treasurer: Sir Richard Weston, Earl of Portland (1577–1635).* Chapel Hill, 1975.

Alfonso, Luigi
1976   "Luciano Borzone." *La Berio* 16, no. 2 (1976).

Alizeri, Federigo
1846–47   *Guida artistica per la città di Genova.* Genoa, 1846–47.

Ancona
1981   *Lorenzo Lotto nelle Marche: Il suo tempo, il suo influsso.* Exhibition, church of the Gesù, Ancona, July 4–October 11, 1981. Catalogue edited by Paolo Dal Poggetto and Pietro Zampetti. Florence, 1981.
1982   *Ancona e le Marche nel cinquecento: Economia, società, istituzioni, cultura.* Exhibition, Palazzo Bosdari, Ancona, January 9–March 21, 1982. Ancona, 1982.
1985   *Andrea Lilli nella pittura delle Marche tra cinquecento e seicento.* Exhibition, Pinacoteca Civica Francesco Posesti, Ancona, July 14–October 13, 1985. Catalogue edited by Giovanna Bonasegale Pittei; contributions by Luciano Arcangeli et al. Rome, 1985.

Anderson, Jaynie
1997   *Judith.* Translated by Bernard Turle. Paris, 1997.

Andretta, Stefano
1994   *La venerabile superbia: Ortodossia e trasgressione nella vita di Suor Francesca Farnese (1581–1651).* Turin, 1994.

Andrews, Keith
1973   "Judith and Holofernes by Adam Elsheimer." *Apollo* 98, no. 139 (September 1973), 206–9.
1977   *Adam Elsheimer: Paintings, Drawings, Prints.* Oxford, 1977.

Anspach
1772   *Verzeichnis der Schildereyen in der Gallerie des hochgräflichen Schönbornischen Schlosses zu Pommersfelden.* 1772.

Antwerp–London
1999   *Van Dyck, 1599–1641.* Exhibition, Koninklijk Museum voor Schone Kunsten, Antwerp, May 15–August 15, 1999; Royal Academy of Arts, London, September 11–December 10, 1999. Catalogue by Christopher Brown and Hans Vlieghe, with contributions by Frans Baudouin et al. London, 1999.

Ascoli Piceno
1992   *Le arti nelle Marche al tempo di Sisto V.* Exhibition, Palazzo dei Capitani del Popolo, Ascoli Piceno. Catalogue edited by Paolo Dal Poggetto. [Cinisello Balsamo], 1992.

Askew, Pamela
1969   "The Angelic Consolation of St. Francis of Assisi in Post-Tridentine Italian Painting." *Journal of the Warburg and Courtauld Institutes* 32 (1969), 280–306.
1978   "Ferdinando Gonzaga's Patronage of the Pictorial Arts: The Villa Favorita." *Art Bulletin* 9 (June 1978), 273–95.

Atlanta
1996   *Rings: Five Passions in the Art World.* Exhibition, High Museum of Art, Atlanta, commemorating the summer Olympics. Catalogue by J. Carter Brown et al. New York, 1996.

Avenel, Denis Louis Martial, ed.
1856   *Lettres, instructions diplomatiques, etc. du Cardinal de Richelieu.* Vol. 2, *1624–1627.* Paris, 1856.

Baglione, Giovanni
1642   *Le vite de' pittori, scultori, et architetti dal pontificato di Gregorio XIII del 1572, in fino a' tempi di Papa Urbano Ottavo nel 1642.* Rome, 1642.
1935   *Le vite de' pittori, scultori, et architetti dal pontificato di Gregorio XIII del 1572, in fino a' tempi di Papa Urbano Ottavo nel 1642.* Facsimile, edited by Valerio Mariani. Rome, 1935.
1995   *Le vite de' pittori, scultori et architetti dal pontificato di Gregorio XIII del 1572 in fino a' tempi di Papa Urbano VIII nel 1642.* 3 vols. Edited by Jacob Hess and Herwarth Röttgen. Vatican City, 1995.

Bailly, Nicolas, and Fernand Engerand
1899   *Inventaire des tableaux du roy, rédigé en 1709 et 1710.* Additions and notes by Fernand Engerand. Paris, 1899.

Bal, Mieke
1996   *Double Exposures: The Subject of Cultural Analysis.* New York, 1996.

Baldinucci, Filippo
1681   *Vocabolario toscano dell'arte del disegno. . . .* Florence, 1681.
1767–74   *Notizie de' professori del disegno da Cimabue in qua, per le quali si dimostra come, e per chi le bell'arti di pittura, scultura e architettura, lasciata la rozzizza delle maniere greca e gotica, si siano in questi secoli ridotte all'antica loro perfezione.* 21 vols. Edited by Domenico Maria Manni. Florence, 1767–74.
1811–12   *Notizie de' professori del disegno da Cimabue in qua. . .* 11 vols. Milan, 1811–12.
1845–47   *Notizie de' professori del disegno da Cimabue in qua. . .* [1681–1728]. 5 vols. Edited by Ferdinando Ranalli (vols. 2–5). Florence, 1845–47.
1974–75   *Notizie dei professori del disegno da Cimabue in qua. . .* [1681–1728]. 7 vols. Edited by Ferdinando Ranalli (vols. 2–5) and Paola Barocchi (vols. 6, 7). Florence, 1974–75.

Banti, Anna
1947   *Artemisia.* Florence, 1947.
1988   *Artemisia.* Translated by Shirley D'Ardia Caracciolo. Lincoln, Nebraska, 1988.

Barcia, Angel Maria de
1911   *Catálogo de la colección de pinturas del excmo. sr. duque de Berwick y de Alba.* [Madrid], 1911.

von Barghahn, Barbara
1986   *Philip IV and the "Golden House" of the Buen Retiro: In the Tradition of Caesar.* 2 vols. New York, 1986.

Baricco, T. Pietro
1869   *Torino descritta.* 2 vols. Turin, 1869.

Barocchi, Paola, comp.
1960–62   *Trattati d'arte del cinquecento.* 3 vols. Bari, 1960–62.
1971   *Scritti d'arte del cinquecento.* Vol. 1. Milan, 1971.

Barocco napoletano
1992   *Barocco napoletano.* Edited by Gaetana Cantone. Proceedings of the conference "Napoli e il Barocco nell'Italia meridionale," held October 28–November 2, 1987, in Naples. Rome, 1992.

Barroero, Liliana
1981   "Orazio Gentileschi, 1599." *Antologia di belle arti* 19–20 (1981), 169–75.
1988   "La basilica dal cinquecento all'ottocento." In *Santa Maria Maggiore a Roma,* edited by Carlo Pietrangeli, 215–315. Florence, 1988.

Barry, James
1809   *The Works of James Barry.* London, 1809.

Barthes, Roland, et al.
1979   *Artemisia: Buren, Charlesworth, Huebler, Kounellis, Kosuth, La Barbara, Lublin, Michals, Paolini, Sonneman, Twombly, Zaza. Textes.* Texts by Roland Barthes, Eva Menzio, Lea Lublin et al. Paris, 1979.

Bartoli, Francesco

1776 *Notizia delle pitture, sculture, ed architetture che ornano le chiese e gli altri luoghi pubblici de tutte le più rinomate città dell'Italia.* 2 vols. Venice, 1776.

Barzman, Karen-Edis

2000 *The Florentine Academy and the Early Modern State: The Discipline of Disegno.* Cambridge, 2000.

Bassompierre, François de

1837 *Mémoires du maréchal de Bassompierre.* Nouvelle collection des mémoires pour servir à l'histoire de France. Paris, 1837.

Bätschmann, Oskar

1998 "Rome, a Cultural and Artistic Power." In Münster–Osnabrück 1998–99, vol. 2, 215–25.

Battisti, Eugenio

1963 "La data di morte di Artemisia Gentileschi." *Mitteilungen des Kunsthistorischen Institutes in Florenz* 10, no. 4 (February 1963), 297.

Baudi di Vesme, Alessandro

1897 "La Regia Pinacoteca di Torino." *Le gallerie nazionali italiane; notizie e documenti* 3 (1897).

1932 *L'arte negli Stati Sabaudi ai tempi di Carlo Emanuele I, di Vittorio Amedeo I e della reggenza di Cristina di Francia.* Atti della Società Piemontese di Archeologia e Belle Arti, vol. 14. Turin, 1932.

Baudouin-Matuszek, Marie-Noëlle

1992 "La succession de Marie de Medicis et l'emplacement des cabinets de peintures au Palais de Luxembourg." *Bulletin de la Société d'Histoire de Paris et de l'Île-de-France* (1990).

Bauer, Linda, and Steve Colton

2000 "Tracing in Some Works by Caravaggio." *Burlington Magazine* 142 (2000), 434–36.

Baumgart, Fritz E.

1955 *Caravaggio: Kunst und Wirklichkeit.* Berlin, 1955.

Baxandall, Michael

1988 *Painting and Experience in Fifteenth-Century Italy: A Primer in the Social History of Pictorial Style.* 2d ed. Oxford, 1988. First published 1972.

Beal, Mary

1984 *A Study of Richard Symonds: His Italian Notebooks and Their Relevance to Seventeenth-Century Painting Techniques.* Outstanding Theses from the Courtauld Institute of Art. New York, 1984.

Becker, Rotraut

1974 "Campori, Pietro." In *Dizionario biografico degli Italiani,* vol. 17, 602–4. Rome, 1974.

Belloni, Venanzio

1973 *Penne, pennelli e quadrerie: Cultura pittura genovese del seicento.* Genoa, 1973.

1988 "1605: F. Fanelli (scultore) e A. Tassi (pittore) nella chiesa di Sant'Agnese." In *Scritti e cose d'arte genovese,* 13–15. Genoa, 1988.

Bellori, Giovan Pietro

1672 *Le vite de' pittori, scultori, e architetti moderni.* Rome, 1672.

1976 *Le vite de' pittori, scultori, e architetti moderni* [1672]. Edited by Evelina Borea. Turin, 1976.

Benedetti, Laura

1999 "Reconstructing Artemisia: Twentieth-Century Images of a Woman Artist." *Comparative Literature* 51 (1999), 43–61.

Benigni, Venanzo, marchese

1924 *Compendioso ragguaglio delle cose più notabili di Fabriano* [ms. 1728]. Edited by Costantino Benigni Olivieri. Tolentino, 1924.

Bentivoglio, Guido

1807 *Memorie del Cardinal Bentivoglio.* Milan, 1807.

Bergamo

2000 *Caravaggio: La luce nella pittura lombarda.* Exhibition, Accademia Carrara, Bergamo, April 12–July 2, 2000. Catalogue edited by Claudio Strinati and Rossella Vodret. Milan, 2000.

Berlin

1975 *Katalog der ausgestellten Gemälde des 13.–18. Jahrhunderts.* Berlin: Gemäldegalerie, Staatliche Museen Preussischer Kulturbesitz, 1975.

1978 *Catalogue of Paintings, 13th–18th Century: Picture Gallery, Staatliche Museen Preussischer Kulturbesitz.* 2d ed. Translated by Linda B. Parshall. Berlin, 1978.

Bernardi, Marziano

1964 *Barocco piemontese.* Turin, 1964.

Berne Joffroy, André

1959 *Le dossier Caravage.* Paris, 1959.

Bershad, David L.

1985 "The Newly Discovered Testament and Inventories of Carlo Maratti and His Wife Francesca." *Antologia di belle arti,* no. 25–26 (1985), 65–84.

Bertolotti, Antonio

1876 "Agostino Tassi: Suoi scolari e compagni pittori in Roma." *Giornale d'erudizione artistica* 5 (1876), 183–204.

Betcherman, Lita-Rose

1970 "The York House Collection and Its Keeper." *Apollo* 92 (1970), 250–59.

Bevilacqua, Mario

1993 "L'organizzazione dei cantieri pittorici sistini: Note sul rapporto tra botteghe e committenza." In Rome 1993, 35–46.

Bilbao

1991 *La restauración de 'Lot y sus hijas' de Orazio Gentileschi.* Bilbao, 1991.

Bionda, Claire-Lise

1992 "Artemisia Gentileschi." *L'Oeil,* no. 442 (June 1992), 20–29.

Birmingham

1960 *Birmingham City Museum and Art Gallery: Catalogue of Paintings.* Descriptions by Mary Woodall. Birmingham, 1960.

Bissell, R. Ward

1966 "The Baroque Painter Orazio Gentileschi, His Career in Italy." 2 vols. Ph.D. dissertation, University of Michigan, Ann Arbor, 1966.

1967 "Orazio Gentileschi's *Young Woman with a Violin.*" *Bulletin of the Detroit Institute of Arts* 46, no. 4 (1967), 71–77.

1968 "Artemisia Gentileschi: A New Documented Chronology." *Art Bulletin* 50 (1968), 153–68.

1969 "Orazio Gentileschi and the Theme of 'Lot and His Daughters.'" *Bulletin of the National Gallery of Canada* 14 (1969), 16–32.

1971 "Orazio Gentileschi: Baroque without Rhetoric." *Art Quarterly* 34 (1971), 274–300.

1974 "Concerning the Date of Caravaggio's *Amore Vincitore.*" In *Hortus Imaginum: Essays in Western Art,* edited by R. Enggass and M. Stokstad, 113–23. Lawrence, Kansas, 1974.

1981 *Orazio Gentileschi and the Poetic Tradition in Caravaggesque Painting.* University Park, Pennsylvania, 1981.

1999 *Artemisia Gentileschi and the Authority of Art.* University Park, Pennsylvania, 1999.

Bissell, R. Ward, and Claudio Strinati

2001 *Orazio Gentileschi Madonna and Child—*

Madonna col bambino, Galleria M. Datrino, Castello di Torre Canavese. Turin, 2001.

Blancher-Le Bourhis, Magdaleine

1939 "Les peintures de Jean Monier au Luxembourg." *Bulletin de la Société d'Histoire de l'Art Français,* 1939 (1940), 204–15.

Blunt, Anthony

1970 *Art and Architecture in France, 1500–1700.* 2d ed. Harmondsworth and Baltimore, 1970. First published 1957.

Bober, Phyllis Pray, and Ruth Rubinstein

1986 *Renaissance Artists and Antique Sculpture: A Handbook of Sources.* London, 1986.

1991 *Renaissance Artists and Antique Sculpture: A Handbook of Sources.* London, 1991.

Boccardo, Piero

2000 "Un avveduto collezionista di pittura del seicento: Pietro Maria Gentile. Un inventario, un Reni inedito, e alcune precisazioni su altre opere e sull'esito di una quadreria genovese." In *Studi di storia dell'arte in onore di Denis Mahon,* edited by Maria Grazia Bernardini, Silvia Danesi Squarzina, and Claudio Strinati, 205–13. Milan, 2000.

Böhmová-Hájková, Hedvika

1956 "Restaurace obrazu 'Zuzana a starci' od A. Gentileschi." *Casopis Moravského musea* 41 (1956), 307–8. Translated into German as "Die Restaurierung des Bildes 'Susanna und die beiden Alten,'" 309–10.

Bold, John

2000 *Greenwich: An Architectural History of the Royal Hospital for Seamen and the Queen's House.* With contributions by Peter Guillery et al. New Haven, 2000.

Boll, W.

1928 "Zur Geschichte der Kunstbestrebungen des Kurfürsten von Mainz, Lothar Franz von Schönborn." *Neues Archiv für die Geschichte der Stadt Heidelberg und Kurprfalz* 13 (1928), 235–36.

Bologna, Ferdinando

1953 "Altre prove sul viaggio romano del Tanzio." *Paragone* 4, no. 45 (1953), 39–45.

1958 *Francesco Solimena.* Naples, 1958.

1992 *L'incredulità del Caravaggio e l'esperienza delle 'cose naturali.'* Turin, 1992.

Bologna

1968 *Il Guercino (Giovanni Francesco Barbieri, 1591–1666): Catalogo critico dei dipinti.* Exhibition, Palazzo dell'Archiginnasio, Bologna, September 1–November 18, 1968. Catalogue edited by Denis Mahon, with contributions by Cesare Gnudi. 2 vols. Bologna, 1968.

1975 *Mostra di Federico Barocci (Urbino 1535–1612).* Exhibition, Museo Civico, Bologna, September 14–November 16, 1975. Catalogue edited by Andrea Emiliani. Bologna, 1975.

Bologna and other cities

1991–92 *Giovanni Francesco Barbieri: Il Guercino, 1591–1666.* Exhibition, Museo Civico Archeologico, Bologna, and Pinacoteca Civica e Chiesa del Rosario, Cento, September 6–November 10, 1991; Schirn Kunsthalle, Frankfurt am Main, December 2, 1991–February 9, 1992; National Gallery of Art, Washington, D.C., March 15–May 17, 1992. Catalogue by Denis Mahon, with contributions by Andrea Emiliani, Diane De Grazia, and Sybille Ebert-Schifferer. Bologna,

1991. English ed.: *Guercino: Master Painter of the Baroque*. Washington, D.C., 1992.

Bologna–Fort Worth

1993   *Ludovico Carracci*. Exhibition, Museo Civico Archeologico, Pinacoteca Nazionale, Bologna; Kimbell Art Museum, Fort Worth. Catalogue edited by Andrea Emiliani, with contributions by Maria Silvia Campanini et al. Bologna, 1993.

Bologna–Los Angeles–Fort Worth

1988–89   *Guido Reni, 1575–1642*. Exhibition, Pinacoteca Nazionale e Accademia di Belle Arti, Museo Civico Archeologico, Bologna, September 5–November 10, Los Angeles County Museum of Art, December 11, 1988–February 14, 1989; Kimbell Art Museum, Fort Worth, March 10–May 10, 1989. Catalogue. Bologna, 1988.

Bologna–Washington–New York

1986–87   *The Age of Correggio and the Carracci: Emilian Painting of the Sixteenth and Seventeenth Centuries*. Exhibition, Pinacoteca Nazionale de Bologna, September 10–November 10, 1986; National Gallery of Art, Washington, D.C., December 19, 1986–February 16, 1987; The Metropolitan Museum of Art, New York, March 26–May 24, 1987. Catalogue translated by Robert Erich Wolf et al. Washington, D.C., 1986. Italian ed.: *Nell'età di Correggio e dei Carracci: Pittura in Emilia dei Secoli XVI e XVII*. Bologna, 1986.

Bordeaux

1959   *La découverte de la lumière des Primitifs aux Impressionnistes: Catalogue*. Exhibition, Musée des Beaux-Arts, Bordeaux, May 20–July 31, 1959. Catalogue by Gilberte Martin-Méry. Bordeaux, 1959.

Borea, Evelina

1966   *Francesco Mochi*. I maestri dalla scultura, no. 43. Milan, 1966.

1974   "Caravaggio e la Spagna: Osservazioni su una mostra a Siviglia." *Bollettino d'arte* 59 (1974), 43–52.

1980   "Date per il Baglione." *Storia dell'arte* 38–40 (1980), 315–18.

Borella, Glauco, and Patrizia Giusti Maccari

1993   *Il Palazzo Mansi di Lucca*. Lucca, 1993.

Borroni Salvadori, Fabia

1974   "Le esposizioni d'arte a Firenze dal 1674 al 1767." *Mitteilungen des Kunsthistorischen Institutes in Florenz* 18, no. 1 (1974), 1–166.

Borsi, Franco, Giuliano Briganti, and Marcello del Piazzo

1962   *Il Palazzo del Quirinale*. Rome, 1962.

1973   *Il Palazzo del Quirinale*. Rome, 1973.

Bösel, Richard

1985   *Jesuitenarchitektur in Italien (1540–1773)*. Vol. 2. Vienna, 1985.

Bosio, Antonio

1650   *Roma sotterranea; opera postvma di Antonio Bosio, nella quale si tratta de' sacri cimiterii di Roma; del sito, forma, & vso antico di essi*. Edited by Giovanni Severani. Rome, 1650.

Boston

1999   *Saints and Sinners: Caravaggio and the Baroque Image*. Exhibition, McMullen Museum of Art, Boston College, February 1–May 24, 1999. Catalogue edited by Franco Mormando. Chestnut Hill, Massachusetts, 1999.

Bottari, Giovanni Gaetano, and Stefano Ticozzi

1822–25   *Raccolta di lettere sulla pittura, scultura ed architettura scritte da' più celebri personaggi dei secoli XV, XVI, e XVII*. 8 vols. Milan, 1822–25. First published Rome, 1754–68.

Bousquet, Jacques

1978   "Valentin et ses compagnons: Réflexions sur les caravagesques français à partir des archives paroissiales romaines." *Gazette des Beaux-Arts*, ser. 6, 120 (1978), 101–14.

Braghirolli, Willelmo

1874   *Notizie e documenti inediti intorno a Pietro Vannucci detto Il Perugino*. Perugia, 1874. Extracted from *Giornale di erudizione artistica*.

Brandi, C.

1930   "Mei, Bernardino." In *Allgemeines Lexikon der bildenden Künstler von der Antike bis zur Gegenwart*, edited by Ulrich Thieme and Felix Becker, vol. 24, 339. Leipzig, 1930.

Brejon de Lavergnée, Arnauld

1987   *L'inventaire Le Brun de 1683: La collection des tableaux de Louis XIV*. Notes et documents des musées de France, 17. Paris, 1987.

Brejon de Lavergnée, Arnauld, and Nathalie Volle

1988   *Musées de France: Répertoire des peintures italiennes du XVIIᵉ siècle*. Paris, 1988.

Brejon de Lavergnée, Barbara

1979   "Une *Sainte Madeleine pénitente* de Claude Mellan." *Revue du Louvre* 5/6 (1979), 407–10.

Brigstocke, Hugh

1982   *William Buchanan and the Nineteenth-Century Art Trade: 100 Letters to His Agents in London and Italy*. London, 1982.

2001   *Oxford Companion to Western Art*. London, 2001.

Brown, Jonathan

1986   *Velázquez, Painter and Courtier*. New Haven, 1986.

Brown, Jonathan, and John Huxtable Elliott

1980   *A Palace for a King: The Buen Retiro and the Court of Phillip IV*. New Haven, 1980.

Brown, Jonathan, and Richard Kagan

1987   "The Duke of Alcalá: His Collection and Its Evolution." *Art Bulletin* 69 (1987), 231–55.

Brummer, Hans Henrik

1970   *The Statue Court in the Vatican Belvedere*. Stockholm Studies in History of Art, no. 20. Stockholm, 1970.

Brunetti, Estella

1956   "Situazione di Viviano Codazzi." *Paragone* 7, no. 79 (1956), 48–69.

Brusco, Giacomo

1781   *Description des beautés de Gènes et de ses environs*. Genoa, 1781.

Brussels–Rome

1995   *Fiamminghi a Roma, 1508–1608: Artistes des Pays-Bas et de la principauté de Liège à Rome de la Renaissance*. Exhibition, Palais des Beaux-Arts, Brussels, February 24–May 21, 1995; Palazzo delle Esposizioni, Rome, June 16–September 10, 1995. Catalogue. Brussels, 1995.

Buchanan, William

1824   *Memoirs of Painting with a Chronological History of the Importation of Pictures by the Great Masters into England since the French Revolution*. 2 vols. London, 1824.

Bulwer, John

1644   *Chirologia; or, The Naturall Language of the Hand . . . Whereunto Is Added Chironomia; or, The Art of Manuall Rhetoricke. . . .* London, 1644.

Burckhardt, Jacob

1855   *Der Cicerone: Eine Anleitung zum Genuss der Kunstwerke italiens*. Basel, 1855.

Burghley House

1797   *A History or Description, General and Circumstantial, of Burghley House, the Seat of the Right Honourable and Earl of Exeter*. Attributed to John Horn. Shrewsbury: J. & W. Eddowes, 1797.

Burke, Marcus B.

1984   "Private Collections of Italian Art in Seventeenth-Century Spain." 3 vols. Ph.D. dissertation, New York University, 1984.

Burke, Marcus B., and Peter Cherry

1997   *Collections of Paintings in Madrid, 1601–1755*. Edited by Maria L. Gilbert. 2 vols. Documents for the History of Collecting, Spanish Inventories, 1. Los Angeles, 1997.

Buscaroli, Rezio

1935   *La pittura di paesaggio in Italia*. Bologna, 1935.

Cadogan, Jean, ed.

1991   *Wadsworth Atheneum Paintings*. Vol. 2, *Italy and Spain: Fourteenth through Nineteenth Centuries*. Hartford, 1991.

Calendar of State Papers, Domestic

1859   *Calendar of State Papers, Domestic Series, of the Reign of Charles I, 1628–1629*. Edited by John Bruce. London, 1859.

1860   *Calendar of State Papers, Domestic Series, of the Reign of Charles I, 1629–1631*. Edited by John Bruce. London, 1860.

Calvesi, Maurizio

1971   "Caravaggio o la ricerca della salvazione." *Storia dell'arte* 9/10 (1971), 93–141.

1990   *Le realtà di Caravaggio*. Turin, 1990.

1996   "A gara con la Roma imperiale." In *I Borghese*, vol. 1, *Storia di una famiglia*, 13–42. Exhibition, Fattoria Medicea, Monsummano Terme, 1996.

1999   "La galleria dei Carracci." In *Arte a Roma: Pittura, scultura, architettura, nella storia dei Giubilei*, edited by Maurizio Calvesi, 126–31. Rome, 1999.

Calvi, Felice

1808   *Notizie della vita e delle opere del Cavaliere Giovan Francesco Barbieri detto Il Guercino dal Cento, celebre pittore*. Bologna, 1808.

1884   *Famiglie notabili milanesi. . . .* Milan, 1884.

Calvi, Giulia, ed.

1992   *Barocco al femminile*. Rome, 1992.

Camboulives, Catherine

1990   "La *Judith* de Pietro della Vecchia du Musée de Grenoble." *Gazette des Beaux-Arts*, ser. 6, 116 (1990), 213–22.

Cammell, Charles Richard

1939   *The Great Duke of Buckingham*. London, 1939.

Campori, Giuseppe

1870   *Raccolta di cataloghi ed inventarii inediti di quadri, statue, disegni, bronzi, dorerie, smalti, medaglie, avorii, ecc., dal secolo XV al secolo XIX*. Modena, 1870.

Cannatà, Roberto, and Vicini, Maria Lucrezia

1992   *La Galleria di Palazzo Spada: Genesi e storia di una collezione*. Rome, [1992].

Cannon, JoAnn

1994   "*Artemisia* and the Life Story of the Exceptional Woman." *Forum Italicum* 28 (1994), 322–41.

Cantelli, Giuseppe

1980   "Mitologia sacra e profana e le sue eroine nella pittura fiorentina della prima meta del seicento." *Paradigma*, no. 3 (1980), 147–69.

Cantone, Gaetana

1984   *Napoli barocca e Cosimo Fanzago*. Naples, 1984.

Capozzi, Frank

1975 "The Evolution and Transformation of the Judith and Holofernes Theme in Italian Drama and Art before 1627." Ph.D. dissertation, University of Wisconsin, Madison, 1975.

Cappelletti, Francesca

1998 "Una nota di beni e qualche aggiunta alla storia della collezione Aldobrandini." *Storia dell'arte* 93–94 (1998), 341–47.

Cappelletti, Francesca, and Laura Testa

1994 *Il trattenimento di Virtuosi: Le collezioni secentesche di quadri nei Palazzi Mattei di Roma.* Rome, 1994.

Carità, Roberto

1946 "La data di nascita di Orazio Gentileschi." *Arti figurative* 2, no. 1–2 (1946), 81–82.

Carletti, Giuseppe

1795 *Memorie istorico-critiche della chiesa e monastero di S. Silvestro in Capite di Roma.* Rome, 1795.

Carloni, Livia

1997 "Il giovane Guerrieri tra Sassoferrato, Fabriano e Roma. Alcuni inediti." In Fossombrone 1997, 19–28.

Carpenter, William H.

1844 *Pictorial Notices, Consisting of a Memoir of Sir Anthony Van Dyck, with a Descriptive Catalogue of the Etchings Executed by Him, and a Variety of Interesting Particulars Relating to Other Artists Patronized by Charles I.* London, 1844.

Castagnari, Giancarlo, ed.

1986 *La città della carta: Ambiente, società, cultura nella storia di Fabriano.* 2d ed. Fabriano, 1986.

Castrichini, Monica, Luca Castrichini et al.

1999 *Arte in Umbria, Todi, i 'rioni' S. Prassede e S. Silvestro.* Perugia, 1999.

Catello, Angela

1991 "De Rosa, Diana (detta Dianella o Annella)." In *Dizionario biografico degli Italiani,* vol. 39, 163–65. Rome, 1991.

Causa, Raffaello

1972 "La pittura del seicento a Napoli dal Naturalismo al Barocco." In *Storia di Napoli,* vol. 5, part 2, *Cava de' Tirreni.* Naples, 1972.

Causa, Stefano

1993 "Risarcimento di Onofrio Palumbo." *Paragone* 44, n.s. 37–38 (January–March 1993), 21–40.

2000 *Battistello Caracciolo: L'opera completa.* Naples, 2000.

Cavaliere, Barbara

1976 "Artemisia Gentileschi: Her Life in Art." *Womanart* 1 (fall 1976), 18–23.

Cavazzini, Patrizia

1993 "New Documents for Cardinal Alessandro Peretti-Montalto's Frescoes at Bagnaia." *Burlington Magazine* 135 (May 1993), 316–27.

1997 "Agostino Tassi and the Organization of His Workshop: Filippo Franchini, Angelo Caroselli, Claude Lorrain and the Others." *Storia dell'arte,* no. 91 (1997), 400–426.

1998 *Palazzo Lancellotti ai Coronari: Cantiere di Agostino Tassi.* Rome, 1998.

2000 "Agostino Tassi Reassessed: A Newly Discovered Album of Drawings." *Paragone* 32 (2000), 3–31.

Celio, Gaspare

1638 *Memoria delli nomi dell'artefici delle pitture che sone in alcune chiese, facciate, e palazzi di Roma.* Naples, 1638.

1967 *Memoria delli nomi dell'artefici delle pitture che sone in alcune chiese, facciate, e palazzi di Roma.*

Facsimile, edited by Emma Zocca. Milan, 1967.

Chambéry

1995 *Du Manierisme au Baroque: Art d'élite et art populaire.* Exhibition, Musée des Beaux-Arts, Chambéry, March 3–May 28, 1995. Catalogue. Chambéry, 1995.

Chantilly

1979–80 *La Madone de Lorette.* Exhibition, Musée Condé, Chantilly, October 16, 1979–January 15, 1980. Catalogue edited by Sylvie Béguin. Paris, 1979.

Chappell, Miles L., and Chandler W. Kirwin

1974 "A Petrine Triumph: The Decoration of the Navi Piccole in San Pietro under Clement VIII." *Storia dell'arte* 21 (1974), 119–70.

Chartier, Roger

1989 "The Practical Impact of Writing." In *A History of Private Life,* vol. 3, *Passions of the Renaissance,* edited by Roger Chartier, 111–60. Cambridge, Massachusetts, 1989.

Chettle, George H.

1937 *The Queen's House, Greenwich, Being the Fourteenth Monograph of the London Survey Committee.* Greenwich, 1937.

Chiappini di Sorio, Ileana

1983 "Cristoforo Roncalli detto Il Pomarancio." In Cinotti and Dell'Acqua 1983, 3–199.

Chiarini, Marco

1962 "Gli inizi del Gentileschi." *Arte figurativa* 55 (1962).

Christiansen, Keith

1988 "Technical Report on *The Cardsharps.*" *Burlington Magazine* 130 (1988), 26–27.

1994 "Orazio Gentileschi and S. Giovanni dei Fiorentini." *Burlington Magazine* 136 (1994), 621.

1999 "Caravaggio's 'Holy Family with the Infant Saint John the Baptist.'" *Paragone* 50, no. 26 (1999), 1–11.

2001 "London and Rome: The Genius of Rome." *Burlington Magazine* 143 (2001), 383–86.

Christie, Nicola

1997 "Technical Examination of Gentileschi's *The Finding of Moses* (ex castle Howard)." *Apollo* 145, no. 424 (1997), 36–37.

Ciardi, Roberto Paolo, Maria Clelia Galassi, Pierluigi Carofano

1989 *Aurelio Lomi, maniera e innovazione.* Pisa, 1989.

Ciletti, Elena

1984 "'Ma questa è la donna terribile!': Artemisia Gentileschi and Judith." Paper presented at the College Art Association meeting in Toronto, February 1984.

Ciliento, Bruno, and Franco Boggero

1983 "Un ciclo inedito di Giovanni Andrea Ansaldo a Genova-Sampierdarena." *Storia dell'arte* 49 (1983), 187–90.

Cinotti, Mia, ed.

1975 *Novità sul Caravaggio: Saggi e contributi. Atti del Convegno internazionale di studi caravaggeschi di Bergamo.* Milan, 1975.

Cinotti, Mia, and Gian Alberto Dell'Acqua

1983 *Michelangelo Merisi detto il Caravaggio: Tutte le opere.* I pittori bergamaschi dal XIII al XIX secolo: Il seicento, vol. 1. Bergamo, 1983.

Cleveland

1971 *Caravaggio and His Followers.* Exhibition, Cleveland Museum of Art, 1971. Catalogue edited by Richard Spear. Cleveland, 1971.

Cleveland–Fort Worth–Naples

1984–85 *Bernardo Cavallino of Naples, 1616–1656.*

Exhibition, Cleveland Museum of Art, November 14–December 30, 1984; Kimbell Art Museum, Fort Worth, January 26–March 24, 1985; Museo Pignatelli Cortes, Naples, April 26–June 26, 1985. Catalogue by Ann T. Lurie and Ann Percy; essays by Nicola Spinosa and Giuseppe Galasso. Cleveland, 1984.

Cochin, Charles-Nicolas

1773 *Voyage d'Italie.* Vol. 1. Paris, 1773.

Cohen, Elizabeth Storr

1991 "No Longer Virgins: Self-Presentation by Young Women in Late Renaissance Rome." In *Refiguring Woman: Perspectives on Gender and the Italian Renaissance,* edited by Marilyn Migiel and Juliana Schiesari, 169–91. Ithaca, 1991.

1992 "Honor and Gender in the Streets of Early Modern Rome." *Journal of Interdisciplinary History* 22, no. 4 (1992), 597–625.

1992a "Court Testimony from the Past: Self and Culture in the Making of Text." In *Essays on Life Writing: From Genre to Critical Practice,* edited by Marlene Kadar. Toronto, 1992.

2000 "The Trials of Artemisia Gentileschi: A Rape as History." *Sixteenth Century Journal* 31, no. 1 (2000), 47–75.

Cohen, Elizabeth Storr, and Thomas V. Cohen

1989 "Camilla the Go-Between: The Politics of Gender in a Roman Household." *Continuity and Change* 4 (1989), 53–77.

Cohen, Thomas V., and Elizabeth Storr Cohen

1993 *Words and Deeds in Renaissance Rome: Trials before the Papal Magistrates.* Toronto, 1993.

Coliva, Anna

1998 "Casa Borghese: La committenza artistica del Cardinal Scipione." In Rome 1998, 391–420.

2000 "Scipione Borghese collezionista." In *Galleria Borghese,* by Paolo Moreno and Chiara Stefani, 16–29. Milan, 2000.

Colonna, F.

1895 "Inventario dei quadri di casa Colonna fatta da Luca Giordano." *Napoli nobilissima* 4, no. 2 (1895), 31, no. 60.

Compin, Isabelle, and Anne Roquebert

1986 *Catalogue sommaire illustré des peintures du Musée du Louvre et du Musée d'Orsay.* Vol. 4, *École française: L–Z.* Paris, 1986.

Confraternite nell'Italia Centrale

1993 *Le Confraternite nell'Italia Centrale tra antropologia musicale e storia.* Atti del Convegno, Viterbo, 1989. Viterbo, 1993.

Coniglio, Giuseppe

1967 *I viceré spagnoli di Napoli.* Naples, 1967.

Connoly, T. H.

1983 "The Cult and Iconography of St. Cecilia before Raphael." In *La Santa Cecilia di Raffaello,* edited by Andrea Emiliani, 121–39. Bologna, 1983.

Constable, W. G.

1929–30 "Dipinti di raccolte inglesi alla mostra d'arte italiana a Londra." *Dedalo* 10 (1929–30), 723–67.

Contini, Roberto

1989 In Gregori and Schleier 1989.

1996 "Giovan Battista Pozzo, iperbole del Baglione." *Nuovi studi* 1 (1996), 95–102.

Conversano

2000 *Paolo Finoglio e il suo tempo: Un pittore napoletano alla corte degli Acquaviva.* Exhibition, Castello Acquaviva d'Aragona, Conversano, and other locations, April 18–September 30, 2000.

Catalogue edited by Silvia Cassani and Maria Sapio. Naples, 2000.

Cornini, Guido, Annamaria De Strobel, and Maria Serlupi Crescenzi

1992   "Il palazzo di Gregorio XIII." In *Il Palazzo Apostolico Vaticano*, edited by Carlo Pietrangeli, 151–68. Florence, 1992.

Corti, Gino

1989   "Il 'Registro de' mandati' dell'ambasciatore granducale Piero Guicciardini e la committenza artistica fiorentina a Roma nel secondo decennio del seicento." *Paragone* 40, no. 473 (1989), 108–46.

Costa, Patrizia

2000   "Artemisia Gentileschi in Venice." *Source* 19, no. 3 (2000), 28–36.

Costanzi, Costanza

1999   *Ancona: Pinacoteca Civica "F. Podesti." Galleria d'arte moderna*. Bologna, 1999.

Couché, Jacques

1808   *Galerie du Palais Royal, gravée d'après les tableaux des differentes écoles qui la composent; avec un abrégé de la vie des peintres et une description historique de chaque tableau*. 3 vols. Paris, 1808.

Craveri, Giovanni Gaspare

1753   *Guida de' forestieri per la real città di Torino: In cui si dà notizia delle cose più notabili di questa città. . . .* Turin, 1753.

Crelly, William R.

1962   *The Painting of Simon Vouet*. New Haven, 1962.

Crinò, Anna Maria

1954   "Due lettere autografe inedite di Orazio e di Artemisia Gentileschi De Lomi." *Rivista d'arte* 29 (1954), 203–6.

1960   "More Letters from Orazio and Artemisia Gentileschi." *Burlington Magazine* 102 (1960), 264–65.

1967   "The Date of Orazio Gentileschi's Arrival in London." *Burlington Magazine* 109 (1967), 533.

Crinò, Anna Maria, and Benedict Nicolson

1961   "Further Documents Relating to Orazio Gentileschi." *Burlington Magazine* 103 (1961), 144–45.

Croft-Murray, Edward

1947   "The Landscape Background in Rubens's *St. George and the Dragon*." *Burlington Magazine* 89 (1947), 89–93.

1962   *Decorative Painting in England, 1537–1837*. Vol. 1, *Early Tudor to Sir James Thornhill*. London, 1962.

Cropper, Elizabeth

1984   *The Ideal of Painting: Pietro Testa's Düsseldorf Notebook*. Princeton, 1984.

1992   "Artemisia Gentileschi, la 'pittora.'" In Calvi 1992, 191–218.

1993   "New Documents for Artemisia Gentileschi's Life in Florence." *Burlington Magazine* 134 (1993), 760–61.

1996   "Michelangelo Cerquozzi's Self-Portrait: The Real Studio and the Suffering Model." In *Ars naturam adivans: Festschrift für Matthias Winner*, edited by Victoria von Flemming and Sebastian Schütze, 401–12. Mainz, 1996.

1996a   "Ritorno alla crocevia." In *Poussin et Rome: Actes du colloque à l'Académie de France à Rome et à la Bibliotheca Hertziana, November 16–18, 1994*, edited by O. Bonfait et al., 257–68. Paris, 1996.

1998   "La réforme de l'art et la deuxième renaissance de Rome des Carrache au Bernin." In *L'art italien de la Renaissance à 1905*, edited by P. Morel, 89–293. Paris, 1998.

Crowe, Joseph Archer, and Giovanni Battista Cavalcaselle

1881   *The Life and Times of Titian, with Some Account of His Family*. 2d ed. 2 vols. London, 1881.

Cummings, Frederick

1974   "The Meaning of Caravaggio's 'Conversion of the Magdalen.'" *Burlington Magazine* 116 (1974), 572–78.

D'Ambrosio, Angelo

1973   *Il Duomo di Pozzuoli: Storia e documenti inediti*. Pozzuoli, 1973.

Da Morrona, Alessandro

1787–93   *Pisa illustrata nelle arti del disegno*. 3 vols. Pisa, 1787–93.

1812   *Pisa illustrata nelle arti del disegno*. 2d ed. 3 vols. Livorno, 1812.

Davies, Randall

1907   "An Inventory of the Duke of Buckingham's Pictures, etc., at York House in 1635." *Burlington Magazine* 10 (1907), 376–82.

D'Azeglio, Roberto

1819   *La Reale Galleria di Torino*. Turin, 1819.

1836–46   *La Reale Galleria di Torino illustrata*. 4 vols. Turin, 1836–46.

De Angelis, Pietro

1950   *L'Arciconfraternita ospitaliera di Santo Spirito in Sassia*. Rome, 1950.

De Caro, G.

1967   "Bevilacqua, B." In *Dizionario biografico degli Italiani*, vol. 9, 786–88. Rome, 1967.

De Dominici, Bernardo

1742–44   *Vite de' pittori, scultori e architetti napoletani. Non mai date alla luce da autore alcuno*. 3 vols. Naples, 1742–44.

1840–46   *Vite de' pittori, scultori ed architetti napoletani*. 4 vols. Naples, 1840–46.

1979   *Vite dei pittori, scultori ed architetti napoletani*. Facsimile ed. 3 vols. in 2. Bologna, 1979. First published Naples, 1742–43.

De Grazia, Diane

1984   *Le stampe dei Carracci con i disegni, le incisioni, le copie e i dipinti connessi: Catalogo critico*. Edited and translated by Antonio Boschetto. Bologna, 1984.

De Grazia, Diane, and Eric Garberson

1996   *Italian Paintings of the Seventeenth and Eighteenth Centuries. The Collections of the National Gallery: Systematic Catalogue*. Washington, D.C., 1996.

De Grazia, Diane, and Erich Schleier

1994   "St Cecilia and an Angel: 'The Heads by Gentileschi, the Rest by Lanfranco.'" *Burlington Magazine* 136 (1994), 73–78.

Del Bravo, Carlo

1967   "Su Cristofano Allori." *Paragone* 18, no. 205 (1967), 68–83.

Dell'Acqua, Gian Alberto, and Mia Cinotti

1971   *Il Caravaggio e le sue grandi opere da San Luigi dei Francesi*, Milan, 1971.

Della Valle, Federico

1627   *Iudit*. Milan, 1627.

De Marchi, Giulia

1987   *Mostre di quadri a S. Salvatore in Lauro (1682–1725): Stime di collezioni romane*. Miscellanea della Società Romana di Storia Patria, no. 27. Rome, 1987.

Dempsey, Charles

1980   "Some Observations on the Education of Artists in Florence and Bologna during the Later Sixteenth Century." *Art Bulletin* 62 (1980), 552–89.

1993   "Idealism and Naturalism in Rome around 1600." In *Il classicismo (Atti del Colloquio Cesare Gnudi)*, edited by Elena De Luca, 233–43. Bologna, 1993.

2000   "Nicolas Poussin between Italy and France: Poussin's *Death of Germanicus*." In *L'Europa e l'arte italiana: Per i cento anni dalla fondazione del Kunsthistorisches Institut in Florenz*, edited by Max Seidel, 320–25. Venice, 2000.

De Rinaldis, Aldo

1929   *Neopolitan Painting of the seicento*. Florence, 1929.

1936   *La Galleria Nazionale d'Arte Antica in Roma*. 2d ed. Rome, 1936.

1976   *Neopolitan Painting of the seicento*. Reprint ed. New York: Hacker Art Books, 1976.

De Rossi, Onorato

1781   *Nuova guida per la città di Torino*. Turin, 1781.

Detroit

1965   *Art in Italy: 1600–1700*. Exhibition, Detroit Institute of Arts, April 6–May 9, 1965. Catalogue entries by Robert Engass et al. Detroit, 1965.

De Witt, Antony

1939   "Ein Werk aus dem Caravaggio-Kreis." *Pantheon* 23 (1939), 51–53.

Di Fabio, Clario

1988   "Gli affreschi della villa Gentile-Bickley di Cornigliano: Contributio al catalogo di Andrea Ansaldo." *Bollettino dei Musei Civici Genovesi* 10, no. 28–30 (1988), 85–97.

Dijon

1982–83   *La peinture dans la peinture*. Exhibition, Musée des Beaux-Arts de Dijon, December 18, 1982–February 28, 1983. Catalogue by Pierre Georgel and Anne-Marie Lecoq. [Dijon], 1983.

Dijon–Le Mans

1998–99   *Éloge de la clarté: Un courant artistique au temps de Mazarin, 1640–1660*. Exhibition, Musée Magnin, Dijon, June 8–September 27, 1998; Musée de Tessé, Le Mans, October 29, 1998–January 31, 1999. Catalogue by Alain Mérot, Emmanuel Starcky, and Françoise Chaserant. Paris, 1998.

Di Monte, Michele

2000   "Gilio, Giovanni Andrea." In *Dizionario biografico degli Italiani*, vol. 54, 751–54. Rome, 2000.

Dirani, Maria Teresa

1982   "Il *Ratto di Elena* di Guido Reni e la *Morte di Didone* del Guercino nella corrispondenza del Cardinale Bernardino Spada." *Ricerche di storia dell'arte* 16 (1982), 83–94.

Donnini, Giampiero

1981   *Guida alla Cattedrale di Fabriano*. Urbino, 1981.

D'Onofrio, Cesare

1963   *La Villa Aldobrandini di Frascati*. Rome, 1963.

Dorati da Empoli, Maria Cristina

2001   *Una guida artistica di Roma in un manoscritto secentesco anonimo*. Rome, 2001.

Drost, Willi

1933   *Adam Elsheimer und sein Kreis*. Potsdam, 1933.

Dublin

1992   *Caravaggio and His Followers in the National Gallery of Ireland*. Exhibition, National Gallery of Ireland, Dublin, February 19–March 24, 1992. Catalogue by Sergio Benedetti, with an essay by Colin Wiggins. Dublin, 1992.

Dubois de Saint Gelais, Louis François

1737   *Description des tableaux du Palais Royal, avec la vie des peintres à la tête de leurs ouvrages*. 2d ed. Paris, 1737.

Düsseldorf–Darmstadt

1995–96   *Die Galerie der starken Frauen: Die Heldin in der französischen und italienischen Kunst des 17. Jahrhunderts.* Exhibition, Kunstmuseum Düsseldorf, September 10–November 12, 1995; Hessisches Landesmuseum Darmstadt, December 14, 1995–February 26, 1996. Catalogue by Bettina Baumgärtel, Silvia Neysters et al. Munich, 1995.

Edinburgh

1994   *Raphael: The Pursuit of Perfection.* Exhibition, National Galleries of Scotland, Edinburgh, May 5–July 10, 1994. Catalogue essays by Timothy Clifford, John Dick, and Aidan Weston-Lewis. Edinburgh, 1994.

Eigenberger, Robert

1927   *Die Gemäldegalerie der Akademie der Bildenden Künste in Wien.* 2 vols. Vienna, 1927.

Emiliani, Andrea

1958a   *Giovan Francesco Guerrieri da Fossombrone.* Collana di studi archeologici ed artistici marchigiani, vol. 7. Urbino, 1958.

1958b   "Orazio Gentileschi: Nuove proposte per il viaggio marchigiano." *Paragone* 103 (1958), 38–57.

1991   *Giovanni Francesco Guerrieri da Fossombrone.* Fano, 1991.

Engerth, Eduard, Ritter von

1881   *Gemälde: Beschreibendes Verzeichniss; Kunsthistorische Sammlungen.* Vol. 1, *Italienische, spanische und französische Schülen.* Vienna, 1881.

1884   *Gemälde: Beschreibendes Verzeichniss.* Vol. 1, *Italienische, spanische und französische Schülen.* Kunsthistorische Sammlungen des Allerhöchsten Kaiserhauses. 2d ed. Vienna, 1884.

Evelyn, John

1873   In *Voyage de Lister à Paris en MDCXCVIII.* Paris, 1873.

Fabriano

1982   *Aspetti e problemi del monachesimo nelle Marche: Atti del Convegno di studi tenuto a Fabriano, Monastero S. Silvestro Abate, 4–7 giugno 1981.* 2 vols. Fabriano, 1982.

Fagiolo, Marcello, and Maria Luisa Madonna, eds.

1992   *Sisto V.* Vol. 1, *Roma e il Lazio.* Corso Internazionale di Alta Cultura, VI, Roma, 1989. Rome, 1992.

Fagiolo dell'Arco, Maurizio, and Maurizio Marini

1970   "Rassegna degli studi caravaggeschi." *L'arte* 11–12 (1970), 117–28.

Fairfax, Brian, ed.

1758   *A Catalogue of the Curious Collection of Pictures of George Villiers, Duke of Buckingham, in Which Is Included the Valuable Collection of Sir Peter Paul Rubens; with the Life of George Villiers, Duke of Buckingham, the Celebrated Poet . . . [1649].* London, 1758.

Faldi, Italo

1956   *La quadreria della Cassa Depositi e Prestiti.* Rome, 1956.

Fanti, Vincenzio

1767   *Descrizzione completa di tutto ciò che ritrovasi nella galleria di pittura e scultura di sua altezza Giuseppe Wenceslao del s.r.i. principe regnante della casa di Lichtenstein. . . .* Vienna, 1767.

Faranda, Franco

1986   *Ludovico Cardi, detto Il Cigoli.* Rome, 1986.

Farina, R. E.

1976   "Artemisia Gentileschi: Italian Artist of the Seicento." Master's thesis, California State University, Los Angeles, 1976.

Farinacci, Prospero

1618   *Opera Omnia.* Antwerp, 1618.

Fassò, Luigi, ed.

1956   *Teatro del seicento.* La letteratura italiana. Storia e testi, vol. 39. Milan, 1956.

Federici, Vincenzo

1899   *Regestro del monastero di San Silvestro de Capite.* Rome, 1899.

Feigen, Richard L.

2000   *Tales from the Art Crypt: The Painters, the Museums, the Curators, the Collectors, the Auctions, the Art.* New York, 2000.

Félibien, André

1705   *Entretiens sur les vies et sur les ouvrages des plus excellens peintres anciens et modernes.* Rev. ed. 4 vols. London, 1705. First published Paris, 1666–88.

Ferrara

1983   *Frescobaldi e il suo tempo: Nel quarto centenario della nascita.* Exhibition, Palazzo dei Diamanti, Ferrara, September 13–October 31, 1983. Catalogue. Venice, 1983.

Ferrara–New York–Los Angeles

1998–99   *Dosso Dossi: Court Painter in Renaissance Ferrara.* Exhibition, Pinacoteca Nazionale, Ferrara, September 26–December 14, 1998; The Metropolitan Museum of Art, New York, January 14–March 28, 1999; J. Paul Getty Museum, Los Angeles, April 27–July 11, 1999. Catalogue by Peter Humfrey and Mauro Lucco, with contributions by Andrea Rothe et al.; edited by Andrea Bayer. New York, 1998.

Finaldi, Gabriele

1999   "Orazio Gentileschi at the Court of Charles I." In London–Bilbao–Madrid 1999.

Finet, John

1987   *Ceremonies of Charles I: The Note Books of John Finet, 1628–1641.* Edited by Albert J. Loomie. New York, 1987.

Fiocchi Nicolai, Vincenzo

2000   "San Filippo Neri: Le catacombe di S. Sebastiano e le origini dell'archeologia cristiana." In *San Filippo Neri nella realtà romana del XVI secolo,* edited by Maria Teresa Bonadonna Russo and Niccolò Del Re, 105–30. Rome, 2000.

Fiorani, Luigi, ed.

1985   *Ricerche per la storia religiosa di Roma: Studi, documenti, inventari.* Vol. 6, *Storiografia e archivi delle confraternite romane.* Rome, 1985.

Fleming, John

1955   "The Hugfords of Florence." *Connoisseur* 136 (1955), 106–10, 197–206.

Florence

1970   *Caravaggio e caravaggeschi nelle gallerie di Firenze.* Exhibition, Palazzo Pitti, Florence. Catalogue by Evelina Borea. Florence, 1970.

1983   *Disegni di Giovanni Lanfranco (1582–1647).* Exhibition, Gabinetto dei Disegni, Florence, 1983. Catalogue by Erich Schleier. Florence, 1983.

1984   *Cristofano Allori, 1577–1621.* Exhibition, Palazzo Pitti, Florence, July–October, 1984. Catalogue edited by Miles L. Chappell. Florence, 1984.

1986   *La Maddalena tra sacro e profano: Da Giotto a De Chirico.* Exhibition, Palazzo Pitti, Florence, May 24–September 7, 1986. Catalogue edited by Marilena Mosco. Florence, 1986.

1986–87   *Il seicento fiorentino: Arte a Firenze da Ferdinando I a Cosimo III: Pittura.* Exhibition, Palazzo Strozzi, Florence, December 21, 1986–May 4, 1987. Catalogue edited by Giuliana Guidi and Daniela Marcucci. Florence, 1986.

1991   *Artemisia.* Exhibition, Casa Buonarroti, Florence, June 18–November 4, 1991. Catalogue edited by Roberto Contini and Gianni Papi. Rome, 1991.

Forcella, Vincenzo

1877   *Iscrizioni delle chiese d'altri edifici di Roma.* Vol. 9. Rome, 1877.

Fortunati Pietrantonio, Vera

1986   *Pittura bolognese del '500.* 2 vols. Bologna, 1986.

Fossombrone

1997   *Giovanni Francesco Guerrieri: Un pittore del seicento fra Roma e le Marche.* Exhibition, Chiesa di San Filippo and Corte Alta, Fossombrone, July 19–October 1997. Catalogue edited by Marina Cellini and Claudio Pizzorusso. Venice, 1997.

Fowle, G. E.

1980   "The Lady Who Got Tassi Thrown into Prison." *Helicon Nine* 2 (summer 1980), 54–63.

Francini Ciaranfi, Anna Maria

1955   *The Pitti Palace and Gallery in Florence: Handbook and Itinerary.* Translated by Hilda M. R. Cox. Florence, 1955.

Frankfurt am Main

1992   *Kunst in der Republik Genua, 1528–1815.* Exhibition, Schirn Kunsthalle, Frankfurt am Main, September 5–November 8, 1992. Catalogue edited by Bernhardt Schwenk and Bettina-Martine Wolter. Frankfurt am Main, 1992.

Fredericksen, Burton B.

1972   *Catalogue of the Paintings in the J. Paul Getty Museum.* Malibu, 1972.

Freedberg, Sydney J.

1975   *Painting in Italy, 1500 to 1600.* Harmondsworth, 1975.

1976   "Gentileschi's 'Madonna with the Sleeping Christ Child.'" *Burlington Magazine* 118 (1976), 732–35.

Freiberg, Jack

1995   *The Lateran in 1600: Christian Concord in Counter-Reformation Rome.* Cambridge, 1995.

Friedlaender, Walter F.

1955   *Caravaggio Studies.* Princeton, 1955.

Frimmel, Theodor von

1894   *Verzeichnis der Gemälde in gräflich Schönborn-Wiesentheid'schem Besitze.* Pommersfelden, 1894.

1913   "Zur Herkunft des neuerworbenen Elsheimer (St. Christoph) im Kaiser Friedrich-Museum." *Studien und Skizzen zur Gemäldekunde* 1 (1913), 45–46.

Fröhlich-Bume, Lili

1940   "A Rediscovered Picture by Artemisia Gentileschi." *Burlington Magazine* 77 (1940), 169.

1954   "Three Unknown Drawings for Famous Pictures." *Gazette des Beaux-Arts,* ser. 6, 44 (1954), 355–60.

Frommel, Christoph L.

1971   "Caravaggios Frühwerk und der Kardinal Francesco Maria Del Monte." *Storia dell'arte* 9/10 (1971), 5–55.

Fuda, Roberto

1989   "Un'inedita lettera di Artemisia Gentileschi a Ferdinando II de' Medici." *Rivista d'arte* 41 (1989), 167–71.

Fumagalli, Elena

1990   "Guido Reni e altri a San Gregorio al Celio e a San Sebastiano fuori le Mura." *Paragone* 1990, 67–94.

1992 "Le fabbriche dei Borghese: Committenza di una famiglia romana nel sei e settecento." Doctoral dissertation, Rome, 1990.

Gabrieli, Giuseppe
1996 *Il carteggio linceo.* Rome, 1996.

Gaeta
1976 *Arte a Gaeta: Dipinti dal XII al XVIII secolo.* Exhibition, Palazzo De Vio, Gaeta, August–October 1976. Catalogue edited by Maria Letizia Casanova. Florence, 1976.

Galante, Gennaro Aspreno
1985 *Guida sacra della città di Napoli.* Edited by Nicola Spinosa. Naples, 1985. First published Naples, 1872.

Galasso, Giuseppe
1982 *Napoli spagnola dopo Masaniello: Politica, cultura, società.* 2 vols. Florence, 1982.

Galilei, Galileo
1929–39 *Le opere di Galileo Galilei.* 20 vols. Edited by Antonio Favaro. Florence, 1929–39.

Gallo, Marco
1998 "Ulteriori dati sulla chiesa dei SS. Luca e Martina e sugli esordi di Jusepe de Ribera." *Storia dell'arte* 93/94 (1998), 312–34.

Gamba, Carlo
1922–23 "Orazio Gentileschi." *Dedalo* 3 (1922–23), 245–66.

Gandolfi, Giovan Cristoforo, ed.
1846 *Descrizione di Genova e del genovesato.* Part 4, *I monumenti e le produzioni delle belle arti.* Genoa, 1846.

Garas, Klará
1969 "La collection de tableaux du château royal de Buda au XVIIIᵉ siecle." *Bulletin de Musée Hongrois des Beaux-Arts,* nos. 32–33 (1969).

Gardner, Elizabeth E.
1986 *Gardner's Art through the Ages, II: Renaissance and Modern Art.* 8th ed. Revised by Horst de la Croix and Richard G. Tansey. San Diego, 1986.
1998 *A Bibliographical Repertory of Italian Private Collections.* Vol. 1, *Abaco–Cutolo.* Edited by Chiara Ceschi, with the assistance of Katharine Baetjer. Venice, 1998.

Garrard, Mary
1980 "Artemisia Gentileschi's *Self-Portrait as the Allegory of Painting.*" *Art Bulletin* 62 (1980), 97–112.
1982 "Artemisia and Susanna." In *Feminism and Art History: Questioning the Litany,* edited by Norma Broude and Mary D. Garrard, 146–71. New York, 1982.
1989 *Artemisia Gentileschi: The Image of the Female Hero in Italian Baroque Art.* Princeton, 1989.
1993 "Corisca and the Satyr." *Burlington Magazine* 125 (1993), 34–38.
2001 *Artemisia Gentileschi around 1622: The Shaping and Reshaping of an Artistic Identity.* Berkeley and Los Angeles, 2001.

Gash, John
1980 *Caravaggio.* London, 1980.
1985 "American Baroque." *Art History* 13, no. 2 (1985), 249–61.
1990 Review of Garrard 1989. *Art in America* 77, no. 5 (1990), 67–69.

Gaynor, Juan-Santos, and Ilaria Toesca
1963 *S. Silvestro in Capite.* Le chiese di Roma illustrate, vol. 73. Rome, 1963.

Genoa
1788 *Description des beautés de Gènes et de ses environs.* Genoa, 1788.

1947 *Mostra della pittura del seicento e settecento in Liguria.* Exhibition, Palazzo Reale, Genoa, June 21–September 30, 1947. Catalogue by Antonio Morassi. Milan, 1947.
1992 *Genova nell'età barocca.* Exhibition, Galleria Nazionale di Palazzo Spinola and Galleria di Palazzo Reale, Genoa, May 2–July 26, 1992. Bologna, 1992.
1997 *Van Dyck a Genova: Grande pittura e collezionismo.* Exhibition, Palazzo Ducale, Genoa. Catalogue edited by Susan J. Barnes. Milan, 1997.
1999– *El siglo de los Genoveses e una lunga storia di*
2000 *arte e splendori nel Palazzo dei Dogi.* Exhibition, Palazzo Ducale, Genoa, December 4, 1999–May 28, 2000. Catalogue edited by Piero Boccardo and Clario Di Fabio, with the collaboration of Raffaella Besta. Milan, 1999.

Gerard, Véronique
1982 "Philip IV's Early Italian Commissions." *Oxford Art Journal* 5, no. 1 (1982), 9–14.

Gere, John A., and Philip Pouncey
1983 *Artists Working in Rome, c. 1550 to c. 1640.* Italian Drawings in the Department of Prints and Drawings in the British Museum, vols. 8, 9. London, 1983.

Germond, Suzan Major
1993 "Orazio Gentileschi and S. Giovanni dei Fiorentini; with Appendix." *Burlington Magazine* 135 (1993), 754–59.

Giacchetti, Giovanni
1629 *Historia della venerabile chiesa e monastero di S. Silvestro de Capite di Roma.* Rome, 1629.

Giffi Ponzi, Elisabetta
1994 "Gentileschi a Genova: Un nuovo dipinto e alcune considerazioni sulla cronologia delle opere." *Bollettino dei Musei Civici Genovesi* 16 (1994), 51–59.

Gigli, Giacinto
1958 *Diario Romano (1608–1670).* Edited by Giuseppe Ricciotti. Rome, 1958.

Gilii, C., and S. Guerrieri
n.d. "Memorie storiche di Fabriano." Ms. 209 [early eighteenth century], Biblioteca Comunale, Fabriano.

Gilio da Fabriano, Giovanni Andrea
1564 *Due dialogi.* Camerino: Antonio Gioioso, 1564.

Giustiniani, Vincenzo
1981 *Discorsi sulle arti e sui mestieri.* Edited by Anna Banti. Florence, 1981.

Glenn, L. A.
1999 "Virtuous Ladies and Melancholic Geniuses." M.A. thesis, University of Victoria, 1999.

Glück, Gustav, and August Schaeffer
1907 *Die Gemäldegalerie Alte Meister.* 2d ed. Vienna, 1907.

Goffen, Rona
1997 *Titian's Women.* New Haven, 1997.

Goldstein, Carl
1996 *Teaching Art: Academies and Schools from Vasari to Albers.* Cambridge, 1996.

Goodman, Godfrey
1839 *The Court of King James the First.* Compiled by John S. Brewer. 2 vols. in 1. London, 1839.

Gorsen, Peter
1980 "Venus oder Judith? Zur Heroisierung des Weiblichkeitsbildes bei Lucas Cranach und Artemisia Gentileschi." *Artibus et historiae* 1 (1980), 69–81.

Gould, Cecil
1976 *The Paintings of Correggio.* London, 1976.

Grabski, Józef
1985 "On Seicento Painting in Naples: Some Observations on Bernardo Cavallino, Artemisia Gentileschi and Others." *Artibus et historiae* 11 (1985), 23–63.

Greer, Germaine
1979 *The Obstacle Race: The Fortunes of Women Painters and Their Work.* New York, 1979.

Gregori, Mina
1962 "Avant-propos sulla pittura fiorentina del seicento." *Paragone* 13, no. 145 (January 1962), 21–40.
1968 "Su due quadri caravaggeschi a Burghley House." In *Festschrift Ulrich Middeldorf,* edited by Antege Kosegarten and Peter Tigler, 414–21. Berlin, 1968.
1990 "Una nota per Artemisia Gentileschi." *Paragone* 41 (1990), 104–6.
1994 as editor. *Pittura a Como e nel Canton Ticino dal Mille al settecento.* Milan, 1994.
1996 as editor. *Come dipingeva Il Caravaggio: Atti della giornata di studio.* Proceedings of a conference held in Florence, January 18, 1992. Contributions by Elisa Acanfora, Roberta Lapucci, and Gianni Papi. Milan, 1996.

Gregori, Mina, and Erich Schleier, eds.
1989 *La pittura in Italia: Il seicento.* 2 vols. Milan, 1989.

Grendler, Paul F.
1989 *Schooling in Renaissance Italy: Literacy and Learning, 1300–1600.* Baltimore, 1989.

Grenoble–Rennes–Bordeaux
1989–90 *Laurent de La Hyre, 1606–1656: L'homme et l'oeuvre.* Exhibition, Musée de Grenoble, January 14–April 10, 1989; Musée de Rennes, May 9–August 31, 1989; Musée de Bordeaux, October 6, 1989–January 6, 1990. Catalogue by Pierre Rosenberg and Jacques Thuillier. Geneva, 1988.

Griseri, Andreina
1961 "L'autunno del Manierismo alla corte di Carlo Emanuele I e un arrivo 'caravaggesco.'" *Paragone* 12, no. 141 (1961), 19–36.

Gronau, Georg
1936 *Documenti artistici urbinati.* Florence, 1936.

Guillaume, Marguerite
1980 *Catalogue raisonné du Musée des Beaux-Arts de Dijon: Peintures italiennes.* Introduction by Jacques Thuillier. Dijon, 1980.

Hagen, Rose-Marie
1988 "Artemisia, die entehrte Malerin." *Art,* no. 8 (1988), 72–84.

Hall, Marcia B.
1999 *After Raphael: Painting in Central Italy in the Sixteenth Century.* New York, 1999.

Harris, Ann Sutherland
1989 "Fresh Paint." *Women's Review of Books* 6, no. 12 (1989), 8–10.
1998 "Artemisia Gentileschi: The Literate Illiterate of Learning from Example." In *Dolcere delectare movere: Affetti, devozione e retorica nel linguaggio artistico del primo barocco romano,* 103–20. Rome, 1998.

Harris, Enriqueta
1967 "Orazio Gentileschi's 'Finding of Moses' in Madrid." *Burlington Magazine* 109 (1967), 86–89.

Hart, Clive, and Kay Gilliland Stevenson
1995 *Heaven and the Flesh: Imagery of Desire from the Renaissance to the Rococo.* Cambridge, 1995.

Hartford

1998   *Caravaggio and His Italian Followers from the Collections of the Galleria Nazionale d'Arte Antica di Roma*. Exhibition, Wadsworth Atheneum, Hartford, April 23–July 26, 1998. Catalogue by Claudio Strinati, Rossella Vodret et al. Venice, 1998.

Haskell, Francis

1963   *Patrons and Painters: A Study in the Relations between Italian Art and Society in the Age of the Baroque*. New York, 1963.

1989   "Artemisia's Revenge?" Review of Garrard 1989. *New York Review of Books*, July 20, 1989, 36–38.

Haskell, Francis, and Nicholas Penny

1981   *Taste and the Antique: The Lure of Classical Sculpture, 1500–1900*. New Haven, 1981.

Haskins, Susan

1993   *Mary Magdalen: Myth and Metaphor*. New York, 1993.

Heiden, Rüdiger an der

1998   *Die Alte Pinakothek: Sammlungsgeschichte, Bau und Bilder*. Munich, 1998.

Held, Julius S.

1980   *The Oil Sketches of Peter Paul Rubens: A Critical Catalogue*. 2 vols. Princeton, 1980.

Heller, Joseph

1845   *Die gräflich Schönborn'sche Gemäldesammlung zu Schloss Weissenstein in Pommersfelden*. Bamberg, 1845.

Herklotz, Ingo

1985   "*Historia Sacra* und mittelalterliche Kunst während der zweiten Hälfte des 16. Jahrhunderts in Rom." In *Baronio e l'arte: Atti del convegno internazionale di studi, Sora, 10–13 ottobre 1984*, edited by Romeo De Maio et al., 23–72. Sora, 1985.

Hermanin, Federico

1924   *Catalogo della R. Galleria d'Arte Antica nel Palazzo Corsini, Roma*. Bologna, 1924.

1944   "Gli ultimi avanzi di un'antica galleria romana." *Roma* 13 (1944), 43–48.

Hersey, George

1993   "Female and Male Art: 'Postille' to Garrard's 'Artemisia Gentileschi.'" In *Parthenope's Splendor: Art of the Golden Age in Naples*, edited by Jeanne Chenault Porter and Susan Scott Munshower, 322–35. Papers in Art History from the Pennsylvania State University, 7. University Park, 1993.

Herz, Alexandra

1988   "Cardinal Cesare Baronio's Restoration of SS. Nereo ed Achilleo and S. Cesareo de' Appia." *Art Bulletin* 70 (1988), 590–620.

Hess, Jacob

1952   "Die Gemälde des Orazio Gentileschi für das 'Haus der Königin' in Greenwich." *English Miscellany* 3 (1952), 159–87.

1967   "Die Gemälde des Orazio Gentileschi für das Haus der Königin in Greenwich." In *Kunstgeschichtliche Studien zu Renaissance und Barock*, vol. 1, 241–57, 421–22, vol. 2, pls. 171–83. Rome, 1967.

Hibbard, Howard

1971   *Carlo Maderno and Roman Architecture, 1580–1630*. University Park, Pennsylvania, 1971.

1972   "Ut picturae sermones: The First Painted Decorations of the Gesù." In Wittkower and Jaffe 1972, 29–49.

Hinks, Roger P.

1953   *Michelangelo Merisi da Caravaggio: His Life—His Legend—His Works*. London, 1953.

Hirst, Michael

1981   *Sebastiano del Piombo*. Oxford, 1981.

Hofrichter, Frima Fox

1980   "Artemisia Gentileschi's Uffizi Judith and a Lost Rubens." *Rutgers Art Review* 1 (January 1980), 9–15.

Honorati, A.

1990   *Ricerche sulla Casa Trionfi di Ancona*. Ancona, 1990.

Hoogewerff, Gottfried Johannes

1938   "Nederlandsche kunstenaars te Rome, 1600–1725. Uittreksels uit de parochiale archieven: I, Parochie van Santa Maria del Popolo." *Mededellingen van het Nederlandsch Historisch Instituut te Rome* 8 (1938), 49–125.

1942   *Nederlandsche kunstenaars te Rome (1600–1725) uittreksels uit de parochiale archieven*. The Hague, 1942.

Houston

1953   *The Samuel H. Kress Collection at the Museum of Fine Arts of Houston*. Annotated by William Suida. Houston, 1953.

1981   *The Museum of Fine Arts, Houston: A Guide to the Collection*. Houston, 1981.

Imparato, Francesco

1889   "Documenti relativi ad Artemisia Lomi Gentileschi pittrice." *Archivio storico dell'arte* 2 (1889), 423–25.

Ingenhoff-Danhäuser, Monika

1984   *Maria Magdalena: Heilige und Sünderin in der italienischen Renaissance. Studien zur Ikonographie der Heiligen von Leonardo bis Tizian*. Tübingen, 1984.

Isella, P. C., and M. Lanza

1991   *Pagine inedite sul monte dei Cappuccini*. Turin, 1991.

Jacobs, Fredrika H.

1997   *Defining the Renaissance Virtuosa: Women Artists and the Language of Art History and Criticism*. Cambridge, 1997.

Jacobus de Voragine

1993   *The Golden Legend: Readings on the Saints* [ca. 1260]. 2 vols. Translated by William Granger Ryan. Princeton, 1993.

Jaffé, Michael

1963   "Peter Paul Rubens and the Oratorian Fathers." *Proporzioni* 4 (1963), 209–41.

1977   *Rubens and Italy*. Oxford, 1977.

Janssen, M.

1974   "Maria Magdalena." In *Lexikon der Christlichen Ikonographie*, vol. 7 (1974), 516–41.

Jones, Pamela M.

1992   *Federico Borromeo and the Ambrosiana: Art Patronage and Reform in Seventeenth-Century Milan*. Cambridge, 1992.

Judson, J. Richard, and Rudolf E. O. Ekkart

1999   *Gerrit van Honthorst, 1592–1656*. Aetas aurea, 14. Doornspijk, 1999.

Jullian, René

1961   *Caravage*. Paris and Lyon, 1961.

Kaftal, George

1948   "Three Scenes from the Legend of Santa Francesca Romana." *Journal of the Walters Art Gallery* 2 (1948), 50–61.

Kahr, Madlyn Millner

1978   "Danaë: Virtuous, Voluptuous, Venal Woman." *Art Bulletin* 60 (March 1978), 43–55.

Kaufmann, Thomas Da Costa

1970   "Esther before Ahasuerus: A New Painting by Artemisia Gentileschi in the Museum's Collection." *Metropolitan Museum of Art Bulletin* 29 (December 1970), 165–69.

Kind, Joshua Benjamin

1967   "The Drunken Lot and His Daughters: An Iconographical Study of the Uses of This Theme in the Visual Arts from 1500–1650, and Its Bases in Exegetical and Literary History." Ph.D. dissertation, Columbia University, New York, 1967.

King, Catherine

1999   "Portrait of the Artist as a Woman." In *Gender and Art*, edited by Gill Perry, 37–60. New Haven, 1999.

Kitson, Michael

1967   *The Complete Paintings of Caravaggio*. New York, 1967.

Kleinschmidt, Hans J.

1976   "Discussion of Laurie Schneider, 'Donatello and Caravaggio: The Iconography of Decapitation.'" *American Imago* 33, no. 1 (spring 1976), 92–97.

Klessmann, Rüdiger

1978   *Herzog Anton Ulrich-Museum, Braunschweig*. Munich, 1978.

1985   "New Acquisitions for the Brunswick Museum." *Apollo* 121 (1985), 383–87.

Koerner, Joseph Leo

1993   *The Moment of Self-Portraiture in German Renaissance Art*. Chicago, 1993.

Köpl, Karl

1889   "Urkunden, Acten, Regesten und Inventäre aus dem K.K. Statthalterei-Archiv in Prag." *Jahrbuch der Kunsthistorischen Sammlungen des allerhöchsten Kaiserhauses* 10 (1889), LXIII–CC.

Kryza-Gersch, Claudia

1998   "Leandro Bassano's Portrait of Tiziano Aspetti." *Burlington Magazine* 140 (1998), 265–67.

Kultermann, U.

1990   "Woman Asleep and the Artist." *Artibus et historiae* 22 (1990), 129–61.

Labrot, Gérard

1979   *Baroni in città: Residenze e comportamenti dell'aristocrazia napoletana, 1530–1734*. Naples, 1979.

1993   *Palazzi napoletani: Storei di nobili e cortigiani, 1520–1750*. Naples, 1993.

La Granja

2000   See Segovia 2000.

Langdon, Helen

1998   *Caravaggio: A Life*. London, 1998.

Lanzi, Luigi

1795–96   *La storia pittorica della Italia inferiore*. 3 vols. Florence, 1795–96.

Lapierre, Alexandra

1998   *Artemisia: Un duel pour l'immortalité*. Paris, 1998.

2000   *Artemisia: The Story of a Battle for Greatness*. Translated by Liz Heron. London, 2000.

Laskin, Myron, Jr., and Michael Pantazzi, eds.

1987   *European and American Painting, Sculpture, and Decorative Arts: Catalogue of the National Gallery of Canada*. Ottawa, 1987.

Lastri, Marco

1791–95   *L'Etruria pittrice; ovvero, Storia della pittura toscana dedotta dai suoi monumenti che si esibiscono in stampa dal secolo X fino al presente*. 2 vols. Edited by Niccolo Pagni and Giuseppe Bardi. Florence, 1791–95.

Lattuada, Riccardo

1991 "De Rosa, Giovan Francesco, detto Pacecco." In *Dizionario biografico degli Italiani* 39, 167–71. Rome, 1991.

2000 *Francesco Guarino da Solofra nella pittura napoletana del seicento (1611–1651).* Naples, 2000.

Laureati, Laura, and Ludovica Trezzani

1993 *Il patrimonio artistico del Quirinale. Pittura antica: La decorazione murale.* Milan, 1993.

Lavagnino, Emilio

1933 *La Galleria Spada in Roma.* Rome, 1933.

Lavin, Marilyn Aronberg

1975 *Seventeenth-Century Barberini Documents and Inventories of Art.* New York, 1975.

Leningrad

1973 *Karavadzho i karavadzhisty.* Exhibition, Hermitage, Leningrad. Catalogue by Svetlana N. Vsevolozhskaia and Irina V. Linnik. Leningrad, 1973.

1975 *See* Vsevolozhskaia and Linnik 1975.

Leonard, Mark, Narayan Khandekar, and Dawson W. Carr

2001 "'Amber Varnish' and Orazio Gentileschi's 'Lot and His Daughters.'" *Burlington Magazine* 143 (2001), 4–10.

Leone de Castris, Pierluigi

1991 *Pittura del cinquecento a Napoli, 1573–1606: L'ultima maniera.* Naples, 1991.

1992 "Stanzione e il Barocco." In *Barocco napoletano* 1992, 545–68.

Le Pas de Sécheval, Anne

1993 "Aux origines de la collection Mazarin: L'acquisition de la collection romaine du Duc Sannesio (1642–44)." *Journal of the History of Collections* 5, no. 1 (1993), 13–21.

Lépine, Laurence

1984 "Récherches sur la collection de tableaux du duc de Liancourt." Dissertation, Université de Paris IV, Sorbonne, 1984.

Lerberg, Ellen

1993 "Judith i Nasjonalgalleriet." *Kunst og Kultur* 76 (1993), 182–91.

Levenson, Jon Douglas

1997 *Esther: A Commentary.* Louisville, Kentucky, 1997.

Levey, Michael

1962 "Notes on the Royal Collection–II: Artemisia Gentileschi's 'Self-Portrait' at Hampton Court." *Burlington Magazine* 104 (1962), 79–80.

1964 *The Later Italian Pictures in the Collection of Her Majesty the Queen.* London, 1964.

1991 *The Later Italian Pictures in the Collection of Her Majesty the Queen.* 2d ed. Cambridge, 1991.

Lippincott, Kristen

1990 Review of Garrard 1989. *Renaissance Studies* 4, no. 4 (1990), 444–48.

Litta, Pompeo

1872 *Famiglie celebri italiane: Savelli di Roma.* Milan, 1872.

Lockyer, Roger

1981 *Buckingham: The Life and Political Career of George Villiers, First Duke of Buckingham, 1592–1628.* London and New York, 1981.

Loire, Stéphane

1996 *École italienne, XVIIe siècle.* Vol. 1, *Bologne.* Musée du Louvre, Département des Peintures: Catalogue. Paris, 1996.

1998 "La Carrière de Jérôme David." In *Claude Vignon en son temps: Actes du colloque de Tours (23–24 janvier 1994),* edited by Claude Mignot and Paola Pacht Bassani, 157–88. Paris, 1998.

Lomazzo, Giovanni Paolo

1584 *Trattato dell'arte de la pittura diuiso in sette libri, ne' quali si contiene tutta la theorica, & la prattica d'essa pittura.* Milan, 1584.

London

1930 *Exhibition of Italian Art, 1200–1900.* Exhibition, Royal Academy of Arts, London, January 1–March 8, 1930. Catalogue edited by W. G. Constable; essays by Adolfo Venturi and Ugo Ojetti. London, 1930.

1931 *A Commemorative Catalogue of the Exhibition of Italian Art Held in the Galleries of the Royal Academy, Burlington House, London, January–March 1930.* 2 vols. Edited by David Lindsay Balniel and Kenneth Clark. London, 1931.

1938 *17th Century Art in Europe: An Illustrated Souvenir.* Exhibition, Royal Academy of Arts, London. Catalogue. London, 1938.

1960 *Italian Art and Britain.* Exhibition, Royal Academy of Arts, London, January 2–March 6, 1960. Catalogue. London, 1960.

1972–73 *The Age of Charles I: Painting in England 1620–1649.* Exhibition, Tate Gallery, London, November 15, 1972–January 14, 1973. Catalogue by Oliver Millar. London, 1972.

1981 *Important Italian Baroque Paintings, 1600–1700: An Exhibition in Aid of Restoration of the Guarino Paintings at Solofra and the Giottesque Frescoes in Sta. Chiara, Naples.* Exhibition, Matthiesen Fine Art Ltd., London. Catalogue. London, 1981.

1982 *Painting in Naples, 1606–1705: From Caravaggio to Giordano.* Exhibition, Royal Academy of Arts, London, October 2–December 12, 1982. Catalogue by Clovis Whitfield and Jane Martineau. London, 1982. Also shown at the National Gallery of Art, Washington, D.C., February 13–May 1, 1983.

1985 *Around 1610: The Onset of the Baroque.* Exhibition, Matthiesen Fine Art Ltd., London, June 14–August 16, 1985. Catalogue. London, 1985.

1986 *Baroque III: 1620–1700.* Matthiesen Fine Art Ltd., London, June 13–August 15, 1986. Catalogue. London, 1986.

2001 *2001, an Art Odyssey, 1500–1720: Classicism, Mannerism, Caravaggism, and Baroque.* Exhibition, Matthiesen Fine Art Ltd., London. Catalogue. London, 2001.

London–Bilbao–Madrid

1999 *Orazio Gentileschi at the Court of Charles I.* Exhibition, National Gallery, London, March 3–May 23, 1999; Museo de Bellas Artes de Bilbao, June 7–September 5, 1999; Museo del Prado, Madrid, September 20–November 20, 1999. Catalogue edited by Gabriele Finaldi. London, 1999.

London–Rome

2001 *The Genius of Rome: 1592–1623.* Exhibition, Royal Academy of Arts, London, January 20–April 16, 2001; Palazzo Venezia, Rome, May–August 2001. Catalogue edited by Beverly L. Brown. London, 2001.

Longhi, Roberto

1915 "Battistello." *L'arte,* 1915, 58–75, 120–37. Reprinted in Longhi 1961, 177–211.

1916 "Gentileschi padre e figlia." *L'arte,* 1916, 245–314. Reprinted in Longhi 1961, 219–83.

1927 "Ter Bruggen e la parte nostra." *Vita artistica* 2, no. 6 (1927), 105–16. Reprinted in Longhi 1967, 163–78.

1935 "I pittori della realtà in Francia ovvero i caravaggeschi francesi del seicento." *L'Italia letteraria* 11, no. 3 (1935).

1943 "Ultimi studi sul Caravaggio e la sua cerchia." *Proporzioni* 1 (1943), 5–63. Reprinted in Longhi 1999, 1–54.

1951 "Sui margini caravaggeschi." *Paragone* 2, no. 21 (1951), 20–34.

1952 *Il Caravaggio.* Milan, 1952. Reprinted in Longhi 1999, 159–223.

1961 *Opere complete di Roberto Longhi.* Vol. 1, *Scritti giovanili, 1912–22.* Florence, 1961.

1963 "Giovanni Baglione e il quadro del processo." *Paragone* 14, no. 163 (1963), 23–31.

1967 *Opere complete di Roberto Longhi.* Vol. 2, *Saggi e ricerche, 1922–1928.* Florence, 1967.

1968 *Il Caravaggio.* Rome, 1968. Reprinted in Longhi 1999, 241–91.

1999 *Opere complete di Roberto Longhi.* Vol. 11, *Studi caravaggeschi, I, 1943–1968.* Milan, 1999.

Loomie, Albert J.

1987 *See* Finet 1987.

1996 "The Destruction of Rubens's 'Crucifixion' in the Queen's Chapel, Somerset House." *Burlington Magazine* 140 (1996), 680–82.

Los Angeles

1976–77 *Women Artists, 1550–1950.* Exhibition, Los Angeles County Museum of Art, December 21, 1976–March 13, 1977, and other cities. Catalogue edited by Ann Sutherland Harris and Linda Nochlin. Venice, California, 1976.

Lukehart, Peter M.

1993 "Delineating the Genoese Studio: *Giovani accartati* or *sotto padre?*" In *The Artist's Workshop,* edited by Peter M. Lukehart, 36–57. National Gallery of Art, Studies in the History of Art, 38. Washington, D.C., 1993.

Lurie, Ann Tzeutschler

1975 "Pictorial Ties between Rembrandt's *Danaë* in the Hermitage and Orazio Gentileschi's *Danaë* in the Cleveland Museum of Art." *Acta historiae artium* 21, no. 1–2 (1975), 75–81.

Luzio, Alessandro

1913 *La galleria dei Gonzaga venduta all'Inghilterra nel 1627–28.* Rome, 1913.

1974 *La galleria dei Gonzaga venduta all'Inghilterra nel 1627–28.* Rome, 1974.

Maccherini, Michele

1997 "Caravaggio nel carteggio familiare di Giulio Mancini." *Prospettiva* 86 (1997), 71–92.

MacGregor, Arthur

1989 *The Late King's Goods: Collections, Possessions, and Patronage of Charles I in the Light of the Commonwealth Sale Inventories.* London, 1989.

Macioce, Stefania

1990 *Undique splendent: Aspetti della pittura sacra nella Roma di Clemente VIII Aldobrandini (1592–1605).* Rome, 1990.

1999 "La sala Clementina." In *Arte a Roma: Pittura, scultura, architettura, nella storia dei Giubilei,* edited by Maurizio Calvesi, 133–41. Rome, 1999.

Maddicott, Hilary

1998 "The Provenance of the 'Castle Howard' Version of Orazio Gentileschi's *Finding of Moses.*" *Burlington Magazine* 140 (1998), 120–22.

Madocks Lister, Susan

2000 """Trumperies Brought from Rome': Barberini Gifts to the Stuart Court in 1635." In *The Diplomacy of Art: Artistic Creation and Politics in Seicento Italy*, edited by Elizabeth Cropper, 151–75. Bologna, 2000.

Madrazo, José de

1856 *Catálogo de la galería de cuadros del Excmo. Sr. D. José de Madrazo*. Madrid, 1856.

Madrid

1970 *Pintura italiana del siglo XVII*. Exhibition, Casón del Buen Retiro, Madrid, April–May 1970. Catalogue. Madrid, 1970.

1972 *Museo del Prado: Catálogo de las pinturas*. Madrid, 1972.

1985 *Pintura napolitana de Caravaggio a Giordano*. Exhibition, Madrid. Catalogue by Alfonso E. Pérez Sánchez and Manuel Mena Marqués. Madrid, 1985.

Maggiori, Alessandro

1821 *Le pitture sculture e architetture della città di Ancona*. Ancona, 1821.

Magnanimi, Giuseppina

1980 "Inventari della collezione romana dei principi Corsini." *Bollettino d'arte* 65, no. 7 (1980), 91–126, no. 8 (1980), 73–114.

Magnuson, Torgil

1982–86 *Rome in the Age of Bernini*. 2 vols. Stockholm, 1982–86.

Mahon, Denis

1947 *Studies in Seicento Art and Theory*. Studies of the Warburg Institute, vol. 16. London, 1947. Reprinted, Westport, Connecticut, 1971.

1952 "Addenda to Caravaggio." *Burlington Magazine* 94 (1952), 3–23.

Malaguzzi Valeri, F.

1926 "I nuovi acquisiti della pinacoteca di Bologna." *Cronache d'arte* 3, no. 1 (1926).

Mallè, Luigi

1970a *I musei civici di Torino: Acquisti e doni, 1966–1970*. Turin, 1970.

1970b *Palazzo Madama in Torino*. 2 vols. Turin, 1970.

Malvasia, Carlo Cesare

1678 *Felsina pittrice: Vite de pittori bolognesi alla maesta christianissima di Luigi XIIII [sic]*. 2 vols. Bologna, 1678.

1841 *Felsina pittrice: Vite de' pittori bolognesi*. 2 vols. Edited by Giampietro Zanotti et al. Bologna, 1841.

Mancini, Giulio

1956–57 *Considerazioni sulla pittura [1617–21]*. Compiled and edited by Adriana Marucchi; commentary by Luigi Salerno. 2 vols. Rome, 1956–57.

Maniello, Sabina

1994 "Orazio Gentileschi: Un documento relativo al 'Battesimo' in S. Maria della Pace." *Alma Roma*, 1992 (1994), 155–60.

Mann, Judith W.

1996 "The Gentileschi *Danaë* in the Saint Louis Art Museum. Orazio or Artemisia?" *Apollo* 143 (June 1996), 39–45.

1997 "Caravaggio and Artemisia: Testing the Limits of Caravaggism." *Studies in Iconography* 18 (1997), 161–85.

Manzoni, Alessandro

1827 *I promessi sposi: Storia milanesi del secolo XVII scoperta e rifatta*. 3 vols. Florence, 1827.

Marangoni, Matteo

1922–23 "Note sul Caravaggio alla mostra del sei e settecento." *Bollettino d'arte*, ser. 2, 1 (1922–23), 217–29.

1945 *Il Caravaggio*. Florence, 1945.

Marcheselli, Carlo Francesco

1972 *Pitture delle chiese di Rimini, 1754; Ristampa anastatica corredata da indici di ricerca, da un commentario di orientamento bibliografico e informativo, da un repertorio illustrato. In appendice, il manoscritto di Marcello Oretti sull pitture nella città di Rimini, 1777*. Edited by Pier Giorgio Pasini. Bologna, 1972.

Marcoaldi, Oreste

1873 *Guida e statistica della città e comune di Fabriano*. Fabriano, 1873.

Marcolini, Giuliana

1996 "Alla ricerca di un Guercino 'perduto': *La Santissima Vergine che va in Egitto* della Galleria conti di Lucca." *Arte documento* 10 (1996), 69–75.

Marcon, Giulio, Silvia Maddalo, Giuliana Marcolini

1983 "Per una storia dell'esodo del patrimonio artistico ferrarese a Roma." In Ferrara 1983, 93–106.

Marini, Maurizio

1974 *Io Michelangelo da Caravaggio*. Rome, 1974.

1981 "Un 'Giaele e Sisara' di Francesco detto 'Cecco del Caravaggio.'" *Antologia di belle arti* 19/20 (1981), 176–79.

1981a "Caravaggio e il naturalismo internazionale." In *Storia dell'arte italiana*, vol. 6, part 1, 347–445. Turin, 1981.

1987 *Caravaggio: Michelangelo Merisi da Caravaggio "pictor praestantissimus." La tragica esistenza, la raffinata cultura, il mondo sanguigno del primo seicento, nell'iter pittorico completo di uno dei massimi rivoluzionari dell'arte di tutti i tempi*. Rome, 1987.

Marrow, Deborah

1982 *The Art Patronage of Maria de' Medici*. Ann Arbor, 1982.

Marshall, David R.

1993 *Viviano and Niccolo Codazzi and the Baroque Architectural Fantasy*. Milan, 1993.

Martinelli, Valentino

1959 "L'amor divino 'tutto ingudo' di Giovanni Baglione e la cronologia dell'intermezzo caravaggesco." *Arte antica e moderna* 5 (1959), 82–96.

Matteoli, Anna

1980 *Lodovico Cardi-Cigoli, pittore e architetto*. Pisa, 1980.

Matthiesen, Patrick

2001 Letter to the editor. *Burlington Magazine* 143 (2001), 162.

Mayer, Hans

1975 *Aussenseiter*. Frankfurt am Main, 1975.

McComb, Arthur

1934 *The Baroque Painters of Italy: An Introductory Historical Survey*. Cambridge, Massachusetts, 1934.

McEvansoneya, Philip

1987 "Some Documents Concerning the Patronage and Collections of the Duke of Buckingham." *Rutgers Art Review* 8 (1987), 27–38.

McEwen, J.

1999 "The Arts: Torchlight Flickers over the Cross." London *Sunday Telegraph*, April 4, 1999.

Meaux

1997–98 *Jean Senelle, 1605–avant 1671*. Exhibition, Musée Bossuet, Meaux, December 13, 1997–March 9, 1998. Catalogue by Sylvain Kerspern. Meaux, 1997.

Mechel, Chrétien de

1784 *Catalogue des tableaux de la Galerie Impériale et Royale de Vienne*. Basel, 1784.

Meissner, William

1999 *To the Greater Glory—a Psychological Study of Ignatian Spirituality*. Milwaukee, Wisconsin, 1999.

Menzio, Eva, ed.

1981 *Artemisia Gentileschi / Agostino Tassi: Atti di un processo per stupro*. Milan, 1981.

Merkel, Kerstin

1992 Review of Garrard 1989 and Florence 1991. *Kunstchronik* 45, no. 8 (1992), 346–55.

Mezzanotte, Antonio

1836 *Della vita e delle opere di Pietro Vannucci da Castello della Pieve cognominato Il Perugino: Commentario istorico*. Perugia, 1836.

Mezzetti, Tilde

1930 "L'attività di Orazio Gentileschi nelle Marche." *L'arte* 33 (1930), 541–51.

Milan

1951 *Mostra del Caravaggio e dei caravaggeschi*. Exhibition, Palazzo Reale, Milan, April–June 1951. Catalogue by Roberto Longhi. Florence, 1951.

1993 *L'Europa della pittura nel XVII secolo: 80 capolavori dai musei ungheresi*. Exhibition, Palazzo della Permanente, Milan, April 6–May 30, 1993. Catalogue edited by Agnes Szigethi. Milan, 1993.

Milicua, José

1970 "Pintura italiana del siglo XVII en el Casón del Buen Retiro." *Goya* 97 (1970), 2–10.

Millar, Oliver

1954 "Charles I, Honthorst, and Van Dyck." *Burlington Magazine* 96 (1954), 36–42.

1958–60 as editor. *Abraham Van Der Doort's Catalogue of the Collections of Charles I*. Walpole Society 37 (1958–60). [London], 1960.

1970–72 as editor. *The Inventories and Valuations of the King's Goods, 1649–1651*. Walpole Society 43 (1970–72). [London], 1972.

Miller, Dwight

1991 *Marcantonio Franceschini and the Liechtensteins: Prince Johann Adam Andreas and the Decoration of the Liechtenstein Garden Palace at Rossau-Vienna*. Cambridge, 1991. First published 1990.

Mochi Onori, Lorenza, and Rossella Vodret Adamo

1989 *La Galleria Nazionale d'Arte Antica: Regesto delle didascalie*. Rome, 1989.

Moir, Alfred

1967 *The Italian Followers of Caravaggio*. 2 vols. Cambridge, Massachusetts, 1967.

1969 "Did Caravaggio Draw?" *Art Quarterly* 32 (winter 1969), 358–72.

1976 *Caravaggio and His Copyists*. Monographs on Archaeology and Fine Arts, no. 31. New York, 1976.

Molajoli, Bruno

1930–31 "A proposito del Gentileschi nelle Marche." *Rassegna marchigiana* 9 (1930–31), 99–106.

1936 *Guida artistica di Fabriano*. Fabriano, 1936.

1955 *Notizie su Capodimonte; Catalogo delle Gallerie e del Museo*. Naples, 1955. Reprinted as *L'arte tipografia*, Naples, 1960.

1990 *Guida artistica di Fabriano*. 3d ed., revised and expanded. Fabriano, 1990.

Molajoli, Bruno, Luigi Serra, and Pietro Rotondi

1936   *Inventario degli oggetti d'arte d'Italia.* Vol. 8, *Le Provincie di Ancona e Ascoli Piceno.* Rome, 1936.

Moltmann-Wendel, Elisabeth

1982   *The Women around Jesus: Reflections on Authentic Personhood.* Translated from German by John Bowden. London, 1982.

Monsummano

1996   *I Borghese.* Exhibition, Fattoria Medicea, Monsummano Terme, September 6–15, 1996. Catalogue, 2 vols. Rome, 1996.

Montaigne, Michel de

1991   *Viaggio in Italia.* Preface by Guido Piovene. Bari, 1991. Translation of *Journal du voyage en Italie*, 1580–81.

Moore, Susan

1999   "Artistic Bloodline of a Daddy's Girl" (review of London–Bilbao–Madrid 1999). *Financial Times*, March 16, 1999.

Morel, Philippe

1999   "Jacopo Zucchi a servizio di Ferdinando de' Medici." In Rome 1999–2000, 115–24.

Mormando, Franco

1999   "Teaching the Faithful to Fly: Mary Magdalen and Peter in Baroque Italy." In Boston 1999.

Moroni, Gaetano, comp.

1854   *Dizionario di erudizione storico-ecclesiastica.* Vol. 61. Venice, 1854.

Mortari, Luisa

1995   *Bernardo Strozzi.* Rome, 1995.

Muller, Jeffrey M.

1989   *Rubens: The Artist as Collector.* Princeton, 1989.

Münster–Osnabrück

1998–99   *1648, War and Peace in Europe.* Exhibition, Westfälisches Landesmuseum für Kunst und Kulturgeschichtes Museum, Münster; Kunsthalle Dominikanerkirche, Osnabrück, October 24, 1998–January 17, 1999. Catalogue, 3 vols. edited by Klaus Bussmann and Heinz Schilling. Münster, 1998.

Murphy, Caroline

1996   "Lavinia Fontana: An Artist and Her Society in Late Sixteenth-Century Bologna." Ph.D. University College, London, 1996.

1997   "Lavinia Fontana and Female Life Cycle Experience in Late Sixteenth-Century Bologna." In *Picturing Women in Renaissance and Baroque Italy*, edited by Geraldine A. Johnson and Sara F. Matthews Grieco, 111–38. Cambridge, 1997.

Murray, Peter

1980   *Dulwich Picture Gallery: A Catalogue.* London, 1980.

Nantes

1983   *Peintures monumentales du Musée des Beaux-Arts de Nantes.* Vol. 1. Nantes, 1983.

Naples

1938   *La mostra della pittura napoletana dei secoli XVII–XVIII–XIX.* Exhibition sponsored by the Italian tourist information bureau. Catalogue by Sergio Ortolani. Naples, 1938.

1984   *Il patrimonio artistico del Banco di Napoli: Catalogo delle opere.* Exhibition, Museo e Gallerie Nazionali di Capodimonte, Naples. Catalogue introduction by Bruno Molajoli; edited by Nicola Spinosa; contributions by Riccardo Lattuada et al. Naples, 1984.

1984–85   *Civiltà del seicento a Napoli.* Exhibition, Museo di Capodimonte and Museo Pignatelli, Naples, 1984–85. Catalogue edited by Silvia Cassani. 2 vols. Naples, 1984.

1991–92   *Battistello Caracciolo e il primo naturalismo a Napoli.* Exhibition, Castel Sant'Elmo, Chiesa della Certosa di San Martino, Naples, November 9, 1991–January 19, 1992. Catalogue edited by Ferdinando Bologna, with contributions by Stefano Causa et al. Naples, 1991.

1992   *Jusepe de Ribera, 1591–1652.* Exhibition, Castel Sant'Elmo, Naples, February 27–May 17, 1992. Catalogue. Naples, 1992.

1994–95   *I tesori dei d'Avalos: Committenza e collezionismo di una grande famiglia napoletana.* Exhibition, Castel Sant'Elmo, Naples, October 22, 1994–May 22, 1995. Coordinator: Pierluigi Leone de Castris. Naples, 1994.

1997–98   *Capolavori in festa: Effimero barocco a largo di palazzo (1683–1759).* Exhibition, Palazzo Reale, Naples, December 20, 1997–March 15, 1998. Catalogue. Naples, 1997.

Nappi, Eduoardo

1983   "Pittori del '600 a Napoli: Notizie inedite dai documenti dell'Archivio Storico del Banco di Napoli." In *Ricerche sul '600 napoletano: Saggi vari.* Milan, 1983.

Nava Cellini, Antonia

1969   "Stefano Maderno, Francesco Vanni e Guido Reni a Santa Cecilia in Trastevere." *Paragone* 227 (1969), 18–41.

Negro, Emilio, and Massimo Pirondini, eds.

1995   *La scuola dei Carracci: I seguaci di Annibale e Agostino.* Modena, 1995.

Neppi, Lionello

1975   *Palazzo Spada.* Rome, 1975.

Neugass, Fritz

1963   "Neuerwerbungen amerikanischer Museen." *Die Weltkunst* 33, no. 17 (1963), 16–17.

New Haven–Sarasota–Kansas City

1987–88   *A Taste for Angels: Neapolitan Painting in North America, 1650–1750.* Exhibition, Yale University Art Gallery, New Haven, September 9–November 29, 1987; John and Mable Ringling Museum of Art, Sarasota, Florida, January 13–March 13, 1988; Nelson-Atkins Museum of Art, Kansas City, April 30–June 12, 1988. Catalogue. New Haven, 1987.

New York

1984   *Italian, Dutch, and Flemish Baroque Paintings.* Exhibition, Colnaghi, New York, April 4–May 5, 1984. Catalogue by Clovis Whitfield and Elaine Banks. New York, 1984.

1985   *Landscape Painting in Rome, 1595–1675.* Exhibition, Richard L. Feigen & Co., January 30–March 23, 1985. Catalogue by Ann Sutherland Harris, with contributions by Marcel Roethlisberger and Kahren Hellerstedt. New York, 1985.

1989   *Old Master Paintings.* Exhibition, Newhouse Galleries, Inc., New York, October–November, 1989. Catalogue. New York, 1989.

1990a   *A Caravaggio Rediscovered: The Lute Player.* Exhibition, The Metropolitan Museum of Art, New York, February 9–April 22, 1990. Catalogue by Keith Christiansen, with contributions by Andrea Bayer and Laurence Libin. New York, 1990.

1990b   *Italian Paintings.* Exhibition, Richard L. Feigen & Co., New York, June 12–July 27, 1990. Catalogue. New York, 1990.

1995–96   *Women in Art.* Exhibition, Wildenstein, New York, September 1, 1995–January 31, 1996. Catalogue. New York, 1995.

1998–99   *From Van Eyck to Bruegel: Early Netherlandish Painting in The Metropolitan Museum of Art.* Exhibition, The Metropolitan Museum of Art, New York, September 22, 1998–January 21, 1999. Catalogue edited by Maryan W. Ainsworth and Keith Christiansen. New York, 1998.

New York–Naples

1985   *The Age of Caravaggio.* Exhibition, The Metropolitan Museum of Art, New York, February 5–April 14, 1985; Museo Nazionale di Capodimonte, Naples, May 12–June 30, 1985. Catalogue by Keith Christiansen et al. New York, 1985.

Nicodemi, Giorgio

1914   "La Pinacoteca dell'Arcivescovado di Milano." *Rassegna d'arte* 14 (1914), 279–88.

1927   *Pier Francesco Mazzucchelli, detto "Il Morazzone."* Varese, 1927.

Nicolson, Benedict

1958   *Hendrick Terbrugghen.* London, 1958.

1960   "Some Little Known Pictures at the Royal Academy." *Burlington Magazine* 102 (1960), 76–79.

1970   "Caravaggesques in Florence." *Burlington Magazine* 112 (1970), 636–41.

1974   "Caravaggio and the Caravaggesques: Some Recent Research." *Burlington Magazine* 116 (1974), 603–19.

1979   *The International Caravaggesque Movement: Lists of Pictures by Caravaggio and His Followers throughout Europe from 1590 to 1650.* Oxford, 1979.

1985   "Orazio Gentileschi and Giovanni Antonio Sauli." *Artibus et historiae* 12 (1985), 9–25.

1990   *Caravaggism in Europe.* 2d ed., revised and enlarged by Luisa Vertova. 3 vols. Turin, 1990.

Novelli, Magda

1974   "Agostino Beltrano, uno 'stazionesco' da riabilitare." *Paragone* 25, no. 287 (1974), 67–82, pls. 49–58.

1974a   "Precisazioni cronologiche su Massimo Stanzione," by Magda Novelli Radice. *Campania sacra*, no. 5 (1974), 98–103.

1989   "Una traccia per Annella de Rosa." *Napoli nobilissima* 28 (1989), 147–54.

Nürnberg

1989   *Die Grafen von Schönborn: Kirchenfürsten, Sammler, Mäzene.* Exhibition, Germanisches National-museum, Nürnberg, February 18–April 23, 1989. Catalogue edited by Hermann Maué and Sonja Brink. Nürnberg, 1989.

Nuttall, W. L. F.

1965   "King Charles I's Pictures and the Common-wealth Sale." *Apollo* 82 (1965), 302–9.

Oertel, Robert

1960   "England und die Italienische Kunst." *Kunst-chronik* 13, no. 4 (1960), 89–97.

1971   "Von Gentileschi bis Boucher—Erwerbungen der Gemäldegalerie." *Jahrbuch der Stiftung preussicher Kulturbesitz* 9 (1971), 235–48.

Orbaan, Johannes A. F.

1919   "Der Abbruch Alt-Sankt-Peters, 1605–1615." *Jahrbuch der Königlich Preussischen Kunst-sammlungen* 39 (1919), 1–139.

1920   *Documenti sul barocco in Roma.* Rome, 1920.

Rome–Siena

2000–   *Colori della musica: Dipinti, strumenti e*
2001   *concerti tra cinquecento e seicento.* Exhibition, Galleria Nazionale d'Arte Antica, Palazzo Barberini, Rome, December 15, 2000– February 28, 2001; Santa Maria della Scala, Siena, April 6–June 17, 2001. Catalogue edited by Annalisa Bini, Claudio Strinati, and Rossella Vodret. Milan, 2000.

Ronot, Henry

1990   *Richard et Jean Tassel: Peintres à Langres au XVIIe siècle.* Paris, 1990.

Rosci, Marco

1965   *Orazio Gentileschi.* I maestri del colore, no. 83. Milan, 1965.

Rosière, François de

1580   *Stemmatum Lotharingiae ac Barri Ducum. . . .* Paris, 1580.

Rossi, Attilio

1907   "Le opere d'arte del monastero di Tor de' Specchi in Roma." *Bollettino d'arte* I (1907), 4–22.

Röthlisberger, Marcel

1995   "From Goffredo Wals to the Beginnings of Claude Lorrain." *Artibus et historiae* 16, no. 32 (1995), 9–37.

Röttgen, Herwarth

1992   *Caravaggio: Der irdische amor; oder, Der Sieg der fleischlichen Liebe.* Frankfurt am Main, 1992.

Rovi, Alberto

1992   "Precocità del Gentileschi di Brera." *Arte lombarda* 101, no. 2 (1992), 107–9.

Ruotolo, Renato

1982   *Mercanti-collezionisti fiamminghi a Napoli: Gaspare Roomer e i Vandeneynden.* Naples, 1982.

Ryley Marshall, David

1993   *Viviano and Niccolò Codazzi and the Baroque Architectural Fantasy.* Milan, 1993.

Safarik, Eduard A.

1996   *Collezione dei dipinti Colonna: Inventari, 1611–1795.* With the assistance of Cinzia Pujia; edited by Anna Cera Sones. Munich, 1996.

Sainsbury, William Noël

1859a   "Artists' Quarrels in Charles I's Reign." *Notes and Queries,* ser. 2, 8 (1859), 121–22.

1859b   as editor. *Original Unpublished Papers Illustrative of the Life of Sir Peter Paul Rubens as an Artist and a Diplomatist. . . .* London, 1859.

Salerno, Luigi

1956   See Rome 1956–57.

1960   "The Picture Gallery of Vincenzo Giustiniani: Inventory," parts 1, 2. *Burlington Magazine* 102 (1960), 93–104, 135–48.

1965   *Palazzo Rondinini.* Rome, 1965.

1977–80   *Pittori di paesaggio del seicento a Roma / Landscape Painters of the Seventeenth Century in Rome.* 3 vols. Rome, 1977–80.

1988   *I dipinti del Guercino.* Rome, 1988.

Salerno

1954–55   *Opere d'arte nel salernitano dal XII al XVIII secolo.* Exhibition, Duomo di Salerno, Aula 'San Tommaso,' September 1954–September 1955. Catalogue by Ferdinando Bologna. Naples, 1955.

Sales, Saint Francis of,

1892   *Oeuvres de Saint François de Sales.* Vol. 10. Annecy, 1892.

Salonika

1997   *Michelangelo Merisi da Caravaggio e i suoi primi seguaci.* Exhibition, Salonika, 1997.

Salvatori, Gaia

1999   "La sindrome delle muse: Motivi, problemi e orientamenti della critica sulle donne artiste del seicento europeo." In *Donne e filosofia nel seicento europeo,* edited by Pina Totaro, 393–434. Rome, 1999.

Samek Ludovici, Sergio

1956   *Vita del Caravaggio dalle testimonianze del suo tempo.* Milan, 1956.

San Severino Marche–Bologna

1988   *Giovan Francesco Guerrieri: Dipinti e disegni; un accostamento all'opera.* Exhibition, Palazzo di Città, San Severino Marche; San Giorgio in Poggiale, Bologna. Catalogue by Sergio Anselmi, Andrea Emiliani, and Giovanni Sapori; appendix by Augusto Vernarecci. Bologna, 1988.

Sánchez Cantón, F. J.

1933   *Fuentes literarias para la historia del arte español.* Vol. 2. Madrid, 1933.

Sandrart, Joachim von

1925   *Academie der Bau-, Bild- und Mahlerey-Künste von 1675: Leben der berühmten Maler, Bildhauer und Baumeister.* Edited by Adolf R. Peltzer. Munich, 1925.

Santi, Francesco

1976   "Una tela di Orazio Gentileschi in Umbria." *Bollettino d'arte,* ser. 5, 41 (1976), 43–44.

Santini, G.

1969   *Gente anconetana.* Fano, 1969.

Santoni, Alessandro

1884   *Guida di Ancona.* Ancona, 1884.

Santore, Cathy

1991   "Danaë: The Renaissance Courtesan's Alter Ego." *Zeitschrift für Kunstgeschichte* 54 (1991), 412–27.

Saracini, Giuliano

1675   *Notitie historiche della citta d'Ancona gia termine dell'antico regno d'Italia con diuersi auuenimenti nella Marca Anconitana, & in detto regno accaduti.* Rome, 1675.

Sarrazin, Béatrice

1994   *Catalogue raisonné des peintures italiennes du Musée des Beaux-Arts de Nantes, XIIIe–XVIIIe siècle.* Paris, 1994.

Sassi, Romualdo

1889   *Il "chi è?" Fabrianese.* Fabriano, 1889.

1923–24   "Sonetti di poeti fabrianesi in onore di Gentile da Fabriano." *Rassegna marchigiana* 2 (1923–24), 273–82.

1926   "Le origini e il primo incremento del monastero olivetano di Santa Caterina di Fabriano." *Rivista storica benedettina* 17 (1926).

1926–27   "Arti e storia tra le rovine di un antico tempio francescano." *Rassegna marchigiana* 10 (1926–27), 105.

1928–29   "Chiese artistiche di Fabriano: S. Lucia." *Rassegna marchigiana* 7 (1928–29), 13–19, 45–53, 90–110.

1932   "Chiese artistiche di Fabriano: San Benedetto, II." *Rassegna marchigiana* 10 (1932), 143–66.

1939   *Il culto di S. Carlo Borromeo e de S. Venanzo Martire a Fabriano.* Excerpted from vol. 14 of *Studia Picena.* Fano, 1939.

1951   *La prima Università dei Cartari di Fabriano e la sua chiesa di Santa Maria Maddalena.* Milan, 1951.

1952a   "Echi degli Anni Santi a Fabriano." *Studia picena* 25 (1952).

1952b   "I primi documenti della cattedrale e del capitolo di San Venanzio." *Atti e memorie della Deputazione di Storia Patria delle Marche* 7 (1952).

1954   "La fine del monastero olivetano di Santa Caterina di Fabriano." *Rivista storica benedettina* 33 (1954).

Sassoferrato

1990   *Giovan Battista Salvi, "Il Sassoferrato."* Exhibition, Chiesa di San Francesco, Sassoferrato, June 29–October 14, 1990. Catalogue by François Macé de Lépinay, Pietro Zampetti, and Silvia Cuppini Sassi. Milan, 1990.

Scavizzi, Giuseppe

1963   *Caravaggio e i caravaggeschi.* Naples, 1963.

1974   "La teologia cattolica e le immagini durante il XVI secolo." *Storia dell'arte* 21 (1974), 171–212.

Schiller, Gertrude

1971–72   *Iconography of Christian Art.* 2 vols. Translated by Janet Seligman. Greenwich, Connecticut, 1972.

Schleier, Erich

1962   "An Unknown Altar-piece by Orazio Gentileschi." *Burlington Magazine* 104 (1962), 432–36.

1970a   "Panico, Gentileschi, and Lanfranco at San Salvatore in Farnese." *Art Bulletin* 52 (1970), 172–77.

1970b   "Pintura italiana del siglo XVII." *Kunstchronik* 23 (1970), 341–49.

1971   "Caravaggio e i caravaggeschi nelle gallerie di Firenze." *Kunstchronik* 24 (1971), 85–102.

1989   "La pittura del seicento a Roma." In Gregori and Schleier 1989, vol. 1, 399–460.

1993   "Orazio Gentileschis 'Verspottung Christi.'" *Pantheon* 51 (1993), 196–200.

2000   "An Unknown *St. Catherine of Alexandria* by (or after?) Orazio Gentileschi." *Gazette des Beaux-Arts,* ser. 6, 135 (February 2000), 167–70.

Schloder, John E.

1982   "Un artiste oublié: Nicolas Prévost, peintre de Richelieu." *Bulletin de la Société de l'Histoire de l'Art Français,* 1982, 59–60.

Schnapper, Antoine

1990   "La cour de France au XVIIe siècle et la peinture italienne contemporaine." In *Seicento: La peinture italienne du XVIIe siècle et la France,* 423–37. Paris, 1990.

1994   *Curieux du Grand Siècle, Collections et collectionneurs dans la France du XVIIe siècle.* Paris, 1994.

Schütze, Sebastian, and Thomas Willette

1992   *Massimo Stanzione: L'opera completa.* Naples, 1992.

Segovia

2000   *El Real Sitio de La Granja de San Ildefonso: Retrato y escena del Rey.* Exhibition, La Granja de San Ildefonso, Segovia, June 23–September 17, 2000. Organized by Delfin Rodríguez Ruíz. Madrid, 2000.

Sella, Domenico

2000   *L'Italia del seicento.* Rome, 2000.

Sestieri, Giancarlo, and Brigitte Daprà

1994   *Domenico Gargiulo detto Micco Spadaro, paesaggista e 'cronista' napoletano.* Milan, 1994.

Settis, Salvatore

1985   "Danae verso il 1495." In *I Tatti Studies: Essays in the Renaissance,* vol. 1, 207–37. Florence, 1985.

Seville

1973   *Caravaggio y el naturalismo español.* Exhibition, Sala de Armas de los Reales Alcazares, Seville, September–October 1973. Catalogue by Alfonso E. Pérez Sánchez. Seville, 1973.

Shapley, Fern Rusk

1973   *Paintings from the Samuel H. Kress Collection. Italian Schools, XVI–XVIII Century.* London, 1973.

1979 *Catalogue of the Italian Paintings. National Gallery of Art, Washington.* Washington, D.C., 1979.

Shearman, John

1979 "Cristofano Allori's *Judith.*" *Burlington Magazine* 121 (1979), 3–10.

Siena

1978 *Rutilio Manetti, 1571–1639.* Exhibition, Palazzo Pubblico, Siena, June 15–October 15, 1978. Catalogue edited by Alessandro Bagnoli. Florence, 1978.

Sinisi, S.

1963 "Il Palazzo Santacroce ai Catinari." *Palatino* 8 (1963).

Skrine, Henry Duncan

1887 *The Manuscripts of Henry Duncan Skrine, Esq. Salvetti Correspondence.* Historical Manuscripts Commission 11th Report, Appendix 1. London, 1887.

Slap, Joseph

1985 "Artemisia Gentileschi: Further Notes." *American Imago* 42, no. 3 (1985), 335–42.

Sofri, A.

1979 "La vedova, il generale e la metà del regno." *Lotta continua,* December 10, 1979, 16–17.

Solerti, Angelo

1905 *Musica, ballo e drammatica alla corte Medicea dal 1600 al 1637.* Florence, 1905.

Soprani, Raffaele

1674 *Le vite de' pittori, scoltori, et architetti genovesi. . . .* Genoa, 1674.

1768 *See* Ratti 1768.

Spear, Richard E.

1971 "Caravaggisti at the Palazzo Pitti." *Art Quarterly* 34, no. 1 (1971), 108–10.

1982 *Domenichino.* 2 vols. New Haven, 1982.

1989a Review of Garrard 1989. *Times Literary Supplement,* June 2–8, 1989, 603–4.

1989b "Re-viewing the 'Divine' Guido." *Burlington Magazine* 131 (1989), 367–72.

1994 "Guercino's 'Prix-fixe': Observations on Studio Practices and Art Marketing in Emilia." *Burlington Magazine* 136 (1994), 592–602.

1997 *The "Divine" Guido: Religion, Sex, Money, and Art in the World of Guido Reni.* New Haven, 1997.

2000 "Artemisia Gentileschi: Ten Years of Fact and Fiction." *Art Bulletin* 82 (2000), 568–79.

Spezzaferro, Luigi

1975 "Una testimonianza per gli inizi del caravaggismo." *Storia dell'arte* 23 (1975), 53–60.

1975a "Ottavio Costa e Caravaggio: Certezze e problemi." In Cinotti 1975.

1981 "Il recupero del Rinascimento." In *Storia dell'arte italiana. Parte seconda: Dal cinquecento all'ottocento,* vol. 1, *Cinquecento e seicento,* edited by Federico Zeri, 185–274. Turin, 1981.

1985 "Un imprenditore del primo seicento: Giovanni Battista Crescenzi." *Ricerche di storia dell'arte* 26 (1985), 50–73.

Spike, John

1991a "The Gentileschi Papers." *Journal of Art* 4, no. 9 (1991).

1991b Review of Florence 1991. *Burlington Magazine* 133 (1991), 732–34.

Spinosa, Nicola, ed.

1984 *La pittura napoletana del '600.* Milan, 1984.

1994 *Museo Nazionale di Capodimonte.* With contributions by Luisa Ambrosio et al. Naples, 1994.

Sricchia, Fiorella

1963 "Lorenzo Lippi nello svolgimento della pittura fiorentina della prima metà del '600." *Proporzioni* 4 (1963), 242–70, pls. 162–99, figs. 1–68.

Sricchia Santoro, Fiorella

1974 "La Madonna di Pistoia e l'attività romana di Anastasio Fontebuoni." *Commentari* 25 (1974), 29–46.

Stassi, Maria Gabriele, ed.

1995 *Opere di Federico Della Valle.* Turin, 1995.

Stefaniak, R.

1991 "Raphael's *Santa Cecilia:* A Fine and Private Version of Virginity." *Art History* 14, no. 3 (1991), 345–71.

Sterling, Charles

1958 "Gentileschi in France." *Burlington Magazine* 100 (1958), 112–21.

1964 "Une nouvelle oeuvre de Gentileschi peinte en France." *La revue du Louvre et des musées de France* 14 (1964), 217–20.

Stocker, Margarita

1998 *Judith, Sexual Warrior: Woman and Power in Western Culture.* New Haven, 1998.

Stolzenwald, Susanna

1991 *Artemisia Gentileschi: Bindung und Befreiung in Leben und Werk einer Malerin.* Stuttgart, 1991.

Stoughton, Michael

1985 Review of Cleveland–Fort Worth–Naples 1984 –85. *Burlington Magazine* 127 (1985), 193–94.

Strinati, Claudio

1974 "Gli anni difficili di Federico Zuccari." *Storia dell'arte* 21 (1974), 85–116.

1980 "Roma nell'anno 1600: Studio di pittura." *Ricerche di storia dell'arte* 10 (1980), 15–48.

2000 "Per una storia del *naturalismo* a Roma, in attesa del Caravaggio." In *Il cinquecento lombardo: Da Leonardo a Caravaggio,* edited by Flavio Caroli, 51–61. Milan, 2000.

Stryienski, Casimir

1913 *La Galerie du Régent Philippe, duc d'Orléans.* Paris, 1913.

Suida, Wilhelm

1906 *Genua.* Leipzig, 1906.

Sutton, Denys

1959 *Christie's since the War, 1945–1958: An Essay on Taste, Patronage, and Collecting.* London, 1959.

Sykes, Susan Alexandra

1991 "Henrietta Maria's 'house of delight.'" *Apollo* 133 (1991), 332–36.

Symonds, Henry

1913 "English Mint Engravers of the Tudor and Stuart Periods, 1485 to 1688." *Numismatic Chronicle and Journal of the Royal Numismatic Society,* ser. 4, 13 (1913), 349–77.

Szigethi, Agnes

1979 "Quelques contributions à l'art d'Artemisia Gentileschi." *Bulletin du Musée Hongrois des Beaux-Arts,* no. 52 (1979), 35–44.

Tagliaferro, Laura

1995 *La magnificenza privata: "Argenti, gioie, quadri e altri mobili" della famiglia Brignole Sale, secoli XVI–XIX.* Genoa, 1995.

Tanfani-Centofanti, Leopoldo

1897 *Notizie di artisti tratte dai documenti pisani.* Pisa, 1897.

Taylor, John Russell

1999 "Father in the Spotlight" (review of London–Bilbao–Madrid 1999). *The Times* (London), March 15, 1999.

Teodosiu, Anatolie

1974 *Catalogul Galeriei de Artă Universală.* Vol. 1, *Pictura italiană.* Bucharest, 1974.

Testa, Laura

1998 "Presenze caravaggesche nella collezione Savelli." *Storia dell'arte,* no. 93/94 (1998), 348–52.

2000 "Le collezioni Aldobrandini all'inizio del seicento." Ph.D. dissertation, Università di Roma "La Sapienza," 2000.

Thuillier, Jacques

1960 "Poussin et ses premiers compagnons français à Rome." In *Nicolas Poussin,* vol. 1. Paris: Centre National de la Recherche Scientifique Colloques Internationaux, 1960.

1998 "The Thirty Years' War and the Arts." In Münster–Osnabrück 1998–99, vol. 2, 15–27.

Tiberia, Vitaliano

1973 "Una notizia sul Gentileschi e sugli pittori alla Madonna dei Monti." *Storia dell'arte* 17 (1973), 181–84.

Titi, Filippo

1675 *Studio di pittura, scoltura, e architettura, nelle chiese di Roma.* Rome, 1675.

Toesca, Illaria

1960a "Un documento del 1595 sul Gentileschi." *Paragone* 123 (1960), 59–60.

1960b "Due telle del 1607 in S. Silvestro in Capite a Roma." *Bollettino d'arte* 45 (1960), 283–86.

Topper, David, and Cynthia Gillis

1996 "Trajectories of Blood: Artemisia Gentileschi and Galileo's Parabolic Path." *Women's Art Journal* 17, no. 1 (spring/summer 1996), 10–13.

Torriti, Piero

1971 *Tesori di Strada Nuova: La via Aurea dei Genovesi.* Genoa, 1971.

Trapier, Elizabeth du Gué

1967 "Sir Arthur Hopton and the Interchange of Paintings between Spain and England in the Seventeenth Century." *Connoisseur* 164, no. 662 (1967), 239–43.

Tufts, Eleanor

1974 *Our Hidden Heritage: Five Centuries of Women Artists.* New York, 1974.

Turin

1963 *Mostra del Barocco piemontese.* Exhibition, Palazzo Madama, Palazzo Reale, Palazzina di Stupinigi, Turin, June 22–November 10, 1963. Catalogue edited by Vittorio Viale. 3 vols. Turin, 1963.

Turner, Richard

2000 *Roman Baroque Drawings (Italian Drawings in the Department of Prints and Drawings in the British Museum).* London, 2000.

Tyndale, William

1848 "The Obedience of a Christian Man." In *Doctrinal Treatises, . . .* edited by Henry Walter. Cambridge, 1848.

Urbino

1953 *Antichi dipinti restaurati della Soprintendenza alle gallerie delle Marche: Catalogo e presentazione.* Exhibition, Palazzo Ducale, Urbino, March 29–April 11, 1953. Catalogue by Pietro Zampetti. Urbino, 1953.

1968 *Mostra di opere d'arte restaurate.* Exhibition, Palazzo Ducale, Urbino. Catalogue edited by Filippa Maria Aliberti Gaudioso. Urbino, 1968.

1992 *Piero e Urbino: Piero e le corti rinascimentali.* Exhibition, Palazzo Ducale, Urbino, July 24–October 31, 1992. Catalogue edited by Paolo Dal Poggetto. Venice, 1992.

Utrecht–Braunschweig

1986–87   *Holländische Malerei in neuem Licht: Hendrick ter Brugghen und seine Zeitgenossen.* Exhibition, Centraal Museum Utrecht, November 13, 1986–January 12, 1987; Herzog Anton Ulrich-Museum Braunschweig, February 12–April 12, 1987. Catalogue by Albert Blankert and Leonard J. Slatkes, with contributions by Marten Jan Bok et al. Braunschweig, 1986.

Valdivieso, Enrique

1978   *Catálogo de las pinturas de la Catedral de Sevilla.* Seville, 1978.

Valentiner, William R.

1935   "Judith with the Head of Holofernes." *Detroit Institute of Art Bulletin* 14, no. 8 (May 1935), 102–4.

Valletta

1949   *The Madonna in Art.* Exhibition, Valletta, Malta, 1949.

Valli, F.

1988   "Saint Catherine of Alexandria." In Bologna–Los Angeles–Fort Worth 1988–89, 186.

Vannugli, Antonio

1991   "Stanzione, Gentileschi, Finoglia: Serie de San Juan Bautista para el Buen Retiro." *Boletín del Museo del Prado* 10, 1989 (1991), 25–33.

1994   "Stanzione, Gentileschi, Finoglia: Le Storie di San Giovanni Battista per il Buen Retiro." *Storia dell'arte* 80 (1994), 59–73.

Varriano, John

1999   "Caravaggio and Violence." *Storia dell'arte* 97 (1999), 317–32.

Vasari, Giorgio

1568   *Le vite de' più eccellenti pittori, scultori, e architettori. . . .* 2d ed. 3 vols. Florence, 1568.

1878–85   *Le vite de' più eccellenti pittori, scultori, ed architettori. . . .* Based on the 1568 ed., with annotations and comments by Gaetano Milanesi. 9 vols. Florence, 1878–85.

1962–66   *Le vite de' più eccellenti pittori, scultori, et architettori. . . .* 9 vols. 1568 text, edited and with notes by Paola Della Pergola, Luigi Grassi, and Giovanni Previtali. Milan, 1962–66.

Vaudo, Erasmo

1976   *Scipione Pulzone da Gaeta, pittore.* Gaeta, 1976.

Venditti, A.

1979   "Cavagna, G. B." In *Dizionario biografico degli Italiani*, vol. 22, 560–63. Rome, 1979.

Venturi, Adolfo

1882   *La R. Galleria Estense in Modena.* Modena, 1882.

1921   *Guida alle gallerie di Roma.* Rome, 1921.

Venturi, Lionello

1910   "Studi su Michelangelo da Caravaggio." *L'arte* 13 (1910), 268–84.

Vertue, George

1931–32   *Vertue Note Books.* Vol. 2. Walpole Society, vol. 20 (1931–32). Oxford, 1932.

1935–36   *Vertue Note Books.* vol. 4. Walpole Society, vol. 24 (1935–36). Oxford, 1936.

Vicini, Maria Lucrezia

1992   "L'eredità Veralli e Rocci." In Cannatà and Vicini 1992.

1998   as editor. *Guida alla Galleria Spada.* Rome, 1998.

1999   *La famiglia Spada Veralli: Ritratto della Marchesa Maria Veralli e di cinque suoi figli.* Rome, 1999.

2000   *Orazio e Artemisia Gentileschi alla Galleria Spada: Padre e figlia a confronto.* Rome, 2000.

Vienna

1954   *Gemälde-Galerie: Die italienischen, spanischen, französischen und englischen Malerschulen.* Vienna, 1954.

1991   *Die Gemäldegalerie des Kunsthistorisches Museum in Wien: Verzeichnis der Gemälde.* Vienna, 1991.

Villari, Rosario

1976   *La rivolta antispagnola a Napoli: Le origini (1585–1647).* Rome, 1976.

Viotti, L.

1979   Review of Greer 1979. *Lotta continua*, December 12, 1979.

Visceglia, Maria Antonietta, ed.

1992   *Signori, patrizi, cavalieri in Italia centro-meridionale nell'età moderna.* Edited by Maria Antonietta Visceglia, with contributions by Renata Ago et al. Rome, 1992.

Volpe, Carlo

1970   "Caravaggio e caravaggeschi nelle gallerie di Firenze." *Paragone* 21, no. 249 (1970), 106–8.

1972   "Annotazioni sulla mostra caravaggesca di Cleveland." *Paragone* 23, no. 263 (1972), 50–76.

Voss, Hermann

1911   "Spätitalienische Bilder in der Gemäldesammlung des Herzoglichen Museums zu Braunschweig." *Münchner Jahrbuch der bildenden Kunst* 6 (1911), 235–55.

1911a   "Kritische Bemerkungen zu Seicentisten in den Römischen Galerien." *Repertorium für Kunstwissenschaft* 34 (1911), 119–25.

1912   "Italienishe Gemälde des 16. und 17. Jahrhunderts in der Galerie des Kunsthistorischen Hoffmuseums zu Wien." *Zeitschrift für bildende Kunst* 23 (1912), 62–67.

1920a   "Gentileschi, Orazio." In *Allgemeines Lexikon der bildenden Künstler von der Antike bis zur Gegenwart*, edited by Ulrich Thieme and Felix Becker, vol. 13, 410–12. Leipzig, 1920.

1920b   *Die Malerei der Spätrenaissance in Rom und Florenz.* Berlin, 1920.

1925   *Die Malerei des Barock in Rom.* Berlin, 1925.

1929   "Elsheimers 'Heilige Familie mit Engeln'—eine Neuerwerbung der Gemäldegalerie." *Berliner Museen* 50, no. 2 (1929), 20–27.

1959   "Orazio Gentileschi: Four Versions of His 'Rest into Egypt.'" *Connoisseur* 144 (November 1959), 163–65.

1960–61   "La Cappella del Crocifisso di Orazio Gentileschi." *Acropoli* 1, no. 2 (1960–61), 99–107.

1960–61a   "Venere e Amore di Artemisia Gentileschi." *Acropoli* 1, no. 1 (1960–61), 79–82.

Vsevolozhskaia, Svetlana N., and Al'bert G. Kostenevich

1984   *Italian Painting* [in the Hermitage]. Leningrad, 1984.

Vsevolozhskaia, Svetlana N., and Irina V. Linnik

1975   *Caravaggio and His Followers.* Translated by V. Vorontsov and Y. Nemetsky. Leningrad, 1975.

Waagen, Gustav F.

1843–45   *Kunstwerke und Künstler in Deutschland.* 2 vols. in 1. Leipzig, 1843–45.

1854   *Treasures of Art in Great Britain.* London, 1854.

Wachenfeld, Christa, and Roland Barthes

1992   *Die Vergewaltigung der Artemisia: Der Prozess.* Freiburg, 1992.

Waddingham, Malcolm R.

1961   "Alla ricerca di Agostino Tassi." *Paragone* 139 (1961), 9–23.

1972   "Elsheimer Revised." *Burlington Magazine* 114 (1972), 600–611.

Wagner, Hugo

1958   *Michelangelo da Caravaggio.* Bern, 1958.

Walpole, Horace

1826–28   *Anecdotes of Painting in England with Some Account of the Principal Artists and Incidental Notes on Other Arts; Collected by the Late Mr. George Vertue.* With contributions by the Reverend James Dallaway. 5 vols. London, 1826–28.

Warsaw

1990   *Opus Sacrum: Catalogue of the Exhibition from the Collection of Barbara Piasecka Johnson.* Exhibition, Royal Castle, Warsaw. Catalogue edited by Józef Grabski. Warsaw, 1990.

Washington

1991   See Bologna and other cities 1991–92.

1998   *Lavinia Fontana of Bologna, 1552–1614.* Exhibition, National Museum of Women, Washington, D.C., February 5–June 7, 1998. Catalogue by Vera Fortunati. Washington, D.C., 1998.

Washington–Cincinnati

1988–89   *Masterworks from Munich: Sixteenth- to Eighteenth-Century Paintings from the Alte Pinakothek.* Exhibition, National Gallery of Art, Washington, D.C., May 29–September 5, 1988; Cincinnati Art Museum, October 25, 1988–January 8, 1989. Catalogue by Beverly Louise Brown and Arthur K. Wheelock Jr. Washington, D.C., 1988.

Waźbiński, Zygmunt

1994   *Il Cardinale Francesco Maria Del Monte, 1549–1626.* 2 vols. Florence, 1994.

Weber, Christoph

1994   *Legati e governatori dello Stato Pontificio (1550–1809).* Rome, 1994.

Weizsäcker, Heinrich

1952   *Adam Elsheimer: Der Maler von Frankfurt.* Vol. 2, *Beschreibende Verzeichnisse und geschichtliche Quellen.* Edited by H. Möhle. Berlin, 1952.

Weston-Lewis, Aidan

1997   "Orazio Gentileschi's Two Versions of *The Finding of Moses* Reassessed." *Apollo* 145 (1997), 27–35.

Whinney, Margaret Dickens, and Oliver Millar

1957   *English Art, 1625–1713.* Oxford, 1957.

White, Christopher

1982   *The Dutch Pictures in the Collection of Her Majesty the Queen.* Cambridge, 1982.

Wiedmann, G.

1979   "Il conte Simone Alaleona marchigiano al seguito dei principi Savelli." *Studi Picena* 46 (1979), 67–83.

Wilson, Michael I.

1994   *Nicholas Lanier: Master of the King's Musick.* Aldershot, Hampshire, and Brookfield, Vermont, 1994.

Wittkower, Rudolf

1958   *Art and Architecture in Italy, 1600–1750.* Baltimore, 1958.

Wittkower, Rudolf, and Irma B. Jaffe, eds.

1972   *Baroque Art: The Jesuit Contribution.* New York, 1972.

Wittkower, Rudolf, and Margot Wittkower

1963   *Born under Saturn: The Character and Conduct of Artists. A Documented History from Antiquity to the French Revolution.* New York, 1963.

Wood, Carolyn H.

1992   "The Ludovisi Collection of Paintings in 1623." *Burlington Magazine* 134 (1992), 515–23.

Wood, Jeremy

2000– "Orazio Gentileschi and Some Netherlandish
2001   Artists in London: The Patronage of the Duke
    of Buckingham, Charles I, and Henrietta
    Maria." *Simiolus* 28, no. 3 (2000–2001), 103–28.

Woods-Marsden, Joanna

1998 *Renaissance Self-Portraiture: The Visual
    Construction of Identity and the Social Status of
    the Artist.* New Haven, 1998.

Wrede, Kristina von

1978 "Braunschweig erwarb einen Gentileschi."
    Weltkunst 45 (1978).

Wurzbach, Alfred von

1910 *Niederländisches Künstler-Lexikon; auf Grund
    archivalischer Forschungen bearbeitet.* Vol. 2.
    Vienna and Leipzig, 1910.

Zampetti, Pietro

1990 *Pittura nelle Marche.* Vol. 3, *Dalla Controriforma
    al Barocco.* Florence, 1990.

Zarucchi, J.

1998–99 "The Gentileschi Danaë: A Narrative of Rape."
    Woman's Art Journal, fall 1998–winter 1999, 13–16.

Zeri, Federico

1954 *La Galleria Spada in Roma: Catalogo dei dipinti.*
    Florence, 1954.

1957 *Pittura e Controriforma: L'arte senza tempo di
    Scipione da Gaeta.* Turin, 1957.

1959 *La Galleria Pallavicini in Roma: Catalogo dei
    dipinti.* Florence, 1959.

1970 *Pittura e Controriforma: L'arte senza tempo di
    Scipione da Gaeta.* Turin, 1970.

Zonghi, Aurelio, ed.

1990 *Documenti storici fabrianesi.* Statutas artis lanae.
    Rome, 1990.

Zuccari, Alessandro

1981a "La politica culturale dell'Oratorio romano
    nella seconda metà del cinquecento." *Storia
    dell'arte* 41 (1981), 77–112.

1981b "La politica culturale dell'Oratorio romano
    nelle imprese artistice promosse da Cesare
    Baronio." *Storia dell'arte* 42 (1981), 171–93.

1984 *Arte e committenza nella Roma di Caravaggio.*
    Turin, 1984.

1992 *I pittori di Sisto V.* Rome, 1992.

1993 "La Biblioteca Vaticana e i pittori Sistini." In
    Rome 1993, 59–76.

1995 "Cultura e predicazione nelle immagini
    dell'Oratorio." *Storia dell'arte* 85 (1995), 340–54.

1999 as editor. *La storia dei Giubilei.* Vol. 3, *1600–1775.*
    Florence, 1999.

2000 "I Toscani a Roma: Committenza e 'riforma'
    pittorica da Gregorio XIII a Clemente VIII." In
    Storia delle arti in Toscana: Il cinquecento, edited
    by Roberto Paolo Ciardi and Antonio Natali,
    137–66. Florence, 2000.

Zuccari, Federico

1607 *L'idea de' pittori, scultori et architetti.* Turin,
    1607.

Zucchini, Guido

1938 *Catalogo delle collezioni comunali d'arte di
    Bologna.* Bologna, 1938.

Zürich

1958 *Die Frau als Künstlerin: Werke aus vier Jahr-
    hunderten.* Exhibition, Helmhaus, Zürich, July 2–
    August 31, 1958. Catalogue by Ursula Isler-
    Hungerbühler. Zürich, 1958.

General Index

Sampierdarena, 167–68; Palazzo Gentile, 166, 189; Palazzo Lomellini, 168; Palazzo Negroni, 167; Palazzo Spinola, 166

Gentile, Pietro Maria I, 11, 97, 98, 166, 170, 179, 189

Gentile, Pietro Maria III, 97, 189

Gentile da Fabriano, 126, 136, 152

Gentileschi, Artemisia: artistic training, 27, 255, 288–89, 313; character and stereotypes of, 249–50; collaborations, 290, 384–86, 408; as diplomat, 270; in England, 230, 258–59; fame of, in her own time, 263, 268–69, 270–71, 275, 278–79, 283; feminist interest in, 249–51; in Florence, 269–70, 283, 313–19, 328–30, 335–43; husband and children of, 335; illiteracy of, and education, 289–90, 313, 314, 326; learned friends of, 314–15; marriage of, 264; as a model, possibly for her father, 11, 98, 188, 274–75, 286, 290–91; models, use of, 273–75, 288–89; in Naples, 258–59, 269, 270, 283, 342, 379–91; portraits of, 11, 188, 268, 283, 315, 320, 322, 339, 418, figs. 95, 119; rape of, by Agostino Tassi, accusation, trial, and consequences, 3, 11, 18, 98, 119, 249, 254, 263, 264, 272, 274, 284, 286, 287–88, 296–98, 302, 310, 432–44; in Rome, 283–95, 335–43; in Venice, 268–69, 317–18, 335, 342

Gentileschi, Francesco, 4, 10, 30, 167–68, 198, 225, 226, 238, 286, 288; art of, 230; Man Playing a Guitar (Carige collection, Genoa), 170

Gentileschi, Giulio, 168, 225, 226, 227

Gentileschi, Marco, 225, 226

Gentileschi, Orazio, 45, 337; and antiquarianism, 82, 150, 198; appearance, 3, 10; and Baglione's libel suit, 88, 255, 275; and Baroque style, 31–36; and Caravaggio, friendship and collaborations, 255; character of, 4–5, 216; collection of prints, 27; collectors and patrons, 12–19, 117–26, 251; colorito, 8–9; as diplomatic agent, 223–24, 270; and earlier art, 35, 68, 126, 148, 152; in England, 217, 223–31; Florentine art, relation to, 118; in France, 203–13, 216; in Genoa, 165–71, 172, 218, 256–57, 337; gesture, use of, 240, 242–44; households of, 134, 274–75, 283–95; light, use of, 8, 20, 67–68; models, use of, 9–12, 20, 62, 66, 68, 91, 94–96, 98, 109, 130, 153, 200, 235; multiple versions of compositions, 20–27; patrons of, 12–19, 117–24, 165–68, 224–27; portrait of, 3, 5, 230, fig. 1; recycling of figures, 154, 183; religious art, character of, 34, 66–70, 126–27, 148–50, 152–53; studio of, 9–10, 288

Gerbier, Balthazar, 203, 217–18, 225–27, 232, 241

Ghidoni, Giovan Battista, various works, 315

Gigli, Giacinto, 339

Gilio da Fabriano, Giovanni Andrea, 68, 136, 152, 200

Giordano, Luca, 386

Giorgione, 19, 244; Portrait of Laura (Kunsthistorisches Museum, Vienna), 246

Giovanni d'Ancona, 118

Giovanni da San Giovanni, 372

Gisberti, Michele, 118

Giustiniani, Cardinal Benedetto, 7, 46, 339

Giustiniani, Marchese Vincenzo, 7, 21, 27, 46, 47, 80, 94, 130, 339

Giustiniani collection, 89

Giustiniani family, 44, 284

Goltzius, Hendrick, 408

Gonzaga, Cardinal Ferdinando, 176, 206

Gonzaga, Vincenzo I, fourth duke of Mantua, 10, 20, 67, 91, 119–21, 146, 225

Gonzaga family, 205

Goujon, Jean, 235; Nymphs, 205

Gramatica, Antiveduto, 46, 284, 337, 339, 341; Judith and Her Maidservant with the Head of Holofernes (Nationalmuseum, Stockholm), 46, 84, 342, 342, fig. 120

Gregory XIII Boncompagni, Pope, 39

Gregory XV Ludovisi, Pope, 19, 172, 256–57, 335–36, 337, 341

Griffio, Orazio, 110–12, 123

Guarini, Giovanni Battista, 386; Il pastor fido (play), 397

Guarino, Francesco, 255, 382, 387, 408, 426; works: copy after Stanzione's Annunciation to Zacharias, 407; Saint Agatha (Museo di San Martino, Naples), 388; Saint Cecilia (private collection), 387; Saint Christina (Museo Civico, Pesaro), 387, 387, fig. 136

Guercino, 9, 21, 113, 162, 166, 178, 188, 208, 223, 242–44, 257, 258, 337, 339, 340, 356, 395, 424; works: Jael and Sisera, copy after (location unknown), 346, 346, fig. 122; Lot and His Daughters (Escorial), 180–81; Madonna of the Rosary (San Marco, Osimo), 152; Prodigal Son (Galleria Sabauda, Turin), 181; Saint Mary Magdalene with Two

Angels (Pinacoteca Vaticana, Rome), 338, 339, fig. 118; Susanna and the Elders (Museo del Prado, Madrid), 181; various works, 189, 338

Guerra, Giovanni, 39–40, 284

Guerrieri, Giovanni Francesco, 125–26, 134, 156, 299, 315, 422; works: Circumcision (San Francesco, Sassoferrato), 66, 125, 125, 127, 153, fig. 55; Mass of Saint Nicholas (Santa Maria del Ponte, Sassoferrato), 124, 125, fig. 54; Saint Charles Borromeo (San Venanzio, Fabriano), 122, 125, fig. 52; attributed to, Madonna and Child (Palazzo Pitti, Florence), 300, 302, fig. 107

Guicciardini, Piero, 4, 5, 12, 18, 98, 119, 137, 140; judgment of Orazio's art, 12, 18, 264–65

Guzmán, Manuel de, 407

Hapsburgs, 336

Harrach, Aloys Thomas von, 377

Henrietta Maria, queen, 3, 13, 203, 232, 235, 238, 240, 270; marriage of, 216, 217; as patron, 223, 228

Henry II of France, 235

Henry III of France, 268

Henry IV of France, 41

Hernandes, Pietro, 274

Honthorst, Gerrit van, 46, 94, 118, 138, 227, 228, 232, 234, 236, 255, 298, 324, 335, 337, 338, 366, 368, 370, 382; works: Christ Crowning Saint Teresa (Santa Anna, Genoa), 170; Mercury Presenting the Liberal Arts to Apollo and Diana (Royal Collection, Hampton Court), 229, 234, 235, fig. 89; Mocking of Christ (Brentwood Holdings Assets Ltd., Spier Collection, London), 368, 370, fig. 129; Saint Francis (Cassa di Risparmio, Cosenza), 138; Smiling Girl, a Courtesan, Holding an Obscene Image (Saint Louis Art Museum), 324, 324, fig. 116

Houghton, Robert, 244

Hugford, Ignazio, 320

Ignatius of Loyola, Saint, 64, 118, 336

Imperiale, Davide, 270

Imperiali, Giovanni Vincenzo, 165

Isabella, archduchess, 227

Jabach, Everard, 376

Jacobus de Voragine, Golden Legend, 70, 325, 350–52, 384

Jacopo da Empoli, 206

James I of England, fig. 90

Januarius, Saint (San Gennaro), 383, 411–13

Jerome, Saint, 94

Jesuits, 13, 39, 41, 64, 66, 68, 117, 118–19, 184, 336, 379

Jones, Inigo, 225, 228–29, 238

Julius III, Pope, 283

Laer, Pieter van, 271

La Granja palace, Spain, 427

La Hyre, Laurent de, 113, 160, 210; Allegory of Arithmetic (Hannema-de Stuers Foundation, Heino, Netherlands), 207, 210, fig. 81

Lallemant, Georges, 205

Landriani, Marchesa Vittoria Malatesta, 118

Lanfranco, Cardinal, 285–86, 339, 342, 383, 384, 413

Lanfranco, Giovanni, 13, 34, 44, 46, 74, 88, 143, 156, 166, 182, 208, 269, 288, 338, 380, 445; Orazio's work with, 102; works: Agony in the Garden (San Giovanni dei Fiorentini, Rome), 150; Buongiovanni chapel (Sant'Agostino, Rome), 147–48; Pentecost (Pinacoteca Civica, Fermo), 117; various works, 86

Lanier, Nicholas, 225

La Tour, Georges de, 365

Laureti, Tommaso, 44

Lazzari, Dionisio, 380

Le Brun, Charles, 208

Le Nain, Antoine, 210–12

Le Nain, Louis, 210–12; works: Holy Family (private collection), 209, 211, fig. 83; various works, 211

Le Nain, Mathieu, 208, 210–12

Le Nain brothers, 160, 210–11, 235

Leonardo da Vinci, 130, 235, 273, 430

Leòn y Càrdenas, Martín de, 383, 411

Leopold Wilhelm, Archduke, 217

Le Sueur, Eustache, 208

Liancourt, Roger du Plessis de, duke of La Roche-Guyon, 204, 227, 235

Liechtenstein, Prince Johann Adam Andreas von, 113

Liechtenstein, Prince Karl von, 269

Ligozzi, Jacopo, 206, 326

Lilio, Andrea, 40, 43, 118, 119

Lippi, Filippo, 198

Liss, Johann, 257

Livy, 361

Lomazzo, Giovanni Paolo, 352

Lomi, Aurelio, 6, 40, 123, 170; comparison with Orazio, 169; works: Annunciation (Santa Maria Maddalena, Genoa), 169, 169, 200, 372, fig. 65; Last Judgment (Santa Maria in Carignano, Genoa), 165; Resurrection of Christ (Santa Maria in Carignano, Genoa), 165

Lomi, Francesco, 360

Lomi, Giulio, 360

Lomi family, 6, 326, 346, 347

London, Queen's House, 228–30, 232, 238; Artemisia's work in, 270; Whitehall, 232, 421; York House, 10, 225

Longhi, Onorio, 15, 275, 284

Longhi, Roberto, 1916 article on the Gentileschi, 6, 19–20, 102, 198, 246, 249, 265

Lopresti, Lucia (under the pseudonym Anna Banti), novel about Artemisia, 249, 265–66

Loredan, Gianfrancesco, 279

Loreto, 117

Lotto, Lorenzo, 35, 152

Louis XIII of France, 205, 268

Louis XIV of France, 376

Ludovisi, Ippolita, 146

Ludovisi, Cardinal Ludovico, collection of, 356, 358

Ludovisi family, 338, 339, 341

Luini, Bernardino, 130, 430

Luti, Benedetto, 298, 356

Maderno, Carlo, 15

Maderno, Stefano, 43; Saint Cecilia (Santa Cecilia in Trastevere, Rome), 350

Maggiori, Alessandro, 117

Magno, Giovanni, 20, 91

Maino, Juan Bautista, 73, 212

Malvasia, Carlo Cesare, 101

Mancini, Giulio, 11–12, 21, 46, 287, 340; on Orazio, 8–9

Manet, Edouard, Olympia (Musée d'Orsay, Paris), 11

Manetti, Rutilio, 244, 315, 377, 424

Manfredi, Bartolomeo, 7, 8, 12, 46, 104, 255, 337, 340, 342; Allegory of the Four Seasons (Dayton Art Institute), 92

Mannerism, 8, 40, 48–50, 52, 66, 68, 77, 80, 88, 91, 137, 146, 216, 255, 284, 337, 354, 424

Mantegna, Andrea, 332

Maratta, Carlo, 62, 166

Marches, the, 117–29; Orazio in, 136, 144, 152, 257, 287 (see also Ancona and Fabriano in the location index)

Maria Maddalena of Austria, 269, 313

Maringhi, Francesco, 257, 316–17, 346, 446, 447

Marino, Giambattista, 84, 279, 339, 379

Marriage of the Virgin (subject), fig. 78

Marucelli, 206

Masaccio, 126, 148

Massei, Pietro, 162

Massimi, Cardinal, 21

Master of the Annunciation to the Shepherds, 382

Master of the Judgment of Solomon, 382

Mattei family, 44, 284, 339

Medici, Cardinal Alessandro de', 42, 43, 313

Medici, Averardo de', collection of, 426

Medici, Cosimo II de', 98, 119, 137, 257, 314, 317, 330, 347, 372; Artemisia's letter to, 346

Medici, Ferdinand II de', 41, 203, 269–70, 317, 406

Medici, Giovanni de', 119

Medici, Marie de', 3, 21, 183, 203, 204, 205–6, 210, 212, 214–16, 218, 227, 271

Meleghino, Jacopo, 79

Mellan, Claude, 177, 181, 209; works: Cleopatra (engraving), 403; Lucretia (engraving), 362–64; Saint Mary Magdalene in Penitence (engraving), 177, 209–10; Samson and Delilah (engraving), 181, 205, 209, fig. 79

Mellin, Charles, 380

Michelangelo, 158, 276; works: Annunciation, drawings for, 137–38; Apollo (Museo del Bargello, Florence), 80; Battle of Cascina (destroyed), 182; frescoes in the Sistine chapel, 152, 158, 296, 298, figs. 105, 376; various works, 84

Sannesi, Jacopo, 13
Sansovino, marble *Madonna* (Sant'Agostino, Rome), 290
Santacroce, Francesco, 121
Santi di Tito (Gamba), 152, 198, 346
Saraceni, Carlo, 3, 7, 8, 34, 44, 46, 105, 142–43, 284, 286, 288, 337, 338, 437; landscapes, 76, 142
Sassoferrato, 68, 152, 387; *Holy Family*, 74
Sauli, Anton Maria, 165–66, 172
Sauli, Domenico, 166, 172
Sauli, Giovan Antonio, 3, 19, 21, 98, 165–66, 172, 251, 256, 362
Savelli, Bernardino, 122
Savelli, Federigo, 18
Savelli, Cardinal Giulio, 18, 121–22
Savelli, Paolo, 13, 15–18, 66, 119, 137, 284
Savelli family, 15–19, 70, 113, 114, 121–22, 137, 138, 158, 287
Savoy, 337; court of, 198
Savoy, Cardinal Maurizio of, 196, 198, 217
Scarpellino, Francesco, 10, 18, 19, 109
Schönborn collection, 356
Sebastiano del Piombo: *Christ Bearing the Cross* (Museo del Prado, Madrid), *58*, 60, fig. 41; *Madonna del velo* (Museo di Capodimonte, Naples), 144, 146–47
Seghers, Gerard, 337
Selva, Francesco, 124
Serodine, Giovanni, 46, 339
Sfondrato, Cardinal Paolo Emilio, 15, 42, 48, 72, 73, 118, 127, 144, 192
Sirani, Elisabetta, 113, 390
Sixtus V Peretti, Pope, 6, 118; patronage of, 39
Solari, Giovan Antonio, 8
Soprani, Raffaele, 203; biography of Orazio (1679), 3, 15, 166, 172–73
Soragna, Camilla Lupi di, 86
Spada, Lionello, 117
Spada collection, 104, 299, 350
Spadarino, 337, 338
Spain, 41, 224, 336, 340, 342, 379; occupation of Naples, 380
Spinola, Paolo Agostino, 165
Stanzione, Massimo, 255, 269, 342, 380, 381–82, 383, 384, 387, 389, 404, 414; works: *Assumption of the Virgin* (North Carolina Museum of Art, Raleigh), 381; attribution to, 386; *Cleopatra* (Pushkin Museum, Moscow), 387, 388; collaboration with Artemisia, 384; *Life of Saint John the Baptist* (Museo del Prado, Madrid), 382, *383*, 406, fig. 133; *Orpheus Beaten by the Bacchantes* (Banca Manusardi, Milan), 386
Stella, Jacques, 210
Stelluti, Francesco, 15, 122–23, 148
Stiattesi, Palmira, 360
Stiattesi, Pierantonio, 264, 288, 360
Streeter, Robert, ceiling in Sheldonian Theatre, Oxford, 230
Strozzi, Bernardo, 21, 168, 170, 191, 299, 318; *Paradise* (*modello;* Accademia Ligustica, Genoa), 96, 168, *168*, fig. 64
Stufa, Angelo, 119

Symonds, Richard, 27
Tassel, Jean, *Penitent Magdalene*, attributed to (Musée des Beaux-Arts, Dijon), *174*, 177, 372, fig. 69
Tassi, Agostino, 3, 4, 10, 34, 98, 100, 118, 143, 165, 249, 263, 275, 285–88, 289, 310, 337, 338, 339, 342, 432; character of, 264, 285; friendship and collaboration with Orazio, 102, 285–86; influence on Artemisia, 291; influence on Orazio, 105
Tassi, Nicolò, 98, 119, 122
Tasso, Torquato, 314
Tavarone, Lazzaro, 168
Tempesta, Antonio, 39, 44, 370
Terbrugghen, Hendrick, 244, 337
Teresa of Avila, Saint, 336
Theatines, 39, 379
Tiarini, Alessandro, 60
Tibaldi, Pellegrino, 79
Titian, 19, 225, 235, 258, 272, 350, 358, 404; works: *Bacchanals*, 273; *Bacchus and Ariadne* (National Gallery, London), 80; *Crucifixion* (San Domenico, Ancona), 117, 148; *Danaë* (Museo del Prado, Madrid), 100, 178, 306, *306*, fig. 108; *Madonna and Child with Saints Maurice and Jerome* (Musée du Louvre, Paris), 302; *Penitent Magdalene* (Galleria Palatina, Florence), 134, 174–76, *174*, 325, 372, fig. 68; *Self-Portrait* (Gemäldegalerie, Berlin), 418, *420*, fig. 145; various works, 200; *Venus with a Lute Player* (Museo del Prado, Madrid), 371
Tolentino, 117
Torriani, Francesco, 79
Tournier, Nicolas, 255, 337
Townshend, Aurelian, 229
Trionfi, Camilla, 118
Trisegni, Filippo, 275, 284
Trotta, Mario, 288
Turchi, Alessandro, 147, 338, 339
Tyndale, William, 361

Urban VIII, Pope, 257, 337, 340
Urbino, 117
Ursino, Valerio, 287
Usimbardi, Lorenzo, 285

Vaccaro, Andrea, 388
Valentin de Boulogne, 34, 46, 255, 337
Valentin, Moïse, 339, 340, 341, 342
Vallemani, Antonio, 126
Vallemani family, 123–24, 148
Vanni, Francesco, 43, 50, 62, 337
Vannini, Ottavio, 315; *Allegorical Figure* (Palazzo Pitti, Florence), 315, *316*, fig. 111
Vanvitelli, Luigi, 67
Varin, Quentin, 205
Vasari, Giorgio, 84, 176, 381
Vatican, 336–37; Biblioteca Apostolica (Biblioteca Sistina), 6, 40, *41*, fig. 31; Sistine chapel, 46, 79, 84, 298

Vecchi, Giovanni de', 39, 337
Velázquez, Diego, 267, 340, 380, 381
Veneziano, Agostino, *Cleopatra*, 304
Venice, 257, 273, 337; art of, 19, 114, 234, 342
Veralli family, 104, 299
Vermeer, Johannes, 20; *Allegory of Faith* (Metropolitan Museum, New York), 20; *Girl with a Pearl Earring* (Mauritshuis, The Hague), 244–46; *Study of a Young Woman* (Metropolitan Museum, New York), 244–46
Veronese, Paolo, 50, 225, 229, 234, 238, 240; *Finding of Moses* (Museo del Prado, Madrid), 238; various works, 296
Veronese, workshop of, *Esther and Ahasuerus* (Musée du Louvre, Paris), *374*, 376–77, fig. 130
Vespignani, Virgilio, 299
Vesuvius, 342, 379, 383
Vezzo, Virginia da, 255
Vico, Enea, *Judith and Her Maidservant* (engraving after Michelangelo), 84, *84*, fig. 45
Viola, Giovanni Battista, 339
Viviani, Antonio, 122–23
Volpi, Ulpiano, 73
Volterra, Daniele da, 79
Volterrano, 278
Vouet, Simon, 34, 167, 176, 208–9, 228, 235, 255, 257, 335, 337, 338, 341–42, 366, 380, 381, 387, 388, 394, 398; works: *Allegory of Wealth* (Musée du Louvre, Paris), 208; *Birth of the Virgin* (San Francesco a Ripa, Rome), 182, 406; *Circumcision* (Museo di Capodimonte, Naples), 339, 381, 406, 426; *Fortune-Teller* (National Gallery of Canada, Ottawa), 208; *Holy Family with a Bird* (etching), 398; *Jael and Sisera*, attributed to (Whitfield Fine Art, Ltd., London), 346, *346*, fig. 123; *Lucretia* (Národni Galerie, Prague), 362–64, *364*, fig. 127; *Saint Francis Taking the Habit* (San Lorenzo in Lucina, Rome), 382; *Temptation of Saint Francis* (San Lorenzo in Lucina, Rome), 335, *336*, 368, 381, fig. 117; *Time Vanquished by Hope, Love, and Beauty* (Museo del Prado, Madrid), 394; *Virgin Appearing to Saint Bruno* (San Martino, Naples), 384; workshop of, 418
Vouillement, Sébastien: engravings by, 428; *Virgin Sewing* (engraving), *427*, 428, fig. 147

Wael, Cornelis and Lucas, 168
Waldmüller, Ferdinand Georg, 142
Wals, Goffredo, 76, 143; *Rest on the Flight into Egypt* (National Museum of Western Art, Tokyo), 143
War of Mantuan Succession, 337
Weston, Sir Richard, 227
Wilson, Andrew, 190
Wynn, Sir Richard, 228

Xavier, Saint Francis, 336

Zuccari, Federico, 44, 47, 58, 275, 337; writings, 44
Zucchi, Jacopo, 41
Zurbarán, Francisco de, 61

Index of Works by Orazio Gentileschi

Italic page numbers indicate illustrations. **Boldface** numbers indicate principal discussions of works.

473

Index of Works by Artemisia Gentileschi